THE SECRET
LIFE OF CHOCOLATE

THE SECRET
LIFE OF CHOCOLATE

Marcos Patchett

AEON

First published in 2020 by
Aeon Books Ltd
12 New College Parade
Finchley Road
London NW3 5EP

British Library Cataloguing in Publication Data

A C.I.P. for this book is available from the British Library

ISBN-13: 978-1-91159-706-3

Typeset by Medlar Publishing Solutions Pvt Ltd, India
Printed in Great Britain

www.aeonbooks.co.uk

For

Luke, Joe, and Sam.

In the hope that even when life tastes bitter, it's still good.

CONTENTS

DISCLAIMER

The information in this book should be used responsibly. The author does not endorse the use of any illegal substances. Any attempt to replicate the formulas in this book or to utilise the information contained herein is undertaken at the discretion of the reader, and is their responsibility; the author accepts no liability for any harm arising from medicinal or culinary uses of chocolate or other substances described in this book. All medicinal recommendations should be checked with your physician, qualified medical herbalist, or accredited health professional.

Every attempt has been made to ensure that sources are properly cited and acknowledged. I've endeavoured to present the historical, scientific, anthropological, and philosophical information in this book accurately, although some of it (particularly the neurophysiology in Chapter 5 and the philosophies of consciousness in Chapter 10) were pushing the limits of my competence, so any mistakes, misapprehensions, or non sequiturs are unlikely to be the fault of the cited authors.

A WORD ON ANIMAL EXPERIMENTS

When I began researching this book in 2006, I was omnivorous. In 2014 I became vegan. Since then I debated removing all the research based on non-human animal experimentation from the book, but that would have obviated years of research and eliminated a lot of the evidence, particularly the already-sparse support for the central hypothesis of Cacao's psychoactivity beyond its accepted role as a sort of vegetable caffeine-and-polyphenol delivery system. I also consider that, while I disapprove of the method, the results of non-human animal experimentation are still valid. Similarly, I have not excluded unethical experimentation on humans from the mid-twentieth century, such as force-feeding chocolate to inmates of mental asylums to test its effects on their teeth, or performing fake surgery on angina patients without their consent to test the effectiveness of the operation. Information isn't invalidated by immoral methodologies.

It's unfortunate that animal torture is still used to test medicinal substances, particularly in the case of plants and foods such as Cacao which are known to be safe for human consumption, simply because such experiments are much cheaper than human clinical trials. There are also fewer restrictions on the type of testing which can be done, because non-human animals are considered to be expendable. It's my hope that in future, we will move towards a more ethical and sustainable diet and cease to see similarly sentient* beings as food, now that the majority of people living in developed countries have no morally or technically defensible reason for continuing to consume them, and a plethora of ethical and environmental reasons for ending the factory farming of livestock. Eventually, lab-grown human organs and other developments may enable us to replicate conditions inside human bodies and allow testing on non-sentient living tissue, and experimenters will adopt more ethical forms of experimentation—if the scientific paradigm itself hasn't been superseded by then.

---

*I suspect that eventually, plants will be recognised as sentient too, albeit in a different way from humans: see recent excellent books by Monica Gagliano and Stefano Mancuso for research evidence of consciousness in plants. That doesn't invalidate the general ethical argument for a plant-based diet, though, as plants don't appear to feel pain, at least not as we know it, and many more plants are required to sustain cattle than would be necessary if we just ate the plants. Nor does plant agriculture contribute to environmental damage and pollution on anything like the same scale as livestock farming. Admittedly, though, scientific proof that plants are self-aware could cause more intensely ethical vegans to have a bit of a crisis.

INTRODUCTION

Mrs Doyle: "... and speaking of cake: I have cake!"
Father Ted: "I'm fine for cake, Mrs Doyle."
Mrs Doyle: "Are you sure, Father? There's cocaine in it!"
Father Ted: "There's what!?"
Mrs Doyle: "Oh no, not cocaine! What am I on about ... No, I meant, erm—what do you call them—raisins."

(from *Father Ted*, Series 2, Episode 1, "Hell")

Sadly, Mrs Doyle's cocaine would be a poor choice of cake adulterant. It would taste bad, and have very low bioavailability—when swallowed, cocaine is swiftly broken down in the liver before it gets into the general circulation, so has greatly reduced effects when consumed orally. Hence the practices of snorting, smoking, or injecting various preparations of the drug, to bypass the stomach and get it straight into the bloodstream, with increasing potency. So cocaine would be a bad baking choice for these reasons, not to mention its expense or toxicity. Ideally, Mrs Doyle's stimulant-laced cake should incorporate a different drug, one which is more widely available, and cheaper; a substance which also produces a "high" or subjectively improved mood when orally consumed, and may improve sociability if eaten regularly; a drug which tastes good, has low toxicity, and benefits health so much that it may even extend the human lifespan. In other words, she should have used chocolate.[i]

Chocolate is made from the toasted seeds of the tree known by the botanic name *Theobroma cacao*. In common with other psychoactive cash crops like tobacco, nutmeg, and opium, wars have been fought for control of the regions where this plant can be cultivated. Chocolate, in one form or another, has been historically associated with contracts and celebrations, with medicinal virtue and poisonous vice, and at least as much with slavery and sacrifice as with sex and romance. Actually Mrs Doyle's drug of choice, tea, has a similar back story in many respects,

---

[i] It should however be pointed out that cake is not the best medium for delivering drugs which are sensitive to heat, oxygen, or the presence of protein, as many of the compounds in chocolate are. Chocolate cake, even more than tablet/ bar chocolate, sacrifices pharmacological potency for the sake of flavour and texture; the stimulating compounds caffeine and theobromine survive, but most of the antioxidant polyphenols will not. Which admittedly is a sacrifice many are willing to make.

both chocolate and tea being caffeine-containing stimulants over which (amongst other reasons) nations brawled, and whose traditional reputation for possessing health-enhancing properties are now being ratified and defined by experimental science. But tea just doesn't have the *sexy* reputation that chocolate has. The words which occurred to a sample of people to describe chocolate included "delectable", "luscious", "intoxicating", and "delicious", but also "guilt producing" and "sinful"![1] My summary of the two main themes chocolate elicits for people would be first: pleasure, and second (sometimes): guilt—in that order. See what I mean? Sexy.

So why is Mrs Doyle's improbable cocaine/raisins mix-up amusing? It's probably because of the extreme contrast between the illegal stimulant cocaine, a notorious chemical isolated from the leaf of the generally rather benign Andean shrub *Erythroxylum coca*, and the innocuous raisin, dried fruit of the grape vine *Vitis vinifera*, not to mention the excellent comic performances of Pauline McLynne and Dermot Morgan. But this distinction raises another interesting question—where does food stop and drug begin? This isn't as simple to resolve as it may seem. Many foods and condiments contain compounds which act in drug-like ways, in other words they mimic or interfere with the various substances produced by the human body that regulate its function, such as hormones, neurotransmitters, or enzymes.

Examples of such interactions are plentiful, such as the isoflavones genistein and daidzin from soy beans interacting with oestrogen receptors,[2] peptides derived from gluten in wheat[3] and casein in milk binding to opiate receptors,[4] or compounds found in garden sage (*Salvia officinalis*) that affect a neurotransmitter (messenger chemical between nerve cells) called acetylcholine.[5] Food can also be preventive or curative of medical conditions, from gross nutrient deficiency syndromes such as scurvy or pellagra (vitamin C/ascorbic acid and vitamin B3/niacin deficiency, respectively), to more subtle imbalances such as essential fatty acid intake possibly linked to changes in inflammatory pathways.[6] Hence that old Greek doctor Hippocrates' famous injunction, sadly often ignored or distorted to faddish and foolish extremes: let food be your medicine and medicine be your food. In fact, the pleasure we take in eating and our desire for food itself is a product of internal neurochemical messages; sugars and fats, for example, both trigger the release of pleasure-giving endorphins in the brain when they are eaten.[7] So in this sense, every food is a drug. Even—and perhaps especially, given their high concentration of natural sugars—raisins.

We now perceive chocolate as a sweet, a naughty indulgence, and more recently as an "antioxidant-rich" health food too. While chocolate is still highly regarded, at least in the sense of being appreciated, its modern status is much reduced from the revered substance it once was in pre-Colombian Central America. The fruits and seeds of *Theobroma* species were transformed into numerous beverages by the inhabitants and used for many different purposes—secular, religious, celebratory, ceremonial, medicinal, and magical. Central America is one of the most bio-diverse regions in the world, with a panoply of different medicinal and psychoactive plants. So it's not as if there weren't stronger drug plants available, yet Cacao assumed the culturally pre-eminent place among Mesoamerican peoples' use of psychoactive flora, analogous to coca leaf (*Erythroxylum coca*) in the Andes, or kava (*Piper methysticum*) in Polynesia. What made Cacao, of all plants, so precious?

As a chocolate consumer by inclination and medical herbalist by trade, I'm fascinated by the pharmaceutical history and medicinal properties of *Theobroma cacao*, the "cocoa tree", and its associate plants: how chocolate was made and consumed in the past by the societies it came from, what medicinal and magical properties it was thought to have, and how modern pharmacological investigations into Cacao and its associate plants (e.g., the vanilla vine) can help to explain chocolate's continuing allure. I want to peel back the layers of European historical adaptations to Cacao, and reveal more of the cultural significance of Cacao throughout history and prehistory, and its substantial medicinal properties. My epicurean interest in chocolate is born from a desire to improve a pleasurable substance—to make it both more healthful *and* more gratifying, as a food and as a drug. Instinct, experience, and information led me to conclude that the best way to improve chocolate would be to investigate its origins and the oldest, time-tested traditional methods of preparation and use. Although the stronger forms of commercially processed Cacao, such as "dark chocolate", do possess notable, sub-coffee stimulating effects, and have vaunted potential health-promoting qualities, the traditional forms were more potent, being made with the finest quality beans, toasted and ground by hand, without added fat, sugar, or milk, and spiced with native herbs. A conquistador's account describes the effect of traditional Cacao drinks at the time of the Spanish conquest:

> This drink is the healthiest thing, and the greatest sustenance you could drink in the whole world, because he who drinks a cup of this liquid, no matter how far he walks, can go a whole day without eating anything else. (Anonymous Conqueror, 1556, quoted in Coe & Coe, 1996)

a bit stronger than a cup of cocoa, then. Some commentators have speculated that a combination of malnutrition and caffeine naivety (tea or coffee had not yet gained a foothold in Europe) meant that the native drinks affected the Spanish conquistadors much more than they would affect a contemporary caffeine-tolerant European; those hardy men were used to marching on empty stomachs in the most abject conditions, so a fat-rich low-caffeine emulsion in the form of a Cacao-based beverage would have had an inordinately noticeable effect. This may be so, but it's my personal and oft-repeated experience that traditionally made chocolate drinks are much more pleasurable and potent than factory-processed chocolate. My own attempts to recreate traditional pre-Colombian chocolate drinks in the process of researching and writing this book led me to conclude that the anonymous conquistador's account is largely accurate: traditional Cacao-based drinks are psychoactive and sustaining drugs, more intense and delectable than their mass-produced sweet bastard offspring which we call "chocolate".

Research into the polyphenols found in chocolate, wine, tea, and many other foods has uncovered a multitude of hitherto undiscovered health benefits, and dark chocolate in particular is now suspected of being one of the most protective foods against heart disease and stroke.[8] But no natural product, be it food or drug, is a panacea. A great many health claims have been extrapolated from research findings, and the "raw food" movement in particular has latched on to the exceptionally high levels of polyphenols in raw, untoasted Cacao, thereby claiming that chocolate produced from untoasted beans is healthier and tastier than cooked forms.[9] I wanted to investigate the veracity of these claims, and simultaneously explore the pharmacology of the bean as thoroughly as I possibly could to try to pin down the truth about chocolate's purported health benefits. While this book does propose some hypotheses about Cacao's pharmacological activity and sociocultural utility which may be considered far-fetched, I've taken care to state my sources and outline my reasoning, so that readers may make their own decisions on whether to follow me round some of the tighter intuitive U-bends.

I also have a personal reason for wanting to root out the facts here. I'm a recovered binge-eater and former recreational drug user, and a chocophile. My days of regular pharmaceutical drug use are confined to my time as an art student, a three-year period in my late teens and early twenties. I was accustomed to using MDMA or amphetamine (and alcohol, cannabis, LSD, etc.) most weekends, eating very little, and a favourite Sunday night post-clubbing dessert was a bowl of sliced banana with melted dark chocolate. Shortly after quitting weekend pharma drug use completely, I went through what in retrospect was a couple of months' acute psychosis, convinced that someone was living in my attic, creeping out and moving my stuff around when I was out of the house, along with an endearing facial tic (eye twitching) and a habit of grinding my teeth constantly.

A binge-eating disorder developed insidiously about a year and a half after going cold turkey on pharmacological revelry (except for occasional recreational or ceremonial use of natural products of geographically variable legality such as cannabis, khat, or *Psilocybe* mushrooms), and lasted for eight months of escalating intensity. That eating disorder was subsequently resolved, with amazing speed, through the intervention of a very close wise friend and a sensible nutritionist. But my curiosity was piqued when, three years later, during my herbal medicine BSc, I came across a journal article detailing several case histories of binge eating of "carbohydrates" associated with chocolate craving, which developed up to three years following regular MDMA use.[10] Coincidence? I had experienced every manifestation of the cases' problems, from social paranoia and outbursts of anger to sleep-wake cycle inversion. The real question for me, though, was this: why chocolate?

Finally, I wanted to look at the mythology of chocolate, because it came from an area of the world whose history I've always been drawn to. From childhood I was obsessed by Mesoamerican history: the Aztecs and Montezuma, the Maya, the tales of the savage, sophisticated, beautiful, and brutal empires discovered and destroyed by the conquistadors in the sixteenth century. It was never taught at school—all our history was *boring* old Tudors,[ii] or the more interesting but still familiar Greeks and Romans, so I spent hours of my pre-teen life in the school library reading about the Maya and the Aztecs and their mysterious, alien civilisations; drawing costumes and weapons and cities and inventing armies and imagining what it must have been like to live in such a time and place. Part of the long journey of writing this book has been self-funded solo travels round Mexico and Guatemala in search of the remnants of the past, to get an authentic echo of the cultures who pioneered the use of the "cocoa bean" as a drug and a food.

So this book is an effort to dispel the ersatz glamour of confectionery adverts, to moderate the unremittingly positive spin of the food industry or diet gurus, and to delve into the historical,

---

[ii] Childhood opinion. I quite like them now.

pharmacological, and mythological roots of chocolate. It's my attempt to rediscover the drugs made from Cacao in their original form, without added milk, fat, sugar, or commercial elaboration: the rich dark heart of chocolate, stripped of Europe's and America's sickly sweet, off-white confectioner's refinements. I'd be glad if, in some small way, this book helped to restore *Theobroma*'s rightful prominence as the "food of the gods"—the demanding, ruthless gods of ancient Mesoamerica, who knew that life is brief, bitter, and beautiful, and required reciprocal dedication and sacrifice in exchange for the world they immolated themselves to create.

PART I

CHOCOLATE ROOTS

A potted history of chocolate

"[Cacao] was [like] jimson weed;[iii] it was considered to be like the mushroom, for it made one drunk, it intoxicated one. If he who drunk it were a common person, it was taken as a bad omen. And in past times only the ruler drank it, or a great warrior, or a commanding general … If perhaps two or three lived in wealth, they drank it … they drank a limited amount of Cacao, for it was not drunk unthinkingly."

(Sahagún, quoted in Coe & Coe, 1996)

"Money doesn't grow on trees."

(my mum, many times)

The seeds of the Cacao tree, *Theobroma cacao*, are the essential base ingredient in all forms of chocolate. The tree originates from Central and South America—the part of the globe which came to be known as the New World back in the day of plagues, religious sectarianism, witch burning, and rampant imperialism (now we have HIV, religious or secular ideological fundamentalism, scapegoating of minorities, and ethically challenged multinational corporations; *plus ça change*). In order to understand Cacao's place in the world better, it's necessary to look at a bit of history. Specifically, the bit before the gringos arrived on the eastern shores of Central America in their "floating houses". It won't be necessary to do this in great detail—other books do that—just enough to get a sense of the order of events which led to the cultivation of Cacao and its use in medicine, drinks, and food.

BC (Before Chocolate)

It's currently thought that people first arrived in North America via Siberia, around 14,000 years ago (12,000 BCE). There are two theories how this may have happened. The older theory, sarcastically called the "follow the reindeer" theory by its detractors, supposes that people hunting

---

[iii] Jimson weed, aka thornapple (*Datura stramonium*), a deliriant and true hallucinogen, is an important plant in New World shamanism, considered to be of a somewhat malevolent character. It contains powerful tropane alkaloids, analogous to the Old World "witching plants", deadly nightshade (*Atropa belladonna*), henbane (*Hyoscyamus niger*), and mandrake (*Mandragora officinarum*).

mammoth and other mobile woolly edibles followed them through an "ice-free corridor", an area of land not covered in glaciers and ice sheets down the middle of North America. As the animals moved south, people followed. The other, newer theory—which has not yet been dignified with a derogatory epithet by its critics—suggests that people may have migrated down the western (Pacific) coast of North America even earlier than 12,000 BCE. Warm ocean currents from the south kept coastal temperatures relatively balmy, and it's surmised that people may have travelled by sea as well as by land, even then. So there would have been lots of edible plant life available onshore, and enough seafood offshore to satisfy the enterprising, possibly raft-borne, prehistoric hunter-gatherers.

Having discovered the continent of America, people began living there. In Central America, they took the trouble to begin domesticating and cultivating maize (corn on the cob, *Zea mays*), which they first genetically engineered using selective reproduction. They took the scrawny wild grass now known by the name *teosinte*, or another similarly runty undomesticated plant of the same type—archaeologists disagree exactly which wild grass species was used—and, by careful seed selection over a few human generations, turned it into a high-yield sustenance crop. This happened in the present-day Tehuacan and Oaxacan valleys in central Mexico, some time between 8000 and 5000 BCE. Archaeologists have discovered graves dating back to 6000 BCE, containing baskets, blankets, and nets, sophisticated tools of civilisation.[11] As the corn cobs grew larger, people began to settle into villages as fixed communities evolved to tend the crops. This age of early settlement and agriculture, from 7000 to 1500 BCE, is now referred to by academic types as the Archaic Period of Mesoamerica (Mesoamerica simply means "middle America", referring to the central American continent.)

The development of agriculture—and, by extension, culture—throughout the world had much to do with ensuring and controlling the supply of highly valued plants, including those with intoxicating or psychoactive properties. Most psychoactive plants are prized for their medicinal, magical, sacramental, and pleasurable uses. Many such plants have since become worldwide cultural phenomena, with varying degrees of perceived beneficence or harmfulness (examples: tobacco, tea, cannabis, Cacao). Tobacco in the New World, and mandrake, henbane, and belladonna in Stone Age Jericho are examples of early cultivation of psychoactive plants which may have influenced the movement towards farming practices and settled communities.[12] Another, less homocentric view, would acknowledge that all species and their environments mutually influence each other in their evolution, structurally or behaviourally, and many plants which humans use could equally be said to be making use of *us*, to further *their* evolutionary agendas.

No culture before our materialistic society believed that nature is purposeless, and there is some scientific evidence to suggest that it may not be. The unjustly controversial scientist Rupert Sheldrake's books *Morphic Resonance* and *The Science Delusion* (*Science Set Free*) describe experiments demonstrating apparent purposefulness and cohesion in nature and supposedly random natural phenomena, and other "anomalies". Even if we assume that current scientific consensus is correct, and that nature has no inherent purposes, it's still unclear which species ultimately has the upper hand in many human-plant relationships. Objectively, mass cultivation of particular crops by human agents is an evolutionary triumph for which species, exactly? Pharmacognosy—the pharmacology of natural substances—has revealed that wheat, for example, contains various types of glutens, some of which are *exorphins*.[13] These substances bind to opiate receptors in the mammalian central nervous system, and have weak sedative and euphoriant effects[14] in the human brain that are likely to enhance the mood-raising effect of eating any carbohydrate-based food on the brain's uptake of the amino acid known as 5-hydroxytryptophan, or 5-HTP, which is converted into serotonin, a feel-good neurotransmitter (chemical messenger in the brain). Bread cravings explained. Which species "cultivates" the other?

As an obviously psychotropic (mood-altering or mind-affecting) plant, Cacao could also be hypothesised to have mutually influenced human (agri-)cultural development in this way. The seeds' psychoactive properties, and their perceived embodiment of powerful spiritual forces, could have been the impetus for their dissemination and ritual usage by pre-Colombian Mesoamericans.[15] Viewed from this through-the-looking-glass perspective, many cultivated plant species can be seen as prehistoric versions of the mythical apple[iv] from the Biblical tree of knowledge of good and evil. Once such plants began being consumed by humans, things changed—people needed a regular supply of the good stuff, these seductive fruits of the earth which altered their vision of reality: after all, the word psychedelic means to clear (*delos*) the mind (*psyche*). Psychoactive and edible plants precipitated humanity's fall towards civilisation from the less sophisticated hunter-gatherer societies which preceded agriculture. Cacao's psychotropic properties, and the issue of whether or not Cacao in any of its forms can be considered addictive, are discussed fully in Chapters 5 and 7, and Cacao's symbolic role as an entheogenic substance and vehicle of dangerous knowledge are revisited in the third section of this book. The term *entheogen* refers to plants or drugs with profound consciousness-altering properties, typically used for sacramental or ritual purposes.

Two thousand BCE onwards has been described as the "formative period" in Mesoamerica, where people began living in villages sustained by agriculture. Archaeologists have dug up or discovered pottery and ceramic figurines from this period, little "zoomorphic" half-human, half-animal statues[16] of gods, spirits, or humans channelling supernatural beings in shamanic worship, all signs of civilisation—but early ballcourt alleys have been found dating from 5000 BCE,[17] indicating that the Mesoamericans may already have been living in larger, static communities by this time. These ancient ballcourts are early versions of the stone-walled courts for the popular game with religious significance that became famous throughout the Mesoamerican world, which in the timeless tradition of such games involves opposing teams knocking a ball around a court. In this case it was a very heavy rubber ball, and the aim was to shoot it through the opposing team's hoop high up on the side wall of the ballcourt, using only one's upper arms and thighs, without using the hands or feet. As these ballcourt ruins show, the first organised settlements may have preceded the "formative period" estimate by a few thousand years.

Before we resume our timeline, it's worth mentioning the method of growing crops that the people of prehistoric Mesoamerica devised in these early centuries. The system came to be known in post-colonial times as the *milpa*, or "maize field". They would grow several types of interdependent edible and medicinal plants together, on the same patch of land, like a mixed-up vegetable garden. These plants were selected because they are agriculturally and nutritionally complementary, in other words they helped each other grow better, and made complete meals.

[iv] More likely a mistranslation of the more probable fig. Apple trees are a north European fruit, and weren't cultivated in ancient Judea.

For example, beans, maize, avocados, squashes, melons, tomatoes, and chillis would be grown in the same plot. The beans would use the maize stalks to climb up, while the bacteria in their roots fertilised the soil by fixing nitrogen. The fields were burned in preparation for planting, then the earth was dug up and maize and beans were sown together, with squashes between the rows; useful medicinal "weeds" which benefitted the soil or plants around them were left alone. Earth was piled up around the roots as the crops grew, and the mix of plants prevented soil erosion and almost guaranteed a harvest, no matter the rainfall pattern.[18] Nutritionally, there was a good mix of carbohydrates (maize), proteins (beans) and sometimes fats, too, in the form of avocado tree fruits. While maize lacks the amino acids lycine and tryptophan, beans lack cysteine and methionine, but each contains what the other omits. So for the farmer, a *milpa* constituted the basis of a sustainably produced balanced diet. How sustainable? Some present-day *milpas* have been in continuous cultivation for more than four thousand years, providing sustenance for hundreds of generations. The Mesoamericans cracked large-scale permaculture approximately three thousand years ago.

Between 2000 and 1500 BCE, the first big civilisation aggregated in Mesoamerica. Not knowing what they called themselves, they have been named the "Olmecs", which is confusing because the Mexica (otherwise known, also inaccurately, as the "Aztecs", the dominant culture in Meso-america at the time of the Spanish conquest) referred to another group of people inhabiting an entirely different region over a millennium later by the same name. The original Olmecs inhabited the lowlands on the east coast in Mesoamerica, in modern Veracruz and Tabasco. The first city they built has been named "San Lorenzo" (1200–900 BCE), which was eventually superseded by a second city, "La Venta" (1150–300 BCE). It's thought that the Olmecs' belief system evolved from a shamanic perspective, whereby everything was infused with spiritual power, similar to the *chi* of Chinese culture, the *prana* of Ayurveda, the *pneuma* of the Greeks, or the *mana* of Oceanic cultures.

In this animist world view, nothing of natural origin lacks life, whether or not it is sentient: rocks, winds, and streams are as full of life as birds or humans. Olmec art contains many representations of inter-species transformations, representing natural and magical changes of state between the "elements" which formed the world; human, jaguar, eagle, and serpent forms are often mingled. Jaguars were particularly revered as they hunt by day and night, on land and in rivers—they crossed symbolic boundaries of earth and water, human (daylight) and spirit (nocturnal) worlds. The Olmecs developed political organisation and a hierarchical, class-based society; they traded goods over long distances; they invented a form of hieroglyphic writing (by 750 BCE) and the concept of mathematical zero (before 32 BCE), which has only happened twice in recorded history (by the Olmecs in Mesoamerica and the Hindus in ancient India);[19] they created a detailed and accurate astronomical calendar, probably for divinatory (astrological) purposes. It's thought that they also drank a form of chocolate.

Cacao cultures

1. The Olmecs (1500–400 BCE)

In fact there's no hard evidence that the Olmecs used *Theobroma cacao*, the Cacao tree, from whose seeds chocolate is made. They almost certainly did though, because the Maya word for the seeds, *kakaw*—from which we derive the word Cacao, and thence cocoa—is of Olmec origin.[20] The Olmecs were one of the first civilisations in Mesoamerica known to have developed trade networks for precious substances such as jade. They attributed religious significance to caves and mirrors, and practised bloodletting and human sacrifices. They had a four-directional or "quadripartite" concept of the world, analogous to Old World compass directions[21] (the principles behind these developments are discussed in Chapter 9). The Olmecs are known to have used various entheogenic plants and substances in their worship and medicine, including secretions from the parotid glands of the toad *Bufo marinus*, which have hallucinogenic effects.[22]

Olmec bowls and calabashes thought to have been used for drinking *kakawa* (the later Maya name for Cacao-based beverages) have been found on the Pacific coast of Chiapas and the gulf coast of Tabasco, two traditional Cacao-growing regions. The earliest definitively *kakaw*-tainted relics are fragments of broken pottery discovered in other Cacao-cultivating districts such as the Soconusco, west of Lake Atitlan on the Pacific coast of Guatemala and Mexico, and the Olmec region on the Gulf Coast of Mexico in contemporary Tabasco, which suggest truly ancient origins of Cacao as a beverage. The pottery fragments from the Soconusco date as far back as 1900 BCE.[23] These tableware remnants are coated with residues of Cacao, measured by testing for traces of theobromine, a chemically stable compound that in Central America is only found in *Theobroma* species (although theobromine is present in many other plants worldwide). It's thought that Cacao became the pre-eminent commercial crop in south-eastern Mesoamerica from 1000 BCE, and was traded for other valued commodities such as salt, feathers, hides, and obsidian.[24]

The oldest intact spouted pottery vessel containing traces of chocolate was found in Belize (a non-Olmec region) and dates from around 600 BCE. Similar artefacts have been found in the Ulua valley in Honduras and dated from 1000–700 BCE, but they lack detectable residues of Cacao. Vessels of this type, resembling a slightly flattened teapot with a short spout and a tall, wide neck without a lid, were used by later Maya societies for serving Cacao-based drinks. These vessels are a bit of an enigma, as almost all later depictions of chocolate drinks and most contemporary Central American versions of ancient Cacao-based beverages call for a substantial head of foam, to which their design appears unsuited: pouring foamy *kakawa* through the spout would presumably have involved much bubble-squashing, and on many of these vessels there's a fixed bucket-type handle on the top which would hinder stirring, easy pouring from a height or other foam-raising and skimming activities. So it's possible that at this stage the foam which was depicted on the pottery, murals, and carvings of later Mesoamerican cultures was not yet a feature of *kakawa* at all.

On the other hand, the drinks could have been pre-frothed, then poured into the "Cacao teapot" so that the bubbles would build up in the high necks of the vessels. The froth could then have been ladled or skimmed from out of the neck, then the body of the beverage may have been poured from the spout and the bubbly bit subsequently replaced on the finished *kakawa*, though this assumes a very durable sort of spume (we'll revisit this foam conundrum in later chapters). It's also been proposed that the spouts may not have been for pouring but for blowing: forcing air through the liquid to raise a head of foam. In which case, *Cappucino* may not be such a modern concept after all. Later *kakawa* drinking and storing vessels were "easy pour, easy froth" wide-necked tripods, and long-legged tripod pots from 100 CE have been found in Costa Rica, possibly for heating the *kakawa* from below to keep it warm—the "hotplate" design.

The first confirmed representations of *Theobroma* in Mesoamerican archaeological relics are high-relief Cacao pods on a clay vessel from Peru, dating from 1100–700 BCE. The vessel also

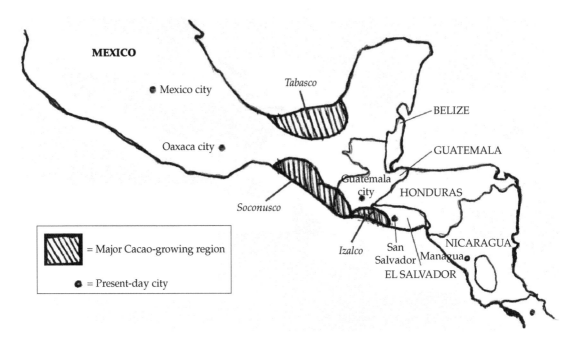

Figure 1. Traditional Cacao cultivation zones in Mesoamerica.

depicts spider monkeys, which are known to be natural agents of the tree, as they eat the fruit pulp in Cacao pods, scattering and distributing the seeds in the process. It's surmised that the original human use of *Theobroma* may have been consuming the sweet pulp and/or using it to make alcoholic beverages (this is still done today), and the Peruvian vessel may have been a container for a type of Cacao fruit beverage or "wine". But the seeds appear never to have been made into sophisticated Cacao drinks in the southern continent as they were in Central America. The Olmecs are thought to have greatly influenced Mesoamerican cultural development, and although nothing is currently known about their use of chocolate, the Maya—known Cacao users—adopted big slices of Olmec cultural and religious influence, including their word for the plant. Significantly, the humid, verdant lowland climate of the Olmec area is a perfect natural habitat for *Theobroma cacao*, and parts of the region, such as the modern state of Tabasco, are Cacao-growing territories to this day (see Figure 1 above).

2. The Zapotecs, Teotihuacan, and the pre-Classic Maya (600 BCE–200 CE)

The Zapotecs were the real new kids on the block in Mesoamerica in 600 BCE. Their society coalesced from several small villages in Mexico's Oaxaca valley around 500 BCE, when they built a city, which has been named "Monte Alban". The Zapotecs also had complex systems for recording time; their grasp of astronomy can be seen from the orientation of many of their temples towards stars or constellations at specific (and presumably ritually significant) times of year.[25] The Zapotec capital became a political power for a thousand years, before finally being abandoned in 600 CE. Monte Alban was Central America's first true imperial power—it commanded a 10,000 square mile empire, had a caste-based society in the Olmec mould, and a population of between fifteen and thirty thousand. Helpfully, they also labelled their monuments using the Olmec-derived trick of hieroglyphic writing, so archaeologists could discover that Monte Alban is older than the ruined Maya cities. Monte Alban is also the source of the oldest record of the Mesoamerican 260-day ritual calendar, to be discussed in Chapter 10. The calendar itself is likely to be even older, perhaps dating back to Olmec times, as some of the animals and plants which are used as day names are of lowland origin,[26] and wouldn't be found in the sierra of the Zapotec heartland.

Theobroma species don't grow in the relatively arid environment of Oaxaca valley, despite the fact that modern Oaxaca City is famous for its chocolate in food (such as *molés*, the generic name for a wide variety of complex sauces, some of which contain Cacao) and drink. It's likely that the Zapotecs imbibed Cacao-based beverages too, perhaps trading for the ingredients using the exchange networks that had existed across Mesoamerica since the so-called Archaic period. While the Olmecs and Zapotecs were inventing Mesoamerican city living, the Maya were a large and disparate group of country bumpkins, affectionately known as the "pre-Classic Maya" (1500 BCE to 200 CE) by archaeologists. They used *milpa*-style agriculture in the forests of the Yucatan peninsula adjacent to the Olmec heartlands, and they began building villages and adopting Olmec ideas about social order, emphasising kingship, nobility, and caste systems (albeit on a smaller scale). The Maya obstinately continued to not build any of modern Mexico's or Guatemala's tourist attractions throughout the rise of the Zapotec empire, but they did develop the most complex system of time reckoning in Mesoamerica, the "Long Count" (detailed in Chapter 10), and a shared foundation of myth and ideology;[27] burials in the caves at Loltun in Yucatan may date back to 6000 BCE, suggesting that the origins of the Maya civilisation may be older than was previously thought.[28]

In order to leave no large gaps in this outrageously condensed history (as no one wants a chocolate advent calendar with open doors and missing pieces), we must mention the great city Teotihuacan (population 200,000 in its heyday) in central Mexico, north of present-day Mexico City. Teotihuacan grew up from 50 BCE and flourished until a great fire razed the city in around 725 CE, and it never fully recovered, although it limped on for another quarter century.[29] Unlike the Maya, the Teotihuacanos appear to have adopted a more democratic or community-based rather than dynastic rule, and—in common with other Mesoamerican peoples—viewed time as cyclical rather than linear.[30] They were also the first group known to have worshipped the "feathered serpent" central to later Mexica ("Aztec") theology, who evolved into the deity known as Quetzalcoatl, and who the Mexica deemed responsible for the discovery of Cacao and many other foodstuffs.

The Teotihuacano feathered serpent god was less human than later iterations, a water-sky deity (an uncanny combination of sea snake and bird, denizens of both domains) more akin to ancient Chinese dragons, an elemental being of great power. This entity eventually came to be known as the *waxak-lahun-ubah-kan* or "feathered serpent of war" of the Classic Maya, a god who was ritually "housed" in special battle standards which could be carried with the army, bringing the potent force of a portable war god onto the battlefield. The magical Teotihuacan battle standards were a feather-rimmed disc on top of an orb or globe, mounted on a staff. Often a war-owl was depicted, the owl being a messenger bird of the underworld; the disc at the top of the standard may have been made with a flayed human hide stretched over a wooden frame. The Teotihuacanos either invented or elaborated older beliefs into this new, potentiated ritual warfare, which they bequeathed to the Maya and subsequent cultures. This has been described as the "Venus-Tlaloc" style of war, because it was calendrically determined by the phases of the planets Venus and Jupiter and the end of the rainy season—Tlaloc being the name of a rain god from the much later Mexica (Aztec) pantheon.[31]

Teotihuacan formed the centre of many of the trade networks in Central America, and is now famous for its spectacular ghost-town ruins, an awesome parade of monumental temple pyramids. Cacao distribution was a major part—or even *the* most important part—of Mesoamerican merchandise, being a high-status, high-demand product, which only grew in select regions, often distant from major centres of consumption such as Teotihuacan, situated in the dry heartland of Mexico. Cacao was both trade and tribute, and tithes of Cacao were paid to the pre-eminent city by vassal states from Cacao-growing zones. The Cacao trade was dominated by Teotihuacan for a couple of centuries, before the Tlaxcalans assumed control of the supply when the declining Teotihuacan civilisation eventually collapsed, for reasons unknown, in around 750 CE. Eventually their monopoly would pass to the Mayan polities in the Chontal region, in present-day Tabasco in Mexico. At all times, pre-Colombian ownership of Cacao-growing regions was a coveted prize, and the areas from which the best Cacao beans came were hotly contested; the contemporary regions of Chiapas in Mexico and Suchitequepez in Guatemala, where *criollo* Cacao is grown, were a perpetual focus of skirmishes and territorial disputes.[32] But the acquisition of rich Cacao-growing land was merely another sign of favour from the gods, who were to be repaid with sacrifices. It may be that Teotihuacan's ascendancy magnified the importance of ritual warfare and sacrifice in Mesoamerica, and consolidated the template of trade, ritual warfare, and tribute-based expansionism which shaped Mesoamerican culture for the next thousand years.

3. The Classic Maya (200–900 CE)

Centuries before the conquest, the Maya became the world's first archaeologically certified society of chocoholics. Although, strictly speaking, they weren't chocoholics, because chocolate—as we know it—is a modern invention. Neither the Maya nor any other pre-conquest American society consumed *kakawa* principally as a sweet, although sweetened forms of the beverages made from it did exist. In any case, the Maya comprised various culturally similar but politically separate peoples who inhabited the Yucatan peninsula and its environs (Chiapas state in Mexico, and the modern nations of Guatemala and Belize) from 1500 BCE onwards. The ancestral Maya's descendants live there today, but archaeologists and historians get particularly excited about the period from 200–900 CE, which they call the Classic Maya era, as during this time the Maya finally got around to building beautiful cities in the inhospitably vegetative terrain of the Yucatan.

This environment has been described as "geochemically hostile"[33] due to low rainfall and very salty groundwater; essentially the Maya had to "terraform" their environment before crops could be grown, making the "Maya heartland … a network of artificially habitable terrestrial islands".[34] The Maya adapted this environment by using crushed limestone to "cap" sediments beneath their settlements and filter rainwater in sinkholes or natural wells called *dzonots* (or *cenotes*, in Spanish rendering of native dialect), thereby making it drinkable; in many of these wells, fresh water from above sits atop a layer of salt water at sea level. Towns and cities aggregated around these natural and modified reservoirs, which were sacred places. Each of the Classic Maya polities in the Yucatan was ruled by a patrilineally descended king and royal family, with a governing council of chiefs, priests, and advisors. After each twenty-year cycle, or *katun*, new governors were chosen by the ruling elites; so even though noble status was heredi- tary, positions of administrative power had to be decided by consensus among the ruling class. War commanders, or *nacom*, were chosen every three years, as the post carried a heavy weight of secular and religious responsibility: the *nacom* was expected to remain celibate and maintain a strict diet for the duration of his tenure.[35]

The Maya elaborated earlier technologies and discoveries such as writing, mathematics, astronomy, architecture, and the production of Cacao-based beverages. Classic era Mayan writ- ing is a mix of phonetic and logographic,[36] in other words a combination of symbols representing sounds and stylised picture-writing; so the word for "tree" could be written as symbols which made the sounds for the Mayan word for "tree", or a picture of a tree, or a picture of something else that reminded the Maya of their word for "tree", such as an allegory, rhyme, or metonym. They also made use of many medicinal and entheogenic plants, including "magic mushrooms"; even before the Classic era, sculptures of mushrooms have been found together with small grinding stones of the sort used by twentieth-century Mixtec shamans to grind *Psilocybe* mush- rooms, indicating the great age of this practice.[37]

Theobroma cacao doesn't grow particularly well in most of the Maya region due to low rain- fall, although small quantities were cultivated around the *dzonots* with their fresh water supply, evidenced by murals and carvings depicting Cacao pods hanging from the ceiling of sinkholes. *Dzonots* were considered to be portals into the underworld, which was conceived by the Maya and later Mesoamerican peoples as a watery domain—not unreasonably, given that the entrances to the earth, to which all things revert in death, were filled with water. Inland Maya living in more arid regions traded for Cacao grown in coastal plantations by such groups as the Chontal Maya on the east coast, in present-day Tabasco, who also exported Cacao via the Tlaxcalan city of Cacaxtla, established on the trade route to the hub of ancient Mesoamerican civilisation, Teotihuacan. The Maya are the earliest native population known to have used Cacao beans as money: a small, portable exchange system whereby a set number of beans could be swapped for particular items. Offerings of counterfeit Cacao beans have even been discovered in an ancient temple in Guatemala; the beans are perfect replicas made of clay, though it's not clear whether the cache of painstakingly realistic fake beans is evidence of piety or forgery.

Vases from the Early Classic period (250–600 CE) depict feasts with large cylindrical pots of frothy *kakawa* drinks; other representations show liquid being poured from one of these vessels into another from a height for the purpose of creating a desirable head of foam on the bever- age. By the Late Classic period (600–800 CE) the Maya began using spouted vessels for serving *kakawa* akin to the "Cacao teapots" in use almost a millennium earlier, which does suggest that these vessels were used for frothing the drink in some way, as the Mayans liked their chocolate well aerated. The forms of *kakawa* also evolved: specific pottery vessels for serving different types of *kakawa* have been identified, often labelled with hieroglyphic inscriptions describing their contents, such as "tree-fresh *kakawa*" (a beverage made from Cacao fruit pulp, perhaps) or "honey *kakawa*" (a form of sweet chocolate drink). Some inscriptions contain instructive descriptions or phrases, such as *"takan kel"*—to roast Cacao well, in order that beverages made from it would produce a lot of *"yom kakawa"*, or foam. Some of the storage vessels were of an ingenious "lock-top" design, having a twist-on lid with a handle to enable the transportation and storage of pre-prepared *kakawa*.

The Maya usually drank from hemispherical clay bowls, and consumed both hot and cold *kakawa* potions; but, like cocoa-drinkers today, they mostly ingested Cacao in hot drinks. Moreover, although *mole negro*—a complex sauce for turkey made in contemporary Mexico, in which Cacao is a key ingredient—is supposed to have been invented by seventeenth-century Mexican nuns, there is archaeological evidence that the Classic Maya were using Cacao in food, too, and are the likely originators of this tradition. Plates and pots in royal tombs have been found with remnants of savoury dishes, such as fish and turkey bones, and traces of Cacao. The Spanish chronicler and early anthropologist Friar Bernardino de Sahagún documented the culture and geography of the "New World" after the conquest; he noted the Mexica (Aztec) use of a sauce called "*chiltepitl molli*", among many other sauces and stews, in feasts that were typically rounded off with a cup of chocolate.[38] Unfortunately he didn't specify the ingredients of this sauce, although we know that *chiltepitl* is a variety of chilli. We also know that what the Mexica referred to as "*atolli*", the generic name for a type of thin gruel made with boiled corn in water, is known in contemporary Mexico as "*atole*"—as *atolli* is to *atole*, so *molli* is to *mole*, perhaps. In any case, Cacao was central to Mayan societies, and freely traded between cities. Its status was such that the last three rulers of the great city of Tikal, located in modern-day Guatemala, were given the title "Lord *Kakaw*".[39]

The Maya region was made up of shifting "power blocs" of cities and tribal alliances, in which the merchant class—trading commodities such as salt, Cacao, and cotton across the region—eventually superseded the priestly elite as the dominant earthly powers. In the "Terminal Classic" period (800–900 CE) the Maya began abandoning their cities. In fact, between 750 and 950 CE, all the main power blocs in Central America—Monte Alban, Teotihuacan, and the Classic Maya cities—imploded, for unknown reasons. Eco-theories suggest that the inhabitants overtaxed their environment and then failed to cope during an extended period of drought, leading to starvation, rebellion, and anarchy. But that doesn't completely explain events, as we know that Mayan cities in areas with the highest rainfall were the first to go. Recent historical speculation suggests the main failures may have been administrative or political: perhaps too much attention was paid to warfare rather than feeding the population, leading to generalised civil unrest following a long period of reduced crop yields. Historian Charles Mann compared this situation to the political climate in the Soviet Union in the 1970s and 1980s, but played out over two centuries rather than decades,[40] owing perhaps to the partisan and fragmented nature of the kingdoms; the dominos took longer to fall, not being lined up next to each other, but the winds of change eventually blew almost every one down.

It's possible that the religious beliefs of the Classic Maya also had a role in their eventual collapse. The Classic Maya had adopted the *waxak-lahun-ubah-kan*, the feathered "war serpent" deity also known as Kukulcan from Teotihuacan, and its associated ritual and seasonal warfare tied to the astronomical cycles of Venus and Jupiter. Tikal may have been the first Mayan city to absorb this deity when the Teotihuacanos brought a war-standard "ensouled" with their serpent war god to the city, and, in 378 CE, empowered by the new weapons and ritual protocols imprinted by Teotihuacan, Tikal decided to attack its neighbouring city Waxaktun: the Mayan "star wars" had begun. Once this style of war was taken up, special astronomical events, such as eclipses, could also trigger hostilities as the need for captives to propitiate the gods and ensure good fortune became urgent—even in the rainy season,[41] which was traditionally "time off".

The patronising Victorian perception of the Maya as a peaceful society of "noble savages" has been dismantled by more recent discoveries. As in many ancient (and not so ancient) societies, slavery was commonplace; it was the standard sentence for theft, and both prisoners of war and orphans often ended up as slaves. People could also be sold into slavery, and their children, too, would be slaves, because like many Mesoamerican social roles, the position was hereditary.[42] Maya kings did public ritual dances holding the sacred war staffs, wearing costumes "festooned with the shrunken heads of past captives".[43] The Classic Maya sometimes used prisoners of war in brutal ways: archaeological evidence has shown that they could be ritually tortured, trussed up and used as living "balls" during ballgames, scalped, burned, or disembowelled before being decapitated in religious ceremonies. Living offerings may have accompanied the noble dead, so the death of a king was a bad day for POWs.[44] As with earlier forms of worship in Mesoamerica, bloodletting was also important to the Maya, for which purpose they used stingray spines, sharp obsidian blades, carved bones, or cords knotted with thorns. Males drew blood from the penis, females from the elbows, earlobes, or tongue; stingray spines were especially suitable for this purpose, because, once inserted, it was easier to pull them through than to retract them. The blood was collected on specially made bark-paper strips, and burned as offerings to the gods.[45] The significance and purpose of such gory rituals is discussed in Chapter 9. So it turns out that the Maya were just as complex and crazy and capable of state-sanctioned malevolence as any other human society.

A mural at the Classic Maya site Bonampak in present-day Chiapas, Mexico, depicts king Chan-Muwan ritually consecrating the temple in 790 CE at the heliacal rising of Venus (Venus' first appearance in the sky as the morning star rising before the sun, after several months of invisibility). This "ensouling of the temple" was accompanied by bloodletting, ritual dances, and feasts, and followed by the obligatory ritual war to acquire captives for sacrifice. Battle was joined, the mural records, when Venus and the sun lined up with each other in the middle of the sky at noon[46] (Venus' inferior conjunction with the sun on the *medium coeli*, when Venus is closest to the Earth.) As the Maya cities expanded and grew, and their populations swelled, the Venus-Tlaloc "star wars" style of warfare coupled with the demands of an expanding population on suboptimally fertile land gradually consumed the region in a near-constant, grinding state of war between the ancient dynasties. By the eighth century, the Maya cities had "unparalleled wealth and unprecedented problems";[47] the obligation to fight may have annulled treaties, severed bonds forged by marriages and alliances, disrupted farming and cultivation in a fragile ecosystem, and produced a completely unsustainable state of pan-Mayan conflict which resulted in eventual collapse.[48] This systemic failure as a result of an ideologically driven, expansionist lack of co-operation and consequent ecological mismanagement should be a salutary lesson for the world today.

4. The Toltecs and post-Classic Maya (900–1168 CE)

While the big cities were fragmenting, smaller city states survived, such as Cacaxtla in Tlaxcala and Xochicalco near Morelos, both in central Mexico. A new political power appeared in central-eastern Mexico in the form of the Toltecs, about whom little is known. They had a distinctively geometric and imposing architectural style which influenced the later Mexica (Aztec) culture, and is most evident in the ruins of the city of Tula (c.950–c.1170 CE), located in the northern region of the Yucatan peninsula. The Toltecs' first king assumed the name Quetzalcoatl, and it is thought they were a militaristic society, inheriting the ritual "star wars" style of combat from the Maya but with a more Teotihuacan-type expansionism. Toltec culture strongly influenced post-Classic Mesoamerica, particularly the later Mexica, who venerated the Toltecs and believed that the fourth creation of the world had begun in Tula. The Toltec style appears in the monolithic architecture of the Mayan cities Chichen Itza and the later site known as Mayapan, both located in the Yucatan. These sites are often referred to as post-Classic Maya or Toltec-Maya sites.

It's unknown whether Chichen Itza or Tula itself was the centre of expansion, but in either case the rise of Tula represented a newer and more aggressive Toltec-Maya state emerging from the dissolution of the old order in the peninsula. Chichen Itza appears to have been an imperial city, run by the nobility, who seem to have had far more military and strategic influence than they did in the theocratic Classic Maya civilisations. Unlike the Classic Maya polities, Chichen Itza was governed by a council of lords rather than one divinely-mandated ruler.[49] The city subsisted on a diet of warfare and commerce, which included the exchange or seizure of large quantities of much-prized Cacao; but the Toltec religion was even more sacrifice-oriented than the Classic Maya theocracies had been, and heart sacrifice—where a person had their still-beating heart cut out of their chest—became a central feature of worship.[50] Meanwhile, the Mixtecs took over Monte Alban, becoming famous for their metalwork and mosaic art, although they never achieved the dominant status of the earlier Zapotecs.[51]

The Yucatan Maya grew Cacao in the traditional Mayan way—in *cacaotales*, "Cacao orchards" which were biodiverse, multicropping systems, like large *milpas* established on high ground (much like tree-sized "raised beds" for better drainage). More than six hundred and twenty-five Cacao trees could be grown on a hectare of land, and the first Cacao pods would be ready to harvest three to four years after planting; many different varieties were grown, identifiable by the colour of the ripe fruits: yellow, white, red, black, and purple Cacao. As in other Maya regions, Cacao was the basis of a number of different hot and cold drinks, and was used as an admixture in various maize gruels—these being the basic, subsistence-level food of the people. Cacao was even consumed as a toasted snack,[52] in addition to being traded for salt and metal tools. Now, however, Cacao is scarce in this region: it is a fragile tree, and many of the tricks of cultivation (proper companion planting and "organic" soil maintenance techniques, for example) have been lost as the native population dwindled and became increasingly Europeanised.

The city-state of Mayapan came to prominence following Chichen Itza's demise in 1221, when the first Toltec-Maya city's subjects revolted. Mayapan was governed by ruling noble families for over two hundred years with the consent and assistance of local Maya lords, but it too succumbed to insurrection in 1441, initiating another descent into tribal warfare in the Yucatan. Incidentally, the remnants of the Yucatan Maya were the last native Mesoamerican culture to submit to Spanish rule after the conquest. A small band of Spanish explorers arrived in 1519. After fighting their way to the Mexica capital, they were received as guests by the emperor in 1521; the Spanish took him hostage and seized power, plunging the Mesoamerican universe into chaos and war, and opening the floodgates for colonisation from Europe once the population had been decimated by imported diseases. Many Maya polities in the Yucatan remained independent of Spanish control after the conquest because of the ease with which guerrilla warfare could be conducted in the relatively inaccessible jungle terrain they inhabited. The last Maya group to succumb to the Spaniards were the Itza of Peten, in 1675.

5. The Mexica (Aztecs) (1300–1521 CE)

Meanwhile, in twelfth-century pre-conquest Mesoamerica, while Europe was enjoying the ongoing Crusades just prior to the first outbreak of the Black Death, the Toltec-Mayan city states were fragmenting, and the Mexica (Aztecs) had been busy colonising the valley of Mexico. In 1325 they established the soon-to-be city of Tenochtitlan on an island in the centre of lake Texcoco. They formed an alliance with two cities on the edge of the lake, Texcoco and Tlacopan, and over the next two centuries this Triple Alliance, increasingly dominated by Tenochtitlan, proceeded to subjugate large swathes of Central America. Tenochtitlan grew to become a remarkable city, with aqueducts bringing fresh water into the city centre, good food sold in the marketplaces, and floating *milpa*-style gardens built up out of the lake criss-crossed with canals. Most people lived in clan or family-based neighbourhoods, called *calpulli*, while foreigners had their own districts or ghettos[53] (much like Chinatown or the Jewish quarter in many Old World cities). Mexica writing had devolved from the Classic Maya era to basic picture-writing, just as their calendrical and astronomical reckoning wasn't as advanced (see Chapter 10). Mexica books were used as mnemonic devices, helping students learn the words of songs, histories, and divinatory processes in a predominantly oral tradition. Books of ritual or divination were referred to collectively as *teoamoxtli*, "god-books", and the wise men who could interpret and use them were referred to as *tlamatini*, "ones who know".[54]

The so-called "Aztec empire" of the Mexica wasn't a single unified territory; it was a complex tribute-collecting network of conquered states, an imperial power governed by a trade-based hegemony. (The term "Aztec" was invented by the German naturalist Alexander von Humboldt in 1810. It is derived from *aztecatl*, a native Mexican (Nahuatl language) term meaning "from Aztlan", Aztlan being the mythical homeland of the Mexica.) "Flowery wars"—in the pattern of the "star wars" style of ritual warfare established by Teotihuacan and the Classic Maya—were regularly fought between the armies of the Triple Alliance and non-imperial regions or vassal states to obtain ritual human sacrifices required by the gods. When foreign kings and nations submitted to Mexica rule, they were allowed to keep their throne and national identity so long as they paid tribute and engaged in regular holy wars as the calendar required;[55] the customary aim was to incapacitate and capture enemies, not just kill them, because the blood of captured warriors was more pleasing to the gods.[56]

Like the Classic-era Maya, Mexica kings were often deified after their death, but unlike the Maya, the Mexica king or *tlatoani* ("speaker") was elected by nobles from a noble family. The *tlatoani* had to be a male blood-relative of a previous incumbent, but one who was chosen based on competence and who had proven himself in battle. Noble children and gifted commoners were educated in the *calmecac*, schools where theology, history, oratory, singing, the calendar, astronomy, and astrology were taught—and, after the age of fifteen, Mexica boys from the *calmecac* and the regular schools, the *telpochcalli*, were given military training.[57] One of the most famous personages in pre-Colombian Mesoamerican history is Tlacaelel, the cunning advisor to five successive *tlatoani* during the expansion of the empire, and the embodiment of the "power behind the throne". Tlacaelel created a sort of military aristocracy, providing a powerful incentive to fight on behalf of the state by making it possible for commoners to acquire noble status through distinguished military careers. He also had many history books burned, and mandated a new history of the Mexica people, featuring them as the chosen people of their patron sun-war god, Huitzilopchtli,[58] demonstrating the truth of two maxims of the philosopher Walter Benjamin: "History is written by the victors," and "There is no document of culture which is not at the same time a document of barbarism."

Like the Maya, the Mexica used Cacao as currency, as well as the base material for elaborate chocolate drinks. Half a bean would buy you a piece of fruit, a prostitute's services could be acquired for eight to ten beans, and a human slave was available to those with a hundred beans to spend.[59] Because Cacao doesn't naturally grow in the valley of Mexico, it had to be imported from far-flung parts of the empire. The Mexica never managed to completely subdue the Mixtec peoples in Oaxaca valley, but by dint of strategic alliances with Zapotec chiefdoms there, they secured their principal aim—to control the trade route from the capital cities of the Triple Alliance through Mixtec territory and down the isthmus to Soconusco,[60] all for the purpose of safeguarding their supply and control of Cacao imports. Incidentally, the Mixtec were known for their three-footed ceramic bowls, used as drinking and offering vessels; in some surviving codices, Mixtec elites are depicted drinking foaming Cacao-based drinks or *pulque*, a milky-looking alcoholic beverage made from fermented Maguey cactus sap, from these tripod cups at important meetings or marriage ceremonies.[61]

De Sahagún said of Soconusco in 1525 that "the whole province is a garden filled with Cacao trees", with over 1,600,000 Cacao trees in that region alone.[62] Cacao was brought to Tenochtitlan by trade caravans, travelling on foot through enemy territory, so its cultural cachet was greater among the Mexica than the Yucatan Maya.[63] A *xiquipil* was a unit of Cacao, approximately eight thousand beans; three *xiquipiles*, or twenty-four thousand beans,[64] weighing around 23kg (coincidentally, the upper weight limit for separate items of baggage decreed by many airlines today) was the most one person could carry, and the typical load of a Cacao porter in a caravan. The merchants who arranged these caravans came from a prestigious caste, known as *pochteca*, "men of the land of the Ceiba"—the Ceiba (*Ceiba pentandra*) being the national tree of modern-day Guatemala, an extraordinarily tall tree producing a water-resistant fibre called kapok. Being a merchant was a high-risk profession, as the caravans were frequently attacked by bandits or war bands from neighbouring hostile states, and the *pochteca* fulfilled important roles as ambassadors, explorers, spies, and even warriors as well as traders;[65] they were the scouting vanguard for Mexica territorial expansion. The principal routes of the Mexica trade caravans ran from Tochtepec in central Mexico (close to modern-day Oaxaca city) to Tenochtitlan, Texcoco, and Tlacopan.

Consequently Cacao was a luxury commodity in the Mexica capital, and its consumption was restricted by law to nobles and warriors, the *pochteca*, and the royal household. Soldiers may have occasionally been provisioned with Cacao in dried tablet form, but priests would probably not have partaken of it, just as getting drunk on communion wine would be taboo for Christian clergy today. Mexica law decreed that women and children were not permitted to drink Cacao, and any man who didn't go to war—even if of royal blood—was forbidden to wear cotton, feathers, or flowers, to eat rich food, drink Cacao, or smoke; the good life was only to be enjoyed by those who contributed to the Mexica's militaristic society.[66] Like other Mesoamerican cultures, the Mexica used entheogens such as *Psilocybe* mushrooms and the seeds of morning glory (*Turbina corymbosa*) vines, or *ololiouhqui* ("ollow·lee·ock·wee"). These plants were venerated as gods and accorded ritual respect; the small baskets used to store *ololiouhqui* seeds were passed down through many generations.[67] At the accession celebration for the last Mexica emperor, Motecuhzoma III (also known as Moctezuma or Montezuma), over two thousand dancers ingested entheogenic mushrooms as part of the festivities, which lasted for four days.[68] The purpose of this mass consumption of psychedelics was religious: to communicate with the gods, plunging the celebrants into a state of visionary ecstasy to sanction the *tlatoani*'s sacred purpose.

The Mexica also notoriously practised human sacrifice and cannibalism, religious acts which had historical precedents throughout Mesoamerica, but which became more central to post-Classic religious practice following the Toltec era. Human sacrifices to the principal gods of the Mexica pantheon, Tlaloc and Hutizilopochtli, were killed by heart extraction on the altar at the top of the great twin-temple pyramid in the centre of Tenochtitlan. Their decapitated heads were mounted on the *tzompantli* or skull-rack in the square.[69] As part of his duty, the *tlatoani* had to participate in important religious festivals, and was sometimes required to impersonate deities; but he had a relatively easy time of it. For some important occasions in the ritual calendar, a person was selected to "live as a god" before being sacrificed: one such festival, held in the month called Toxcatl, had a handsome, blemish-free young man live as the god Tezcatlipoca for one year, during which he played the flute and ocarina every day, and lived lavishly. At the appointed hour, he ceremonially smashed the instruments and climbed the stairway of the great temple to be sacrificed, leaving the broken fragments at the foot of the steps.[70] After such sacrifices, the corpse would sometimes be flayed so that priests or warriors could wear the skin for a designated period of time, as in the ceremonies of the Mexica god of spring, Xipe Totec, "the flayed one".[71]

For the Mexica, human flesh could transmit the powers of the gods. If a sacrificial victim impersonated a god, those who ceremonially ate his flesh would absorb some divine essence into themselves. This belief recalls the words of the Catholic Eucharist: "Take this, all of you, and eat of it, for this is my body, which will be given up for you …" Prisoners of war could be sacrificed by heart extraction, or occasionally pitted against opponents in gladiatorial contests with a handicap (such as a club studded with feathers rather than obsidian blades). Captives in such contests were often chained to a post, and fought against a properly-armed opponent; if they prevailed, against all odds, they were sometimes set free. Human sacrifices were made every day at the principal shrines of major deities, but multiple sacrifices were only performed at major ceremonies such as key points in the astronomical-agricultural cycle or the accession of a new *tlatoani*.[72]

By the time Hernán Cortés and his band of Spanish fortune-hunters arrived on the eastern shore of Mexico in 1519, the royal household at Tenochtitlan consumed copious quantities of Cacao. The Mexica deity Quetzalcoatl is apocryphally associated with the story of the conquest of Central America, as he was the god allegedly prophesied (by the later Toltecs) to return in the year one reed—the very year the Spanish conquistador Hernán Cortés landed in

Mexico. The forked tongue of prophecy is purported to be one reason why Cortés was wel-comed into the Mexica capital, as the god's legendary appearance—pale skin, bearded—lent so much extra mystery to the grubby Spaniards, with their strange four-legged beasts and alien technology, that they were welcomed with awe and strategic caution. Their recipro-cal gifts of treachery and smallpox helped them to claim a continent. Curiously, all the pre-conquest native sources and legends mention no specific date for Quetzalcoatl's return; only accounts of the legend written *after* the European invasion specifically mention the year one reed, with the implication of fate and divine retribution against the native population that the prophecy's apparent accuracy suggests.

It's not recounted whether or not the Mexica used Cacao in food, but it's noteworthy (and another nail in the coffin for the "Spanish nuns" origin story for Cacao's use in savoury dishes) that the Mexica word for stew, *mulli*, is the root of the modern Mexican word *molé*, the elaborate spiced sauces and stocks which sometimes contain Cacao, such as *molé negro*. The conquistador Bernal Diaz described one of the emperor Motecuhzoma's meals:

> From time to time [the servants] brought him, in cup-shaped vessels of pure gold, a certain drink made from Cacao, and the women served this drink to him with great reverence [...] As soon as the great Moctezuma had dined, all the men of the Guard had their meal and as many more of the other house servants, and it seems to me that they brought out over a thousand dishes of the food [...] and then over two thousand jugs of Cacao all frothed up, as they make it in Mexico, and a limitless quantity of fruit, so that with his women and female servants and bread makers and Cacao makers his expenses must have been very great. (Diaz del Castillo, 1632)

At the average Mexica lord's banquet, smoking tubes of tobacco were served before the meal, while *cacahuatl* (the name for Cacao-based beverages in the native Mexica language, *Nahuatl*) was served in painted or decorated gourds at the end of the meal. The gourd was held in the right hand, with a stirring stick and gourd rest placed at the left hand of each guest. Less prestigious guests would receive their *cacahuatl* in clay cups.[73] Unlike the Maya, who liked it hot, the Mexica drank their chocolate at room temperature—which in the valley of Mexico is tepid, not cold. Otherwise the Mexica and Maya Cacao drinks were similar—mostly bitter or savoury, spiced, and foamy concoctions with many ingredients and variations.

Cacao was the first item on the list of necessities for large, one-off banquets given by success-ful merchants. The shopping list for such feasts also included hallucinogenic mushrooms, to be consumed with *cacahuatl* by members of the warrior caste, for the dual purposes of divination and recreation. Ethnopharmacologist Jonathan Ott proposes that the Mexica may well have mixed the sacred mushrooms into *cacahuatl*, actually incorporating the fresh mushroom juice into the beverages at these feasts as a pleasant means of consuming them.[74] For the Mexica, *caca-huatl* consumption was reserved for men only—women had to make do with beverages made from chia seeds and water, or gruels of maize, water, and spices (*atolli*). The standard alcoholic beverage at these occasions was *octli* (now known as *pulque*), or other mead-like products of fer-mented honey, water, and herbs. *Octli* was restricted for all except the elderly, who had earned the right to drink more. But *octli* was a drink for commoners, who couldn't afford to drink *cacahuatl*; only the richest merchants, warriors, lords, and princes consumed Cacao, because to drink Cacao was to literally consume money.

There are also accounts of a Mexica Cacao-based drink called *itzpacalatl* which allegedly translates as "water from the washing of obsidian blades".[75] This was a special form of Cacao-based beverage, made by priests for the specific purpose of jollying up a slave who was due for sacrifice, and perhaps unsurprisingly failing at the task of joyously dancing while pretending to be the god Quetzlcoatl as part of a forty-day ritual which would culminate in his death. The drink was made from Cacao and water in which sacrificial obsidian knives had been washed— in other words, bloody water—and it made the slave dance happily again, and gladly go to be sacrificed.[76] It seems likely that this drink contained some potent botanical additives, which will be discussed more thoroughly in the following chapters.

Chocolate spreads

After the conquest, the Spanish took over the practice of taking Cacao beans as tribute or tax from the natives, and imposed European farming practices in many areas. Disease and enslavement had decimated the indigenous population, and Cacao production dwindled as both land and people were exhausted. Central America was flooded with European settlers and their Afro-Caribbean vassals, and these early colonists adopted the custom of using the beans as money, finding them to be an effective means of bartering with the natives, but were slow to take up the consumption of Cacao themselves. The Italian expatriate chronicler Girolamo Benzoni's account of his *cacahuatl* habit is representative of the gradual shift in European attitudes as they were exposed to this new drug-food:

> It [*cacahuatl*] seemed more a drink for pigs, than a drink for humanity. I was in this country for more than a year, and never wanted to taste it, and whenever I passed a settlement some Indian would offer me a drink of it, and would be amazed when I would not accept, going away laughing. But then, as there was a shortage of wine, so as not to be always drinking water, I did like the others. The taste is somewhat bitter, it satisfies and refreshes the body, but does not inebriate, and it is the best and most expensive merchandise, according to the Indians of that country. (Benzoni, quoted in Coe & Coe, 1996)

The Spanish introduced the *encomienda* system, whereby a representative of the Spanish monarch invested individuals with the right to own land—and the indigenous people on that land, who were then used as slave labour. At the time of the conquest, a Cacao orchard such as Izalco in El Salvador had 33,570 trees each producing 400,000 beans annually;[77] after a few years of indentured slavery, enforced mismanagement of the land, overtaxation and corruption, Izalco's output was reduced to almost nothing. The colonists almost exclusively used slave labour to cultivate Cacao, which increased production at the cost of human suffering and diminishing returns from traditional Mesoamerican sources, obliging Europeans to seek new locations to cultivate Cacao in the West Indies and South America.[78]

Nevertheless, as the Europeans became accustomed to Cacao, they started to modify the drinks containing it. The Spaniards began to consume *cacahuatl* as a hot drink, in the manner of the Yucatec Maya; they added sugar to sweeten it; they substituted most native spices (with the notable exception of vanilla) with cinnamon from Sri Lanka, black pepper from the Indies, and aniseed from Europe; and they elaborated the *molinillo*, a beautiful type of wooden hand whisk for frothing the drinks, still in use in Mexico today. I suggest elaborated, not invented, because there is second-hand evidence that the Mexica, at least, used some kind of utensil for frothing *cacahuatl*: an inventory of requirements (ingredients and equipment) for a Mexica banquet includes "chocolate beaters … two or four thousand of them".[79] The Spanish also changed the name of the drink: *cacahuatl* became *chocolate*. Theories abound, but the etymology of the new name is unclear. The reason for the change may be quite basic—it's possible that the Europeans were discomfited by their growing preference for consuming a gloopy aromatic brown liquid known locally as *caca*-something. *Caca* (a word used colloquially in French, Spanish, Italian, German, and Romanian, and the basis of the modern Spanish word *cagar*) is derived from the Latin word *cacō*—"to defecate, shit, or pass excrement".[80] Definitely more of a niche market name.

Cacao was, as yet, alien to most of Europe; English and Dutch pirates seized two Spanish ships with a cargo of Cacao in the late 1500s and burnt it all, allegedly mistaking the brown beans for dried sheep dung.[81] But by the mid-seventeenth century, chocolate had gone transatlantic—it became "the first drink to introduce Europe to the pleasures of alkaloid consumption".[82] Alkaloids are the given name for a group of nitrogen-containing chemicals found in plants, many of which have potent pharmacological effects on the human organism. But it's untrue that Europeans were unfamiliar with alkaloid-containing beverages, as there are thousands of alkaloid-producing medicinal herbs native to Europe, some of which were drunk as decoctions or tisanes or brewed into beer centuries before chocolate arrived from the New World, such as the medieval European almost-panacea wood betony (*Stachys officinalis*), which contains the alkaloids stachydrine and betonicine, to name just one plant. But chocolate *was* the first popular drink to introduce European courts to the pleasures of consuming the group of stimulating alkaloids known as the *xanthines* (the famous trio of theophylline, theobromine, and the Diana Ross of the group, caffeine), preceding tea and coffee. Chocolate became very fashionable at the Spanish court, and even had a new item of crockery invented in its service: the *mancerina* was a silver or porcelain saucer with a raised ring in the centre for holding a small cup, to facilitate genteel, spillage-free socialising with appropriate doses of chocolate.

Relatively libertarian religious orders such as the Jesuits, and Jewish refugees from racial and religious persecution in Spain were responsible for introducing Cacao consumption to the rest of Europe in non-aristocratic circles.[83] By the late 1660s Cacao had made its way to France, via Italy. Cacao was one of the exciting new "imported drugs" from the New World, so it was principally recommended by well-heeled physicians as a medicinal tonic for the gentry. The fact that this sweet chocolate was extremely palatable—and exotic—and expensive—didn't hinder its burgeoning popularity in the least; special silver *chocolatières* were invented for its consumption at the French court, with a side handle and a hole in the lid for a built-in *molinillo*, and a little spout for pouring the prepared drink. This gave rise to a whole range of porcelain and metal *chocolatières* of great craftsmanship and beauty, so the upper crust could enjoy their morning chocolate in an appropriately civilised fashion.

By the time chocolate arrived in England, it had been further bastardised to suit European tastes. Served in the new coffee, tea, and chocolate houses in London it would be boiled in water, and sometimes prepared with milk and eggs. Such adaptation was nothing new in the history of Cacao, while boiling the bean or tablets made from it in water would liberate the flavour and many of the active compounds in the seeds, but it must have produced a decidedly inferior product when compared to the much more laborious traditional process of making *cacahuatl*. This richer, sweetened, attenuated, milk- or egg-enriched chocolate became the starting point for the modern confection. A contemporary author noted that the flour and eggs often added to the drinks

> makes the Chocolate never the better; and without such addition, it is excellent good, and very agreeable, strengthening Nature exceedingly […] And truly, what we now use in England, is but a compound of Spices, Milk, Eggs, Sugar &c., and perhaps there is in it a fourth or fifth part of the chiefest ingredient, the Cacao […] So it is no wonder if this Drink be not found of that virtue and efficacy as hath been noised abroad, or as many expect: But doubtless if Physitians did but narrowly pry into the secrets of the nature of it, they would quickly finde (the right use thereof being made) that it can scarcely be too much commended. (Hughes, 1672)

Chocolate had an impressive—though controversial—medicinal reputation at this time, particularly as an aphrodisiac. Dr Henry Stubbe's 1682 pamphlet, for one, described its many venereal virtues in lyrically euphemistic prose. But Cacao's novelty and association with wealth, privilege, decadence, and the heathen "Indians" of Mexico had earned the drug some ecclesiastical enemies, particularly the Dominicans, who regarded its growing consumption during Lent and other fasting periods with horror. Other religious sects, such as the Jesuits, consumed it with gusto, claiming its status as a drink obviated any classification of chocolate as a nutritious food, thereby permitting its consumption during fasting—this despite the fact that one of the native medicinal uses of Cacao in Mexico was to encourage weight gain! In Mexico, it had become the custom for Spanish ladies to consume chocolate during Mass; when one bishop attempted to ban this practice, threatening excommunication to anyone flouting his decree, he died shortly afterwards in a grotesque manner, "allegedly from a cup of poisoned chocolate slipped into his house by one of the angered ladies".[84]

From the late 1500s, slave ships would make a three-way trading trip from Europe to the coast of Africa, where they would barter manufactured goods for human slaves; the slave ships then sailed to the West Indies and the New World, where they would sell the slaves and collect slave-farmed crops such as sugar and Cacao, and return to Europe.[85] Sometime in the seventeenth century, the Spanish took Cacao to the Philippines, and thence to Sri Lanka. The French acquired Cacao seeds and established plantations in Martinique, St. Lucia, and Bahia in 1660, and by 1778 the Dutch had transplanted seedlings to East India, and set up an experimental Cacao garden in Jakarta.[86] Meanwhile, England began growing *Theobroma cacao* to service the coffeehouses of London on its slave-worked plantations in Jamaica. Other European nations followed suit, establishing Cacao cultivation in Africa in the 1800s, when the Spanish colonies began to assert their independence. Spanish missionaries established Cacao plantations on the island of Fernando Po off the coast of West Africa, and African natives—slaves and freed men and women—transported seeds to the mainland on their own initiative. Ghanaian lore relates that a blacksmith called Tatteh Quashie, a member of the Ga tribe, smuggled seedlings back to Africa from Fernando Po, and produced the first African Cacao crop in 1883.[87] Cacao's global expansion correlated with declining production in its place of origin, with the eventual result that almost all the chocolate sold in today's market is produced outside Central America.

Cacao wasn't the only Mesoamerican crop to be adopted overseas. Tomatoes, chillies, and corn were all diffused over the globe, but it was corn—the staple Mexican starch, their "staff of life", and erstwhile accompaniment to Cacao in food and drink—that caused some trouble. At some point in prehistory, the Mesoamericans had invented a process of boiling maize with wood ash and lime to soften it; the maize was then rinsed, dried, and ground to make flour, known nowadays as *masa harina*. This process, called *nixtamalization* (from the word *nixtamalli* in Nahuatl) has been found to even out the balance of essential amino acids in corn, the protein building substances that must be acquired from food, and to liberate niacin, also known as vitamin B3, making it available for use. Without nixtamalization, the niacin isn't bioavailable— it can't be absorbed. Europeans eschewed the "barbaric" traditional nixtamalization process, but with widespread cultivation of maize a new disease appeared, causing skin lesions, diarrhoea, lassitude, and cognitive decline. Called "pellagra", meaning "rough skin", two hundred years of epidemics occurred in Italy, France, Egypt, and other parts of Africa, resulting in widespread suffering and death. Pellagra was known to be linked to the consumption of corn, but was thought to be due to some contaminant; it wasn't until the twentieth century that the cause was determined to be niacin deficiency.[88] Maize *masa* was the basis of tortillas and many a liquid meal in Mesoamerica, and while there are a few recipes which call for un-nixtamalized maize, they are exceptions to the general rule. The early modern pellagra pandemics are a not-so-shining example of how we ignore traditional processes, however strange or superfluous they may seem, at our peril.

In 1727 Nicholas Sanders manufactured the first "official" milk chocolate drink for Hans Sloane, surgeon to King George III, who had tasted chocolate while visiting Jamaica and found it unpleasantly sharp, so he added milk. Sloane and Sanders marketed the milky drink as a treatment for consumption (tuberculosis), the bacterial lung disease which attacks white blood cells, and was a common cause of gradual weight loss, feverishness, declining lung function, and eventual death in the pre-antibiotic era. Although Cacao has no systemic antibiotic action, particularly against an organism as resilient as *Mycobacterium tuberculosis*, the drink may have done some good simply by providing extra nutrients and calories, perhaps improving resistance to the disease in dietetically defective Londoners. As we shall see in Chapter 4, laboratory (*in vitro*) research suggests Cacao may stimulate part of the adaptive immune system which helps protect against microorganisms such as bacteria, and it helps to soothe chronic coughs. Whether or not Sanders's milk chocolate achieved the goal of allaying symptoms or promoting weight gain for its consumptive purchasers, sales of the drink certainly fattened Sir Hans's bank balance.

By the 1800s, consumption of chocolate drinks in Europe had declined in popularity, giving way to coffee, partly as a consequence of Cacao's expense but principally because of the amount of labour required to turn the beans into a drink; simple grinding and boiling was inadequate because the beans had to be worked to the consistency of a liquid and whisked into hot water. The prohibitive cost of the raw material and the time taken to prepare drinking chocolate largely restricted its regular consumption to the sedentary classes, those who could afford servants. In 1828, the Dutchman Coenraad van Houten invented the process that came to be called "Dutching"—treating the unroasted, shelled, and fragmented cocoa beans or "nibs" with alkali to make the final product more miscible with water, then roasting and pressing them to extrude the fat, or "cocoa butter", and grinding the resulting de-fatted roasted seed cake to powder. The result of this process is cocoa powder—darker, drier, and lighter than Cacao bean mass (so-called "cocoa liquor"), much easier to mix with water, but also markedly less flavoursome. The industrialisation of Cacao processing and the invention of cocoa powder was an important step in the worldwide distribution of Cacao, because cocoa is a useful ingredient in many recipes and products, in addition to being (in marked contrast to whole Cacao beans) easy to make into a beverage. Nonetheless, cocoa was yet another step removed from the rich, labour-intensive, full-bodied, and full-flavoured Cacao-based drinks of Mesoamerica.

The British Victorians enhanced the global dissemination of Cacao by transporting live trees around the world in "Wardian cases", miniature greenhouses which were invented in London for culturing ferns, then adapted to solve the problem of loss of viability in seeds and living plants on long sea journeys.[89] In 1847, Joseph Fry invented the world's first "chocolate bar" by combining cocoa powder, cocoa butter, and sugar. This wasn't the world's first eating chocolate, however—the Maya and the Mexica both produced portable "tablets" of spiced Cacao for use by their travelling merchants and warriors. The tablets were pulverised and beaten into water to produce a drink when required, but it's unlikely that they weren't eaten as a simple food source and ready-made stimulant in the absence of the time or equipment necessary to produce a beverage—a Mexica legend, transcribed shortly after the conquest, describes Cacao as being "drunk and sometimes eaten".[90] Incidentally, similar use has been made of coffee beans in Africa: the Oromo tribe of Abyssinia in present-day Ethiopia shaped dried coffee beans mixed with fat or salted butter into billiard ball shaped rations, which would be eaten on long overland journeys. Cacao has a relative advantage here, as it already has a high fat content—no need to adulterate the bean to get a good balance of calories and caffeine![91]

When Henri Nestlé produced evaporated (powdered) milk in 1867, it was only a matter of time before someone took the next logical step, and that someone was the Swiss manufacturer Daniel Peter, who in 1879 became the first person to oversee the production of edible milk chocolate, the delectable combination of cocoa liquor (Cacao bean paste), milk powder, sugar, and extra cocoa butter. The final step in the transformation of Cacao from bitter beverage to sweet confection—and another step down in potency and purity from the handmade plant-based drinks of ages past—was the invention of the conching process in the same year by Rudolphe Lindt. Conching is the term applied to the repeated beating of cocoa liquor by mechanised rollers over many hours or days to reduce any particles in the liquid to the smallest possible size and make it as smooth as possible, so that the finished chocolate has a completely grit-free and orally pleasing texture.

So Cacao, the sacred seed which was the basis of various elaborate beverages for the New World elite, became a commonplace pleasure of the Old World masses: a sweet, secular snack. In Chapter 2, we will look more closely at all the guises *Theobroma cacao* has assumed during its journey so far, as a prelude to investigating its medicinal properties. We'll see how we may benefit from reviving some of the ancestral, time-consuming ways of preparing the seed to make old-school Maya *kakawa* or Mexica *cacahuatl*, the real contenders for the food—or, rather, drinks—of the gods.

Table 1. Theobroma cacao timeline

Date	Chocolate timeline	Mesoamerican timeline	"Old World" timeline
9000–7000 BCE		8000–7000 BCE: Maize developed from *teosinte* and cultivated in Tehuacan & Oaxaca valleys	Wheat cultivation begun in Syria & Mesopotamia; barley in the Indus valley
3200 / 3000 BCE			3200 BCE Sumerian tablets written in cuneiform "alphabet"
3000–2000 BCE		3000–2000 BCE: Villages, farming, early trade networks began to form	Indus Valley Aryans, Ancient Egyptian cultures
2500 BCE			
2000 BCE			Minoan civilisation in Crete
1900 BCE	1900 BCE: Soconusco region cultivating **Cacao. Beverages being made from the seeds?** Pottery fragments with traces of theobromine found		
1800 BCE		1800 BCE–300 CE: **Olmec** culture on E. Coast of Mexico	
1800–1200 BCE		1800–1200 BCE: **Olmec** sites San Lorenzo & Veracruz	
1600–1045 BCE			1600–1045 BCE: China: Shang dynasty
1500 BCE–200 CE	**Peruvian** vessel depicting Cacao & spider monkeys made	1500 BCE to 200 CE: **Pre-Classic** Maya settlements in the Yucatan	
1200–400 BCE	**Ulua Valley, Honduras – Theobroma** cultivation begins; entire drinking vessels found		
1150–300 BCE	1200–400 BCE: Olmec Cacao use (?)	1150–300 BCE: **Olmec** site La Venta	
1000 BCE			Assyrian empire; Greek settlement in Ionia & development of Greek city states begins
			Persian empire; China divided into separate states under Chou dynasty
c.600 BCE	600 BCE – **earliest complete vessel with detectable Cacao residues** (a "Cacao teapot") from Belize, spouted & wide-necked		c.600 BCE Roman republic founded, slow expansion
500 BCE–600 CE		500 BCE–600 CE	Classical Greece: Athenian empire comes into ascendancy
334–323 BCE			334–323 BCE: Alexander the Great

Chocolate history	Mesoamerica	World history
CE1	**CE1**	**CE1**
		27 BCE, foundation of the Roman Empire under Octavius — Birth of Jesus Christ
	Zapotec city of Monte Albán in Oaxaca	
435–551 CE: Copan tomb–food remains with Cacao, & a scoop stained with	50–700 CE Teotihuacan in Central Mexico	410 & 455 CE: Rome sacked by Visigoths and Vandals
	250–900 CE: Classic Maya period in the Yucatan – cities such as Copan, Palenque, Uxmal, Tikal, & many others	
500	**500**	**500**
cinnabar & Cacao; "lock top" vessel for pre-prepared drinks containing Cacao residues found at Rio Azul in Guatemala, dated c.500 CE. Similar Late Classic Maya vessels have hieroglyphic inscriptions for specific types of Cacao drink; Maya pottery & murals depict preparation & consumption of Cacao	600–900 CE: post-classic Zapotec	570 CE: birth of Prophet Muhammad — China: 581–618 CE: Sui Dynasty unites China
		896–927: First Bulgarian Empire
	950–1170 CE Toltecs	Founding of Baghdad; growth of the Arab caliphate; 1095–1291, the Crusades
	950–1250 CE: Toltec-Maya in the Yucatan: Chichen Itza, and Mayapan	1088: University of Bologna founded.
1000	**1000**	**1000**
1500–1521 CE: Post-Classic Maya wide-necked vessels with traces of Cacao found, similar to ones from Formative era (900–700 BCE)		1206–1227: Ghengis Khan & the Mongol Empire
	1323–1519 CE:	Baghdad sacked by Mongols, 1258
		1492: Columbus' voyage to America — 1347–1351: peak of the Black Death
	Growth of the Mexica empire from Tenochtitlan, C. Mexico	
1500	**1500**	**1500**
1580: Spanish chronicler Hernández uses word "chocollatl"; molinillos invented; European documentation of Mexica and native Cacao consumption methods; addition of sugar, and substitution of native spices; Cacao travels to Europe	1519–present:	1543: Copernicus publishes *De Revolutionibus Orbium Coelestium* — 1519–1522: Magellan circumnavigates the world
1727 CE: Hans Sloane "invents" milk chocolate drink; 1753 CE Carl von Linné (Linnaeus) names *Theobroma cacao*	European invasion, partial genocide, and re-colonisation of Mesoamerica; cultural hybridisation.	18th century: beginning of the Industrial Revolution — 1756–1763: the Seven Years' war: British world dominance — 1776: American independence
1828: Coenraad van Houten makes cocoa; 1847: Joseph Fry manufactures eating chocolate; 1879: Daniel Peter invents solid milk chocolate & Rudolphe LIndt develops the conching process	1821: Mexican independence	1820: discovery of Antarctica — 20th century: World Wars I & II
2000	**2000**	**2000**

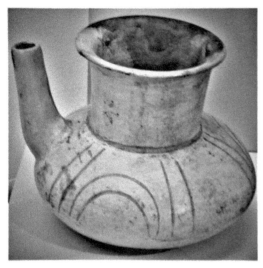

Ancient spouted chocolate pot, Popol Vuh
museum, Guatemala city, 2011

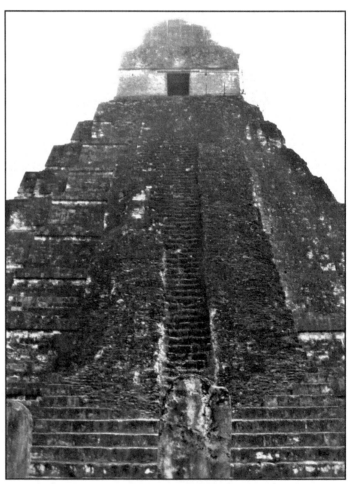

Ruined temple of Ha'Kakaw,
'Lord of Cacao', Tikal, Guatemala,
2011

CHAPTER TWO

Bodies of chocolate

sophisticated (sə'fɪstɪkeɪtɪd) *adj.* **1.** having refined or cultured tastes and habits. **2.** appealing to sophisticated people: *a sophisticated restaurant*. **3.** (of machines or methods) complex and refined. [Latin *sophisticare* 'tamper with', from *sophisticus* 'sophistic']
sophisticate (sə'fɪstɪˌkeɪt) *vb.* **1.** to make (someone) less natural or innocent, as by education.
(Collins Pocket Dictionary, 1989, & Compact Oxford English Dictionary, 2008)

In fact, people do not really know what good chocolate is.

(Telly, in Szyogi, 1997)

*K*akawa, to use the Mayan name, or *cacahuatl* as the Mexica called them, are old-school pre-Colombian Mesoamerican drinks made with Cacao. These traditional chocolate beverages are interesting concoctions, physically speaking. Unlike tea or coffee, they're not simple infusions, that is, products of steeping plant material in water to extract flavour and pharmacological properties in the form of water-soluble chemicals. Nor are they only suspension-infusions, like a cup of cocoa, wherein tiny dried particles of plant matter float suspended in a liquid (such as hot water or milk) while their water-soluble chemicals diffuse into the surrounding menstruum. Some are infusion-emulsions, like *kava-kava*, the psychoactive drink of Polynesia, or the more familiar (to Westerners) *espresso* coffee, from which solids are strained out, leaving fats or fat-soluble compounds from the plant material mixed into the water in the form of microscopic globules, together with dissolved water-soluble substances such as caffeine.

In the case of kava-kava this emulsification is achieved by pulping roots of kava plants (*Piper methysticum*) and repeatedly squeezing the root mash in water through some kind of sieve or cloth, forcing resinous substances from the root into the liquid; with espresso, a jet of steam is blasted through roasted and ground seeds of the coffee plant (*Coffea arabica*), driving fats from the bean to mingle with the resultant concentrated infusion. Most old-school chocolate drinks are suspension-emulsion-infusions, combining elements of all three modes of distribution: the fatty Cacao seeds are well ground, with other ingredients, then mixed with hot or tepid water. The mixing process is carried out gradually when tepid (room temperature) water is used, to prevent separation of the emulsified fats, and the finished drinks are then frothed by pouring from a height or beating with a whisk to keep the particles in suspension

27

and the fats in emulsion, to facilitate infusion, and raise a head of aromatic foam. (On the subject of froth, more later.)

This laborious method of preparation was favoured for most of chocolate's history. The probable pharmaceutical and practical reasons are that this method of preparation maximised the pharmacological effects and flavour. Lighter aromatic compounds such as essential oils from the toasted beans, or vanillin, the main molecule in vanilla (and a trace flavour compound present in the Cacao bean itself), burst free from the bubbles of foam popping in the mouth and hit the palate quickly; water soluble compounds in infusion are likewise detected by the tongue or nose relatively quickly. (After all, taste is mostly a matter of aroma, managed by olfactory receptors in the nose which detect smells. Anyone who wishes to test this for themselves should try eating a banana while wearing a nose clip.) Fat-soluble substances such as capsaicin, the "heat-bearing" chemical from chilli, yield their flavours more slowly, lingering on the palate, providing depth and interest by introducing "layers" to the flavour of the drink, which is less achievable with a simple infusion. Finally, the particulate matter in the beverage—the suspended solids from Cacao and the other ingredients—take a little longer to break down in the gut, providing a "timed release" component to the pharmacological action of the drink. The physiological effects resulting from different preparations of Cacao are discussed in Chapter 4. In this chapter, we will look at the evolution of Cacao products in history, walking backwards through time from the present-day chocolate manufacturing industry to early Mesoamerican botanical beverages. But let's begin with a closer look at the Cacao plant itself.

The "chocolate tree"

Theobroma cacao is a short, sturdy, understorey equatorial tree, growing in narrow bands of latitude around twenty degrees north and south of the equator, and is native to the Americas. It likes high humidity, ample rainfall, the shade and humus-enriched soil provided by taller trees. Valentine's Day chocolates are a token of desire, a kind of symbolic down-payment on sexual attraction; and, appropriately enough, the Cacao tree seems to thrive in moist and fertile crevices. Wild Cacao grows on riverbanks and was cultivated in the Mayan *dzonots* or *cenotes* of the Yucatan peninsula, sink-holes that penetrate deep below the surface and expose the water table, providing perfect warm, damp, and sheltered Cacao-growing microclimates. Cacao enjoys such shady places on the borders and apertures of the watery Mesoamerican underworld. The tree won't tolerate temperatures much lower than 16°C (64°F) for any length of time,[92] and prefers ambient temperatures above 27°C (81°F).[93] Unlike the Asian tea plant *Camellia sinensis* or the South American coca bush *Erythroxylum coca*, the botanical source of our archetypal Central American stimulant prefers lower altitudes, and won't grow more than 700 metres above sea level.[94]

There are three principal varieties of Cacao: *criollo*, which is the original Mesoamerican cultivar; the hardier, more fertile *forastero*, which originated in South America; and the hybrid *mestizo* or *trinitario*, so named because it was developed in Trinidad. A tree of any type can grow up to fifteen metres tall, with a deep taproot drawing nutrients and moisture from several metres down. Because Cacao is an understorey tree, its photon-catching organs—glossy leaf blades, darkly flushed with chlorophyll—are highly effective; nevertheless, having traded light for shelter, subsoil strategies to absorb more nutrients are necessary. As with so much about *Theobroma cacao*, there's a lot going on beneath the surface. The rich leaf litter of the forest floor sustains various fungi, some of which are symbionts with Cacao: lateral "feeder roots" from the tree spread out and collude with fungal mycelia, each organism supplying the other with sustenance, much like the microbiome ("gut flora") in humans. Soil fungi help *T. cacao* absorb minerals, while the tree provides waste products such as carbon which the moulds thrive on. *Theobroma* has a high mineral requirement, and this collaboration maximises mineral uptake in suboptimal conditions; the presence of *mycorrhizae*—the technical name for a plant-fungus symbiosis around the roots—has been shown to increase the duration of flowering, the number of seeds, and the number of fruits which make it to maturity.[95] So the use of chemical anti-fungals to treat Cacao crops may have unforeseen detrimental effects further down the line.

The Maya chose trees in the pea family (*Leguminosae*) to act as shade cover for Cacao, which is no accident, as these plants "fix" nitrogen in the soil, greatly assisting plant growth.[96] Biodiverse multicropping systems known as *cacaotales* or "Cacao orchards" are established on elevated ground. These *cacaotales* consist of Cacao trees, their companion plants, and shade trees, being an arboreal equivalent of the Mesoamerican *milpa* farming system with its large-scale companion planting. They have a high density of Cacao trees, at least 625 trees per hectare.[97] They're also efficient carbon sinks, storing up to a hundred times more carbon dioxide than equivalent areas of farmland.[98] Within three to four years of planting out, the young Cacao trees begin to fruit, and in a few more years are festooned with multicoloured pods—yellow, white, red, purple, and black fruits slowly ripening in the warm shade of the *cacaotale*.

Theobroma's leaves are glossy green ellipses with a heart-shaped base and a pointed tip, up to 35cm (13.8") long and 8cm (3.1") wide.[99] The tree produces new leaves two or three times a year, or more during dry periods, or if inadequately sheltered.[100] *Theobroma cacao* flowers and fruits directly from little mounds called "cushions" on the trunk, an atypical form of growth referred to as *cauliflory*;[101] early post-colonial European illustrators who hadn't seen the tree frequently depicted it inaccurately, autocorrecting the fruits and flowers onto the branches in their prints and woodcuts. The Cacao tree produces thousands of tiny white nocturnal blooms growing directly from the trunk, each barely the size of a fingertip. They begin to open in late afternoon, and maximal blooming occurs at around five a.m., so *Theobroma's* chief pollen-porters are semi-nocturnal insects.[102] Perversely, the Cacao tree begins flowering when insect populations are low, at the onset of the wet season. Its main pollinators are midges, tiny flies which emerge from the humid shade of the subtropical forest leaf litter. This is why the Cacao tree flowers—and therefore fruits—using cauliflory: the mossy trunk can hold moisture and acts as a bug highway direct from the forest floor, with deluxe motel accommodation. The tree has adapted itself to the seasonal scarcity of pollinators. Nevertheless, from the profusion of flowers, only one to five per cent in a cultivated Cacao crop are fertilised and develop into fruits; the rest wither and drop off.

Cacao doesn't flower all at once—clusters of flowers open at different times during the year.[103] As far as sex goes, *Theobroma* seems to value consistency, preferring a conservative "little and often" approach. Being a tree which likes to dwell on the threshold of the Mesoamerican under-world, it should be no surprise that Cacao's flowers are most receptive to pollination at dawn and dusk, and that the tree's chosen pollen-envoys are barely visible insects which dwell in decaying matter. Some of them "bite"; in other words, they drink blood. The flowers are scent-less only to humans: for their insect emissaries, they produce a cocktail of seventy-eight subtle aromatic compounds which draw in mostly female midges from a handful of insect families such as the *Ceratopogonidae*,[104] as well as tiny stingless bees.[105] It's unclear whether any of the blood-drinking insect species which fertilise Cacao flowers are vectors for human illnesses,[106] but similar midges have been found to transmit parasites to humans in South America.[107] It's a curious thought that the reproductive agents of the tree which gives us chocolate may extract a small tithe of blood, and even offload some pathogenic passengers.

Cacao trees only begin to produce fruits after four to six years of life, and they continue fruit-ing for approximately fifty years.[108] The fruits begin life as fertilised flowers, which turn into tiny green pods called "cherelles" or "chilios" in contemporary Central America, that grow to their full size over five or six months. In the rare event of a surplus of embryonic fruits, trees often suffer from "cherelle wilt", when a number of the baby pods shrivel and blacken while still attached to the tree.[109] Cacao aspires to fecundity but ultimately conserves its energy, and produces relatively few fruits; *Theobroma*'s wild ancestors put far more energy into simple cloning, or vegetative reproduction[110]—the elaborate business of pollen and fruit is a fallback strategy. When Cacao does invest in sexual reproduction, it's important that there are no little accidents: its flowers are incompatible with gametes from the same tree, so they can only be fertilised by insects bearing pollen-parcels with different genetic material.[111] Cacao demands a lot from its human cultivators, because the tree is environmentally sensitive, highly susceptible to pests and diseases, and co-dependent with other trees and plants—it can't be successfully mono-cropped for any length of time—and is not naturally bountiful. It's fortunate, then, that the pre-Columbian Mesoamericans had three thousand years to interact with the plant and perfect their cultivation techniques.

Mature Cacao pods can weigh anything from 200 grams to a kilo, and are ribbed, vaguely pointed ovals, mottled green, yellow, purple, or red, with a waxy finish. They're tough; when hacked open with a machete, their inch-thick rind holds an average of thirty to forty-five beans packed in a five-pointed star arrangement in cross-section, and coated with a sweet, white, mucilaginous fruit pulp. Ripe pods don't fall like coconuts—they need to be manually cut off the trees, as (apart from its arrangement with *Homo sapiens*) the plant naturally relies on crea-tures such as rats, squirrels, parrots, or monkeys seeking the sweet pulp inside to propagate itself. Wild animals gnaw into the pods while they're still attached to the trees and discard the unwanted, bitter seeds on the forest floor. The bright colours of mature Cacao fruits attract visual feeders such as parrots and monkeys, and rotting, hollow pods—still attached to the tree—are a perfect breeding ground for the insects which pollinate the tree, particularly during the rainy season, when Cacao is in flower.[112] The mucilaginous fruit pulp contains a germina-tion inhibitor, so only once the pod is opened and the seed is removed from its fruity matrix—whether by animals of the four- or two-legged kind—can it begin to germinate.[113] Cultivated seeds are propagated by soaking them in water overnight to pre-germinate them, and removing any fruit pulp. Then they are planted in soil with the top half of the seed exposed, and watered; a shoot soon emerges.[114]

Criollo Cacao, botanically designated as *Theobroma cacao ssp.* (subspecies) *cacao*,[115] is the indigenous Mesoamerican variety, originally cultivated in the region of present-day Tabasco on the east coast of southern Mexico, and Soconusco on the west coast of northern Guatemala.[116] *Criollo* fruits are a little more elongated, with a noticeable point at the end of the pod, and more "knobbly" skin.[117] The immature fruits are green, turning red or yellow when they ripen,[118] with a slightly soft, "dentable"texture, and contain twenty or thirty seeds per pod. The flowers are entirely white.[119] *Criollo* seeds contain fewer astringent polyphenols and more caffeine than other varieties, making them less sour and more stimulating. They're ivory or pale purple in cross-section. *Criollo* is the most delicate, disease-sensitive variety of Cacao, but it's also the longest lived, with a lifespan of a hundred to a hundred and fifty years.[120] There are at least four known cultivars of *criollo* Cacao: a Mexican variety, another called *lagarto* ("lizard") for its knobbly, warty appearance, "Cacao real" from Nicaragua, and a Colombian cultivar.[121] Sadly, owing to hundreds of years of interbreeding and government-sponsored initiatives to increase production through hybridisation, pure *criollo* is now a rarity, genetically speaking;[122] most "*criollo*" trees in Central America are actually, to some extent, *mestizo* (mixed), although small, scattered groves of pure *criollo* Cacao still exist. *Criollo* accounts for 20% of contemporary Central American Cacao production,[123] and only 5% of the world's Cacao population.[124]

Forastero, known by botanists as *Theobroma cacao ssp. sphaerocarpum*, originates from South America, is more robust than *criollo*, and fruits year-round. This variety usually has green pods which are somewhat rounder and harder than those of its northern sibling; the pods are often red when immature (unlike *criollo*), and they have a smoother surface with no "nipple" at the end.[125] *Forastero* seeds have a flatter appearance,[126] a sourer taste, and a deeper purple blush when cut in half, due to their higher polyphenol content.[127] *Forastero* most likely originated in the Amazon basin, but only began being cultivated in Amazonia from the seventeenth century onwards[128] to meet growing international demand. *Forastero* Cacao produces more fruits, with larger and more numerous seeds than *criollo*: *forasteros* have up to thirty or forty seeds per pod—ten more than *criollo*, on average.[129] The third variety of Cacao, *mestizo* or *trinitario*, is a hybrid. Created to mingle the better flavour profile characteristics of *criollo* with the hardiness of *forastero*, they truly more closely resemble *forastero*.[130] Ninety-five per cent of the world's Cacao is *forastero*, owing to the subspecies' greater disease resistance and higher crop yields.[131]

Enterprising Central American farmers have developed means of increasing crop yields from sensitive *criollo* trees. One such method is grafting: in Alta Verapaz, Guatemala, the hardiest *criollo* trees are chosen to be "hosts", and young, fruiting branches from *criollo* or *mestizo* saplings are selected as "donors", cut, and tied onto the host tree. After twenty days, the ligature is removed, and the grafted branch usually begins to grow within five weeks. The type of fruit the grafts produce depends on the donor, but the host provides longevity and disease resistance. Clones of the most prolific trees are selected as donors on the basis of the high yield of their fruits, and Cacao pods from grafted *mestizo* or *criollo* clones may contain up to fifty or sixty seeds per pod—almost double the average *criollo* seed count.[132] But this cloning-and-grafting method of increasing output is not without cost: flowers from a wild-type Central American *criollo* Cacao variety—determined to be genetically close to the ancestral native trees—have an elaborate aroma which draws more midges than the less complex scent of hybridised Cacao cultivars.[133] Generations of cloning and grafting appear to dilute the reproductive chemistry of the plant, which may account for the very low fertilisation rate of farmed Cacao. The other side effect of cloning is increased disease susceptibility: even when a plant is selected for its hardiness, any genetic weaknesses it has will be passed on to its identical offspring. And Cacao is afflicted by many diseases: pests such as the cocoa borer moth and capsids, or fungal infections like "black pod disease" or "witches' broom disease" to name but a few.[134]

The most destructive pathogen of Cacao is the witches' broom fungus, *Moniliophthora perniciosa* (formerly known as *Crinipellis perniciosa*), first identified on Cacao trees in the Amazon rainforest in 1785. It principally affects *criollo* Cacao. For anyone who prefers to maintain delusions of nature's essential benevolence, look away now: spores from the fungus infect living Cacao trees though scratches and wounds, and the growing fungus parasitises the tree for a few months, causing it to mutate—the name "witches' broom" comes from the multiple growths of frondy, useless, broom-like shoots produced by tumours on infected trees. *Moniliophthora* draws nutrients from the tree; eventually, after several months, it turns lethal, causing leaves to wither and pods to rot and the tree to die. The fungus then feeds off the corpse, producing little mushrooms which look like parasols designed by H. R. Geiger, that release new spores.[135] Epidemics of witches' broom have devastated Cacao production, turning Brazil from a major exporter to a net importer of Cacao in the 1980s; plagues of the fungus thirty years ago decimated the crop, reducing commercial yields to anything from fifty to ten per cent of former outputs worldwide.[136] Africa has so far been spared, which is why it is now the world's largest Cacao exporter.

Primordial chocolate

Although *Theobroma cacao* was first cultivated in Mesoamerica, it's thought that the tree's wild ancestor may have originated from South America, and was originally harvested for the sweet gooey pulp inside the pod, rather than the bitter seeds. From there, it was a short step to the production of fermented beverages—a kind of rudimentary Cacao wine.[137] At some point, fermentation of the seeds along with the fruit may have taken place, and some bold experimenter noticed salutary effects after eating them; or, perhaps, someone received inspiration in a dream, or through shamanic means, via some otherworldly experience. In any case, the established theory is that seeds of an ancient wild variety of Cacao from present-day Colombia were transported by human agency northward into Mesoamerica, where the tree co-evolved with humans into the *criollo* subtype, which was bred to produce potent and better-tasting seeds; other varieties, meanwhile, were distributed south and east into Amazonia and present-day Venezuela, where they became *forastero*.

Populations of *criollo* Cacao, indigenous to Central America, appear to be very ancient, just like the *forasteros* in South America. Some researchers contend that the variants may have evolved separately, at two centres of origin.[138] But there are actually many more than just three types of Cacao; genetically speaking, ten subgroups or "clusters" have been identified: *criollo*, *Marañon*, *Curaray*, *Iquitos*, *nanay*, *Contamana*, *amelonado*, *Purús*, *nacional*, and *Guiana*. Every genotype but *criollo* is generally lumped in under *forastero* or *trinitario*, but some of them, such as *amelonado*, can be identified by physical characteristics: *amelonado* pods are rounder. As this book is focused on exploring the Mesoamerican development of Cacao, for the sake of convenience we will continue to refer to all non-*criollo* Cacao as *forastero* or *trinitario*. The *criollo* genotype is the only Cacao cluster to be found growing wild in Central American forests, while all ten clusters—including *criollo*—occur in South America, which supports the theory that human agents took an ancestor of *criollo* Cacao from South America and transported it north of the Andes.[139]

Recent research has dated the "domestication" of the *criollo* cluster—the story of its agricultural symbiosis with man—to approximately three thousand six hundred years ago, although the association may go back as far as ten thousand years. That breeding process selected for higher disease resistance in the tree, lower antioxidant polyphenols, and increased xanthine production in its seeds (xanthines, such as caffeine and theobromine, are the main stimulating compounds in Cacao). It's also apparent that the selective breeding of *criollo* resulted in lower crop yields[140]—presumably because selecting for desirable characteristics shrunk *criollo*'s gene pool, so the cluster became less adaptable. *Criollo* Cacao is favoured by chocolatiers for its milder flavour, owing to the seeds' lower polyphenol content; in other words, the human dialogue with the plant resulted in a Cacao cluster which produced more stimulating, less sour seeds. Seeds, not fruit: the inescapable conclusion is that maybe as far back as ten thousand years ago, humans had already discovered the use of Cacao seeds, and had formed an intimate and somewhat controlling relationship with the plant, based on hunger for its babies. They bred the plant to live longer, taste better, and give a good buzz—and made it more dependent, lower-yielding, and less adaptable in the process. *Criollo* Cacao is somewhat of a geisha: in exchange for a sheltered life in partnership with humans, the plant was refined, cultivated, and controlled—to maximise the pleasure of the consumer.

The jaguar tree

There is one other *Theobroma* species in common use in Central America. Its seeds are milder in flavour, less stimulating, and cheaper than Cacao. This is *Theobroma bicolor* or the jaguar tree, so called because its fruit pods, which are more globular than Cacao's, have a mottled appearance which has been likened to the patterns on a jaguar pelt. *T. bicolor* was known to the Mexica as *pataxtle* ("pat·asht·lay"), and its seeds are used as a Cacao substitute in various regions. They're ivory coloured when raw, and become golden brown once toasted, with a savoury, nutty flavour. To the Mexica, *pataxtle* was a decidedly inferior replacement for Cacao, "fit only for low people,"[141] donated to the poor by the royal household, though when mixed with Cacao it was said to produce more foam.[142] The seventeenth-century English physician Henry Stubbe, chocolate enthusiast and author, described *"patlaxt"* or, as the natives called it, *"quauhpatlahtli"* as "not so useful as the ordinary, yet … used by the meaner sort".[143] In present-day Tuxtepec, Mexico, they're known as *cacao cimarrón,* and used in place of Cacao in a local variant of the beverage known as *popo*; in San Antonio Suchitequepez, Guatemala, they're used to make the local version of the pan-Mesoamerican maize-based *atole*—a gruel based on nixtamalized corn and water—called *pinole*; and in San Andres Tuxtla, Oaxaca, Mexico, they're fermented to produce a unique product called *cacao blanco*.

To make *cacao blanco*, the light brown *pataxtle* seeds are soaked for one week in a large clay pot, then a deep rectangular pit is dug in a place where the earth isn't too soft and has more stones in it for slower drainage. The hole must be one and a half metres deep, and one and a half metres long by two metres wide. First, the pit is filled with water and left for a couple of days, to saturate the earth. Then the bottom is lined with a layer of sand to deter insects, before a hundred kilos of *pataxtle* seeds are added, and immersed in water; the whole lot is covered with a woven mat called a *petate*, then protected with a wooden lid. The pit is inspected at least every other day, and the water topped up as necessary. After three months the pungent, rotting beans are taken out, washed, and put back into the pit, with fresh water. After six months the plutonian process is complete; the exhumed beans no longer smell bad, but have shrunk to half their former size: fifty kilos of seeds emerge, with blackened, shrivelled seed coats splitting to reveal chalky white flesh. They're washed well, then spread out to dry in the shade on large *petates*. The drying process, too, should be slow, and takes about a month in a well-aerated place such as a covered porch.[144] The *cacao blanco* is shelled prior to use; the naked, fermented seeds are soft, white, and slightly rubbery, like crumbly eggs or chalk-dry feta cheese, with no discernible odour. They are an irreplaceable ingredient and the principal foaming agent in a local beverage called *chocolate atole*.

Germination hijack: seed processing

Newly harvested Cacao seeds undergo several steps to make them into raw material for beverages and foodstuffs. Like *cacao blanco*, the process is a sort of necromantic alchemy, killing the seeds and biochemically transforming what would have been the next generation of trees into an epicurean pleasure. First, the pods are cut off the tree, split open, and the seeds and flesh are scooped out. If the fruit pulp is the desired crop, the pods are harvested when slightly unripe; the sweet pulp is still occasionally eaten (mainly by plantation workers), or used to make beverages (see below).[145] After harvesting the ripe pods, the seeds are fermented, with the pulp still attached. Owing to their sourness, purple *forastero* beans require fermentation for up to a week, while the milder *criollo* seeds only need one to three days.[146] A special process, known as Cacao *lavado* ("washed Cacao") in contemporary Mexico, is used to produce beans with a milder flavour; here, *criollo* seeds are fermented for one day only before the beans are rinsed, and set out in the sun to dry.[147]

There are several methods for fermenting the beans, the simplest of which is "heap fermentation". As the name would suggest, the beans are simply raked into heaps, covered to protect them from rain, and left to nature's devices for a few days. This method is the most common in traditional processes and for smaller producers, as heaps range in size enormously, from twenty-five to twenty-five *thousand* kilos. Some industrial producers prefer "box fermentation", wherein the seeds are tipped into a box raised off the ground, with outlet holes in the base to allow liquids to drain; this method is preferred for larger quantities of one or two tonnes of raw seeds.[148]

After fermentation, the seeds are washed to remove any traces of pulp, excess acids, microbes, and fermentation by-products. Traditionally, they were then sun-dried, by spreading them out on *petates* (or nowadays on concrete), raking to turn them occasionally. Artificial methods such as air-dryers are sometimes used in modern times and wetter countries, although sun-dried beans have been rated the most highly by taste.[149] Fire-drying is unsuitable, as Cacao beans are highly flavour-absorbent and easily tainted by the smell of smoke.[150] After drying, the beans are toasted: this process was traditionally carried out on a *comal*, a slightly concave clay dish which is perched on stones or bricks above a fire; clay retains heat and diffuses it somewhat, and the curved surface helps food fall back towards the centre of the dish, while deflecting smoke from the fire around the edges. The *comal* facilitates a deeper and more even toasting of the beans than a flat metal surface, which may tend to superficially scorch them without completely cooking the centre; moreover, a flat surface more readily allows beans towards the edges to come into contact with smoke. Despite this, metal cooking surfaces are often used to toast Cacao in contemporary Central America.[151] Industrial chocolate production utilises large roasting machines or ovens, which attain much higher temperatures, the result of which is greater uniformity in taste and appearance—but the lower temperature and variable heat exposure in open-air *comal*-toasting produces more depth of flavour and a better pharmacological profile, as we shall see in Chapter 4.

The beans are then shelled by hand, usually while still warm. Roasting causes the husks to become papery and brittle, so shearing the beans between thumb and forefinger with gentle pressure is often enough to separate the skin from the toasted seed. Roasted Cacao beans are fragile, and may crumble, falling apart along their natural fault lines; so hand-shelling is an art, and accomplished Cacao-makers can shell several beans a minute, while novices often end up painstakingly picking fragments of shattered shell out of palmfuls of bean bits. A simple process of separating the two is to blow gently across the palm, causing the lighter shell fragments to scatter. Industrial processing makes use of this fact by blowing air up through vibrating sieves: the shaking mesh shucks off the seed coats, and the air blows them upward, while the denser seed fragments fall into the maw of the machine for further processing.[152] Traditional Cacao processors accomplish the same thing after hand-shelling the bean by pouring the beans from one large bowl into another from a height on a windy day; the breeze carries away any shell fragments, while the denser beans all end up in the bowl.[153]

The next step, grinding the beans, is traditionally carried out using the *metate*, a uniquely Mesoamerican piece of kit. The *metate*—known as the *metatl* by the Mexica—is a chunky stone quern or grinding surface, used in conjunction with a *mano*, the Spanish term for what the Mexica called a *metlapil*,[154] a rolling-pin-like stone. The *metate* is the static surface and the *mano* or *metlapil* is the moving, hand-held element. The type used for processing Cacao is a squat grinding table with three or four short legs, usually made of granite or hard volcanic rock; it has a rectangular grinding surface, very slightly concave, which slopes downward in a shallow gradient away from the human operator, with a slight upward tilt or lip at the other end. The *metate* is the standard grinding instrument used in food preparation in pre-Columbian Central America, and remains in use today—a testament to its functional utility. Its Old World equivalent is the mortar and pestle, with its pounding-and-grinding action, which the Mesoamericans also used, and which goes by the name of *molcajete y mano*. Unlike a mortar and pestle, the back-and-forth shearing action and broad surface area of a *metate* are uniquely suited to manually grinding Cacao, which liquefies and spreads out as it is ground. When ambient temperatures are low, a small fire or hot coals can be set beneath the *metate* to keep the surface warm, so that ground Cacao remains in a liquid state. The *metate*'s slightly concave surface prevents liquefied Cacao from running over the sides too readily before it can be scraped back towards the centre, and the action of dragging the beans back and forth across a rough hot stone surface incrementally smashes them into a lacquer of liquid chocolate—it feels like weaving chocolate on a stone loom. Cacao may be ground two or three or even more times on a *metate* to achieve a smooth consistency. Once Cacao beans have been roasted and ground—by hand or by machine—the liquefied ground beans are referred to as "cocoa liquor".

After grinding, cocoa butter may be extracted. The fat is also used in traditional medicine in Central America (see Chapter 3), and there are two traditional methods for extracting it from the seeds—a "cold method", and a "hot method". Both methods require the addition of water to cocoa liquor. Factory production utilises much greater quantities of beans and generates far higher yields, as cocoa butter is an essential ingredient in chocolate manufacture, whereas cocoa butter was principally extracted for medicinal purposes in Mesoamerica. The "cold method" is the oldest: cocoa liquor is mixed with a little tepid water in a calabash and whipped by hand until the cocoa butter separates. The calabash is held in one hand, and the other hand is used like a paddle or scoop to agitate the liquid. Like all manual Cacao processing, this method is labour-intensive and time-consuming, and relies on higher ambient temperatures, and the water used must be at room temperature to begin with, so the cocoa butter can melt: on a cool, misty day in Guatemala, the method failed to work at all.[155] The "hot method" is used for extracting larger quantities of the fat: a huge pot of cocoa liquor and water is placed over the fire and stirred constantly to bring it to a simmer without burning—two to three litres (68–100 fl. oz. [US]) of water are added to one kilo (2.5lb) of Cacao.[156] The key is the ratio: too much water, and the fats will emulsify: the ratio of fat to water must not exceed 1:4 (of course, the opposite is the case for making drinks with Cacao). After some time—an hour or more—the cocoa butter begins to separate; it's skimmed off with a small gourd, more water is added to the mix, and the process is repeated. Eventually the cocoa butter, collected in a half-gourd, can be placed in a container of water to cool—the gourd floats on the surface of the water, a little coracle with a puddle of opaque, off-yellow fat in the centre, like a yolk, or a cataracted eye.

Once the beans are ground, the traditional processing of Cacao for making beverages markedly diverges from the modern, mechanised process for making candy; in both cases, making cocoa liquor is essential. At this stage, ground spices may be added and ground with the Cacao on the metate once more, to incorporate their flavour, and then used to make drinks immediately; or, the cocoa liquor can be puddled or poured into moulds, with or without added spices, and allowed to cool. These Cacao tablets may be stored at room temperature for many months before using them. Traditionally-processed beans have a more complex taste and chemistry as a result of smaller-batch heap fermentation, lower-temperature open-air toasting, and less intense grinding on a metate, but the end products of both will be at least passingly similar—although anyone who tastes drinks made from hand-processed Cacao will no longer make the mistake of thinking that industrially produced chocolate is an adequate substitute.

Cacao in the Old World

Perhaps *criollo*'s wild ancestors sacrificed their seeds for human consumption to co-opt *Homo sapiens* as guardians, just as aphids feed ants honeydew in return for their protection.

After all, Cacao's primary natural reproductive strategy is non-sexual, so giving up a few seeds in exchange for guaranteed territorial expansion and protection seems like more than just a happy accident in terms of species survival. Thanks to its relationship with humans, Cacao now grows on four of the seven continents (excepting only those beyond its natural range 20° north or south of the equator: North America, Europe, and Antarctica are too cold). Currently, more than 40% of the world's Cacao is grown in Africa; specifically, on the equatorial west coast of the continent, in Côte d'Ivoire, Ghana, Nigeria, and Cameroon.[157] Brazil was once the world's main supplier, before witches' broom (*Moniliophthora*) decimated the country's output; and the South-East Asian suppliers, specifically Malaysia, have been hit by outbreaks of the cocoa pod borer moth, and many plantations have been replaced by more reliably remunerative oil palms.[158]

Central America barely exports any Cacao, although growers are seeking an international market. Representatives of collectives such as APROCAV[v] in Alta Verapaz, Guatemala are desperate to find an economic incentive to continue farming Cacao,[159] which is relatively high-risk and labour-intensive; they have developed cloning and grafting techniques to maximise yields of high-quality *criollo* Cacao, so it's a pity no one's biting (literally)—their prices may be higher, but Central America has a direct line to the original strains of *criollo*, genetically speaking. More economically persuasive, perhaps, is the pleasure principle: online surveys suggest that Venezuela, which does have some export market for Cacao, produces the best-tasting beans in the world.[160] But there are more reasons than just historical elitism, fair trade, or gastronomic considerations for supporting Central American *criollo* farmers, particularly those using traditional methods to conserve genetically authentic ancestral strains of the plant.

We know that varieties of the same plant or species grown in different parts of the world can exhibit enormous pharmacological variation, presumably as an adaptation to altered microbial and environmental terrains. This variable chemistry in a psychoactive plant such as Cacao can result in changed effects; historic examples abound, such as unsuccessful British efforts to grow superior Virginia tobacco (*Nicotiana tabacum*) in Rhodesia (present-day Zimbabwe),[161] or the enormous decline in morphine yields from opium poppies (*Papaver somniferum*) transplanted from Afghanistan to a cottage garden in the Cotswolds, or even the vineyard-specific taste of grapes and their fermented output, particular and distinguishable by variety, microclimate, and the dusting of wild yeasts on the skin of the fruit. So relocation causes many inward changes: perhaps part of the diminished reputation of Cacao from a superb, exotic New World medicine to a sweet pabulum suitable for children owes as much to geography as it does to historical hyperbole, or the confectioner's art.

In the last ten years, there has been a trend towards "raw chocolate" production, products made from unroasted Cacao beans, often substituting "agave nectar" for white sugar, and coconut oil for cocoa butter. The claim is that raw Cacao beans and raw chocolate are more healthful than roasted beans and conventional chocolate candy. Raw beans do contain more antioxidant polyphenols, but there's more to the story: the transformations effected by toasting the beans develop flavour, and appear to alter the effects (see Chapter 4 for more details). Many "raw chocolate" vendors claim that their product is more uplifting—this is contrary to my experience,

[v] APROCAV = *Asociacion de PROductores de Cacao de Alta Verapaz.*

at least. While very pleasant, raw chocolate doesn't compare to properly processed traditional drinking chocolate made from roasted beans, in terms of either flavour or effect. There's also the issue of dubious health claims for coconut oil, which contains similar quantities of saturated fat to cocoa butter, and "agave nectar", a partly or wholly refined syrup with a high fructose content, and not very healthy at all. "Raw Cacao powder", produced by milling de-fatted uncooked Cacao seeds, is much higher in antioxidants when manufactured, but may rapidly lose its antioxidant properties when stored due to the loss of protective fats (see Chapter 4), so its vaunted health benefits may be much reduced by the time of purchase or consumption. None of which is to say "raw chocolate" is bad—there are some excellent products available—but when all's said and done, it's still a confectioner's toy.

In any case, chocolate confectionery is big business. According to the Food and Agriculture Organization of the United Nations data from way back in 1995, Cacao seeds—in their denatured, consumer-friendly guise as cocoa—were most avidly imbibed in Austria, France, and the United Kingdom, with 2.98, 2.94, and 2.52 kg consumed per person each year, respectively. The British appetite for tea exceeded that of all other countries except Kuwait, but only in the UK did cocoa consumption exceed the per capita consumption of coffee *and* tea combined.[162] This is a bit surprising, considering the reputation of the British as a nation of tea drinkers; it appears that something in the British temperament inclines us to a clandestine preference for cocoa. In 2010, annual chocolate consumption in Switzerland was 10.4 kilos (23lb) per person, with the UK in second place at 9.9 kilos (22lb), followed by Belgium, then Austria, and Australia in fourth place.[163] In 2015, Switzerland, Ireland, and the UK were the world's top three countries for *per capita* spending on chocolate, with a marked preference for milk chocolate; by contrast, Iran and Israel were the only countries where dark chocolate made up more than 50% of chocolate sales. It's a curiosity that the biggest consumers of Cacao are not the producers, but perhaps it was ever thus: in Mesoamerica, Cacao was consumed by nobles, royals, and on special occasions, and great quantities were traded to cities like Teotihuacan and Tenochtitlan, far to the north of where it grew; now, it's produced in Africa and Asia, and mostly consumed in Europe. Cacao has always been a special substance of affluence, and it has always travelled; it has always been attended by vassals, harvesting its produce for the privileged—like drones bringing nectar to the sequestered queen of the hive. The history of the plant is curiously bound up with themes of privilege, luxury, hierarchy, and serfdom, even to the present day.

So some of the most affluent countries in the world spend a lot of money on chocolate: three quarters of them are European countries, as 45% of the world's Cacao market is based in Western Europe; most of this chocolate is bought in the winter months, and chocolate consumption peaks between eight p.m. and midnight.[164] Darkness, dampness, and cold are conducive to sales: it's almost as if having had their hibernatory impulses hijacked by living in artificially neon-lit winter darkness and the grind of a relentless twenty-four-hour clock, consumers are trying to import the warm, vital, teeming shade of the tropical understorey forest. There are more prosaic explanations, of course—"comfort food" being one of them. But it's worth considering possible links between Cacao consumption, seasonal affective disorder (SAD), and serotonin, as well as fat, sugar, and milk: these ideas and connections are explored in Chapters 5 and 7.

Mechanised Cacao: chocolate, as we know it

We left off discussing the transformation of Cacao seeds at the stage of hand-grinding them, with two traditional methods of extracting cocoa butter. Industrial Cacao processing deals with enormous volumes of beans, so various types of mechanised mill are necessary for grinding them; these, of course, achieve a much smoother final consistency than is possible by hand, which is preferable when making confectionery: nobody wants a "gritty mouthfeel". Impact mills use pistons to pound the beans to a paste; disc mills have two circular grinding surfaces, a rotary surface above a stationary one, and they shear the beans apart, in the manner of an old-school stone flour mill; and ball mills employ a rotating drum partially filled with heavy metal balls which tumble around, bouncing off each other, smashing the beans.[165] All three types will effectively liquefy Cacao, but the last is the most commonly used. In all cases, the temperature is monitored so that the Cacao only gets hot enough to keep its fats melted—to facilitate grinding—while not overcooking it.

After roasting and grinding the beans, the next stage in industrial processing is "conching", a process whereby open vats or "conches" of cocoa liquor are continually beaten, mixed, and ground with mechanised rollers for up to several days, to make the texture of the chocolate extremely smooth by further reducing particle size. Conching is considered to be essential for manufacturing eating chocolate. The "long conche" was invented by chocolatier Rudolphe Lindt in 1879, and consists of a granite trough with a roller that continually grinds and stirs the cocoa liquor, making the texture smoother and mellowing the flavour[166]—while causing further chemical changes (discussed in Chapter 4). Conching machines have now become sophisticated so that many of them have cooling sleeves to prevent further "cooking" of the chocolate; some operate in a vacuum, which reduces overheating even more, and the most advanced capture escaping aromas and fractionally distil these vapours, so that desirable scents can be added back in to the cocoa liquor at the end of the process.[167]

An important part of modern chocolate confectionery and cocoa powder production is the removal of the fat, or "cocoa butter" from the roasted seeds. Industrially, this is often done with hydraulic presses, which generate a lot of heat and may further cook the Cacao, but they do extract around two-thirds to three-quarters of the fat from the seeds.[168] An alternative method, called the "Broma process", was developed by the American chocolate manufacturer, Ghirardelli. According to its website, a bag of cocoa liquor is suspended in a very hot room, the molten fats drip out,[169] and a vessel is left beneath it to capture the cocoa butter. This method is reputed to create "more flavoursome" cocoa butter,[170] but the process is poorly documented—the temperature of the room and the materials for the bag are not publicly recorded. Presumably the room would need to be around the mid-30°C to low 40°C range (around 95–110°F) so the cocoa butter remains molten, and the bag would have to be made from a tight weave cloth such as linen to retain very fine particulates in the cocoa liquor, while allowing the fat to leak through.

After de-fatting the seeds, they can be ground into cocoa powder. If the "Broma process" has been used, the remaining cocoa mass is just ground up and sold as "natural cocoa powder"; most often, though, whole seeds are "Dutched". Standard, Dutched cocoa powder is one of the most processed forms of chocolate, apart from chocolate cakes, biscuits, and so on. To make it, the shelled and crumbled beans or "cocoa nibs" are soaked in a highly alkaline solution of potassium carbonate before roasting them, which apparently causes less clumping in the finished product, so that when hot water is poured onto cocoa powder, you don't get lumpy cocoa. The process is referred to as "Dutching" because it was invented by Coenraad van Houten, a nineteenth-century Dutch chemist and chocolatier;[171] it was his father who pioneered the use of the hydraulic press to extract cocoa butter from Cacao seeds. Surprisingly, however, van Houten's process is still technically somewhat dubious: it's known only that the colour is darkened and the flavour made milder, but the anti-clumping effects—rather amusingly known in the chocolate industry as "anti-caking" properties—are uncertain.[172]

To produce commercial eating chocolate, the two essential ingredients—found in all types of chocolate candy—are cocoa butter and sugar. Cocoa liquor and sometimes also cocoa powder may be added to make dark or milk chocolate, and dehydrated full-cream milk is used in addition to make milk chocolate. Occasionally, small amounts of an emulsifier such as lecithin are added. Proportions vary, but eating chocolate has a minimum of 5% sugar and 50%–60% fat, for the very darkest, bitter black chocolate. Most dark chocolate, listed as 70%–80% cocoa solids, may contain around 50% cocoa liquor, 20%–30% additional cocoa butter (cocoa liquor itself is around 50% fat), and the remainder is sugar. With dark chocolate, it's useful to remember that the "remaining percentage" is entirely sugar: for example, a "70% cocoa solids" bar could just as easily be labelled "30% sugar"—so for the health-conscious, darker is better.

Milk chocolate, for the most part, has far less cocoa liquor, sometimes only 20%, and even more sugar and fat. White chocolate barely deserves to be called chocolate at all—it takes the name because of its high cocoa butter content, but it really is just fat, sugar, and milk powder. These ingredients are combined while the cocoa liquor and butter are still molten, before the tricky part of chocolate candy manufacture: setting the chocolate. If done badly, the chocolate will "bloom"—which sounds nice, but it means that it acquires a mottled appearance and grainy texture, with white, mould-like patches on its surface. These are just tiny crystals of fat extruding from the surface, but it spoils the look and feel of the confectionery. Bloom often spontaneously occurs in old and out-of-date chocolate, but can also appear during the setting phase.[173] So great pains are taken in the industry to cool melted chocolate in a controlled manner, a process referred to as *tempering*.

This means cooling melted chocolate to the correct temperature and keeping it there while it sets. The process can be expedited by adding some "pre-set" cocoa butter (which must have been solidified at around 30°C/86°F) to the chocolate, to "seed" it with the correct sort of fat structure (see Chapter 4 for more details).[174] Traditionally, a portion of the molten chocolate would be poured onto a cool marble surface and worked with palette knives until it achieved a viscous texture at 28°C (82.4°F), then this properly cooled chocolate would be re-added to the still-molten remainder.[175] In industrial processes, the whole body of chocolate is heated to a uniform temperature of 45°C (113°F) to melt, then cooled to 27°C (80.6°F) degrees, then agitated or stirred and gently heated to the correct temperature[176]—perhaps with the addition of a small amount of "pre-cooled" liquid chocolate or cocoa butter crystals—then it's allowed to rest and begin to set. Dark chocolate is set at 31–32°C (87.8–89.6°F), milk chocolate at 29–30°C (84.2–86°F), and white chocolate requires a setting temperature of 28–29°C (82.4–84.2°F).[177] The delicacy and labour-intensiveness which Cacao requires in cultivation is reflected in its processing—the plant and its products are as much Goldilocks as geisha: things need to be "just right".

Well-made chocolate doesn't require any other additives. Sometimes, the emulsifier lecithin is used to help incorporate the sugar and fat in chocolate, as it reduces costs by lowering viscosity in the liquid stages of manufacture without necessitating the addition of extra cocoa butter, which is relatively expensive.[178] Small quantities of lecithin are present in Cacao beans anyway, so adding it isn't a great crime. But inferior chocolate frequently incorporates various undesirable "extras"—aspartame, corn syrup, refined agave or glucose syrup, denatured alcohol, maltitol, hydrogenated fats, or the excitingly named tertiary butylhdroquinone [THBQ][179]—all variations on the theme of nutritional abomination. These adulterants are inveigled into the chocolate for economic reasons—they're cheap, and may be used to increase sweetness or shelf-life, aiding commercial enterprise. Not one of them is necessary, and they occur on a sliding scale of questionable to objectionable in terms of long-term effects on human health. But "the West" and, especially, northern Europe, are thoroughgoing devotees of industrially processed forms of Cacao. As with the invidious transformations of tobacco to cigarettes or the coca leaf to cocaine, the Old World converted another revered New World substance into, and made it synonymous with, a pleasurable, sophisticated, and denatured commodity. So far, most of the Europeanised versions of Cacao don't appear to be in any way harmful (though this issue is discussed further in Chapter 7)—in fact, as far as dark chocolate goes, quite the reverse. Of all the economically significant Old-World-transmuted, New-World-origin psychoactive drugs, chocolate is arguably the most successful, being the least in need of an image consultant, or a lawyer.

Colonial Cacao

Anthropologist Sophie Coe describes the post-colonial trajectory of the tomato, devolving from a powerful-tasting sour fruit to "a monotonous and uninteresting sweetness, more suitable to the palate of a three-year-old than that of an adult appreciating complexity".[180] The same thing has happened with Cacao, but from the very first, Europeans sweetened it by mixing it with their other slave-grown pleasure, sugar. The effect that European sophistication had on Cacao was to make it sweeter, blander, and denser. Even before the era of mechanised chocolate production, Cacao was already significantly altered. By the time it was introduced to North America in the early nineteenth century by missionaries and travellers in California, they were accustomed to taking hot chocolate as their daily breakfast, made in the European style with a large quantity of added sugar and milk; for these early American settlers, coffee was a "make-do" substitute. In Canada, European immigrants were so desperate to replicate chocolate's unattainable luxury that they invented "wild chocolate", a vaguely passable (and considerably more toxic) imitation made from decocted (boiled) fresh bloodroot (*Sanguinaria canadensis*), sugar, and milk.[181] *Sanguinaria* is a valuable medicinal plant which does contain alkaloids, chemicals in roughly the same class as caffeine from Cacao, but the alkaloids in bloodroot are structurally quite different and potentially hazardous. Short-term ingestion of the whole plant extract is most likely safe, although the beverage could be quite literally nauseating, and the maximum serving was one teacupful.[182] So chocolate, not coffee, was the stimulating beverage of choice for the first colonial Americans and Canadians.

Early North American chocolate aficionados recognised the need for proper processing of Cacao, noting the hazards of under- or over-roasting the bean, leading to either "harshness" of taste in the one case, or a complete loss of medicinal effect in the other.[183] But America was pick-ing up where three centuries of European familiarity with Cacao left off: chocolate had become popular in seventeenth-century London coffeehouses, where it took a further step away from Mesoamerican chocolate, and towards cake and candy. Dr Stubbe inveighed against the adul-teration and over-spicing of chocolate, decrying those who have

> sophisticated and spoiled one of the most excellent and healthful drinks in the world [...] Chocolata made up with so great a proportion of sugar [...] no physician will promiscuously, and without distinction of persons, allow it [...] and the obstructiveness of [these drinks] ... arises not from any particular badness of the Cacao-nut, but from the general unwholesome-ness of all confects, and sweet-meats. (Stubbe, 1662)

His contemporary, Dr William Hughes, similarly decried the attenuation of Cacao with sugar, eggs, and milk (see previous chapter). Dr Stubbe also reported the hand-grinding of chocolate on iron tables with iron rollers—metal *metates*, which remained in vogue with chocolatiers until the early twentieth century. Stubbe recommended the use of traditional stone grinding tools, and points out that a stone *metate* allows the heat of the fire underneath it to be more easily mod-erated and controlled, and that the iron implements "work the Chocolata blacker"[184] than stone utensils do, no doubt signifying oxidative processes taking place as a result of the equipment used to process the cocoa liquor being made from a reactive metal. In contemporary manufac-ture, any surfaces in chocolate-processing equipment that come into contact with cocoa liquor are made from non-reactive materials such as stainless steel, stone, or ceramic.

Juan Badiano's sixteenth-century translation of a Nahuatl herbal into Latin,[185] and Dr Francisco Hernández de Toledo's comprehensive early seventeenth-century book on native New World medicinal plants,[186] *Index Medicamentorum*, were translated into several European languages. Thanks to Hernández and his translators, and the dissemination of early anthropo-logical accounts of New World flora and fauna, European doctors now had information about the medicinal uses and categorisation of Cacao and its indigenous flavourings, so they began advocating traditional means of processing the beans, and the addition of Mesoamerican spices. As Cacao diffused through the courts of Europe, the traditional additives—with the one excep-tion of vanilla—were gradually usurped by more familiar, but equally exotic and aromatic ingredients. European nobility had developed an appetite for elaborate new formulations of Cacao-based beverages, and many Old World spices were used in these ostentatiously expen-sive concoctions. One Italian recipe from Dr Francisco Redi, the physician to Cosimo III de Medici, incorporated ambergris, musk, jasmine, cinnamon, citron, and lemon peel, in addition to vanilla[187]—the only Mesoamerican spice in the formula.

Meanwhile, post-colonial European epicures, experimenters, and apothecaries were busy working out the best techniques for producing high-quality drinking chocolate. Several authors concur that after Cacao had been prepared and allowed to set, the tablets should be aged for a month or more before being made into chocolate, as this produced a superior drink.[188] One Spanish recipe reflects this early European experimentation: a Cacao tablet was grated into hot water and boiled, then more water and sugar were to be added; the mixture was brought back to a boil and simmered until the cocoa butter separated out on top, and this was to be drunk.[189]

This preparation was thought to be tastier, but less healthy than the more standard foamy chocolate. Perhaps having a slick of fat on top of the drink appealed in an age when starvation was still an issue among poor country folk and in the slums of Europe—or it may have been tastier than it sounds (see *tejate*, described below and in Chapter 8).

In general, though, the Spanish colonial-era style of making chocolate remained closer to Mesoamerican methods: the prepared Cacao—either as cocoa liquor, or as crushed or grated tablets, spiced or not—was whisked into room-temperature water with a *molinillo* to make a head of foam, which was then transferred to another receptacle; the remaining de-frothed chocolate was heated with sugar, then the foam was replaced on top. This froth-making-and-replacing is highly reminiscent of several traditional Mesoamerican recipes. Another procedure called for mixing the Cacao with hot water in a cup, bit by bit, and once the liquid was very thin, the rest of the water and sugar was added.[190] Both methods beg some questions. The foam on plain chocolate mixed with water is relatively shallow and not so stable that it easily survives transfer, so some botanical foaming agent may have been added. It's also not clear why Cacao may have needed to be mixed with water bit by bit—unless the drink is made with cool water, dumping a grated Cacao tablet into a sufficient quantity of boiling water and whisking it well will produce excellent hot chocolate.

In fact both of these methods would make more sense if there was ground maize in the drink, as in the native *atoles*—in the first instance, because starch from the maize dissolved in the water can help create more stable bubbles (see Chapter 4), and in the second, because gradually mixing a powder with water in order to achieve a liquid consistency is a standard cook's trick for avoiding lumps in similar suspensions, such as béchamel sauces. Dr Stubbe made the same observation, that unless maize meal were added, the froth on plain chocolate would not be prodigious or durable.[191] So there seem to be some missing steps or ingredients in the reported methods—but aside from the addition of sugar, post-colonial Spanish hot chocolate appears to have borne a much greater resemblance to its predecessors than later European permutations, which makes sense, given that the Spanish had a direct line to the source of Cacao, as the conquerors of Central America.

Dr Hughes also recounted a "plantation chocolate" recipe, which was the daily breakfast of workers and household staff on the colonial plantations in Jamaica, "without which, servants or others are not well able to perform their most laborious employments".[192] The recipe calls for a fifty-fifty mix of native cassava bread and grated Cacao tablets. The bread should be crumbled into warm water, allowed to dissolve, then boiled; the Cacao is added, the broth is simmered for fifteen minutes, then sweetened with a little sugar.[193] This is a Creole recipe, a starch-swapping Caribbean version of the mainland maize-based *atole*, substituting the locally available cassava bread for nixtamalized maize. But Hughes also refers to the narratives of "American travellers" through post-colonial Central America, who tell of "the magnificent Collations of Chocolate that the Indians offered him in his Passage and Journies through their Country".[194]

Contemporary cacahuatl

The official chronicler for the sixteenth-century Spanish court, Gonzalo Fernández de Oviedo y Valdes, observed the traditional processing of Cacao beans in Mexico. He noted several fine points, which were lost in subsequent years. For example, the beans were taken out to dry in the sun several times each day and not left out all day, as they are now; and, once the roasted beans were ground into cocoa liquor, the little "cakes" were left to stand and set for at least five or six days, to improve the quality of the beverage.[195] There may be a pragmatic reason for this recommendation: in Central America, cocoa liquor may take up to seven cooler nights to set completely.[196] But the basic procedures used in non-industrial processing of Cacao beans has remained the same since ancient times, and in modern-day Central America, many of the pre-Columbian recipes and formulae incorporating Cacao also survive largely unchanged. They have, of course, been influenced by European tastes—sugar, milk, wheat, and cinnamon being the expatriate additives. But while a lot of the details of pre-conquest Cacao recipes are missing, historical descriptions from conquistadors, chroniclers, and colonists, or from Mesoamerican art and archaeology, line up very closely with contemporary recipes.

For the past millennium, the best Cacao in the world has been reputed to grow in the Soconusco region on the west coast of present-day Guatemala. The famous eighteenth-century French gastronome, Brillat-Savarin, declared as much two hundred years ago,[197] and it remains the case today—though few outside the country now get the opportunity to partake of Cacao grown there. Brillat-Savarin commended the Cacao from two locations in Venezuela, at the top end of South America, as well; but Mesoamerica was the cradle of *criollo*, the birthplace of the unique domesticated plant-drug-product originally conceived in a partnership between *Homo sapiens* and *Theobroma cacao* on the upper waters of the Napo, Putumayo, and Caqueta rivers in South America, somewhere between three and ten thousand years ago.[198] So it is to Central America that we must look for the most accomplished and authentic Cacao compositions.

In contemporary Mexico, Cacao is made into drinking chocolate tablets, called *chocolate por la mesa* ("chocolate for the table"), usually made up with sugar and cinnamon. These tablets are broken up and whisked into hot water or milk to make drinking chocolate; sugar often comprises more than half of the volume of the tablets, and even a "semi-bitter" Mexican *chocolate por la mesa* tablet is 40% sugar. In Oaxaca city, Mexico's culinary epicentre, one must request "chocolate for diabetics" to be given an unsweetened chocolate drink. So, while the processing of the beans is Mesoamerican, and the chocolate has an exquisitely intense flavour, the drink itself is a post-Enlightenment cultural hybrid. Oaxacan chocolate is an essential ingredient in the famous *mole negro*, a multi-ingredient sauce for savoury chicken dishes, normally consumed on festival days, particularly the Mexican "day of the dead". The recipe is extremely complex and variable, usually calling for several different types of chilli pepper and tomatoes, Oaxacan chocolate tablets, peanuts, avocado leaves, and salt, in addition to Old World imports such as onions, garlic, pecans, almonds, thyme, cinnamon, cloves, raisins, bread, plantain, and lard;[199] the preparation is lengthy and intricate, and the result is a highly aromatic, rich brown-black paste used to make a distinctive sauce with a characteristic taste. *Mole negro* itself is clearly a colonial hybrid, but the culinary use of Cacao with savoury dishes—as we saw in Chapter 1—dates back to Maya times, at least, and it's likely that the combinations of Mesoamerican ingredients in the sauce, including Cacao, were familiar to pre-conquest cooks; a recipe using similar ingredients may have been adapted by the Oaxacan nuns who are alleged to have invented the state's signature dish.

The most popular Cacao-based beverages in Central America are various *atoles*. Today, as in ancient times, these are the subsistence foods of the poor, often drunk for breakfast and dinner or lunch, with one solid meal every day, at midday or in the evening.[200] The gruels and pottages of medieval and early modern Europe served the same purpose, providing budget-stretching basic fuel in the form of some carbohydrate and vitamins, which could be supplemented with one high-protein meal every day. By adding Cacao, *atoles* are made much more pleasant and sustaining (see Chapter 5 for research on Cacao's effect on mood, and Chapter 7 for effects on appetite). Of course, Cacao itself is quite expensive; but by padding it out with maize flour, a little can go a long way. In the regions where it's regularly consumed in *atoles*, Cacao is grown and processed by people who make their living selling the beverages, and these are bought and consumed in pre-mixed forms from street and market vendors, as powders or balls that can be mixed with water. More elaborate *atoles* may only be made for special occasions, or sold only once or twice a week at specific locations; regulars turn up at the appointed times, sometimes gathering in the town square or market hall even before the vendor arrives to set up shop.

As in pre-Columbian times, only the rich in major cities or the poor in Cacao-growing regions drink it without added maize, because only they can afford to; and even then, it's rarely a daily indulgence. The standard forms of Cacao-based drinks are those made from home-made tablets, or purchased *chocolate por la mesa*, prepared with hot water (*chocolate de agua*) or milk (*chocolate de leche*). *Atoles*, however, are almost infinitely variable; the basic *atole de Cacao* is made with nixtamalized maize, toasted ground Cacao, spices (such as chilli), water, and—according to taste—some *panela* (unrefined sugar, made from dehydrated sugar cane juice). The Mexican drink *champurrado* is a highly sweetened, Europeanised version of *atole de Cacao*, often made with added milk, cinnamon, aniseed, or cloves, and frequently drunk for breakfast. Some more traditional Cacao-based *atoles* are variants of Mexican *pozol* (or *posol*, or *posolli*), and the Guatemalan *panecito* and *pinole*, drunk by K'iche and Ladino Maya.[201] These are very similar, being made from the basic *atole* formula of maize and water, with added Cacao. Both *pozol* and *pinole* are only sometimes made with Cacao, and *pozol* can be cultured, a kind of sourdough maize: the kneaded maize *masa* (dough) is shaped into a ball, then allowed to "sour", or ferment slightly through microbial action.

Pozol balls are wrapped in leaves to keep them fresh, and the same leaves are used many times, transferring microbes to new dough, so the leaf wrapping acts as a starter for the souring process. In Oaxaca, "*pozole* leaves" refers to the large, tough leaves of *Calathea lutea*, a variety of "prayer plant". Fermentation of the *masa* creates a more nutritious drink: lab rats fare better on *pozol masa* than ordinary maize *masa*.[202] Often *pozol* is a basic subsistence food, made from only nixtamalized maize and water, with or without salt; farmers go to the fields carrying a ball of *pozol* dough, and dissolve it in a gourd of water for breakfast, adding salt or licking some from the back of their hand.[203] Likewise, many Cacao-based *atoles* are staple foods, often sold as dried powders in markets, ready to be mixed with water, and European influence appears with the addition of sugar—to *pozol*, *panecito*, and *pinole*—and cinnamon, to *panecito* and *pinole*. *Panecito* tends to have a higher sugar content, though this varies with the vendor. One version of *pinole* is made with toasted *pataxtle* seeds (*Theobroma bicolor*) instead of Cacao. It should be added that these are the ingredients of *pinole* in present-day Soconusco; a hundred years ago in northern Guatemala, the name *pinole* referred to a beverage more like the Mexican *pozol*, made from maize, Cacao, cinnamon, sometimes aniseed, and the native plant known as *orejuela* or "ear-flower"[204]—on which, more shortly.

Other simple variations on the theme of *atole* are the Guatemalan *taxcalate* and *tiste*. These beverages are stored and sometimes sold in powdered, "instant" form, ready to mix with water, or by the glassful. They incorporate *achiote*, a Hispanicised version of *achiotl*, a Nahuatl name referring both to the seeds of the native plant known as annatto (*Bixa orellana*), and to the brick-red cakes of food dye which are made from them. This little tree grows much like the completely unrelated butterfly bush or *Buddleja*, though it has its own plant family (*Bixaceae*), with bright blousy pink flowers and burgundy seed pods that look like frondy Martian testicles growing at the end of the branches. The seeds are soaked in hot water to extract the dye, then the blood-red liquid is evaporated over heat until it thickens; modern cooks add fat and salt and other spices to flavour the concentrated red liquid, making round red patties called *pasta de achiote* for storage and use in cooking. *Taxcalate* is made from maize, Cacao, and ground annatto seeds added to water or milk;[205] *tiste* has a more pronounced European influence, being more than three-quarters white sugar, in addition to which it contains Cacao, roasted rice, cinnamon, and ground annatto, with or without a little vanilla. The taste is described as a little "insipid" but "palatable", and not strongly Cacao-flavoured.[206]

Some *atoles* made with Cacao are more elaborate, and likely to be older because they incorporate more native plants. Several feature a head of foam—a traditional way of serving the most prestigious Cacao-based beverages—but some skimp on the Cacao, using it only to generate a separate layer of froth to top a plain (and much less expensive) maize-and-water *atole*; the bland gruel topped with an aromatic foam makes a pleasurable contrast of flavours and textures. Food writer and researcher Diana Kennedy (in *Oaxaca al Gusto*, 2010: ©University of Texas Press) recounts several Cacao-based *atoles* from modern-day Oaxaca. The foam on *atole colorado* from central Oaxaca is deep red, owing to its annatto content. A fine powder is made from toasted wheat and cinnamon—the Old World imports—plus toasted Cacao, and *achiote*; this powder is then soaked in sweetened water, and frothed with a *molinillo* in a clay bowl called an *apastle* until large red bubbles form. These bubbles are used to top a plain *atole*. A generation or two ago, yellow corn *masa* was used instead of wheat,[207] but a pragmatic substitution was made, as wheat makes better bubbles than corn (see Chapter 6 for discussion on the composition of foams). *Chocolate atole*, similarly, is a plain, pale *atole* with a head of Cacao-flavoured foam; in this case, the white *atole* is made from un-nixtamalized corn, and the foamy head is made from toasted corn, wheat, or rice—or sometimes a mixture of these grains—*cacao blanco* (fermented and roasted *pataxtle* [*Theobroma bicolor*] seeds), toasted Cacao *lavado* seeds, and, sometimes, toasted cinnamon, all finely ground and whisked in water to produce a stable froth.[208]

Bu'pu is an *atole* made in the isthmus region (the narrowest part of Central America) of Oaxaca. Like *chocolate atole*, un-nixtamalized corn is used, and the foam is made separately and placed on top. The corn is cooked without lime, rinsed, and immediately made into a *masa*, which is mixed with boiling water and filtered to make a smooth *atole*. Substantial quantities of both fresh and dried Frangipani (*Plumeria rubra*) flowers are used to make the bubbly head on this *atole*, along with toasted Cacao and raw sugar, made from evaporated sugar cane juice, known as *panela* in Central America. *Bu'pu* was originally made with the flowers of another tree indigenous to the region, *Bourreria huanita*, which have a powerful jasmine-like aroma when fresh.[209] Kennedy describes another regional drink from San Mateo in Oaxaca, called *chaw popox*—translated as "foamy [*Popox*] atole [*chaw*]". This *atole* is usually drunk on special occasions such as weddings, and, much like *chocolate atole*, consists of a plain maize-and-water *atole* topped with a Cacao-flavoured foam.

But not all traditional *atoles* relegate Cacao to the top of the bowl. The Maya *atole de puzunque*, very unusually for a native recipe, incorporates raw Cacao, using half-and-half raw and roasted Cacao seeds, with toasted tortillas, vanilla, water, and the usual non-native addition of cinnamon. This is evidence that raw Cacao wasn't unheard of in Mesoamerica, as it's improbable that the inclusion of raw seeds is a modern addition—the recipe is a traditional *atole* of the K'iche and Ladino people, and unlikely to have been much influenced by confectionery trends. Other variations on the theme include *atole de sapuyul*, made with the ground seeds of *sapuyul* or sapodilla fruits (*Manilkara zapota*).[210] *Saka* is a ceremonial *atole*, made for agricultural and healing rituals. Unusually, it's made from un-nixtamalized maize gruel, with the addition of Cacao, with or without sugar, and "botanical foaming agents"[211]—plants such as the mysterious and unidentified *sugir* or *suguir* (on which, more later).

Tejate is a classic *atole* made and sold in Oaxaca, Mexico. It's probably the most familiar *atole* to tourists in Oaxaca city, as *señoras* who have been up since before dawn preparing the beverage are dotted around the city centre, tending their trestle tables dominated by a large bowl filled with beige liquid, with what looks like a scum of congealed suds floating on top. This unappealing-looking brew is sold by the half-gourd (*jicara*) or served in plastic cups, with syrup added to taste, and has a somewhat nutty, savoury taste; the gloop floating on it turns out to be a soft, fatty substance which melts in the mouth quite pleasingly, releasing a subtly sweet flavour, analogous to toasted nuts and cream. *Tejate* is made from only native ingredients: a *masa* is prepared from the best quality white nixtamalized maize, well cooked with lime and wood ash, together with several fatty *guacoyules*, the seeds of a local palm tree species, *Attalea cohune*. The recipe incorporates toasted flowers of *rosita de cacao* (*Quararibea funebris*), an aromatic flower with a sweet, rich scent, in addition to Cacao seeds and a crushed, toasted almond-scented *mamey* (*Pouteria sapota*) fruit pit.

In some recipes, several *mamey* seeds are used instead of the *guacoyules*, but in this case the *mamey* seeds, referred to as *pixtles*, must be soaked in water for one hour beforehand,[212] presumably to extract some of the cyanide-containing compounds they contain—the same compounds which are responsible for their almond-like flavour—and reduce their toxicity. The Cacao *masa* with the ground flowers and seeds is then added to the maize *masa* and re-ground on the *metate* to thoroughly mix the two, and the resulting beige-brown mixture is put in a large clay or plastic bowl. Water is added slowly, and mixed in by hand, one cupful at a time, producing a thick, cake-mix-like consistency;[213] as more water is added, the fats from the palm seeds begin to precipitate as lumps on the surface, and at this point the water is poured bit-by-bit into the mix from a great height to raise a better head of "foam". It is this aromatised, aerated fat which floats atop the finished beverage.

Another popular *atole* is *popo*, possibly the foamiest, frothiest *atole* of all. Chef and food writer Susana Trilling says, "One has to inhale the *popo*—the original chocolate mousse!"[214] Actually, *popo* isn't one beverage, but several—there are at least three different regional variants of this *atole*, made with different botanical foaming agents, and the path to producing the bodacious bowls of Cacao-flavoured foam differ. In Diana Kennedy's research, the recipe for *popo* made in La Chinantla, Oaxaca, called for the peeled, toasted, and crushed young shoots of a sarsaparilla species (*Smilax spp.*), mixed with some partly re-fermented Cacao beans—the only instance of this double fermentation of Cacao I am aware of. The Cacao seeds are washed and wrapped in a *pozole* leaf while still damp, then left to ferment for eight days. When the seeds are unwrapped, they are covered with "feathery white mould growth";[215] they're then sun-dried, toasted, shelled, and ground with the cooked *Smilax* shoots to make the drink. Don't try this at home, unless you live in Mexico and have access to all the proper ingredients and preferably direct tuition from someone who makes the drink! There's no guarantee that the mould which grows on your moist Cacao seeds at home will be the same as that above, even if it looks white and feathery; wild ferments are often highly variable, and microbe populations vary enormously in different environments.

Sarsaparilla (*Smilax spp.*) is a traditional Cacao additive, but the plant is better known as a flavouring in soft drinks. The roots of many species are used for this purpose and in traditional medicine, but in Mesoamerica it was the stems and petioles—the stalks connecting stems to leaves—that were (and are) used as foaming agents. Only young stalks are used—the shoots that emerge from the ground, resembling etiolated asparagus. They're stripped of any leaves, then put on hot ashes to cook very briefly, for no more than a minute or two, before being chopped and ground with toasted Cacao or *pataxtle* (*Theobromoa bicolor*) seeds—depending on which region of Mexico the *popo* is from. Sarsaparilla was known as *cozolmecatl* ("koz·oll·meh·cat·ul") to the Mexica, and is called *cocolmeca* or *azquiote* in contemporary Mexico.

Susana Trilling describes a completely different process used to make *popo* in Tuxtetpec, Oaxaca. Here, the young shoots of a different plant are used; this plant is also known as *cocolmeca*, but in this instance a species of birthwort, *Aristolochia laxiflora*, is described. Nixtamalized maize and toasted *cocolmeca* (*A. laxiflora*) are ground together, then ground Cacao is added and worked into the *masa*, sugar is added, then the *masa* is dumped into a sack and squeezed in water many times. The resulting emulsion-infusion is then frothed for an hour, continually, to produce a towering head of foam, which is served on its own in *jicaras* (half-gourd bowls).[216] *Smilax aristolochiifolia* grows in the same regions as *A. laxiflora*, and both plants are sold as *cocolmeca* in the marketplaces of central Mexico.[217] The botanical abundance of Central America's highly bio-diverse terrain makes such substitutions and variants common; given a choice, *Smilax* species may be preferable, as *Smilax* is non-toxic, whereas *Aristolochia* species contain aristolochic acid, prolonged or repeated consumption of which has been linked to kidney failure and urinary tract cancers.[218]

A third, more Europeanised variant of *popo* from Acuyacan in Veracruz calls for rice and cinnamon, toasted Cacao, *panela*, and the fruit rind or fresh, peeled root of *chupipe*, a local species of milkweed vine (*Gonolobus niger*). The rice and cinnamon are soaked, then ground with the Cacao and the *chupipe* skin or root; as in the last *popo* recipe, the resulting mass is mixed with water and strained through a cloth, before frothing it well.[219] According to one source *G. niger* sap is sometimes expressed, dried, and rolled into balls which can be refrigerated, and small amounts of this crude extract are used as foaming agents too.[220] Another variant of *popo* from Ojitlan in Oaxaca calls for toasted, unfermented seeds of "Cacao *cimarrón*"—actually *pataxtle*, or *Theobroma bicolor*—ground with lightly toasted fresh *cocolmeca* (*Smilax sp.*), then mixed with maize dough, stirred into water, filtered multiple times, sweetened, and frothed well.[221] Although the recipes vary considerably, their basic format is a combination of a ground starch-source (maize or rice), Cacao, sugar, and a specific botanical foaming agent, all ground together and dispersed in water. Two of the three formulas explicitly call for filtration of the whole beverage before frothing, making *popo* more of a beverage, an *aperitif*, or dessert rather than a meal replacement.

A few traditional Cacao-based drinks are made without the nutritional and financial benefit of attenuating the drink with maize. *Batido* is drunk by some contemporary Mayan people in northern Guatemala, and is made from Cacao and the native spice *orejuela* ("little ears"), the resinous and peppery dried flowers of the ear flower tree (*Cymbopetalum penduliflorum*) known as *muc'* to the K'iche Maya.[222] Sometimes toasted *mamey* seed, vanilla, or *achiote* are added; occasionally, cinnamon or black pepper. Toasted and shelled Cacao beans are ground on a *metate* to a coarse powder, then half is set aside and the remainder is ground so that it liquefies, then the two portions are mixed together. Then, the ground Cacao is placed into a *guacal* or half-gourd, equivalent to the Mexican *jicara*, a little tepid water is added, and the mixture is agitated by hand until the cocoa butter separates. This suggests that the "cold water" method of extracting cocoa butter mentioned earlier in this chapter may be of pre-conquest origin, and that the amount of water used should not be greater than three times the volume of the Cacao, or else the method will not work. Once the "thin paste" made of partly liquefied Cacao, spices, and a small amount of water has been created, and the fat has separated, a teaspoonful is added to a *guacal* containing approximately half a litre of hot water. No frothing or mixing is mentioned, though surely this must take place. After drinking it, natives allegedly crunch up the gritty residue of any partly-ground Cacao at the bottom of the vessel. As the anthropologist Wilson Popenoe pointed out in 1919, on the basis of its ingredients this beverage resembles pre-conquest Mexica *cacahuatl*,[223] although the portions seem rather parsimonious and the beverage itself quite insipid by comparison.

In parts of Guatemala, Cacao beverages are still made and drunk without the addition of sugar—just toasted Cacao, water, and spices. Unsurprisingly, given the cost of Cacao, these are regions where *Theobroma* grows naturally, such as Alta Verapaz and Soconusco. The most common addition is allspice (*Pimienta dioica*), and the drinks are made with locally grown *criollo* Cacao, and drunk hot, much as the Classic Maya did.[224] They're frothed with a *molinillo*, so they have a modest head of foam. But hardly anybody outside Central and South America takes real, traditional chocolate as a drink any more, and even within those countries, the number who drink it without added milk and sugar is small and ever-diminishing. Likewise, the younger generation in Oaxaca prefer Pepsi to *tejate*. Don Mateo Poptchu, a Mayan spiritual guide and diviner in San Luis, Peten, north Guatemala, related that in his youth, Cacao beverages were drunk at every occasion, celebratory or ceremonial, and were the first thing to be made for both secular and religious festivities. The older women prepared it in the early hours of the morning so that the aroma of toasted Cacao filled the air like a "perfume", and the beverage was ready when the village woke up. "We did not have diseases when we only drank Cacao, since it is the cure for illnesses on earth," he said, "[but] today we drink these sodas and many things, and now there are diseases."[225] Don Mateo himself has since been diagnosed with type II diabetes, a rarity in his grandparents' day. Cacao has been usurped by sugary pretenders in the place of its birth.

A question of froth

The highest class of Cacao drinks prepared by the Mexica, known as *tlaquetzalli* ("tul·ack·et·zall·ee"), meaning "precious thing"[226]—referencing the iridescent plumage of the *quetzal* bird that the Mexica prized—all had an enormous head of foam. In fact, the "drinks" may have been at least 50% foam, to be eaten with a spoon: an account by one of the *conquistadors*, the first European witnesses to native Mesoamerican practices, describes how the Cacao and spices were mixed with water in "basins with a point"—possibly spouted clay vessels—then poured back and forth from one vessel into another to raise a head of foam, which was set aside; then,

> when they drink it, they mix it with certain spoons of gold or silver or wood, and drink it, and drinking it one must open one's mouth, because *being foam* [my italics] one must give it room to subside, and go down bit by bit. (the "anonymous conqueror" of 1566, quoted in Coe & Coe, 1996)

As described earlier, many contemporary Central American *atoles* feature a substantial layer of transplanted bubbles, which often comprise more than half the volume of the beverage. If Cacao alone is mixed with water in the correct ratio and frothed, a modest head of level foam can be created, but illustrations from some Mexica codices show conical caps of froth protruding from goblets of Cacao. The *atole* formulas suggest that certain mixtures of Cacao, water, and starch-sources such as maize or wheat may produce more foam, but to achieve big, Mr. Whippy-esque stacks of bubbles probably requires filtration in addition to botanical foaming agents—plants which produce a lather.

The "correct" ratio of Cacao to water to generate foams appears to be around two parts Cacao by weight to eleven or twelve parts water, by volume—e.g. 20g (¾oz) Cacao in 110–120ml (four fluid ounces) water. The Cacao must be toasted and well ground, and if the water isn't too cold, then vigorous agitation with a *molinillo* will eventually raise a small but stable layer of foam. Technique is very important: the *molinillo* should be held firmly between flat palms, at a ninety degree angle to the liquid with the head of the whisk under the surface, and the palms rubbed briskly back and forth to rotate the *molinillo* rapidly. A bowl or other receptacle with a larger surface area and high sides is required, so that splashes are contained and the foam has room to spread out and build up, without the bubbles being broken by the continual rotary action of the *molinillo*. Persistence is key, for most of the foamy Cacao-based *atoles* require continuous or repeated frothing to generate a good head of foam.

Foaming agents exponentially increase the volume of the froth, but working out which plants they are in a recipe is a process of deduction. For example, fresh frangipani flowers (*Plumeria rubra*) appear to be the principal foaming agent in the *atole* known as *bu'pu*. That frangipani flowers have foam-making attributes is probable, because the foam of *bu'pu* is very large and stable—and because of some compounds in the plant, discussed further in Chapter 6.[227] More-over this froth is quite simple—made from Cacao, *piloncillo* sugar, and both fresh and dried *cacalosúchil* or *flor de mayo* (aka frangipani), so the frangipani flowers must be the volumising additive (in addition to contributing their scent and medicinal properties—see Chapter 8 and Appendix B). (*Piloncillo* or *panela* are simply boiled and evaporated sugarcane juice. It's essentially identical to Indian *jaggery*, has a complex caramel sweetness, and is sold in the form of blocks or cones, ranging in colour from amber to a dark brown-black.) Although *bu'pu* is frothed with a *molinillo* today, in the early twentieth century the foam was created with a *pala*, a special beating implement of simple design[228]—another clue that, like *mole* sauce, perhaps the *molinillo* isn't so much a Spanish innovation as an improvement or adaptation of a pre-existing indigenous invention.

There's an alternative explanation for the bubbly towers protruding from Cacao drinks in pre-conquest illustrations: it could be aerated fat, not foam. The floating scrambles of blancmange-like aromatic suet atop *tejate*, produced when the fats in the boiled palm (*Attalea cohune*) seeds or toasted *mamey* (*Pouteria sapota*) pits separate and precipitate in the water, are delicious: light, dissolving on the tongue, and infused with delicate flavours. Several pre-Colombian illustrations depict Cacao-based beverages being poured from a height to raise a head of foam, and this technique is employed in the latter stages of making *tejate*, to increase the volume of the fatty froth, whereas most other contemporary foamy Cacao-containing drinks use the *molinillo* or a hand whisk to generate bubbles. The deliberate separation of fat prior to adding the rest of the water in descriptions of the northern Guatemalan beverage called *batido* is interesting, too, as it suggests that the separation of fat in Cacao beverages wasn't localised to Oaxaca, or specific to *tejate*; and that the post-colonial Spanish liking for Cacao-based beverages with a layer of separated fat on top wasn't a purely European idiosyncrasy. Pre-Colombian "foam" may have been light and airy or much denser, and more akin to whipped cream, depending on the formula used. For the most part, though, it seems likely from the abundance of contemporary *atoles* that require froth that the majority of toppers were (and are) true foams.

The hardware is another story. Various clay bowls and dishes are used in present-day Oaxaca, Mexico, including beautiful glazed jugs with flat bases, fat round bottoms, and wide cylindrical necks, to facilitate whisking and foaming, or the more commonly used *cazuelas*, plain or enamelled wide clay bowls, which allow for a larger surface area to generate a separate stock of foam for topping *atoles*. Beautiful examples of elaborate lathe-turned *molinillos*, or chocolate whisks, are currently sold in Central American markets, with rattling wooden hoop-rings around one of their many tapered waists. But they were initially made without rings, which can destroy foam even as the rotary motion of the whisk creates it; it seems the elaborate rings may be a triumph of form over function.[229] The earliest examples of *molinillos* simply have notched heads, in a star shape—perhaps reminiscent of the cut ends of a branch, such as the "wild *molinillo*" made by my guide and friend Juan-Pablo in the Soconusco: having carefully selected a straight branch from a Cacao tree with several smaller branches radiating from one joint, he sawed it off, deftly stripped the bark from it, then amputated the radiating branches—producing a long, smooth stick, with five protruding stumps at one end. There are many such "wild *molinillos*" in houses of the poor in Guatemala, which adds a little circumstantial evidence to my theory that the *molinillo* isn't truly a Spanish invention, and, like 53*uri* sauce, it's more likely to be an elaboration of a much earlier native tradition, as the use of "chocolate beaters" in the emperor Motecuhzoma's household suggests (see Chapter 1).

The *popo* recipes described above made use of three different botanical foaming agents: *Aristolochia laxiflora*, a *Smilax* species (possibly *S. aristolochiifolia*) and *Gonolobus niger*. One Oaxacan *atole* relies on the foam-forming properties of *cacao blanco*, the fermented seeds of *pataxtle* (*Theobroma bicolor*). This is *chocolate atole*, which Diana Kennedy recounts is made in Teotitlan del Valle.[230] Large quantities of fermented *pataxtle* seeds are required: the ratio of *cacao blanco* to Cacao is 1:2, or even 1:1.[231] In any case, a whole mythology has built up surrounding the tricky process of making *chocolate atole* foam—if a woman can't raise a head of foam, she is assumed to be afflicted by the evil eye, or be using unclean or greasy equipment, and a pregnant woman—presumably with cleaner utensils—is brought in to froth the beverage, so that her life force will invigorate the beverage and help it foam. As Kennedy reports, "a woman's prestige is at stake!"[232]

Chaw popox utilises the bark of a climbing plant referred to locally as *n'ched* as a foaming agent. This climbing, ornamental plant grows on walls in the town of San Mateo del Mar, and is another *Gonolobus* species, which I identified as possibly *G. barbatus*—"barbatus" meaning "bearded", referring to the small, furry-looking five-petalled, star-shaped flowers. The outer bark of *n'ched* is used in its raw state, a single 50cm length of stem being stripped and pulverised on the metate with eighty toasted Cacao beans and a substantial quantity of cinnamon;[233] the mixture is ground a ritual eight times to ensure a very smooth paste with no lumps or gritty granules.[234] This paste is then mixed with water and frothed to create the foam.

The Coes also mention the Lacandon Maya use of a "grass called *aak'*" as a foaming agent. *Aak'* is ground with Cacao to make the base for their sacred drink, given as an offering—consumed only by the gods, not by man.[235] Why is *aak'* used only in the sacred drink? Could it be toxic to men, but harmless to the gods? Until this plant is positively identified, and any other uses documented, we don't know. Another foam-raising plant known as *sugir* or *suguir* was located by chocolatier Dominique Persoone, who went in search of the foaming agent used by the Lacandon Maya people of the Yucatan peninsula. The process was described by Sophie and Michael Coe, who reported that a length of the vine called *sugir* was cut, then separated into tough and tender parts; the tough part was infused in water, and strained out, then the tender part was ground with Cacao and toasted corn to make a masa which was then added to the *sugir*-infused water, stirred, and frothed.[236] Persoone was able to locate a plant used in Cacao beverages known locally as *suguir*, finding a thorny, climbing vine with little red berries; his guide verified that they had the correct plant by making a foaming Cacao beverage with it, which he photographed.[237] Unfortunately his account doesn't include a photograph the plant itself or a description of which part of the plant was used, the manner of its preparation, or any details of the recipe.

Another piece of the puzzle was added by Boris, a helpful tour guide at Tikal, one of the most famous and tourist-choked ruined Mayan cities in the Yucatan jungle. Boris was able to show me one of the trees growing there, known locally as *palo de tzol* or *sibul*; he alleged the red berries are dried and used in Cacao "like allspice" by local women.[238] The tree is *Blomia prisca*, a member of the *Sapindaceae* or soap-berry family: the clue's in the name—it could well be a foam-raising ingredient. I wondered if this might be one and the same plant as Persoone's *suguir*, with its red berries; but this is a tree, that is a vine—and the Coes recount that the stem of *sugir* is the required ingredient, not the fruit. This could be a "common name problem"—a plant's vernacular name can differ in various places, or be the same for different plants, as we have seen with the name *cocolmeca* referring to both *Smilax* and *Aristolochia* species; *sugir* and *suguir* could be two different plants with similar common names. But Señor Reginaldo Huex, a herbalist and director of a group dedicated to the conservation of traditional Itza Maya knowledge and medicinal plants in Peten, Guatemala, averred that while the fruit flesh (epicarp) of *palo de tzol* seeds was edible, the "pip" or "stone" was intensely bitter, and inedible, and would spoil any beverage it was added to.[239] So the identity of *sugir* or *suguir* currently remains a mystery, and the use of *Blomia prisca* as a foaming agent, uncertain.

So there are a great variety of additives and techniques used to produce drink-toppers in Central American *atoles* and Cacao-based beverages, ranging from fat precipitation to foam generation, and employing a wide armamentarium of botanical additives which we have only begun to investigate and describe. These beverages are complex, labour-intensive, and sophisticated: like many other highly valued plants, Cacao is a spur to human inventiveness.

Cacao in Mesoamerica

The earliest non-native descriptions of Cacao-based beverages were created by Hernández, Badiano, Sahagún, and the Dominican friar Diego Durán, author of *The History of the Indies of New Spain*. These early ethnographers documented indigenous uses of plants soon after the Spanish occupation of Central America, and before the ravages of slavery, disease, missionary activity, waves of colonisation, and all the miseries of imperial subjugation had completely decimated the local population and obfuscated traditional practices. There are also hints from archaeological finds, illustrations from murals and codices (those not burnt or destroyed by minions of the Church), and the living tradition of *atoles* and Cacao-based drinks from which some reconstruction may be attempted. The best records are accounts of sixteenth-century native recipes, as these primary sources are taken from eyewitness accounts and living traditions, many of which have long since atrophied. Even though these texts are often filtered through a European lens of Christianity, Galenic medical doctrine (see next chapter), and unfamiliarity with native technologies, they nevertheless have a more natural understanding of pre-conquest indigenous perspectives than modern readers might, as the native population, too, was fervently religious, utilised an analogous medical theoretical framework, and existed in a civilisation that was just as handcrafted as any other in the era before mass production and mechanisation. The great divisions of dogma, socialisation, and circumstance were arguably more easily intellectually bridged then than now; we post-Enlightenment folk have a better mechanical and theoretical understanding of the past, but subjectively inhabit a different world altogether.

We know from Hernández's account that the Mexica graded Cacao into four types (all of which would now be recognised as *criollo* subvarieties: *forastero* had yet to be imported from South America). These were *cuauhcacahuatl* ("koo·aw·kaka·hoo·attle"), or "eagle/wood Cacao", the largest and highest quality available; *mecacahuatl* ("meh·kaka·hoo·attle"), or "maguey Cacao", a medium-sized variety; *xochicacahuatl* ("soh·chee·kaka·hoo·attle"), a smaller variety of high quality, with a "reddish" seed coat, perhaps analogous to the high-quality "red *criollo* Cacao" grown in contemporary Chiapas, Mexico; and, finally, *tlalcacahuatl* ("klal·kaka·hoo·attle"), "earth Cacao", the smallest variety, which was preferred for culinary use—the larger three were most often used as currency.[240] Belgian chocolatier Dominique Persoone claims that Cacao *lavado*, or even unfermented Cacao, was the standard form of Cacao used in pre-conquest Mesoamerica.[241] It seems unlikely that completely unfermented beans were used, given the amount of traditional *atole* recipes and ingredients which call for fermentation, or even double-fermentation of ingredients (as in soured *pozol* containing Cacao, or putrefied Cacao beans used in one *popo* recipe)—and the current hypothesis for the discovery of Cacao seeds as a viable foodstuff depends on the fermentation of the fruit making the seeds more palatable. The Maya are known to have fermented Cacao beans in hollow logs;[242] but it's true that many of the more traditional *atoles* made with Cacao in both Mexico and Guatemala preferentially utilise Cacao *lavado*; and in the city of Coban, Alta Verapaz, Guatemala—one of the few regions in Central America where some people do still drink Cacao beverages such as *batido* without maize or added sugar—the only Cacao available for purchase in the marketplaces is barely fermented.[243]

The first known instance of the word *chocolatl* is found in Hernández's account of an eponymous Cacao-based drink made by the Mexica, which utilised the seeds of the majestic *Ceiba pentandra*, the tall, straight kapok tree, known today as the national emblem of Guatemala. Kapok fruit pods split to reveal seeds surrounded by white fluffy fibres, which are light, buoyant, and water-retardant, and have many industrial uses. The round, pea-sized seeds, called *pochotl* ("poh·choh·tul") by the Mexica according to Hernández's sixteenth-century testimony, were used in equal proportion to Cacao to make a foaming drink.[244] Nobody I spoke to in Mexico or Guatemala today knows of such a use of ceiba seeds, so the use of *pochotl* with Cacao may have died out, or be far less widespread than it once was; which is ironic, given that the word for the drink made from them appears to have become the ubiquitous term for products made from Cacao.

But *tlaquetzalli xochicacahuatl* beverages—those of royal quality—contained no "extenders" such as maize or *pochotl* (*Ceiba pentandra* seeds), and were made using only high-quality toasted Cacao beans, spices or other botanical additives, and water. Their characteristic head of foam was made separately or removed-and-replaced, and, as we have seen, this tradition is preserved in many contemporary Cacao-containing *atoles*. But the Maya were less classist in their categorisation of *kakaw*; *posolli* or *pozol* was, and remains, a basic foodstuff of the poor, and is frequently enhanced by the addition of Cacao. This is perhaps a function of geography as much as society—the Classic Maya polities were separated from the Mexica by a span of hundreds of years as well as miles, and much of the verdant Maya heartland, unlike the more arid climate of central Mexico, is Cacao-cultivating territory: like as not the Mayan poor—then as now—could grow their own.

Sahagún lists Mexica *cacahuatl*-preparing equipment including clay jars, presumably used as tureens or vessels for mixing, storing, and dispensing the prepared drink; a large painted gourd vessel for hand-washing; "richly designed drinking vessels", and "the strainer with which was purified the chocolate".[245] The strainer is an interesting addition, though no details are given as to its composition or manufacture—whether it was fine cloth, mesh, or a sort of sieve or colander, for example. It seems likely that the most highly valued of the pre-conquest Cacao drinks were filtered, as Hernández reports, then foamed by agitation, turning the entire beverage into a light, aromatic froth, like a maize-free version of *popo*. A "smooth mouthfeel" is an important quality-control criterion for contemporary confectioner's chocolate, as it appears that a well-filtered, smooth *cacahuatl* was also a significant consideration for the Mexica.

According to Sahagún, the Mexica served their *tlaquetzalli cacahuatl* in gourds called *xicalli*, painted inside and out,[246] sometimes with a stopper—made of what material, he doesn't say— and a separate beater. This is remarkable, as the Mexica were alleged to have raised the foam by pouring the prepared chocolate back and forth from one vessel to another,[247] according to pictures in codices and vases and frescoes, as well as accounts by post-conquest documentarians like Sahagún and Hernández. We don't know if the little beaters or stirrers provided with individual servings of *cacahuatl* resembled the later *molinillo*, allegedly a Spanish invention, or if they were of a different design. Perhaps the beaters were only served with the *cacahuatl* in case it was set aside for a while and "went flat", so the guest (or a servant) could refresh the foam?

Because gourds have a naturally round base, circular jar rests like stuffed doughnuts of cured leather or ocelot skin were provided at banquets,[248] and positioned at the left hand of important guests, while the *xicalli* was conventionally held in the right hand, and the beaters were placed on the same side.[249] Simple wicker circles and carved or painted hemispherical gourd-bowls are still sold in the markets of Oaxaca today, although the gourds used as drinking vessels by the Mexica sound like they were sawn off much higher, so they tapered from a wider base to a narrower opening, which could be stoppered to keep the *cacahuatl* fresh. The Mexica also served their *cacahuatl* with "small spoons of gold or silver or wood"[250] for eating the foam—a practice which is retained today with Oaxacan *chocolate atole*, giving purpose to the miniature wooden spoons sold in local markets with beautifully carved, painted animals on the handles—too small for adults and too fancy for babies, but perfect for savouring delectable mouthfuls of froth.

"Green" Cacao

In present-day Nicaragua, one local *refresco*—a cool, sweet drink, the traditional and less sugary version of a soda—is made using Cacao fruit pulp, mixed with water (and, of course, added sugar), producing a frothy, "refreshing" drink with a "citrus-like flavour" (Young, 1994).[251] Cacao fruit pulp contains a little caffeine, which probably accounts for the "refreshing" effect; but the interesting thing here is that such beverages—minus the added sugar—appear to be of ancient origin, and that some of their forebears may have been fermented for an ethanolic kick. In South America, a form of *chicha*, or alcoholic beverage, is made from Cacao fruit, and it has been speculated that the original fermentation of Cacao seeds—which develops their flavour, as well as many interesting trace compounds (see Chapters 4 and 5)—may have been a serendipitous consequence of the fermentation of the fruit pulp to produce ethanol. It may just have been easier to ferment the gluey fruit flesh while it was still attached to the seeds.[252]

Adding weight to this theory, a contemporary Guatemalan *refresco* called *refresco de pocha*—*pocha* being a term referring to whole Cacao pods—utilises the seeds and pulp scraped out of the pods, stirred well with a little added water and sugar, and drunk; but sometimes this *refresco* is allowed to ferment for up to thirty days, presumably with some kind of airlock to prevent it turning to vinegar, in order to create an alcoholic beverage.[253] Whether this is a modern innovation or not is unclear, but we do know that the human tendency to alcoholic innovation is of ancient origin, as is the consumption of Cacao fruit pulp. Inscriptions on Classic Maya ceramic vessels indicate their contents of "tree-fresh Cacao", possibly the ancient equivalent of a modern *refresco*, and "honey Cacao", which may have been a sweetened Cacao beverage—or, knowing the Maya predilection for drinking unsweetened *kakawa*, "honey Cacao" could just as plausibly have been a fermented Cacao fruit beverage, given the traditional use of added sugar in the form of honey or concentrated *maguey* cactus (*Agave americana*) sap, also known as agave nectar, to assist fermentation. Many scholars have puzzled over the report by Sahagún, describing how the "green Cacao" drunk by the Mexica at their feasts makes one drunk … makes one dizzy, confuses one, makes one sick, deranges one. When an ordinary amount is drunk, it gladdens one, refreshes one, consoles one, invigorates one. (Sahagún, quoted by Henderson & Joyce in McNeil, 2006)

While this could be an account of the effects of strong *cacahuatl* spiked with more powerful psychoactive plants (see below), it sounds more like the effects of an alcoholic drink. Researchers John Henderson and Rosemary Joyce point out that in Nahuatl, the Mexica language, the word for "green", *xoxohqui* ("shoh·shoh·kwee"), also means unripe, or sour.[254] Alcoholic beverages made from fermented fruit are sour-tasting: what has been translated as "green Cacao" could actually mean "soured Cacao", a fermented Cacao fruit drink. But drunkenness was frowned on in Mexica society; it was tolerated in the elderly, who had earned the right to a certain amount of public dissipation, and *octli*, especially, was regarded as a vulgar drink—*cacahuatl* was the libation of the privileged.[255]

Intoxicating flowers

Perhaps unsurprisingly for one of the most biodiverse regions on Earth, the Mesoamerican peoples had an extensive *materia medica*, and their use of flowers in medicine and gastronomy was as elaborate as any Old World culture. In Mesoamerican cultures, flowers were a metaphor for elegance, sophistication, and artistry, and, from the time of Teotihuacan onwards, they also came to represent the soul, life force, spiritual and magical potency, and the visible effects of these things in terms of status, charisma, and acquisition of worldly goods (the symbolism of flowers in Mesoamerica is discussed further in Chapter 9). Aside from their striking and diverse beauty, their evocative aromas, their profusion, and their transience—noted by poets and artists across all cultures and throughout history as a perfect allegory for life's joys—many native flowers are powerfully psychoactive. Mexica poetry speaks of "intoxicating flowers"; the Mesoamericans included mushrooms and cacti under this umbrella, and psychedelic *Psilocybe* mushrooms were referred to as "little flowers".[256]

Floral spices and medicines were arguably more highly regarded in Mesoamerica than in the Old World. True, saffron (*Crocus sativum*) and damask roses (*Rosa damascena*) were very expensive and held exalted positions in the canon of Arabic and European medieval medicine, and Old World cultures recognised the handiwork of the divine in plants which served as both food and medicine. But there is a definite chain of command in monotheistic ideology: god, human, animal, plant, mineral; and, in lieu of God's direct intervention, humans call the shots. But the pre-Columbian cultures of Central America took their flowers very seriously, as they were extensions of the divine: some flowers, properly employed, could be a hotline to revelation; plants were not merely products, they were ensouled beings. Even the most mundane healing plant hosted spiritual power and presence—the Mesoamerican universe was polytheistic, and abundantly god-haunted. So the addition of flowery spices or medicines to the favoured psychoactive drugs in Mesoamerica, the drinks made using Cacao, was more than just flavour enhancement: it was a form of sacrament, and a magical act.

The favoured "chocolate spice" used by the Mexica in their *cacahuatl* was ear flower (*Cymbopetalum penduliflorum*). Ear flower is a direct translation from the Nahuatl name *xochinacaztli* ("shoh·chee·na·kaz·tlee"), and the plant was also known as *hueinacaztli* ("way·na·kaz·tlee"), ("great ear") and *teonacaztli* ("tay·oh·na·kaz·tlee"), ("divine ear") because the leathery dried petals of *Cymbopetalum penduliflorum* look—with a little imagination—a bit like ears.[257] Ear flower is still the principal spice in contemporary *batido*, but was reported by Hernández to "inebriate like the mushrooms" when added to Cacao-based drinks,[258] and Dr Stubbe wrote that they "improve chocolate far beyond its selfe"[259], and Hernández reported that "There is nothing else in the … markets of the Indians more frequently found nor more highly prized than this flower."[260] Dried ear flowers may still be found today in some Guatemalan marketplaces. A more familiar Cacao spice, which has by now retained this role for upwards of two thousand years and across the globe, is the humble vanilla pod.

Actually, vanilla isn't very humble at all. The Mexica name for vanilla was *tlilxochitl* ("clil·soh·chul") or "black flower",[261] because after harvesting the ripe seed pods of the climbing, vine-like orchid, the pods must be scalded, fermented for several months so they blacken, and carefully dried to develop the flavour.[262] Fresh, green vanilla just smells fresh and green; as with Cacao, only once the microscopic microbial chemists have had at it during fermentation are the aromatic breakdown products produced. Vanilla pods sometimes have a visible fur of crystallised vanillin, the principal odour compound in the fermented fruit, so profuse that it sweats out of the drying plant material and rimes the desiccated pod with an aromatic frost. The plants must be hand-pollinated, so cultivation is highly labour intensive, making vanilla the second most expensive spice in the world (after saffron). This process was developed by the Mesoamericans, and the origins of the classic pairing of vanilla with Cacao—two fermented, aromatic products gloriously enhancing each other—is lost in the mists of time. Like that phrase, vanilla itself seems to have become a cliché, transformed into a one-note synthetic flavouring used in cheap icing and available for pennies in the baking aisles of supermarkets. Accept no substitutes: the real thing is vastly superior.

While vanilla doesn't seem particularly "intoxicating", the smell of vanilla pods is almost universally appealing. Estate agents will tell you that the smell of vanilla helps sell houses faster; but whether it shifts real estate or not, vanillin alone—the main odour compound in the fermented pods—has distinctly antidepressant and behaviour-changing properties, at least in rodents (see Chapter 6). The other familiar botanical additives to Cacao can't claim any notable psychotropic effects: neither chilli, annatto, or allspice have significant mood-altering effects. Because of their firm association with Asian cuisine, many people don't realise that chillies (*Capsicum spp.*) originate in Central America. The Mesoamericans developed many different varieties of chillies for use in food and medicine, from large sweet ones to tiny fiery fruits; they're still used in herbal medicine as a circulatory stimulant, and to enhance the effectiveness of other medicinal plants in a formula.[263] Allspice berries were also known as *xocoxochitl* ("shok·oh·shoh·chittle") by the Mexica, and the dried seeds have a long history of use in Cacao-based beverages. The tree has a pale trunk with twisting, mangrove-like sculptural roots, and distinctively aromatic leaves and berries. Their flavour is reminiscent of cloves, nutmeg, and cinnamon, hence the name bestowed on it by Europeans; the seeds and leaves have several medicinal properties (see Chapters 3, 6, and Appendix B]. Today the seeds are used as an occasional spice in Guatemalan hot chocolate, and are a key ingredient in *batido*.

Holy leaf (*hoja santa*, or *Piper auritum*) was known to the Mexica as *mecaxochitl* ("meh·ka·soh·tchul") and has been referred to as the root beer plant, owing to its distinctive flavour. This plant is related to the Asian black pepper (*Piper nigrum*) and the Polynesian kava-kava (*Piper methysticum*). The Mexica and the Maya used the leaf for cooking and medicine, but used the dried flower spikes, which look like little black threads, as a Cacao spice. It was used to enhance both high-class and less exclusive drinks by the Mexica, who—along with every pre-Colombian civilisation—drank *atolli* (now Hispanicised to *atole*). Hernández describes one such recipe, called *atextli*, which called for a hundred toasted Cacao seeds, properly ground, with "two hands' worth" of cooked, nixtamalized maize, vanilla pods, ear flowers, and the dried fruits of the root beer plant.[264] While its use with Cacao is based on its agreeable and slightly spicy taste, *hoja santa* appears to have fallen into disuse as a Cacao additive, though the leaves are still used in Central American cooking to wrap *tamales* and fish before steaming them, infusing them with their particular, green-plant-spice flavour; and the plant is still used medicinally (see Chapters 3 and 6].

Because of their use in *atoles*, pink and yellow frangipani (*Plumeria rubra*) flowers are known as *flor de maiz tostado* ("Flower of Toasted Maize").[265] The tree flowers in spring, so they're also referred to as *flor de Mayo* (May flower) in the Mexican isthmus; each type has a distinctive fragrance, the smell of the yellow flowers being both sweeter and more rubbery, the pink flowers having a deeper, more rose-like scent, though both are often used in combination. There is also a white-flowered variety. The flowers are almost the size of an open palm, and are to be found in the markets of the Oaxacan isthmus strung onto garlands. The Mexica called the tree *cacaloxochitl* ("kaka·low·soh·chul"), and the Zapotec name for the plant is *guie-chachi*, meaning "brilliant flower". The Mexica had different prefixes for this tree, depending on the colour of its blooms: *itzac* for white flowers, *tzapaltic* for red flowers;[266] the spectacular blooms have enamoured gardeners everywhere so that, like its compatriot Cacao, Frangipani now engirdles the world, growing on every tropical continent. The Maya knew it as *baak nik'te* ("bone flower")[267] because the latex from the tree was used to accelerate bone healing,[268] but it has also come to be known as temple tree because of its popularity in Asian temple gardens.

Other common plants added to Cacao-based beverages were popcorn flower (*Bourreria huanita*), known to the Mexica as *izquixochitl*[269] ("is·key·soh·tchul"); *eloxochitl*, or *yolloxochitl* ("yoll·oh·soh·tchul"), Mexica names for varieties of the spectacular Mexican magnolia tree (*Magnolia dealbata* and *Magnolia mexicana*, formerly known as *Talauma mexicana*); and hand flower (*Chiranthodendron pentadactylon*), also known as "devil's hand flower" in some parts of Mexico today, listed by Hernández as a spice used with Cacao. Popcorn flower is so named because its white flower clusters very vaguely, with a lot of artistic licence, resemble white popcorn kernels. Its contemporary Spanish name is *Jasmin del Istmo* ("Isthmus Jasmine"), a much more fitting name than the English one: the tree grows in the humid Isthmus region of Oaxaca, and the flowers smell very like Jasmine, although their scent, like Jasmine, is evanescent—when dried, the aroma becomes a shadow of its former self. Like the effects of desiccation on the perfume of the fresh flowers, their use in *cacahauatl* has faded from memory in present-day Mexico.

Dried magnolia flowers are still sold as medicine in Central American marketplaces, and have a subtle aroma, which can be enhanced by lightly toasting them; but the scent is much stronger when they're fresh.[270] There are, however, three varieties of magnolia sold in central

Mexico: *flor de corazon* ("heart flower"), *magnolia*, and *Yolosúchil*. All three are clearly different: *flor de corazon* (uncertain species) is a hard, grey-brown petrified-looking dried flower; *magnolia* (*Magnolia dealbata*) is orange, with faintly scented petals, looking aylittle like strips of dried mango; and *yolosúchil* (*M. mexicana*) is bright yellow when dried, with a stronger floral scent. All three are used for similar indications. *M. mexicana* was the *yolloxochitl* of old, used in Cacao-based drinks.[271] These were alleged to be emperor Motecuhzoma's favourite *cacahuatl* spice,[272] conveying a slight melon-like flavour to the *cacahuatl*. The devil's hand flower, or *macpalxochitl* ("mack·pal·soh·tchul")—literally, "hand flower"—in Nahuatl, is a bat-pollinated tree from the same plant family as Cacao. The name derives from its distinctive flowers with five long, shiny stamens, like curling carmine hands emerging from sharp-petalled stars. They have a very astringent taste, and may have been added to Cacao for medicinal effects, or, somewhat in the style of molecular gastronomy, to enhance the perceived "dryness" of the beverage, perhaps in contrast to an oily "foam".

There are several other known or suspected botanical additives to Cacao—pine nuts (from *Pinus edulis*); the Mayan spice *itsim-te*, thought to be *Clerodendrum ligustrinum*; carry crate flower or *Philodendron pseudoradiatum*, referred to as *huacalxochitl* in Durán's lists of additives used by the Mexica, and many more (see Appendix B for a non-definitive list). One colonial-era reference describes the flower of a "pitchy or rosiny tree, which yields a gum like that of the *Styrax* [*benzoin*], but of a finer colour; its flower is like that of the orange tree, of a good smell, which they mix with the chocolate."[273] This tree still hasn't been positively identified, though some think it may be funeral tree (*Quararibea funebris*)—a tree not known for producing resin. It could be the Frangipani, which has aromatic flowers vaguely similar to orange tree blossoms, though much larger; but that exudes a milky latex, not a resin.

The funeral tree itself (*Quararibea funebris*) was second only to ear flower (*Cymbopetalum*) in its traditional significance as a Cacao-drink spice. It's called *rosita de cacao* ("Little Rose of Cacao") in contemporary Mexico, and the Mexica knew it as *cacahuaxochitl* ("kaka·wah·soh·tchul"), or "flower of Cacao" in Nahuatl. The tree blooms profusely after the rains, and the dried flowers have a heady, deep perfume, somewhat sweet like vanilla but with a woodier note; the scent is incredibly persistent, and lingers in dried specimens for many years. Toasted, they are still used in contemporary Oaxaca as the principal spice in *tejate*. *Cacahuaxochitl* was so important to the Mexica that it appears to be carved on the base of the statue of Xochipilli ("soh·chi·pill·ee"), one of the Ahuiateteo ("ah·wee·ah·tey·teo"), the five Mexica "gods of excess". Xochipilli was a god of love, ecstasy, games, dancing, feasting, flowers—and venereal disease. His statue was embellished with representations of four other notably psychoactive plants: tobacco (*Nicotiana tabacum*), morning glory (*Turbina corymbosa*), "magic muchrooms" (*Psilocybe aztecorum*), and the lesser-known but amusingly named shrubby yellowcrest (*Heimia salicifolia*).[274]

Ethnobotanist Jonathan Ott refers to Sahagún's identification of *Q. funebris* as *poyomatli*, entheogenic flowers.[275] Sahagún describes a smoking mixture made with *poyomatli*, other flowers, "mushrooms", tobacco, and an unidentified resin, although Ott's self-experiments ingesting funeral tree flowers produced no discernible psychoactive effects.[276] But as author Dale Pendell points out, *poyomatli* is a generic term meaning "befuddling" or "intoxicating", and there's little strong evidence linking it to *Q. funebris*.[277] So there's some doubt as to the identity of the flower carved on the Xochipilli statue, and it has been suggested that the flowers represented may be those of *Solandra grandiflora*, the snowy chalicevine,[278] or even the dream-enhancing herb *sinicuichi* (*Calea zacatechichi*),[279] and not—as current consensus holds—*Quararibea funebris*. In any case, it appears that *Q. funebris* flowers don't have powerful mind-altering properties on their own, so perhaps they were venerated for other reasons, or for an ability to enhance the properties of other plants; their probable association with four other powerfully psychoactive plants is a conundrum, which will be explored further in Chapter 6. But the psychedelic properties of *Psilocybe* mushrooms aren't in doubt, and Mesoamerican people certainly used them with Cacao.

God flesh and serpent vines

From Sahagún's account of a Mexica banquet:

> They ate the mushrooms before dawn when they also drank Cacao. They ate the mushrooms with honey and when they began to feel excited due to the effect of the mushrooms, the Indians started dancing, while some were singing and others weeping. (from Rudgley, 1993)

Likewise, Durán reports that the coronation of the Mexica emperor Ahuitzotl was accompanied by drinking Cacao beverages and eating psychoactive mushrooms.[280] Pharmacological reasons for this combination are discussed in Chapter 6, but it's clear that Cacao and mushrooms were consumed together, though as far as we know the mushrooms were eaten separately, after the *cacahuatl* was drunk, and not incorporated into the drinks themselves. But the mushrooms were often dried and powdered, or ground with water on a *metatl* to make "mushroom juice",[281] so the addition of either powdered mushrooms or the juice extract to Cacao-based drinks is entirely possible. The Mexica even made an alcoholic mushroom-based *pulque* called *nanacaoctli* ("nana·ka·ocked·lee").[282] *Psilocybe* mushrooms were known as *kaiz'alaj okox* ("kaiz·allaj·ock·osh") to the Maya,[283] and *teonanacatl*—meaning "god flesh"—to the Mexica, because consuming them enabled communion with the gods. They were referred to as "intoxicating flowers" in Mexica poetry, and were associated with music, both recreationally and functionally, when music was used to aid in spirit work—or, as some may prefer, to "alter consciousness". Mesoamerican use of psychoactive mushrooms appears to be ancient, as more than two hundred mushroom-shaped stone effigies dating back to the first millennium BCE have been found in Central America, including a sculpture of a ring of figures dancing around a giant mushroom, and murals in Teotihuacan show priests bearing mushrooms in the presence of the rain god Tlaloc—which makes sense because mushrooms, as we know, emerge after rain.[284] Accounts of Mexica mushroom use indicate that they were taken at celebrations by warriors, merchants, and other socially distinguished men for divinatory purposes—an experience which could be exhilarating or disturbing, as Sahagún's account illustrates.

There is reason to suspect that other psychoactive plants were sometimes used with, or even added to Cacao-based beverages. First, there is the curious assertion by Sahagún that *cacahuatl* was "like the mushroom … it made one drunk; it intoxicated one".[285] Second, there is the extraordinary effect of *itzpacalatl* to consider—the drink made by Mexica priests which caused a human sacrifice to forget his plight and dance happily. This response—tantamount to a kind of possession or takeover of the will—is far more than mere mood-modification, and beyond the powers of Cacao alone. The magical and ritual elements of the drink's administration would have greatly magnified its influence, and it's possible that this may explain its extraordinary potency; altered states can be induced through the placebo effect, which Daniel Moermann asserts should be renamed the "meaning effect", as its magnitude depends on the degree of meaning that both recipients and administrators of a drug or treatment attribute to it (see Chapter 4 for a fuller discussion of this phenomenon). Examples of this include surgery performed using hypnosis or acupuncture rather than anaesthetic, and a startling anecdote by the pharmacologist Alexander Shulgin, who recounted being rendered unconscious by a white powder partly dissolved in orange juice, which he believed to contain a potent drug, but actually turned out to be plain sugar.[286] The intense ritual and symbolic significance of *itzpacalatl* in the context of the Mesoamerican belief system would no doubt have encouraged extreme psychological responses, but even so, as with drugs, the placebo effect doesn't work the same for everybody, so it's likely that some sort of pharmacological enhancement was used in the form of botanical additives to the drink.

So, what may have caused Cacao-based drinks to be perceived as potently psychotropic? And, more specifically, what could have been added to *itzpacalatl* to produce such remarkable effects? First, it's just possible that Sahagún's description of the "intoxicating" properties of *cacahuatl* were due to the psychotropic action of Cacao itself. Consider that at the time, caffeine was almost unknown in Europe: tea and coffee had yet to become ubiquitous, and the effects of stimulants, which today are commonplace, seemed marvellous. It's also the case that Cacao prepared in the traditional way, without added sugar and undiluted by maize or other "extenders", is more potent and noticeably affecting than one might think: real Cacao can produce more than a "buzz", it can even generate euphoria, and may be used to facilitate altered states induced by other substances or rituals, exemplified by the "Cacao ceremonies" pioneered by Keith Wilson (see Appendix C, Interview 3), or the consumption of dark chocolate as a potentiator for some contemporary psychoactive drugs, discussed in Chapter 5. The "anonymous conqueror" described how drinking a single cup of *cacahuatl* enables a man to walk as far as he likes in a day without feeling hungry[287]—a potent stimulant indeed, and one which would be all the more noticeable to a half-starved soldier who had never ingested caffeine in his life.

But even though *cacahuatl* may have been more appreciably "drug-like" in its intensity than we may expect, Cacao alone doesn't have psychedelic, "hallucinogenic", or inebriating properties. So it's probable that other additives were responsible for these effects. As we have seen, at least two of the native spices already mentioned, ear flower (*Cymbopetalum penduliflorum*) and the funeral tree (*Quararibea funebris*), are suspected of enhancing Cacao's own psychoactivity. While it's possible that Sahagún confounded the effects of concurrent *Psilocybe* mushroom and *cacahuatl* ingestion with the effects of the spices added to the drink, he actually states that ear flowers "inebriate *like* the mushrooms"; he knew the difference between a mushroom and a flower. So that leaves the possibility that he was right: *Cymbopetalum* plus Cacao equals psychedelic effects—or, alternatively, that there may have been another additive in some *cacahuatl* drinks, of which he was unaware.

One candidate is the seed of the morning glory plant, *Turbina corymbosa* (a climber with larger seeds) or *Ipomoea violacea* (a climber with smaller, black seeds). *Turbina corymbosa* was the substance known as *ololiuhqui* in Nahuatl or *xtabentun* ("shtah·ben·toon") to the Maya, and *Ipomoea violacea* was *tlitliltzin* ("clit·lilt·zin") in Nahuatl or *yaxce'lil* ("yash·cheh·lil") to the Maya.[288] The seeds of both plants have effects very similar to *Psilocybe* mushrooms, although with a more sedative aspect and a greater tendency to induce nausea. The Mexica referred to these climbing, sprawling plants in the bindweed or *Convolvulaceae* plant family as *cohuaxihuitl* ("co·wah·shee·wittle") ("herb of serpents") or *coatlxoxouhqui* ("co·attle·shoh-shoh·uh·kwee") ("green snake"),[289] and both have a long history of medicinal and magical use in Mesoamerica, which continues to the present day, where they are still employed by Mixtec and Zapotec healers. The seeds are ground and infused in cold or tepid water, the infusion is strained, and drunk[290]—so to make a Cacao-based beverage using them is relatively simple, as this infusion may become the liquid for the drink, to which ground Cacao and other ingredients are added.

Both morning glory plants were used in a straightforwardly medicinal fashion, as well as for shamanic divination and healing; but in contrast to mushrooms, they were often used in one-on-one sessions rather than in group ceremonies, because of their sedative effects.[291] It's this aspect of their use, rather than other issues—such as the need to prepare the seeds in tepid or cold water, or their nauseating taste, or there being no accounts of morning glory seeds being used with Cacao—which suggests that *ololiuhqui* and *tlitliltzin* are less likely to have been additives in *cacahuatl* at feasts and public occasions. On the other hand, Cacao is exceptionally good at masking bitter or unpleasant flavours, and the presence of *ololiuhqui* on Xochipilli's plinth bespeaks its importance as both a sacred medicine and a potentially recreational substance. It's possible to produce a palatable, room-temperature Cacao-based beverage which is mildly psychedelic and doesn't induce nausea or sedation using a cold-water infusion of the seeds.[292]

Another possible additive to Cacao drinks, at least in the Oaxacan region of Mexico, are the leaves of *Salvia divinorum*, or *pipiltzintli* ("pip·ill·tsin·tlee") in Nahuatl[293]—which indicates that the plant was known to the Mexica, although it was (and is) principally used by the Mazatec people. It's a type of sage in the lavender-mint plant family (*Lamiaceae*), mainly used in Central American magico-medical practice for divination-assisted diagnosis. Also known as *ska pastora* in present-day Mexico, the fresh leaves were traditionally chewed, or ground with water on the *metate* to extract the juice, which was drunk; their ingestion produces a mild altered state which the ethnobotanist Gordon Wasson described: "dancing colours in elaborate, three-dimensional designs", but "It did not go beyond the initial effect of the mushrooms."[294] Even so, *S. divinorum* has acquired a fearsome reputation as a hallucinogen due to the intense psychotropic activity of concentrated extracts from the leaves when smoked—a non-traditional manner of use.

As with morning glory seeds, there are no records of *Salvia divinorum* being incorporated in Cacao-based drinks; but the Maya, particularly, were known to mix-and-match various psychoactive substances and brews for ceremonial or recreational purposes, sometimes having enemas of mind-altering (or spirit-accessing) plants, while also—and, according to the anonymous conqueror's account, simultaneously—consuming psychoactive brews (he refers to both the enemas and the drinks as "wine",[295] which is conquistador shorthand for anything psychoactive). Tobacco was often smoked, usually mixed with other plants, often at feasts, or ingested in much higher doses for shamanic purposes. Cacao would have been consumed in both sacred and secular situations. So other psychoactive plants such as morning glory seeds or *Salvia divinorum* could have been ingested alongside Cacao, even if they weren't incorporated into the beverages themselves.

But a highly potent additive would have been required in *itzpacalatl* to overcome the awareness of imminent death. It's possible that this additive could have been the *teonanacatl* themselves: *Psilocybe* mushrooms' principal active constituent, psilocybin, has been administered to people dying of advanced cancer,[296] as the psychedelic effects help to transmute pain and relieve existential dread by revealing or inducing a sense of underlying unity and meaning. So this combination could powerfully alter the perspective of soon-to-be-sacrificed captives, although the effects of mushrooms plus Cacao seems likely to have been somewhat unpredictable; those who ingested mushrooms at feasts could end up laughing or crying, and therapy groups of cancer patients who have been given psilocybin typically aren't overwhelmed with joy—the benefit is rather one of increased acceptance of impending death.[297]

The post-conquest Spanish chronicler Fray Juan de Torquemada wrote that ingesting *itzpacalatl* left the slave "blazing with spirit and courage",[298] though it should be noted that Torquemada was recording eyewitness accounts second-hand, over half a century after the fall of the Mexica empire, so some distortion or exaggeration is possible. But in this age of scepticism or agnostic doubt, the effects of *itzpacalatl* might well be quite different than it would have been for a Mexica slave or captive who held similar beliefs to his captors; the effects of a mushroom-infused Cacao drink, enhanced with potent blood from living human hearts, would be to directly connect them with the gods; if even now, in this secular age, psilocybin-induced visions can help people accept imminent death, what could they have done under such circumstances? It may very well have been sufficient to convert an unwilling victim into a collusive participant, convinced of their own imminent apotheosis after an *itzpacalatl*-induced revelation.

Another possible additive is the plant *Datura innoxia*, known as *toloaxihuitl* ("tollow·ashy·wittle") to the Mexica, and nowadays as *toloache*, jimsonweed, or the Devil's herb.[299] The Nahuatl name means "nodding head",[300] and refers to the pendulous, spiked fruits, but also perhaps to its soporific or narcotic effects. Like the European "hexing herbs" henbane, mandrake, and deadly nightshade, *Datura* species produce extremely potent and toxic tropane alkaloids, substances which cause distinctive effects such as accelerated heartbeat, dilated pupils, difficulty urinating, easier breathing (airway dilation), flushing, and dry mouth. But the most remarkable effects are mental: lower doses induce mild sedation and poor memory retention—for this reason, some tropane alkaloids are often used in pre-surgical injections. But higher doses result in total delirium, a dissolution of the boundary between dream and waking consciousness, extreme physical discomfort, lethargy, and true hallucinations that can be felt, seen, heard, spoken to, and interacted with, often of a dark or disturbing nature. The genus *Datura* has representatives in Africa and Asia, too, and everywhere these plants grew they were respected or even feared as potent spirit medicines and entheogens.

All varieties of *Datura* have similar properties, and even though physical discomfort, frightening experiences, and lethargy don't sound like they'd be especially useful in *itzpacalatl*, the plants' ability to induce suggestibility, amnesia, and delirium make *Datura* a strong contender. Ethnobotanist Richard Schultes relates that a Mexican *Datura* species, *D. ceratocaula*, was known as the "sister of *ololiouhqui*" in pre-Colombian Mexico, and that *toloaxihuitl* (*D. innoxia*) is added to *mescal*—a distilled beverage rather similar to tequila, made from fermented *Agave* cactus sap—as a "catalyst", to "induce good feeling and visions".[301] The most telling suggestion that perhaps *toloaxihuitl* may have been an essential ingredient of *itzpacalatl* comes from the sixteenth-century

Chinese herbalist Li Shih-Chen's account of the effects of pharmacologically similar *D. metel* flowers. Shih-Chen recounts that someone under the influence of the plant will mimic laughing or dancing in others, and is drawn to imitate such movements and gestures.[302] In the twenty-first century, the tropane alkaloid called scopolamine—present in *Datura* species—has been used by criminals in major cities, principally Bogota in Colombia, to "spike" drinks or cocaine (itself a tropane alkaloid, albeit with quite different effects) and render people suggestible, pliable, and forgetful so that they can be directed to reveal their secrets, give away their money, and remember nothing.[303] So *toloaxihuitl*, or a related *Datura* species, is a strong candidate for being the "business end" of *itzpacalatl*, perhaps on its own, or in combination with *ololiouhqui* or other plants. But, if *toloaxihuitl* is the main active ingredient of *itzpacalatl*, why even add Cacao? Other than its ceremonial significance, and its ability to disguise harsh flavours, it's possible that Cacao could modify the effect of the *Datura*—a speculation which will be revisited in Chapter 6.

So traditional Cacao-based beverages were both structurally unique, and highly variable in their composition. Chocolate confectionery is equally elaborate in its construction, but differs from native Cacao-based drinks in the same way that store-bought pre-sliced white bread differs from home-made sourdough, or methadone from opium, or rubbing alcohol from champagne; chocolate candy is the packaged, processed, sweetened, sophisticated, densified, and degraded offspring of Cacao. The Cacao tree itself is a fragile shade-dweller, dependent on the protection of other trees, susceptible to disease, and—from the human point of view—very demanding of its cultivators. That the tree is pollinated by bloodsuckers and insects almost invisible to the human eye seems appropriate, given that Cacao has a long association with blood and unseen powers, from hearts cut out in sacrifice in offerings to the gods, to sugar-moulded Valentine's Day confections for propitiating potential lovers—associations discussed in more detail in Section III of this book.

In present-day Central America, the living tradition of *atoles* made with Cacao preserves many ancient methodologies and ingredients, such as the construction of foams (e.g., *popo*, *bu'pu*, *chaw popox*) or aerated fat "toppers" (*tejate*), the use of native floral spices and flavourings (e.g., magnolia, ear flower, funeral tree), or additionally fermented ingredients (e.g., *cacao blanco*, vanilla, soured maize). There's evidence from historical accounts that ancient Cacao-based beverages were equally variable in their construction. Botanical additives could enhance foam, flavour, and psychotropic or medicinal effects; Cacao itself was valued as a preserver and promoter of good health, and its many additives enhanced or modified its virtues, and these health-enhancing properties are being rediscovered today. In Mesoamerica and post-conquest Europe, Cacao had high value as a drug, in both senses—for pleasure and medicine. And it's the latter of these identities to which we shall now turn in the next chapter, to take a closer look at Cacao as the high-status Mesoamerican elixir, the wonder-drug from distant lands in post-Columbian Europe, and a useful item in any contemporary Latin American "kitchen pharmacy".

PART II

MEDICINAL CHOCOLATE

CHAPTER THREE

The chocolate apothecary

"Preserving health entire, purging by Expectorations, and especially by the sweat-vents of the body, preventing unnatural fumes ascending to the head ... driving from the centre to the circumference, or external parts of the body, all that is obnoxious, or may turn to putrefaction [...] Exceeding nourishing to all such as require a speedy refreshment after travel, hard labour, or violent exercise, exhilarating and corroborating all parts and faculties of the body [...] and all aged people may safely take it, especially in the heat of Summer, when the skin and pores are relaxed by a great expense of Spirits, causing a faintness [...] And certain it is, that a man may live longer with it, than with any kinde of Wine whatsoever."

(Hughes, *The American Physitian [...] a discourse on the Cocoa-nut-tree*, 1672)

"Mental persuasion or willpower works for the perfectly rational, but for those of us who are imperfectly rational: Chocolate."

(from "Curing Irrationality with Chocolate Addiction" by Catherine S. Elliott, in Szogyi, 1997; © Hofstra University, New York)

Cacao and its botanical admixtures have a long history of medicinal use, and the vast majority of that history—a few thousand years of it—occurred before the development of biomedical science. The evidence-based-medicine approach is very helpful, assisting us to discriminate what works pharmacologically from what doesn't, and to determine precisely why: for example, citrus juice cures scurvy and vinegar doesn't because scurvy is caused by vitamin C (ascorbic acid) deficiency, and citrus fruits contain ascorbic acid and vinegar doesn't. Powerful antibiotics help tuberculosis but bleeding (exsanguination) doesn't, because TB is caused by a bacterial infection. The enormous practical use of the scientific method and its demonstrable effectiveness, producing rapidly acting drugs and procedures, has ensured its success. But there is the danger of "throwing the baby out with the bathwater"; if not thoroughly tested and examined over time, older and more complex cures, being less immediate, and often lacking a clear mechanism of action (which isn't to say they don't have one), may be passed over or rejected wholesale by the medical establishment. This has resulted in the transformation of many plant-based and traditional medicines into attenuated, novelty weight loss or skin-clearing pills and pre-packaged products of dubious value, following their relegation to the shelves of "health food stores" in richer countries—even though much of the world's popu-lation is still heavily reliant on medicinal plants for primary health care.[304]

Human nature predisposes us to seek certainty, and then, illogically, to reject all that we are uncertain about. We seek to define who we are by what we believe, and then set ourselves against those who see the world differently. The same innately clannish tendencies give rise to team spirit, national pride, and patriotism—which are all fine and healthy, in due measure—but can lead to xenophobia, imperialism, and even genocide if the swelling isn't treated in time. This may seem bizarrely irrelevant to a discussion about the medicinal uses and formu-lations of Cacao, but a lot of the plants used as spices with Cacao were replaced by Old World imports (primarily cinnamon) because the alien flora of Mesoamerica were less familiar to Europeans than the Old World spices. Even after the New World flora were medically classi-fied, history has edited out many of the native spice plants for no better reasons than conser-vatism and happenstance. We tend to make our collective ideological or intellectual positions highly defined—"black and white"—for the sake of making decisions, which is pragmatic: one can't act decisively when feeling uncertain. But these positions usually become ossified into dogma. In matters of ideology, it's said that "the masses are asses", because group preju-dices cause us to make unwise decisions—but it's also the case that the masses are made up of many individual asses: our individual prejudices are based on conditioning and reinforced by biological drives to belong (which will be discussed in Chapters 5 and 7), and it's these persuasive undercurrents that may cause us to "go with the flow", out to sea or over a cliff. Not everyone who lived in Nazi Germany and failed to shelter their Jewish neighbours was a monster; most people were just not resisting the prevailing cultural narrative, turning a blind eye or caught up in their own lives. We often make Pinocchio's choice, and remain on pleasure island, following the herd, sometimes until it's too late, and everybody becomes a donkey in a cage.

A simple and very benign example of our craving for certainty in dogma is the adoption of the arbitrary "five-a-day" fruit and veg consumption guideline—more vitamins, more fibre, etc. This is a common-sense dietary measure for nations increasingly dependent on highly processed, nutritionally abominable fast foods, and is therefore a Good Thing. Yet traditional medicine sys-tems the world over classify most fruits and raw vegetables as very Cooling, and less suitable for people with Cold constitutions—weak digestion, low vitality. The seventeenth-century apoth-ecary Nicholas Culpeper termed fruits and vegetables "bulky foods of little nourishment"[305]—what we would now describe as "low calorie" and "low protein". Most fruits were classified as Phlegmatic food, being Cold and Moist in quality, more suitable for Hot types, warmer weather, and people with Hot—Choleric or Sanguine—constitutions, rather than Colder constitutions or climates. Recent research on the obesity-promoting and potentially liver-damaging effects of high added sugar diets[306] provides some scientific corroboration for this ancient medical model. Whole fruit doesn't appear to be a problem, but fruit juice, concentrate, or isolated sucrose or fructose may cause long-term problems, so the adage "an apple a day keeps the doctor away" still holds, but "apple juice every day keeps the doctor well paid" might also be true. High intakes of free sugars appear to increase obesity and non-alcoholic fatty liver disease,[307] so it shouldn't surprise us that in traditional European medicine, excess fat often signified a Cold,

Phlegmatic constitution. Importing radical "detox" notions involving juice fasting or fruitarian diets may not be appropriate for winter in cold or damp climates; and Phlegmatic types (pale, put weight on easily, weak digestion, slow metabolism, low energy levels) may be perplexed by the failure of their "healthy" fruit-based "juice cleanse".

None of which is to say that fruit is bad—it clearly isn't, because fruits contain an array of compounds with excellent preventive value for many of the biggest killers of the twenty-first century, such as diabetes, heart disease, and some cancers—to say nothing of their vitamin C content preventing scurvy, one of history's great scourges. This is just an illustration of the fact that reality is complex, and we shouldn't be too quick to dismiss or cherry-pick the advice of traditional, pre-scientific systems, as their holistic perspective can be a useful counterpart to contemporary science's analytical brilliance. Likewise (to digress a little longer, but not pointlessly), mainstream medicine is heavily weighted towards diagnosis and treatment of acute disease and providing symptomatic relief, rather than health maintenance or disease prevention. In the contemporary medical model, treatment and prevention alike often involve expensive and lucrative pharmaceuticals. Isolated or synthesised drugs are powerful and life-saving in the short to medium term, but to dismiss empirical mixtures of whole plants and foods as useful medicines as some self-proclaimed avatars of "rational scientific thought" do is foolish. It contradicts behavioural and biological evolution, and the complex living webs of chemical interactions on which life depends.

The argument most frequently used to bolster our growing dependence on single, powerful drugs (or isolated hormones, enzymes, antibodies, genes, whatever) is that their effects are more "predictable" because, unlike whole plants or foods, they are only one chemical substance (or process, or unit), affecting one specific thing, administered in a measured and controlled dose or manner. In short, mainstream medicine, like mainstream science, has chosen a linear, mechanistic model over a non-linear, holistic one. To a great extent, the aim of achieving greater control over disease by refining drugs and reducing their pharmacological complexity is derived from ideology, not experience; while this model has produced many notable successes, its failures—especially in terms of degenerative and age-related diseases such as heart disease, cancer, and diabetes, once relatively rare, and now tragically common—are often excused as side effects of lower infant mortality and an aging population. This may be partially true, but we know that insulin resistance, high cholesterol, high blood pressure, and weight gain are strongly linked to dietary and lifestyle factors, and these factors substantially increase the incidence of degenerative and age-related diseases.[308] But unhelpfully dismissive attitudes towards traditional and holistic medical models in the medical establishment are beginning to change, with more research into medieval treatments[309] (inspired by bacterial resistance to antibiotics) and the appearance of functional medicine and psycho-neuro-immunology, which study complex interactions in biological systems in order to prevent and treat diseases on multiple levels. But these disciplines are still in their infancy, and the prevailing ideology will take time to adapt.

There have very been few clinical trials comparing the efficacy of long-term traditional herbal treatments to their pharmaceutical equivalents. A typical revisionist claim, usually parroted without substantiation, is that prior to the twentieth century there were no effective treatments for bacterial infections. None? The research referenced above has already revealed that to be inaccurate; it's much more likely that knowledge was simply more localised and less well disseminated in the past, so that one herbalist's effective treatment for pleurisy (or whatever) was unknown in the next village. This situation holds true today in many poorer countries—the effective remedy known to *this* village healer may be unknown and unused in *that* village only a few miles away. William Withering's discovery of digitalis from foxglove (*Digitalis purpuraea*)— now used to treat chronic heart failure—is a classic example of this "niche knowledge" issue: Withering deduced that *Digitalis* was the most active component of a poly-herbal remedy for dropsy (swollen ankles); the formula was non-standard, passed on through several generations of the family, and unknown elsewhere.[310]

It's true that serious bacterial infections are very challenging to treat without recourse to antibiotics, but many of the great epidemics in history such as plague or cholera were associated with pre-Germ Theory standards of hygiene, a lack of adequate sanitation in urban centres, and perhaps low disease resistance in the general populace owing to poor diet and squalid living conditions, in addition to great variation in access to effective medical care. But it's untrue that our ancestors were all filthy and ignorant; the most prestigious medieval medical schools taught the importance of hand-washing and sanitation,[311] and even a cursory study of the natural pharmacopoeia (through reading old herbals and accounts of treatments) reveals thousands of antimicrobial and immune-modulating plants, many with long and well-documented histories of medicinal use. One example among many is holy thistle (*Cnicus benedictus*), which is cited in Parkinson's compendious sixteenth-centurycentury herbal, *Theatrum Botanicum*, as a treatment for plague, boils, "itch", and the "venom" of dog or animal bites (bacterial infections).[312] *Cnicus* contains several antibacterial (bacteriostatic, or "bacteria-stopping" and bactericidal, or "bacteria-killing") compounds; among this antibiotic bouquet is the bitter sesquiterpene lactone named *cnicin*, first discovered in this plant, which has a unique broad-spectrum bactericidal mechanism of action, and is accompanied by several other antimicrobial compounds.[313] When herbal treatments are tested, they often perform admirably, sometimes exceeding the performance of their "drug replacement" over time;[314] very often, however, there is far less clinical evidence available for herbs than for conventional drugs, mainly because the financial motivation for conducting expensive, time-consuming research on non-patentable medicines is lacking.

Another pervasive myth is that Galenical medicine and humoral theory, the gold standard of medical knowledge for almost two thousand years in Europe and the Middle East, was useless in practice. Hippocrates, the "father of medicine", an ancient Greek doctor whose teachings are still used as the basis of the physician's oath, and Galen, a Roman physician, were the luminaries of Classical and medieval medical theory. Their teachings emphasised proper diet, lifestyle modification, appropriate use of medicinal plants, and mild purges. While no match for a well-equipped, clean modern hospital in terms of emergency care, when such treatments were administered in relatively hygienic settings such as monasteries or the houses of the rich, they were likely to have been much safer and more effective than post-Enlightenment medicine in the early days of pharmaceutical experimentation, with the gross overuse of mercury salts and the lancet.

This gung-ho approach is often cited as exemplifying "medieval ignorance", but owed much more to early modern experimental willingness to reject strict Hippocratic and Galenic treatment ideals than over-adherence to them. Recall the Hippocratic maxims: "Let food be your medicine, and medicine be your food", and "First, do no harm".[315] Post-Enlightenment medicine, transitioning from the old Vitalist, herbal, and humoral models to the emergent Materialist, chemical, and biomedical world view, clung to the established practices of using large doses of medicines (which is often necessary when using less potent plant drugs to treat acute diseases) and older treatment methods such as purging and bleeding, which were supposed to be used sparingly and judiciously, while simultaneously adopting the new scientific approach of experimenting on the living with bold surgical and chemical interventions. Adopting without adapting: this medical chimera of old and new paradigms utilised antimonial and mercurial purges, copious and repeated bleeding irrespective of the patient's constitution or condition, and doses of chemicals in quantities as large as those used for the much weaker and less concentrated old-school herbal preparations, with disastrous and sometimes horrific consequences. These cautionary tales survive to give us the false impression that ancient medicine was all bleed, hack, or puke, with no subtlety whatsoever.

If anything, exposing human bodies and communities to high doses of isolated compounds, as we often do in medicine today, is counter to our design specification (or evolutionary adaptation requirements, if you prefer a less teleological turn of thought). The inordinate side effect profiles, vastly higher level of documented adverse reactions from isolated pharmaceutical compounds as compared to non-proprietary herbal medicines, and the development of microbial resistance to most synthetic drugs all testify for this "alternative" perspective. Of course this is playing devil's advocate—to a point. Modern medicine is lifesaving: contemporary drugs are indispensable when used knowledgably in crisis situations, to maintain life in those for whom no apparent (or currently known) natural cure exists, or to effect rapid change, though sometimes at the risk of generating longer-term problems—"robbing Peter to pay Paul", colloquially known as side effects, drug resistance, and "superbugs" such as MRSA. On the other hand, popular and indiscriminate advocacy of vitamins, food supplements, the newest "natural miracle medicine", or fad diets, usually touted in a caricatured, one-size-fits-all manner as a panacea to resolve or prevent health problems, isn't a viable alternative. The ultimate point of this introductory tangent is that oversimplification in the cause of ideology, or intellectual dogma—which partisans of both orthodox and complementary medicine, the political left and right, and religious and atheist perspectives (in fact, most humans) are guilty of—is not to our ultimate benefit. Applying things or ideas in isolation or oversimplified forms to treat or prevent chronic problems in a complex being, community, or ecosystem will ultimately cause as many problems as they solve.

So, reviewing the historical uses of Cacao and its admixtures in medicine is more than a curiosity. The virtue of recounting old formulations and applications of Cacao, and their rationale, is that we might actually learn something. Sometimes, that may be to confirm that "we do it best"; but sometimes it may be "they did it best". We should attempt to understand the theoretical mindset of the era we're examining before reviewing those uses and "claims" through a modern, biochemical lens, being aware that a great many things we believe to be certain and true today may be regarded as almost comically absurd errors in a few hundred years—a mere handful of generations. If history tells any tale, it's best described by Percy Shelley's poem "Ozymandias", where the inscription at the base of a ruined statue, a pair of colossal legs with no upper body standing in a desert, reads "My name is Ozymandias, King of Kings;/Look on my Works, ye Mighty, and despair! […] Round the decay/Of that colossal Wreck, boundless and bare/The lone and level sands stretch far away."[316] While it's impossible not to be creatures of our time, it's a good idea to remember that "assume makes an ass of u and me". We'll begin with an exploration of contemporary folk uses of *Theobroma cacao* in Central and South America, moving backwards in time through post-colonial European applications to pre-Columbian applications, finally exploring how the other native plants used in Cacao-based beverages are paired with *Theobroma cacao*, like vanilla vines winding their way up and around a shady tree trunk, growing towards the light.

Chocolate folk medicine

Theobroma cacao has many applications in contemporary Latin America and other Cacao-growing regions. All parts of the tree are used, from roots to leaves and everything in-between. The uses of the whole seed—being the principal theme of this work—include stimulant, or anti-fatigue properties; to assist weight gain; as a prophylactic for general disease prevention, and—specifically—for snakebite.[317] Cacao seeds are also used for calming or anti-anxiety effects—perhaps these could be generally described as "mood regulation"—and to improve digestion, specifically elimination of wastes via bowels and kidneys.[318] Cocoa butter, the fat extracted from the seeds, is also widely used to help heal and prevent damage to the skin. Add in the other parts of the plant, and these applications can be expanded to include treatments for urinary tract problems, menstrual disorders, diabetes, headaches, various aches and pains, stings in general, and several other medicinal functions when combined with other plants.

The stimulant effects of the seeds require no lengthy explanation—we now know that Cacao contains caffeine, and this property is common to all caffeine-containing plants. Their use as a mood regulating agent does require investigation, though—see Chapters 5 and 7 for a pharmacological exploration of the possibilities. The Nahua in Mexico still drink chocolate as an aid to weight gain in wasting diseases, and as a supportive item of diet in Hot ailments such as fevers; they also use Cacao seeds as the smaller part of a prescription comprised mostly of *olli*,[319] roasted Panama rubber tree (*Castilla elastica*) gum, used to treat dysentery.[320] Cacao's role in the latter formula may be partly as a flavouring agent, but Cacao seeds frequently appear in folk treatments for digestive issues, suggesting it brings some medicinal assets of its own to the table. Cacao is generally perceived as a Cooling agent in Central America, beneficial in hot weather and when feeling overheated, hence its use as a tonic (often combined with other, more specific plants) in feverish ailments.

The use of Cacao in envenomation—the seeds against snakebite, in particular—perhaps also reflects its Cooling nature, as reactions to snakebite may include fever, fits, and local inflammation. The "anti-venom" idea is a consistent theme in Central America, although the cultural memory of this usage appears to be waning. In post-conquest Nicaragua, it was thought that drinking chocolate in the morning would provide some immunity from the ill effects of snake-bite in the afternoon[321]—this hypothesis will be examined in Chapter 4. Other twentieth-century uses of Cacao seeds and chocolate from the Dominican Republic include anti-anaemic proper-ties, to improve kidney function, and to "ease the brain when overexerted".[322] In present-day Oaxaca in Mexico, drinking chocolate is thought to help relieve symptoms of bronchitis, and even afford some protection from wasp, bee, and scorpion stings.[323] The use of Cacao or choco-late for lung ailments is controversial in some quarters, though: herbalist and teacher Mario Euan from Merida in Mexico's Yucatan peninsula described how Cacao's Cooling nature makes it inadvisable in coughs, as it may prevent phlegm from being "spat out" (expectorated, or coughed up).[324] But there's some scientific rationale for all of these uses, including for lung ail-ments, which will also be discussed in the following chapters.

Another application of Cacao seeds, recounted separately by two Guatemalan women, one of whom is a midwife of over twenty-five years' experience, is to encourage lactation in breastfeed-ing mothers, either taken as drinking chocolate or consumed in the form of an *atole* made with maize and Cacao for at least two months to increase the milk supply.[325] An additional benefit of chocolate here, whether for new mums or not, is for "wasting" or malnutrition, and drinking it is seen to "protect" a woman when "the body is wasting, [it] has nothing, no food"[326]—the consumption of Cacao as a beverage is reputed to prevent drastic weight loss. This is a very practical consideration in some parts of Guatemala, where inadequate nutrition is a real issue for many people, and becomes especially problematic when breastfeeding, as malnutrition can stop breast milk production. Because Cacao and maize are both dried products, they can be stored for some time, and may therefore be available when fresh produce or meat is not. In the Mexican state of Morelos, drinking chocolate is also used on its own as a parturient—that is, to help a mother give birth—which makes sense, as a stimulant with some anti-anxiety and pain-relieving properties[327] could be quite useful!

For most gynaecological applications, Cacao is combined with other medicinal plants, some indigenous to the Americas, and some of Mediterranean or Middle Eastern provenance—many of which, after five centuries of cultural ferment, have been naturalised and fully incorporated into the Central American pharmacopoeia. While chocolate on its own may help a woman through labour, the addition of rue (*Ruta chalapensis*) creates a more active, contraction-enhancing brew to accelerate the birth; basil (*Ocimum basilicum*) and feverfew (*Tanacetum parthenium*)—all three are Old World plants—may also be added to enhance the effect. For a really potent accelerant, drinking chocolate is made with an infusion of the native herb known as zapoatle (*Montanoa tomentosa*) and a little cinnamon, or, alternatively, the chocolate may be spiked with *tlatlascametl* (*Montanoa frutescens*) and allspice (*Pimienta dioica*): these concoctions allegedly induce such rapid contractions that "no injection is required".[328] Intriguingly, chocolate is also infused with rue to *prevent* abortion, administered as a one-off dose to stop premature contractions, unless the bleeding is very heavy, in which case stronger medicine is required. But high doses of rue have been used as an abortifacient—a remedy to *cause* abortion—in both the Old and New Worlds, and in fact chocolate made with rue, lemon juice, and cinnamon is a remedy to induce contrac-tions and abort a foetus.[329] So the effects of the chocolate/rue combination appear to be very context-dependent!

Other chocolate-based remedies to assist lactation include an *atole* made with Cacao, maize, oats, and peanuts—a slightly "beefed up" version of standard *pinole*, in other words; but, rather more intriguingly, the froth from chocolate made with an infusion of rue is to be regularly applied to the shoulders as well. So the idea for the internal use of rue'd-up chocolate seems to be that the chocolate itself is used as a general tonic and restorative—as well as a flavour-disguiser and vehicle for more bitter herbs—while rue, being a significantly Warming herb, can give a little extra Heat to a womb which is too Cold to hold on to a baby (as cramps were seen as a Cold symptom), but could also be used to give more Heat to a womb which needs the energy to keep contracting, or even to over-Heat a perfectly well-functioning womb, and induce premature labour, or abortion! The reasoning behind the external application of rue-chocolate foam is a little more mysterious, but as Cacao is generally associated with female fertility, and rue is perceived as a circulation-enhancing remedy with a reputation as a "holy" herb, the rationale for the prescription could be magical and symbolic, or empirical, or some combination of the two.

In Cuba, raw *forastero* Cacao beans are mashed into alcohol or gasoline together with chilli and ginger—two notably Hot plants—and applied to arthritic joints.[330] This is the only recorded instance of Cacao being used to treat arthritis, so the seeds may be present to help buffer or activate the other ingredients in this fiery liniment. The use of ethanol or petrol as a vehicle is understandable from the perspective of herbal pharmacy, as these solvents would extract many of the fat-soluble compounds with pain-relieving and anti-inflammatory properties in chillies and ginger, while drawing out much of the water (and, therefore, all of the water-soluble compounds) from the fresh plant material too. They would also dissolve the high quantity of fat in the Cacao seeds (see next chapter), which may protect the skin from the worst damage caused by applying neat ethanol or gasoline. But even the harshness of petrol or ethanol themselves could be useful in arthritis, creating what's called "counter-irritation"—artificially induced superficial tissue inflammation which may help to alleviate deeper pain in the joints, as in the rather robust ancient European prescription to relieve arthritic pain by whipping inflamed joints with fresh nettles. But the use of Cooling purple *forastero* beans in this prescription is interesting; perhaps the high antioxidant polyphenol content of the seeds may add anti-inflammatory properties of their own, or perhaps they are added to balance the extremely Heating nature of the other ingredients.

Cocoa butter is used both internally and externally. In San Antonio Suchitequepez, western Guatemala, it's used in the treatment of stomach "infections" or the folk disease called *empacho*, characterised by nausea, diarrhoea, or vomiting. After a two-day water fast, three tablespoons of liquid cocoa butter are administered with manna tablets (made from the desiccated sap of the manna ash, *Fraxinus ornus*, which contains the laxative sugar named mannitol) and half a cupful of olive oil, to promote a full bowel movement; a third of this dosage is used to treat children.[331] This quantity of liquid fat taken on a completely empty stomach in conjunction with a mild laxative (manna) would certainly stimulate digestion and cause the bowels to empty, which—following a fast to allow any gut trouble to subside, by giving the body an opportunity to "clean house"—may well prove effective at clearing up temporary gut disturbances. Small quantities of liquid cocoa butter are also taken as a soothing cough medicine. Cocoa butter may be massaged into the scalp as a kind of "hair gel", and is recommended as a good remedy for treating smelly hair.[332]

Another important use of cocoa butter is as a massage oil, specifically in the hands of a skilled midwife, to turn a baby: when a baby is in breach position, with its feet rather than its head pointing towards the exit, a traditional midwife can diagnose the problem by manual palpation. Once the baby's position has been determined, she greases the woman's belly with cocoa butter and uses deep abdominal manipulation to turn the baby around[333]—an impressive procedure, demonstrating skills unknown to conventional medicine. These skills are passed down through generations of midwives in Latin America and must be taught directly—so don't try this at home! For all these uses, the cocoa butter must be in liquid form—and, given that it only stays liquid at temperatures above 25°C, this is only practicable at tropical latitudes.

Some *curanderos* (healers) use *Theobroma cacao* leaves externally, and for a wide variety of problems. *Curandero* Don Antonio Xoc' of Ya'al Pemech, Alta Verapaz, recommends bathing children who "cry too much, and begin to lose their hair" in water infused with Cacao leaves.[334] *Curandero* Santiago A'echis of Lanquin, Peten, makes a plaster from ten fresh leaves to be applied to the head every evening to treat chronic headaches, and prescribes a bath made from an infusion of dried leaves to cure dogs of mangy skin problems.[335] More generally, the fresh leaves may be pulped and applied to cuts and abrasions in Central and South America, as antiseptic remedies and to stop minor bleeding.[336] Internal uses of Cacao leaves include a water infusion (what we call a "tea"), taken as a "heart tonic" and diuretic in Colombia, and the tisane is given to "listless" children in Cuna, Panama.[337] Unsweetened Cacao leaf tea is also taken as a remedy for type 2 (adult onset) diabetes in Guatemala.[338]

Señor A'echis also recommends a decoction of Cacao leaves in a much lower dose of one cup for three successive days to treat "stomach pain" and loss of appetite.[339] (A "decoction" is apothecary-speak for "boiled in water", usually for a few minutes or a specified amount of time.) Likewise, Don Xoc' uses Cacao leaves for digestive issues, recommending a cold water infusion made from "a handful" of fresh young Cacao leaf tips, bruised and squeezed so that their juice is expressed into the liquid, then taken with the juice of a whole lemon against persistent "heartburn" (reflux)—although this recipe is used for digestive issues accompanied by heart pain, so it's possible that it may also be for treating angina: heartburn and actual heart pain can be surprisingly hard to tell apart, as emergency room medical staff will attest. Don Xoc's regimen requires that two glasses of this lemon-fresh infusion be taken twice daily, for three days, and repeated if necessary.[340] Meanwhile *Curandero* Diego of San Antonio Suchitequepez has completely different uses for Cacao: he recommends a decoction made with five Cacao leaves boiled in half a litre of water for ten minutes, to be divided into three doses, drunk once every six hours, to reduce heavy menstrual flow and period pain. He also favours a very specific prescription for treating "weak vision", made by harvesting only the third pair of leaves on three branches, counting backwards from the growing tips—three being a number with magical significance. This gives a total of six leaves, to be sun-dried for two days, pulverised, and boiled in a litre of water, which is divided into several doses, with eight hours between doses (approximately twice a day).[341]

Curandero Diego also uses Cacao flowers to treat urinary tract infections such as cystitis, especially when such problems are chronic and resistant to other forms of treatment. Once again, the number of flowers used was ritually specific: eighteen fresh white Cacao flowers were to be infused in twelve ounces (355ml) hot water for six minutes—so the symbolism of this formula relates to the number six (eighteen flowers, twelve ounces, six minutes). The infusion is made in the manner of a *tisane*, appropriate to delicate flowers: they aren't decocted—boiling water is poured onto them and they are allowed to steep.[342] Other *curanderos* in Latin America employ Cacao flower infusion to treat apathy and timidity—what we may recognise as mild depression and anxiety—as well as applying them externally to small cuts or scratches on the feet, in the same way that the leaves are used to remedy minor abrasions on other parts of the body.[343] The Kuna in Panama have a very specific external use for Cacao flowers, using them to treat "screw-worm of the eye",[344] though how this is done is left to the imagination in the source text. Diego's use to treat urinary tract infection is the most interesting from a pharmacological perspective, as it implies the presence of hitherto-unidentified anti-microbial or immune-modulating properties in the flowers. If caffeine is found to be present in the flowers, as it is in other parts of the plant, then the uses for screw-worm, apathy, and timidity may well be partially explained by low doses of this compound, because caffeine acts as a stimulant in humans, but is toxic to most insects.

Cacao fruit pulp finds more general use as a plantation snack—a little reward for the hard labour of harvesting Cacao beans—and as an ingredient in *refrescos*, cold drinks which are the Latin American equivalent of fruit cordials. *Refrescos* are usually made with fruit pulp mixed into cold water, often with added sugar. These soft drinks are available on almost every roadside in Central America, although *refrescos* made with Cacao fruit are uncommon. If allowed to stand for a little longer, Cacao-fruit *refrescos* may also be fermented to make vinegars or alcoholic beverages,[345] which involves a similar process—in the first case, free circulation of air is permitted, but for the second, an airlock or a tight lid is required. In some regions the fruit pulp is decocted and taken as a parturient[346]—an aid to giving birth—possibly with a similar rationale to Cacao seeds or chocolate, to prevent exhaustion. In Cuba, Cacao shells are boiled with indigo dye, and the decoction is applied to treat body lice[347]—again, possibly with a similar pharmacological explanation to the use of Cacao flowers to treat worms in the eye, where caffeine contained in the shells may weaken the parasites. In Nigerian medicine, Cacao tree root decoction is taken to treat anaemia (a decreased oxygen-carrying capacity in the blood, giving rise to fatigue, shortness of breath, and other symptoms, depending on the cause)—and, when tested, the root extract stabilised red blood cell membranes in the laboratory, which suggests that the plant may indeed be helpful in some forms of anaemia.[348] So the tree is utilised from top to bottom, but the leaves and seeds are the most medicinally used parts of the plant in modern ethnomedicine.

Galenical chocolate

When Cacao was first brought to Europe, the dominant medical model was very different from today's "molecules and mechanisms" approach. Humoral medicine was also known as Galenic medicine, after its godfather, the Roman physician and author Claudius Galen, who "wrote the book"—literally, he wrote several—laying down the theory and ground rules for the practice of medicine. Humoral medicine is named after the "humours" or fluids from which the body was believed to be made, and has much in common with other traditional medicine systems worldwide. For example, traditional Chinese medicine describes the bodily functions in terms of five elements (Wood, Metal, Fire, Earth, and Water), whereas Indian Ayurvedic medicine recognises three *dośas* or predominant types of elemental combinations (*Vata*, *Pitta*, and *Kapha*, made from Air and Ether, Air and Water, Water and Earth, respectively).

Humoral or Galenic medicine recognised only four "visible" elements, these being Earth, Air, Fire, and Water, each represented in the human body by a fluid. These fluids could be described as a group of functions: blood contained the largest quantity of the Air element, and was known as the Sanguine humour; it was Warm and Moist (like Air), and nourished the body. Melancholy or black bile had a greater concentration of Earth, and was therefore Cold and Dry, and helped retain necessary substances. Hot, Dry Choler or yellow bile incorporated a lot of Fire, which helped with digestion, appetite, and motivation; while Cool and Moist Phlegm contained a lot of Water, and its function was to lubricate the body and remove waste products. Each element corresponded to a season, a time of day, and a portion of life, too—thus infancy, springtime, and morning were likened to the warmth, motility, and moisture of Air, and the Sanguine humour; youth, summertime, and afternoon to the Heat and Dryness of Fire, or Choler; middle age, autumn, and dusk to midnight were Cold and Dry Melancholic-Earthy phases; old age, winter, and the small hours of the night were Cold, Moist, Watery, and Phlegmatic.

The system was a complex, holistic model which sought to encompass every level of experience. Physically, individual organs and functions were allotted different norms and values— for example, the brain was mostly Phlegmatic (Cool and Moist), while the heart was Hot and Dry (Choleric); memory, being retentive, was Melancholically Cold and Dry, while judgement, requiring the assimilation and balance of information, was Hot and Moist like the Sanguine humour. These classifications seem arcanely nonsensical to those trained in biomedical sciences, but, like most traditional systems, the categories were based on observation and allegory: a Hot disease or organ was one which showed signs of warmth, redness, heat, and activity, while Cold implied paleness, inactivity, or induration—thus memory, being a "fixing-in-place", was a Cold function, while fevers and inflammation were Hot symptoms.

The purpose of medicine, then, was to keep the body and its organs in order by maintaining or restoring their proper temperature and function; and, just as organs differed, so did individuals—a Melancholic person would have a much Colder and Dryer baseline temperament than his Sanguine colleague, and Coldness and Dryness may manifest both in the symptoms he may have when ill, and his personality. Thus Melancholic types may tend to weight loss, constipation, stiffness, or depression, though they may have long memories (all the better for bearing grudges), while Sanguine types—all else being equal—may tend to more robust health and equable mood, though with some tendency to weight gain and being "scatter-brained". As in Ayurvedic medicine, most people were composites—that is, a few people were pure Phlegmatic, pure Sanguine, etc., but most would have a secondary temperament such as Sanguine-Melancholic, a happy-go-lucky type with a serious or depressive streak, or a Choleric-Phlegmatic, the ambitious go-getter who secretly enjoys being a couch potato.

Note that symptoms and susceptibility—the presentation of disease, and who is most likely to get what—are the focus here, not finding the cause of disease—at least, not as we would understand it, as a specific physical agent or process. From a modern perspective, the cause or aetiology of the same disease is always the same in different people, so symptoms of that same illness will be correspondingly similar; but, as Hippocrates is alleged to have said, pre-modern cultures generally believed that "It's far more important to know what person has the disease than what disease the person has."[349] The Mexica and Maya had a similar outlook, classifying diseases into Hot and Cold symptoms and categories. There was a "fifth element" in humoral medicine, too—the "quintessence" or *pneuma*, meaning "breath"—the life force, or animating, organising principle. This, too, finds its equivalents in all cultures save our own: *chi* or *qi* in China, *prana* in Ayurveda, *mana* in Polynesia, *ch'ulel* to the Maya—an invisible vitalising force, which imparts life and purpose.

The greatest contrast between traditional medicine and post-Enlightenment materialist bio-medicine is that the traditional systems are *teleological*, whereas modern science isn't: traditional philosophies assume that things are as they are for a reason, that matter is mindful, and nature has purposes. We still talk about things that way, discussing genes and the like as if they have intentions, but the party line of science today is that nature is impersonal, and evolution is driven solely by Darwinian mechanics. But when Cacao arrived in Europe, a logical first step was to determine what its natural temperature was, how it affected the temperature of the organs, and whether it had any hidden faculties or properties—to work out how this New World drug fitted into the greater scheme. On the face of it, this may seem little different to the taxonomising of botanists, or the chemical classification of a new drug, but what sets these things apart from the ensouled philosophy of pre-modern medicine is that Cacao's place in this scheme would be taken to reveal something of its divinely ordained *purpose* regarding human existence.

But this aim wasn't so easy to accomplish: Cacao's character was controversial. As with any new substance, there were disagreements as to how it should be classified, and these issues are magnified with subjective systems such as humoralism, when the "Temperature" of a thing is determined by its apparent effects. In the days before databases, statistical analysis, and rapid knowledge transfer, arriving at a consensus based on observation could take some time. Unlike other foods and remedies with centuries of recorded human interaction, Cacao was a novelty, so European physicians were keen to stick their fingers in the chocolate pot to help them deduce its nature and applications. Following native Mesoamerican tradition, Hernández classified Cacao as Cool and somewhat Moist, declaring its usefulness to "temper heat and burning", especially in those afflicted by a "hot distemper".[350] As other European doctors also noted, according to Hernández Cacao also "fattens noticeably", a useful property in serious diseases and possibly the origin of its later usage in "consumption".

European sixteenth-century aficionados concurred that raw, unadulterated Cacao is some-what Cold, and while some physicians—particularly those who had acquired a chocolate habit—commended Cacao as a gently Cooling drug, useful in fevers and inflamed states, others averred that it could be excessively Cold, exacerbating Melancholic and Phlegmatic conditions, creating "thick humours" and even "obstructions".[351] Some physicians, such as the seventeenth-century Spanish physician and author Antonio Colmero de Ledesma, advocated the use of Cacao but nevertheless cautioned that it shouldn't be taken with cold water due to its essentially Cooling nature. Tepid chocolate was okay in Mexico, de Ledesma reasoned, due to the ambient warmth and humidity, but consuming the drug in this state could cause harm in more northern climes, unless Heat was added in the form of hot water or spice.[352] While some physicians, such as the French Dr Moreau (not the fictional one with the island) saw Cacao itself as a little too Cooling to be healthful, de Ledesma described warm, spiced chocolate as Temperate, of moderate Heat, and somewhat binding.[353]

Dr Moreau believed that prepared Cacao tablets made from cocoa liquor ground with spices were best aged for at least one month prior to consumption, allowing their Hot-Cold qualities to achieve "balance", making them easier to digest.[354] Likewise, de Ledesma reports that the best chocolate "is that which hath been made some months", and "the new doth hurt by loosening the stomach"[355]—he opines that this is because the "unctuous fat parts" aren't properly "corrected" and mingled with the Earthy, Melancholic parts in Cacao, and long storage helps this. Many foods undergo secondary chemical and physical transformation in storage, sometimes due to slow, ongoing chemical reactions, and sometimes to microbial activity; a gradual diffusing of aromatic substances into the fats, or chemical alterations during storage may be responsible for this mellowing, improving effect of a few months' aging of Cacao tablets. In Cacao's case, microbial activity is less likely, as the negligible moisture content of Cacao tablets makes them inhospitable to microbes.

Negative effects of excessive Cacao ingestion were "stopping" (constipation), over-fattening, or—bizarrely—overheating, perhaps as a result of the alleged "obstructing" effect causing a build-up of inflammatory wastes, a state known as "cacochymia", loosely translated as "crappy fluids", in the terminology of the day. Spices, being Hot, could help to expel excess heat and wastes through sweating, thereby cooling the body; one reason, perhaps, why very spicy foods are popular in hot countries (the other being, potentially, the anti-microbial properties of many spices: food "goes bad" faster in hot weather, and spices may help protect against food poisoning to some extent). One interesting side effect of Cacao's classification as a Cold substance was the recommendation that women should drink less of it, because women were "Wetter"— Water being the Cold and Moist element symbolically associated with fertility, "ripening", and pregnancy—therefore making women Colder than men,[356] and less suited to Cooling foods and medicines. One way of making Cacao more healthful for Colder types—or the entire female sex—was to grind the toasted seeds with Warming spices, to make the drink with hot water, and to add sugar, which was thought to be slightly Warm and Moist: in other words, to make it into drinking chocolate.

Many of de Ledesma's contemporaries likewise regarded spiced hot chocolate as inclining towards Heating and Drying properties. The American physician Dr Hughes described Cacao fruit pulp as Phlegmatic—a characteristic shared by most watery, sweet fruits—but he noted chocolate's ability to "concoct excess Phlegm",[357] meaning it helps digest and process excess waste products, and maintain good health, usually a property of more "warming" drugs. In 1687 Dr de Blegny wrote that chocolate could "heat a cold stomach" but also refresh people who were overheated.[358] These seventeenth- and eighteenth-century scholarly debates about Cacao's humoral nature may have been a consequence of all the different formulations of chocolate which were proliferating in Europe at the time. Separating the Temperature of Cacao itself from the interference created by other ingredients in chocolate would be a challenge, even if the humoral system weren't a non-standardised, largely subjective art. Whatever its Temperature, a moderate intake of chocolate was thought to be tonifying, supporting the "vital spirits"—life energy, or vitality—and, unusually for something made from a Cold plant, these liquid preparations of Cacao helped to expel excess Melancholy, a surfeit of which could cause depression, stiffness, anorexia, or constipation.[359]

Although unprocessed Cacao was thought to be predominantly Cold and Dry (Melancholic) or Cold and Moist (Phlegmatic), it had other qualities, too: the dominant Cold, Dry, Earthy part was counterbalanced by an oily, Warm and Moist part, and a very Hot and Dry component.[360] The Melancholy humour was associated with sourness, Sanguine with sweet or fatty tastes, and Choleric with bitterness, so the Cold and Dry part may be analogous to what we now recognise as the astringent polyphenols; the fat in the seeds may be the Warm and Moist part, and the stimulating alkaloids, including caffeine, comprise the bitter-tasting Hot and Dry elements (the chemical composition of the seeds will be fully discussed in Chapter 4). The Spanish physician Dr Juan de Cardenas reckoned Choleric elements in Cacao to be responsible for its "warm and penetrating" effects, which give rise to perspiration and "expulsion of excrement", or even headaches at high doses. As we might have guessed, he identified its Sanguine or airy parts with Cocoa butter, and quite reasonably deduced that this was responsible for Cacao's fattening properties. Like de Ledesma, de Cardenas reckoned that the fatty parts also had "opening" properties which helped to offset the obstructive coldness of the seeds,[361] but he too argued that excessive intake of Cacao could be harmful through its Earthy, Melancholic components—not by producing obstruction, but by causing anxiety with "faltering of the heart, as if the soul of the person who has eaten it, has left him".[362] In fact it may be the bitter alkaloids—the caffeine, in particular—which are responsible for this effect, rather than the sour and astringent polyphenols; so de Cardenas should perhaps have blamed Choler, not Melancholy, for these hazards of chocoholism.

Dr de Cardenas recommended that chocolate be taken in the morning, before breakfast, as its gentle warmth "helps to spend all that phlegm which has remained in the stomach from … dinner and supper";[363] and he suggests a second serving at five or six p.m. The fitness of this depends on caffeine sensitivity, as for some people this later use of chocolate will guarantee insomnia. Dr Stubbe similarly recommended that chocolate be taken for breakfast, or at four or five o'clock in the morning, suggesting that it would only "prejudice … sleep" if taken "late at night, and not so early, as is here recommended".[364] De Cardenas was also vehemently opposed to the use of raw Cacao, which would cause constipation, retention of urine, poor digestion, shortness of breath, fatigue, menstrual problems, and other issues due to its "obstructing" nature—none of which there is any evidence for, but it was firmly believed at the time. So various additives were used for modifying chocolate to suit different constitutions and seasons, and the reasoning sometimes appears to be inconsistent; like de Ledesma, the early American physician Dr Hughes cautions that spiced chocolate should be avoided in very cold weather as it may cause some "overheating" and exhaustion.

Other physicians recommended that chocolate, as a gently Heating remedy, be taken in winter and old age[365]—the Phlegmatic season and phase of life—so Hughes's proscription of spicy chocolate in winter seems illogical. But in humoral medicine it was considered that the body adapted to the seasons: in summer, the "internal fire" of digestion was weak, but in winter, it grew strong, increasing the appetite, which indeed parallels our understanding of annual fluctuation in thyroid hormone levels: thyroid hormones stimulate metabolism, and levels rise a little in winter.[366] So the recommendation to consume less Heating stimulants in cold weather may not be completely unsound—the traditional advice was to consume warm, moist foods in winter, and to exercise sufficiently to assist digestion and general health, but over-consumption of Heating foods (such as fatty cheese, wine, and spices), too much exercise, and overuse of stimulants were not recommended, as winter was a season for conserving resources, and preserving one's internal Heat. Over-consumption of Heating foods could cause sweating and heat loss, leading to a net Cooling effect, which was unwise—especially in English winters in the days before central heating. Hughes's conclusion is based on this logic, and therefore applies only to very Heating forms of chocolate, made with lots of spices.

Dr Hughes also commends chocolate for its ability to prevent "unnatural fumes ascending to the head … causing a pleasant sleep and rest",[367] referring to its ability to allay Melancholy. When the spleen was overheated, Melancholic "fumes" rose, like smoke, to disturb the brain; chocolate could help to vent those fumes. One nineteenth-century doctor also commended chocolate for the treatment of "spasmodic afflictions", claiming that it calmed the nerves and would help decrease "violent movements".[368] While this isn't a property Cacao is known to have, there is some budding research on the effect of Cacao on degenerative conditions of the nervous system such as Parkinson's disease and Alzheimer's, which will be described in the following chapters. Chocolate was also used as a treatment for scurvy in the days before vitamin C was discovered.[369] While it couldn't have cured the disease, it would certainly have helped symptoms a bit: vitamin C deficiency stops collagen repair and causes connective tissue destruction, and Cacao seeds do contain minimal amounts of vitamin C, which would be of some help, but not enough to prevent or treat deficiency. The antioxidant compounds in Cacao may also have retarded the breakdown of collagen, and some of the compounds in chocolate, the flavanols and procyanidins, have been shown to increase the level of vitamin C in the blood,[370] although any treatment with chocolate in the absence of additional dietary vitamin C would only have slowed down deterioration.

Chocolate's medical uses extended to kidney disorders, including urinary "gravel" (tiny stones or grit in the urine),[371] sunstroke, and sores[372]—for all of which there is at least some pharmacological justification. As we shall see in Chapter 4, the polyphenols in Cacao have antimicrobial action, so the use of Cacao as an external wound-wash may be justified as a means of preventing infection. Cacao rapidly improves circulation when taken internally, so it may plausibly be useful for recovery from sunstroke and accelerating wound healing for that reason; its circulation-enhancing properties extend to protecting the tiny blood vessels in the kidneys, and dark chocolate is still recommended as part of a dietary protocol for reversing declining kidney function.[373] The caffeine in chocolate also has a diuretic effect—it increases urination—so greater expulsion of "gravel" is possible.

Just as *cacahuatl* was consumed after meals by the Mexica, de Ledesma recommends it as "an excellent help to digestion" which "cleanseth the teeth and sweeteneth the breath",[374] and chocolate similarly developed a reputation as a *digestif* in France; Dr Dufour commended chocolate made with water to treat diarrhoea and flatulence.[375] Conversely, de Cardenas and other Spanish doctors recommended it be taken on an empty stomach, to avoid "overloading" digestion, and to maximise its stimulating or tonic effects. The pragmatic solution to this question proposed by one French physician was that chocolate be drunk fasting if required for work, or taken after food to assist digestion.[376] In the seventeenth century Dr de Blegny advised that chocolate should not be used in the presence of "corrupt humours … in the stomach which diminish the appetite",[377] meaning that poor digestion was a contraindication for its use, and another French physician called Dr Duncan cautioned that chocolate can damage "nerves lining the stomach", impair digestion by destroying the lining of the intestines, and increase the risk of dysentery and colic! So the effect of chocolate on digestion is one area where physicians were truly divided—and with good reason, as Cacao's influence on the digestive system is complex and still not fully understood. While there's no evidence that chocolate increases the risk of dysentery, both Duncan and Dufour may be partly correct: Cacao appears to benefit the microbiome and inhibit the growth of "bad bacteria" which can cause diarrhoea, while—paradoxically—it may simultaneously thin the lining of the gut and lower its immune defences, as we shall see in Chapters 4 and 7.

Dr Hughes advised that one should rest for a while immediately after taking chocolate, "because it is apt to open the pores, and thereby it causeth the greater expense of Spirits … and consequently nourishes the less".[378] The explanatory pores and Spirits may be alien to us, but Dr Hughes's suggestion that a brief rest after taking chocolate will improve its effects is good advice. Cacao's high fat content means it may sit in the stomach a little longer than less fatty foods, so a short period of relaxation will help digestion; de Blegny's caution here is correct, in that the high fat content of chocolate makes it a poor choice with an unsettled stomach. Another retrospective reason for heeding Dr Hughes's advice is the "caffeine nap" effect—caffeine (the primary stimulant compound in Cacao) takes about thirty minutes to take effect after consuming it, so having a short nap after drinking chocolate will give the drug time to work, combining the restorative effect of stimulant and siesta. Caffeine also increases digestive secretions, so the *digestif* reputation of chocolate as an aid to digestion—at least in a healthy digestive system—is another accurate observation.

In the days before caffeine's existence was known, the French physician Dr Duncan classified tea, chocolate, and coffee as healthful in moderation and harmful in excess, noting that over-consumption of any one of these drugs made the blood too Hot, "sharp", and "thin". He argues, in agreement with many other physicians of his time, that plain chocolate was bad for Hot-natured Sanguine and Choleric people, though not as bad as coffee. His implication is that excessive consumption of chocolate—even without spices—could become "overheating", just as de Ledesma suggested, causing restlessness, sweating, anxiety, palpitations, and other symptoms which we would now recognise as side effects of high caffeine intake. In other words, the Choleric component of Cacao could exceed the Melancholic parts of the drug when it was consumed in quantity—or, put another way, high caffeine intake causes problems. Contemporary medical practitioners would also advise that anxious, stressed, busy, or very active people consume less caffeine: the language and explanations may differ, but the recommendation is the same.

Because of its fattening properties, Dr de Caylus declared that overweight and sedentary people, or—as he tactfully put it—persons "accustomed to good food" should avoid chocolate. Other physicians advised caution with chocolate for those troubled with "hot intestines" (doesn't bear thinking about), active young folk, and "hypochondriacs". This isn't a reference to people with excessive health anxiety: it's a humoral diagnosis of hypochondriacal Melancholy, meaning a depressive or brooding state of mind accompanied by digestive trouble and pain or wind beneath the ribs, sometimes associated with weight loss. Many people diagnosed with irritable bowel syndrome today might fit these criteria, but in humoral medicine the symptoms were taken as evidence of the cold Melancholic humour accumulating in the spleen and liver.

Doctors continued to debate the finer points of Cacao's humoral identity in print for three centuries after chocolate's arrival in Europe. Dr Moreau suggested that maize shouldn't be mixed with Cacao, because of maize's "windy" and Melancholic nature[379]—the result would be to over-Cool the stomach and the body, upsetting digestion and producing undesirable wastes. But Dr Dufour had quite the opposite opinion, contesting that Cacao's admixture with maize in the form of warm gruels was very healthful, "softening the chest", helping fevers and intestinal transit, and easily digested. Given Cacao's native combination with maize in innumerable *atoles*, Dr Dufour's opinion seems to be nearer the mark. De Ledesma commended native Mesoamerican chilli above the more fashionable black pepper for the purpose of Warming chocolate, and proposed a solution to the maize good/maize bad conundrum: he recommended nixtamalized, or lime-treated maize, as a healthful admixture, and informs us that only uncooked maize husks or untreated maize—like polenta, or corn flour—cause Melancholy.[380] As we saw in Chapter 1, there may be more than a grain of truth (pun intended) here, as nixtamalized maize yields niacin or vitamin B3, while untreated maize doesn't, and one of the many symptoms of niacin deficiency is depression. Most native *atoles* are made with nixtamalized maize, so they pass de Ledesma's corn test—and help to prevent pellagra, the disease caused by niacin deficiency. But *atoles* are decidedly Mesoamerican collations; Europeans, for the most part, preferred to adapt their chocolate with a variety of more familiar ingredients.

Elixirs of chocolate

Early European accounts of Cacao's medicinal value and high status in Mesoamerica fuelled the development and consumption of chocolate drinks by the elite and privileged in the Old World. Gonzalo Fernández de Oviedo y Valdés, King Philip II's official chronicler in New Spain, recorded the native uses of Cacao to satisfy both hunger and thirst, to protect the complexion from sun damage (on which theme, more in Chapter 4), as a protection against snakebite, and—not least—as a refreshing tonic.[381] Testimonials like that could hardly fail to incite medical and popular interest.

To address the problem of chocolate's constitutional suitability, Dr Stubbe advised that Choleric or Hot types—and teenagers, who are Hotter as a group—should make their chocolate with distilled water of endive or chicory (*Chicorium intybus*), a cooling plant. If a Choleric person has a Cold liver—as evidenced by "hypochodriacal" symptoms of weight loss, poor digestion, and aching or pain under the ribs on the right-hand side—then rhubarb root (*Rheum palmatum*) water was recommended, as rhubarb Heats the liver, but nevertheless also expels excess Heat: in the terminology of the day, it was *choleretic*, meaning "bile-expelling". Dr Stubbe commended temperate, lightly spiced chocolate for active, healthy, Sanguine types, but suggested that Phlegmatic people—those who Dr de Caylus would deprive of chocolate, being prone to weight gain, coldness, sluggish digestion, and inactivity—should take it less frequently, with strong spices and very hot water, and only gradually increase the richness or concentration of the drink.

People suffering from "hypochondriacal Melancholy" were advised to make chocolate plain, with water only, strictly no chillies or strong spices excepting those of a "sweet smell" (such as vanilla or musk), no eggs or milk, and only a little sugar, so that it was neither too Hot nor too Cold. Made too Hot, with excess spice, chocolate could end up dispersing remaining Heat through sweating, and have a net Cooling effect, or stir up Melancholy fumes to disturb the brain; made too Cold, with no spice, untoasted Cacao, or cold water, it would aggravate the condition. If they were "deeply hypochondriacal" then the chocolate had to be taken without sugar, and with a little gently Warming spice such as "sandalwood, sassafras, or aniseed in powder", or a "stomachic preparation of antimony".[382] Given that sassafras contains a signifi-cant concentration of safrole, a known carcinogen, and antimony is a highly toxic heavy metal, these recommendations may be best followed in spirit, and not to the letter.

The Galenical reasoning for Stubbe's prescription is that additional, mild Warmth was required—hence the use of gentler spices, lacking the greater Heat of chilli or pepper, which could overheat the spleen and stir up "Melancholic vapours". Although sugar was Warm and Moist, and therefore hypothetically helpful, in "deep Melancholy" the Moisture it con-tained may cause "putrefaction", because excess Melancholy inhibits digestion, and Moisture caused corruption—from the observation that damp things go mouldy. This is one example of a pre-modern perception that sugar could exacerbate digestive issues or mood disturbances in some people. Antimony was recommended as a purge, to "clear out" the excess humour—toxic metals aside, not so crazy a notion as one might think, as the state of the gut has a direct bear-ing on mood: constipation is much more common in people with depressive disorders,[383] and the gut flora (the microbiome) has a complex but deep influence on mental health which we are only just beginning to understand.[384] Previous generations of physicians may have recom-mended a milder botanical laxative such as polypody root (*Polypodium vulgare*) to expel excess Melancholy, but Stubbe was writing in the seventeenth century, during the dangerous crossover period from Galenic to pharmacological medicine. Stubbe's use of antimony shows us he was as much a fashion victim as the pre-Colombian Mexica who practised human sacrifice to help the sun rise every day, or contemporary proponents of "palliative chemotherapy" in advanced and incurable cancer: he was using the best available knowledge.

Dr Pinelo suggested various amendments and formulations of chocolate for women of differ-ing temperaments. It's unclear whether he didn't describe any chocolate formulations for men because they would simply have entailed the addition of less Warming spices, or whether he was catering to his market: women, then as now, were the most avid consumers of chocolate. Sanguine women of robust build and in good health were recommended to drink chocolate *atole*, made with a little aniseed, pepper, and sugar: Warm and Moist, to match their more wholesome temperament, but not too rich, to counteract their natural tendency to put on flesh. Overweight, "sleepy" and pale Phlegmatic women were advised to use strong chocolate made with tepid water and more balanced spices such as cinnamon, pepper, musk, and *achiote*—as we will see, *achiote* or annatto was regarded as a Cold spice, whereas the other additives were Hot, so the overall effect of this chocolate formula would be very slightly Warming, and somewhat more Drying. Lean, dark, "crazy", and insomniac Melancholic women were advised to drink warm chocolate with *atole*, a little anise and musk, and no overheating spices: a gently Warm and Moist preparation, to offset their naturally depressive dispositions.[385] Hot-tempered Choleric women were advised to avoid chocolate completely, as it could be too Heating—which seems rather unfair, especially as Cacao was, by nature, deemed to be somewhat cooling, and most physicians concluded that it only became Heating when taken to excess; fortunately, Dr Stubbe had them covered with his Cooling endive-water chocolate.

For those with chronic lung ailments such as tuberculosis, milk—regarded as a Warm, Moist substance, like sugar—was recommended as an additive, although some doctors considered milk too "rich … and difficult to digest", and therefore inadvisable.[386] Twentieth-century chocophile Dr Robert commends the combination of oats (*Avena sativa*), milk, and chocolate as the most beneficial combination for enfeebled patients, helping to remedy physical debility and wasting "of women and children".[387] Dr Robert doesn't reveal why these women and children are especially sensitive to "wasting", or why men may not find similar benefit—he perhaps alludes to the seventeenth-century use of chocolate to treat the "green sickness" in women, a type of lassitude or debility which may have been iron-deficiency anaemia, anorexia nervosa, or chronic fatigue.[388] Dr Happenland, a physician to the Russian court, commended a breakfast of chocolate made with milk as a calmative for "nervous, excitable and violent" types, as well as a good tonic for the elderly, debilitated, or fatigued persons.[389]

These divergent opinions on the benefits—or otherwise—of adding milk to chocolate may be reconciled in the words of the apothecary Nicholas Culpeper, who described milk as a "windy meat … not profitable in head-aches, yet … it is an admirable remedy for inward ulcers in any part of the body … but it is very bad in diseases of the liver, spleen, the falling-sickness [epilepsy], vertigo or dizziness in the head."[390] In the Galenic system, milk was regarded as a good food for the very old and very young and a useful article of diet in Hot, Dry wasting conditions such as consumption, with weight loss and "inward ulcers" (characterised by pain with coughing, urinating, or spitting of blood), the commonest example of which was tuberculosis (TB). But milk was also hard to digest, and to be avoided in all other diseases.[391] Such nuance is important for understanding old medical texts, because on first reading the information seems contradictory—which it sometimes is, but context is crucial.

The European taste for that other exotic status symbol, sugar, is also evident in many post-colonial chocolate prescriptions. The eighteenth-century French Doctor Pierre Buc'hoz commended the addition of a bit of sugar to chocolate taken after a meal to "facilitate digestion and stop hiccups"![392] Although the medical fraternity may have been fond of a little sweetness, there was a recognition that sugar intake should not be excessive; as we have seen, some medical chocophiles such as Drs Stubbe and Hughes inveighed against the overuse of sugar and other additives in chocolate. In general, though, owing to its more "balanced" nature, bespoke chocolate was regarded as a tonic, especially beneficial for the elderly, being "strengthening, restorative … [it] helps digestion, allays the sharp humours that fall upon the Lungs: it keeps down the fumes of the wine, promotes Venery, and resists the malignity of the humours"[393] according to the eighteenth-century French physician Dr Lemery. "Keeping down the fumes of wine" seems like a caffeine-related effect, as caffeine's stimulating properties can undo some of the torpor that excess alcohol intake induces, though being dosed with it does nothing for the intoxication in other respects—you just get a livelier drunk.

Cacao's effects on the lungs have already been mentioned. Chocolate candy or—exceptionally—raw chocolate ("*chocolat cru, ou en confiture*") was commended by Dr Pinelo in the seventeenth century as helpful for those who are housebound or bedbound with chronic lung problems[394]—presumably as it was convenient to take, and required no special preparation. Dr Pinelo was ahead of his time in this regard—most of his peers subscribed to the belief that raw Cacao was harmful, and if anybody lacked the time (or servants) to prepare elaborate, expensive, and exotically spiced hot chocolate, that was just too bad. European doctors were more united in their commendation of chocolate preparations for ongoing breathing issues like TB or ingrained pulmonary problems of the sort we would now diagnose as COPD (chronic obstructive pulmonary disease, or emphysema). De Blegny recommended chocolate made with vanilla and skimmed milk taken several times a day to allay violent coughs with bloody sputum—most likely symptoms of tuberculosis—while Drs Lemery and Navier thought the oily or airy parts of Cacao helped to counter "bitter humours" and reduce catarrhs, or contained some sort of "antiseptic … essential salt".[395] Asthma, too, was said to be relieved by it.[396]

"Venery", or increased sexual appetite, is an alleged attribute of chocolate which certainly helped its popular image with everyone outside the Church, who were naturally opposed the use of "aphrodisiac" foods and drugs, but is now regarded as a myth—to be discussed further in Chapter 5. De Ledesma put it well in rhyme, suggesting that Cacao "creates new-motions of the flesh", referring both to its ability to reinvigorate the elderly and to reignite the sexual appetite. Although chocolate was thought to enhance libido, this is partly a subtext of its reputation as a tonic and geriatric medicine, a substance that could "speedily and readily refresh the bodily strength"[397] whether due to fatigue, debility, or old age—the suggestion being that Cacao and chocolate augmented the "vital spirits" or life energy and acted as a "cordial"—broadly speaking, an antidepressant—and may thus help impotence or reduced sex drive due to exhaustion or "low spirits".

Chocolate preparations were also used in gynaecology, as promoters of fertility[398] and, as is still the case today in Central American folk medicine, as parturients.[399] Then as now, chocolate may have been somewhat helpful to assist conception in the event of any nutritional deficiencies, as Cacao is a good source of several dietary minerals, most notably copper, magnesium, and iron;[400] but it has not been found to possess specific fertility-enhancing properties, despite dubious claims from some doctors that it caused pregnancies in old women, and the like. Other doctors advised that chocolate be avoided during pregnancy as "hazardous to the embryo" as it "heats and dries the womb";[401] another faction commended chocolate as being good for pregnant women, "nourishing the Embryo" and "preventing fainting Fits."[402] As with its effects on digestion, the dispute here may be justified: epidemiological and clinical research reveal that Cacao and chocolate do appear to have some benefits in pregnancy, affording some protection against dangerously high blood pressure (pre-eclampsia). Eating chocolate while pregnant does seem to affect the child, for good or ill; these findings are discussed in Chapters 4 and 7. Chocolate, being somewhat Heating, was also alleged to "provoke sweat and the menses"[403]— not an odd pairing of effects in humoral medicine, as both sweating and menstruation were seen as cleansing operations, so in apothecary terminology Cacao would be a "depurative", an agent which helps the body clean itself, thereby reducing the risk of developing other health problems.

Cacao had another specific virtue in medicine (or murder): its taste could disguise many other flavours, making it an excellent vehicle for nasty-tasting substances. Corrosive sublimate, or mercuric chloride, was the standard remedy for syphilis at the time, and highly toxic—it could cause permanent nervous system and tissue damage, and, much like cancer chemotherapy today, the effects of the treatment were often hard to distinguish from the symptoms of the disease. Also like chemotherapy, the treatment was probably effective often enough to merit its continued use—many commentators assume that it wasn't, but in fact mercuric chloride kills *Treponema pallidum*, the organism that causes syphilis, at dilutions of 1:100,000; by comparison, arsphenamine ("Salvarsan"), the first effective antibiotic used to treat syphilis (since supplanted by penicillin, which is less toxic) is only effective in concentrations up to 1:7500.[404] Corrosive sublimate is highly poisonous though, so even though mercury salt treatment may have saved or prolonged many lives, it came at great cost in terms of human suffering. One eighteenth-century French recipe calls for 420g cocoa liquor, 60g of sugar, and 800mg of corrosive sublimate, to make thirty-two Cacao tablets each containing 32mg of mercuric chloride.[405]

While it was known that chocolate alone wasn't a cure for syphilis, it was thought to be beneficial in venereal diseases. Dr de Blegny referred to chocolate's "cordial properties" which strengthen nature against poisons. Aside from its facility for disguising and carrying other drugs, this was the logic of using chocolate in anti-syphilitic medicines: its anti-venom qualities made it a useful supportive tonic, and it may have been intended to reduce the toxicity of mercury or some of the even more dubious compounds used to treat the pox. De Blegny himself formulated an anti-syphilitic chocolate with marcasite, or iron sulphide, which he claimed resolved symptoms within a month. Syphilis is a tricky disease though, as secondary symptoms such as rash, fever, joint pain, and malaise can vanish, and the disease may lie dormant—the "latent" stage—for years before the final, fatal, tertiary symptoms emerge. De Blegny's marcasite chocolate may have been symptomatically helpful, at least cheering up his patients, but was probably useless against *Treponema pallidum*—although in fairness, marcasite has never been tested for anti-syphilitic properties. Chocolate, a venereal drug which originated from the same part of the world as syphilis itself, being used to administer and disguise toxic anti-syphilitic compounds: a more ironic moral metaphor for the consequences of hedonism in the early modern period would be difficult to find.

Brillat-Savarin, the French gastronome, endorsed a chocolate formula containing ambergris, a bizarre substance. Occasionally found washed up on beaches, and much sought out by perfumiers, it's a sort of fatty sperm whale (*Physeter macrocephalus*) furball, produced in the whale's digestive tract in response to the sharp, indigestible beaks of the giant squid (*Architeuthis dux*) in their diet. These greasy gutballs are coughed up or defecated (nobody knows for sure which) and bob about on the surface of the ocean, sometimes for decades, putrefying and transforming in salt water and sunlight, until they wash up on a beach and make dog walkers who discover them a lot of money (from the UK's *Daily Mirror* newspaper, 31 January 2013, "Dog walker finds smelly lump of whale vomit on beach that's worth £100,000").[406]

Ambergris was used in medicine as a tonic to the vital spirits; according to Culpeper, it "Heats and Dries, strengthens the brain and nerves exceedingly, if the infirmity come of Cold, [and] resists pestilence".[407] So ambergris was a kind of antidepressant, stimulant, and immunomodulator; like saffron, its expense owed as much to its perceived value in medicine as to its scarcity. Brillat-Savarin's recipe is given in Chapter 8, and his testimonial glows like a Ready Brek commercial:

> When I get one of those days when the weight of age makes itself felt—a painful thought—or when one feels oppressed by an unknown force, I add a knob of ambergris the size of a bean, pounded with sugar, to a strong cup of chocolate, and always find my condition improving marvellously. The burden of life becomes lighter, thought flows with ease and I do not suffer from insomnia, which would have been the inevitable result of a cup of coffee taken for the same purpose. (Brillat-Savarin, quoted in Robert, 1957)

Modern readers may raise an eyebrow or two at the colourful descriptions of "ambered chocolate's" salutary effects, but there may be several reasons for such high praise—other than just marketing hyperbole by well-heeled private doctors touting their exotic nostrums, or the fantasies of the idle rich. In addition to any pharmacological effects of ambergris itself (see Chapter 8), the quality of chocolate drinks made with whole Cacao and spices is much higher than modern cocoa; second, caffeine and the drugs containing it were a novelty, so the effects of the alkaloid (described more fully in the next chapter) seemed almost miraculous. Third, the vitamin, mineral, and phytonutrient content of Cacao may have been more noticeably beneficial to those suffering from nutritional deficiencies owing to a less vegetable-rich or varied diet, particularly in winter, when fresh produce was less readily available. Fourth, and not least, is the matter of dosage: back in the day, serving sizes were significantly larger. Most doctors recommended a pint (approximately half a litre) of chocolate at one sitting, sometimes to be repeated twice daily; each serving may have contained anything from twenty to sixty grams of Cacao, equivalent to approximately 40–120g of dark chocolate. Assuming two servings daily, as many physicians recommended, this would bring daily intake to a ludicrously expensive total of somewhere between forty and one hundred and twenty grams of Cacao—a significant dosage, and far greater than the puny 5–15g of attenuated Cacao in a cup of cocoa. At these levels, pharmacological effects would be much more apparent—as will be discussed in the following chapters.

Chocophobia: the corrupting influence of Cacao

Cacao's Cold nature meant it could "thicken the humours" if eaten to excess, or raw and unprocessed. Hernández described the medical effects of seventeenth-century chocoholism as "vitiating the complexion", causing a "bad habit of the bowel", and contributing to "a thousand ailments and illnesses" due to the obstructing nature of Cacao, when taken immoderately.[408] It's hard to say if this allegation was a native Mesoamerican perception which he recorded, or a European doctor's assessment of a novel heathen drug, to be regarded with some caution—and suspicion. Even as late as nineteenth-century America, chocolate was seen as unhealthy at certain times of year—but by this time, seasonal chocolate censure had shifted from summer (due to overheating in dry climates) or winter (due to overheating in cold climates, causing sweating and over-cooling) to spring: apparently "romances, chocolate, novels and the like inflamers" were now "dangerous to be made use of" in the season of rising sap, due to their tendency to incite immoderate and immodest thoughts.[409]

It's clear that by this time the rationale for this advice was only superficially Galenic, and more austerely Puritan: this is, strictly speaking, a moralistic anti-venereal argument rather than a humoral one, taking issue with chocolate's reputation as an aphrodisiac. The logic of temperament is lacking; after all, chocolate being overall somewhat Warming and Drying should present no trouble if taken in a Warm and Moist season. The extra Warmth would simply help dispel excess Moisture, using de Ledesma's logic of why chocolate and Cacao are beneficial in tropical climes: he proposed that ambient moisture in the tropics prevented one from drying out, so the Hot and Dry properties of spiced chocolate only became enervating in the arid heat of Spanish summers.[410] It's amusing that the only season for which chocolate was permitted by all physicians and health commentators was the Melancholic season of autumn, the season which is—supposedly—closest in nature to the natural, un-doctored (in this case, literally) Cool and Dry temperature of the Cacao bean; this is perhaps because moderate intake of chocolate was thought to be useful for expelling Melancholy.

Chocolate's counter-intuitively Heating property was thought to enhance its action as an exotic venereal drug in unsavoury ways, as we saw from its scandalous association with romances and novels. Dr Stubbe notes that "very hot and aromatical", that is, spiced choco-late, can "exstimulate Nature to excessive Venery",[411] but some doctors alleged that cold (room temperature) chocolate was worse, creating "a burning internal fever, an acceleration of the pulse, and an exaggerated tendency to voluptuousness, leading men to a life of indolence and debasement."[412] So cold chocolate could un-man or effeminise, unlike more wholesome, manly hot chocolate. But Stubbe goes on to propose that Melancholics, or those with "salty" humours in the blood caused by diseases such as "the Itch, and Leprosie" can have an unhealthy sex drive; and indolent, luxurious lifestyles increase the tendency to venereal excess: "Lying long, and on soft beds, and living idly doth render men lascivious."[413] Retention of wastes caused by temperamental imbalance, idleness or illness generated Heat in men, creating a kind of false libido with "morbid matter" in the sperm, so that "hereby Diseases are transplanted oftentimes, as the Pocks, and Consumptions".[414]

Similarly, after the Mexican conquest, excess consumption of chocolate was blamed for the epidemics which decimated the indigenous population: chocolate was a predisposing cause, which fattened and weakened the people, and made them susceptible to "incurable diseases".[415] This particular myth was most likely propagated by both conquerors and subjects—the Spanish needed to inoculate against potentially dangerous native nostalgia by denigrating the most valued native customs and products associated with the beliefs and values of the old order, such as Cacao; and the enslaved indigenous population sought an explanation for their current predicament, even if the price of that interpretation was bitter self-recrimination, or culpability.

In Europe, excessive consumption of chocolate was believed to increase the urge to mastur-bate. Aside from religious condemnation of the sin of onanism, masturbation was considered to be unhealthy, particularly for men, because ejaculation caused them to waste their "seed", expending their Natural Spirits or procreative power, which depleted life-giving Warmth and Moisture and increased Melancholy; this, in turn, potentially accelerated the aging process, altered the complexion and could even cause "cachexia"—wasting diseases![416] Wanking was a serious business. But contemporary debates about the harmful effects of porn addiction sug-gest that these ideas, however absurd they seem, may yet turn out to contain a kernel of truth. It's very unlikely that depleting Natural Spirits will turn out to be biologically accurate, and the slippery slope argument (cursing and masturbation leading to drugs, to petty crime, and thereon to a life of moral turpitude) is highly debatable, but as a metaphor for the ultimate effects of compulsive hedonism, there is merit in the observation that excess venery produces Melancholy. Our ancestors certainly believed that chocolate could be an enabler of venereal excess, and this proposition will be explored in Chapters 7 and 10.

The Old World critique of chocolate as a potentially harmful pleasure-drug fascinatingly parallels pre-conquest Mexica reservations about *cacahuatl*. Although European misgivings about chocolate had a sexual spin, there were strong taboos in Mexica society against the consumption of *cacahuatl* by women, children, and ordinary folk, and a legend that overuse of Cacao could be enervating (recounted in Chapter 9). After all, in its homeland Cacao was a powerful, precious substance, and *cacahuatl* was reserved for males in the Mexica elite: royalty, and those with life-endangering professions. Its use by merchants, warriors, and the nobility in Mexico was both a caste-based privilege and a socially sanctioned reward for shouldering potentially life-threatening responsibilities. As we shall see in Chapter 5, Cacao may be pharmacologically useful for stress management, and is perhaps capable of diminishing some specific long-term effects of trauma. So if Cacao is a drug which helps to loosen the bonds of certain anxieties and enhance pleasure, could it ultimately affect the whole structure of society, potentially undermining the existing order?

While this seems unlikely—this is chocolate we're talking about, after all, not opium, heroin, or crack cocaine—a similar anxiety underlies all legislation and social taboos concerning the use of psychoactive drugs. Psychotropic substances do change perspectives and alter behaviour, so the more conservative the government or prevailing ideology, the more carefully circumscribed the social rituals and availability of such substances tends to be. Perhaps a more prosaic explanation for early modern European condemnation of Cacao's "Venereal" properties and the Mexican restrictions on Cacao consumption would be that, despite their enormous ideological differences, both pre-Columbian Mexica and Renaissance European societies had deeply patriarchal and rigidly religiously influenced hierarchical class structures, which decried unearned pleasures, and idealised productive work for the glory of those above, whether regal or divine; so, in both societies, Cacao became a symbol of a luxurious and privileged life, but its mythos carried a warning note about the dissipative dangers of luxury. We'll return to this theme of Cacao, society, and attitudes to pleasure in Chapters 5 and 10. But for now, note that in European medicine, Warming the Cacao with sugar, spices, or literal heat was alleged to enhance vitality and mental well-being—the application of (masculine) Heat dispersed the Phlegmatic (or feminine) attributes of Coldness, and rendered the drug more wholesome.[417]

Three centuries of debate couldn't resolve all the incongruities in the humoral conceptualisation of Cacao. Despite chocolate's Warming faculty, it might yet Cool the liver and cause "stoppings"; chocolate helped expel Melancholy and waste substances, but its allegedly obstructing nature meant that Melancholics must never take it made too strong, or—conversely—with too much spice. Chocolate was considered less suitable for women, who consumed it the most; it was less good in the heat of summer, or the cold of winter—depending who you believed—but in either case, it could be adjusted to a more fitting Temperature, by adding Cooling ingredients in summer or by omitting very Heating spices in winter. Chocolate was a vehicle for other drugs, including those used to treat venereal disease, but could also incite lust and even create the preconditions of chronic venereal disease; it could help or harm fertility, the female reproductive system, and the unborn child.

In many cases, such apparent contradictions can be resolved by quantity or formulation. Most of the problems that were seen to arise do so because in excess, chocolate was regarded as potentially over-Heating—whether this was blamed on "obstructions" causing bad blood, a Choleric component in Cacao, or over-spiced chocolate, in all cases the answer was to adjust the formulation of the chocolate with other ingredients, or to reduce its consumption. Dr Stubbe noted that "uncertainty of compounding *Chocolata*" lay behind many misadventures with the drug: "Several have experienced the consequences of this variety of mixtures … for, having taken *Chocolata* of Antwerp for Hypochondriacal distempers, by using that of Spain they have instantly been molested by the haemorrhoids."[418]

Haemorrhoids notwithstanding, it seems temperance is the watchword: immoderate use of chocolate, or over-liberal application of spices and additives could induce "dyscrasias", or humoral imbalance. That Cacao was inherently Cold, yet could produce Hot ailments if taken to excess seems odd, but isn't a sign that the humoral system was broken, or that Cacao was mis-categorised—although certainly Galenic classifications were often idiosyncratic. Rather, the humoral system contained built-in explanations for these things, such as Cold drugs which could obstruct, and lead to over-Heating, or which incorporated some Hot elements which could build up and surmount the Cold when the substance was over-consumed, and both explanations were applied to Cacao. From a biochemical perspective, the second reason appears to be the truer one, as Cacao's caffeine content means it can indeed become over-Heating (in the Galenic sense) when consumed to excess. Cacao itself is somewhat contradictory. Looking at its history, the food-drug was always a restricted luxury, a gift of the underworld; its European transformation into an exotic nostrum for aristocratic ailments is merely an intriguing plot twist.

Pharmacacahuatl: *Mesoamerican chocolate, and other drugs*

Like Galenic medicine in Europe, Mesoamerican theories of health and disease were temperature-based. Pre-Colombian systems recognised four elements (Water, Earth, Fire, and Wind) comprising the world, each relating to a season and a compass direction—almost identical to the European humoral scheme—but the core of their medicine was binary, focusing on Hot and Cold as primary states, rather than the Aristotelian concept of Heat, Cold, Damp, and Dryness that constituted the elements in the Greco-Roman humoral model. Like other traditional medicine systems, health was a state of balance between opposites, and deviations from personal norms led to disease.[419] Also in common with humoral medicine, Warmth was life-giving and Cold was potentially harmful, although necessary for fertility—which, as in the Galenic system, was perceived as a Cold function, being Watery. This is a natural analogy, as the body swells when pregnant, milk is produced in the breasts, and just before birth the amniotic fluid leaves the body—the "waters break"; and more broadly, water is a necessary precondition for growth and life. Fertility deities are often associated with rain, which allows life-sustaining crops to grow: consequently, many cultures around the world associate fertility with Water.

Like the Galenists in Europe, the Mexica believed that life energy, or *teyolia*, the animating force, dwelt in the human heart—the equivalent of *pneuma* being converted to Vital Spirits and distributed from the heart in the humoral system. The Mexica also believed that there were three primary causes of disease: natural, magical, and divine.[420] In contemporary highland

Maya cultures, illnesses are loosely categorised in this way as good (natural)—deriving from "upset social relations"—or bad (magical): due to witchcraft.[421] As in humoral medicine, natural causes of disease arose from temperamental imbalances, either due to external conditions such as climate or weather, behavioural considerations like diet, sleep, and exercise, or internal influences like emotional disturbances and the interaction of one's innate constitutional balance with environmental factors.[422] Such disturbances could be the result of accidents, or patterns of deficiency or excess: all illness was seen as disharmony, reflecting a person's relationship with society, the gods, the ancestors, or the environment, so divining the root cause of such imbalances—often supernatural, such as a failure to pay proper respects to ancestors, or behavioural—was most important.[423]

Magical causes were due to the intervention of other human beings, either deliberate—cursing, or casting spells—or accidental, like the "evil eye", wherein an envious person with "strong vision" may unknowingly harm another, a belief which persists in Latin American folk medicine, or *curanderismo*, to this day.[424] Evil sorcerers might send diseases in the form of insects[425]—a belief which perhaps parallels a microbial truth, as many biting insects are vectors for potentially lethal or disfiguring diseases such as malaria or leishmaniasis. Divine causes were fated and mystically ordained,[426] and the gods of the underworld were generally responsible for them; each of the nine Maya Lords of Xibalba, the underworld, were named after a different set of disease symptoms, and many diseases were regarded as sentient underworld entities, much like demons in the Judaeo-Christian tradition.[427] Treatment modalities for various illnesses included sweat baths, confessions, and both external and internal treatment with medicinal plants, accompanied by prayer and ritual.[428]

Diagnostic divination is described in Chapter 10, but the physical aspect of the procedure likely involved pulse reading, a technique which survives in some contemporary Maya cultures. In this case, though, the pulse isn't simply interpreted as a guide to physiological processes, it's seen as an expression of the patient's own spirit and their ancestor spirits which reside in the blood, and may be interrogated: a diviner-medic asks questions, and interprets the pulse to get answers to those questions in an attempt to reveal the nature of the illness which affects the patient, and by extension their family and society. A medical consultation is a kind of "socioscopy", and the cure is effected through ritual to rebalance or restore the patient's relationship to family, society, nature, and the cosmos.[429] But medicines are important, too, and like many traditional medical systems, plant, mineral, and animal remedies may be employed; after determining which spirits may be responsible for causing an illness, a Mixtec diviner may ask questions such as "What animal should be roasted and applied?"[430]

Like the Spanish after them, the Mexica regarded Cacao as a Cooling and nourishing tonic, and its role in the magical and mystical aspects of Mexica medicine will be discussed in Chapter 10. Hernández recorded that Cacao beverages were temperate, agreeable to "all the people of this land, and even the whole world", and "often given to those who have serious diseases, unmixed with any other thing, which is very useful to temper heat and burning".[431] Cacao's Cooling nature and its tonifying, restorative effect were highly valued by the Mexica, as was its ability to temporararily relieve existential angst: Mesoamerican poets repeatedly speak of Cacao in the context of inducing exhileration, the "intoxicating" properties of "flowery" (foaming, precious) Cacao associated with singing, dancing, splendour and celebration of life, despite a continual sorrowful awareness of inevitable death.[432] Cacao-based drinks were served during the making of treaties and contracts; this use of Cacao to seal a deal could infer some pharmacological property, such as stimulant, cognition-enhancing or anti-anxiety properties which may be useful during negotiations, or perhaps imply nothing more than Cacao's valued status as a drink, analogous to the serving of champagne in the modern West at important social functions.

Mexica high-class *cacahuatl* was made from Cacao, *heuinacaztli* (*Cymbopetalum penduliflorum*) or ear flower, vanilla pods or *tlilxochitl* (*Vanilla planifolia*), and *mecaxochitl* or the dried fruits of holy leaf (*Piper auritum*). Hernández described this royal beverage as a cordial with an agreeable taste, which "warms the stomach, perfumes the breath, combats all poisons, and alleviates intestinal pains", but, according to Sahagún, an "excess … can intoxicate, derange and disturb".[433] The Mexica incorporated Cacao in treatments for physical ailments such as fevers, "skin eruptions" (unspecified), diarrhoea and bloody dysentery, indigestion and flatulence, "lung problems" (also unspecified), exhaustion, impotence, to delay hair growth, to clean the teeth, and as a prophylactic against snakebite. They also used it in treatments for ailments we would now consider to be mental health issues, such as agitation, vision-quest hangovers, insanity, to encourage or prohibit sleep, and to increase courage and reduce fear.[434]

Just as the Mexica used *cacahuatl* with psychoactive mushrooms, there are accounts of indigenous men in Nicaragua shortly after the Spanish conquest using chocolate drinks to recover from a shamanic ritual in which some unidentified plants were smoked in a pipe, accompanied by dancing and drumming. The men "fell senseless on the ground or ran amok weeping … and had to be carried off to bed by their wives or friends".[435] In the aftermath of this psychic assault, they were left suffering from "stupidity of mind" for a week or so, which was treated with chocolate. The ingredients of the smoking mixture are speculative, but it sounds like the pipes may have contained tobacco and *Datura*, which the Mexica referred to as *toloaxihuitl*—the plant which possibly featured in *itzpacalatl* (see Chapter 2), and which can have lingering physical and mental side effects. If so, this may be a second instance of Cacao being used to antidote some of the negative effects of *Datura* intoxication, only—in this instance—to help recovery after the event, and not administered simultaneously. (There would, after all, be little point offering anything to help recover sanity after taking *itzpacalatl*, as the beverage was only used as a preparative for human sacrifice). The pharmacological ramifications of this possibility will be discussed in Chapter 6.

Medical sorcery and flowery mojo

Cacao would rarely have been used alone in medicines, or in as clinically prescriptive a manner as the list of physical and mental ailments and indications for which the Mexica used it makes it sound. After all, it was a Cooling herb employed within a magico-medical system based on humours and mystically-induced infirmities, not tightly defined biomedical diagnoses. Nevertheless, Spanish chroniclers recorded Mexica use of Cacao for these issues, and many of those uses survive today in Latin American folk medicine. The original Mexica formulations incorporated many other plants in prescriptions that made use of ritual and sympathetic magic (discussed further in Chapter 10). Sympathetic magic is when something is utilised because it allegorically invokes the desired qualities or effects; for example, incorporating flowers in a prescription to magically induce happiness or love because their perceived beauty, appealing scent, and transience reminds us of these emotional states. Mexica formulae featuring aromatic flowers used in Cacao-based beverages include a potable infusion and an unguent for removing fear and cowardice, a body wash to help "the fatigue of those who administer the republic and discharge a public duty", an amulet to protect travellers, and another potion to treat "insanity, or losing one's mind".[436] All require multiple ingredients—and some of the same ingredients show up repeatedly, many of them being key constituents in Cacao-based beverages.

It may be assumed that the properties of reducing fear, fatigue, disordered thinking, and, somehow, providing protection were all associated with Cacao and its admixture plants. In the days before the effects of drugs were explained by chemistry, there was no logical reason to assume that ingestion was required to obtain benefit from a drug; if a substance was able to induce certain effects, then merely carrying it, or its image, or even just saying its name, could—with the correct supernatural assistance—transmit its virtues. The aromatic flowers which feature in many Cacao-based beverages are a prominent feature of these formulae: *cacaloxochitl* (yellow or pink frangipani, *Plumeria rubra f. typica*), *necuxochitl* (white-flowered frangipani, *Plumeria rubra f. acutifolia*), *cacahuaxochitl* (funeral tree flowers, *Quararibea funebris*), *mecaxochitl* (holy leaf, *Piper auritum*), *tlilxochitl* (vanilla), *yolloxochitl* (*Magnolia mexicana*), and *heuinacaztli* (ear flower, *Cymobpetalum penduliflorum*) all occur in multiple prescriptions; *izquixochitl* (popcorn flower, *Bourreria huanita*) and *eloxochitl* (*Magnolia dealbata*) both occur in only one formula.

The two internal formulae are (1) an infusion of aromatic flowers in spring water, including both types of frangipani, and funeral tree flowers, mixed with white clay (kaolin) and other medicinal herbs, and used to treat fear or cowardice; and (2) the expressed juice of fresh funeral tree and magnolia (*yolloxochitl*) flowers, bark, and roots, used to treat "losing one's mind".[437] The presence of funeral tree (*Quararibea funebris*) in both prescriptions is suggestive of psychoactive effects, and implies specific value in mentally debilitated states. Funeral tree flowers were also boiled as a cough remedy by the Zapotecs, and in fact the juices of *Q. funebris* and *Magnolia mexicana* in this prescription are supposed to "remove the bad humour in the chest", making breathing easier or less laboured.[438] As magnolia flowers are commonly used to treat heart pain or palpitations,[439] an anti-anxiety effect seems likely for them too; perhaps the juicy part of the insanity prescription combines the probable anxiolytic effects of both plants with possible cough relieving (anti-tussive) properties from funeral tree and the heart-regulating (anti-arrhythmic) effects of magnolia flowers, which have also been traditionally used to treat asthma (discussed further in Chapter 6).

These two prescriptions also perfectly illustrate the dovetail between pharmaceutical and magical elements in Mexica medicine. The plant juice part of the anti-crazy prescription was to be taken for a few days, then followed with a more overtly magical mixture of "stones" taken from the crops of various birds, together with semi-precious jasper and pearls, which were dropped into water. Some of this water was to be decanted and administered to the patient, and the remainder was used to wash their head, while they held an owl's gall bladder and another stone from a bird's crop in their hand. Likewise, the "fear" prescription goes on to state that the infusion of flowers with kaolin is to be mixed with laurel leaves, the blood of a vixen, swallow's excrement, sea foam, and a specific type of worm; this by-now less delightful-smelling paste was applied to the head and neck, while a stone from the crop of a swallow was worn as a pendant.[440]

The stones from birds' crops may represent tough humours being removed from inside the body. The owl is also a herald of the underworld, and the semi-precious stones have chthonian symbolism: jasper is the colour of blood, and pearls are associated with water, the element of the underworld. Some of the ingredients may have active pharmaceutical properties, too—some animal tissues, like many medicinal plants, contain physiologically active substances. But for magical purposes, the vixen is a nocturnal predator, and therefore also associated with the underworld; the sea was the primordial water from which all gods and creation emerged,[441] and foam was the most rarefied part of that creative chaos, merging the elements of water with wind/air. The most recognisable piece of sympathetic magic appears in an addendum to the prescription against fear: for those who are "frightened by lightning or sparks", the paste must incorporate the juice of a tree recently struck by lightning, and some of the plants grow-ing nearby—thereby infusing the patient with a sort of homœopathic, like-cures-like magical remedy for that specific fear. Magnolia flowers also feature in the external amulet used for travellers, both as a powder and as the case of the amulet itself: a single dried magnolia flower is to be filled with all the other pulverised ingredients and worn around the neck. The aromatic botanicals used include vanilla and ear flower, as well as a few other ingredients such as copal resin. The anti-arrhythmic properties of magnolia flowers may be relevant here as a symbol for "fortifying the heart"—bringing much-needed courage and support to a traveller.

Despite its classification as a Warming plant, Hernández commended the "glutinous and astringent" *yolloxochitl*—the large, extra-aromatic *Magnolia mexicana*—for its ability to "comfort and cool the heart" and "bind the belly", so its principal medicinal use was to reduce fever, resolve palpitations, and treat diarrhoea. For severe diarrhoea the flowers could be adminis-tered in powdered form.[442] In contemporary folk medicine, *M. mexicana* flowers are known as *yolosúchil*, and used to treat stomach, heart, and chest pains, "melancholy", and *espanto* or "fright sickness",[443] otherwise known as *susto*. *Susto* or *espanto* is a folk illness caused by extreme fear or shock, sometimes referred to as "soul loss", and is treated with ritual and herbs.[444] It's characterised by symptoms such as depression, nightmares, craving solitude and darkness, lack of motivation and appetite, diarrhoea and vomiting. The symptoms resemble a Galenic diag-nosis of hypochondriacal melancholy with obstruction, and a contemporary diagnosis of IBS with anxiety and depression, or even a rare physical issue known as Addison's disease, caused by low adrenal function. The milder and more common *eloxochitl* (*Magnolia dealbata*) flowers are sold as *Magnolia* in Mexican markets, and used to remediate anxiety, headaches, and high blood pressure.[445] *Yolloxochitl* flowers were also used to treat female sterility, in combination with four other plants including the Cacao spices *tlilxochitl* and *mecaxochitl*, vanilla (*Vanilla planifolia*), and holy leaf (*Piper auritum*), respectively.[446]

For the latter purpose the five herbs were boiled and the infusion was applied as a vaginal douche. It's hard to say if this treatment would have any pharmacological benefit, as there would be little systemic absorption of compounds in the herbs from this method of use, and lack of fertility can have many causes; it's plausible that the mixture may have had some degree of pharmacological efficacy for some of those causes. But once again the magical symbolism of the prescription—washing the vagina with an extract of aromatic flowers to enhance fertility—is likely to be a key part of its effectiveness. There were no dividing lines between the medicinal action of a thing and its magical properties: the associations between flowers and female sexuality, for instance, were not just a human concept, but a divinely ordained affiliation in a world created by the gods for humans. A key difference between many ancient and traditional cultures and the modern West is the unselfconscious way that magical associations were assumed to be innate, not "made up"—because if humans could think it, then those thoughts arose from divine inspiration, or the fact that we ourselves are products of divine power, and therefore possessed the ability to perceive or make such connections for ourselves, albeit on a much smaller scale.

Cacao features alongside its additives in the complex external prescription against "the fatigue of those who administer the republic". Given the expense and number of its ingredients, which included plant and animal parts from all over the empire, the prescription had to be used by royalty; no one else could have afforded it, or even been able to access all the ingredients simultaneously. All of the flowers mentioned above, together with Cacao seeds and fruit pulp, and a generic recommendation of "all other good-smelling summer flowers" were to be infused for "one day and one night" in clean spring water, together with a list of specific medicinal plant leaves. The wood of *Heamatoxylon brasiletto*, another potential Cacao additive known to the Mexica as *huitzcuahuitl* ("hoo·itz·kwa·wittle"), was steeped in the water to turn it blood-red, before actual blood from several animals was added: the magical symbolism is striking, as all the animals are predators at the top of the food chain—the red jaguar, the albino jaguar, the wolf, the mountain cat, and the ocelot. Being nocturnal, these animals trod the boundary between the world of the living and the dead, and, like the lion in Africa, jaguars represented royal power. The whole body was to be anointed with this gory perfume, and then washed off—after one sticky night—with another infusion of precious stones, kaolin, and stones from birds' crops.[447]

While some aromatherapeutic benefit from the flowers can't be ruled out, the prescription is clearly magical, and through the lens of biomedical science, it appears both messy and pointless. In fact it was a complex invocation for an exalted state of mind (flowers and precious stones) and dominant spiritual and earthly power (the blood of nocturnal apex predators). Washing off the gory paste with jewel-, clay-, and gastrolith-infused water after a night spent caked in dried feline blood and floral sap must have been a relief—a feeling of rinsing away unwanted "stuff", a cleansing and renewal, reminiscent of sponging the diluted gore and bodily fluids off a newborn child. Cacao's association with the other ingredients in this prescription clearly links it with symbols of strength, exaltation, and mortality: flowers are short-lived, and here mixed with blood. The gladdening and empowering symbolism of flowers, jewels, and regal beasts is also an implicit reminder of the transience and the precariousness of life and authority. This ritual potion incorporates both carrot and stick, symbolically empowering the subject of the ritual while reminding them of the precarious and brief nature of existence. Cacao is the only seed and fruit in the formula, mixed with other botanicals and blood; the prescription was said to give "the endurance of a gladiator; banish fatigue, dissipate fear, and give vigour to the heart".[448] These qualities may also be inferred to reside in Cacao, as the basis for many drinks containing the specific flowers listed in the formula, and the only plant other than maize mythologically linked to both the underworld and the human heart (see Chapter 9 for more details).

Materia Mexica

Hernández's descriptions of Cacao and the plants used with it introduced many doctors and learned folk in Europe to their virtues, and were instrumental in the dissemination of knowledge about chocolate through the Old World. His descriptions of the plants represent a cultural intersection, describing native uses and largely following the lead of his indigenous informants on their Temperature and properties, but slotting them into the existing European humoral system: thus *xochinacaztli* or *hueinacaztli*, the ear flower (*Cymbopetalum penduliflorum*) is "Hot and Dry in the fourth degree", equivalent in "heat" to chillies or garlic.[449] As well as being "cordial", helping the heart, and heating a cold stomach, ear flower was used to treat asthma, says Hernández, particularly when combined with chilli. "Cordial" is Galenic terminology meaning a remedy which strengthens vitality in some way and helps to alleviate depression or low mood, but the specific applications and temperatures of all the native Mesoamerican flora he documents are based on information provided by indigenous sources.

The admixture plants which Hernández describes can be divided into two categories: Heating and Cooling. The Heating plants include *Cymbopetalum penduliflorum*, *Vanilla planifolia*, *Pimienta dioica*, *Magnolia mexicana*, and *M. dealbata*, chillies of all kinds (*Capsicum spp.*), *Piper auritum*, and *Quararibea funebris*, as well as tobacco (*Nicotiana tabacum*)—not generally used in Cacao, but widely consumed alongside it—and the hallucinogenic morning glory seeds, *Turbina corymbosa* or *Ipomoea violacea*. These remedies were Hot because they tasted bitter or spicy, they caused sweating or increased circulation, or they remedied Cold symptoms and diseases. They ranged from the Galenic "first degree" of Heat—barely Warm, such as the funeral tree, *Quararibea funebris*, which has subtle relaxing effects, a pleasant aroma, and doesn't cause sweating—to those placed in the fourth and most intense degree of Heat and Dryness, such as chillies (*Capsicum spp.*), which taste very spicy, cause redness when applied to the skin and flushing if eaten, and produce an immediate and notable discharge of Phlegm from the body in the form of watering eyes, a runny nose, and perspiration. Tobacco (*Nicotiana tabacum* or *Nicotiana rustica*) was placed one point lower, at the third degree of Heat, as its capacity when chewed or ingested to apparently chase away headaches, catarrh, and sensations of cold were all properties of a Hot drug. Again, though, caution was advised: overuse of tobacco resulted in "the gravest ills"—history suggests Hernández's admonition was warranted in this case.

Another Hot drug which may have been used with or alongside Cacao was *ololiuhqui* (*Turbina corymbosa*), the principal morning glory species used for divinatory and healing purposes in Mesoamerica. The plant was attributed the fourth and highest degree of Heat in the Galenic system; Durán recorded that both *picietl* (tobacco) and *ololiuhqui* had "the strange ability of causing fainting and dizziness, and when applied as a poultice, of desensitising one's flesh",[450] so it was sometimes used to treat migraine, vertigo, or joint pain. It's certain that the psychoactive mushrooms, *teonanacatl* (*Psilocybe cubensis*) were used alongside Cacao, but while their ritual use is recorded by the Spanish, their medicinal use isn't. Given their important ceremonial role and cultural significance, the psychoactive mushrooms were likely to have been used with Cacao for magico-medical purposes, but the records are non-existent: they may have been expunged by the Church, along with the thousands of Mesoamerican statues that were smashed and books that were burnt in a systematic destruction of "diabolical" indigenous lore.

Presumably the mushrooms were beyond the pale to be considered for medicinal use, as the "mushroom cult" was a powerful inducement to idolatry; after all, the natives could communicate with their gods using the mushrooms, which constituted a substantial threat to the Spanish missionaries' holy commission to eradicate native belief systems.

Europe in general was also quite mycophobic at the time—a few mushrooms, such as the medicinally important "agarick" (*Fomitopsis officinalis*)[451] were used in Galenical treatments, but most mushrooms were lumped together under suspicion of toxicity. Culpeper refers to mushrooms as a subset of the category "Things Bred From Plants" (alongside the parasitic herb mistletoe), and describes them as "under the dominion of Saturn … [they] do as much harm as good",[452] before alluding to poisoning; his attitude is fairly representative of the European mindset on mushrooms outside the Baltic regions. Although *ololiuhqui* was also tainted by heretical associations—Hernández reports its use by "old priests [who] ate this plant to see a thousand phantasms" and "speak with demons"[453]—at least it wasn't a mushroom. *Ololiuhqui* was less potent than the psychoactive fungi, its use was more specialised, and it wasn't used "recreationally" as the mushrooms used to be at Mesoamerican feasts and celebrations. So it could safely be placed in the drug cabinet alongside other well-known psychoactive European plants, such as the "hexing herbs", henbane (*Hyoscyamus niger*), mandrake (*Mandragora officinarum*), and belladonna (*Atropa belladonna*): like them, it was still suspect, being somewhat toxic and associated with witchcraft, but recognised for its medicinal utility. The plant was reputed to be an effective treatment for the "French Disease"—syphilis. The pox had different names, depending on what country you were from: the French disease, the English disease, the Spanish disease, etc.: usually the disfiguring STD was named after a despised rival nation.

Turbina corymbosa has no known anti-syphilitic properties, but New World drugs were often seized on as possible remedies for this New World malady; it's feasible that *ololiuhqui* may have alleviated some symptoms of syphilis, at least. The plant was administered to relieve Cold pains such as cramps, to relieve "chills", resolve "wind" and "swellings"—the "wind" Hernández refers to is unlikely to be flatulence, as "wind" was a Galenic term for what would now be thought of as nervous system issues such as tics, twitches, and shooting nerve pains. It was also used as a remedy for "the pelvic troubles of women" and to treat "dislocations and fractures",[454] implying some analgesic properties, effective against menstrual cramps or the pain of musculoskeletal injuries. *Ololiuhqui* was also used topically and internally to treat "eye ailments", for which purpose the seed decoction was to be drunk, or made into a poultice with milk and chilli, and applied to the head.[455] Given the lack of direct application to the eye, and the use of fresh chillies, this sounds like a remedy for eye pain or visual disturbances rather than inflammation or injury to the eye itself; application around the eye would permit transdermal absorption of pain-relieving substances, whereas putting raw chilli and boiled seeds directly into the eye would probably be counterproductive.

The milder *tlitliltzin* or *Ipomoea violacea* seeds are still used in folk medical practice in the Mexican state of Morelos, where a plaster or poultice of the fresh plant material is used to treat minor wounds, and a tea made with one or two leaves steeped in a glass of water is prescribed as a mild stimulant to alleviate fatigue.[456] Both *T. corymbosa* and *I. violacea*'s sole link to Cacao comes from the plants' association with the Mexica deity *Xochipilli* (see Chapter 2), and a pharmacological similarity with *teonanacatl*—both psychedelics have tryptamines as active constituents (see Chapter 6), although no combinations of *ololiuhqui* with Cacao are explicitly mentioned by Hernández or other authors.

As the Mesoamerican *materia medica* became known in Europe, thanks to the work of Hernández, Sahagún, and other enterprising medical anthropologists and documentarists, other European doctors weighed in on the virtues of native Mesoamerican flora. Many just parroted Hernández, but some clearly took the time to experiment and observe the effects of various compositions for themselves. For example, Dr Moreau reiterated Hernández's assertion, derived from native Mesoamerican medicinal lore, that vanilla was a good "antidote to poisons" and strengthened the heart (in the Galenic sense of strengthening vitality and resilience), but Dr de Blegny added a novel use, recommending vanilla as a helpful addition to chocolate in "chest ailments"[457]—presumably the chronic type for which Cacao was thought to be indicated. But vanilla was "insupportable" for "hysterics and hypochondriacs" (in the humoral sense), who could get "violent headaches", tremors, or vertigo if they took chocolate with vanilla.[458] This seems a little ludicrous to the modern eye, but chocolate—and perhaps, by association, vanilla—is still under suspicion in migraine and Parkinson's disease, although it seems likely to be exonerated for both (see Chapter 7).

The botanical ingredients in *cacahuatl* that Hernández cites as Cooling are *Bourreria huanita*, *Bixa orellana*, *Plumeria rubra*, and *Theobroma cacao* itself. Their Cool natures could be observed in their power to lower fever or lessen subjective symptoms of heat, to reduce appetite, or in some way slow down the system. Cacao, for instance, helped weight gain, *Bourreria huanita* is a sedative used to treat dental pain,[459] and *Bixa orellana* was used to help control dysentery and reduce swellings.[460] The popcorn flower *Bourreria huanita* was also used to help digestion and treat coughs, though its mild Coldness made it more suited to feverish conditions, or over-Heated situations such as a dry cough or heartburn.[461] The Cold flowers of *Plumeria rubra*, cacalosúchil—*cacaloxochitl* in Nahuatl—or frangipani, are still used in *bu'pu*, the foamy *atole* made in the Isthmus region of Oaxaca, where *Bourreria huanita* also grows. The Maya referred to frangipani, with its gorgeously aromatic, Day-Glo pink, yellow, or pure white flowers as *baak nik'te* or "bone flower" because the milky white sap or latex from the trunk was used externally to accelerate bone healing, by soaking a cloth with it and applying it to the affected limb.[462] Hernández gives another use for the "cold and glutinous" exudate, as an external application to the chest to "take away pain", and describes how a bark decoction was also used to remove pain and visceral obstructions.[463] The tree was medicinally valuable, but it was the aromatic flowers which were—and still are—prized for the subtle perfume they lend to Cacao, as well as the prodigious foam they help to generate.

The latex and flowers of aromatic pink- or yellow-flowered *cacalosúchil* (*Plumeria rubra*) are also used to treat various superficial infections and inflammations in Mexican folk medicine, including ringworm, verrucae, inflamed eyes, and vaginal discharge; for most of these purposes, the latex or pulped flowers can be applied neat—except for treating the eyes, for which a flower infusion is preferred, and vaginal discharge, for which a decoction is used as a douche. The latex may be applied directly to the teeth to treat toothache, or used in a more elaborate treatment for ear or pelvic pain: branches from the tree are roasted over an open fire and cotton balls are dipped in the latex which sizzles out of the broiling tree limbs; the cotton balls are then inserted into the ears or the vagina.[464] White-flowered *cacalosúchil* (*Plumeria acutifolia*), known as *itzaccacaloxochitl* by the Mexica, is treated similarly, but in this case the cotton sponges with cooked latex are applied to stop bleeding, and the flower decoction is also used to clear the skin of pimples, wash wounds, and treat scabies. The most flexible and tender young branches may also be roasted, pulped, and applied to the small of the back as a poultice to reduce fertility and prevent having children,[465] a use which is interestingly contrasted by the traditional recommendation that the flower infusion may be drunk as a galactagogue: an agent that increases breast milk production.[466]

By the logic of the Old World's Galenic medical system, Cacao's traditional use to help weight gain could only be possible were it only very mildly Cold—no more than Cold and Moist in the first degree, to be exact, like most fruit—as things which were too Cold could quench the appetite and weaken digestion. The Coldest of the three cooling plants associated with Cacao which Hernández catalogued is *achiote* or annatto (*Bixa orellana*), which was Galenised as Cold in the third degree, the same level of Coldness as cucumbers (*Cucumis sativus*), of which Culpeper wrote, "If they were but one degree colder, they would be poison."[467] The "third degree" implied a potent, but non-toxic cooling effect, whereas drugs which were Cold in the fourth degree were stupefying narcotics or numbing toxins such as opium, henbane, or hemlock.

A concentrated hot water infusion of annatto seeds was used with an unidentified "resin" to treat scabies, and Hernández commends *achiote* for its ability to heal swellings, treat bloody dysentery, reduce thirst and urinary tract inflammation—it "comforts and provokes urine", and is especially good with Cacao: "Made with chocolate [it] will not harm in whatsoever quantity and is good, because it often causes speedy digestion without danger of indigestion,"[468] perhaps by offsetting the Warming effects of properly prepared chocolate. This assertion is contested by later European commentators such as Stubbe, who agrees with Hernández's opinion of *achiote* "in due proportion" but also notes that annatto seeds could provoke nausea or headache when mixed with Cacao, an observation I can attest to first-hand; ever the empiricist, Stubbe observed that this is most likely the result of using older seeds, which gradually darken in colour from a vibrant red to a deep, dried-blood burgundy colour.[469] Hernández, being based in New Spain, had access to the good stuff, freshly prepared and readily available—as he recounts, "The natives think highly of it, and grow it near their dwellings."[470]

Conversely, *mecaxochitl* (holy leaf, or *Piper auritum*) was one of the Hottest herbs; it was ranked as Hot in the fourth degree, alongside *ololiuhqui* and chilli peppers, though one point less Dry. Hernández recounts its use to flavour Cacao, counter halitosis—no doubt a useful property given the lack of dental services in those times, and the growing appreciation for sugar— to assist weight loss, "comfort the heart", reduce colic or gastrointestinal pains, and induce menstruation.[471] A common flavour combination in *cacahuatl* was *mecaxochitl* with *tlilxochitl* or vanilla, and this formula was used to help expel the placenta after childbirth—or to deliver a stillborn child, in the event that the mother needed some assistance to go into labour.[472] Because *mecaxochitl* is in the black pepper family its long, dried fruits impart a somewhat peppery taste; they have fallen out of use, replaced with black pepper by the Spaniards and since then displaced entirely by the ubiquitous (and delicious) *canela* (cinnamon) as a primary Mexican chocolate spice. *Piper auritum* was also used to treat headaches and fevers, and is an antidote for the condition known as *susto* ("fright") in contemporary Latin America. These uses suggest some effect on the brain and nervous system, and in rats the water extract of *Piper auritum* leaves does have anxiety-relieving and painkilling properties;[473] perhaps these qualities pleasantly enhance the effects of Cacao.

Chillies (*Capsicum spp.*) were a staple food and medicine in Mesoamerica. Notably Hot, they were used in many external applications to treat pain and inflammation, and internally to help digestion, improve appetite, and induce menstruation;[474] they were generally regarded as a helpful tonic herb in Mesoamerican medicine because of their non-toxic Heating properties. In contemporary folk medicine, a variety of chilli whose fruit points phallically upward, the *chili parado*, is used alongside annatto seeds, which grow in furry bollock-like fruits, to treat male impotence.[475] Both fruits are notably bright red, as if flushed with blood: magical symbolism is alive and kicking in folk medicine. Nowadays, though, chilli is usually only combined with Cacao in the famous Oaxacan *mole* sauces, and rarely added to Cacao-based beverages; spicy has been usurped by sweet.

Allspice (*Pimienta dioica*) or *xocoxochitl* was a Heating herb, mainly used as a carminative—to reduce "wind" in the modern sense of bloating and flatulence, to help phlegmy coughs and menstrual pain.[476] In contemporary Guatemalan folk medicine, Don Angel Chiac of San Luis, Peten, uses the leaf infusion to treat "heart pain" and diarrhoea.[477] Reginaldo Huex, herbalist and head of the Itza Maya traditional medicine association in San Jose, Peten, recommends an infusion of young allspice leaves to dispel Cold and help sleep, and advises that the fresh leaf or seed pulp can be placed on a painful tooth to anaesthetise it; he also prescribes a decoction of ten allspice seeds to treat "internal pains".[478] Allspice has been used externally for this purpose as well: the Mexica made a paste from allspice berries, *ololiuhqui*, and other botanical ingredients and applied this to the shoulders as a poultice to treat pains caused by "wind and cold".[479] In the past, flannel soaked in allspice extract was used in European pharmacy in a similar way, as an external application for back pain,[480] and today, in Guatemala, the crushed fresh berries are still applied to treat bruising or alleviate muscle and joint pain.[481] In Costa Rican folk medicine, allspice leaf tea is drunk to treat diabetes, whereas in Jamaica it's principally used in the treatment of high blood pressure, colds, and to obtain relief from menstrual cramps.[482]

Another Warming herb, and occasional *cacahuatl* additive, was *macpalxochitl* or Devil's hand flower (*Chiranthodenron pentadactylon*). This plant was—and still is—used on its own to treat diarrhoea and insomnia, or mixed with other plants to treat epilepsy.[483] One Mexica prescription for "pubic pain" calls for three stones—obsidian, flint, and another unidentified rock—to be added to the juice of four herbs, including *macpalxochitl*, *toloaxihuitl* (*Datura innoxia*), and brambles (*Rubus fruticosus*), mixed with the blood of a swallow, a lizard, and a mouse. This mixture is to be warmed, then the liquid applied to the affected area.[484] The stones and animal blood have magical significance, but the three known herbs have clear pharmacological properties. *Datura* is a powerful antispasmodic pain-reliever, and both hand flower and brambles contain high levels of tannins, which are frequently used in botanical medicines to arrest secretions, dry tissues, and inhibit infectious microorganisms. Because tannins bind to proteins, the animal blood may have impaired the astringent properties of the brambles and hand flower in the gory unguent, although the powerful alkaloids in *Datura* no doubt made a significant contribution to its effects. The Mexica also cooked hand flower leaves with honey and applied them to haemorrhoids, or infused the flowers, leaves, and bark in water to make an eye wash[485]—and in these cases, the drying, anti-microbial, and anti-inflammatory properties of the compounds in the plant (discussed further in Chapter 6) are unimpeded by added proteins, and likely to have made a more noticeable contribution to any medicinal effects.

The seeds of the *mamey sapote* fruit, *Pouteria sapota*, are used in the beverage known as *tejate* in present-day Mexico, and the fibrous-crystalline-textured *mamey* fruits, somewhat resembling a cross between a melon and a mango with the skin of a baby lizard, are common in Central America today. The large, ovoid seeds are employed in Mexican folk medicine to make an oil to treat dandruff and hair loss;[486] the expressed seed oil is also applied to treat joint pain,[487] or taken internally as a diuretic.[488] The powdered seeds are used as a wound dressing,[489] and may be taken internally to treat kidney stones, arthritis, and as a preventive tonic for heart disease;[490] the leaf decoction is drunk to treat alcoholism.[491] Hernández mentions only the unrelated white sapote, *Casimiroa edulis* or *cochiztzapotl* in Nahuatl, and another tree he calls *quauhtzapotl* (identified as *Annona cherimolia*[492]), but not the *mamey*—which is odd, as the fruit originates from Central America.

The palm nuts known in Oaxaca as *guacoyules* are also sometimes used in *tejate*. These are the seeds of *Attalea cohune*, an indigenous palm variety, also not explicitly mentioned by Hernández, though he does reference another palm tree by the name of *coyolli*. His description of *coyolli* sounds like the African and Micronesian psychostimulant, the "Betel nut", actually the fruit of the Areca palm (*Areca catechu*)—Hernández says that *coyolli* is a tough-skinned nut with white, red, and dark spots inside, an astringent taste, and usually "a fifth part" of the seed is mixed with "half a part of the leaf of the plant called *buyo*" and, Hernández says, the two are carried about in the mouth by natives, staining the lips red, preventing bad odours in the mouth, comforting the stomach and the brain, and preventing vomiting due to Cold illnesses.[493] Areca nuts are sucked wrapped in the leaves of the betel vine (*Piper betle*)—hence the common name "betel nut"—and have similar effects, acting as a somewhat addictive stimulant, but they originate from Asia.[494] The *guacoyules* are from a different genus, and appear to lack the flavour, colour, and medicinal qualities of *coyolli*, but their similar-sounding name may have a common ancestral root.

Of the additives used in Cacao, the foaming agent known to the Mexica as *cozolmecatl* would become the most internationally famous and celebrated medicine, if only for a while. The plant goes by the names *cocolmeca* and *azquiote* or *axquiote* in present-day Mexico, and the reason for its fame was the extremely unpopular success of that other New World export, syphilis. *Cozolmecatl* is a *Smilax* or sarsaparilla species, possibly *Smilax aristolochiifolia*, but several *Smilax* species were, and are, used in medicine. While the young shoots are the part of the plant used to help Cacao or *pataxtle*-based beverages foam, it is the roots that are employed medicinally. The Mexica employed it in a magical formula to repel scabies, but it had a reputation as a Heating "blood cleanser" when taken internally, so it was used as a treatment for chronic skin problems and to help recovery from snakebite, as these conditions were thought to represent variations on a theme of "dirty blood" or "poisons in the blood". For similar reasons, *Smilax* was used as a treatment for gonorrhoea and syphilis in Europe, and was used to treat the latter problem from the late sixteenth to the nineteenth centuries.

Both Mexican sarsaparilla (*Smilax aristolochiifolia*) and oriental sarsaparilla (*Smilax glabra*) were used as anti-venereal medicines in Europe but their initial popularity waned, because effecting a complete cure required long seclusion, a strict diet, keeping warm, and chastity for weeks to months while taking the medicine.[495] Despite sarsaparilla's lack of side effects by comparison with the most widely used anti-syphilitic drug, mercuric chloride, the mercury salts were at least known to have some effects whatever you did, whereas sarsaparilla came to be seen as a chancy cure. It was still used medicinally until the invention of specific anti-syphilitic antibiotics in the twentieth century, but never regained its reputation as a powerful anti-syphilitic. *Smilax aristolochiifolia* roots are still used in Mexico to treat urinary tract and kidney problems, and employed more generally to treat rheumatic conditions and liver disease;[496] *Smilax* species roots are considered to be a specific treatment for psoriasis in European herbal medicine.[497] The Chinese classify *Smilax glabra* as a herb that "clears heat and relieves toxicity", and use it to remove "damp-heat from the skin", helping issues such as sores, other Hot skin lesions, as well as joint pain, jaundice, or symptoms of urinary tract infection,[498] which shows remarkable continuity with both European and Mexican traditional uses.

Like Old World Galenic-humoral medicine, native Mesoamericans categorised medicines on a Hot-Cold spectrum, and incorporated their use in magical and religious ritual contexts so that the plants' spiritual attributes augmented their physical effects—although in truth, the division between physio-chemical properties and magical virtues is a post-Cartesian concept that would have been alien to them. Despite the enormous theological differences between the pagan Mesoamericans and their Christian invaders, it wasn't too much of a stretch for the Europeans to fit Cacao and its botanical additives into their humoral classification and therapeutic system, particularly as they too believed in spiritual causes of disease and the natural magical properties of plants, minerals, and animals. After three hundred years of debate on the correct application of Cacao and its admixtures—what adjustments needed to be made for each season, stage of life, innate temperament, and different infirmities—Galenic-humoral theory was abandoned by the medical elite in favour of the new sciences of biology and chemistry, with their less subjective and more evidence-based experimental procedures and proofs.

Nevertheless, five hundred years after the conquest of Mexico, Cacao and many of its admixture plants are still used in Central and Latin American folk medical practices, and their manner of use is commonly a hybrid of the contemporary disease-drug model and traditional, magical, and temperature-based approaches: a Hot plant may be prescribed for anaemia or *susto*, a Cool plant applied to an angry-looking skin infection or used to wash away bad luck. Some of the more potent magico-pharmacological prescriptions of the past appear to have been forgotten, for good or ill; nobody is making psychoactive pastes of flowers and blood to smear exhausted politicians, police chiefs, or gangster bosses with—at least not openly, or (probably) literally. But the old ways remain relevant to daily living in many parts of Central America, and the value of seeing medicines as rebalancing agents and adjusters of temperature is that their use becomes less limited and more flexible; on the other hand, when a specific pharmacological property is revealed or confirmed by science—such as magnolia flowers' anti-arrhythmic effects on the heart[499]—then that's likely to become a key indication for prescribing the plant.

In practice, all forms of medicine combine qualitative information with objective facts to decide the best treatment. Despite our ancestors' very different ways of seeing the world and verifying those facts, practising the art of medicine at the highest level required the same qualities of observation, experience, and ingenuity. But with new technology came new truths—and the revelations of pharmacology, which would quantify and explain how medicines worked as never before. So, in the next chapter, we put Cacao under the microscope—or the chromatograph, to be exact.

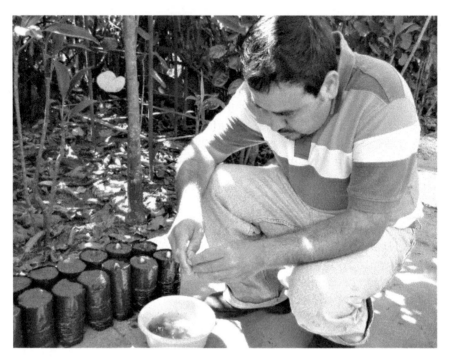

Juan-Pablo Porres Esquina sowing Cacao seeds at Don Angel's farm, San Antonio Suchitequepez, Guatemala, 2011

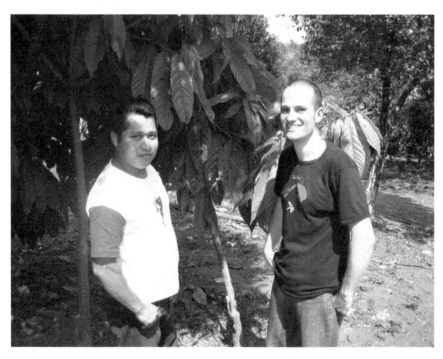

Curandero Diego and the author with Theobroma cacao tree, San Antonio Suchitequepez, Guatemala, 2011

CHAPTER FOUR

Pharmaceutical chocolate

"The pharmaceutical industry has spent tens, probably hundreds of millions of dollars in search of a chemical that would reverse ... [or ward off vascular diseases]. And God gave us flavonol-rich cocoa which does that."

(Norman Hollenberg, quoted in Paoletti et al., *Chocolate and Health*, 2012)

"Enumerate the parts of a carriage and you have not defined a carriage."

(excerpt from the *Tao Te Ching*, trans. McCarroll, 1982)

L ike most other medicinal plants and foods, Cacao contains an array of pharmacologically active chemicals. In the natural pharmacopoeia, there's no sharp division between foods and drugs; these distinctions are flexible, and often based on the use to which a plant is put—food or medicine—rather than its chemistry alone. Medicinal plants such as chamomile (*Chamomilla recutita*) or white willow bark (*Salix alba*) contain fewer toxic compounds than the poisonous leaves and shoots of the common potato plant (*Solanum tuberosum*), or other culinary staples such as cassava or manioc (*Manihot esculenta*), the tropical tuber which is a staple food in parts of South America and Africa, or kidney beans (*Phaseolus vulgaris*), which require soaking and thorough cooking to make them edible. Plants such as carrots, garlic, fennel, and barley have both edible and medicinal uses. Foods can have profound effects on health, positive or negative—witness research into the health-promoting effects of so-called "phytoestrogens" in soya beans, capillary-strengthening antioxidants in bilberries, and compounds in tomatoes and pumpkin seeds which retard the onset of prostate enlargement in men (amongst other things).[500]

Many interactions between plant and *Homo sapiens* chemistry are fundamentally important to human health or disease, such as the requirement for vitamin C from fruits and vegetables to prevent scurvy, or, on the flip side, the inherited sensitivity to gluten in some cereal crops which causes the digestive disorder known as coeliac disease, to name but two. These effects are a result of our co-evolution with plants. Plants are our primary and original source of food and medicine, as well as building material, paper, various fabrics, and dyes (to say nothing of oxygen); they have influenced us chemically, metabolically, environmentally, and behaviourally from the start. We are plant-interdependent organisms.

The point of all this is that the original Hippocratic maxim "let food be your medicine" is poorly understood in this pharmacophilic era. Population studies show that

> Cardio-vascular disease [CVD], including stroke, is the leading cause of death and disability in developed countries. [...] Diet is a major factor contributing to the onset and development of CVD [...] Defining specific modifications of dietary habits in a population can have a major impact on CVD, especially during the long period in which the disease is silent. (Galleano, Oteiza, & Fraga, 2010)

This is to say nothing of the presumed longer-term influence of diet and lifestyle on diabetes, cancer, senile dementia, or a host of other interlinked "Western" diseases of affluence. The bio-medical model's preventive strategy for dealing with these issues is to provide generic dietary and lifestyle advice (eat fruit and vegetables, don't smoke), or to use powerful, potentially harmful drugs to reduce single risk factors for specific health problems, leaving commercial enterprises to market various "alternative" novelty pills as unproven magic bullets for disease prevention in the form of the multi-million dollar vitamin and supplements industry.

Our pharmacophilic mentality originates in large part from the post-Paracelsan[vi] conceit that any medicinal plant is equivalent to its "main active principle", a notion which has been dis-proved time and again by clinical and pharmaceutical research into the effects of medicinal plants versus their chemical offspring. It now seems laughably simplistic to say of a plant, "This is the bit that makes it work—the rest of it's garbage," a bit like saying that apples are only vitamin C with packaging. It is naïve to dismiss some compounds as irrelevant on the basis that they are "inert" (they have no apparent pharmacological activity on their own) or "trace" (there's too little to have any biological relevance). The intricacies of metabolism may mean that what at first appears to be so much chemical filler actually turns out to influence the effect of the whole plant once ingested, by interacting with other compounds in the drug or in the living body (*"in vivo"*), sometimes in surprising ways. The most pharmaceutically active compounds produced by plants are referred to as "secondary metabolites", which were

> once regarded as simple waste products of a plant's metabolism. However this argument is weakened by the existence of specialist enzymes, strict genetic controls, and the high meta-bolic requirements of these compounds ... Today most scientists accept that many of these compounds serve primarily to repel grazing animals or destructive pathogens. (Pengelly, 2004)

Even this is a reductionist view. These compounds are so variable in type and quantity, from spe-cies to species and even intra-species, that is, from daisy to daisy, or nettle to nettle—depending

---

[vi]"After Paracelsus", aka Philippus Aureolus Theophrastus Bombastus von Hohenheim (1493–1591), the surgeon, alchemist, astrologer, and lecturer who is credited with originating the pharmaceutical obsession with using powerful and specific chemicals or drugs in medicine, as a result of his advocacy for mineral remedies and alchemically 'puri-fied' plant extracts. He was a notable empiric, despised tradition to the extent of publicly burning the collected medical works of Galen and Avicenna, and was one of the early pioneers of antisepsis in wound dressing, advocating cleanliness first and foremost in wound healing.

on the age and location of the plant, its growing conditions, and many other factors—that they represent a kind of pharmacological "fingerprint".

When medieval alchemists distilled volatile aromatic compounds from medicinal plants they characterised these so-called Essential Oils as the physical vehicle of the Soul or Spirit of the herb, because of their distinctive and penetrating smell, so intensely redolent of the source plant. In a similar way, secondary metabolites in general may be seen as a plant's "chemical character", its unique molecular personality profile. Their physical effects when ingested by different organisms are as much a product of their co-evolution with other species as the behavioural adaptations of humans and other animals to their environment, reflecting levels of interactive complexity in survival strategies which go far beyond chemical warfare. For example, plants such as the opium poppy or the Cacao tree which humans find useful may be cultivated, and this cultivation will often maximise production of those much-desired "secondary metabolites"—ensuring the plant species' survival, dissemination, and adaptation through involvement with the aggressively expansionist mammal, *Homo sapiens*. To what extent this may be thought coincidental when one can observe incredibly complex inter-species evolutionary survival tactics throughout nature is debatable.

So examining the chemistry of foods or medicines (and Cacao has a branch in both camps) can help us understand them further, as an aid to defining their nutritional or medicinal uses, as long as this pharmacognostic approach is used alongside traditional knowledge, and filtered by common sense. It also demonstrates very clearly the remarkable and irreproducible, irreducible complexity of natural pharmacy, and the need to evolve from our current medical-pharmaceutical model towards a more integrative and holistic approach.

Scientific objectivity, clinical research, and chocolate in action

"The placebo effect … one of the most powerful forces in our lives—the biological consequences of social, human, and meaningful interaction—[has] been tossed into the ash [*sic*] can." (Moerman, 2002)

Most research on medicinal plants and foods is limited to one condition, or focused on one outcome, such as blood pressure, pain, or whatever factor the researchers are interested in. The evidence-based medical research model for testing drugs begins with lab research (*in vitro*, meaning "in glass", i.e., in the laboratory), progresses to live test animals such as rats (*in vivo*—meaning "in life"), and—finally, if the substance is shown to be useful—in human clinical trials. The "gold standard" clinical trial model is the randomised double-blind placebo-controlled clinical trial. In these trials the substance or treatment in question is given to one group, another group is given a fake "placebo" treatment, and there is often a third group, the "control" group, which is given no treatment at all. The participants are matched in terms of participation criteria such as age, weight, sex, etc., then randomly split into groups. Most important, steps are taken so that neither the researchers nor the participants know who is taking the real treatment and who is taking the placebo until after the trial is over, to prevent the researchers accidentally or deliberately influencing the participants. This type of design is used to verify "real" effects of treatments, as most interventions will produce strong *placebo* or *nocebo* effects, that is, the belief of the participants—or the researchers—about who is receiving the "active" treatment will create some medicinal benefits (placebo) or unpleasant side effects (nocebo), so it's important to distinguish these *psychosomatic* (mind-body) effects from the "genuine", "objective" effects of a treatment.

Sometimes a double-blind trial isn't possible, for example if you were testing, for reasons best known to yourself, the effects of bungee jumping on hair growth—it can be hard to fake the real thing. In such cases, to give more reliable results, no placebo is used; instead, larger numbers of people may be recruited into the trial, all partaking of the "real" treatment, and compared to an equal-sized group of participants receiving no treatment at all. Because these "open" trials don't reduce the impact of the mind-over-matter placebo effect as much as double-blind trials, they often give stronger positive results for the treatment under scrutiny. But what tends to be forgotten is that this doesn't reduce the *practical* importance of positive results in less well controlled studies. Pragmatically, it doesn't matter if the effectiveness of a drug is pharmacological or psychological, so long as the results are *consistent* and *replicable*. Placebo is a fancy way of saying "genuine medical effects of non-pharmacological origin". What placebo does *not* mean is "ineffective". In his penetrating book on the placebo effect, Professor Daniel Moerman argues that the phrase "placebo effect" should be changed to "meaning effect", as the seemingly magical powers of placebo depend largely on the depth and nature of the cultural, symbolic, and emotional *meaning* which the treatment has for patients and therapists.[501]

The inner workings of the meaning (placebo) effect can be mind-blowing. In the case of angina, a condition where blood flow to the heart is restricted and causes chest pain, physicians who are enthusiastic about their treatment cure 70%—90% of their patients, whereas those who doubt its efficacy cure only 30%—40% of their patients, using identical treatments. Old drugs and surgical procedures become measurably less effective the moment new treatments come along. Advertising and branding increase the medicinal effectiveness of all drugs. The colour and shape of a pill alter its effects on people, and the nature and magnitude of effects vary in different locations and cultures. Placebo treatments produce measurable physical changes just like a "real" drug, such as opiate release (painkilling), and can cause other physical changes identical to a "real" drug, including side effects, and this can happen *even when patients are unaware that these effects would normally occur*. Simply including patients in a study—just putting them under observation—improves health outcomes. Patients with a view of plants or greenery from their hospital room have better recovery rates than patients with a plant-free hospital experience.[502] These are all examples of the meaning effect at work.

The "number needed to treat" in a placebo-controlled clinical trial of a pharmacologically effective drug varies, but the phrase refers to the number of patients who benefited in the group who received the "real drug" as compared to the "placebo"—and this number is often surprisingly small. It's thought that, like hypnosis, being susceptible to the placebo effect must depend on individual psychology or beliefs, perhaps to some sort of suggestibility or credulousness—but it turns out, that isn't the case, and all of us are equally susceptible to its benefits. What does matter, greatly, is the belief of the doctor or treatment administrator: as in the angina trial above, their degree of confidence will be mirrored in their results. The often remarked-upon "arrogance" of top surgeons, doctors, and charismatic therapists, it turns out, may be an essential ingredient of their success, and not simply because they are tirelessly (or tiresomely) self-promoting.[503] Placebo has become a dirty word; we of the modern, post-industrial world are so hung up on finding out how a medicine or procedure is "really working", that we sometimes minimise the most important matter, which is how well a given medicine or treatment works *in real life*.

Additionally, the biomedical model of drug testing—from lab, to animal, to human trials—sometimes misses important things. Say a plant is traditionally used in the treatment of cancer, and researchers apply an extract of that plant to some cancer cells in the laboratory, and it doesn't have any effect on them. The plant is then discarded, and not investigated any further. But what if that plant only produces effects on cancer in living human bodies, and doesn't act on cancer cells directly? It may work through secondary mechanisms, such as enhancing the immune response to specific cancer cells, or even more indirectly, by altering the composition of microbes in the gut which may in turn influence the immune response or produce cancer-retarding compounds. If cancer is an armed robber, the lab screening will find all the plants who are like trainee policemen. It won't detect the plants which are like surveillance camera operators, or like people who call the police to tell them a robbery is in progress, or like effective prosecution lawyers—only the ones which may eventually be directly involved in the process of stopping cancer, if they pass the tests!

So what, then? How are plants or substances that were traditionally used for a condition, but may not act directly, tested? In the current system, they often aren't. The issue of the questionable relevance of some research is public knowledge. Frankie Boyle said it well: "Shall we have a go at curing cancer? No. I'm going to see how many fruit pastilles it takes to choke a kestrel."

So reality isn't found in the artificially restricted conditions of a laboratory experiment or a clinical trial. "Evidence-based medicine" tests should be used as a method to help determine which of two treatments is *more effective*, and what *proportion* of a treatment's measurable benefit is down to the drug or procedure, in other words how much of its effectiveness depends on the meaning ("placebo") effect. Whether it's effective or not can simply be determined by a statistical analysis of a given treatment's real-life performance: whether the majority of patients so treated feel better and live longer, or not. Put over-simply, randomised double-blind placebo-controlled clinical trials reveal how much of a given medicine's effect is mind over matter—aka the *vis medicatrix naturae*, nature's inherent healing power, or the sum total of reparative psychobiological processes—which we call "placebo". The medical reality is to be found in the real world, under real conditions, in which the perceived character and symbolic qualities of all medical interventions of any kind are integral to their effectiveness.

We also know that drug plants are complex entities, producing complex effects. The chemicals in a substance such as Cacao can interact in the body in several ways. Some compounds of plant origin may not be found in the whole plant at all, but are created in the human body from the original plant chemicals; these original compounds may be utterly transformed by metabolic processes in the digestive system or liver, or by some of the billions of microscopic organisms living in the gut, for example. Very simply put, the different pharmacologically active compounds in a single medicinal plant can inhibit, enhance, or do nothing at all to affect how they work together. Enhancement can occur in two ways: it can be *additive*, meaning that chemicals simply add their effect to one another (1+1 = 2), or it can be *synergistic*, meaning that the total effect of the two chemicals is far greater than would have been expected (1+1 = 11). Likewise, they can inhibit each other by *antagonism*—they simply cancel each other out, one activates and the other deactivates (1+ –1 = 0)—or by *competitive inhibition*, where both chemicals are trying to do the same job in the same place at the same time and they get in each other's way, like two footballers on one team trying to kick the ball simultaneously and tripping each other up (1–1 = 0). So the overall effect of a medicinal or pharmacologically active plant in the body is the result of how all its constituents work together. In other words, every plant has a sort of chemical personality, and where the "ingredients" all mesh well as regards a particular action on human physiology, they can produce noticeable effects. Because of this complexity, most medicinal plants alter bodily functions with brush strokes and mixed colours, rather than the relatively straight lines and primary colours of pharmaceuticals.

Cacao, too, contains many different compounds, which contribute to its nutritional profile, its flavour, and its medicinal effects. So to attain a better understanding of chocolate, we will look at the chemical composition of Cacao and its botanical accomplices.

Filleting the bean

Before enumerating Cacao's parts, we should keep in mind that looking at individual substances from any natural product is often quite misleading, because there are so many compounds in one plant (or animal, for that matter). Not all of the chemicals in Cacao will be absorbed from the human digestive tract, depending how the bean is ingested, and not all of those which are absorbed will remain chemically active for very long once the liver does its work; and some will enhance or inhibit the absorption or effectiveness of others. How, in what form, and when the Cacao is consumed will also influence matters, as (most importantly) will the state of the organism consuming it: for example, whether they have a full or empty stomach, what else they have recently eaten or drunk, their age, weight, sex, baseline mood, etc.

Clinical science gets round this problem by using statistics and controlled conditions to arrive at average outcomes and attain consistent, reproducible data for each component, disregarding "anomalous" results. Averages and controlled situations don't always reflect reality though, otherwise all Western adults would be married and live in a semi-detached house with 2.5 children and half a pet with a stable income of whatever the current national bell curve suggests. As described in the last chapter, traditional medical systems account for individual differences by observing and classifying different plants, people, illnesses, ages, times of year/day, etc. in terms of their different characteristics, in order to predict outcomes and guide treatments, but often do so in allegorical, empirical ways, such as describing particular organs of the body or foods or drugs as Hot and Dry or Cold and Wet, or making connections between illnesses and the time of year, the weather, or personal temperament. The drawback of such traditional medical systems is that inappropriate or ineffectual treatments are harder to spot, because they are based on subjective results which can depend on many different factors, and are concerned only with individual outcomes, not with statistical evidence. Nevertheless it should be recognised that from a real-world, individual perspective, reality is much more idiosyncratic than statistics suggest. With this caveat, the chemical compounds in Cacao seeds are to be analysed using the following categories:

- **Pharmacodynamics (pD)**—what they do in the body
- **Pharmacokinetics (pK)**—how well they're absorbed and distributed around the body, and what factors affect this, and
- **Interactions**, which may be synergistic, additive, or inhibitory.

For a detailed account, please see the monograph in Appendix A: this chapter will gloss and summarise the findings, so as to be more digestible. After that, it will be useful to look at other plants used alongside Cacao in traditional chocolate drinks, and how they are likely to affect each other's pharmaceutical activities and the overall quality of these preparations. Some of the conclusions are speculative and based on a combination of observation, known chemistry and pharmacology, anecdotal reports, and logical deductions, *in lieu* of comprehensive clinical data; but, as the saying might as well go, you can't make chocolate without shelling a few beans.

Cacao chemistry

Chocolate chemistry, like that of many natural products, is extremely complex. Cacao contains a large number of biologically active and bioavailable compounds ("bioavailability" refers to the capacity for a substance, whether nutrient, drug, or toxin, to be absorbed and reach its site of action or use in the body, the "target tissue"). When human volunteers' urine was analysed 24 hours after consuming chocolate,

> 27 metabolites related to cocoa-phytochemicals, including alkaloid derivatives, polyphenol metabolites (both host and microbial metabolites), and processing-derived products such as diketopiperazines were identified. (Paoletti et al., 2012)

Translating the pharma-jargon, this tells us that many of the various plant chemicals ("phyto-chemicals") in Cacao had made their way through the body, some of what remained was still being excreted in the urine twenty-four hours later, and many of the chemicals were created by microbes in the human gut, using the chemicals in the plant.[504] In other words, the eventual effects of Cacao, or of any medicinal plant, are not only dependent on the chemicals the original drug contains, but on the complex array of chemicals produced by our bodies, and the smaller microbial bodies inhabiting them.

The following chart is a visual representation of the different groups of chemical compounds found in toasted Cacao seeds.

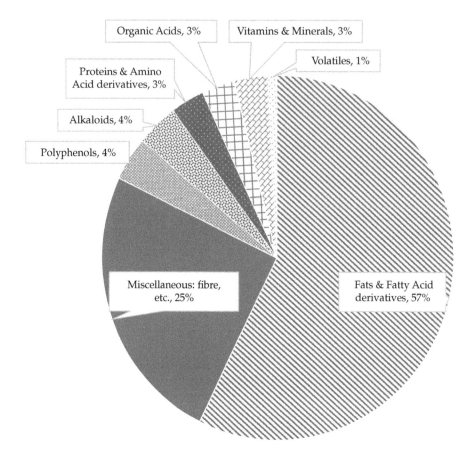

Figure 2. Approximate chemical composition of toasted *Theobroma Cacao* seeds, as % dry weight.

Over half of the seeds are composed of fats and related substances, with approximately 15%–25% carbohydrate (standardised to 18% in Figure 2)—these carbohydrates are "fibre" such as cellulose and pectin, and naturally occurring sugars. This "filler" may still affect the properties of the seed once ingested, by modifying the absorption of other constituents, or providing food for gut microbes. The more pharmacologically "active" material—the alkaloids, polyphenols, amino acid-based compounds, organic acids, vitamins, and minerals—comprise up to a third of the seeds' dry weight.

Bulking: fats and miscellaneous constituents

The combination of fatty acids in Cacao, collectively referred to as "cocoa butter", has the useful property of being liquid at body temperature but solid below 25° Celsius (77° Fahrenheit), enabling chocolatiers to produce chocolate that melts in your mouth (or your hand, or your pocket, or on a hot day). Fats are calorie-dense, and provide some rationale for Cacao's traditional reputation as a food-drug for weight gain and convalescence. Approximately 34%

of Cacao's fat content is made up of "bad" saturated fats, the kind linked to heart disease—except in this case, just over half that is *stearic acid*, a type of saturated fat which lowers "bad" LDL cholesterol. When applied to the skin of tortured mice, stearic acid sped up the healing of burns,[505] which corroborates the traditional usage of cocoa butter for healing damaged skin. The remainder comprises "heart-healthy" mono- and poly-unsaturates. It should be noted that the fatty acids in cocoa butter tended to increase blood coagulation and blunt insulin sensitivity in the lab, effects which are outweighed by the potency of Cacao's polyphenols. Nevertheless this is another good argument for consuming traditional Cacao beverages rather than eating chocolate bars, with their added fat content.

The fatty portion of the seeds also contains a small quantity (about 0.2%) of *phytosterols*, hormone-like compounds which help to prevent several types of cancers and reduce cholesterol absorption from the intestines. The quantity of these compounds in Cacao is not exceptionally high, but 20mg of the phytosterol *β-sitosterol* taken three times daily, equivalent to the amount found in 40–80g Cacao seeds (comparable to the daily dose found in high-potency Cacao beverages), has been found to reduce the symptoms of prostate enlargement in older men.[506] These compounds also improve immunity and reduce the immediate stress effects of hard exercise on the body and the immune system.[507] A tiny proportion of Cacao's fats are made up of compounds called *phospholipids*, which are surfactants (a kind of emulsifier, or "soap", which helps make water-soluble compounds more fat-soluble, and vice versa). These phospholipids, though small in quantity, increase the absorption and effectiveness of some of the polyphenols in Cacao[508]—another example of how the pharmacological actions of a drug plant are the sum of its parts.

Buffering: polyphenols

"One serving of dark chocolate is thought to impart a greater antioxidant capacity than the average amount of antioxidants consumed daily in the United States." (Castell et al., from Watson et al., 2013, my italics)

Much has been made of Cacao's "antioxidant" properties, resident in the *polyphenols*, a group of compounds which collectively comprise about 4% of the toasted beans' weight. Antioxidant properties are measured by a scale called oxygen radical absorbance capacity (ORAC), and polyphenols are a large group made up of tannins (sour- and dry-tasting molecules which make the inside of your mouth pucker when you drink black tea without milk) and many smaller compounds. Chocolate contains the highest weight of polyphenols in any food,[509] and freshly prepared un-Dutched cocoa powder (the powdered and de-fatted bean) has a higher ORAC level by far than blueberries, red wine, and many other foods.[510] But the antioxidant effects of Cacao, which are often touted as its main benefit, should be viewed with caution—because many of the medicinal effects of the polyphenols in Cacao may turn out to be independent of their antioxidant properties *per se*.

"Antioxidant" is a bit of a sloppy generic term for a very wide range of natural and synthetic substances, all of which share that one common feature but may be quite different in terms of their effects in the living human organism. Antioxidants are substances that mop up *free radicals*. Despite the name, free radicals are not in fact tiny Che Guevaras; they are molecules with missing electrons. This means they lack one negatively charged particle, and are electrically unbalanced, so they steal electrons from other atoms to stabilise themselves. Free radicals are generated like dirty smoke by ordinary cellular activity, causing damage as they rip electrons away from other atoms and ultimately destabilise the cells those atoms are part of; they degrade cell structure "one brick at a time". Antioxidants are substances with spare electrons, so they donate an electron to a hungry free radical, and rebalance it.

A theory called *mitohormesis* proposes that free radicals (or "reactive oxygen species" [ROS], to give them their proper name) are actually necessary to promote long life. By acting as stressors produced by the engine of the cell (the *mitochondria*, after which the theory is named), free radicals/ROS induce the cell's energy production to become more efficient.[511] Just as oysters make pearls as a result of the irritation produced by grains of sand, so the mitochondria require just enough—and not too much—free radical activity to prolong the cell's life. So seeing free radicals only as "bad guys" to be zapped by antioxidants is too simplistic.

Cacao compounds exert antioxidant activity in several ways: they directly neutralise free radicals by donating an extra electron to them in the usual way; they inhibit enzymes which produce reactive oxygen species (a type of free radical); and they "chelate metal ions"—in other words, attaching themselves to little electrically charged metal atoms and smothering their charge, like little brown fire blankets. Some other compounds in Cacao, the xanthine alkaloids (theobromine, caffeine, and theophylline) play a role here too, as they are also metal ion chelators.[512] The theory goes that the antioxidants in Cacao neutralise free radicals and promote release of nitric oxide from the linings of blood vessels, causing them to dilate, and improving blood flow.[513] In fact these effects are all mediated by very specific sequences of interactions between particular polyphenols and enzymes in the body; you couldn't just chuck some "antioxidant-rich" blueberry/acai/whatever juice into a blood vessel and expect exactly the same effect. One example of this is the well-researched flavonoid (a type of polyphenol) called epicatechin, found at high levels in Cacao and green tea. Epicatechin protects heart cells from injury not by antioxidant means, but by binding to opiate (endorphin) receptors in the heart, which blocks some injury-causing chemical chain reactions that occur when cells are deprived of oxygen.[514]

We do know that Cacao, once eaten, significantly increases the antioxidant level and reduces lipid (fat) oxidation in the blood, which is generally good: this indicates that Cacao most likely counteracts tendencies to *atherosclerosis*, or "furring up" of arteries and blood vessels, and may therefore reduce the risk of developing heart disease. But, interestingly, excessively high levels of Cacao flavanols can become *pro-oxidant*, especially in the presence of metals which react with oxygen (any metal which tarnishes or rusts, e.g., iron or copper). This fact will become especially relevant when looking at possible links between Cacao and Parkinson's disease in Chapter 7. Moreover, some studies showed that Cacao appeared to have significant health benefits, even in the absence of any obvious antioxidant effects.[515] This also suggests that the undoubtedly high antioxidant capacity of Cacao may not be directly related to its health benefits; the fact that some of Cacao's most "health-promoting" compounds may turn out to be antioxidants doesn't necessarily suggest that Cacao can be substituted with other high-antioxidant foods or substances in the expectation of achieving the same results, just as forcing a vet to stand in for a professional lion tamer may not go well, even if they are both used to handling cats.

The greater proportion of Cacao's polyphenols (see Figure 3 below) is made up of *lignin*, a form of indigestible fibre which helps to feed good bacteria in the gut. Lignin is a common compound found in many types of plant material, which probably exerts few direct effects, although some anti-viral activity has been noted in the laboratory.[516] Of the remainder, the procyanidins and flavan-3-ols are the subject of intense research. *Criollo* Cacao (the "posh" variety, traditionally used by the Maya and Mexica) contains no *proanthocyanidins*, red-purple compounds which break down to yield smaller *procyanidins*, but it does contain high levels of *flavanols* (technically, flavan-3-ols) and the procyanidins themselves, so its antioxidant properties are the same, in effect, as the other varieties with higher levels of polyphenols and the sourer-tasting proanthocyanidins.[517] Cacao polyphenols as a whole, if consumed regularly, have been shown to prevent or delay the development of several types of cancer in animal experiments, including prostate cancer in rats, at levels of intake which may be achievable with traditional Cacao beverages.[518] The polyphenols also increased lab animals' lifespans, improved their memories, protected them from heart disease, lung damage, and peptic ulceration, and reduced clotting risks.

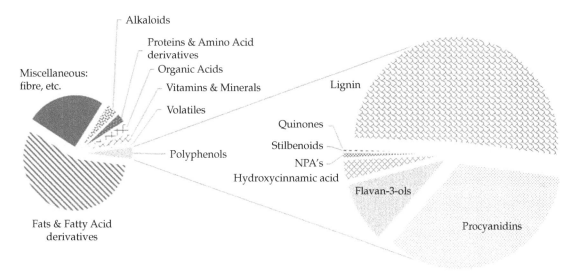

Figure 3. The polyphenols in *Theobroma Cacao* seeds.

In addition to being associated with a reduced risk of heart disease and stroke in humans, the flavanols may also improve cognition. In animal studies, they accumulate in parts of the brain associated with learning and memory, and in human studies, higher levels of dietary flavanol intake are linked to better brain function in aging and age-related diseases such as dementia and stroke.[519] Lab research into the procyanidins show potential anti-cancer activity, and complex, modulatory effects on the immune system and inflammation.[520] Lab and animal research suggests that the flavanols in Cacao also reduce inflammation, alter immune system protection of the lining of the airways and digestive tract, enhance levels of "happy" brain chemicals such as dopamine and phenethylamine by reducing the rate at which they are broken down, protect the heart, thin the blood like aspirin, and reduce the risk of developing gum disease.[521] These compounds have been shown to get into the system after ingesting Cacao, and blood levels peak two hours after consumption.[522]

Many of the smaller polyphenols such as the flavanols and procyanidins are manufactured from larger molecules (*flavonoids* and proanthocyanidins, respectively) by gut microbes, so the exact effects of whole chocolate in each person's case will be modified by the state of their digestive tract. The terrain of the gut, as is often the case, influences the effect of the medicine— and vice versa, as the polyphenols' effects on immunity and the gut lining will affect the microbes living there. However, milk almost halves the level of Cacao flavanols detectable in the bloodstream after consuming chocolate, because the proteins in milk bind to the polyphenols and reduce their absorption. Conversely, sugars and starches increased their absorption significantly[523]—although added sugars (glucose, fructose, sucrose, honey, or even fruit juices) are known to reduce the immune response for several hours after consumption (specifically, the ability of some "first-line" immune cells, white blood cells known as neutrophils, to ingest or "phagocytose" bacteria is suppressed for several hours following the consumption of these sugars, an effect which doesn't occur with whole fruit).[524] On the other hand, complex carbohydrates such as *masa harina* flour will break down and yield sugars in the gut, where they may assist the absorption of Cacao polyphenols, while also providing beneficial insoluble fibre to feed "friendly bacteria" in the large intestine—without flooding the system with free sugars, which may spike insulin, reduce immunity, and encourage the overgrowth of less beneficial gut microorganisms. Yet more reasons to take chocolate without milk and with only complex carbohydrates such as maize, or with very little added sugar, in the traditional Mesoamerican style.

Some of Cacao's trace polyphenols, such as *caffeic acid*, also help to protect liver and blood vessel cells from injury,[525] and the *phenolic acids*—formed during fermentation of the bean—may provide some protection for the pancreas (the organ which controls blood sugar), the stomach lining, the heart, and the kidneys, and contribute to Cacao's pain-reducing and anti-inflammatory properties[526] if the lab results and animal experiments are anything to go by. The *hydroxycinnamic acids* in Cacao have similar effects in the test tube, reducing blood sugar, protecting immune cells, and brain cells, and liver cells from injury.[527] However, the principal hydroxycinnamic acid in Cacao, *chlorogenic acid*, may also inhibit vitamin B1 (thiamine) absorption from foods when Cacao is consumed with them, although this is disputed.[528] Trace compounds known as *NPAs* (N-phenyl-propanoyl-l-amino acids, to give them their full title) also protect brain cells from injury, reduce blood clotting and inflammation, and dilate the airways.[529] Pharmacologically active levels of NPAs have been found in the bloodstream of humans two hours after eating chocolate.[530]

The *stilbenoids* include the well-researched *resveratrol*, red wine's much trumpeted "miracle" health-promoting compound. Resveratrol raises the level of stimulating brain chemicals such as dopamine and phenethylamine by preventing their breakdown (of which more later), but its predicted anti-aging, brain- and heart-protecting, and anti-cancer properties from results in the lab don't seem to translate well to real-life trials using the isolated compound.[531] That said, resveratrol administered to human volunteers over a one-year period in combination with other polyphenols did reduce blood markers of inflammation.[532] So it's possible that the stilbenoids in Cacao have measurable effects in conjunction with the other phenolics, even though the amount is small. While there are very tiny, sub-active amounts of *quinones* in Cacao, these substances have the rare property of being able to rejuvenate old cells by stimulating the mitochondria—the cell's energy-producing battery—to repair themselves, and have been shown to reduce harmful effect of stress in humans.[533] It's unknown how all these compounds interact, but it's striking that many have similar effects, and the possibility of these effects "stacking up" and adding up to something considerable is very real, particularly if the results from human trials with whole chocolate, detailed later in this chapter, are anything to go by.

Accelerating: alkaloids

One of the most notable (and popular) groups of compounds in Cacao are in the class known as alkaloids, so named because these molecules contain nitrogen, giving them an alkaline pH. They're popular because they're principally responsible for Cacao's stimulating, mood-lifting effect, though there are other components at work here, too. Alkaloids are found in (and extracted from) many other world-famous recreational plant drugs such as coca leaf, coffee, khat, kratom, opium, tea, and tobacco, although alkaloids in general are a very diverse group of chemicals: not all plants that contain alkaloids affect the brain, and not all chemicals that affect the brain are alkaloids. The alkaloids comprise around 4% of the weight of toasted Cacao, neck-and-neck with polyphenols (see Figure 4).

The primary alkaloids in Cacao are the three so-called *xanthine alkaloids*, theobromine, caffeine, and theophylline, plus a sprinkling of other trace compounds—salsolinol, the tetrahydro-beta-carbolines (THβC's), the pyrazines, and trigonelline. Of these, *caffeine* is the most stimulating, acting by blocking a sedative brain messenger (neurotransmitter) called adenosine so that "signal amplification" occurs in various parts of the brain. Caffeine is partly responsible for many of Cacao's mind-altering effects, as lower doses (up to 250mg), such as may be found in coffee, tea, or a real chocolate drink, generally increase feelings of sociability, confidence, and good mood, raise pain thresholds, and provide a weak generalised stimulation to the pleasure and habit-forming regions of the brain. Caffeine enhances the action of the brain chemical *dopamine* in these areas, which generates both pleasure and motivation. Despite this, only lower doses of

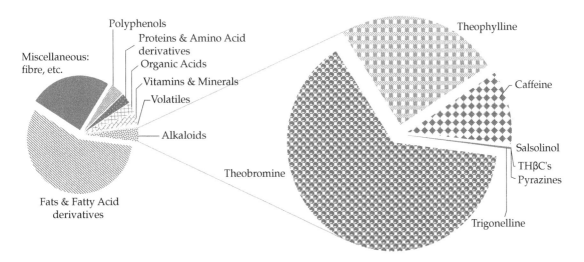

Figure 4. The alkaloids in *Theobroma Cacao* seeds.

caffeine (such as those found in Cacao) resemble the effects of more powerful dopamine-releasing drugs such as cocaine or amphetamine in the principal brain region involved, the *nucleus accumbens*. Higher doses of caffeine—as anyone who has overdone the coffee can testify—don't have such a pleasurable effect, and end up making the user feel uncomfortably overstimulated, anxious, and jittery. In science lingo, higher doses of caffeine become aversive.

Cacao contains around 0.2% caffeine,[534] but a 40g dose of Cacao seed which may be consumed in a traditional Cacao-based beverage contains 84mg of caffeine, greater than the amount in a cup of tea. *Criollo* Cacao beans, the variety of Cacao with the longest pedigree, and still the preferred variety for chocolate connoisseurs and makers of traditional chocolate drinks, contain more caffeine than *forasteros*.[535] One might assume that varieties of psychoactive plants are appreciated on the basis of the quantity of the most potent psychoactive compound they contain, as seems to be the case with Cacao, where the higher-caffeine *criollo* is preferred to *forastero*. But this is often not the case; khat (*Catha edulis*) chewers from Somalia favour tender green-leafed khat over the stronger, higher-cathinone water-stressed "red" varieties; South American coca leaf aficionados prefer the lower-cocaine Peruvian *Erythrolylum novogranatense* to the Bolivian *Erythroxylum coca*; in Fiji and Vanuatu, milder but more pleasurable varietals of kava kava (*Piper methysticum*) are preferred to super-strong, high-kavalactone types such as the "tudei" cultivar (so-called because it knocks users out for two days); and in China and Japan, green, white, or fermented *pu-erh* teas (*Camellia sinensis*) may be preferred to black tea varieties, with variable levels of caffeine. In many cases the more esteemed varieties often contain lower levels of the so-called principal active constituents, but higher levels of other constituents which modify the drug's action—such preferences are dictated by perceived quality of effects, flavour, and tradition, rather than "strength" of stimulation, as measured by one compound only.

Xanthine alkaloids act as "positive reinforcers", meaning that they increase taste preferences for foods or beverages which contain them,[536] and caffeine is the most potent of the three. Even though it's often assumed that Cacao products, such as cocoa or chocolate, are not strongly stimulating, even 12.5mg of caffeine from only 8g Cacao, the amount found in a 25g bar of milk chocolate, has been shown to noticeably affect human behaviour.[537] Caffeine can increase anxiety, and actually reduces blood flow to the brain up to 30%, while simultaneously increasing brain activity. Despite this, longer-term low caffeine intake has been linked to reduced incidence of depression, and adaptation to its use means caffeine habitués move around *less* than those who don't use it at all. Caffeine levels peak in the bloodstream approximately thirty minutes after ingestion, and its stimulating effects are blunted by sugar.[538] Caffeine habituation also produces a well-known withdrawal syndrome on breaking the habit, with headache, lethargy, and low mood which can last for up to two weeks unless caffeine is consumed again.

At 1.2% of the seed's weight, *theobromine* is the most plentiful alkaloid in Cacao. It's also produced in the body as a breakdown product of caffeine. Theobromine is a stimulant, but people's sensitivity to it varies much more than with caffeine; it may even decrease caffeine's stimulating properties, although it makes no difference to caffeine's effect on mood.[539] Theobromine's effects on the heart (increasing the rate and force of the pulse) and the kidneys (increasing urination) are stronger than its effects on the brain, and it dose-dependently increases heart rate.[540] It also has the interesting property of strengthening tooth enamel.[541] Theobromine weakens some cancer cells—most strikingly, a highly aggressive form of brain cancer called glioblastoma—and helps to protect blood vessels.[542] In this regard, its actions complement those of the polyphenols in Cacao. However, high doses of theobromine can also damage the testes and inhibit sperm production, and may suppress immune function;[543] high intakes have been linked to prostate cancer in older men.[544] Theobromine also reacts with copper to produce cell-damaging free radicals.[545] Although Cacao's highly antioxidant, cell-protecting polyphenols may reverse and offset these effects, high intakes of cocoa powder (5% of the diet) have been shown to cause fertility problems in male rats,[546] so this issue should not be ignored. Like the flavanols, theobromine levels peak in the bloodstream approximately two hours after ingesting Cacao.

The third sister xanthine alkaloid to caffeine's Diana Ross is *theophylline*, comprising 0.4% of the seed. Theophylline is more stimulating than theobromine, but less so than caffeine. It does have a few unique effects though—it reduces coughing, dilates the airways, and increases the anti-inflammatory potency of steroid drugs,[547] so it's sometimes used as a medicinal drug in the treatment of asthma. It also dilates the blood vessels in the heart.[548] It has some anti-cancer effects in the lab, which may not translate to real life, but it has been shown to increase the potency of the chemotherapy drug Doxorubicin.[549] Incorporating Cacao or tea (both of which plant-drugs contain theophylline) into the diet while undergoing Doxorubicin-containing chemotherapy treatments or implementing cancer prevention strategies may be a good idea in general, as discussed later in this chapter.

Finally, there is a sprinkling of trace alkaloidal compounds in Cacao, each comprising a fraction of a percentage of the seed. Many of these trace compounds are produced by microbial action during fermentation, or by roasting the seeds, and may be found in other aged, fermented, or roasted foods, such as cheese or coffee. The quantity is small, but tiny doses don't always mean tiny results—if the compounds make it into the brain, or combine their effects with other chemicals, or build up over time, their effects can be disproportionate. These trace alkaloids are shown in Figure 5, below, as the amount found in a 40g serving of Cacao. The doses really are miniscule: to give a sense of scale, a 1mg dose is smaller than a grain of fine

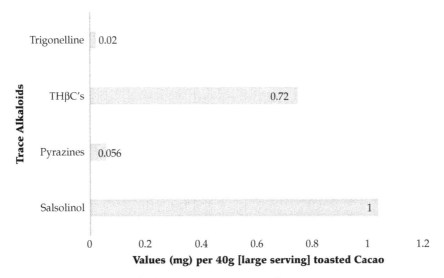

Figure 5. Trace alkaloids in toasted *Theobroma Cacao* seeds.

sand. Although, it should be noted that the strength of the individual chemicals is of enormous importance: 1mg of LSD, for example, is extremely potent.

The most plentiful of these trace alkaloids is *salsolinol*, amounting to 1mg in every 40g of Salsolinol is a trace alkaloid found in small but appreciable amounts in fermented Cacao seed (and presumably less in partially fermented varieties, such as Cacao *lavado*). Salsolinol is produced by microbes during fermentation of the seeds, and is also present in white wine and some aged cheeses, such as emmenthal.[550] Salsolinol easily crosses into the brain from the bloodstream, and has been noted to build up in nerve cells in the brain, so may have cumulative effects. It inhibits the breakdown of stimulating brain chemicals such as dopamine and noradrenaline (norepinephrine), and greatly enhances the release of the stimulating brain chemical glutamate (of which more shortly). Salsolinol is also manufactured by dopamine-releasing cells in the brain when there are high levels of ketones or aldehydes in the bloodstream, as may occur with carbohydrate-restricted diets, fasting or starvation, alcoholism, and diabetes.

Salsolinol strongly activates dopamine-releasing nerve cells in an area of the brain which plays a role in habituation and addiction,[551] so it's possible that the weak habit-reinforcing properties of caffeine may be shored up by the addition of salsolinol to Cacao's alkaloid cocktail. Interestingly, salsolinol's effects on dopamine-producing cells are strongest at very low concentrations, and taper off as the dose increases,[552] and it has been shown to accumulate in the same cells. Salsolinol may also reduce the release of endorphins (opioids) in the brain over time, causing a gradual anhedonia or loss of pleasure, as in chronic alcoholism.[553] But in the presence of endorphins or opiates, salsolinol may enhance the release of a hormone called *prolactin*,[554] which induces lactation in breastfeeding women (from the Latin *pro lactis*, "for milk"), and has a complex role to play as a brain messenger hormone in social bonding.

It's currently not possible to know exactly how much salsolinol contributes to Cacao's physical and mental effects—especially as the mental effects have, so far, only been crudely studied (as we will see in Chapter 5). Given that salsolinol is found in other non-mind-altering foods such as sardines, we may assume it has little relevance. However, we know that it has stronger effects at lower concentrations, and that it makes its way into the brain. We also know that other compounds in Cacao affect dopamine and opiate release at specific sites in the brain (polyphenols, xanthines, and other trace constituents). This means that the small but measurable quantity of salsolinol in each dose of Cacao could hypothetically be contributing to the effects of the whole drug by subtly modulating the action of other constituents, especially over time, as it builds up in dopamine-releasing cells. In the presence of heavy metals, however, salsolinol is converted into a toxic compound which damages these same dopamine-producing cells, and has been linked to the movement disorder, Parkinson's disease.[555] This issue will be further discussed in Chapter 7.

The next alkaloidal supporting cast members worthy of mention are the *tetrahydro-beta-carboline* alkaloids, or THβCs, and *trigonelline*. Like salsolinol, THβCs are products of fermentation, occur in many other foods, and can be manufactured in the human brain. Also like salsolinol, THβCs have been found to strengthen opiate and alcohol dependency in primates and rats in lab experiments,[556] activating dopamine and opiate signals in the brain,[557] and several THβCs inhibit the breakdown of the "happy" brain chemical serotonin, although the precise activities of the THβCs in Cacao are unknown. Presumably the THβCs and salsolinol act on the same brain circuitry controlling motivation and habit formation. So although present in very small quantities, these compounds could be acting in tandem to modify Cacao's effect on the brain. Closely related compounds called beta-carbolines are known to be strongly psychoactive, and some THβCs may be converted into beta-carbolines following ingestion, although this is currently uncertain.

Beta-carbolines are also found in coffee beans (another fermented, caffeine-containing seed)—but the types and quantity of THβCs per serving is different (see Table 2, below). Many THβCs are known to activate areas of the brain associated with pain relief and psychedelic responses. *Trigonelline* is present in Cacao at very low levels, and is produced from ingested niacin (vitamin B3, also found in Cacao seeds), and helps lower cholesterol and blood sugar. It also ferries the mood-elevating compound phenethylamine directly into the brain—on which subject, more to come …

Table 2. Relative beta-carboline and THβC alkaloid content in coffee and Cacao

β-Carbolines in toasted Cacao:		*β-Carbolines in roasted coffee beans:*	
Absolute:	Large serving size (40g prepared beans in approx. 60ml water)	Absolute:	Large serving size (Grande size coffee = 16oz)
0.87–7.86mcg/g beans	0.03–0.72mg	0.21mg/L prepared coffee	≤ 0.1mg
Including:		Including:	
• 6-Hydroxy-1-methyl-1,2,3,4-tetrahydro-β-carboline • 1,2,3,4-tetrahydro-β-carboline-3-carboxylic acid • 1S,3S-1-methyl-1,2,3,4-tetrahydro-β-carboline-3-carboxylic acid • 1R,3S-1-methyl-1,2,3,4-tetrahydro-β-carboline-3-carboxylic acid • 1-methyl-1,2,3,4-tetrahydro-β-carboline		• 9H-β-carboline (Norharman) • 7-Methoxy-1-methyl-9H-pyrido [3,4]-β-carboline (Harman)	

Provisioning: proteins, amino acids, and derivatives

Proteins and related compounds (see Figure 6 below) comprise around 11% of the fermented, toasted and dried seeds. Some of Cacao's proteins do have interesting anti-tumour activity in lab experiments,[558] although whether this translates to similar action in the human body is unknown. The proteins and their constituent amino acids—the bricks from which proteins are made—mainly have nutritional value, forming the building blocks for tissue and hormones and other materials the body needs to function. If free amino acids are like individual Lego® bricks, proteins are like large structures made of Lego®. The ratio of free amino acids in any food can 'push' the body towards greater production of particular proteins and compounds, much as an excess of yellow Lego® bricks and relatively few red, blue, or green ones will result in the finished Lego® projects being mostly yellow.

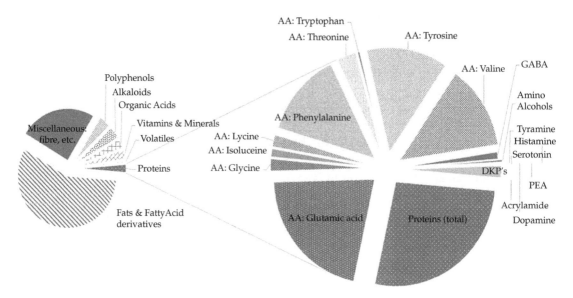

Figure 6. Breakdown of amine-based compounds in *Theobroma Cacao* seeds.

Cacao's prinicpal amino acids are *glutamic acid, phenylalanine, tyrosine,* and *valine.* Interestingly, three of these are building blocks for stimulating brain chemicals or 'neurotransmitters': glutamic acid is used to make glutamate, a common, stimulating neurotransmitter; phenylalanine is used to make the mood-raising nuerotransmitter phenylethylamine, and is converted into tyrosine if need be. Tyrosine is used to make the amines dopamine, adrenaline (epinephrine), and noradrenaline (see below). Of the four amino acids, valine and phenylalanine are essential— they can't be manufactured in the body, and have to be eaten—and Cacao contains a very high level of phenylalanine, in particular. In other words, the cocktail of amino acids in Cacao is particularly suited to the creation of stimulating and mood-raising compounds.

Amino acids themselves are made up of *amines,* many of which are used as chemical messengers in the brain. These include *dopamine, serotonin, tyramine, phenethylamine [PEA],* and *histamine.* Their effect when eaten all mixed together in food is thought to be negligible, although their relative quantities in a food or drug, and the co-presence of other compounds can affect how they are absorbed and distributed in the body and increase their pharmacological potency. Mood-raising serotonin and stimulating, inflammatory histamine in Cacao are present at very low levels relative to the other amines, although Cacao is quite high in histamine in comparison with other foods. As a result of both its histamine content and having the capacity to promote histamine release, Cacao is a known trigger of nettle rash or *urticaria* in some people,[559] a condition where itching and heat in the skin can occur spontaneously. The condition is named after *Urtica* plant species, commonly known as nettles, as nettle stings contain a cocktail of chemicals including histamine and serotonin. Most people can eat chocolate without experiencing this unpleasant side effect, but it's possible that Cacao's histamine content may contribute in some small way to its stimulating effects.

Tyramine, dopamine, and phenethylamine (PEA) are broken down in the body by enzymes—naturally occurring catalysts—called monoamine oxidases. When tyramine-containing foods are eaten with compounds known as monoamine oxidase inhibitors (MAOIs), which have the property of blocking monoamine oxidase, even a low dose of 6–10mg tyramine can cause unpleasant flushing, vomiting, and high blood pressure. Several compounds in Cacao inhibit this type of enzyme, which could allow these amines to build up, and, as noted above, the trigonelline in Cacao can ship PEA directly into the central nervous system (the brain and spinal cord). Tyramine is also found in hard cheeses and some wines, and because tyramine intake is a known migraine trigger, its presence in these foods makes them a risk factor for migraine headaches. It's interesting to note that there is just over 4mg tyramine in a large 60g dose of Cacao, and when this dose is exceeded Cacao starts to produce uncomfortable symptoms such as headache, nausea, and vomiting in some individuals, effects which closely resemble a tyramine overdose.

Even more tellingly, it's been noted that low tissue concentrations of PEA increase the motivational and excitatory (stimulating) effects of dopamine and other stimulating chemicals in the brain.[560] Both tyramine and PEA act on specific receptors in the brain called trace amine associated receptors or TAARs. TAAR activation is strongly linked to the effects of several mind-altering drugs such as amphetamine ("speed") and MDMA ("ecstasy")—an intriguing link.[561] Tyramine and PEA have been described as "neuromodulators"—they have no effect on their own, but modify the effects of other brain chemicals on mood, perception, and behaviour.[562] Even though these compounds are found at infinitesimal dose levels in Cacao, it appears that these trace compounds may make a difference, after all, despite being relatively insignificant in potency and quantity. A secretary equipped with a gun and the correct access keys could assassinate a powerful dictator, where an entire army may fail: profound results are not always dependent on power or number, but can result from being given access to the right areas. The issue of Cacao's possible effects on TAARs will be discussed more thoroughly in Chapter 5.

Cacao contains a small amount of *gamma-amino butyric acid* (GABA), which, like tyramine, is also manufactured from glutamate. GABA has anti-anxiety and sedative properties in adults, although in children's brains it acts as a stimulant. GABA has some activity when taken orally, and can make it into the brain, so it's quite possible that the GABA found in Cacao contributes to its overall effects, particularly as it's present in small but appreciable doses.[563] Some compounds called *amino alcohols* are also present, and these include *anandamide*, which reduces pain, anxiety, and fear, as well as promoting weight gain and controlling milk production during breastfeeding.[564] Anandamide occurs naturally in the human brain, and binds to cannabinoid receptors—it's the natural substance which is mimicked by compounds from *Cannabis* plants, and is often referred to as an *endocannabinoid* (the prefix *endo-* comes from a Greek root word meaning "within"). Anandamide is normally broken down very quickly after ingestion, so it has been suggested that it has no relevance to the effect of Cacao or chocolate on mood or cognition. But it's active at tiny doses,[565] and the other amino alcohols in Cacao, the *n-acylethanolamines*, inhibit its breakdown at very low levels.[566] A fat-based substance called phosphatidylethanolamine in Cacao seeds is also a precursor of anandamide. So, again, the combined effect of these trace substances may be greater than their quantity might suggest. Cacao's history of use to allay fear and anxiety, gain weight, and promote lactation all suggest that GABA and the amino alcohols may contribute to the seeds' activity, despite their low profile.

The *diketopiperazines* (DKPs) are produced during fermentation and toasting of the seeds, so they are found in traditional Cacao beverages and mass-produced eating chocolate, but aren't present in unfermented and uncooked "raw chocolate". They have a bitter taste which contributes to Cacao's overall flavour, and very little is known of their physiological effects, except that they can get into the brain.[567] There are many types of DKP, and some varieties protect nerve cells from damage, inhibit cancer cell growth, lower blood sugar, or inhibit the growth of harmful microbes; but precisely what the DKPs in Cacao do once ingested has yet to be determined. Some of the DKPs may reduce morphine dependency and withdrawal, or alter sensitivity to hormones.[568] Like the THβC alkaloids, also produced during fermentation and heating, a few of the DKPs in Cacao are also found in coffee beans.

Acrylamide is a cancer-causing toxin produced during high-temperature roasting of the beans, although its content in Cacao is low and decreases with storage.[569] The quantity of acrylamide in cocoa powder is up to thirty times higher than in Cacao seeds or cocoa mass, owing to the extra processing—perhaps another argument for adopting traditional Cacao beverages over industrially processed, low-quality cocoa. See Figure 7 below for a graphic representation of the quantity of various trace amines in a 40g serving of Cacao.

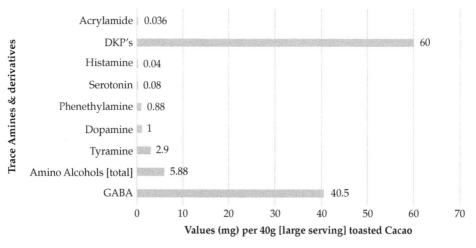

Figure 7. Trace amines and derivatives in toasted *Theobroma Cacao* seeds.

Vitalising: vitamins, minerals, and essential oil

Cacao contains significant levels of the dietary minerals *copper* and *magnesium*. A single 40g serving of Cacao contains more than the entire daily nutritional requirement of copper for an adult. Copper is used to convert dopamine to noradrenaline, a stimulating and euphoriant brain chemical, although an excess of copper may build up and eventually cause damage to dopamine-producing nerve cells, which can result in the movement disorder known as Parkinson's disease. Subjects with depression often have relatively high blood copper levels,[570] and excessive copper intake is known to be detrimental to mood regulation. On the other hand, adequate copper intake is important for dietary iron absorption, and Cacao is a high-iron plant too. So Cacao's copper content may be beneficial for anaemic persons or those with a low-copper diet, but may become harmful over time if the diet is otherwise high in this mineral.

Adequate dietary magnesium contributes to preventing health problems such as high blood pressure, migraines, fatigue, and cramps, and reduces the risk of heart disease and stroke.[571] Very low magnesium levels are associated with depression, and dietary sources of this mineral are important for people prone to mood disorders; supplementation with magnesium has rapidly reversed some cases of major depressive disorder.[572] So here's another rationale for Cacao's heart-protective properties and history of use as a mood-altering food-drug. Cacao is also relatively rich in the trace mineral *manganese*, which is incorporated into many enzymes used in various chemical reactions throughout the body, one of which (superoxide dismutase, or SOD) has the important function of preventing free radical damage. The manganese in Cacao also has a supportive role in maintaining good blood sugar control,[573] which may bolster the hypoglycaemic activity of Cacao's polyphenols. As with copper, excess manganese can become toxic to dopamine-producing cells in the brain by increasing oxidation and overstimulating them, giving rise to Parkinson's disease and other cognitive or behavioural problems.

The *criollo* variety of Cacao is "highly aromatic" and considered to have the best flavour.[574] This suggests that it may have a higher volatile oil (aka essential oil) content. Being very small, airborne molecules, volatile compounds are generally inhaled and sometimes influence brain function directly, via a signalling pathway that links smell to the reactive, emotional, and instinctual part of our brain. This is one reason why specific smells can strongly evoke certain feelings and memories. The molecules in Cacao's complex aroma individually resemble burnt meat, peanuts, maple syrup, cinnamon, coconut, sweat, sulphur, and pepper, and their complex blend produces the uniquely evocative aroma of chocolate. Several of the compounds in Cacao's perfume may directly affect brain cells. Three are known to be stimulating and dopamine-increasing (3-methylbutanal, hexanal, and phenylacetaldehyde). Others inhibit the growth of various microorganisms such as bacteria and yeast, which may play a role in the long shelf life of Cacao products and the seeds' traditional use for treating diarrhoea (dimethyl trisulphide, 2-phenylethanol, nonanal, and ethyl cinnamate). Two compounds in the essential oil, 2–4 nonadienal and ethyl cinnamate, also reduced cancerous transformation of skin cells stimulated by ultraviolet light and inhibited melanoma growth,[575] which may infer a potential use for Cacao as topical after-sun skin treatment—particularly with the burn-healing properties of the stearic acid in cocoa butter.

The chemistry of chocolate making

During **fermentation**, *phase one* of Cacao's transformation, microbes change the flavour of Cacao—making it less astringent (dry) and more acidic (sour), and turning the white-purple beans brown and more recognisably "chocolatey" in smell and taste. Fermentation is, of course, "controlled rot". Many of humanity's favourite foods and drugs such as chocolate, cheese, coffee, wine, beer, bread, yoghurt, and soy sauce are products of deliberate decay. In Cacao's case, nature is almost given free rein: the freshly harvested beans are piled up or contained in the prescribed manner (as described in Chapter 2) and the microbes left to do as they will, for one to eight days, depending on the variety of bean and intended results, established over centuries or millennia of experience. This mess of microbial and chemical activity entails multiple complex chemical reactions. The heat and moisture of fermentation initiate seed germination, then sterilise the seeds; microbial by-products, and the changes wrought in the seed, create a slew of precursor chemicals which are further transformed by toasting to create the characteristic flavour and odour of Cacao.[576] Without at least partial fermentation, important trace compounds are omitted (see Table 3, below). The fermentative microorganisms excrete organic acids such as acetic acid (the main acid in vinegar) and alcohols, permeating the beans and dissolving cell walls.[577] Because more air gets into box-fermented beans, more aerobic bacteria proliferate, as opposed to the greater quantity of yeasts in heap fermentation. Bacteria tend to produce more acids, which gives the bean a vinegary taste, whereas yeasts produce more ethanol, which is less sour;[578] this explains why well-managed smaller heaps generate better flavours. In a sense, the fermentation of Cacao is only partial, as the microbes don't get into the beans' innards—their activity is restricted to the outer shell, but the acids and alcohols they excrete do penetrate the shell and infuse the seeds, changing their chemistry and flavour. The heat, acidity, and variable exposure to oxygen reduce many of Cacao's polyphenols into smaller, sometimes inactive components.

Table 3. Gain and loss of known compounds whose presence and quantity differs in raw, fermented, and toasted Cacao

Compounds present:		Unfermented, dried Cacao	Raw, fermented, & dried Cacao	Fermented, dried, & toasted Cacao
Alkaloids	Indoles [THβCs]	–	**GAIN**: Present—produced during fermentation.	NO DATA
	Pyrazines	–	–	**GAIN**: Pyrazines formed during toasting; increase with longer roasting and higher temps.
Phenolics	Procyanidins Flavan-3-ols N-phenylproanoyl-l-amino acids	Total phenolics = 6–8% dry weight of bean.	**LOSS**: occurs due to oxidation with cell wall (parenchymal) dissolution in fermentation, plus heat generation.	**LOSS**: due to heat-induced oxidation. Total phenolics = 126 pprox. 1.2% dry weight of bean. NPA ≤ 60% decrease during toasting. Longer roasting and higher temps. = greater loss.

(Continued)

Table 3. (Continued)

Compounds present:		Unfermented, dried Cacao	Raw, fermented, & dried Cacao	Fermented, dried, & toasted Cacao
Proteins, etc.	Albumin	Present. ≤ 1.5% dry weight.	**LOSS + CHANGE**: semi-fermented Cacao albumin has *in vitro* anti-tumour activity.	**LOSS**: 13% albumin loss after 42 mins toasting at 150°C; thereafter, rapid decline.
	Amino Acids	Present.	**GAIN**	**LOSS**
	Amino Alcohols	Present.	NO DATA	NO DATA
	Biogenic Amines	Present.	**GAIN**—levels increase during fermentation with proteolysis.	**LOSS**—variable, dependent on length and temp. of toasting.
	Diketopiperazines	–	**GAIN**—produced during fermentation.	**GAIN**—heat increases formation.
	Acrylamide	–	–	**GAIN**: produced during toasting proportional to temperature, but decomposes with longer toasting and in storage.
	Volatile compounds	Present.	**GAIN**: new volatile compounds produced during fermentation.	**GAIN**—net gain, some loss by volatilisation and oxidation. Transformation and production of many new volatile compounds.

It's been observed that so-called Cacao *lavado* from Chiapas and Tabasco in Mexico (and used as standard in Alta Verapaz in Guatemala, though not referred to by this name), the variety of Cacao bean which is fermented for one day only before being washed and dried, has a much higher content of the "antioxidant" compound epicatechin than fully fermented seeds. Epicatechin is one of the most studied compounds in Cacao, not least because it's also thought to be one of the main "healthy" constituents in *Camellia sinensis*, the tea plant. Many of the proteins in Cacao are denatured into amino acids during fermentation, some of which are themselves disassembled into amines such as 2-PEA (phenethylamine). Many of the polyphenols and amines created by fermentation are later decreased by roasting and even further by alkalisation, if the Cacao is made into cocoa powder.[579] Fermentation also generates tiny quantities of tetrahydro-β-carbolines, diketopiperazines, and rafts of new volatile compounds, all of which contribute to the complex pharmacology and flavour of chocolate. So Cacao *lavado*, fermented for only a day, contains a higher level of polyphenols but fewer trace amines and trace alkaloids; Cacao *fermentado*, the reverse.

Phase two, **drying**, can either be done artificially (if the weather is rainy or unpredictable), or in the sun. Sun-dried beans taste best. Fresh Cacao seeds are up to 65% water[580] but after fermenting and drying, this is reduced to 6–8%.[581] Paradoxically, fermentation has antimicrobial effects; the weak acids produced during fermentation inhibit the growth of contaminants such as *Aspergillus* fungus species.[582] A few traditional chocolate drink formulas call for raw, lightly fermented beans, but they are in the distinct minority. One of the reasons for this may be hygienic—as contemporary "Cacao shaman" Keith Wilson points out, if the raw beans are laid out to dry in the sun after fermentation in many country farms in Central and South America they often get "rinsed with barnyard tea" by various domesticated animals wandering about (see Appendix C, Interview 3). Research has found that if fermenting Cacao is inoculated with *Salmonella* bacteria, the *Salmonella* count will actually continue to increase during drying, whereas if beans are exposed to *Salmonella* during drying, there was very little increase in *Salmonella* counts.[583] What this suggests (other than the advisability of not permitting microbiologists access to your fermenting Cacao beans) is that while dirty conditions during drying (Keith's "barnyard tea" scenario) may not be so critical, any exposure to microbial contaminants during the fermentation process could be disastrous—and many small producers in poorer regions have less than perfect sanitation.

Phase three is **toasting** the beans: one of the consistent features of traditional chocolate drinks, as described in Chapter 2, is that they were almost universally made from *toasted* Cacao beans. The heat kills off any remaining unsavoury microbes on the beans, so toasting is an important step in sterilising Cacao before consumption, in addition to catalysing more obvious changes in taste and savour. Toasting the beans (or industrially roasting them) lowers moisture levels even further, to 2–3% of the beans' weight,[584] also decreasing acidity levels and altering the volatile oil content, creating many new aromatic compounds, such as the diketopiperazines. It's known that theobromine forms "chemical adducts" with diketopiperazines during roasting,[585] creating new combination compounds, with as-yet unknown effects on their pharmacological properties.

The characteristic "chocolate" aroma and flavour are properly developed during toasting through a series of chemical transformations known as Maillard and Strecker reactions. Maillard reactions occur in foods when they are cooked to the point where they "brown"—heat causes intrinsic sugars to break down and react with proteins in the presence of water, generating new flavours. The brown colour of the toasted beans comes partly from compounds called melanoidins, generated from sugars and proteins in Maillard reactions.[586] The first molecules formed in Maillard reactions are referred to as "Amadori compounds", composed of free amino acids and sugars; in Cacao's case, Amadori compounds are produced from reactions between phenylalanine (which the beans contain a lot of) and fructose, which create many characteristic chocolate flavours.[587] Strecker reactions specifically refer to the formation of aldehydes (chemical compounds related to alcohol) from amino acids;[588] in fact the characteristic "roasting chocolate" smell is produced when the amino acids leuceine, threonine, and glutamine react with glucose, creating new volatile aromatic compounds, or "Cacao essential oil" as an aromatherapist would say—the distinctive fragrance or perfume of chocolate, basically. Strecker reactions are very important in Cacao processing, as they also cause the formation of trace alkaloids known as *pyrazines* which contribute significantly to chocolate flavour.

One of these pyrazines (tetrahydromethylpyrazine, or THMP) produced during roasting of Cacao seeds improves blood flow through the brain and spinal cord, reduces inflammation in blood vessel walls, and protects nerve cells from damage caused by temporary oxygen deprivation[vii] in high doses—such damage occurs in stroke, heart attack, or accidents where blood supply to cells may be interrupted. Although the amount of THMP in Cacao is very small, its properties complement those of Cacao's flavanols and procyanidins, present in much greater quantities, which have similar effects. The interesting thing is that roasting causes the formation of other pyrazines, such as trimethylpyrazine when Cacao is toasted at above 120°C, as in traditional processing methods (toasting on a *comal*), and two forms of dimethylpyrazine, created with higher-temperature cooking, associated with industrial processing to make eating chocolate and cocoa powder. Little is yet known about the pharmacology of these other pyrazine compounds produced during cooking, and what specific effects they may have in the human body after ingestion.

It's estimated that around 69% of all Cacao used in eating chocolate may be "overcooked"— being UHT (ultra-high-temperature) treated, baked in giant ovens or even smoked,[589] seriously denuding its content of polyphenols and other probable actives such as biogenic amines, and thereby greatly reducing its medicinal value. However, if the roasting temperature is kept around the 100°C (212°F) mark, it's possible to maintain 90% of Cacao's flavanols intact.[590] Optimal toasting temperatures and times for the preservation of the widest range of chemical components and best flavour have been calculated: temperatures greater than 150°C produce more of the carcinogenic product *acrylamide* and destroy more of the polyphenols, while toasting for less than forty minutes preserves the bulk of the proteins which remain after fermentation.[591] Fortunately, most chocolate manufacturers roast at temperatures from 110–140°C (230–284°F);[592] less fortunately, the roasting is usually continued for forty-five minutes to an hour. The "optimal" toasting temperature and duration for generating a good flavour profile while conserving oxidisable constituents has been calculated as twenty-three minutes at 116°C (241°F)! This time and temperature minimises acrylamide production, preserves polyphenols, and generates flavoursome (and biochemically active) pyrazines.[593]

In general, research indicates that lower temperatures and shorter roasting times are best for optimal Cacao chemistry—another reason for respecting the traditional method of toasting the seeds on open-air clay *comales* at lower temperatures, not roasting them by the kilo in huge metal ovens. It must be remarked that in present-day Mexico and Guatemala there is huge variation in the degree to which Cacao is toasted. I witnessed relatively brief toasting of beans with a low flame on clay *comales* for preparation of *tejate* in Oaxaca (see Chapter 8 for recipe); I also witnessed Cacao being charred to a coffee-like finish in smoky huts in Guatemala. Production quality was strongly influenced by individual preferences. Whether this was the case five hundred or a thousand years ago in the same region before the arrival of Europeans is open to speculation.

[vii] Ischaemia-reperfusion injury.

Preparing the toasted beans for making traditional Cacao beverages also causes chemical changes to take place, altering both flavour and pharmacology. This is even truer for "candy bar" chocolate, owing to the additional processes required to produce it. *Phase four*, **shelling** the beans, involves no notable pharmacological changes, but reduces the quantity of lignin—the major component of wood—in the final product, as well as the quantity of carcinogenic acrylamide in the burnt shell casings. The differing methods employed in *phase five*, **grinding** the beans to make chocolate, also affect the final product's chemistry and taste. Grinding can involve either shearing or pounding. The favoured industrial and traditional method is shearing, wherein the beans are crushed between two sliding surfaces. For industrial production of chocolate, disc mills are used, which sandwich the seeds between one rotating surface and another fixed one, breaking the seeds up most effectively. This is akin to the traditional Mesoamerican method of grinding the beans on a *metate*, or the European practice of grinding grains in a round mill. The other, less favoured method is to pulverise the beans with repeated impacts, as with mechanised pistons or "impact mills" where the nibs are pounded to a paste by hammer-pins, or by hand in a mortar and pestle, known as a *molcajete* in contemporary Latin America. In both scenarios, heat generated by the friction causes the fat in the beans to liquefy and coat the diminishing particles of solids as they are pulverised, transforming the solid beans into unadulterated cocoa liquor.[594]

Using a mortar and pestle is much slower work than grinding on a *metate*, and produces a slightly inferior drinking chocolate, as does simply grinding the beans in a machine (called a "melangeur") using granite rollers. One reason for this may be that drawing the fresh cocoa liquor up and down the flat surface of a hot *metate*, repeatedly spreading a film of chocolate over a broader surface area, allows more of the sour-tasting organic acids produced during fermentation to evaporate, thereby mellowing the flavour. By contrast, grinding the liquid in a bowl or even mixing large volumes in a machine will not allow as much acid to vaporise and escape.

Cocoa liquor consists of tiny particles of plant fibre such as cellulose and lignin suspended in liquid cocoa butter, and is very prone to pick up odours.[595] So, as per traditional recommendations (see Chapter 2), any aromatic spices such as vanilla or allspice should be added to chocolate when it is ground, before it's made into a drink or allowed to cool and solidify. Solid chocolate (whether factory-made slab for eating, or Cacao discs and tablets for making drinks) retains some of this odour-absorbing tendency, which is one reason why chocolate should never be kept in the fridge unless it's stored in an odourless, airtight container. One might surmise that the process of grinding Cacao beans must inevitably cause some decline in the quantity of active compounds in the cocoa liquor. The repeated back and forth motion involved in grinding beans on a *metate*, for example, must expose some polyphenols in the film of warm chocolate to oxygen, with which they may react, and also inevitably cause some volatile oils to disperse. So this would have the effect of making the flavour milder and more pleasant, by virtue of liberating some of the acids, but may simultaneously diminish some of the pharmacological effects of the polyphenols.

The first few hours of industrial conching cause a steep decline in complex polyphenols, which break up into smaller, still-active flavonols, as the continuously moving surface of the cocoa liquor comes into contact with the air, and presumably air is also beaten into the mixture. The amount of volatile compounds which can be detected in the air above a conche declines by over 80% over those first few hours.[596] During conching the cocoa liquor's moisture content is reduced by a further 30%, and several flavour compounds have been noted to diminish during this operation,[597] modifying the chocolate aroma and its pharmacological profile. Less-intensive traditional manual processing of Cacao (such as toasting on a *comal* and grinding on a *metate*) is likely to be less detrimental to the polyphenol content than industrial conching.

But even industrial processing produces relatively little change in the overall flavonoid content of the cocoa liquor unless the fat has been removed—as occurs in the production of "Dutched" cocoa powder, for instance. Dutching may help to mix cocoa powder with water as the alkaline potassium carbonate added to the beans *saponifies* fats in the seed, in other words it produces soapy compounds, in the same way that lye added to fat makes soap. Too much potassium salt causes the cocoa to taste soapy;[598] just right, and it will help residual fats in the powdered seed mix with water, and prevent clumping. Pharmaceutically speaking, though, Dutching has a high cost: the reason that Dutched cocoa is darker in colour and milder in flavour than Cacao, "natural" cocoa, or cocoa liquor, is that another 10–30% of the flavanols are lost to oxidation during the alkalising process, diminishing the flavour and potency of the finished product. It seems that the high fat content of Cacao—the "cocoa butter"—protects many compounds in the seeds from exposure to the air, and therefore to oxidation, during grinding and conching. Cocoa powder still contains around 12% to 22% fat,[599] but because some of that fat is saponified, the lipids aren't an effective barrier against water any more, and can no longer protect delicate compounds from oxidative chemical reactions. Only baked chocolate goods have lower medicinal potency than cocoa powder—so chocolate cake should not be excused as medicine, at least not on pharmacological grounds, as most of the remaining flavanols will be lost on baking. Its value as a comfort food, however, may be a different matter.

The key "ingredients" for deterioration in Cacao's flavanol content are high temperatures, reduced fat content, exposure of dry and de-fatted seed matter to air, and the presence or addition of moisture. All these elements are maximised in the production of industrial cocoa powder; the "alkalisation" step involves water, with the result that processed cocoa has very low flavanol content, eating chocolate has variable flavanol content, and traditional chocolate drinks made from comal-toasted Cacao have high flavanol content. "Raw chocolate" products made from untoasted Cacao potentially have the highest flavanol content of all—so long as they are made from the whole bean, not de-fatted Cacao bean powder, which many of them are; in the latter case, the flavanols will slowly oxidise with exposure to air. But raw chocolate products lack some of the other molecules produced during toasting such as the pyrazines and volatile compounds, to say nothing of the increased risk of unwelcome microbial guests as a consequence of omitting the cooking process (see above re contamination). Unfermented raw beans also lack the biogenic amines, including the much-discussed PEA, and several interesting trace psychoactive alkaloids and amine-based compounds such as the THβCs and DKPs, which may be crucial for enhanced psychoactive and medicinal effects. Fermented but uncooked Cacao has the highest levels of amines, but lower levels of pyrazines, DKPs, and volatile oils than toasted Cacao (see Table 3 below).

Phase six, **setting** the Cacao, that is, allowing the cocoa liquor to solidify for storage, is optional in traditional chocolate manufacture, and depends on whether the Cacao-based beverage is to be drunk immediately or later on. In this case, no sugar or extra fat is added, so there are no complicated processes involved. "Bloom", the bane of the chocolatier's existence, occurs when cocoa liquor melts and resets without temperature control, and is caused by the fat having separated out owing to the different "crystallisation forms" cocoa butter can take. Cocoa butter set at lower temperatures has an "unstable" structure, but if set at temperatures of around 30–34° Celsius (86–93.2°F), then the crystalline structure of the solidified fat will be stable.[600] If the cooling process isn't carefully controlled by tempering, or if you keep chocolate somewhere it will be exposed to heat then cool down again (e.g., near a sunny window, or the stove), still-liquid fat is squeezed out of the solidifying matrix of cooling cocoa butter onto the surface of the chocolate, giving your chocolate bar eczema. Bloom is a non-issue for traditional forms of drinking chocolate, as it is destined to be dissolved in hot water before consumption, so uniform texture and colouration makes no difference.

The cooled and set Cacao is now ready to make into drinks. Many books have reported the difficulty of getting solid chocolate to dissolve in hot water as a reason why traditional whole-bean drinking chocolate fell from favour, claiming that the high fat content of the bean meant such drinks were tricky to prepare, and likely to separate. But this is a fallacy: as long as drinking chocolate is made from well-ground whole beans—"well ground" meaning worked to the consistency of a smooth liquid before setting—they will readily and easily disperse when beaten or whisked into hot water. (This isn't true of ordinary "candy bar" eating chocolate, whose added fat content is too high to allow it to disperse easily in hot water.) One reason for this may be Cacao's content of a small amount of lecithin, a natural emulsifier.[601]

Chocolate, the superdrug?

1. Chocolate hearts, sweet blood

The native Kuna of the San Blas islands in Panama are accustomed to drinking five or more cups of traditional, whole-bean drinking chocolate every day—around forty cups of real, full-potency Cacao-based drinks every week. Being made only from toasted Cacao, water, banana, sugar, and spices, these beverages are naturally flavanol-rich; it's estimated that the average Kuna adult consumes about 900mg of Cacao polyphenols per day,[602] equivalent to 22.5–75g (¾–2⅔oz) of high quality Cacao seed. This is approximately the same as 75–150g (2⅔–5oz) dark chocolate per day, but without the added fat, and less highly processed so undoubtedly containing more polyphenols, and probably with a better flavour to activity ratio too. The Kuna living in San Blas experience very little age-related high blood pressure, circulatory disease, or type 2 diabetes, but when they move to other regions and abandon their traditional diet and the copious quantities of ultra-high quality drinking chocolate that entails, these migrated Kuna acquire the same levels of diabetes and cardiovascular disease as any other average city-dwelling, Western diet-consuming population.

This observation is highly relevant because cardiovascular disease (CVD)—including heart attack and stroke—is the main cause of death in the so-called developed world, killing an estimated 17 million people every year.[603] Which makes it interesting that there is now a growing body of clinical research suggesting that Cacao is a highly effective preventive remedy for these disorders. Dark chocolate slightly lowers blood pressure and beneficially affects cholesterol profiles, marginally raising HDL and lowering LDL and total cholesterol, indicating a small reduction in the risk of heart attack or stroke.[604] Far more significant is the effect of Cacao on the "vascular endothelium", the inner lining of blood vessels, and on platelets, components of the blood which are central to the clotting process. The flavanols in Cacao increase nitric oxide production in the vascular endothelium, dilating blood vessels and increasing blood flow throughout the body. The polyphenols also reduce platelet aggregation and clot formation, and stimulate *angiogenesis*—the growth of new blood vessels.[605] Essentially, Cacao appears to be a haemodynamic marvel, simultaneously reducing almost every risk factor for cardiovascular disease: it dilates narrowed blood vessels, decreases the tendency to clot, reduces inflammation in the lining of blood vessels, lowers levels of blood lipids which can accumulate on damaged artery walls, stabilises damaged red blood cells, strengthens the heartbeat, reduces blood pressure, and increases the rate of blood vessel repair. (See Appendix A for full details of the studies conducted on Cacao and chocolate.)

A meta-analysis is a type of study which rounds up all previous studies on the same subjects, filters out the ones that weren't done to a high enough standard or where the results may be inaccurate or biased, and works out what the sum total of the evidence so far is saying. It should be no surprise that a 2011 meta-analysis of Cacao's usefulness for preventing CVD concluded that people who eat the most chocolate were 37% less likely to have a heart attack and 29% less likely to have a stroke than people who ate little or no chocolate, *no matter what else they did*; smokers, the obese, people who didn't exercise, people who ate only fried food—they all had similar reduction of relative risk if they ate more chocolate.[606] This extraordinary finding is derived from several large surveys: in the US a Boston study which used questionnaires and heart scans (cardiac computerised tomography) to assess 2217 participants found an inverse association between frequency of chocolate consumption and coronary artery atherosclerosis, with the lowest risk of arterial disease for those who consumed chocolate two or more times per week.[607] In a separate, questionnaire-only study with 4970 participants from the same population, frequency of chocolate consumption was also found to reduce risk of coronary heart disease (CHD) even more significantly. The greatest reduction occurred for those who consumed chocolate five times or more each week (a 57% relative risk reduction compared to non-consumers); eating chocolate one to four times a week reduced CHD risk by 26%, but those who consumed chocolate only one to three times each month had the same risk as non-consumers.

Interestingly, the latter study also showed that consuming *non-chocolate* candy five times or more each week was associated with a 49% *higher* relative risk of CHD—in other words, higher added dietary sugar intake clearly increased the risk of developing heart disease, if the sugar was not mixed with Cacao in the form of chocolate.[608] This makes sense, given the observation that carbohydrates increase the absorption of Cacao's polyphenols. In both of the Boston studies great care was taken to get a clear picture by adjusting for other factors which could have affected the result, such as smoking, alcohol intake, exercise, calorie intake, BMI, fruit and vegetable intake, age, sex, and education. Another study from Germany suggests that the protective effects of chocolate may be even stronger against stroke than heart and arterial disease. This eight year population study with 19,357 participants showed that the people with the highest levels of chocolate consumption had a 49% relative risk reduction for heart attack and stroke put together, with slightly stronger protective effects against stroke. Most interestingly, the group with the lowest risk—the most avid consumers of chocolate—also had the lowest vegetable intake![609]

To illustrate these results: say forty-two in every 1000 UK residents have CHD: the UK population is 63.7 million, and 2.7 million UK residents have CHD (as of August 2013): a staggering 4% of the adult population with confirmed heart disease. If all adult UK residents consumed dark chocolate five times or more each week, then—if these figures bear out—only eighteen in every thousand UK residents (1.8% of the population) may go on to develop CHD. This is a massive difference; across the whole population approximately 1.5 million fewer UK residents could have CHD. Even if all UK residents were to eat only one to four "servings" of proper (dark, high Cacao-content, preferably 80% or higher) chocolate a week, CHD prevalence could be reduced from 2.7 million to 2 million, meaning that 700,000 fewer people could be living with this severe health problem.

In 2009, the total healthcare costs for CHD in the UK (primary care, outpatient care, emergency care, inpatient care, and medications combined) cost the NHS approximately £1.8 *billion* (approximately US$2.4 billion).[610] Not everybody needs a chocolate prescription to cut these numbers: if people at higher risk were targeted, such as those with a family history of CVD, high blood pressure, high cholesterol, and so on, then by the simple expedient of encouraging everybody in higher risk groups to eat *at least one serving of real dark chocolate every week*, UK healthcare costs could potentially be reduced by up to £468 million for coronary heart disease *alone*. If people at high risk of developing CVD (family history, smoking, no exercise, etc.) ate quality chocolate at least five times a week, the cost could be more than halved, a national saving of over £1 billion effected by chocolate.

One might ask, if this is the case, then why does the UK—one of the world's highest chocolate consumers—have such a high prevalence of CVD? The answers are: quality, distribution, and sugar. Put simply, the people who most need good chocolate (in terms of their dietary and lifestyle risk factors) are not the ones who are eating it; and the "chocolate" they are eating may have only a superficial acquaintance with Cacao. Many of the "chocolate bars" or "chocolate-flavoured" products which crowd the confectionery aisles of supermarkets and the counters of petrol stations are over-advertised pretenders to the name, so loaded with sugar and cholesterol-raising fats that they're more likely to increase the level of CVD risk. Which may explain the bizarre, ironic inanity of a recurrent British Heart Foundation campaign, urging people to "De-Chox"—to be sponsored to give up eating chocolate, *for the sake of their heart health*, to raise money for heart disease research and treatment. The campaign produces mugs and badges with phrases like "balls to chocolate", and "give chocolate the finger".[611] This could be intended to reduce dietary intakes of added sugar and saturated or trans-fats, assuming that most "chocolate" is just cake and low-Cacao confectionery, and that chocolate eaters are likely to have other, less healthy habits, too. But as we have seen, eating real chocolate reduces risk of CVD even when other lifestyle risk factors are present. The campaign is appallingly wrong-headed, demonising the only type of confectionery which has a protective effect!

If every UK resident consumed *only* non-chocolate sweets (to which I would add soft drinks (sodas), biscuits, confectionery, etc., five times or more each week, avoiding chocolate entirely, the prevalence of CHD could *rise* to sixty-three out of every thousand UK residents (6.3%), bringing the total number of people living with heart disease up to four million, and escalating the national bill for coronary heart disease health care to £2.7 billion. To be effective, the use of chocolate for disease prevention must target the correct groups and entail sufficient consumption of high quality Cacao, while *simultaneously* replacing dietary consumption of other refined sugar-containing foods. A bog-standard "chocolate bar" comprising 25% biscuit, 75% refined sugar and fat, 4% highly refined cocoa powder and 1% added god-knows-what just won't cut it, and will—at best—do nothing to reduce CVD risk. The chocolate needed for noticeable effect is dark, rich, and strong.

So our currently high levels of CVD are the consequence of a national diet loaded with added sugar, saturated fat, and a dearth of beneficial botanical compounds. Few of the people who need it are eating enough of the right type of chocolate. Which begs the question—how would disease statistics, and the consequent healthcare costs, be affected if refined sugar was entirely removed from the UK diet, *and* people at risk of heart disease or stroke switched to consuming traditional chocolate drinks, sweetened only a little, or not at all?

What's true of chocolate and heart disease may also be true of diabetes mellitus, or chronically high and uncontrolled blood sugar. In diabetes, the pancreas either stops producing the hormone insulin (in type 1 diabetes, and—eventually—type 2 as well), or the cells become unresponsive to insulin (type 2). Insulin enables all the cells in the body to absorb glucose, which they use for fuel. If insulin isn't being produced, or the cells stop responding to it, blood sugar rises and the cells begin to starve; as Coleridge's ancient mariner said, "Water, water everywhere, nor any drop to drink"—though in diabetes mellitus it's "glucose, glucose everywhere …" Insulin also helps cells take up fats (triglycerides) and proteins, so these rise in the bloodstream too, and the consequences of all the extra sugar and fat in the blood is a gradual clogging-up of the circulatory system, with small blood vessels in the eyes, kidneys, hands, and feet gradually closing up; even larger organs, such as the liver, brain, and heart become more and more congested with fat and unable to function as well. Diabetes effectively silts up the whole body, increasing the likelihood of acute disease and early death.

The mixture of flavanols in Cacao have been shown to rapidly lower the levels of fats (triglycerides) in the blood and reduce fat production (lipogenesis) in mice at high levels of intake,[612] equivalent to around 108g whole Cacao for a human, a high dose but within the realms of possibility for daily human consumption. Human studies have substantiated these results: in several trials, high-polyphenol dark chocolate was found to improve pancreatic function and insulin sensitivity, reduce blood pressure and cholesterol, and improve arterial blood flow over periods of up to twelve weeks, in doses equivalent to an average of 80g Cacao per day.[613] More recent lab and animal research suggests that Cacao may help protect both the liver and pancreas,[614] reducing the risk of developing diabetes and fatty liver disease.

Another potentially serious medical condition which affects the circulatory system is anaemia. Technically, anaemia is a generic term which may have several different causes. The name means "without blood", and refers to symptoms caused by a reduction in the ability of red blood cells to carry oxygen around the body. It's a disease state characterised by shortness of breath, fatigue, pallor, and rapid heart rate; it can also lead to faintness, angina (chest pain brought on by exertion), pains in the legs and calves on walking, and—eventually—heart failure. Causes of anaemia may include blood loss from heavy menstruation, or low dietary iron intake. But two major types of anaemia are caused by specific inherited mutations in the genes coding for haemoglobin, the substance made from proteins and iron which resides inside red blood cells and transports oxygen around the body. These "altered haemoglobin" anaemias are thalassaemia and sickle-cell anaemia, which affect millions of people worldwide. The current prevalence of these disorders is 2.55 per 1,000 births; 56,000 children are born with thalassaemia major and 275, 000 babies are born with sickle-cell disease every year,[615] making them major health issues on a global level.

Thalassaemia is the name given to inherited disorders in which haemoglobin isn't properly formed, causing red blood cells never to mature or to die easily. Severe thalassaemia causes bone deformities, recurrent bacterial infections, leg ulcers, and gallstones, and requires blood transfusions to treat, often leading to toxic iron accumulation. In sickle-cell anaemia, red blood cells (erythrocytes) appear normal until subjected to stress such as low blood oxygenation or inflammation, at which time the mutated haemoglobin polymerises (forms long chains) and deforms the shape of the erythrocytes from blood-vessel-friendly squashy biconcave discs to pipe-clogging crescent ("sickle") shapes. The more this happens, the more inflexible the "sickled" blood cells become; they tend to pile up and block blood vessels, causing upstream tissue damage and severe pain. The "sickle-cell crisis" is usually accompanied by fever, and can present as bone, chest, liver, or kidney pain, epileptic fits, or painful, persistent erections in men (priapism). Without access to good medical treatment, sickle-cell disease usually results in reduced lifespan (death typically occurs at forty to fifty years old).

The relevance of Cacao to these diseases should be obvious: if *Theobroma cacao* can stabilise red blood cells, reduce clotting, and prevent inflammation in the walls of blood vessels while dilating them at the same time, might it not help alleviate sickle-cell disease, reducing the possibility of a crisis? *Theobroma* may also be of use in thalassaemia by improving blood flow and the lifespan of red blood cells, thereby reducing the need for blood transfusions, and could have crisis-averting, lifesaving benefits for people living with sickle-cell disease. So if physicians around the world were trained to prescribe appropriately prepared Cacao or dark chocolate to high-risk groups and (at higher "doses") to premorbid heart disease or diabetes patients, the cumulative reduction in morbidity, and the alleviation of human suffering which could be achieved is huge; the potential reduction to national healthcare costs, almost beyond belief.

2. Intelligent chocolate

Test subjects who ate 85g dark or milk chocolate fifteen minutes before a cognitive function test performed up to 20% better than the control group—but, interestingly, the milk chocolate group did better than the dark chocolate group in this study.[616] This could reflect the greater placebo value of familiar and comforting milk chocolate, or the anti-anxiety effects of exorphin (sedating, opiate-like) compounds in milk pairing with the compounds in chocolate (more on this topic in Chapter 7). It should be noted that fifteen minutes isn't long enough for many of the compounds in chocolate to get into the bloodstream, so all this study shows is that being given chocolate shortly before doing mental work may improve performance by undefined mechanisms.

More recent research into the chocolate eating habits of a community of 968 Americans aged twenty-three to ninety-eight over an eighteen-year period has revealed that habitual *dark* chocolate consumption is strongly linked to improved cognitive function relative to abstainers, bestowing better abstract reasoning, working memory, and visual-spatial memory among chocolate eaters.[617] As with the findings in the cardiovascular studies, these chocolate-related benefits were independent of other factors such as exercise, fruit and vegetable consumption, obesity, and general health. Another four-year study assessing the cognitive functioning of 531 older people aged sixty-five or above found that chocolate intake was associated with a reduced risk of cognitive decline—but only if caffeine intake was less than 75mg per day, suggesting that those who also drink tea or coffee or other caffeine-containing substances on a daily basis may not experience any chocolate-related brain benefits over the long term.[618]

Real-life corroboration of Cacao's possible brain benefit can be surmised from the survey of the Kuna, the group of people living in Panama who consume up to 75g of Cacao on a daily basis. In addition to lower incidence of heart attack and stroke, Cacao-drinking Kuna are noted to have much lower levels of neurological pathologies (such as Alzheimer's or Parkinson's disease) than members of the tribe who move to the city and abandon their traditional diet and lifestyle.[619] This finding will be discussed in more detail in Chapter 7, but for now I'd like to point out that the Kuna's average daily caffeine intake from Cacao is double the daily limit of 75mg caffeine in the study mentioned above, suggesting that while higher caffeine intakes from other sources may prevent Cacao from having longer-term cognition-enhancing effects, the caffeine in Cacao itself is not an issue. As we see time and again, it's inadvisable to reduce the effects of a plant to single chemical compounds when assessing real world effects: it's about the whole package.

Other lifestyle factors which differentiate between city and country living may play a role in the lower incidence of dementia and age-related movement disorders among countryside-dwelling Kuna, but the quality of their Cacao appears to be highly significant. After all, the Kuna aren't eating "sophisticated" chocolate bars, but drinking their toasted bean-based beverages. The higher polyphenol content of their traditionally-processed Cacao may be a contributing factor to their reduced risk of cognitive decline, in addition to other variables such as fewer environmental pollutants and more robust social networks in their homeland, in contrast to their relatively sickly city-dwelling relatives.

Whole Cacao bean extracts prevent Alzheimer's disease proteins from accumulating in mouse brains *in vitro*,[620] and one Cacao polyphenol (called epigallocatechin gallate, or EGCG, also found in green tea) can even halt the progression of the terminal, paralysing neurological disease amyotrophic lateral sclerosis (ALS) in mice.[621] Most interestingly, a single dose of Cacao containing 450mg flavanols, equivalent to a serving of 40g whole Cacao beans in a traditional drink, and even a third of this dose taken every day for five days significantly increased blood flow to the brain as measured by an MRI scan in human volunteers.[622] In a similar experiment, isolated flavanol mixtures from Cacao were administered to volunteers aged between sixty-one and eighty-five over an eight-week period, in a double-blind, placebo-controlled clinical trial. The outcome was that daily doses of the flavanols—equivalent to 13g and 143g of whole Cacao—dose-dependently improved performance in tests of verbal fluency and trail making (the ability to quickly link up dots: mental processing, sequencing, flexibility, and executive function), with concomitant improvements in insulin sensitivity and blood pressure at the higher dose.[623]

Another brain imaging study of blood flow in six healthy adults fed flavanol-rich chocolate showed increased signal intensity during a task requiring concentration compared to scans performed without prior chocolate consumption, although it isn't known whether this reflected increased nerve firing or just increased blood flow to the activated brain areas.[624] The assumption is that the Cacao enabled the brain to increase its blood and therefore oxygen supply as necessary—but as this was such a small trial with no placebo group that we can't be certain whether it was the chocolate or the participants' expectations which caused this response. But these findings may be of interest to people dealing with aging-related cognitive decline and dementia, especially "vascular dementia", where compromised blood flow to the brain is the root of the problem.

So we know that many compounds in Cacao have nerve and brain-cell-protecting or regeneration-promoting activity, at least in the laboratory. We know that many of these compounds get into the bloodstream after ingestion, and that some of them are capable of passing through the blood-brain barrier to reach the brain (e.g., flavanols such as epicatechin, or other polyphenols such as clovamide, resveratrol, and pyrryloquinoline quinone; the diketopiperazines; and many of Cacao's alkaloids, such as tetramethylpyrazine and trigonelline. See the *Theobroma cacao* monograph in Appendix A for detailed studies on each of these compounds and whole Cacao.) Animal experiments in rats and mice revealed that large doses of isolated Cacao polyphenols do indeed improve mental performance in tests of learning and memory, and caused acute increases in the blood level of adrenaline. To achieve such results, these experiments used rats ingesting fairly large doses of these compounds,[625] equivalent to 108–120g of whole Cacao for a human. Although the use of isolated polyphenols in animal experiments means we should be cautious in interpreting these results to infer benefit in a human population, coincidentally this dosage isn't too far from the total daily intake of Cacao for the Kuna people in Costa Rica, who have such low levels of degenerative and neurological disease.

Sleep deprivation is a commonplace cause of less pathological "neurological deficits", in other words it's known to negatively affect performance and various aspects of mental functioning such as mood and working memory. Less well known is that regular sleep deprivation increases risk of heart disease and stroke. In a recent evaluation of the effects of Cacao on working memory and circulation in thirty-two sleep-deprived volunteers, high-flavanol dark chocolate restored good circulation[viii] and working memory performance.[626] So Cacao may be the perfect remedy after pulling an all-nighter! A final interesting link between Cacao and mental functioning is the robust statistical association between higher national chocolate consumption and Nobel prizes—the more chocolate a country eats, the more likely that country is to produce Nobel prize winners.[627] Of course this association may not be causal, at least not directly—it's more feasible that chocolate-consuming countries are richer and have better education systems than non-chocolate consuming countries (generally true), or that some other factor linked to higher chocolate consumption—increased corporate sponsorship, for example—may account for this statistic. But the link is real, and worthy of further exploration.

[viii] As measured by brachial flow-mediated dilation.

While there are no high-quality clinical trials showing that chocolate can significantly impact neurological disease in humans as yet, Cacao shows promise as a nootropic drug—that is, a cognition-enhancing substance—and its circulation-enhancing properties suggest that it may be valuable for the prevention or treatment of vascular dementia and general age-related cognitive decline.

3. Asthmatic chocolate

Several substances in Cacao have anti-asthmatic activity, so in theory Cacao is a useful addition to the diet for asthmatics—which corroborates the traditional use of Cacao as a lung tonic for chronic (long-term) lung problems. A laboratory study using whole Cacao extract showed that it reduced the production of a substance called neopterin in white blood cells, indicating anti-inflammatory effects and the potential for Cacao to affect or "modulate" the immune system, perhaps damping down some types of allergic responses.[628] But this is only a lab test result, so should be taken as an "early days" finding. More potential interactions of Cacao with the immune system are discussed in Chapter 7. Similarly, the phenolic compound clovamide dilates the airways *in vitro* with the same potency as the anti-asthmatic drug Salbutamol (often marketed as Ventolin™). Clovamide was detected in the urine two hours after humans consumed Cacao beverages, indicating that it found its way into the general circulation, and might be expected to affect the lungs;[629] it has been found to allay coughing caused by inhaling chilli fumes, for example.[630] The alkaloid theophylline in Cacao even more strongly inhibits airway spasm and inflammation, as well as impairing histamine release;[631] its effects likely outweigh those of the minute amount of histamine in Cacao. Likewise, Cacao's principal alkaloid theobromine suppresses the cough reflex and slightly dilates the airways, effectively reducing persistent coughing. In children, the airway-dilating effects of both theobromine and theophylline last for two to six hours after ingestion,[632] so these effects are likely to be present in whole Cacao. Even more intriguingly, children born to mothers who consume chocolate during pregnancy have a lower incidence of asthma.[633]

4. Reproductive chocolate

A small human observational ("cohort") study found another advantage for women consuming dark chocolate during pregnancy: a significant reduction in the risk of developing high blood pressure during the pregnancy, which can cause miscarriage and other medical complications, including a serious and potentially life-threatening condition called pre-eclampsia. Higher chocolate consumption was correlated with lower blood pressure and a reduced risk of pre-eclampsia, particularly when it was regularly eaten in the first trimester, and the level of of theobromine in the umbilical cord (indicating chocolate intake before giving birth) corresponded with lower incidence of pre-eclampsia.[634]

Cacao's traditional use as a *galactagogue*—a drug to increase breast milk production, a common folk medicine use in Central America, as described in Chapter 3—hasn't yet been scientifically validated. Horsey types report success using "an old gypsy remedy", feeding cocoa powder to mares to increase their milk supply after they've foaled.[635] Administering the alkaloid salsolinol (one of the trace compounds in Cacao) to sheep increases levels of the hormone prolactin in the bloodstream, which stimulates lactation when natural endorphin levels are high.[636] So it could be that this substance is responsible for the galactagogue effect observed in folk veterinary practice, particularly as the alkaloid accumulates in the brain and has stronger effects on dopamine-releasing cells (which control the levels of prolactin) at *lower* doses. Endorphins create feelings of pleasure and comfort and raise pain thresholds when they bind to mu-opioid receptors in the brain, so when the sheep is bonding with its lamb, perhaps experiencing some discomfort from suckling, the brain releases more endorphins to increase feelings of contentment and closeness and decrease the significance of the pain. In this environment the presence of salsolinol will stimulate more milk production, reinforcing the "feedback loop" between suckling and lactation. This provides a possible mechanism by which Cacao may enhance breast milk production in mammals, as Cacao also contains other constituents which modify endorphin release, as we will see in the next chapter, where we will examine Cacao's traditional reputation as an "aphrodisiac" and its effects on male and female reproductive function.

5. Chocolate for pain control

Chocolate confectionery has been used in army rations for over a century because of its long shelf-life, high calorie density, and mildly stimulating properties. And it has proven to be useful in survival situations: the Arctic explorer Sir John Franklin praised the restorative powers of drinking chocolate, recounting how a single cup taken by a companion "seized with a shivering fit" before he slept staved off hypothermia: "The only inconvenience that he felt the next morning was pain in his limbs."[637] Part of this restorative effect, no doubt, may reside in Cacao's circulation-enhancing powers; but Cacao and chocolate also have a marked effect on pain perception.

Cacao has a long history of use for pain control. At minimum, chocolate's reputation as a palliative food or treat could reinforce a placebo response, which would diminish pain, but the flavonoids and methylxanthines in Cacao also have measurable pain-reducing effects. Caffeine alleviates several types of pain, and the flavanols suppress inflammatory responses by reducing production of inflammatory compounds and improve circulation,[638] such that consuming a flavonoid-rich dark chocolate drink after exercise diminishes next-day stiffness and pain.[639] In addition to Cacao's potential therapeutic value in syndromes which may cause or exacerbate pain, such as type 2 diabetes (as above) and obesity (see below), Cacao flavanols specifically reduce both inflammation and pain perception in *trigeminal neuralgia*, a type of facial pain which may be a result of nerve damage during dental work, for example. Cacao more generally allays pain sensitivity associated with the cranial nerves, including the vagus nerve, which has an important role in regulating digestion; these findings may partially explain Cacao's traditional use for abdominal pain.[640] But there is evidence that Cacao affects opiate signalling in the brain ("endorphins"), and Cacao is often used "unofficially" by people to self-medicate certain types of emotional pain—of which more in Chapter 5.

6. Cacao chemotherapy

Several factors increase the risk of developing cancers, including:

1. Prolonged stress, measured by raised levels of the stress hormone, cortisol, which may reduce the immune response to cancer cells[641]
2. Increased oxidative stress; for example, in smokers[642]
3. Chronic inflammation, from infections, normal aging, poor diet, or alcohol ingestion[643]
4. Carcinogenic (cancer-causing) chemicals from environmental pollutants such as lead in petrol fumes, food contaminants like fungal aflatoxins in peanuts, some medicinal drugs like cancer chemotherapy, hormone replacements like the birth control pill, industrial exposure to asbestos or toxic by-products of some manufacturing processes, etc.

Compounds in Cacao counteract or reduce the effects of all these things. Unlike the isolated polyphenols trialled in lab rats, whole Cacao acutely reduces levels of cortisol and adrenaline after ingestion by adult human males under stressful conditions;[644] it has powerful antioxidant properties, lowering levels of oxidative stress marker compounds in the bloodstream;[645] it assuages inflammation in the lining of blood vessels and elsewhere;[646] and it neutralises or blunts the effects of several carcinogens.[647] The polyphenols in Cacao prevent the transformation, growth, and spread of cancer cells in laboratory tests, although there is currently no proof that they do so in live humans.[648] But added to the diet of rats, Cacao gradually increases the general immune response to viruses and cancers,[649] and if this effect is replicated in humans it suggests that Cacao may be *chemopreventive*: a substance which reduces the risk of developing cancer. Cacao may even, to some extent, be *antineoplastic*: this literally means "against new growth"; in other words, it may stop the development of, or even kill cancer cells.

A few of Cacao's aromatic trace compounds also have anti-cancer properties, such as 2,4-nonadienal, which prevents UV light from turning cells cancerous in the laboratory. This effect is enhanced by a naturally occurring cyanide compound called benzaldehyde.[650] This is of particular interest given Cacao's combination with *mamey* seed (*Pouteria sapota*) in the traditional Cacao-based Mexican beverage known as *tejate*; *mamey* seeds, like bitter almonds, are a source of benzaldehyde compounds.[651] Theoretically, the combination of nonadienal and benzaldehyde in *tejate* in sunny Oaxaca may help protect against UV-induced cancer cell transformation. Cacao extracts also inhibit the growth of human colon cancer cells in the laboratory.[652]

Other parts of *Theobroma cacao* than the seeds are more important in traditional medicine; laboratory testing has shown that a Cacao leaf extract is toxic to one type of breast cancer cell, without affecting healthy liver cells.[653] Whether this result has any relevance to the use of Cacao leaf in traditional herbal medicine is questionable, as the solvent used was methanol, whereas most traditional preparations are made by boiling or steeping in water, or simply expressing the fresh leaf juice, and the investigation was performed in a laboratory, under highly artificial ("controlled") conditions. This kind of testing is conducted with the intent to find new drugs which can then be used to develop patentable pharmaceutical medicines, and may be of limited use to consumers of the original plant and the millions of people worldwide who rely on local herbal medicines for medical treatment. It would be far more helpful to investigate the pharmacological properties and mechanisms of action of the whole plant medicines as they are used "in the field" by the societies which have grown up with them; this would practically benefit the users of such plants, the scientific community, and the human organism at large.

So it's highly plausible that Cacao is a useful agent for reducing the probability of developing cancer. A necessary caveat is that there are many different kinds of cancer, and just because a substance is effective *in vitro*, it doesn't mean it'll be active in living human beings; nevertheless, Cacao has demonstrated a broad range of positive influences on various cancer risk factors. And as mentioned above, Cacao's theophylline content enhances the effectiveness of the chemotherapy agent, Doxorubicin: so patients undergoing Doxorubicin-based chemotherapy may benefit from incorporating Cacao into their diet, subject to their oncologist's approval (as antioxidants reduce the effectiveness of some chemotherapy drugs, so it's always important to check that any dietary changes or complementary medicines being taken are compatible with any prescription drugs).

7. The smoker's frenemy

In terms of cardiovascular disease, lung disease, and cancer risk, one group particularly stands out: smokers. Cacao and tobacco have a long, entwined history. They come from the same continent, after all. Olmec, Maya, and Mexica lords smoked tobacco and drank chocolate at banquets, and both substances had spiritual as well as earthly cachet; tobacco was a highly prized sacrament for many New World peoples, used in shamanic healing, and Cacao was a secular libation and a ceremonial drink (see Chapters 2 and 9 for more details). So perhaps it shouldn't be a surprise that their pharmaceutical interactions are interesting, too. For example, it's known that smokers metabolise (break down) caffeine 30–50% more rapidly than non-smokers,[654] because some compounds in tobacco smoke—polycyclic aromatic hydrocarbons, apparently—require the same liver enzymes to be broken down as caffeine does, so the body ups the production of these enzymes. The consequence of this is that consumers of chocolate, tea, or coffee who smoke need more of their caffeinated drug of choice to achieve the same degree of stimulation as non-smokers. Tobacco smoke also deactivates an enzyme called histone deacetylase type 2 (HDAC-2) which is important for repairing blood vessel walls, but even low doses of the alkaloid theophylline, found in Cacao and chocolate (also in tea) reactivates it, restoring its protective effects.[655]

So the banqueting Mexica, bookending their repast with smoking and chocolate, may perforce have consumed more chocolate to achieve a pleasant Cacao "buzz" than would have been necessary if they had not been smokers. And no bad thing if they did drink more chocolate, because it turns out that Cacao undoes some of the harms of tobacco. Specifically, it improves blood flow—which tobacco reduces, by constricting peripheral blood vessels—and reduces inflammation in the linings of blood vessels, which tobacco smoking aggravates.

There is another, less predictable link between Cacao and tobacco, which goes to show that few natural drug relationships are fully a one-way street. It has been noted that nicotine protects dopamine-releasing cells in an area of the brain called the *substantia nigra* from death induced by exposure to salsolinol, one of the alkaloids in Cacao.[656] Death of these neurons eventually causes the syndrome known as Parkinson's disease, in which chocolate consumption may or may not be implicated as a risk factor (see Chapter 7 for a full discussion). It's long been known that for all its damaging effects, tobacco use decreases the risk of developing Parkinson's disease. So perhaps the Mexica were right to combine tobacco smoking with ingesting Cacao at their feasts: though Cacao is by far the more beneficial of these two psychoactive drugs, and appears to accrete longevity-promoting factors as much as tobacco erodes them, it may yet transpire that each undoes a measure of the other's potential harm.

8. Campesino *antivenom*

As we have seen, Cacao is used in traditional medicine as a preventive of snakebite poisoning, a prophylactic antivenom. This seems ludicrous—what does chocolate have to offer to protect against snakebite? Nothing has been proven, but there are several possibilities. One is that the venom of many poisonous snakes increases blood clotting and inflammation in blood vessels, causing circulatory blockages, pain, and tissue death; and we know that Cacao inhibits clotting, dilates blood vessels, and reduces inflammation in blood vessel linings.

Some of the procyanidins in Cacao also inhibit an enzyme called hyaluronidase which is secreted by many pathogenic bacteria. Hyaluronidase breaks down hyaluronic acid, a component of healthy tissue, allowing bacteria to stick to and burrow into surfaces, and a lot of the compounds generated in the process also promote inflammation, increase blood vessel growth, and modify immune system functions.[657] The hyaluronidase inhibitory activity of Cacao goes some way towards explaining its traditional use as a general or supportive tonic in many illnesses including cancer and lung ailments, and possibly its use as a prophylactic "antivenom" against some types of snakebite—because many snake venoms, too, contain hyaluronidases, and inhibiting this enzyme with plant extracts significantly reduces their morbidity (ability to cause suffering, harm, and death) in experimental animals.[658] But Cacao hasn't yet been tested here, so this is currently an intriguing speculation; it's very doubtful that Cacao ingestion could neutralise snake venom, but it's credible that prior ingestion of Cacao could attenuate the effects of some kinds of snake venom, perhaps even making the difference between life and death.

9. Chocolate for beauty and longevity

Cacao causes blood vessels to dilate, so it should facilitate circulation to the skin, just as it does to other organs such as the brain, heart, liver, and kidneys. And so it does: two hours after ingesting Cacao, blood flow to the skin increases by 70%.[659] This is another reason why Cacao is good for smokers—smoking reduces the blood supply to the skin, and Cacao can restore it! I have an anecdotal example of this effect. Two or three times a week, I drink a half pint of a basic chocolate *atole* (my *champurrado* recipe—see Chapter 8) for breakfast or lunch. In September 2016 I had a small growth on my left arm biopsied: a small chunk was cut out to investigate in a lab. When I returned home two or three hours later, I had my usual *champurrado*-style *atole* for lunch. An hour or so later I was watching a film when I felt warm liquid running down my arm. The wound was bleeding to the extent that the dressing was absolutely soaked and the blood had seeped through it: it looked like a bullet wound. After twenty minutes holding my arm above my head while using my left hand to find and apply the styptic powder in my first aid kit and a suitable dressing, I made a note to myself: do not take strong chocolate immediately after any surgical procedure!

This increase in dermal blood flow has an advantage with more popular appeal: slowing down skin aging. A twelve-week double-blind study testing the effects of high-flavanol cocoa in a group of twenty-four women found that those women ingesting the equivalent of 30–40g whole Cacao per day had a significant reduction in signs of sun (UV light) damage such as reddening of the skin, with measurable improvements in skin texture and hydration, although, sadly, no changes in wrinkles were noted.[660] Another thirty-person double-blind trial confirmed that high flavanol cocoa (presumably equivalent to ordinary, good quality Cacao) increased the skin's resistance to sun damage over a twelve week period.[661]

Apart from the possibility of better skin and a sharper mind as you get older, ingesting Cacao may help you live longer. A retrospective review of a group of 470 men aged 65–84 from the "Zutphen Elderly dietary and lifestyle study" conducted in the Netherlands between 1985 and 1990 found a reduced risk of *all-cause mortality* associated with the *highest* levels of cocoa and chocolate intake. After controlling for BMI, smoking, lifestyle, drugs, diet, and caloric intake, cocoa enthusiasts had a 47% reduction in relative risk of death from *all causes put together* during the study period, as compared with non-chocolate consumers.[662] Consuming chocolate only one to three times a month has been correlated with a whole extra year of life in population studies.[663]

High stress levels, associated with elevated blood cortisol, are known to be associated with a shorter lifespan. With excessive stress we literally age faster. The chromosomes in every cell in our body—the bundles of genetic information in the nucleus of each cell—are protected by buffers or caps at each end, called telomeres. Every time a cell replicates itself, these telomeres get worn away, just a little, and an enzyme called telomerase helps to repair them. One study compared the telomeres of women with healthy children to those who had children with chronic health issues, and found that the more stressed women (mostly those with chronically sick children, this being a cause of ongoing worry and stress) were more likely to have shorter telomeres, much less telomerase, and even looked older.[664] As mentioned above, and as we shall see in the next chapter, Cacao may help to lower blood levels of adrenaline and the stress hormone, cortisol.[665] Although Cacao's effect on telomeres and telomerase hasn't been assessed, its notable effect on stress hormone and its traditional reputation would suggest a positive influence.

Paradoxically, Cacao may also have anti-obesity effects, related to the presence of polyphenols. Laboratory research showed that cocoa powder reduced fat production in fat cells, and inhibited digestive enzymes which help break down starch and fats in the digestive tract prior to absorption.[666] In animal studies, rats fed cocoa as part of their diet had less weight gain, and obese diabetic rats fed a high-fat diet for thirteen weeks had less weight gain when Cacao polyphenols were added to the diet. The polyphenols appear to reduce the expression of genes which allow fatty acids (the building blocks of fat) to be manufactured in the liver; they do the same for some cholesterol-making genes, and increase the production of genes which accelerate fat-burning. These effects seem to hold true in human populations: a random selection of just over a thousand healthy people of between twenty and eighty-five years old showed that regular chocolate eaters had a lower BMI, even though their overall calorie consumption was higher.[667] It's possible that these results may be explained if the chocolate consumers were richer (of "higher socio-economic status") overall, which is positively associated with lower levels of obesity and health problems in general, perhaps due to comparatively lower stress, leading to lower cortisol levels—high cortisol encourages weight gain, producing an "apple shaped" body with abdominal fat accumulation. But, of course, we know that Cacao reduces cortisol levels—so either way, Cacao may help!

Traditionally, though, Cacao was used to "fatten", or gain weight. This isn't necessarily a contradiction: the high fat content and nutritional benefit of adding Cacao to the diet of an underweight person would help them gain weight, while the stress-modulating and metabolism-modifying effects may have a different effect in an overweight population. It's very likely that any "weight-reducing" properties may be nullified by the addition of excess sugar and a high-fat, high-meat diet, if the burgeoning incidence of obesity in contemporary Mexico is anything to go by. All else being equal, it seems that Cacao may contribute to keeping us alive for longer, maintaining a healthy body weight, and even helping us to endure the ravages of time a little better too.

* * *

So ingesting real, traditionally prepared Cacao-based beverages—or even good quality dark chocolate with a high cocoa content—may help to prevent and even treat many of the most significant health challenges of the affluent world. Cardiovascular disease, diabetes, some types of cancer, and many age-related problems such as cognitive decline, chronic pain, or respiratory conditions—even, to some extent, the aging process itself—can potentially be ameliorated by the judicious use of Cacao, albeit preferably in combination with significant lifestyle and dietary adjustments. While Cacao may turn out to be almost as beneficial as our ancestors thought, and far more useful than we believed for the prevention and treatment of many ailments, we should also remember that life is complex, and there's no such thing as a panacea. Even a substance as beneficial and pleasant as Cacao isn't a universal solution. Natural drugs are complex, and the friendliest pharmaceuticals or most flavoursome foods offend some bodies, a subject to which we shall return in Chapter 7. But in the next chapter we'll delve a little deeper into Cacao's reputation as a psychotropic drug and an aphrodisiac, and attempt to tease out the subtle truth of its effects on mood and perception.

Señora Anna Maria Garcia Vásquez winnowing Cacao, Juchitan, Guatemala, 2018

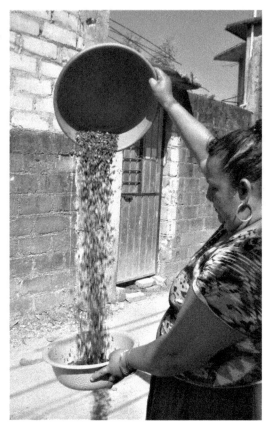

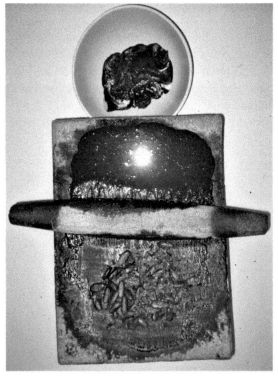

Half-ground Cacao seeds on a metate.

CHAPTER FIVE

Chocolate, love, and bondage (Part I)

Madam Pomfrey: "Well, he should have some chocolate, at the very least!"

Harry: "I've already had some. Professor Lupin gave me some."

Madam Pomfrey: "Did he, now? So we've finally got a Defence Against the Dark Arts teacher who knows his remedies?"

(from *Harry Potter and the Prisoner of Azkaban*: Copyright © J. K. Rowling, 1999)

"People have often asked me whether what I know about love has spoiled it for me. And I just say, 'Hardly.' You can know every single ingredient in a piece of chocolate cake, and then when you sit down and eat that cake, you can still feel that joy."

(Dr Helen Fisher, anthropologist and researcher into the neurobiology of love)

Chocolate is *the* classic food substitute for love in contemporary consciousness. A home remedy for heartache and loneliness, its roles in popular culture range from gifting Valentine's Day chocolates as a token of affection or desire, to a pleasant indulgence, a guilty pleasure, or an unhealthy compulsion. But how much is this public perception of chocolate reflected in the pharmacology of the Cacao bean itself, and how much is poetic licence? Does Cacao really have any effects on the brain and mood beyond placebo? Is it really much different from tea, coffee, or other caffeinated beverages? Is chocolate inherently addictive—is "chocoholism" a product of social or psychological complexes, an imaginary condition, or something else? To what extent do traditional non-confectionery chocolate drinks possess similar properties and attributes to our familiar "candy bar" chocolate? And if chocolate *is* a psychoactive drug, with medicinal properties … could it also be harmful?

In this chapter we set sail for the shores of a new world of scientific investigation into chocolate. We will look at the pharmacology of Cacao on a deeper level, gathering and connecting historical information, anecdotal experience, and research evidence from various disciplines to construct more theories about Cacao's effects on the human brain, social interactions, and society as a whole. As these patterns arise, new therapeutic uses for chocolate and Cacao will be proposed, all of which should provide a rich seam of possibilities for future exploration and experiment.

Chocolate, mind, and mood

For the most part, we are aware of only the grossest changes in our consciousness, because we constantly undergo shifts in mood and perception; we are all habituated to living in our own fluctuating mental landscapes. Some of these perceptual changes originate from within ourselves, in response to external events, such as the hormonal and neuronal cascades induced by angry shouting, or a flirtatious exchange. Others are influenced by external agents, such as drink, drugs, or food. We inhabit an ocean of sensory stimuli conveyed and transacted by constant pharmacological activity in our bodies. The brain and central nervous system are the internal hub of all these interactions, the chief processing unit of perception and response, but in fact the molecular conversations which affect consciousness occur throughout the body, not just in the "central computer" region of our anatomy. Psychoneuroendocrinology (PNEI) is the name given to the science of defining these interactions. It's the discipline of pulling threads from the five-dimensional living Persian rugs of our biochemistry and tracing their paths as individual molecular relays that weave through our cellular biology, influencing our feelings, thoughts, and behaviour.

Perhaps only Buddhist monks, shamans, mystics, prophets, yogis, or psychenauts[ix] whose minds have been temporarily jemmied open by trance techniques or entheogenic drugs are more fully aware of the constant perceptual adjustments which comprise our daily lives—people who by one means or another become attuned by waking exposure to the outer (or inner) limits of human consciousness. For most of us, only the least subtle and most obvious inner shifts are noticed: the perspective-altering consequences of being extremely tired, drunk, sexually aroused, or the effects of people we love or dislike on our mood. Subtler influences, such as that of different types of food upon our temperament and bodily functions, or regular social interactions, may only become apparent with time and contemplation. Many stimuli pass by our notice completely, being the bedrock of our awareness which could only be remarked by their absence, like removing a colour from a picture, or a letter from the alphabet. We mostly discern the forms and feelings of our experiences, not the ground upon which they are based.

Any "drug", therefore, is only a chemical product (or complex of chemicals, in the case of a medicinal plant) falling into the camp of external agents affecting our biochemistry in a more noticeable fashion. Relatively speaking, drugs are blunt instruments, fast-tracking physiological responses on a much grander scale than would usually occur. Psychoactive drugs are those which particularly affect our perceptions. It's arguable that all drugs affect our perceptions in the end, even non-psychoactive medicinal ones, because one thing leads to another. In other words, the consequence of any physical change may be a mental one, and vice versa. A drug which relieves constipation or lowers fever will by default also affect our mental state, both directly (as our symptoms change, so does our mood) and indirectly (emptying the bowel

---

[ix] The usual term is *psychonaut*, but I follow my fellow herbalists Karen Lawton and Fiona Heckels of Sensory Solutions in preferring the more accurate and less implicitly pejorative term "psychenaut". *Psyche*, meaning "mind", originates from the Greek word *psukhē*, meaning "soul"; and the suffix—*naut* comes from the Greek *nautes*, meaning sailor. Although the word *psycho* was originally synonymous with *psyche*, it's now the title of a Hitchcock film about a homicidal maniac.

causes subtle changes in what is reabsorbed from the colon, some components of which may have mood-altering effects; lowering body temperature is accompanied by changes in the circulation, including the circulation to the brain). Body and mind are one unit; that we live with this fact every day means we sometimes overlook its profundity.

The Mexica, as we have seen, used potable formulations of Cacao to reduce fear and timidity, for which purpose it was provided to their warriors to drink on campaigns, and to captives before they were sacrificed to the gods.[668] This historical use of chocolate to increase courage is mirrored in modern-day South American Santeria (a religion similar to Haitian Vodoun or "voodoo" as it's known in popular culture), where Cacao beans are used ritually "to remove fear",[669] and even in pop culture: in the Harry Potter books, chocolate is the best remedy for the after-effects of a Dementor attack. Chocolate is most definitely a psychoactive drug, though in recent years its effects in this category have been relegated by mainstream science to those of a caffeine-based stimulant, and a fairly weak one at that. Its devotees would dispute this on the basis of our perceptions and experiences: no other food or stimulant adequately replaces chocolate. What seems utterly apparent to consumers of traditional toasted, hand-ground Cacao drinks or even the "chocoholic on the street" addicted to the sweet dark brown stuff is that the particular mood alteration experienced following the ingestion of real chocolate can't be attributable to caffeine alone, for the simple reason that neither coffee, tea, or any other caffeine-containing plant seems as desirable as chocolate.

Traditionally prepared drinking chocolate made from the best quality beans may have much greater effects on mood and perception than chocolate candy. Hernández classified Mexica *cacahuatl* as potent psychoactive brews: he likened the effects of *cacahuatl* to the powerfully deliriant plant Jimsonweed (*Datura* sp.), and *Psilocybe* mushrooms (see epigraph in Chapter 1). What follows is a personal report compiled from subjective "drug experience" notes written during and after the consumption of a traditional chocolate drink made with 39.5g hand-toasted *criollo* Cacao *fermentado* beans from San Antonio Suchitequepez in the old Soconusco region in Guatemala, with approximately 0.5g mixed traditional Mesoamerican spices per serving (*Vanilla planifolia, Capsicum frutescens, Quararibea funebris, Pimienta dioica*, and *Magnolia mexicana*).

First, the beans were ground on the *metate*, then the spices were prepared and pulverised in a mortar and pestle and incorporated into the cocoa mass, which was re-ground on the *metate*, then allowed to set in the form of chocolate discs. The solid chocolate was refrigerated for around four months in this form before being made into a beverage with the addition of 10ml maple syrup (a concession to my sweet-addicted contemporary palate) and 55ml hot water, well frothed with a molinillo and consumed at around 9 p.m. in the evening, two to three hours after eating a light meal, while home alone. I wrote down the following impressions:

> An almost immediate sense of pleasure and anticipation from the bitter-sour, rich and slightly sweet taste of the drink. An amplification of feelings of pleasure and comfort in my own skin, first appreciated at 30 minutes and peaking at 2 hours after ingestion [*note*: these times correspond to the peak plasma levels of caffeine and theobromine respectively following chocolate ingestion in pharmacokinetic trials]. There is small but intense literally heart-felt joy, similar to but much less strong than that felt with MDMA, with a paradoxical undertone of sadness akin

to nostalgia, like that produced by daydreaming of a past romance or indulging in a happy childhood memory. Also on looking into a mirror or thinking about life I perceive myself as more attractive, relationships are considered in a more positive light, and life overall seems more full of potential than before. This subtle euphoria lasts around four to five hours with a gradual dissipation, but I am aware of an elevated mood for the rest of the night until I go to bed at around 4am. The following day, after 6 hours' sleep, I am less motivated to work, and feel a little "flat".

When the dose is repeated on the second day, the effects are similar, but with less euphoria. I have previously noted that the effect of a high-quality chocolate drink after a week of daily use, apart from the not inconsiderable pleasure of its consumption, appears to lack the marked comforting, euphoriant and confidence-enhancing effects initially perceived, and may even enhance a feeling of sadness or hollowness felt in the heart region. It seems from my own experimentation that a gap of up to three days may be necessary between "doses" of strong drinking chocolate to fully conserve its unique mood-altering effects, preferably—for maximal effect—abstaining from other sources of caffeine in-between.

These unique effects of real chocolate drinks, at least in myself, are only produced by 40g or so of the best quality Cacao prepared in the traditional manner and ingested as a drink on an almost empty stomach (not less than two or three hours after a meal), and are best experienced in solitude and quiet, or with—at most—relaxed social interaction. Any form of stress or "busyness", such as the requirement to do a lot of physical work, or public socialising, obscures many of the more subtle and pleasant effects on mood which seem to require some mental space for contemplation to be fully appreciated, leaving mainly the "caffeine" aspect of the drug's effect on consciousness, with an increase in alertness and sense of well-being and a potential for increased irritability [...] On the other hand, the drug seems to assist motivation and mental effort, and is very good for generating new ideas. Friends with a higher tolerance for caffeine, such as heavy coffee drinkers, seem to obtain only a mild sense of well-being, sometimes as soon as five minutes or so after ingestion.

Admittedly this account is subjective and based on personal observations, and therefore inadmissible as scientific evidence of psychoactivity, for who's to say that this impression of the mood-altering power of Cacao isn't merely the product of chocolate-addled enthusiasm? However, there's a lot of anecdotal support for Cacao's psychoactivity above and beyond its caffeine and theobromine content. The author of a research paper on the effects of chocolate on pain tolerance noted that "[c]hocolate seems to produce a much more mellow and longer-lasting sense of well-being than marijuana or other drugs" (Eggleston & White, 2013). Observations following the ingestion of traditional Cacao drinks (made with toasted ground Cacao beans, hot water, and Mesoamerican spices, with or without sweetening) which I sold at sporadic market stalls between 2013 and 2017, and dosed friends with at private gatherings, is that the following reactions were noted by other people, strangers or friends, trying real Cacao for the first time:

- An immediate taste-based response, frequently of pleasure ("Ooh"), but occasionally of aversion due to its strong, relatively bitter taste with some sour notes left over from fermentation (when Cacao is hand-toasted at lower temperatures the flavour is more complex).

- Sometimes, around five or ten minutes following ingestion, a sensation of relaxation, with or without a "headrush"; one or two people described a feeling of being a little "stoned", "dizzy", or "spacey". This is too soon for alkaloids and the like to have reached the bloodstream, and may represent the effect of Cacao's volatile constituents, or some compounds absorbed via the oral mucosa.

- About twenty to thirty minutes after ingestion, a feeling of stimulation, enhanced pleasure, sometimes even mild euphoria. This may correspond with peak blood levels of caffeine. Some people—perhaps those who were naturally upbeat, or who had a high tolerance for caffeine—didn't notice anything. At high doses, equal to or more than 60–80g cocoa beans in one "dose" (depending on individual sensitivity, whether the stomach is full or empty, etc.), nausea may occur.

- About 90–120 minutes following ingestion appears to be the "peak effect": perception of enhanced thinking ability and contentment, with a stable, nostalgic mild euphoria, depending on individual sensitivity; this effect is appreciably diminished with frequent consumption of Cacao and, to a lesser degree, other xanthine-containing drugs. Tremor, agitation, headache, nausea, and vomiting may occur with higher intakes (over 60–80g in a single dose). Again, a few people notice or report nothing.

Nothing here is necessarily indicative of anything other than a "caffeine effect" plus placebo, in other words people's perceptions affecting their experiences. But if that's the case, there are many remarkable coincidences in the research on chocolate, brain chemistry, and behaviour.

"'Tasty caffeine"

While there's a lot of information about the biological effects of Cacao's antioxidant compounds and polyphenols, the properties of the trace compounds and volatile oils in Cacao are less well investigated. Most contemporary research focuses on the polyphenols' effects on the heart and circulation, but Cacao was traditionally consumed for its psychoactive attributes— as a mood-raising, anti-fatigue, perception-altering drink. The vascular effects shown by research can hardly have been known as such; although its benefit as a tonifying substance was recognised, this was secondary to the pleasure and stimulation its use occasioned. Ergo, Cacao's traditional consumption at feasts, on important occasions, by kings, nobility, pre-sacrificial victims, warriors, and merchants on long journeys.

Chocolate has been described as "stimulant, relaxant, euphoriant, aphrodisiac, tonic, and antidepressant".[670] To what extent are any of these textbook labels of chocolate's effects true? A 2013 review of the scientific evidence to date concluded that chocolate can improve mood or attenuate negative moods, enhance cognition, and alter brain activation patterns,[671] which suggests that the "tonic" and "antidepressant" labels are at least partially justifiable. What remains uncertain is whether the apparent effects of chocolate on mood are due mainly to an emotional or psychological reaction to consuming delicious chocolate, or to the psychoactive effects of some of the chemical compounds in Cacao. Given the pharmacology of the seeds, it seems likely that mood changes are a consequence of chemistry, not just psychology, and the brain scan studies described in the last chapter which showed increased blood flow following the ingestion of high-flavanol chocolate corroborate this.

Despite the plethora of psychoactive compounds found in Cacao, conventional wisdom has it that Cacao's perceived effects on mood are mainly due to its caffeine content. Caffeine is the most powerful stimulant compound in *Theobroma cacao*, and a 100mg dose, the amount found in approximately 50g of whole Cacao (equivalent to a large serving of Maya or Mexica-style drinking chocolate), or two cups of black tea, produces "alertness, well-being, sociability, willingness to work, energy, and self-confidence" in most people.[672] But compared to caffeine, there is ten times as much of the other major alkaloid in Cacao, theobromine, per serving. Theobromine also has some brain-stimulating effects, binding to similar adenosine receptors on nerve cells in the brain (known as neurons), but much less strongly than caffeine. Theobromine's main effects are on the kidneys (it's diuretic—increasing urine output), heart, and lungs (it stimulates the heart, and dilates the airways a bit). In fact all three xanthine alkaloids in Cacao—theobromine, theophylline, and caffeine—increase preferences for foods or drinks containing them, an effect called *positive reinforcement*.[673] So perhaps caffeine and theobromine are the main reasons for chocolate's appeal, and its purported psychoactive effects?

One small double-blind clinical trial put this to the test. Twenty participants were split into three groups: one group took 11.6g encapsulated cocoa powder, another group took capsules containing 250mg theobromine and 19mg caffeine (approximately the same amount of alkaloid as in the cocoa powder capsules), and a third group took placebo capsules. All the participants were given a mood questionnaire before, during, and after the trial, and their reaction time and visual processing speed (measuring things like how fast an image could be recognised) were tested. The researchers found no differences between the cocoa and caffeine/theobromine groups, and concluded that "[the] psychopharmacological activity [of chocolate] … [is] confined to the combination of caffeine and theobromine."[674] Mixtures of theobromine and caffeine (as found in Cacao) are reported to have no greater effect on mood than caffeine alone[675]—so is Cacao's psychoactivity just down to caffeine, after all?

Caffeine binds ten times more strongly than theobromine to the receptor sites it activates in the brain, yet the high ratio of theobromine to caffeine in Cacao suggests that the stimulating effects of Cacao beans should be far lower than they are.[676] The results of the small clinical trial comparing cocoa powder to an equivalent dose of isolated caffeine plus theobromine may be misleading for several important reasons: 1) the very low doses used; 2) the use of cocoa powder, the most highly processed form of Cacao; 3) a small group size, and 4) the measuring of mood changes with a simple questionnaire, a relatively unsubtle instrument. The design of a mood questionnaire may severely curtail the sensitivity of qualitative evaluation—in other words, if the questions simply asked people to score "alertness" or "well-being", this in no way describes what these people were actually feeling, sensing, or thinking; even a response such as "friendliness" fails to accurately describe the feeling or its intensity.

To unpack each of these issues: 1) the very low dose of cocoa powder used in this trial may mask any differences between the effects of cocoa powder and isolated caffeine plus theobromine. If other, less potent constituents in Cacao have psychoactive effects, these effects may only show up distinctly at higher doses, more representative of the quantities of Cacao in a larger serving of traditional drink, around 40–60g of whole Cacao. 2) Cocoa powder also has a very low polyphenol content, and contains far less volatiles, fats, and fat-soluble compounds than whole Cacao beans; this not only markedly alters the chemical composition of the drug, but alters the pharmacokinetics (substance absorption and distribution in the body). This would reduce any modifying effects of trace constituents, and curtail the impact of fats and lipid-soluble compounds on central nervous system opioid response and amino alcohol absorption (all of which will be discussed more fully later in this chapter, and in Chapter 7). 3) Small sample sizes limit accuracy due to possible skewing of results: if an unweighted dice is thrown ten times, a six may be rolled five times. The conclusion from this limited number of throws would be that "one in two throws of a dice will roll a six". Rolling the same dice a thousand times would produce a score closer to one in six: sample sizes matter.

Finally, 4) the questionnaire used in the trial was limited—it gave a multiple-choice range of physical sensations, such as "heart pounding" and "sweating", and asked participants to mark their "overall mood" on a bad-good scale with either end of the scale representing "the most extreme sensation you've ever felt". It would therefore record gross mood and physical changes but fail to pick up more subtle effects on mood and behaviour, such as fear responses, openness, and self-perception, for example. It's possible that larger trial groups could reveal differences between the whole drug and its isolated principal alkaloids by comparing bigger "doses" of traditional chocolate drinks to similar-tasting liquid caffeine and theobromine-laced beverages, and utilising more in-depth assessments, such as a more detailed questionnaire, psychometric tests, and physical measurements like galvanic skin response to different emotional stimuli (as in a lie detector test).

The previous trial shows that low doses of cocoa powder don't seem to affect gross mood changes any differently from caffeine and theobromine, so if there are any psychoactive properties in Cacao which are not dependent on the xanthines, they are likely to be relatively subtle. Subtle mood effects require subtle tests to measure them. I suggest that future explorations of Cacao's psychoactivity should incorporate the following:

1. A higher *quality* (e.g., ground whole toasted beans, not cocoa powder) and *dose* (e.g., 40–50g) of Cacao tested against an equivalent dosage of caffeine and theobromine, and
2. More detailed methods of assessing various aspects of perception, mood, and emotional processing, including physical measures such as urine output, blood pressure, pulse rate, brachial artery dilation (flow-mediated dilation) and skin response. A validated and comprehensive mood assessment questionnaire may be used, such as the reliable Positive And Negative Affect Schedule-X (PANAS-X) questionnaire. PANAS-X distinguishes between basic positive and negative moods, three positive and four negative emotional states: joviality, attentiveness, and self-assurance (positive) or fear, sadness, hostility, and guilt (negative) as well as four other measures—shyness, serenity, fear, and surprise.

One of the researchers in the group who found no difference between the psychotropic effects of cocoa powder and theobromine plus caffeine commented in another research paper:

> Although the methylxanthines in chocolate appear to represent its pharmacological activity … the list of minor chocolate constituents presented here is not exhaustive, nor does it address potential interactive effects between compounds that are not explained by their individual effects. (Smit, in Fredholm, 2011)[677]

In other words, while caffeine is the primary psychotropic compound in chocolate, there may be more to the story.

Another small uncontrolled (no placebo group) study with 280 participants between eighteen and sixty-five years old tested the effects of consuming controlled doses (12.5g) of white and dark chocolate on Addiction Research Centre Inventory (ARCI) questionnaire responses. The ARCI questionnaire is a 600 item inventory designed to differentiate between the effects of different drug groups, and has a "high degree of reliability and validity".[678] A clear trend was discernible: chocolate-lovers scored higher on the Morphine-Benzedrine Group (MBG) subscale, and the darker the chocolate, the stronger the MBG high-scorers' desire for more chocolate became.[679] The MBG is a scale for quantifying the subjective effects that draw people to use morphine (or other opiates, such as heroin or codeine) or amphetamines ("speed"); the principal characteristics of this group are "feeling more popular", "well-being, euphoria … [and] optimal functioning".[680] The sugar content also had an influence in this direction, though less significant than the Cacao content of the chocolate. Interestingly, more men than women expressed a stronger desire for more of the chocolate—though this could be due to cultural conditioning among some of the women in the group (the "I shouldn't have more, I'm on a diet" effect). The researchers concluded that "multiple characteristics of chocolate, including sugar, cocoa and *the drug-like effects experienced* [my emphasis], play a role in the desire to consume chocolate".[681] However, caffeine alone does modestly increase MBG group score,[682] so this result isn't proof of a non-caffeine-based psychoactive effect for Cacao.

Unfortunately, some researchers appear to be ignorant of the qualitative and pharmacological differences between available types of chocolate: often no distinction is made between chocolate-coated biscuit bars, cheap milk chocolate, or dark chocolate—an error of considerable magnitude. So some researchers found that chocolate-*flavoured* foods, or chocolate containing low doses of Cacao, produced no lasting changes in mood after a single meal; unforgivably, they described all these foods as "chocolate"—a blunder as gross as Sigmund Freud's when he published his paper *"Uber Coca"* ("On Coca") in the late nineteenth century, promoting the therapeutic use of cocaine, confusing the isolated alkaloid with the benign Coca leaf from which it was extracted—a misapprehension for which, arguably, many people are still paying today. (Freud later realised his error after becoming severely addicted to cocaine, and retracted his initial support for the fast-acting wonder drug; but he never cleared up his initial conflation of the isolated substance with its botanical source). Meanwhile, five out of eight studies in a "meta-analysis"—a statistical review of the same type of research to date, which excludes poorly done or low quality research—showed evidence of "either an improvement in mood state or an attenuation of negative mood" after eating chocolate.[683]

Chocolate and depression

Clinical studies on chocolate's effect on mood have produced varying results: according to one experiment, *intention* enhances mood-raising properties of ordinary eating chocolate—in other words, while chocolate could turn the will to happiness into actual happy feelings, it only restored a measure of equanimity to people with the blues in comparison with drinking plain water, which unsurprisingly had no effect on mood. Chocolate apparently boosted subjects' expectations and intentions to feel happy; those who passively awaited a mood boost experienced little improvement.[684] Another study similarly demonstrated that "mindful" consumption of chocolate has a much greater ability to improve mood than "non-mindful" consumption of chocolate, or of dry crackers, whether they were eaten mindfully or not![685] This suggests that some inherent property of chocolate increases its potential to raise mood above that of other foods, but that this potential requires activation through intent.

A group of forty young adults (in their twenties) taking 250mg cocoa both acutely and over a one-month period only experienced a small increase in mental performance and reduction in fatigue immediately after consuming the cocoa, with no cumulative effects on cognition, blood flow, or mood either immediately or after one month.[686] Again, though, the dose is ludicrously low (a quarter of a gram) and the poorest-quality form of Cacao, cocoa powder, was used. To be fair, the assessment methods (clinical tests and validated clinical assessment questionnaires) here were more sophisticated than the basic questionnaire used in the "caffeine and theobromine vs. cocoa" comparison trial. In general, when the drug is low-quality and the dose is too small, the results are of little consequence, but it's still useful to know where the margins lie. Dosage and quality do matter.

By contrast, a small-scale gold standard (double-blind, placebo-controlled) clinical trial using chocolate for patients with senile dementia found that a once-daily dose of chocolate containing 500mg polyphenols over one month significantly improved "self-rated calmness and contentedness", although no improvement in mood or memory and cognition was noted.[687] It's difficult to say how improvement in "calmness and contentedness" isn't an improvement in mood! 500mg polyphenols is equivalent to approximately 40g Cacao, an achievable daily intake and a realistic dosage in terms of traditional Cacao drinks. So chocolate made the demented patients *feel better*, without making them *measurably* happier or better at thinking (by the rubric of this trial). But one month is a very short trial period—if such changes were noted in four weeks, it would be interesting to see what a year's daily intake of high-polyphenol chocolate could do. It should be noted that in this trial, the researchers were very specific about using an adequate dosage of high-quality (high polyphenol) dark chocolate, something which many other investigators have failed to do.

On the other hand, one survey of 1018 Californian adults found that the more depressed people said they were, the more chocolate they were likely to eat.[688] In another online survey of 3000 respondents with a history of clinical depression, just over half (51%) of the women surveyed, and just under a third (31%) of the men reported craving chocolate when depressed.[689] The apparent mood-altering effects of chocolate were ranked higher by cravers than its taste or appearance. The skew towards female 'use' of chocolate in this way may reflect either cultural bias or a sex-linked pharmacological difference in Cacao's effectiveness as a mood modulator in anatomically male and female brains. Uniquely, this survey went even further, to inquire what characteristics set the chocolate-cravers apart from the non-chocophile despondent respondents. What they found was that the depressed chocolate cravers' responses consistently evinced greater *neuroticism*; specifically, they had higher levels of *irritability* and *rejection sensitivity*.[690]

In one sense, these results seems highly predictable, without need of explanation: *of course* people eat more chocolate when they're depressed! But they could be interpreted several ways:

1) The depressives were attempting to "self-medicate" with chocolate
2) Higher intakes of chocolate may *cause* or *aggravate* depression, or
3) The association may be due to the high sugar and fat content of sweet "comfort foods" in general, rather than Cacao in particular (these ideas are investigated in Chapter 7), or
4) It may be an accidental finding due to self-selected samples (there may have been a larger-than-usual proportion of melancholic chocoholics among those who chose to do an online quiz about chocolate and mood).

In other words, was the depressives' increased chocolate intake in these surveys an indication of consequence, causation, or coincidence? As noted in the last chapter, subjects with depression often have relatively high blood levels of copper,[691] and Cacao is a high-copper food-drug, which may imply that regular high chocolate intake could contribute to depressive states (see Chapter 7 for more on Cacao's copper content). On the other hand, another study found that people who "self-medicated" low mood with chocolate or other sweet foods were "more likely to have personality traits associated with hysteroid dysphoria, an atypical depressive syndrome".[692] Hysteroid dysphoria is characterised by low mood associated with a feeling of rejection and sweet craving—or as I like to think of it, "permanently dumped syndrome".

Hysteroid dysphoria is often treated by a class of drugs known as MAOIs (monoamine oxidase inhibitors), and it's intriguing that Cacao contains many substances with this property. There are two types of MAO, known as monoamine-A and monoamine-B. Both types of MAO are enzymes, protein-based substances that catalyse chemical reactions; MAO specifically helps to break down a group of stimulating chemicals called *catecholamines*, which include the brain's most important "desire, excitement, and motivation" chemicals (serotonin, dopamine, adrenaline, noradrenaline, and phenethylamine), so inhibiting MAO enzymes raises the levels of catecholamines in the body or brain. Both types of MAO break down tyramine (a precursor for several other compounds) and the mood-regulating chemicals serotonin and dopamine. As yet there isn't much evidence that chocolate intake modifies levels of catecholamines in the human brain, although huge one-off doses of Cacao polyphenols raised brain serotonin, dopamine, and noradrenaline in rats,[693] and more reasonable doses of whole dark chocolate increased the production and quantity of serotonin in rabbits' brains over two weeks.[694]

Nevertheless there are some indications of real-life "monoamine modification" (adjustments of the brain chemicals listed above) induced by chocolate. In one human clinical trial, a month's daily consumption of 50g dark chocolate significantly raised blood levels of 5-HIAA, a breakdown product of serotonin, which indicates increased serotonin manufacture, release, and breakdown. There was also a not-quite-big-enough-to-be-statistically-significant trend towards increased serotonin and decreasing adrenaline, with an initial increase in noradrenaline after seven days, which receded back to baseline levels after four weeks.[695] In plain English, this implies that the chocolate did at least affect the brain's levels of "happy chemicals", and certainly altered the processing of serotonin. This adrenaline-lowering effect corroborates a finding mentioned in the last chapter, from a placebo-controlled trial wherein a single 50g dose of 72%

dark chocolate administered to men acutely reduced their blood and salivary levels of cortisol and adrenaline in response to stress.[696] In another human trial, thirty people were categorised as having high or low anxiety and given 40g dark chocolate to eat every day for two weeks. The quantity of the stress steroid cortisol and breakdown products of adrenaline in their urine was measured every day. At the end of the trial, all participants' levels of cortisol and adrenaline had *fallen*, but subjects with higher levels of anxiety had a bigger decline in stress markers than their less stressed cohorts.

The study's authors concluded that "dark chocolate … partially normalised stress-related differences in energy metabolism", possibly by modifying host metabolism and gut microbial metabolism.[697] In other words chocolate may have changed the way that the human organism and the tiny organisms living inside the humans operated, to improve stress resistance. So this research indicates an that Cacao has MAO-independent stress-reducing properties, and that this effect may be stronger in more highly stressed individuals. These results suggest that chocolate may have serotonin-conserving, cortisol and adrenaline-depleting activity, by more than one mechanism. There is some *in vitro* support for this hypothesis, as water extracts of Cacao have been found to inhibit the breakdown of an amino acid (a nutrient and building block of protein) called tryptophan, and reduce the production of a substance called neopterin in cells of the immune system. Tryptophan is the main building block of serotonin, and people with clinical depression tend to have high neopterin and low serotonin levels, so the authors of the paper speculate that Cacao may affect mood by regulating these chemicals;[698] in other words, Cacao may be affecting mood by interacting with processes outside the brain as well as within it, providing more evidence that the body is an interactive ecology, not a collection of separate functional units. So the "self-medicating" explanation for some depressives' preference for chocolate may be the correct one, though the jury isn't still out—they are just settling into their seats.

Cacao's traditional assignation of having a "Cold, Dry" nature accords with these results. As we saw in Chapter 3, in sixteenth century European medicine "Cold and Dry" meant having a melancholic nature, yet there are several plant-based medicines in the pharmacopoeia of the time which were said to be "Cold and Dry" and could be used to treat melancholy, such as the plant Fumitory (*Fumaria officinalis*), or Damask Roses (*Rosa uricate*). In modern times we would say that these plants have anti-anxiety, anti-inflammatory, or anti-spasmodic activity; traditionally, it was perceived that they had a definite Cooling effect, for example by reducing fever or relieving itchy skin conditions, yet also relieved melancholy. Cacao could be "warmed" with the addition of sweetening and spices, and was used to treat some forms of melancholy; nevertheless, it could cause "melancholic obstructions" in excess. So early European concepts of Cacao's medicinal actions suggest that it may relieve low mood, especially over the short term, but may exacerbate depression if used immoderately or improperly.

As tangential support for this historical view, in another online survey with 3000 respondents who self-identified as having suffered from clinical depression, 45% of respondents reported chocolate cravings, most of whom referred to chocolate's "capacity to settle 'emotional dysregulation' … and this aspect was ranked above aesthetic factors".[699] Here we have the first piece of non-anecdotal evidence that some depressed people are using chocolate to self-medicate. So it may be that that those of a more "melancholic" disposition—worriers or grumblers—experience more obvious mood-altering effects from Cacao than confident optimists.

An antidote to fear?

So, there are now clinical trials demonstrating that mood can improve after eating chocolate, that chocolate may increase subjective feelings of well-being, that it can modify stress responses over time by diminishing adrenaline and cortisol levels, and that it affects dopamine and serotonin metabolism. Still, solid pharmacological and clinical evidence of conventionally antidepressant effects is lacking. If Cacao has any psychoactivity beyond that of low-dose caffeine, it's not yet been conclusively demonstrated in humans. Tantalisingly, the small feeding trial in rats mentioned above, which drew a blank on acute catecholamine changes, did show that ingestion of larger one-off "doses" of Cacao—equivalent to the upper end of the daily intake for a human, corresponding to an average of around 60–70g whole Cacao daily, more easily achieved through traditional drinks than with eating chocolate—significantly reduced *conditioned fear* responses, even more than a standard tranquilliser drug (intravenous benzodiazepine, 0.1mg/kg). Yet chocolate had no effect on instinctual fear responses in the test animals. Conversely, when given daily over two weeks, the same dosage slightly *increased* conditioned fear reactions, accompanied by a mild rise in brain serotonin levels.[700]

To explain this result, understand that "conditioned fear" is fear which has been trained into a sentient organism (a human or non-human animal) through harsh or unpleasant experiences, and becomes linked to "triggers" associated with those experiences. A backfiring car causing a war veteran to duck, alert to a non-existent threat of bombs or gunfire, is an example of a conditioned fear reaction. Phobias are often—though not always—conditioned fear responses, where a fear-based survival reaction can become magnified or linked to something utterly harmless through a traumatic experience (the "conditioned stimulus"). Instinctive fear responses to such things as snakes or spiders are different—these fears are often hard-wired, primordial reactions, designed to keep us safe, though they can be magnified or reduced by learning and observing other people's behaviours as children; but excessive fear of ordinary things (open spaces, harmless animals) is often conditioned. The word phobia comes from *Phobos*, the Greek god of fear (incidentally, for those who like to contemplate such things, Phobos was the son of the goddess of love and the god of war).

Excesses of conditioned fear result in generalised anxiety disorder or post-traumatic stress disorder (PTSD) in humans, and these responses originate mainly from a primitive but powerful part of the brain called the amygdala. Most interestingly, neither caffeine nor amphetamine has any effect on conditioned fear,[701] indicating a different pharmacological mechanism for Cacao from the conventional "caffeine" explanation for its effect on mood. Moreover, caffeine alone doesn't cause a cumulative increase in brain serotonin. Of course, these experiments were conducted on rats, not people, and the tests used to assess mood effects in animals are much cruder and more brutal than would be permitted in human subjects. But this is the first really solid piece of evidence that Cacao's psychoactivity doesn't depend on caffeine alone, and that the plant may have specific *antiphobic* (fear-reducing) properties.

In support of this hypothesis, research has shown that Cacao may have a direct effect on the amygdala. Some researchers investigating whether chocolate has different effects on the brain chemistry of men and women found that drinking chocolate milk stimulated different brain areas in men and women, and only women had decreased activity in the amygdala.[702] This may suggest that women are more sensitive to Cacao's potential anti-phobic effects, although the Cacao content of chocolate milk is far lower than a traditional Cacao beverage. This research is the first piece of evidence demonstrating that a Cacao-containing food may directly affect the brain's fear response centre. It remains to be seen whether this finding is replicable, and whether higher doses of unadulterated Cacao have a similar effect on men.

A tantalising fact emerges from recent research into PTSD, in which it was discovered that when a fear response was reawoken in male PTSD sufferers, those who were simultaneously taking cortisol in tablet form were much more likely to have their PTSD return.[703] In PTSD there is something called *reconsolidation*, which is another way of saying that when a stress response is replayed, it becomes a habit—it is "re-consolidated", or brought back up and cemented into place. It makes sense that when the background level of stress hormone is higher, the fear response will be more strongly reinforced. Research into PTSD often focuses on something called the *reconsolidation window*, with the aim of stopping the panic response, an outcome called *extinction*—which, in this case, is something we want. The reconsolidation window is a brief period of time when the fear is reactivated, in which there is an opportunity to disrupt or repro-gramme the amygdala's fear response with drugs or therapeutic techniques and break the habit, reducing or extinguishing the PTSD symptoms.[704]

This raises some interesting possibilities: because Cacao lowers cortisol levels and may reduce conditioned fear responses, could it be of benefit to sufferers from PTSD? Note that if the animal trial results on Cacao's effect in conditioned fear turn out to be generalisable to humans, then chronic, daily intake of Cacao—or chocolate—may even slightly increase conditioned fear responses. Larger, one-off doses may be required to reduce conditioned fear, whereas both short and longer-term use may lower cortisol and adrenaline responses. So perhaps an optimal dosing strategy would be a happy medium: regular, but not daily use of larger doses of Cacao, in a therapeutic setting. This accords with the historical use of Cacao by the Mexica as a "reward drug" for warriors and merchants (both very hazardous occupations in fourteenth- and fifteenth-century Mesoamerica) or human sacrificial offerings—what better drug for those in mortal danger than one which may attenuate conditioned fear responses? And the injunction to consume Cacao moderately: it was "not drunk unthinkingly" (Sahagún, quoted in Coe & Coe, 1996). Even the Mexica's recreational use of Cacao drinks laced with "magic mushrooms" (*Psilocybe spp.*) in all-night celebrations had a practical, divinatory function. *Cacahuatl* would not have been drunk every day by any warrior in Mexica society. For the privileged nobles, warriors, and merchants permitted to use the drink, we may speculate that Cacao may have helped them to experience battles, near-death experiences, or intense prophetic visions with-out developing post-traumatic stress. Such properties may underlie Cacao's sacramental status in Mesoamerica.

"Cacao shaman" Keith Wilson's informal "Cacao ceremonies" are intense and interesting.[705] These ceremonies are carried out regularly, usually twice a week, at his home in San Marcos by lake Atitlan in Guatemala, and occasionally in other locations around the world. Keith's process involves administering moderately large doses of Cacao—uricat. 43–45g as a starting dose, equivalent to one serving of traditional Mayan or Mexica-style *kakaw/cacahuatl*—to all the adults present, then talking all participants into a meditative state where they focus on their bodies, and "zone in" on any areas of pain, discomfort, or "blockage", aiming to "release it".

The ceremonies are a "safe space" where participants are encouraged to cry, laugh, move around, or do whatever to "release any blockages" they encounter. The effect of Keith's Cacao is obvious—thirty minutes after everyone drinks their Cacao, the amplifying effect of the guided meditation becomes apparent, with increased excitement, euphoria, mood changes and—in some cases—nausea and physical discomfort; many people became visibly emotional, some laughing, some crying, others sitting as if transfixed. An optional "top-up" of 25–30g Cacao is ingested after an hour or so.

Coincidentally, Keith's total Cacao dosage (57–60g per person, in a mixed group of men and women, average age mid- to late twenties, age range from nineteen to sixty-plus) in the ceremonies approximates, in grams per kilogram of bodyweight, to the amount used in the rat experiment where one-off oral doses of Cacao were found to reduce conditioned fear. Recent research has indicated that if a conditioned fear response is disrupted during the reconsolidation window, it may be erased from the amygdala. This is reminiscent of Keith's process: priming the audience by talking about past trauma, getting people to meditate on and somatise (experience physically) the source of their pain or "blockage", then "releasing" and "transmuting" it with the assistance of high-dose traditional Cacao drinks. The meditation may recall whichever fear or trauma is uppermost in the subconscious by zoning in on physical sensations; hypothetically, Cacao then wedges open the reconsolidation window and partially blocks the fear response by reducing adrenaline and cortisol and perhaps also directly affecting the amygdala. In one experimental session I conducted using guided meditation (a variation of Keith's method with a basic NLP visualisation technique thrown in) with a traditionally prepared Cacao drink for a volunteer subject living with PTSD, this method temporarily helped him overcome the issue (see Appendix D). However, the hypothesis that Cacao has anti-phobic effects requires pharmacological confirmation, as auto-hypnosis or suggestion can powerfully affect outcomes.

Another condition which may be linked to an overactivated or exhausted adrenal response is chronic fatigue syndrome (CFS). CFS is a very debilitating syndrome of unknown cause, suspected to be linked to a combination of issues such as previous infections, immune system dysfunction, and psychological or emotional factors. A very small double-blind placebo-controlled trial tested the effect of a daily dosage of forty-five grams of good quality dark chocolate (85% cocoa solids, containing approximately 1g of polyphenols) on people with CFS over an eight-week period. The trial was a "crossover design", meaning that all ten participants had real chocolate, then were swapped over onto the placebo chocolate halfway through; and because it was double-blind, neither participants nor experimenters knew when the real chocolate was being administered until after the trial. It turned out that when they were taking the real chocolate, all the participants experienced a significant reduction in tiredness and physical handicap, as well as a gradual reduction in anxiety and depression.[706] This correlates well with the reduction in adrenaline and cortisol, together with increased serotonin metabolism recorded in other experiments, though there may be other reasons for these benefits, such as Cacao's beneficial effects on blood circulation and inflammation (see previous chapter). The group size was also very small, and the results would need to be replicated with larger groups, but it's a very encouraging result—particularly as CFS is often seen as an intractable condition.

The possible utility of Cacao as a therapeutic mood modifier, with which people may be self-medicating in the form of confectionery, is underscored by a recent study which compared un-medicated subjects who had recently attempted suicide with people who weren't depressed, measuring the levels of 5-HIAA, cortisol, and the precursor hormone DHEA in their brain and spinal fluid. (DHEA or dehydroepiandrosterone is a hormone manufactured in the adrenals, gonads, and brain, and the body uses it as a precursor for manufacturing the sex hormones oestrogen and testosterone; it's also a hormone in its own right, which modulates behavioural changes in the brain, and affects the immune system.) The result: "Suicide victims [*sic*] tended to have low CSF 5-HIAA and high CSF cortisol."[707] So Cacao's apparent ability to reduce cortisol and increase brain and blood 5-HIAA levels may provide another pharmacological rationale for its traditional use as a food for soldiers, soldiering being a very stressful profession with a high suicide rate among veterans. In Cacao, we may find that not only have we rediscovered a useful ally for the treatment of conditioned fear-related problems such as PTSD, or mind-body-immune system disorders such as chronic fatigue syndrome, but that many of us are already consuming an adulterated form of it, perhaps unaware that we are attempting to self-medicate.

Chocolate for a better personality? (Part 1)

In a study of 305 new mums, women who experienced antenatal stress reported more negative temperaments (fear responses) in their children at six months old. But mothers who ate choco-late weekly or daily during pregnancy rated their children's temperaments more positively at six months postpartum than mums who ate no chocolate. Similarly, mothers who reported high levels of stress during the pregnancy but who also consumed chocolate weekly or daily did *not* rate their children's behaviour more negatively at six months old, unlike chocolate-abstaining mums (although they didn't rate them as highly as the chocolate-consuming women who weren't stressed while pregnant). Remarkably, the effect was also proportional to the quan-tity of chocolate the mums ate: mothers' positive ratings of their children's temperaments at six months old was greater with daily consumption of chocolate during pregnancy than weekly chocolate consumption. The authors concluded that chocolate produced "subjective feelings of psychological wellbeing", but may also "have effects at multiple environmental and psycho-logical levels".[708] To put it another way, the researchers were assuming that the chocolate was affecting the women's perception of their children, but couldn't rule out the possibility that the chocolate may have affected the children's personalities. Importantly, the study was funded by the University of Helsinki, not a chocolate manufacturing company!

As with other social studies, drawing direct conclusions from this data is difficult; the authors caution that there may be "a common denominator that underlies both chocolate consumption and infant temperament".[709] In other words, the dietetically uninhibited mother-to-be who con-sumes chocolate on a daily basis may be the *type of person* who naturally rates her baby's behav-iour more positively, or who would raise a happier baby (whether due to genetic or behavioural influences on the child's personality), and this would be the case even if she lived in a parallel, chocolate-free reality. But it does not accord with the positive correlation between greater choco-late consumption and depression and neuroticism in adults. If the results of this study turn out to be replicable, it's another piece of evidence which suggests that neurotic depressives' greater inclination to consume chocolate may be an attempt at self-medicating their low mood. Unless by some quirk chocolate turns out to exacerbate low mood in some adults but enhance their perception of happiness in their children: chocolate-induced post-natal depression, anyone? "I'm a new mum. I need chocolate."

One social group who may benefit from any stress-relieving potential of Cacao are the elderly. Elderly people in general experience more social isolation and loneliness as a result of the deaths of their peers, and as a consequence of depression and declining health become more "vulnerable to nutritional disorders."[710] A survey of 424 Houston residents over sixty-five years of age found that less isolated elderly people consumed more chocolate-containing foods, possibly "as a means of maintaining social ties"—the "dessert hypothesis" of chocolate-related social integration. But the senior citizens' consumption of chocolate-flavoured foods increased during stressful periods, which again seems to imply using chocolate to self-medicate anxiety or low mood. In another intriguing social study, a survey of 1367 elderly Finnish men of similar income level and social status, averaging seventy-six years old, discovered that men who preferred chocolate to other sweets were found to do more exercise, to have better subjective health, and lower BMI and waist circumference, indicating reduced susceptibility to heart disease and diabetes. They also had significantly fewer feelings of loneliness and depression, rated themselves as happier, and had more plans for the future than respondents who expressed a preference for other types of sweets. As the researchers put it, the chocolate eaters had "better health, optimism and ... psychological well-being".[711] This corresponds with the happy babies, yet contrasts most intriguingly with the picture of chocolate as the neurotic's choice; perhaps this is simply a difference between chocolate preference, and chocolate craving?

As with the well-disposed chocolate-*in-utero* children, it should be noted that these results don't necessarily mean that chocolate increased health, optimism, and well-being among this cohort of elderly gentlemen. It's equally valid to conclude that the men who preferred chocolate may have been *predisposed* to take better care of themselves, or that consumption of *non-chocolate* sweets *reduced* physical and mental health in this group (see last chapter re sweets/candy intake and cardiovascular disease risk). But in the latter case, it would appear that chocolate consumption at least provided some protection from the harmful effects of sugar consumption; and the former possibility, that the chocolate-lovers were a group of "healthy-living" enthusiasts, seems inconsistent with the old-school image of chocolate among previous generations as an indulgence, not a health food.

So, as cause or coincidence, higher chocolate consumption among the elderly (at least those in Houston and Finland) appears to correspond with better mental and social health. Similarly, in a small survey of sixty-five young US university students, chocolate preference was found to be greater in the subset who believed their destiny to be predominantly under their own control than their less chocolate-inclined, more fatalistic fellows—although this sample size is so small as to be of questionable relevance.[712] Again, this doesn't resolve the question of whether greater chocolate consumption is a *consequence* or a *cause* of this more optimistic perspective, but the connection is intriguing.

Fairy dust: the debatable role of Cacao's trace constituents

In European folklore, fairies were supernatural beings of variable form, sometimes quite fearsome to behold, who could be harmed by iron and hated being thanked for good deeds, preferring more permanent guarantees of remembrance. To be "elf shot" in the Middle Ages was to have a wasting disease. In the Victorian era fairies were reinvented as tiny flying people with diaphanous wings who lived in pretty flowers and greetings cards (although it should be noted that the pre-eminent Victorian fairy artist, Richard Dadd, was a schizophrenic who murdered his father in a psychotic episode. He began to paint fairies once he was incarcerated, after his patricidal breakdown, and most of the paintings are umbral works of hallucinatory genius.) Cacao, too, has been reinvented: the Mesoamerican *kakaw*, royal drug and sacramental blood-substitute, and the old European "*chocolatl*", an exotic New World super-drug and controversial aphrodisiac elixir, has gradually morphed into something suitable for children. A tasty morsel of fat, sugar, and a little caffeine doesn't seem very remarkable.

But looking at Cacao's neurochemical and social effects in humans, there is a measurable set of responses following Cacao or chocolate ingestion which can't be attributed to caffeine and theobromine alone: altered serotonin metabolism, improvement in chronic fatigue, stress-dependent reduction in adrenaline and cortisol, mothers' perception of greater happiness in their babies, more sociable elderly people, and more neurotic adults' higher consumption of chocolate—and, as we shall see in Chapter 7, some psychotropic substance users and therapists rate dark chocolate highly as a drug response enhancer. The animal experiments showing chronically elevated central serotonin and acutely decreased conditioned fear responses following Cacao ingestion are also suggestive. These effects constellate chocolate's "fairy dust"—the special magic that many perceive in chocolate, of which there are tantalising hints in its pharmacology, folklore, and clinical research, but are often regarded as mere glamour or erroneously attributed to Cacao's modest caffeine content.

Adding a little circumstantial weight to the notion that chocolate directly affects central serotonin is the observation that chocolate consumption is greater in colder European countries, and US chocolate consumption rises during winter months.[713] This may simply be related to chocolate's high fat and sugar content—as a rule, rich "comfort food" is preferable to salad in wintry climates. But the longer nights of winter and northern latitudes are also associated with lower brain serotonin levels, giving rise to seasonal affective disorder (SAD) in many people during autumn, traditionally known as the melancholic season. As some popular health websites and columnists have pointed out, Cacao does contain tryptophan, the amino acid which is converted into serotonin in the body, and many ascribe the alleged antidepressant effect of Cacao and chocolate to this fact. But a daily dose of more than 1500mg tryptophan is required for antidepressant effects, whereas a serving of 40g whole Cacao (such as may be found in a 100g bar of ordinary dark chocolate, quite a large "dose") contains only 3–7mg of tryptophan; moreover the tryptophan and serotonin contained in chocolate is poorly absorbed due to Cacao's overall protein profile. It's more likely that Cacao's MAO-inhibiting constituents (see below) raise central serotonin levels to some degree, with a little help from the tryptophan; but perhaps it's simply the fat and sugar content of Cacao which are craved in colder weather (of which more in Chapter 7).

In addition to SAD, two other forms of atypical depression are linked to an increased desire for and consumption of chocolate: late luteal phase dysphoric disorder, aka "premenstrual syndrome" (PMS) in women, and hysteroid dysphoria. PMS and SAD involve cyclical low mood, and their depressive phases can be accompanied by excessive sleeping, lethargy, and increased appetite, especially for carbohydrates, sweet foods, and chocolate.[714] Notably, all three conditions appear to improve with serotonin-raising drugs; in PMS, oestrogen dips in the second half of the menstrual cycle, and this decline may trigger a corresponding fall in brain serotonin levels, because oestrogen is thought to increase the manufacture of serotonin in the brain, and the brain's sensitivity to it.[715] This serotonin trough causes PMS-related dysphoria; likewise, brain serotonin declines in autumn as the days shorten and natural sunlight exposure decreases (SAD).[716] But brain serotonin alone is unlikely to be the only factor in Cacao's appeal to people with atypical depression, as the perceived reward from eating chocolate occurs far faster than brain serotonin levels would be expected to rise after eating it—during consumption of the chocolate, and not some time after, once digestion and absorption has taken place.[717] In fact higher chocolate consumption is linked to a later mood "crash", which may be more likely to occur when high-sugar chocolates are consumed than with low-sugar traditional chocolate drinks, although there are at present no studies to confirm or deny this. But chocolate may be craved in these conditions for reasons other than—or in addition to—serotonin-dependent ones, which will be discussed in full in Chapter 7.

Cacao contains much higher levels of phenylalanine (224mg/40g) and tyrosine (228mg/40g) than tryptophan. Phenylalanine and tyrosine are precursors for the manufacture of the stimulating neurotransmitters dopamine and noradrenaline, respectively. On the other hand, there are many other compounds in Cacao which can increase brain serotonin levels, mainly by inhibiting monoamine oxidase A, the enzyme which breaks down serotonin (and dopamine, noradrenaline, and adrenaline). These MAO-A inhibitor compounds include the proanthocyanidins, caffeine, and some of the trace "fairy dust" chemicals such as resveratrol and the tetrahydro-b-carbolines [THbCs]. THbCs may also affect serotonin re-uptake directly.[718] Of the compounds in Cacao, the following constituents are noted to have monoamine oxidase inhibitory effects:

- Inhibiting MAO-A (causing elevation or preservation of serotonin, noradrenaline, dopamine, melatonin, adrenaline, and tyramine): proanthocyanidins/anthocyanins, salsolinol, resveratrol, THβCs
- Inhibiting MAO-B (causing elevation or preservation of phenethylamine, serotonin, tyramine, dopamine): proanthocyanidins/anthocyanins, the flavan-3-ols catechin and epicatechin.

Cacao may have another notable effect on (un)consciousness; several people have said that drinking black Mexican chocolate in the evening gives rise to vivid, brightly coloured, and intense dreams. Mexican cookbook author Susana Trilling records that after eating meals made with *mole negro*, a complex Mexican savoury sauce containing real Cacao: "I have noticed that every time I eat the rich, black, silky smooth sauce … it has a great effect on me—I have fantastic dreams that night!"[719] On one occasion I advised a client to drink a strong dark chocolate beverage every day, made with an infusion of a few other medicinal plants. After a few weeks he reported that his sleep was very disturbed with bright, vivid, and frenetic dreams. I asked him when he was drinking the adulterated chocolate; he told me (as I suspected) that he was taking it every night, just before bedtime. I advised that real drinking chocolate was a stimulant, much stronger than ordinary cocoa, and should be drunk no later than mid-afternoon. At his next visit, he had been drinking his chocolate in the morning only three or four times a week and his sleep was much improved, with no more disturbing dreams.

Incidentally, the neurologist Oliver Sacks noted some side effects of L-dopa, a dopamine precursor medication used to treat Parkinson's disease:

> Alterations in dreaming are often the first sign of response … Dreaming typically becomes more vivid (many patients remark on their dreaming, suddenly, in brilliant colour), more charged emotionally (with a tendency to erotic dreams and nightmares) … Excessive dreaming of this sort—excessive both in visual and in psychic content, and in activation of unconscious psychic content … is common in fever, and after many drugs (opiates, amphetamines, cocaine, psychedelics); during (or at the start of) certain migraines and seizures; and sometimes at the beginning of psychoses. (Sacks, 1990)

So is there any scientific evidence for Cacao having a dopaminergic (dopamine-releasing) effect? Certainly Cacao's most active stimulant compound, caffeine, doesn't affect levels of dopamine very much except at higher dosages, but it *does* enhance the response to normal levels of dopamine or other dopamine-releasing drugs in the brain.[720] Among Cacao's "fairy dust" compounds, there is only one confirmed to be directly dopaminergic: salsolinol, the trace alkaloid produced during fermentation, also found naturally in the human brain. This compound specifically increases dopamine release in the *nucleus accumbens*, the brain's "habituation centre"—and, crucially, it has stronger dopamine-releasing effects at low concentrations,[721] such as the trace amounts in Cacao. Salsolinol also very strongly increases the effects of glutamate, a highly stimulating brain chemical. Very high activity of glutamate has been linked to thought disorder in psychosis or schizophrenia.[722] Low-level stimulation by small quantities of salsolinol may speed up thought association, for example, with possible benefits for flexibility of thought and creativity, although any effects of possible glutamate enhancement from Cacao on mood and cognition in humans have not yet been researched.

MAO-inhibitors prevent the breakdown of dopamine. The one human experiment testing the effect of ordinary dark chocolate on dopamine showed negligible effects for daily dark chocolate over a one month period—although the researchers recorded a consistent rise in brain dopamine levels over the four week period, even if not quite to a level which could be said to be statistically significant.[723] It should be noted that the group size in this experiment was very small, so more data is needed using larger groups, different doses, and variable periods of time (e.g., high-dose, one-off vs. long-term, i.e., a trial period of several months) before any conclusions are drawn. At present, we can't say for sure whether chocolate or Cacao raises dopamine levels in the brain, but it's certainly a possibility—particularly with the higher-concentration traditional Cacao beverages.

Another "fairy dust" compound in chocolate frequently mentioned in popular discussion of Cacao's effect on mind and mood is β-*phenethylamine*, also called phenylethylamine, phenethylamine, or PEA for short. Phenethylamine levels in the brain have been associated with feelings of happiness, and specifically with being "in love", an issue which will be discussed in more detail shortly.

> According to an article in the *Chicago Sun Times*, people who suffer extreme depression as victims [*sic*] of unrequited love have an irregular production of phenylethylamine. Such individuals often go on chocolate binges during periods of depression. Chocolate is particularly high in phenylethylamine, perhaps serving as medication. (Duke, 1983)[724]

Because PEA is rapidly broken down by MAO-B enzymes after ingestion, and doesn't cross over into the brain very easily, the amount required to have any effect on mood or perception after oral administration is very high. In fact over 2,666 times more PEA than the 0.1–0.88mg in a forty gram serving of Cacao is required for oral psychoactivity in humans![725] However, it should also be noted that Cacao contains polyphenols which inhibit MAO-B, and the alkaloid trigonelline in Cacao ferries PEA directly into the brain and greatly enhances its bioavailability.[726] MAO-B inhibitors such as the proanthocyanidins, catechin, and epicatechin in Cacao can increase low levels of PEA in the brain up to a thousand-fold.[727] Cacao also contains high levels of the amino acid phenylalanine, a precursor (building block) of PEA which is easily transported into the brain. So although the PEA *content* of Cacao is very small, other compounds in *T. cacao* seeds boost PEA production, transport, and conservation, such that higher doses of Cacao are likely to substantially elevate PEA levels in the brain, which would, in turn, amplify the stimulating effects of dopamine.[728]

Cacao seeds also contain up to 3mg tyramine per 40g dose. In the presence of MAO-A inhibitors, an oral dose of 6–10mg tyramine can cause a mild hypertensive (high blood pressure) crisis, with side effects such as nausea, vomiting, and headaches. It's noteworthy that larger doses of 60–120g whole Cacao ingested in one go (not when taken in divided doses over the course of a day, like the Kuna), Cacao seeds can cause headaches and vomiting, and it may be that the cocktail of MAO-A inhibitors in Cacao are sufficiently potent to cause *hypertyraminemia* (high levels of tyramine in the blood) at these doses. If so, this would certainly corroborate the notion that the PEA in Cacao contributes to its psychotropic effects, because PEA and tyramine are both broken down by MAO-A. But this has never been clinically tested, and it could be that the side effects experienced from consuming Cacao at this dosage are due to excessive intakes of the xanthine alkaloids: 100g Cacao contains up to 1,900mg xanthine alkaloids, of which 210mg is caffeine and 1,220mg is theobromine. This amount of caffeine—the amount in about three to four shots of espresso coffee—plus over a gram of theobromine, is enough to cause severe side effects in many people. The cumulative strength of the monoamine inhibitors in Cacao and the contribution (if any) of the amines to Cacao's effects at higher doses requires more research. There isn't enough evidence to say that PEA is the cause of the unique "chocolate effect"—first, this effect needs to be better defined, and second, there are many other compounds in the seed which could be contributing to it.

The other trace compounds of debatable significance in Cacao are anandamide and the amino alcohols. In the human brain, anandamide binds to cannabinoid receptors, which when activated help to regulate pain, anxiety, fear, and appetite—and the first three are symptoms for which Cacao appears be beneficial. The tiny quantity of anandamide in 40g Cacao—up to 3.6mg—would ordinarily be orally inactive, and many commentators have dismissed it as a possible factor in chocolate's effects on mind and mood. But, like PEA, the miniscule dosage in traditional Cacao drinks or in larger intakes of dark chocolate may become pharmaceutically relevant due to the presence of other amino alcohols in Cacao which retard anandamide's break-down after ingestion,[729] and, like salsolinol, very low concentrations of anandamide appear to be pharmacologically active, so—hypothetically—only very small amounts would have to make it into the brain for it to do something.[730] And, as is the case with dopamine and phenethylamine, Cacao also contains a precursor compound called *phosphatidylethanolamine*, which is used to manufacture anandamide in the brain.

As with PEA, a conclusive verdict on the relevance of Cacao's "augmented anandamide" content to its psychoactivity is yet to be reached. But most interestingly, cannabinoids have been found to alter dopamine activity and signalling in parts of the brain regulating emotional memory processing: they may help to adapt or change traumatic memories. It appears the natural function of cannabinoids is to "soft-focus" the memory of pain after illness or suffering; without cannabinoids in our brains, time wouldn't heal any wounds. So if Cacao does modulate cannabinoid signalling in the brain—and, especially, if it has a comparable effect on phenethylamine signalling—then this would certainly help to explain chocolate's premier place as a comfort food for the heartbroken.

Chocolate, "opium for the masa"

There is a curious regard for good quality chocolate among recreational opiate users. The following are excerpts from an online forum for users of poppy tea, a source of morphine, codeine, and other opiate alkaloids:

> I've been trying everything lately because it's not easy drinking several large cups of PST every day to get high. [PST = "poppy seed tea", a euphemism for alkaloid-rich poppy head tea—made not only from the seeds, which are low in morphine, but from the seed capsules, which contain morphine and codeine in addition to other opiate alkaloids.]
>
> Grapefruit juice, Cimetidine, diphenhydramine, high-fat meals, etc. … etc. … The winner for me is without a doubt … Cocoa. There's some very real heightened euphoria when I consume cocoa powder with my opiates. I don't know if it's really potentiation, but rather a combination of the effects of the two with synergy, but this has quickly become my favorite combo. (Posted by "Papa Verine", 8 July 2008, http://forum.opiophile.org/archive/index.php/t-17550.html)
>
> On an empty stomach I ate a little less than half a bar of Hersheys dark chocolate. Probably took a 10mg tab about 30 minutes later. 3 hours go by and the effect is wearing off. Then after about another hour when im sitting in traffic, BAM! The pill starts to come on again. This was 3 hours ago and im still feeling it. So 7 hours total. I have never experienced a pill like that come on again so strong. In fact, i have never had a second rush from an opiate before. ever. And i am amazed it happened 4 hours after i took it. It took me some time to figure out what happened as i just put 2+2 together. Note: this is not a placibo [*sic*] effect. I have never heard of or even thought of the possibility of chocolate making opiates stronger. I did do a internet search and while there are some hints that it might, there is no definite clearification on it like there is for grapefruit juice and opiates. I have taken grapefruit juice to potentate pain killers before but i can tell you now, dark chocolate is MUCH better at doing it. At least

it was tonight. If anybody else has had an experience like this with chocolate and opiates i would like to know. (Posted by "ambigroove", 16 December 2011, http://bluelight.org/vb/threads/602275-Chocolate-Opiate-Potentiator)

I actually immediately clicked on this link cause I know what the OP is talking about. Every morning when I take my .5mg of suboxone, I eat a small piece of chocolate, because I swear it potentiates it (does"t make me nod out, but it is noticeable). (Posted by "Znegative", 16 December 2011, http://bluelight.org/vb/threads/602275-Chocolate-Opiate-Potentiator)

Among chocolate's low-level fairy dust compounds, in addition to the cannabinoids, there are some that bind directly to opiate receptors, such as the alkaloids salsolinol and the tetra-hydro-beta-carbolines [THβCs]. There are several types of opiate receptors in the body, named after letters of the Greek alphabet, and different opioid receptors are activated by different endorphins, the body's natural painkilling and pleasure-giving molecules. The main type of opiate receptors in the brain's "reward centre" are called mu- (µ-) opioid receptors. µ-opioid receptor activating endorphins or drugs, such as morphine, can cause sedation, euphoria, analgesia, decreased bowel motility, and itching. Some people report similar responses to chocolate ingestion: for instance, chocolate is contraindicated in chronic urticaria, an itchy red skin condition that looks like nettle stings.[731] Many people describe feelings of "joy" or "relaxation" after eating chocolate, and Cacao was traditionally used to treat diarrhoea. Of course all these reactions could be due to other constituents of Cacao, or may be non-pharmacological placebo responses.

The quantity of these compounds in Cacao is very low, and the strength of any direct endorphin-releasing effects is likely to be correspondingly small. However, Cacao does contain another group of compounds—the polyphenols—which also appear to influence opiate signalling. The polyphenolic compounds in Cacao are present in appreciable, pharmacologically relevant quantities even in ordinary chocolate bars, and some of them activate opioid receptors, such as the flavanols epicatechin and catechin, which bind to delta- (δ-) opioid receptors on heart cells.[732] However, most of the polyphenols in Cacao don't bind directly to opiate receptors, but they do stimulate the release of the gaseous compound nitric oxide (NO), which in turn affects opioid and dopamine pathways in the brain and spinal cord. Several of the polyphenols in Cacao (such as flavan-3-ols and procyanidins) are known to have this effect.

Some of the opiate-activating trace compounds in Cacao are already present in the bean, and some of them are produced by friendly bacteria in the gut from chemical precursors in the bean. This might explain the four-hour delay in amplification of the opiate effect noted by one of the online opiate users, as it would take time for the polyphenols in Cacao to reach the intestines and start to be broken down. These compounds are quickly absorbed, are detectable in the bloodstream after eating (or drinking) chocolate, readily cross the blood-brain barrier, and produce a measurable increase in blood flow through the brain because they trigger NO release in the lining of blood vessels, causing them to dilate. The brain's reward pathways utilise NO as their main neurotransmitter (messenger molecule). Endorphins stimulate NO production and release in the brain's reward pathways, so NO levels in the brain tend to go up during pleasurable activities such as sex, which may in turn affect the release of endorphins. So the THβCs and salsolinol in Cacao are μ-opioid receptor activators, and the polyphenols' enhancement of NO in the brain likely alters opiate responses through a feedback loop.[733]

Because NO is the main signal transducer in the brain's pleasure pathways (of which more shortly), it's thought that an increase in the brain's NO turnover (as may occur, for example, when one has consumed good quality chocolate) would produce a general signal amplification in the neural circuitry of pleasure and desire. And that has ramifications beyond over-the-counter opiate abuse …

Cacao, MDMA, and the TAAR hypothesis

MDMA, or methylenedioxy-N-methylamphetamine, also known as ecstasy, Molly, and sundry other monickers, is a glorious and notorious synthetic psychoactive drug. It's an empathogen; that is, it induces empathy with fellow human beings, changing the perspective for a four- to six-hour window of liberating and fear-destroying synesthetic euphoria. Although MDMA is now mainly used by partygoers, having its heyday in the "rave culture" of the late 1980s and early '90s, it was initially manufactured by Merck pharmaceuticals as a "diet drug" in the early twentieth century, then re-synthesised by the chemist Alexander Shulgin in 1967. Before it was co-opted by rave and acid house subculture, MDMA was used for psychotherapeutic and self-help purposes in the 1970s and '80s, and this usage has continued in an underground, unsanctioned way through to the present day. Today, in the first quarter of the twenty-first century, there is renewed interest in MDMA's potential as a therapeutic agent in post-traumatic stress. A psychiatrist conducting group work using MDMA in the 1990s described a procedure for administering the drug:

> Therapist: We just pass it round and take it. Then we eat some chocolate.
> Interviewer: Oh! Chocolate!
> Therapist: Yes, it *speeds up the effects of the drug* [my italics].
> Interviewer: Really? How is that?
> Therapist: Albert Hoffman (the discoverer of LSD) told me about it with reference to LSD, and he said there are some receptors that it speeds up, and now we do it with MDMA and it seems to me that it works. They always have to take their orange juice, their pills and the chocolate. I think it has something to do with endorphines [*sic*].
>
> (Saunders, 1993. Reprinted with permission)

MDMA increases the release of the brain chemicals serotonin and noradrenaline (norepinephrine), as well as indirectly raising the brain's levels of the hormones oxytocin and vasopressin—to be discussed in more detail shortly. The key points here are that serotonin causes relaxation, noradrenaline is stimulating and pleasure-enhancing, and the hormones oxytocin and vasopressin increase sociability. There are a few key differences between MDMA and other stimulants such as amphetamine—for example, MDMA reduces the brain's fear response to angry or fearful faces, whereas amphetamine increases it. MDMA also reduces identification of negative emotions and enhances identification of positive emotions, whereas amphetamines increase the identification of both positive and negative emotions. MDMA also selectively affects how people rate social images—it increases appreciation for positive social images, but decreases appreciation for non-social images, whereas amphetamine increases appreciation of both. MDMA also increases measures such as authenticity (reduced defensiveness and feeling vulnerable), self-compassion, self-acceptance, pro-social behaviours, and perceptions of empathy from others, but has not been compared to other stimulants for these effects.[734]

There are several superficial similarities and intriguing points of contrast between Cacao and MDMA's psychotropic effects, as compared to other stimulant drugs. Unlike caffeine or amphetamine, MDMA reduces fear responses; also unlike caffeine or amphetamine, Cacao reduces conditioned fear responses in animals, and was traditionally used to dispel fear in humans. MDMA acutely intensifies positive emotions and reduces negative emotions, amphetamine amplifies both, whereas Cacao (dark chocolate, specifically) may have the more nuanced effect of enhancing the effects of intention on positive mood states in the short term, in addition to increasing "calmness and contentedness" and "feelings of … well-being" over the medium term. MDMA rapidly elevates brain levels of serotonin, and reduces the number of serotonin receptors in the brain with continued usage, while former MDMA users have lower levels of serotonin and its metabolite 5-HIAA in the brain and cerebrospinal fluid than people who have never used MDMA.[735] Conversely, regular Cacao use appears to gradually increase the amount of 5-HIAA, the serotonin by-product, in the brain and spinal cord. MDMA immediately enhances sociability, particularly in the young (who are more disposed to take an illegal "party drug"), while regular intake of chocolate is statistically linked to reduced social isolation and greater optimism in the elderly. Blood cortisol levels increase up to 800% in MDMA users,[736] whereas Cacao lowers serum cortisol levels.

A major key to Cacao's "subtle psychoactivity"—what may be an ability to modulate the effects of other psychoactive drugs, and its intention-dependent and nuanced influence on mood and self-assessed contentment—may lie in the discovery of trace amine associated receptors, or TAARs for short. Receptors are like switches on cells in the body which can only be pressed by certain chemicals, and once activated, they begin a chain reaction in the cell. TAARs are found on many nerve cells (neurons) in the brain and spinal cord, several cells in the stomach, and a few locations in the kidneys, lungs, and small intestine. There are also many TAARs in the nose, on neurons which directly access the area of the brain that governs instinctive emotional responses, the *limbic system*. TAARs occur in the brain on neurons which have "amphetamine-like" effects on activation, such as increasing alertness, causing euphoria, tremor, sweating, even headache, nausea, or vomiting at high doses. TAARs are activated by trace amines: most strongly by β-phenethylamine (PEA) and some forms of tyramine. These trace amines are so small that many of them are volatile, in other words they can float in air and be inhaled. And here's the important bit: *TAARs can be activated by tiny doses of these trace amines—sub-micromolar quantities*—and at these concentrations, tyramine and PEA activate the TAARs and cause a reaction in the neurons which magnifies their response to the stimulating brain chemicals dopamine and noradrenaline, and decreases the effect of the sedating brain chemical GABA.[737] The net result is a brain *primed to react to positive stimulation*.

Substances such as amphetamine cause neurons to release lots of dopamine and noradrenaline, like turning up the volume on a sound system. Substances such as cocaine which prevent the breakdown of dopamine and noradrenaline, so that they temporarily build up in the brain, are like using an amplifier to boost the signal—the net effect is much the same as turning up the volume, but the mechanism is different. These drugs typically produce euphoria (at least in the short term). But substances which activate TAARs, such as PEA and tyramine, are like using the EQ on a mixing desk to modify or adjust sound frequencies, for example by enhancing the bass or tuning out background noise: it doesn't make anything louder, but it changes the overall sound balance. Activating TAARs won't cause euphoria, but may strengthen any "feelgood" signals which are already occurring.

Cacao is particularly high in tyramine and the amino acid phenylalanine, which the body uses to make PEA; and, as mentioned earlier in this chapter, Cacao also contains PEA and several compounds which elevate the level of PEA in the brain. The presence of TAARs in the lining of the nose is particularly intriguing given some anecdotal consumer reports of a "headrush" within five minutes of drinking traditional Cacao beverages. Hypothetically, volatile trace amines in Cacao may be inhaled as part of hot chocolate's aromatic bouquet; 90% of taste is, in fact, smell, and smell is the result of tiny volatile chemicals activating receptors on the sensory nerves in the nose. These volatiles from Cacao may be inhaled, activating TAARs which directly access the limbic system, giving rise to a rapid-onset modulation of pleasure-stimulation signals in the brain—hence, a little "headrush".

Now we have a working hypothesis for Cacao's appeal to people who rank highly on the morphine-benzedrine affinity scale, and for the anecdotal synergy between chocolate and MDMA, or chocolate and opiates: Cacao contains several compounds which modulate opiate signalling, and inhibit the monoamine oxidase (MAO) enzymes that break down tyramine and PEA in the brain. The most likely net result: increased levels of NO, PEA, and tyramine, and altered serotonin metabolism in the brain, resulting in amplified opiate signalling and increased TAAR activation. Add to this the possible effects of anadamide and the anadamide-enhancing trace compounds in Cacao, which operate more strongly at low concentrations. Cacao's "fairy dust" compounds may have more to them than meets the eye. So there's much objective evidence for Cacao having profound effects on mind, mood, and behaviour beyond its basic "caffeine-containing drug" status. Here's a bullet point list of what we've determined so far:

- Many compounds in *Theobroma cacao*, not just caffeine and theobromine, cross the blood-brain barrier after oral consumption of chocolate, and the pharmacology of several compounds in chocolate suggests the possibility of additive or synergistic effects
- There's a heightened proclivity towards dark chocolate consumption by a subset of people prone to emotional dysregulation, and a distinct preference for chocolate by men scoring highly on the morphine-benzedrine subscale of the Addiction Research Center Inventory
- Infant children of new mothers who consumed chocolate during their pregnancies were rated as being better-tempered than the children of non-chocolate consumers
- Elderly people who consumed more chocolate had better psychological health and were less socially isolated

- Chocolate has acute intention-responsive effects on mood in human subjects, and causes improvement in calmness and feelings of well-being in people with dementia after one month's daily consumption in clinical trials
- Larger acute doses of Cacao reduce conditioned fear in non-human animals, whereas caffeine exacerbates it
- MDMA and Cacao share several superficial similarities in their effects on mood, and anecdotal reports of Cacao intensifying the effects of MDMA and opiates may hypothetically be explained by both direct and indirect activation of μ-opioid and trace-amine-associated receptors in the human brain by several compounds in the fermented, toasted seeds
- There is measurable modulation of serotonin metabolism after consuming Cacao, leading to elevated levels of 5-HIAA in the spinal fluid of human and non-human animal subjects
- A net reduction in plasma adrenaline and cortisol levels and increased urinary excretion of these substances have been measured following both acute and medium-term Cacao ingestion in humans
- There were significant improvements in chronic fatigue syndrome symptoms with regular dark chocolate consumption in a double-blind placebo-controlled crossover clinical trial.

Table 4, below, summarises and compares known properties and effects of MDMA and Cacao on mood, behaviour, and brain chemistry.

Table 4. Functional comparison on the apparent acute and chronic effects of MDMA and *Theobroma cacao* ingestion on neurophysiology and psychosocial outcomes

	MDMA	*Roasted* T. cacao *seed or chocolate*
Behavioural effects and associations	Acutely reduces human fear response; recently used in the treatment of PTSD.[738]	Acutely reduces conditioned fear in rats; traditional use in humans "against fear".
	Acutely enhances positive emotions in humans, no effect on negative emotions.	Acutely enhances the effect of intention on positive mood states in humans, no effect on negative emotions.
	Chronic/regular use associated with paranoia and negative emotional states, but also reported by some to have improved emotional well-being.[739]	Chronic/regular use higher in depressives, but also increasing "calmness and contentedness" and "feelings of psychological well-being" in demented subjects, relative to placebo.
	Acutely enhances pro-social behaviour in young users.	Acute effects on social behaviour in humans not assessed.
	Regular use linked to increased risk of psychopathology and cognitive deficits, possibly permanent.[740]	Regular consumption linked to less social isolation and greater optimism in the elderly; equivocal evidence for positive effects on cognition.

(Continued)

Table 4. (Continued)

	MDMA	Roasted T. cacao seed or chocolate
Pharmacological effects/ mechanisms	Acutely increases serotonin, dopamine, and noradrenaline release in the human brain; strongly actives TAARs.	No recorded acute effect on serotonin and noradrenaline levels in humans; high doses of polyphenols enhance brain serotonin levels in rats. *May activate TAARs (hypothetical).*
	Chronic use leads to reduction of serotonin receptors and turnover in the human brain.	Chronic use leads to increased levels of the serotonin metabolite 5-HIAA in the brain and spinal cord.
	Acute and chronic use elevates blood cortisol levels up to 800%.	Acutely and chronically lowers blood cortisol and adrenaline levels in humans, though very high doses of flavanols acutely increase adrenaline levels in rats.
	No μ-opioid mediated effects noted in mice;[741] negligible opioid receptor activity in *in vitro* testing.[742]	Increases brain nitric oxide turnover; trace alkaloid salsolinol binds to brain μ-opioid receptors—*may modulate opiate responses (hypothetical).*
	Endocannabinoids involved in reinforcing (habit-forming) effects.[743]	Contains tiny amounts of endocannabinoids and "buffering" compounds which inhibit their breakdown; *may enhance brain anandamide activity (hypothetical).*

Is chocolate an aphrodisiac?

Cacao has an ancient reputation for enhancing libido and sexual pleasure. There is the conquistador Bernal Diaz's famous account of the Mexica emperor Motecuhzoma (Montezuma) taking a meal: "From time to time they brought him some cups of fine gold, with a certain drink made of Cacao, which they said was for success with women."[744] The twentieth-century physician and author Dr Hervé Robert elegantly describes chocolate's popular use as a "panacea of love", while the sixteenth-century Spanish physician Juan de Cardenas declared of chocolate, "This food leads to sins of the flesh."[745] De Cardenas's view was typical of European medical concepts of Cacao at the time, but in this day and age we've largely dismissed chocolate's aphrodisiac reputation as a myth-driven placebo effect. Nevertheless chocolate's association with love, sex, and romance persists in the public imagination.

Dr Robert suggested that chocolate's psychoactivity accounts for its reputation as an aphrodisiac: he averred that the theobromine, serotonin, and phenethylamine it contains exert a "tonic effect", so that chocolate provides an "anti-stress action, antidepressant properties and [the power to] resist fatigue, giving it energising and euphoriant attributes which can only promote the flowering of intense sexual activity."[746] But as we've seen, Cacao's effect on mood seems to be more complex and nuanced than a simple "antidepressant" label would suggest. Dr Robert's suggestion that Cacao has an "anti-stress action" appears to be correct, in that it lowers cortisol and adrenaline levels, although the precise roles of phenethylamine and serotonin in Cacao's effects on brain and behaviour are not yet defined. And there are many euphoriant and anxiolytic (stress-reducing) psychoactive drugs that have precisely the opposite effect, where elevation of mood is accompanied by loss of sexual drive (for many prescription antidepressants or anti-anxiety drugs, "loss of libido" is a common side effect). In fairness Dr Robert does concede that "[t]he chemistry of love is a very complex area."[747]

Considering its historical reputation, and the cultural association of chocolate with sex and romance, there's remarkably little research on this aspect of Cacao's capabilities. One small study on the effect of chocolate on "female sexual function" in 163 women between twenty-five and forty-five years of age was inconclusive. Female sexual function is defined by a questionnaire called the Female Sexual Function Index, assessing six aspects of sexual interaction, namely "desire, subjective arousal, lubrication, orgasm, satisfaction, and pain".[748] In this group of women, chocolate consumption was positively correlated with higher sexual function, but this result is of questionable relevance, because the younger women in the study consumed more chocolate than the older women, so youth, rather than chocolate, could have been responsible for their higher ranking. There were no differences in scores for depression, arousal, sexual satisfaction, or distress between the high-chocolate and low-chocolate groups.[749] The second methodological issue is that the quality of chocolate would need to be better defined and controlled to ensure that all participants were consuming the same amount of high quality—high Cacao content—dark chocolate. This study needs to be replicated with a larger group of women and quality-controlled dark chocolate, ensuring that chocolate consumption is the same across age ranges, before any tentative conclusions regarding the effect of chocolate on female sexual function can be drawn.

Despite Cacao's aphrodisiac reputation, two compounds in *Theobroma cacao* are known to *inhibit* testicular function, reducing sperm count and male fertility. These are Cacao's principal alkaloid theobromine, and the trace alkaloid salsolinol. A diet containing 0.6% theobromine reduces sperm production in rats,[750] and in the laboratory salsolinol has a blocking effect on two enzymes responsible for producing male hormones (androgens).[751] While it's true that isolated chemicals aren't synonymous with the action of the whole plant, and that rats don't always have the same biological responses to chemicals, drugs, or foods as humans, it's troubling to note that cocoa powder fed to rats at 5% of their diet caused irreversible testicular atrophy, permanently damaging the male rats' fertility.[752] Given this information, it may be prudent for men for whom fertility is a concern to limit their Cacao and chocolate consumption, or at least not to consume large quantities on a daily basis.

So far, so unimpressive ... is there *any* pharmacological truth to Cacao's aphrodisiac reputation? Perhaps, and by two means. The first, via the circulatory system; the second, via the brain and central nervous system. The first may be a result of Cacao's well-documented effects on circulation, specifically increasing blood flow and reducing inflammation in the lining of blood vessels, and principally affecting male sexual function. Difficulty getting or sustaining an erection, known as erectile dysfunction (ED) can have many causes, both psychological and physical, but it's common knowledge that male capacity to sustain an erection, and the degree of erections (literally), decline with age.[753]

Part of the reason for this age-related loss of potency is circulatory disease—arteries and blood vessels gradually "silt up" due to low-grade inflammation in the walls of blood vessels, owing to lifestyle factors such as poor diet, smoking, and the aging process; the body's attempts to patch up the damage with plugs of cholesterol and so-called "foam cells" thickens the walls of the blood vessels, and makes them less flexible. This process, known as *atherosclerosis*, is the underlying cause of circulatory disease, heart disease, and stroke: narrowed blood vessels can lead to clot formation, cause elevated blood pressure, or stiffen, weaken, and eventually rupture.

As discussed in the last chapter, Cacao has many positive effects in heart disease because it helps to counter some of the mechanisms underlying this process. What's less well known is that ED is an early warning sign of heart disease and stroke—even in younger men.[754] This makes sense, as the penis is supplied with blood by the pudendal artery, no thicker than a pencil, which splits into three smaller arteries. Atherosclerosis reduces blood flow, making erections weaker. So Cacao's capacity to rapidly increase arterial blood flow, and to reduce inflammation in blood vessel linings, may be expected to have a positive impact on erectile dysfunction by increasing the strength of erections. As yet, no studies have been carried out, but there is some anecdotal information out there; one blogger on a dating website recounts:

> K, I admit that my sexual functioning has been in a decline since 30 years of age. A few weeks ago, during a renovation project, I bought a Waterbridge Belgian Dark 500g chocolate bar from the local Wal-Mart (not intending to solicit, but just for clarification, in case researchers are interested). I would eat two or three chunks of the chocolate bar on my drive home from work. Well, embarrassing as it is, I started getting my daily morning erections again! (Posted by "albino_dino", 4 April 2008, https://forums.plentyoffish.com/datingPosts9675597.aspx)

Dr Eric Ding of Harvard University is quoted as saying that "Erectile dysfunction is also fundamentally a circulation problem—Viagra® is also shown to improve flow-mediated dilation, similar to cocoa."[755] It's noteworthy that one of Cacao's major traditional additives, chilli pepper, is also used as a circulatory stimulant; chilli pepper has become one of the most commonly prescribed plants in African herbal medicine for treating erectile dysfunction[756] and is used in a similar way in contemporary Mexican ethnomedicine,[757] although this usage hasn't yet been clinically tested.

The second means by which Cacao may be aphrodisiac relates to possible effects on the brain and hormones (neurohormonal activity). Cacao has a traditional reputation as a libido-enhancing substance—not simply a Viagra-like, erection-enhancing product, but something which actually increases the appetite and desire for sex. This is closer to the fundamental meaning of the word *aphrodisiac*, a substance which arouses love or desire. The word derives from Aphrodite, the Greek goddess of love. Unlike the existence of erectile stimulants, the existence of true aphrodisiacs is considered to be highly questionable, even apocryphal. But many drugs are known to enhance libido: methamphetamine, for example, increases sexual appetite and the pleasure derived from sex, albeit at very high cost in terms of mental and physical health.[758] Some of the mechanisms by which Cacao may work as a "true aphrodisiac" are proven, others are hypothetical, yet all are based on the known pharmacology of Cacao and the chemical activities of its constituents. To truly investigate chocolate's romantic reputation, first we need to understand the biological basis of desire and attraction. Only then can we examine the ways that Cacao may or may not be manipulating those hidden levers.

The chemistry of attraction: love is a drug (or several)

According to the research of Dr Helen Fisher, formerly of Rutgers University, New Jersey, it seems that love and sexual attraction can be placed into three broad neurochemical categories, based on *Lust* (sex drive), "romantic" *Infatuation* (attraction), and *Bonding* (attachment).

Lust in mammals is principally under the control of the preoptic area of the anterior hypothalamus in the brain (see Figure 8 overleaf). Positioned right in the centre of the head, at the top of the brain stem (an extension of the spinal cord up into the meat of the brain) and approximately in line with the brow, the hypothalamus may be loosely described as the brain's "hormone thermostat", monitoring and adjusting hormone levels all around the body. The pre-optic area is a small region towards the front of the hypothalamus. The hypothalamus is the control centre for a cascade of hormonal events which govern sexual functions: it produces gonadotrophin releasing hormone (GnRH), with which it prompts the anterior pituitary gland, positioned just behind the gap between the eyes, to release hormones which then stimulate the gonads (the testicles or ovaries) to produce sex hormones such as testosterone, oestrogen, or progesterone. There is a strong positive correlation between testosterone (in men and women) and oestradiol, aka oestrogen (in women) and libido; so Lust, at its core, is a hormone-driven state.

The second category, *Infatuation*, involves the activation of highly dopamine-driven brain regions associated with the "primitive" area of the brain that we call the limbic system (see Figure 8). This area of the brain evolved into our emotional processing network (amongst other functions) from an earlier role as a smell-sensation processing unit, and is attached directly to sensory inputs from the nose. There are many reasons why this should be—the volatile compounds which are the source of odours become associated with feelings; for example, the smell of clean sheets or our favourite childhood food may evoke feelings of comfort and safety, whereas the smell of an overflowing drain or burning plastic may remind you of our parents' or guardians' reactions of disgust or alarm. Having these smells wired directly into the limbic system rapidly triggers emotional responses which can help survival, impelling us to move towards pleasant things and away from potentially harmful things; and pheromones, volatile molecules produced by living organisms, are part of this picture. Studies have shown that part of adults' sexual attraction to each other is pheromone-based, possibly hard-wired through genetics or developed through experience, for example the pheromone signature of trusted adults from our childhood—the smell of being wrapped in a comforting hug—may be replicated in the intimate partners we choose as adults.[759]

Infatuation is Hollywood-style "love at first sight" or seemingly magnetic sexual attraction, and is culturally revered in the West, synonymous with "romantic love". Yet behaviourally speaking, Infatuation has been described as "primarily a motivation system"[760]—arguably its main purpose is as an instigator of reproduction, and perpetuation of the species. Infatuation could even be categorised as a self-generated endogenous (meaning "within ourselves") drug addiction, as it involves the dopamine-driven reward pathways linked to natural drives for food and sex—the same brain pathways which are hijacked by stimulant drugs of abuse such as amphetamines and cocaine. Just like these substances, a state of Infatuation is characterised by elevated levels of the "exciting" neurotransmitters dopamine, noradrenaline, and phenethylamine (PEA), and low levels of "calming" serotonin. This blend of brain chemicals gives rise to obsessive thinking and behaviour patterns, exhilaration, suppression of the amygdala's fear response, and the *unstable intensity* characteristic of such a state. One blogger covering this research into the brain chemistry of attraction noted that "Romantic love exists in 150 societies, even though it is discouraged in many of them,"[761] presumably due to its inherent instability.

The third type of "love" is *Bonding*, driven by two neurohormones—hormones which also affect nerve cells in the brain—known as *vasopressin* and *oxytocin*. Bonding infers feelings of "calm, security, social comfort, and emotional union".[762] Oxytocin was once thought to be important only in the delivery of babies as a hormone which increases the strength of uterine contractions during childbirth, but research has revealed its crucial role as a brain hormone affecting behaviour. The level of oxytocin in the blood and brains of women rises during labour, but it remains elevated during breastfeeding to promote emotional bonding between mother and baby. Oxytocin is colloquially known as the "cuddle hormone", and levels in the blood-stream of men and women rise on close and affectionate bodily contact; high levels are linked to reduced appetite and food intake.[763] Because increased oxytocin release in the brain correlates with the feelings of comfort in a breastfeeding baby and attachment to its mother, it makes sense that this hormone is associated with feelings of comfort and satiety. A hug can calm raging emotions and prevent the desire to eat more biscuits than is good for you, and a spike in central (brain) oxytocin release induced by the hug is linked to this outcome; post-break-up ice cream binges may be partly reframed as "oxytocin withdrawal".

Animal behavioural research shows that infants which are given consistent maternal care—regular oxytocin boosts—have lower cortisol (stress hormone) levels and less intense stress responses, stronger immune systems, and themselves become more nurturing as adults, whereas the reverse is true for animals that are given inconsistent care or placed in high-stress environments during infancy. Consequently, badly nurtured animals (or humans)—those that have less regular oxytocin-promoting interactions—are more likely to raise less secure, badly nurturing offspring. A neurohormone-mediated intergenerational cycle of parental negligence or abuse can be perpetuated.[764] Higher scores in human adults partaking in the US based Adverse Childhood Experiences (ACE) study are strongly correlated with lower life expectancy, substance abuse, mental health problems, and serious illnesses such as cancer or heart disease.[765] Put simplistically, higher levels of youthful oxytocin and lower levels of cortisol from more consistently demonstrative care incline mammals to better social skills, stress tolerance, emotional and physical resilience, and decreased impulsiveness in adulthood. In addition to oxytocin, tactile affection also causes the release of dopamine, which "hard-wires" the brain to desire more of whatever it's associated with, and opioids, which provide feelings of comfort, security, and reduced pain sensitivity. Love *literally* takes pain away.

Oxytocin administered to healthy adult males reduced snacking and lowered levels of cortisol and its trigger, the hormone ACTH, and reduced blood sugar following a meal.[766] Other effects of oxytocin include increasing feelings of trust and decreasing anxiety around those with whom we are physically (but not necessarily sexually) intimate, impairing learning memory (facts) but improving social memory (faces), as well as inhibiting physical tolerance to drugs of abuse: affection reduces liability to addiction. Interestingly, higher brain levels of oxyctocin also correlate with aversion to unfamiliar people, so it strengthens emotional bonding to familiar people, as opposed to the "excitement-reward" neurotransmitter, dopamine, which promotes novelty-seeking behaviour. Oxytocin receptors in the brain occur in various places, including the "instinctive emotional response" centre, the amygdala, and the brain's major "pleasure and motivation" area, the nucleus accumbens.

All pleasurable social and sexual interactions are mediated by a cocktail of neurotransmitters, neuropeptides, and neurohormones such as serotonin, dopamine, noradrenaline, adrenaline, opioids (endorphins), vasopressin, sex steroids such as testosterone and oestrogen, the "stress steroid" cortisol, and oxytocin. As with many hormone systems, there are intricate networks of feedback loops conveying the messages which affect and translate emotional drives. Even if stress levels are high so that cortisol and noradrenaline or adrenaline levels rise, so long as the stress is associated with forming new social or personal bonds, oxytocin release also occurs in the brain. Thus stressful events such as dating or socialising have a built-in antidote to stress in the form of oxytocin: this is how strangers become friends or lovers. Without a burst of oxytocin to provide a feeling of security and comfortable familiarity, unstable relationship patterns and behaviours may arise, as the dopamine-driven, novelty-seeking rewards of new sources of stimulation prompt moving on from one new partner or group to another.

Conversely, a hermit-like aversion to socialising may develop if dopamine and oxytocin levels remain low. So lower levels of adult dopamine and oxytocin as a result of less consistent affection during childhood promote apathy and transience in adult relationships, and it may be that the root of many subcultures or countercultural movements (club kids, gangs etc.) are neurochemically deficient teens or adults who seek instant thrills from activities which are associated with the feeling of being part of a like-minded crowd, thereby elevating the stimulating neurotransmitters (with or without chemical assistance in the form of psychotropic drugs) and obtaining an immediate hit of dopamine—and a longer-term elevation of oxytocin, the real, underlying motivator. The risks, the novelty, and the thrills may be, to some extent, simply a paradoxical means to an end: the biochemical reward of *belonging*.

To return to our theme, the three modes of attraction (Lust, Infatuation, and Bonding) are interlinked, and may complement or conflict with one another. Orgasms temporarily boost oxytocin, as well as endorphins, strengthening Bonding, while raised testosterone (as in Lust) elevates dopamine levels and suppresses oxytocin release, increasing the chances of falling into a state of Infatuation, while weakening Bonding. A requited love is likely to be moderated by the calming influence of oxytocin, via physical contact—hugs, cuddles etc.—which increase Bonding, while an unrequited love, or a love affair gone bad (Infatuation without Bonding) is likely to display increasing instability as its purely stimulating, obsessional neurochemical character of elevated dopamine levels precipitates a similar kind of mood rollercoaster as the cocaine addict may experience, lacking the stabilising action of oxytocin and its congruent high serotonin level. Infatuation possesses many characteristics reminiscent of drug addiction. As one paper puts it,

> The psychological sense of love can be interpreted as referring to a satisfaction of a yearning, which may be associated with the obtaining of certain sensory stimulation. Love therefore possesses a close connection not only with reward and pleasure phenomena, but also with appetitive and addictive behaviours. (Esch & Stefano, 2005)

The authors of this paper argue that clear distinctions can be made between what they call "natural love" (Infatuation, in this case) and "artificial" elation induced by drugs. In both cases there is a desire, drive, or appetite—mainly dopamine-driven—which, if satisfied by sexual consummation in one case or ingestion of the drug in the other, would temporarily satisfy that desire. I'd suggest that the level of satiation or satisfaction achieved, have less to do with whether the object of desire is drug-, human-, or other-based; what happens next mostly depends on the degree to which the person in question is developmentally *capable of satiation* with regard to that desire. This is why one person can take methamphetamine once or twice recreationally, and never use it again, some slide into gradual dependency, but others become instantly addicted. The drug itself is only half the story.

In other words: whether the desire-driven pursuit is of love, money, alcohol, cocaine, or whatever, it's the brain chemistry of the human involved that determines whether or not a cycle of craving will begin. As we know from research into the effects of oxytocin on the growing brain, an adult human who received consistent affection in childhood will naturally possess a brain chemistry more resistant to addiction, psychotropic drug use, mood disorders, and so on—and, I would argue, be more resistant to irrational Infatuation—than a child who did not. The popular appeal of Hollywood romances may say a lot about our collective experience of childhood: a culture so addicted to the instant gratification of Infatuation-based love may be suffering from a chronic deficiency of childhood Bonding.

Another set of "love neurotransmitters" worthy of mention are the endorphins, specifically *enkephalin* and *beta* (β)-*endorphin*. Located at the top of the brainstem, the ventral tegmental area (VTA) of the brain processes emotional outputs from the amygdala, and utilises dopamine as a neurotransmitter. This area of the brain generates and regulates motivation and desire. Dopamine signals in the VTA are triggered by endorphins (such as enkephalin and β-endorphin) binding to opiate receptors. Endorphins mainly bind to μ-opioid receptors in the *cortex* (complex reasoning), the *nucleus accumbens* (motivation and desire), and the *amygdala* (emotional control, fear, and safety) (see Figure 8) as well as other regions of the brain such as the VTA and brainstem, and outside the brain in the intestines. Endorphin activation causes euphoria, sedation, feelings of security, and pain relief. We are hard-wired to seek out things which bring us comfort and joy. Activation of some of these receptors in the brain is crucial for functional relationships. Without μ-opioid receptor rewards, forgiving a loved one for their shortcomings and transgressions would be harder; μ-opioid receptor activation performs a kind of emotional smudging, whereby negative emotions are blunted and bad memories are blurred, so that happier associations may float to the surface of consciousness. These receptors "allow one to make rational short-cuts … and they may trigger feelings of wellness, which are essential for positive motivation, lasting relationship, and attachment".[767]

Interestingly, dopamine and endorphins not only affect each other's release (which isn't surprising: desire and pleasure go hand-in-hand), they also share a common biosynthetic pathway (chemical assembly line) in the brain. Mu-opioid receptor activation induces feelings of well-being, but also drives appetite, and these receptors are particularly triggered in states of Infatuation, such that animals without them are more sensitive to pain, but *less prone to addictions*. That μ-opioid receptor stimulation is also induced by loving maternal care has been demonstrated by separating animals from their mothers, whereupon they cry out, and their cortisol (stress hormone) levels rise, but they become relaxed and quiet and their cortisol levels return to normal when they are given μ-opioid receptor stimulating drugs (opiates).[768] So are all mammals addicted to love? Perhaps. But this logic may be inverted: an absence of affection is at the root of adult addictions, as mammals with a history of unstable Bonding or deprivation of care will be drawn to more emphatic, accessible, reliable, and immediate means of raising their chronically low endorphin levels—such as opiates, or dopamine-raising drugs such as cocaine or amphetamines—than the precarious affection of other living beings.

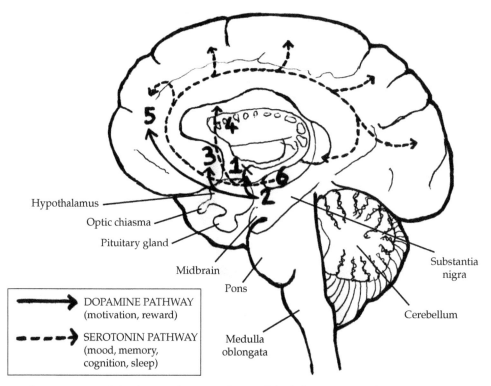

Figure 8. Cross-section of the human brain with simplified dopamine and serotonin pathways.

Figure 8 illustrates the relative positions and neuronal (nerve) pathways of the brain's motivation, pleasure and reward circuitry in the limbic system. The numbered regions are as follows (names in bold are referred to in the main text):

1. The *amygdalae* (singular: **amygdala**) encode emotional reactions, and generate emotionally driven learned responses based on pleasure, trauma, fear, or desire; the feelings generated in the amygdalae dictate whether an experience is pleasurable or aversive.
2. The **ventral tegmental area (VTA)** near the base of the brain filters emotional output signals from the amygdalae, and is the principal motivation and reward control centre. The VTA projects dopamine-releasing neurons to the nucleus accumbens.

3. **Nucleus accumbens** (NA), located in the basal forebrain: this is the main pleasure centre, providing reward and incentive. The NA is the brain's "desire engine", having important roles to play in behavioural reinforcement, as well as fear and addiction.
4. *Caudate nuclei* in the midbrain regulate goal-directed movement, learning, memory, and sleep.
5. The *prefrontal* **cortex** generates or permits conscious processing of inputs—governs behaviour, decision-making, and personality. Receives emotional and desire-based "information" from the limbic system.
6. The **hippocampus**: regulates emotional responses, stores long-term memories.

Cacao, hormones, and brain chemistry

Just as oxytocin induces feelings of comfort while lowering cortisol and blood sugar levels, Cacao and chocolate perform similar actions: regular Cacao consumption reduces cortisol and blood sugar, and chocolate is regarded as a "comfort food" *par excellence*. A disrupted balance of dopamine and oxytocin has been linked to depression, sexual dysfunction, addictions, and eating disorders,[769] all issues for which chocolate has been used or resorted to as a remedy or may even (in the case of binge eating and bulimia nervosa) feature as an element of the compulsive behaviour. Coincidence? Possibly. But we've noted that Cacao contains some trace compounds which bind directly to μ-opioid receptors, and others that trigger the release of nitric oxide (NO) in the brain, which alters opiate signalling. In the absence of opiate-triggering rewards, NO increases the sensitivity of opiate receptors, making the brain more pleasure-sensitive; so when a reward is *not* present, sensitivity to that reward *increases*. Repeated release of NO also increases the number of opiate receptors (as assessed by testing nerve cells in the laboratory with the dopamine-releasing drug, cocaine);[770] this greater number of receptors means that it takes less of the stimulus to produce the same pleasurable reward, making the brain *more pleasure-sensitive*. Paradoxically, in the presence of much opiate stimulation, NO *decreases* opiate receptor sensitivity, *reducing* the pleasure response—so when a reward is present, NO will accelerate the development of tolerance and diminishing returns.[771] In other words, NO will enhance sensitivity to rewards in their absence, but reduce sensitivity to the same rewards once acquired.

So NO may be described as a kind of "hedonic regulator molecule" in the brain's pleasure pathways, a sort of pleasure gatekeeper compound—if dopamine and opiates are molecular sheep, NO is a molecular sheepdog. NO amplifies short-term reward or analgesia (two sides of the same opiate-based coin), but curbs long-term gratification or pain relief if the pleasurable or painful stimulus is continued. NO may be one neurochemical reason why many pleasurable activities, such as sex, become more appealing and intense after a period of abstinence, yet have diminishing returns, becoming less and less fulfilling over time if the activity is repeated without taking a break. Similarly, NO may reduce pain signals in the short term, but could increase pain sensitivity in chronic pain by decreasing opiate signalling.[772]

Following the hypothesis of Cacao's "fairy dust" effects of activating TAARs and enhancing opiate sensitivity, this implies that the motivating, appetitive stimulus of dopamine, as when one is craving a "fix" of sugar, or sex, or drugs, or shopping, or whatever, may be enhanced by Cacao via its effects on TAARs. In the absence of reward, Cacao's property of increasing NO release in the brain may also enhance the endorphin-pleasure response that will be initially experienced. Interestingly, blocking the action of the enzyme histone deacetylase (HDAC) in the brain also increases opiate receptor numbers in response to repeated dopamine stimulus, much as NO does,[773] but the theophylline in Cacao induces and reactivates this enzyme.[774] Perhaps, then, once gratification is accomplished, if the reward is experienced repeatedly (eating cake, having sex, taking drugs, maxing out the credit card), elevated levels of NO and HDAC induced by Cacao may act together to cumulatively dampen the pleasure response. Thus the action of Cacao may be to enhance pleasure responses via the polyphenols (acute effects of elevated NO) plus salsolinol and the THβCs (activating μ-opioid receptors) in the short term, while also increasing tolerance to gratifying stimuli over the long term (chronic effects of elevated NO, and theophylline enhancing HDAC).

So, as far-fetched as it may sound, habitual consumption of Cacao or chocolate may subtly intensify the natural cycle of *desire—gratification—tolerance* (whether the final stage brings disillusion or contentment depends on character and circumstances) that drives human behaviours and characterises many relationships. This is fascinatingly synonymous with the traditional picture of "venery" or sexual activity as something which, in moderation, is a source of joy, but in excess produces melancholy; thus Cacao's characterisation as a Cold, Dry melancholic substance which can relieve melancholy but may, perhaps, increase it over time in certain people, or with continuous use.

Bonding with chocolate

Despite the potentially pleasure-normalising or boredom-accelerating effect of NO release in the brain, enhanced activity of NO (as experienced following ingestion of Cacao) is thought to be crucial in "love", perhaps especially in Bonding, because it "helps to keep or facilitate a state of calmness and contentment … resembling morphine signalling" (Esch & Stefano, 2005).[775] The action of NO on the main "Bonding hormone" oxytocin may be comparable to its action on opiates, in that NO may serve a dual purpose in both scenarios, helping to consolidate or diminish pleasure responses and control Bonding, depending on the circumstances. The brain's natural endocannabinoid, anandamide (also present in, and perhaps boosted by Cacao) triggers release of NO in specific neurons in the *posterior pituitary gland*, the control organ for sex hormones, to switch off vasopressin and oxytocin release, while it also stimulates oxytocin release through another, non-NO dependent pathway.[776]

Activation of serotonin (5-HT1A) receptors elevates oxytocin levels, too; and we know that Cacao contains serotonin-sparing (MAOI) compounds, we've seen evidence from animal studies that larger quantities of Cacao may raise central serotonin levels, and we know that regular chocolate intake measurably alters brain serotonin metabolism in humans. So here, as with endorphins or opiates, Cacao may have a sensitising or modulating effect, which could result in either increasing or decreasing endorphin, oxytocin, and vasopressin levels in the brain in a "state-dependent" manner. In other words, the chemistry of the brain before Cacao may partially determine the effect of Cacao on the brain, at least as regards these two sets of neurohormones.

Corroborating these speculations, surges of enkephalin (an endorphin which binds to μ-opioid receptors) more than 150% above baseline levels have been recorded in the brains of lab rats while eating chocolate.[777] Arguably, the immediate change in the rats' brain chemistry in this experiment may have had more to do with chocolate's fat and sugar content than the effects of polyphenols or alkaloids or any of the other chemicals in Cacao, because the brain responds to the taste of sugar and fat immediately (to be discussed in Chapter 7), whereas the more pharmacologically active compounds in Cacao take longer to get into the bloodstream. If the rats in the experiment had eaten chocolate before, this may also be evidence of a *conditioned reward response*, where the chemical reward of ingesting chocolate became associated with its taste, so that ingesting it produced an immediate reaction in the brain. Habitual drug users experience a similar reward phenomenon, whereupon taking the drug produces immediate relief before the active constituents reach the brain—a regular drug user who is accustomed to injecting drugs may experience their first rush of excitement and pleasure on loading the syringe, before the drug is even injected. The first sip of tea or coffee in the morning produces a popular version of this effect, sometimes accompanied by a satisfied sigh: "Aaah." But the endorphin surge in the brains of chocolate-eating rats was far stronger than that produced by other sweet and fatty foods. Perhaps the smell of chocolate—in other words, Cacao's volatile oils, which may be tickling the TAARs in the rats' limbic systems directly via olfactory receptors in the nose—enhanced the rodents' endorphin response? It would be interesting to test this in humans with and without a sense of smell.

Beta-endorphin dampens male sexual arousal and libido,[778] and if animal studies are any guide, blood levels of β-endorphin may rise following ejaculation,[779] although no changes were noted in the circulating blood levels of endorphins in men or women after orgasm. However, blood levels of the hormone prolactin rose during arousal and remained elevated in the bloodstream for at least thirty minutes after orgasm.[780] Mu-opioid receptor agonists (activators) such as β-endorphin are known to stimulate prolactin release by lowering levels of dopamine in neurons which normally prohibit its release,[781] providing indirect evidence that a burst of pleasurable β-endorphin release during orgasm may trigger the prolactin surge. In other words, turning on μ-opioid receptors (as may occur during lovemaking or orgasm, or—as discussed in Chapter 4—during breastfeeding, or perhaps through regular ingestion of Cacao) turns off dopamine in those pathways, which causes the release of prolactin. Like oxytocin, prolactin was formerly known only as the female reproductive hormone which induces milk production during and after pregnancy, but is now known to be an important Bonding and mood-modifying neurohormone, perhaps influencing the post-ejaculatory sleepy-relaxed state experienced by many men. Prolactin plays a role in parent-child Bonding, particularly in men,[782] and reduces the anxiety levels of pregnant rats both during and after pregnancy, even *affecting their offspring's personality*—infant rats born to mothers with low prolactin levels in the first third of pregnancy showed greater anxiety, and entered puberty later than others.[783]

We know from animal studies that salsolinol in Cacao (one of the compounds which binds to μ-opioid receptors) is an important, naturally occurring trigger for prolactin release in the brain,[784] although it's been shown that a single cup of cocoa doesn't raise prolactin levels in women.[785] However, as noted in Chapters 2 and 4, drinking cocoa (made from cocoa powder) is a very low-quality form of Cacao, and more importantly there's a big difference between a one-off dose and regular intake—particularly as salsolinol can accumulate in dopamine-releasing neurons in the brain,[786] some of which regulate prolactin release. Anecdotally, Cacao does seem to possess prolactin-modulating potential, given its traditional use as a galactagogue (increasing breast milk production), and the study of the infant children of the new mums who ate more dark chocolate during pregnancy and reported happier babies at six months post-partum than those who didn't.

Thus Cacao may lead to an immediate anticipatory surge of endorphins in the brain and/ or an enhanced dopamine-serotonin-phenethylamine response triggered by TAAR-activating volatile compounds, creating a little "rush" and perhaps accompanied by a feeling of satisfaction. We can further speculate that these effects may be sustained by subsequent absorption of compounds in Cacao which affect endorphin (mu-opioid) receptors, TAARs, and perhaps also cannabinoid receptors which regulate the output of oxytocin and prolactin, replicating or enhancing some of the brain chemistry of Bonding. While scientific proof of this hypothesis is lacking, the gifting of chocolates on Valentine's Day may be more than a coincidence.

Lust for chocolate

Nitric oxide also has other important functions in the brain chemistry of "love". When administered directly to cells in the amygdala, the limbic system's "emotional response drive", NO facilitates conditioned sexual arousal. This means that NO is one of the brain's main signals for learned or habitual pleasure responses. It works like this: the amygdala may have its switches tripped by the brain chemicals of excitement, desire, or relaxation—noradrenaline, dopamine, or serotonin—giving rise to sexual arousal. This arousal triggers the release of NO from neurons in the amygdala, which cause recall of sensations from previous sexual encounters. So NO is the messenger for powerful sense-memories in sex, which develops and ingrains what we find pleasurable and arousing (in this case, NO could be spelt Y-E-S). So Cacao may facilitate or enhance a state of arousal and Lust.

The sex steroids ("hormones") produced by the gonads, such as testosterone and oestrogen, also influence brain development in the womb, during childhood, and throughout adolescence. Changes in the brain's neural wiring that hormones affect during growth and development are likely to alter adult behavioural predispositions in the three modes of "love" (Lust, Infatuation, and Bonding). Among many other actions, gonadal hormones affect the distribution and density of receptors in the brain for oxytocin and its "partner hormone", *vasopressin*. Physically, vasopressin helps to retain water and raise blood pressure, but behaviourally—in the brain— it works alongside oxytocin to enhance social behaviours and attachments while reducing anxiety; but, unlike oxytocin, vasopressin tends to increase territoriality and may also increase aggression, particularly in males. As we've seen, Cacao may modulate oxytocin and vasopressin release via its effects on anandamide, serotonin, NO, dopamine, and endorphin receptors— so, hypothetically, Cacao taken during pregnancy may rewire the developing brain by changing its sensitivity to these neurohormones.

This web of chemical interactions gets very complicated. In short, a lot of the brain chemicals which may be influenced by Cacao and chocolate appear to be intimately involved in the control of areas of the brain which govern our sexual behaviours (see Figure 9 overleaf). Essentially, as anyone alive who has been in relationships can testify, there aren't three neat categories of "love". Lust, Infatuation, and Bonding are convenient labels, grouping certain behavioural responses and hormone-neurotransmitter cascades for the sake of dissecting a phenomenon which constantly crosses boundaries. Just ask Romeo and Juliet (they were Infatuated).

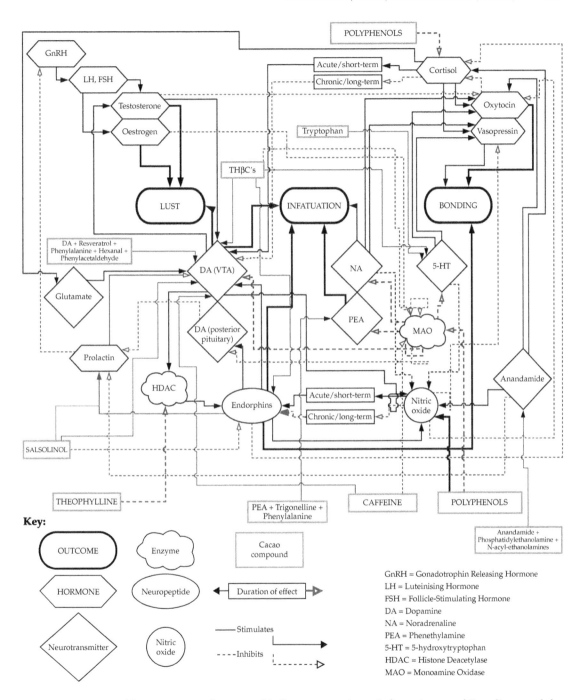

Figure 9. A map of known neuro-hormonal influences on Lust, Infatuation, and Bonding, and the hypothetical influence of Cacao's phytochemicals on these categories of "love" (constructed at www.lucidchart.com).

Chocolate for a better personality (Part 2)

Higher antenatal levels of the "stress steroid" cortisol are also linked to altered behaviour patterns and sexual behaviours in adult offspring,[787] tending to decrease Bonding and increase aggressive or avoidant behaviours. Counter-intuitively, cortisol enhances oxytocin release, which we would expect to have a calming, pro-social effect, because oxytocin suppresses cortisol release in a negative feedback loop. But it may be that without enough hugs and friendly human contact, we don't produce enough oxytocin to shut down the cortisol. So, given the self-replicating nature of good (well Bonded, attentive, and caring) or bad (poorly Bonded, abandoning, or unstable) nurturing, and the long-lasting effects of how happy, safe, and cared for we feel during our formative years, even from *within the womb*, these findings have far-reaching ramifications for adult social interactions, relationships, and even the function of society as a whole.

In other words, hormones in the pregnant mother's blood and in one's own system during childhood have profound effects, as does the nature of the bond between parents and children. Thus a low-stress childhood environment with securely bonded child-parent relationships increases children's baseline β-endorphin levels and μ-opioid receptor stimulation in the brain, and lowers their cortisol levels. These chemical changes positively influence the way those children experience relationships during adulthood; and conversely, a stressful childhood with a low-opiate, high-cortisol neuro-hormonal profile tends to produce adults with more insecure attachments. So a pregnant mother-to-be involved in an unhappy sexual relationship will have an entirely different neurochemical profile from a new mum in a stable but relatively asexual relationship, and chemical differences in these mothers' systems will influence their offspring's "brain wiring" even from before birth, as hormonal changes in the mother's bloodstream influence the unborn child's brain development.

We know that Cacao can lower levels of cortisol and adrenaline in adult humans, and that Cacao contains NO-elevating compounds which may modulate the brain's sensitivity to endorphins, and some compounds that bind to μ-opioid receptors. And we have seen that through its content of salsolinol and its complex interactions with endorphins that Cacao may—possibly—affect prolactin release. We may speculate that Cacao's content of "buffered anandamide" may be sufficient—if mum drank or ate enough chocolate—to reduce the territoriality-promoting hormone vasopressin during infancy. We also have a batch of antenatally chocolate-marinated Italian babies who appear to be happier than their chocolate-naïve gestational cohorts. So there is some foundational evidence that chocolate or Cacao ingested during pregnancy and breast-feeding may modify hormonal influences on personality development, and perhaps even adult sexual behaviour and pair bonding, although this speculation is yet to be investigated.

But even if regular Cacao intake is found not to affect oxytocin, μ-opioid receptor binding, prolactin, and vasopressin in living humans, or not to modify other neuro-hormonal developmental influences after all, its scientifically validated properties of lowering blood levels of cortisol, modulating serotonin metabolism, and increasing NO levels in the brain strongly suggest that Cacao could alter developmental factors which influence adult personality. These effects may provide retrospectively rational, non-religious reasons for the Mexica taboo on women and children consuming chocolate. Aztec society was predicated on aggressive imperialist expansion fuelled by the powerful deific magic of human sacrifice. A perk for men in the warrior and merchant classes—in exchange for regularly putting themselves in mortal danger—was permission to drink *cacahuatl*. Cacao beans were universally available as common currency, but preparing and consuming them as beverages was legally restricted to the emperor, and male members of the nobility, warrior, and merchant classes. If consumption of Cacao during pregnancy inclines towards less fearful, less stressed, less territorial, perhaps ultimately less *warlike* offspring, would it not then be prudent for the state to restrict its consumption to adult males in the ruling classes? Cacao was certainly perceived as a pre-battle courage-instilling (or post-battle *trauma-mollifying*) reward for adult men already religiously conditioned into patriotic war, and kept well away from the developing minds of future tools of state expansion, whether *in-* or *ex-utero*, and forbidden to any member of the theocracy's proletariat. Perhaps this culture, for which Cacao was such an important commodity, understood its sacred drug on subtler levels than we are currently aware of.

In a beanshell

Cacao preparations were traditionally used in Mesoamerica to ameliorate hallucinogenic "vision quest" hangovers, to treat "agitation" and some forms of mental illness.[788] There's a common thread in the consumption of *cacahuatl* by Mexica warriors to increase bravery, contemporary magico-religious use of chocolate to "dispel fear" in Santeria, and the interesting work of "chocolate shaman" Keith Wilson with his cathartic New Age "Cacao ceremonies". Given this recurrent theme, the known pharmacology of Cacao, and the studies cited in this chapter, it may be that higher quality *Theobroma* products such as traditional Cacao-based drinks have profound and largely untapped psychotherapeutic potential, perhaps specifically as an *anti-phobic* substance for reducing conditioned fear and ameliorating certain atypical depressive or anxiety disorders. Issues such as PTSD may respond to the incorporation of medicinal doses of Cacao in a therapeutic context, and Cacao's value as a dietary supplement or medicine in chronic fatigue syndrome or other complex psycho-neuro-endocrine-immunological illnesses needs further investigation.

If Cacao increases the signal amplitude but not necessarily the volume in the brain's pleasure pathways then it's no surprise that chocolate, as the Marquise de Sévigné wrote nearly four centuries ago, "acts according to [my] intention".[789] The intention-dependent effects of chocolate on mood—whereby mindfulness during chocolate consumption significantly improves mood in ways that other foods don't—provides tacit support for the hypothesis proposed in this chapter that Cacao is a kind of *hedonic modifier*, enhancing or lubricating the brain's pleasure circuitry without greatly increasing the amplitude of the signals in that circuitry. This is rather like the difference between oiling an engine and putting your foot on the accelerator: while Cacao may cause a little acceleration due to its low caffeine content, its main power may lie in subtly "greasing the wheels" of pleasure responses, while diminishing the physiological stress response, and perhaps even attenuating fear reactions in the amygdala.

The historical, anecdotal, and pharmacological information provided in this chapter points to specific modification of serotonin and endorphin pathways, which may justify the niche enthusiasm for chocolate by some MDMA and opiate users, as well as Cacao's historical consumption with *Psilocybe* mushrooms (psilocybin binds to serotonin receptors). Cacao's pharmacological profile and documented uses imply that it could also be useful for improving the effectiveness of treatments like cognitive-behavioural therapy in depressive or anhedonic (pleasure-lacking or joyless) states of mind. We saw that chocolate consumed during pregnancy appeared to produce better-adjusted babies, at least by their mothers' accounts; could early exposure to Cacao have given their brain chemistry a little boost, a head start on the journey to becoming emotionally secure adults? And if so—did it last as they grew up?

Cacao's "aphrodisiac" reputation may also be justifiable, partly because of its longer-term positive effects on circulation which may help to improve male erections, and partly due to the potential for complex interactions between the chemistry of Cacao and the neuro-hormonal control systems underlying the three subtypes of love, namely Lust, Infatuation, and Bonding. Many brain regions activated by these three physiologically defined subcategories of love— which can be distinct, but are often co-present to varying degrees in any sexual relationship— are the same as those affected by "drugs of abuse", principally the "reward system", and there is an intricate web of feedback-controlled links between the various neurotransmitters, hormones, and brain regions involved. Cacao's distinct effects on cortisol (reducing) and NO (increasing), in addition to possible modulatory effects on trace amine associated receptors, serotonin, dopamine, PEA, anandamide, and opiate receptors in the brain, provide ample means for Cacao to modify the neurochemistry of love.

Hypothetically—following the rabbit all the way down the hole—Cacao has the potential to amplify and possibly accelerate the course of Infatuation and Bonding, increasing the predilection for romantic attraction, and perhaps even hastening disillusionment in sexual relationships. Could regular consumption of Cacao increase the appetite for romance and sexual interactions, yet shorten the honeymoon period in relationships? Could we go further, almost absurdly, and infer that the enormous popularity of chocolate in the West may parallel soaring divorce rates? Or maybe, as the scant clinical evidence suggests, Cacao's influence on mood is neutral or mostly benign, so any effects on human interaction are non-existent or wholly beneficial? Of course this could be statistically evaluated—do high chocolate consumers (*sic*) have more or less stable and satisfying sexual relationships? Cacao may even turn out to be both angel and devil depending on the situation—the brain chemistry of the persons consuming it, their life experiences, or the stage of life at which they are exposed to chocolate. All of these are potentially fruitful avenues for statistical and pharmacological inquiry.

Perhaps the most prevalent psychoactive drugs in any society both reflect and affect it, chicken-and-egg style. If Cacao does influence personality and behaviour—just like other psychoactive drugs can, and as some of the evidence and conjecture presented in this chapter suggests that it might—then perhaps any culture which embraces Cacao will be transformed by it in both subtle and obvious ways, as with any other psychoactive substance, from coffee to tobacco to heroin. Despite its contemporary reputation as a mild caffeine-containing stimulant, and its attenuation and relegation to the confectionery aisles of supermarkets, it should be recalled that Cacao was once the royal drug of the Mexica, subject to stringent taboos and ritual proscriptions, regarded as a divine plant growing out of the mouth of the underworld throughout pre-Colombian Mesoamerica. No matter how absurd it may seem, the mass consumption of Cacao, and the nature of its transformation from an exalted bitter beverage to a cheap sweet treat, may reflect—or affect—the trajectory of those societies which consume it. The meaning of this dialogue between Cacao and those societies which favour its products will be discussed in part III of this book.

When we are upset, lonely, insecure, or heartsick, chocolate is often our go-to remedy—and there's enough evidence to suggest that this may be more than a matter of "comfort food". Cacao, like other psychotropic drugs, partially hijacks some of the brain's reward systems. It achieves this so subtly and quietly that, almost without our conscious intent, many of those who taste chocolate find that Cacao becomes a default remedy for romantic disillusionment: aspirin for headache, chocolate for heartache. This hypothesis casts a rather different light on the spread of this apparently benign food-drink-drug across the world, and its symbolic (and, it turns out, quite literal) association with matters of the heart. The possibility of invisible associations between the pharmacology of Cacao and food cravings, addictions, and mental or physical health issues will be explored further in Chapter 7. But next, we'll take a look at the pharmacology of some of Cacao's most distinguished botanical collaborators.

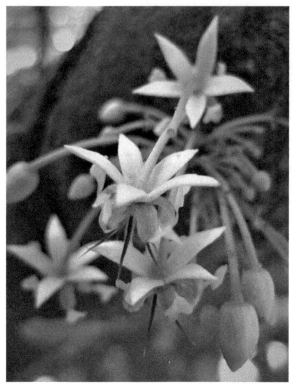

Criollo Cacao flowers, Guatemala, 2011

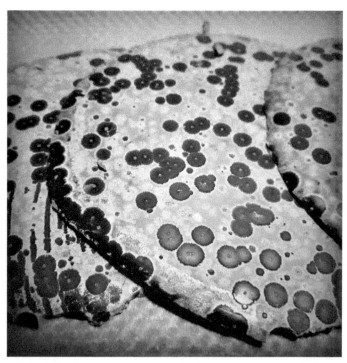

Natural bloom patterns in
homemade Cacao discs.

CHAPTER SIX

Associates and accomplices

"All have come
from where the flowers arise.
The flowers that confuse the people,
which cause their hearts to whirl.
They have come to scatter, to make them fall like in a rain,
garlands of flowers,
intoxicating flowers.

Who stands
on the flowery mat?
Indeed your home is here,
in the midst of the paintings.
Xayacamach speaks, sings,
inebriated with the heart of the Cacao flower."

(Mexica poet-ruler Xayacamach of Tizatlan,
fifteenth century CE, from Léon-Portilla, 1992)

Historically, as we have seen, Cacao was rarely consumed on its own. The word "spice" implies merely flavouring, an appealing additive; but the majority of spice plants contain an impressive array of compounds and have useful medicinal properties that complement and augment Cacao's own pharmacological attributes. Some of these Cacao beverages were drunk for pleasure, but many were consumed for medicinal or tonic effects as well. There are detailed monographs describing Cacao's commonest additive plants in Appendix B, but these companions are too important to relegate to the back of the book. They include international culinary superstars such as chilli peppers and vanilla, supporting cast members like allspice, sarsaparilla, and annatto, and undeservedly obscure aromatics such as holy leaf, popcorn flower, funeral tree, and ear flower. These lesser-known spices still have a local fan base in some Central American indigenous recipes, but they were unjustly supplanted as mainstream Cacao additives by the Spanish colonists' favourite Asian imports such as cinnamon, black pepper, or nutmeg. The indigenous ingredients contributed distinctive characteristics and effects when combined with Cacao. There's also the small matter of the Mesoamerican custom of drinking Cacao with "magic mushrooms" (*Psilocybe spp.*) at feasts and important ceremonies to consider …

Medicinal flowers

Heart flower, blood sugar

For the sake of convenience, Cacao's traditional admixture plants can be grouped by matching them with the different health-promoting properties and medicinal uses of Cacao. Perhaps unsurprisingly, a great number of the spices may be useful in cardiovascular disease. The lesser-known, fragrant popcorn flower (*Bourreria huanita*), a favourite Maya *kakawa* additive, may lower blood pressure;[790] and several other additive plants may reduce blood fats or cholesterol levels. These include the red food colouring agent known as annatto or *achiote*, made from the seeds of *Bixa orellana*; aromatic frangipani flowers (*Plumeria rubra*); the familiar vanilla pods (*Vanilla planifolia*); melon-tasting Mexican magnolia flowers (*Magnolia mexicana* and *Magnolia dealbata*); the almond-scented seeds of the fruit *mamey sapote* (*Pouteria sapota*), and the pre-eminent Mexica *cacahauatl* ingredient, the resinous, spicy ear flower (*Cymbopetalum penduliflorum*). Of these, magnolia flowers contain flavone glycosides which appear to act directly on heart muscle, and are specifically used to treat palpitations, dizziness, high blood pressure, and anxiety;[791] the Mexica name for this beautiful, spectacularly flowering tree was *yolloxochitl*, meaning "heart flower", and it's still known in Mexico as *flor del corazon*.[792]

Ear flower and annatto, too, are reputed to be "heart tonics". Annatto (*Bixa orellana*) seeds contain the carmine-red pigment bixin, which protected rats fed a high-fat diet from developing heart inflammation and cardiac fibrosis (scarring in the heart muscle).[793] Although annatto was not traditionally used for heart problems, it's prescribed in contemporary folk medicine for type 2 diabetes and erectile dysfunction,[794] both of which may be associated with heart disease. Magnolia and ear flower also contain the alkaloid liriodenine, a known anti-arrhythmic agent that increases the production of nitric oxide in heart muscle.[795] This has the effect of protecting the heart from injury when its blood supply is temporarily cut off and reinstated, as in a heart attack—most of the damage after a heart attack (or stroke, in the brain) occurs not when the blood flow is cut off, but when it returns: the flood of blood into oxygen-starved tissue catalyses destructive oxidative, free-radical reactions, like a starving person wolfing down a three-course meal and becoming very sick—it's too much for the weakened state of the tissues. Liriodenine from ear flower and magnolia may help buffer this effect, if its laboratory action is anything to go by; magnolia flowers have also demonstrated beneficial effects in heart disease in humans in uncontrolled trials.[796]

Several other spices may be useful additives to Cacao in prevention or dietary assistance in type 2 diabetes: cayenne (*Capsicum spp.*), allspice (*Pimienta dioica*), vanilla, and the so-called root beer plant or holy leaf (*Piper auritum*). Cayenne, also known as the familiar hot chilli pepper, increases the secretion of insulin from the pancreas; allspice and vanilla enhance the sensitivity of insulin receptors; and holy leaf, a species of pepper, does the same thing, but also inhibits the production of advanced glycation end-products (AGEs).[797] This is the technical term for compounds formed when glucose combines with fats or proteins, which it does all the time when blood sugar is high: AGEs are the stuff that "silts up" the system in diabetes. The acronym AGE is appropriate, as they are a factor in aging, and have been linked to Alzheimer's disease as well as atherosclerosis.

The dried flower spikes of holy leaf (*Piper auritum*), which were used in Cacao-based drinks, presumably have a similar chemical make-up to the better-investigated leaves of the same plant, and certainly contain similar aromatic constituents if their smell and taste are anything to go by. The leaves give the plant their other English name, as their high content of a volatile compound called safrole (which can be carcinogenic in isolation) creates an appealing, root-beer-like smell, and the fresh leaves are used in cooking, to wrap *tamales* or as essential ingredients in green *mole* sauces. Their ability to prevent formation of AGEs turns out to be higher than the isolated chemical, gallic acid, which is used as the benchmark or "reference compound" in tests—*Piper auritum* beats the best. This property suggests that holy leaf may have powerful abilities to prevent diabetes-related complications such as organ damage, peripheral neuropathy (loss of sensation or tingling in hands and feet), deterioration of eyesight, and so on. So far the leaf has only been tested in diabetic rats, with very positive results: when it was incorporated into their food for twenty-eight days, the rats' blood sugar fell, and their cholesterol profiles, liver chemistry, and stores of glycogen (fuel reserves) in the liver and muscles returned to healthy values.[798]

Pain-relieving plants

Holy leaf was also traditionally used to relieve pain and fatigue, and has marked anti-anxiety, pain-relieving, and anti-inflammatory effects, at least in rats—perhaps not surprisingly, as in addition to containing flavonoids and a complex volatile oil, the plant produces powerful aporphine alkaloids, a type of compound known to have central nervous system activity.[799] The addition of *P. auritum* dried flower spikes to Cacao may therefore be expected to augment Cacao's own pain-relieving, stress-reducing properties. Several other additive plants have pain-relieving properties too. Cayenne has this effect when applied externally, in the same way that chillies make food taste hot: the compound capsaicin triggers the release of a pain-signalling chemical given the B-movie name "substance P". A single application of capsaicin produces the familiar chilli "burn", and can be used to test the effectiveness of pain-relieving drugs—in fact injections of capsaicin were used in tests to induce trigeminal neuralgia (facial nerve pain) in rats that Cacao was shown to alleviate![800] But with repeated application of cayenne, or isolated capsaicin, the production of substance P incrementally dwindles. This process of gradual desensitisation, called *tachyphylaxis*, is the reason why chilli fans can eat hotter and hotter chillies, eventually—if they keep "scaling up"—to the point of tolerating whole raw chilli peppers. Tachyphylaxis also explains why repeated application of cayenne or capsaicin is an effective treatment for nerve pain on the surface of the body (e.g., peripheral neuropathy). Cayenne is no help for internal pain though—but popcorn flower, frangipani—and even, to a lesser extent, allspice—appear to have those bases covered.

Allspice (*Pimenta dioica*) berries, so-named because their scent is redolent of cloves, nutmeg, and cinnamon combined, contain a high percentage of volatile compounds ("essential oil") and polyphenols. They were traditionally used in poultices to treat neuralgic or rheumatic pain, and taken internally for colic (cramping abdominal pain) or to assist childbirth—both to speed up the process (a "parturient") and, presumably, to help pain relief. In rats, at least, allspice berry water extracts have analgesic effects.[801] It appears that another Cacao spice, popcorn flower (*Bourreria huanita*), the highly-perfumed flowers of a tropical tree in the Borage plant family, may be a more potent painkiller: an infusion of the flowers was traditionally used in combination with other plants to help accelerate recovery from internal injuries and relieve pain, and in animal trials alcoholic (ethanol) extracts of unspecified parts of the plant had sedative, anti-anxiety and antidepressant properties.[802] Although traditional drinks were made with water, not ethanol, whole dried pulverised flowers were used in Cacao-based beverages by the Mesoamerican peoples, so any alcohol-soluble constituents—which are also fat-soluble, and therefore extracted by liquid fats, such as melted cocoa butter, from ground Cacao dispersed in hot water—would have easily made it into the drinks.

Frangipani (*Plumeria rubra*) may be even more potently analgesic and anti-inflammatory than *B. huanita*. This striking tree with its distinctive, five-petalled aromatic flowers has been exported all around the world. While it is the flowers that were—and are—used in some Cacao-based drinks, frangipani bark was used as an analgesic; traditionally, it was decocted (boiled in water) to treat "internal bruising", diarrhoea, and arthritis. Dr Francisco Hernández de Toledo, the famous Spanish sixteenth-century royal physician and chronicler of indigenous remedies in Mexico, recommended drinking six to eight ounces of the decoction twice daily to treat dropsy (oedema, or fluid retention in the lower legs), to dissolve "obstructions" causing abdominal pain in the stomach, liver, and spleen, and to help recovery from long illnesses.[803] Frangipani bark has since been found to contain a potent cocktail of alkaloids, sterols, polyphenols, and steroid-like terpenoids,[804] and has antimicrobial activity against a variety of bacteria and fungi[805,806]—which may be the basis of its traditional use in diarrhoea and dysentery. When administered to mice, bark extracts had analgesic and anti-inflammatory effects, in addition to anti-ulcer and anti-diabetic properties.[807]

Frangipani flowers also have anti-anxiety activity, and appear in a traditional Mexica formula against fear or cowardice,[808] as well as being used in contemporary folk medicine to treat diabetes.[809] So, although they may be less potently anti-inflammatory and analgesic than the bark, the flowers' use with Cacao may add another layer of potency and complexity to Cacao's own analgesic, anti-diabetic and psychotropic activities. Interestingly, the flowers were also used as an aphrodisiac[810]—another crossover with Cacao's traditional reputation. Perhaps their anti-anxiety effects could be useful here, to counter "performance" problems, where anxiety may be a factor in sexual performance issues.

Anti-sickling blooms

Cacao's possible usefulness as a treatment in sickle-cell anaemia was mentioned in Chapter 4, and some of its botanical associates may be very helpful here. Cayenne stimulates the circulation, and the antioxidant carotenoids it contains penetrate red blood cells and accumulate in them,[811] which is likely to reduce their susceptibility to sickling. In rat studies, cayenne reduced dangerous blood clotting, and a lower incidence of medically dangerous spontaneous blood clotting (thromboembolism) has been noted in populations consuming large quantities of hot *Capsicum* varieties.[812] These properties suggest that cayenne could be a useful additive to Cacao as part of a sickle-cell anaemia management strategy. Annatto, too, may be useful, as the heart-protective properties of its chief carotenoid, bixin, and its anti-inflammatory, antioxidant attributes suggest it may improve overall circulatory health. Frangipani flowers could be beneficial additives for their anti-inflammatory, pain-relieving properties. But the number one Cacao spice for sickle-cell treatment must be vanilla.

Traditionally, vanilla was used against fatigue and "cold poisons",[813] the symptoms of which would be cramping and pain—coincidentally, much like the symptoms of a sickle-cell crisis. In a small (thirty participants) eight-week placebo-controlled double-blind clinical trial, isolated vanillin—the main odour compound in vanilla—was given to sickle-cell patients as capsules of 250mg taken every six hours. At the end of the trial, the number of sickled red blood cells had declined by 20% in the vanillin group, and the "sickling time"—the time it took for the red blood cells to change shape under stress—increased by 50%.[814] This is an exciting finding, but the bad news is that it would take daily ingestion of *twenty-eight grams* of dried vanilla pods to achieve similar blood levels of isolated vanillin! This would be both very expensive and most likely toxic. The potentially good news is that although vanillin is only 1–3.4% of the bean's dry weight, there are other, structurally similar compounds in the essential oil, and polyphenols and alkaloids in the whole bean too,[815] so it's feasible—likely, even—that the whole plant has stronger effects than may be expected from its vanillin content alone.

Frustratingly, researchers have so far only ever tested isolated vanillin for anti-sickling effects (the old profit-driven drug development model again)—although, more positively, vanillin is quite cheap to synthesise whereas vanilla beans are expensive, so good results for vanillin may mean cheaper medicine! The other bit of good news is that non-oral dosing of vanillin may be much more effective. When taken by mouth, vanillin is rapidly broken down in the liver before getting into the blood, but taking it rectally in suppositories would bypass the liver and deliver it straight into the bloodstream. Suppositories are often more effective than taking drugs orally because when a drug comprised of smaller molecules—which aromatic substances such as vanillin are—is taken rectally, it's absorbed directly into the bloodstream through the lining of the colon, and doesn't get broken down in the liver for a while (as anything taken orally does). Vanillin and the other essential oils in *V. planifolia* are all fat-soluble, so they are readily taken up by melted cocoa butter, as any chocolatier knows. Cocoa butter is often used for making suppositories because it's solid at cooler temperatures but readily melts at body temperature, and is easily absorbed by epithelial tissue (linings, such as the skin externally or mucous membranes internally). So one experimental protocol for attempting to improve well-being and avert crises in sickle-cell anaemia could be to drink *cacahuatl* made with Cacao, added vanilla, annatto, and cayenne every day, with or without added frangipani flowers, while also using cocoa-butter-based vanilla suppositories.

The cordials: mood medicine

Vanilla's other assignation by early European colonists was, along with several other chocolate spices, as a "cordial"—to benefit mood and general vitality. A great many traditional *kakawa* spices shared this designation: popcorn flower (*Bourreria huanita*), ear flower (*Cymbopetalum penduliflorum*), magnolia (*Magnolia mexicana*), holy leaf (*Piper auritum*), allspice (*Pimienta dioica*), frangipani (*Plumeria rubra*), and funeral tree (*Quararibea funebris*)—all of which, according to animal testing, have some psychotropic activity, evidenced by antidepressant (*B. huanita*, *V. planifolia*), anti-anxiety, sedative (*B. huanita*, *M. mexicana*, *P. rubra*, *Q. funebris* [possibly], *C. penduliflorum* [possibly]), or anodyne/analgesic (*P. dioica*, *B. huanita*, *P. auritum*, *P. rubra*) properties. Vanilla is the only one of these plants to have been tested for antidepressant activity. Rats exposed to chronic unpredictable mild stress in the form of tilting cages, suddenly being forced to swim in cold water and similar non-lethal forms of torture developed depression, and chronic unpredictable stress is a standard means of inducing depression in animal models (a useful thing to remember when dealing with depression in humans). Rats whose cages were "fumigated" with vanillin developed fewer signs of depression—they moved more, and didn't lose their appetite for sucrose (table sugar—ironically, itself a problematic food for depressed animals, as we will see in the next chapter!).

When they were killed, the vanillin-exposed rats' brains had higher levels of the mood-elevating compounds serotonin, dopamine, and noradrenaline than all the other rats living without the benefit of vanilla-scented living quarters—including the rats not exposed to extra stress! Significantly, the antidepressant effect of vanillin vanished when rats' olfactory bulbs were removed, so that they had no sense of smell.[816] As discussed in Chapters 4 and 5 with relation to the TAARs, the effective drug delivery route here is from the nose, via the olfactory nerve and straight into the limbic system, the brain's emotion-regulating, memory-forming, and motivation-producing centre. Because flavour is mostly smell, the Mesoamerican preference for Cacao-based drinks with a tall head of aromatic foam, and bubbles that pop in the mouth, takes on a new dimension when considered in this light: the highly aerated foam is a sort of central nervous system drug delivery apparatus for aromatic, low molecular weight (i.e., small and floaty) compounds.

Ear flower and funeral tree, two of the other "cordial" flowers used with Cacao, may also be very useful to combat long-term negative effects of stress. While there is very little—or no—scientific research into the pharmacological effects of both plants, they were two of the most highly regarded *kakawa* spices in pre-Columbian Mesoamerica. Known as *flor de oreja* or *orejuela* in Mexico today, ear flower (*Cymbopetalum penduliflorum*) blooms contain resins, flavonoids, steroid-like triterpenoids, and a cocktail of alkaloids, including liriodenine, also found in *Magnolia mexicana* flowers. Liriodenine is known to have sedative and nerve-protective activity, at least in the laboratory.[817]

Funeral tree flowers feature in the Mexica prescription against "losing one's mind" (see Chapter 3)—schizophrenia, or dementia, perhaps?—and are used in contemporary Mexico to treat "fear".[818] Hypothetically, they may be a valuable adjunct to Cacao for stress reduction, and preventing or treating certain forms of dementia, or in PTSD or other syndromes associated with conditioned fear or anxiety. Vanilla may be useful for protecting the brain itself, if the action of vanillin in rats is anything to go by. When a 5% solution of ethanol was injected into rats pre-dosed with oral vanillin, the vanillin prevented brain cell injury in the now-intoxicated rodents.[819] In a rodent model of Parkinson's disease, injections of vanillin dose-dependently alleviated symptoms and helped conserve the action of an enzyme called *tyrosine hydroxylase* in the rats' brains which helps produce dopamine,[820] the substance which becomes depleted in the brain and causes symptoms of Parkinson's. This fits with the higher levels of dopamine in the rats living in vanillin-scented cages. Perhaps Cacao flavoured with vanilla and funeral tree flowers might be a useful preventive for some forms of neurological disease?

The cordials: cancer

Aside from their mood-modifying actions, "cordial" plants are a pharmacologically diverse group. Another meaning of the Galenic term "cordial" is something which strengthens vitality. "Cordial" plants typically combine mild psychoactivity of the antidepressant-anxiolytic variety with other longevity-promoting properties, such as immune-system modifying, or *immuno-modulatory* activity. Nowadays we might describe such plants in terms of anti-inflammatory, antioxidant, cholesterol-lowering, or anti-cancer activity. Vanilla may have cancer-preventing activity if *in vitro* tests with isolated vanillin are verified in living humans, as vanillin inhibits chromosome damage caused by ultraviolet light and inhibits formation of some types of lung cancer cells (unfortunately not the most aggressive type, small cell lung cancer).[821] Of course, this is one isolated constituent in the proverbial test tube, not the whole plant in the human body, but the antioxidant polyphenols in the dried seed pods are likely to assist rather than hinder this action, if anything, based on the anti-neoplastic (preventing cancer cell growth) action of many polyphenols.

Allspice extracts, too, have inhibitory effects on prostate, breast, and pancreatic cancer cells,[822] and suppressive effects on breast and prostate cancers have been demonstrated in mice, where large doses of allspice berries inhibited tumour growth.[823] While the doses used in this experiment were achievable in human terms, they are much larger than standard doses when allspice is used in Cacao-based drinks; but the existence of such properties suggests that allspice berries would contribute positively to Cacao's anti-cancer activity. Interestingly—with reference to its property of "dissolving obstructions"—frangipani (*P. rubra*) leaf extracts had significant anti-cancer activity in mice, reducing the volume of abdominal tumours and normalising blood test results. The leaf extracts didn't increase the overall survival time of the mice, but did significantly improve their symptoms and quality of life, and showed strong liver-protecting properties.[824] Capsaicin in cayenne alters the expression of genes associated with cancer cell survival, growth, and spread *in vitro*, weakening cancer cells,[825] so even chilli pepper may turn out to be a useful chemopreventive addition to Cacao. Cayenne is used in herbal medicine to increase the effectiveness of other medicinal plants by maximising their absorption and distribution, so a delectable chemopreventive or anti-neoplastic *cacahuatl* recipe could feature frangipani flowers, allspice, vanilla, and a hit of chilli.

Flowers vs. Snakes

Some Cacao additives may enhance its prophylactic powers against snake venom. Arguably, this is more of an imaginal exercise than of practical use—given that the Cacao beverage would need to be drunk before, not after a snake bite, and who knows in advance when they may be bitten by a snake? (Zookeepers working in reptile houses, wildlife documentary makers, or game reserve poachers?) And, what sensible person would rely only on spiced chocolate for protection? Nevertheless, the information may come in handy for somebody, somewhere, and drinking spiced *cacahuatl* is no penance! Certainly, for the Mesoamerican Mayan civilisations, literally surrounded by snake-infested jungle, the danger of snakebite was a constant reality; the central importance of snakes in Mesoamerican iconography and mythology in such guises as "the mouth of the underworld" (see Chapter 9) testifies to a deep cultural awareness of, and respect for, the fearsome danger that poisonous snakes represented. For those privileged elements of Mesoamerican society who could afford to drink Cacao regularly, it isn't too far-fetched to imagine that a greater chance of survival after being bitten may have been a valued advantage conferred by their most prized beverage.

Annatto (*Bixa orellana*) has been tested against snake venom. When annatto leaf extracts were mixed with the venom of *Bothrops asper*, the pit viper known as fer de lance, and injected into mice, there was much less swelling than if only the viper venom was injected; but, if the annatto leaf extract was administered orally, the effects were negligible.[826] Given that the seed, not the leaf, is used in Cacao-based drinks, and such drinks are typically consumed orally, this experiment may be of little relevance to Cacao-based drinks. But the three "cordial" plants mentioned above—*Bourreria huanita*, *Piper auritum*, and *Vanilla planifolia*—all had traditional recommendations for use against "poisons affecting the heart", meaning they may confer some life-preserving properties against any toxin of external origin, be it venom or infection (the two were not clearly distinguished, both often resulting from animal bites and having similar features). Could they be any help?

There isn't enough research on *B. huanita*, though its Cold nature and reputation as a fever-lowering agent suggest possible use in recovery from inflammatory conditions, such as perhaps may be caused by snakebite. *P. auritum*'s demonstrable anti-inflammatory and analgesic properties may be of some use, too, and the familiar "black flower" of the Mexica, *V. planifolia*, may offset the effects of venoms which cause nerve damage, if the rat research mentioned above holds up in humans. So, depending on the type of snake venom—as different snake venoms have different effects—these spices may benefit. But, we don't know for sure; in lieu of more experiments, we can only speculate that these plants may enhance any protective, snake-venom-attenuating properties of real Cacao-based drinks. So far, nobody has volunteered to test this theory.

Spice up your lungs

Cacao's potential benefits in asthma may be enhanced by ear flower, frangipani, and the seed of the common Central American fruit, the *mamey sapote*, known in English as marmalade plum. Ear flower (*Cymbopetalum penduliflorum*) contains liriodenine, the alkaloid also found in *Magnolia mexicana*. Liriodenine is antispasmodic in tracheal muscle[827]—in other words, it reduces airway narrowing, one of the two pathological responses in asthma, the other being inflammation in the lining of the airways. *C. penduliflorum*'s largely un-investigated resin content may also be relevant here, as some resinous plants, such as pine (*Pinus spp.*) or tar weed (*Grindelia camporum*) have antiseptic and expectorant activity—that is, they inhibit infectious microbes, and stimulate proper secretion and expulsion of mucus from the lungs—although it must be said that the precise properties of the resins in *C. penduliflorum* are currently unknown. *Plumeria rubra*, the frangipani, is also traditionally used to treat asthma, and although its anti-asthmatic activity hasn't been tested, its proven anti-inflammatory properties may be relevant. *Mamey sapote* seeds, used in the Oaxacan beverage *tejate*, contain *cyanogenic glycosides* (cyanide-yielding compounds, bound to sugars), which give the seeds their amaretto-like flavour, and tiny doses of these molecules assuage airway irritability and reduce coughing; the bark is used for this purpose in Mexican folk medicine, being higher in cyanogenic glycosides, but the seeds are also active.[828]

Sex with spice

As discussed in the last chapter, Cacao may also help to relieve erectile dysfunction in men due to its positive effects on the circulatory system. Circulation-stimulating cayenne may be useful here, as may annatto, which was traditionally used to treat male impotence.[829] Blood-sugar and blood-fat lowering properties have been detected in annatto seed extracts in animal experiments,[830] and oral capsaicin from chilli peppers attenuated atherosclerotic damage in rats,[831] which suggests that both plants may be specifically useful in combination with Cacao if used in erectile dysfunction associated with cardiovascular disease.

On the other side of the biological gender binary, frangipani flowers were used with Cacao to increase breast milk production, but this may be more magically than pharmaceutically justifiable. Cacao pods grow directly from the tree trunk like breasts, and the frangipani tree weeps a milky white latex when cut, so these plants in combination symbolically evoke breast milk. The combination of fruit and flower in one nutritious, uplifting, and somewhat pain-relieving beverage would be a logical choice when breastfeeding. In fact *P. rubra* flower extracts have *anti-fertility* effects when administered to rats, reducing sex hormone production in the ovaries;[832] so while frangipani probably does affect female sexual function, regular consumption could have the opposite result from the one intended! That said, the existence of an effect on female sex hormone production in rats suggests the need for further investigation on its action in humans. On closer inspection, frangipani's milk-making reputation may turn out to be more than symbolic—or not.

More brown liquid

Perhaps recovery from diarrhoea isn't the first thing that comes to mind when chocolate is mentioned. But the quantity of polyphenols in Cacao suggests that it may be beneficial, as polyphenols often inhibit pathogenic microbe growth, and sure enough it turns out that the flavanols in Cacao decrease levels of systemic inflammation and improve the microbe balance in the gut when given to humans in sensible doses (equivalent to 40g of Cacao per day) over a four-week period.[833] The high fat content of Cacao probably makes it unsuitable for treatment of acute diarrhoea, but one traditional Cacao spice—the devil's hand flower, *Chiranthodendron pentadactylon*—would amplify Cacao's power to rectify loose bowels. *C. pentadactylon* has a high flavanol content, and is also regarded as a "cordial" in Mexican folk medicine, having sedative and anti-anxiety properties, so it may be another useful anti-stress additive.

The plant is astringent, binding the bowels, because it contains *tannins*. Tannins are a type of polyphenol, and some tannins are hydrolysable—meaning they may be hydrolysed, or "split apart" using hydrogen ions, to make other compounds. Generally this job is done by microbes in the gut, where the hydrolysed tannins yield smaller polyphenolic substances like flavanols and anthocyanins of the sort we find in Cacao. Hydrolysable tannins are a kind of flavanol pro-drug, and it is this sort which predominates in *C. pentadactylon*. As one might expect, non-hydrolysable tannins (the other sort) don't break down, but both types share the property of cross-linking proteins, pulling these molecules closer together, making a tougher, less flexible surface, like a woollen garment shrinking in a hot wash. It's this property that gives "tannins" their name, as these are the compounds traditionally used to tan leather. When ingested, tannins produce the "dry-mouth" feeling of black tea or red wine; this same protein-linking property affects many gut microbes and reduces secretions in the bowel, helping to stop diarrhoea. It also explains hand flower's application to ulcers and haemorrhoids, as astringents cicatrise wounds by sealing off the surface, tightening tissues, and reducing superficial swelling and inflammation.

Research has validated hand flower's reputation for treating bum trouble, as flower extracts inhibit eight bacteria known to cause diarrhoea, including *E. coli* and *Salmonella* species;[834] they also significantly inhibit the protozoa *Entamoeba histolytica* and *Giardia lambla*,[835] the cause of amoebiasis and giardiasis, respectively. Amoebiasis and giardiasis are common types of dysentery, often a source of misery for travellers, and of much suffering worldwide. Hand flower's inhibitory effect on *Entamoeba histolytica* is as potent as the standard drug, Emetine, *in vitro*.[836] Water extracts of *C. pentadactylon* leaves fed to rats at very high doses for twenty-eight days caused no signs of toxicity—on the contrary, all the animals gained weight,[837] so if the leaves contain similar compounds to the flowers—and we know that they do—perhaps the flowers' addition to Cacao may assist weight gain in humans? The flowers also inhibited intestinal over-secretion caused by cholera toxin in rats and mice,[838] and slowed down excessive intestinal movements (hyperperistalsis) in rats as effectively as the standard over-the-counter drug, Loperamide.[839] One of the side effects of dysentery is rapid weight loss, so Cacao with added *C. pentadactylon* flowers may be a useful aid to recovery from dysentery or indeed any condition with chronic or recurrent infectious diarrhoea and consequent weight loss, such as HIV infection or other immunosuppressed states. Annatto, too, contains tannins and was traditionally used to treat dysentery,[840] as were allspice berries, which also contain tannin in addition to their antimicrobial, antispasmodic essential oil.[841]

The spice of life

Cacao's powers as a potential life-extending (anti-senescent), cognition-enhancing (nootropic), old-person-benefitting (geriatric tonic) drug may be enhanced by particular spices. Vanilla, as we have seen, may be of benefit for improving mood, protecting brain cells, and perhaps even be of benefit in Parkinson's disease; circulatory disorders may respond well to Cacao spiked with cayenne, annatto, and holy leaf—and for many of the other diseases which may emerge with age, such as heart disease, diabetes, cancer, and respiratory problems, many of the traditional Cacao spices already discussed may be of benefit in reducing risk and slowing deterioration.

But what about the aging process itself? As we know, Cacao lowers cortisol levels, which may reduce the rate of aging. But which traditional spices may help here? One stands above the rest: root beer plant, or holy leaf, *Piper auritum*. This plant's remarkable ability to inhibit the formation of advanced glycation end products (AGEs) marks it out as a spice which could slow down the inevitable "silting up" of the microcirculation, helping to sustain blood flow through tiny capillaries which are so necessary to conserve function, such as those in the retina of the eye or surrounding the glomeruli (tiny filtering tubes) in the kidneys.

Speaking of the eyes—as cataracts or other forms of visual deterioration such as macular degeneration, which causes blindness, are a common pest of age—the carotenoid pigment called nor-bixin in annatto reduced retinal damage when fed to mice over a three-month period.[842] A whole annatto seed extract also protected retinal cells from toxic damage in live mice,[843] and we know from both rat and human studies that nor-bixin is well absorbed from the gut and gets into the circulation.[844] So there's reason to suppose that annatto may be beneficial for some forms of visual impairment related to the aging process. Cayenne, too, with its blood-thinning, circulation-stimulating powers may be more generally useful as we age—indeed, aayenne is the only plant mentioned here (in addition to Cacao) which has the distinction of some statistical correlation with reduced mortality. A six-year survey of more than 16,000 adults in the US found that higher dietary chilli pepper consumption was linked with a 13% reduction in relative risk of all-cause mortality.[845] This is, of course, much more modest than the 47% relative risk reduction in all-cause mortality produced by high levels of dark chocolate intake found in the smaller Dutch study on elderly men,[846] but we can infer that the Mesoamerican innovation of adding chilli peppers to Cacao was probably, as they say, "on point".

Getting into a lather

The famous foam of ancient Cacao drinks is a tradition which persists today on the most prized *atoles* in Central America; this foam has various formulations, described in Chapter 2. The emulsification of cocoa butter from ground Cacao seeds mixed into water is a key part of this process, not only for the obvious "thickening" effect this has on the liquid but, more importantly, because the phospholipids in Cacao are natural emulsifiers. Emulsifiers are substances whose molecules are half water-loving/fat-hating, and half fat-loving/water-hating, so they "zip together" small globules of fat surrounded by water (or the reverse). Emulsions can only form when there is no more than a quarter of the volume of oil-in-water or water-in-oil; more than 25% of one of the two phases will result in separation.

In *cacahuatl*, the tiny particles of fibre from ground Cacao beans held in suspension in the liquid also help to keep the fat and water mixed, through something called the Pickering effect, or Pickering emulsion—named after a Mr Pickering, one presumes—whereby little particles of solids in a liquid adhere to the interfaces between water and fat globules (or, again, vice versa), and help them stay separate. Emulsifiers also enable bubbles to form more easily. When air is whipped into water, the surface tension of the water—created by the water molecules' strong mutual attraction—normally prevents a foam from forming. But once some soap-like emulsifying agent is added, bubbles can form: air remains trapped in spheres of liquid, where films of water molecules are held between outer "walls" of emulsifiers. The water-loving "heads" of the emulsifying substance molecules stick into the water and their water-hating tails stick out of it; this pushes the water molecules closer together on one side ("heads"), and further apart on the other ("tails"), curving the plane of the film of water.[847] Bubbles are spherical because a sphere is the most space-efficient way that the film of water can contain the trapped air.

Even the presence of hydrolysable tannins (the larger polyphenols) in Cacao may assist foam formation,[848] as they interlink protein molecules, providing a "trellis" which helps stabilise bubbles. Hence toasted, liquefied Cacao seeds and water can produce a small but stable foam. The foam of Cacao and water alone, or with minimal additives, has small bubbles and is mostly a product of fat emulsion, which can be seen when light reflects off the foam: pearlescent rainbows on every bubble, like the psychedelic visual effect of a thin film of oil on a wet road surface. But to produce the towering cumulonimbi of aromatic froth we see in Mesoamerican artistic depictions of Cacao-based beverages and atop many contemporary *atoles*, additives are needed to amplify the foaming effect. These botanical foaming agents are still not fully documented, but several different techniques and additives are used to produce foam.

Of those mentioned so far, a water extract of annatto seeds produces a modest froth, which—in sufficient quantity—enhances Cacao's natural frothiness. Annatto seeds can be ground whole and used in Cacao drinks, but a more concentrated form of annatto is found in Mexican *pasta de achiote*. This condensed annatto extract is the principal foaming agent (in addition to emulsified Cacao) in contemporary *atole colorado* (red atole), fully described in Chapter 8. It's likely that the tannins in annatto help, but the starches in corn or wheat used for *atoles* also contribute, because they dissolve in water and polymerise—that is, form long chains—making a kind of molecular mesh which stabilises bubbles, along with any tannin-linked proteins. Señora Mecinas, who provided the recipe for *atole colorado*, said that wheat was easier to use in the recipe than the corn used by her grandmother; might this be because wheat also contains the protein gluten, which would be cross-linked by tannins, producing a stronger "trellis" for bubble formation? Although gluten is insoluble in water, the wheat is ground into tiny particles which are held in suspension so that the starch dissolves into water and polymerises, thickening the liquid. Proteins are relatively large structures—molecularly speaking—and the effect of first finely grinding the wheat, then beating it in water, will cause some of the gluten proteins to unravel (denature), and the water-hating parts of the unravelled protein strands will begin to stick to fats in the liquid. The polyphenols from Cacao in the water would also connect them, forming a stronger trellis than starch alone. It's certainly the case that the bubbles on *Atole Colorado* can be quite large, opaque-looking, and stable—as well as being brick-red, due to the Annatto.

The complex method of producing *cacao blanco* from *pataxtle* (*Theobroma bicolor*) seeds is recounted in Chapter 2, and the long fermenting process has not yet been pharmacologically analysed. It would likely denude the beans of many polyphenols and water-soluble constituents due to the long decomposition in water with successive changes of liquid, no doubt generating other compounds due to the microorganisms involved. Even though *cacao blanco* mixed with Cacao produces a prodigious foam on *chocolate atole*, if *cacao blanco* seeds are crushed and infused in water, the water doesn't foam at all when poured or whisked, suggesting that whatever foam-making properties they give to the *atole* are not dependent on water-soluble saponifying (soap-making) compounds. The foam-promoting properties of *cacao blanco* may be down to the physical composition of the fermented seed and emulsifiers it contains, as with Cacao and its modest quotient of phospholipids and its high fat content: Cacao seeds, too, do not produce a foam when simply infused in water—they must be ground into it, and physically present in high concentration in suspension-emulsion. This makes sense, as of course *cacao blanco* is made from a close relative of *Theobroma cacao*.

The ladies who make *chocolate atole* grind the white *cacao blanco* seeds on a cold *metate*, as, they claim, if the fats in the seed melt and exude before it is mixed with Cacao and wheat and the other ingredients, "… the Cacao will not produce the required foam."[849] Given that the ground *cacao blanco* is then mixed with the other ingredients on a warm *metate* set over hot coals and reground, this initial cold-grinding suggests that perhaps fermented *Theobroma bicolor* seeds contain some heat-reactive compound which must be carefully liberated from within the seeds first before mixing with the other ingredients. Could it be that the fermentation of *T. bicolor* seeds produces enzymes as products of microbial action? Enzymes are compounds which catalyse chemical reactions, and are heat-sensitive, being inactive at low temperatures and deactivated by very high temperatures. This may explain the need to initially cold-grind the *cacao blanco* seeds on their own, to liberate the enzymes from within the seeds without activating them, then—after mixing them with the other ingredients—grind them again on a *metate* over a low heat, to catalyse whatever reactions must take place, which presumably help bubble formation in the beverage. Or perhaps the explanation is more prosaic, as the ladies suggest: that the seed is "greasy" and the oil in it mustn't melt before mixing with the other ingredients, rather as the order in which ingredients are added to a cake mix or sauce may be crucial to avoid clumping. In any case, the specially processed *cacao blanco* is highly effective in combination with Cacao's own modest frothing potential, and the skill of the cook.

The addition of fresh frangipani flowers (*Plumeria rubra*) to the extremely foamy *atole* known as *bu'pu* may be necessary because, perhaps, some constituents in the flowers break down during the drying process—whether this is loss of aromatic flavour constituents such as volatile oils by oxidation or evaporation, or loss of foaming agents is unknown. The precise nature of any foaming agents which may occur in frangipani flowers in uncertain, but based on their chemistry, they are likely to be *triterpenoid glycosides*, which are *saponins*—triterpenoids are compounds which have a steroid-like structure (and therefore often exert pharmaceutical effects), and glycosides possess a sugar moiety (moiety = part, or attached molecule); saponins means they have some soap-like, foam-forming properties. The triterpenoid part would be fat-soluble, and the sugar part would be water-soluble, fulfilling the basic functional requirements of an emulsifying agent. The triterpenoids have only been officially identified in the bark,[850] but it's likely that the flowers also contain them. Similarly, the use of sarsaparilla (*Smilax spp.*) or *cocolmeca*/*azquiote* as a foaming agent in some variants of the *atole* known as *popo* is unsurprising from a pharmacological standpoint, as the plant also contains high levels of steroidal saponins, the hormone-like, soapy emulsifying compounds.

Sarsaparilla roots are used medicinally to treat urinary tract problems, "burning feet" (perhaps plantar fasciitis, an inflammation of the soles of the feet, or possibly gout), and to enhance weight loss, as well as being used in treatments for inflammatory disorders, as a "blood cleanser" for skin and joint conditions, in liver disease, and as a general "tonic".[851] Sarsaparilla's most famous historical use is as an anti-syphilitic remedy. Startlingly, there has been almost no pharmaceutical investigation of this—despite the fact that research into *Smilax* species has demonstrated neuroprotective, anti-inflammatory properties, inhibition of several cancer cell lines *in vitro*,[852] benefits for arthritis, high blood sugar, liver function, and breast cancer in rats and mice,[853] and positive results in poorly controlled human trials for kidney damage, leprosy, and psoriasis.[854] Certainly the whole genus, and particularly its most commonly used medicinal species, deserves further investigation.

Susana Trilling's source from Tuxtepec in Oaxaca recounts the use of *cocolmeca* in *popo*—only in this case, the name refers to "the other *cocolmeca*", *Aristolochia laxiflora*. Trilling explicitly cautions that *A. laxiflora* must be toasted or it will "scratch your throat", and—reminiscent of the instructions for preparing *cacao blanco*—that "no greasy hands can touch it or it will ruin the foamy froth".[855] Diana Kennedy's *popo*-making connection from Usila in Oaxaca similarly recommends toasting the *cocolmeca*—in this case, *Smilax sp.*, or sarsaparilla.[856] Presumably toasting either wilts physical hairs on the stem which could cause throat irritation—although the uncooked *Smilax* stem, at least, is perfectly smooth—or maybe the heating causes some chemical transformation that neutralises an inflammatory compound in the fresh plant. But it seems strange that this specific cooking process should be necessary for two such accidentally similar but taxonomically unrelated plants (*Smilax* is in the Lily family, whereas *Aristolochia* is in the Pepper family). Perhaps the toasting procedure is necessary for only one of the two species sold as *cocolmeca*, and the processing was applied to the coincidental doppelganger by default; or perhaps there are other, more basic taste- or hygiene-related reasons for toasting the stems, such as generating sugars or destroying microbes.

The strict instruction to avoid contaminating the *cocolmeca* with grease prior to adding it to Cacao is also intriguing, given the high fat content of Cacao. The suggestion that grease or fat coming into contact with the *cocolmeca* during processing, prior to mixing it with Cacao, should suppress its saponifying (suds-making) properties, is only made for the recipe containing *A. laxiflora*, not for the *Smilax spp.* version: perhaps the saponifying properties of *Smilax spp.* are greater, and less "fragile"? Or perhaps Kennedy's source did not explicitly mention this aspect of preparation? Unfortunately, neither account gives quantities of the plant material used, although evidently a large quantity of *A. laxiflora* is required, as the amount of ground and toasted vine mixed with corn *masa* prior to the addition of Cacao makes the mixture look like "black mud" with a "nutty and aromatic" smell.[857]

The third plant to be used in *popo* is the milkweed vine known as *chupipe* (*Gonolobus niger*). According to different recipes, either the fruit peel or the root of this vine are used as saponifiers (soap-making, or foaming agents) in *popo*, but the chemistry of the plant is largely unknown—although some of its foam-making properties appear to reside in its slightly toxic, sweet-tasting milky latex, from which the genus takes its name. The same caution about frothing *popo* with equipment which is scrupulously grease-free is repeated by sources who use this ingredient too,[858] which suggests that the foam-breaking quality of unwanted grease in a recipe has less to do with the specific formula and more to do with a general need for clean, non-greasy surfaces to avoid the emulsifiers in any frothy formula being diverted from their delicate water-fat balancing act in the bubbles by a layer of grease on the side of the mixing bowl. In any case, the saponification (suds-making) property of a sufficient quantity of *cocolmeca*/*azquiote* or *chupipe* is impressive, and combined with the maize or rice starches, emulsified fats and Cacao polyphenols in the *popo* liquid, raises a very stable, sudsy head of foam, though to do this the *popo* mix must be beaten continually with a *molinillo* for some time.

There's also the question of filtration: in all the *popo* recipes, the prepared *masa* of Cacao, toasted *cocolmeca* or raw *chupipe*, boiled corn or soaked rice, *panela* and additional spice must be squeezed into water through a sack, or stirred into water and then strained.[859] The use of a sack to filter the *masa* is interesting, reminiscent of the preparation of the Polynesian beverage kava-kava. As with kava-kava, manually squeezing the *masa* in water would force insoluble fat parti-cles out into the liquid, forming an emulsion; but because of the presence of saponin-containing emulsifiers in *popo*, fats from the seeds would disperse into the infusion in any case. This is important because the presence of fats not only thickens the beverage and makes it more palat-able but also acts as a vehicle for other fat-soluble compounds such as essential oils. Straining the liquid would exclude any larger particles, producing an emulsion-infusion: a much lighter, less grainy liquid, containing starches from the grains, fats, and saponins, but reducing the surface-disrupting presence of bulkier insoluble solids—leaving only the Pickering effect of the most finely ground particles, more conducive to producing a voluminous but durable foam.[860]

There are other unexplored and possible foaming agents used in traditional Cacao-based beverages. An infusion of *Ceiba pentandra* seeds doesn't foam at all, so here, again, we have an ingredient which apparently lacks saponins. (Ceiba seeds, you may recall from Chapter 2, were also known to the Mexica as *pochotl* and used, according to Hernández, in a recipe with toasted Cacao to make a foaming drink, the original *chocolatl*.)[861] Ceiba's foam-making properties—if they exist—may depend on grinding the seeds to make an emulsion (as the seeds have a high fat content)[862] or concentrated starch solution, or utilise any proteins it contains in combina-tion with Cacao's polyphenols, necessitating larger quantities of the pulverised seed and more determined and persistent agitation to raise a head of foam. Likewise, the seeds of the tree known in the environs of Tikal, Guatemala as *palo de tzol* (*Blomia prisca*) (see Chapter 2) may contain a large amount of saponins, as its plant family (the soap-berry family) would suggest, so only a very small quantity may be required for creating a foam—the objection against their use is their extremely bitter taste, but perhaps if only very tiny quantities are necessary this may be tenable. Another plant cited by Diana Kennedy as the principal foaming agent in the *atole* known as *chaw popox*, made in the Isthmus region on the Western coast of Oaxaca, is the bark of the plant known as *n'ched*, which I identified as *Gonolobus barbatus*, a close relative of *chupipe* (*G. niger*) used on the opposite coast. Again, one can only speculate as to the exact chemical composition of its latex, but the presence of saponins is highly likely.

The results suggest that funeral tree flowers had very mild froth-promoting properties, but only the cold-water extract of annatto seeds have significant foam-enhancing activity, so *pasta de achiote* is likely to help Cacao drinks froth. The lack of notable activity in the other tested spices doesn't necessarily mean they don't help, though; as with the Frangipani flowers, it's possible that any foam-enhancing constituents are present only in the fresh plant material, or are fat-soluble. Fat-soluble constituents in fresh plant material will be expressed with the juice when the plant is crushed, and naturally get blended and emulsified with Cacao when ground with it, but once the plant is dried they don't readily mix with cold water. Likewise, some constituents may only have foam-forming properties when combined with Cacao, as is the case with *cacao blanco*, the anaerobically fermented and dried seeds of *Theobroma bicolor*.

All of these plants have their own medicinal properties and uses in local herbal medicine (see Appendix B for monographs), and their pharmaceutical attributes are largely un-investigated. Unfortunately I was unable to test three of the major foaming agents—the two *Gonolobus* species (*chupipe* and *n'ched*), and *Smilax aristolochiifolia* shoots (*cocolmeca* or *azquiote*)—as these need to be used fresh; only dried plants were available, as the samples had to be brought back to my home in the UK from Mexico and Gautemala. A small table of the "frothing capability" of various Cacao spices in water infusion is shown in Table 5 below. This is crude kitchen science, using 100ml room temperature water, to which 1g of finely ground dried plant matter was added.

Table 5. Foam-producing properties of various Cacao admixture plants in cold water infusion

Plant [Common names, Botanical name]	Part Used	Foam, Y/N?	Foam Height in mL	Persistence in Seconds
Annatto, Achiote, Lipstick Plant (*Bixa orellana*)	Dried seeds	Y	9ml	< 450
Kapok, Ceiba (*Ceiba pentandra*)	Dried seeds	(Y)	3ml	< 2
Devil's Hand Flower, Flor de Manita, Macpalxochitl (*Chiranthodendron pentadactylon*)	Dried flowers	Y	5ml	≤ 10
Ear Flower, Flor de Oreja, Hueinacaztli, Xochinacaztli, Muc' (*Cymbopetalum penduliflorum*)	Dried flowers	Y	3ml	< 7
Mexican Magnolia, Eloxochitl (*Magnolia dealbata*)	Dried flowers	(Y)	2ml	< 2
Frangipani, Yoloxochitl, Baak' Nik'te, Guie Chachi (*Plumeria rubra*)	Dried flowers	(Y)	2ml	< 2
Marmalade Plum, *mamey sapote* (*Pouteria sapota*)	Seed	(Y)	3ml	< 3
Marmalade Plum, *mamey sapote* (*Pouteria sapota*)	Seed, toasted	(Y)	3ml	< 2
Funeral Tree flower, Rosita de Cacao, Cacahuaxochitl (*Quararibea funebris*)	Dried flowers	Y	5ml	≤ 20
Funeral Tree flower, Rosita de Cacao, Cacahuaxochitl (*Quararibea funebris*)	Dried flowers, toasted	Y	4ml	≤ 18
Jaguar Tree, Pataxte, Pataxtle, "Cacao blanco" (*Theobroma bicolor*)	Fermented dried seed powder	N	–	–
Sarsaparilla, Cocolmeca (*Smilax aristolochiifolia*) (?)	Fresh young shoots		UNTESTED	
Chupipe (*Gonolobus niger*)	Fresh fruit skin, fresh root pulp		UNTESTED	
N'ched (*Gonolobus barbatus*)	Fresh outer stem bark		UNTESTED	

The mixture was left to steep for two minutes, stirred gently (so as not to raise a froth), then left to steep for twenty minutes, stirring gently every five minutes to help the plant matter infuse, before being carefully filtered through clean muslin. The liquid was decanted into a jug, then poured from a height (non-standardised—approximately 50cm) into a clean 250ml measuring cylinder. Any resulting foam was measured from the top of the meniscus (upper border of the water level), and the time it took for the foam to disappear completely was measured. Allspice, chillies, and vanilla weren't tested, as my familiarity with these spices led me to conclude they weren't foaming agents.

Psychedelic chocolate

Cacao was drunk at feasts and ceremonial occasions in Mesoamerica much as we may drink champagne today—to lighten mood, to celebrate, and as a social lubricant. But it was also consumed in ritual contexts, and as the obligatory accompaniment of any occasion whereby inner constraints needed to be loosened. This is a bit like the different ways that wine is used: one might consume alcohol socially as "Dutch courage", or to "loosen up", but it takes on a different significance in the Christian eucharist, where it becomes a sacrament. As we saw in the first part of the book, *Psilocybe* mushrooms were consumed with *cacahuatl* at Mexica feasts, and there is evidence that psychedelic mushrooms and morning glory (*Turbina corymbosa* and *Ipomoea violacea*) seeds were important entheogenic plants throughout Mesoamerica. Certainly there was a link between Cacao and "magic mushroom" use in Mesoamerica, but the question is—why? Both plants are psychoactive, both had sacramental value, and both were ingested on important occasions; is there any pharmacological significance to this association, or is it just a coincidence?

Psilocybe mushrooms and the seeds of *I. violacea* and *T. corymbosa* are classified as hallucinogens, capable of inducing visionary states, but in addition to the phylogenetic differences between the fungi and the plants, the magic mushrooms and the sacred seeds were used in different ways (described in Chapters 2 and 3), and their effects are qualitatively distinguishable, too. The psychoactivity of *I. violacea* and *T. corymbosa* is principally dependent on the indole alkaloid called *lysergic acid amide* or LSA, which is structurally similar to the synthetic alkaloid *lysergic acid dimethylamide*, commonly known as LSD. LSA has the same effects as LSD, but it's much less potent and has a shorter duration of action than its synthetic cousin. The seeds of both Morning Glory varieties also contain a cocktail of other alkaloids and substances, which together produce some nausea and sedation in addition to the psychedelic effects. *Psilocybe* species, on the other hand, owe their psychoactivity to the alkaloids *psilocybin* (4-phosphoryl-dimethylamide) and *psilocin* (4-hydroxy-dimethylamide), although they also contain other alkaloids such as *baeocystin* and *norbaeocystin*, which have barely been pharmacologically investigated.[863]

The "dimethylamide" bit of the mushroom alkaloids' chemical names can be abbreviated to DMT, which is one of the main active constituents in the now-famous Amazonian psychedelic brews known as *ayahuasca*. DMT is a chemical naturally produced from serotonin in the central nervous system, and presumably its existence is the reason that compounds such as psilocybin have activity in the human brain—they are similar enough to bind to some of the same receptors. DMT, the *Psilocybe* alkaloids, and LSA all belong to a class of compounds known as phenethylamines, named after PEA because of their common structural elements. When chemically isolated and smoked, DMT characteristically propels the user into another dimension populated with entities apparently separate to oneself. Under normal circumstances, DMT is rapidly broken down upon oral ingestion, but in the presence of monoamine oxidase inhibitors, DMT is conserved and makes its way into the brain. Orally ingesting DMT-containing plants with MAOI-containing plants doesn't produce quite the same dramatic effect as smoking isolated DMT, but is still reputed to be one of the most intense psychedelic experiences. Although there are many different *ayahuasca* recipes, their common denominator is that they're made with plants containing DMT, such as *Virola* species, mixed with other plants, such as the vine *Banisteriopsis caapi*, which contain powerful β-carboline alkaloids that function as MAOIs, which make DMT orally active.

As we noted in the last chapter, there are MAOI compounds in Cacao, too, albeit lower in potency (the polyphenols, caffeine) or quantity (salsolinol and the THβCs), and, just as these compounds likely potentiate the PEA in Cacao and in the human brain, they may also interact with phenethylamines in other plants. In Amazonia, close botanical relatives of *Theobroma cacao*, specifically *Theobroma subincanum* and *Herrania* species, are used in *ayahuasca* brews and to make snuffs with DMT-containing *Virola* species.[864] Researchers have also noted that another Central American plant with hallucinogenic properties, *Salvia divinorum*, may operate by activating kappa-opioid and cannabinoid receptors in the brain,[865] which suggests that Cacao—with its trace levels of cannabinoids and cannabinoid modulating compounds—may enhance its effects. *S. divinorum* is a relatively subtle psychedelic when the leaves are used in the traditional manner. While it's interesting to speculate that Cacao may have been used with *I. violacea*, *T. corymbosa*, or *S. divinorum*, we know for certain that it was used alongside *Psilocybe* mushroom species.

Psilocybin and psilocin have very low physical toxicity, but exert profound effects on the mind. An oral dosage of 12–20mg psilocybin will reliably produce an altered state of consciousness in an adult human. Around 50% of the alkaloid psilocybin makes it into the bloodstream twenty to forty minutes after ingestion, the drug peaks in the blood at fifty minutes, then is slowly metabolised, and is completely cleared from the system after about six hours. The effects of the drug, though, are experienced for three to six hours in total, and the commonest physical symptoms of inebriation are dilation of the pupils (*mydriasis*), increased reflexes, and elevated heart rate. Almost one in two people who take mushrooms or psilocybin also experience nausea. The nausea is a result of serotonin receptors in the gut being activated by the drug; the other common effects are due to adrenaline-type (*sympathomimetic*) effects, which are mainly confined to the brain and central nervous system, not so much the whole body: so even though the pupils are dilated and the mind is racing, the blood pressure can go up or down, and a few people (approximately 13%) even have a slower heart rate than normal when under the influence of mushrooms.[866]

The main "thinking" region of the brain, the cortex, is absolutely lit up by psilocybin. Brain metabolism on psilocybin is up to 25% higher in the cortex, particularly the right side of the brain, which is more linked to creativity, inspiration-intuition, and non-linear thought processes. The only part of the brain to have its metabolism reduced in a bemushroomed state is the thalamus, one of the brain's main relay stations, whose job it is to edit and filter information going to and from the cortex. The serotonin receptors activated by the drug in the brain are of the 5-HT2A type, which trigger secondary dopamine release in an area of the brain called the *dorsal raphe nucleus*, a huge cluster of serotonin-releasing neurons at the top of the brainstem. The dopamine signals from the dorsal raphe nucleus in turn trigger noradrenaline release in another region called the *locus coeruleus*, a part of the brainstem governing stress responses, and part of the larger *reticular activating system*, which helps to filter and integrate sensory inputs.[867] Because psilocybin turns down thalamus activity and activates pathways from the reticular activating system in the brainstem, it hugely enhances sensory inputs to the cortex, effectively turning off filtering systems and amplifying input channels. Psilocybin opens the gates—or, as Aldous Huxley famously put it (referring to its chemical cousin, mescaline), it opens the doors of perception.

The psychedelic properties of mushrooms, morning glory seeds, or LSD are subjectively very similar, but best experienced rather than described, as they are hard to put into words. Psilocybin's effects have been characterised as stimulated senses, enhanced capacity for intro-spection, and more correlative thinking reminiscent of dreams, with perceptual changes, altered time sense, and synaesthesias: experiencing one sense as another, for example, hearing smells, or seeing sounds.[868]

This description is rather dry, though; the mushroom effect is characterised by amplification of external perceptions and sensations so that colours are bright and numinous, surfaces ripple and shift, and the world becomes a skein of breathing fractals. The most profound change is inward, as the walls that normally block awareness of one thought process from another seem to dissolve or are surmounted, so that one becomes aware of "self" as a narrative of separate thoughts, impressions, and shifting domains. The inner defragmentation that psilocybin, LSA, or LSD accomplish means that one sees the "familiar" room, face, person, event, object, or situa-tion as a living tapestry of fresh information and impressions. The subjective effect on mundane thought processes is similar to—but stronger and more sustained than—the jarring, momentary perception of a place-as-itself that one may get when returning home after a long time away and suddenly seeing one's house or street as a stranger might; or, conversely, when visiting an old school, and finding the buildings both smaller and different than one remembered: things are seen with fresh eyes, but with simultaneous awareness of old meanings and memories. A very high dose is utterly (and, potentially, terrifyingly) ego-dissolving, as "context"—which, after all, is a product of mental editing and circumscription—is subsumed into the experience of all-that-is-happening-now; and, as with DMT, at a certain dosage level the inner floodgates to the domain of the subconscious (or, perhaps more accurately, supra-conscious) are so open that "entities" or other-worldly intelligences may be—apparently—encountered.

Psilocybin is somewhat effective for treatment of PTSD, and may be very effective in treatment-resistant depression. Two separate doses of psilocybin given in a "controlled set-ting" with psychological support in an open clinical trial produced significant improvements which were still evident six months later; the drug created a sense of "connectedness" which alleviated the so-called "mood disorder".[869] In addition to its modest MAOI properties, if the TAAR-activating hypothesis of Cacao outlined in the last chapter is accurate, then there are at least two mechanisms by which Cacao may amplify the *Psilocybe* alkaloids' psychoactive effects, providing a pharmacological rationale for the consumption of Cacao-based beverages prior to ingesting *Psilocybe* mushrooms. Even if we attribute only modest MAOI potency to

Cacao, the increase in cerebral circulation effected by Cacao polyphenols, as observed in CAT scans of human trial subjects,[870] would surely deliver more of any co-administered drug to the cortex. So if, as the historical record and some contemporary research suggests, Cacao proves to be a hedonic modifier with antiphobic properties, it is also a logical companion to boundary-dissolving, connection-enhancing psychedelics.

Other potentially psychoactive additives to Cacao include the funeral tree (*Quararibea funebris*) or *cacahuaxochitl*, a contender for the identity of one of the flowers on the statue of Xochipilli. As noted in Chapter 3, funeral tree flowers feature in two Mexica prescriptions for mental health issues ("fear" and "insanity"), which suggests some degree of psychoactivity. The funeral tree does contain several alkaloids which are still barely investigated, as well as a complex essential oil, and several sterols. *Q. funebris* essential oil contains aminolactones which are structurally very closely related to gamma-butyrolactone,[871] otherwise known as GHB, a substance which is used recreationally as a disinhibiting sedative, and medicinally for its anticonvulsant activity. Ethnobotanist Jonathan Ott reports that the seeds of another *Quararibea* species known locally as *espingo* are used as an inebriant in Peru, and possibly as an optional additive to the psychedelic brew ayahuasca.[872] Perhaps, in ayahuasca-like fashion, these innocuous-seeming flowers act as a catalyst for more potent psychoactive effects when combined with certain other plants. But *ayahuasca* is often a kind of soup of drugs anyway, so a great many plants get added to the brews, and not all of them are central to its effects.

But the *Quararibea* and Cacao-containing beverage *tejate* isn't noticeably psychoactive, so it could be that *Q. funebris* was valued only for its sublime scent. If Sahagún's identification of *Q. funebris* as *poyomatli* is correct (see Chapter 2), then *cacahuaxochitl* flowers were smoked at banquets, according to Sahagún, mixed with other "aromatic flowers, a type of bitumen called *chapopotli*, mushrooms … and others", together with tobacco, all dried and finely chopped and inserted into hollow reeds.[873] But *poyomatli*'s identity is yet to be confirmed, and it's possible that its inclusion in these "festival cigars" was nothing more than a way of aromatising the tobacco to improve its taste—although the inclusion of dried mushrooms suggests that these "smoking tubes" weren't just an early form of cigarette.

It's also worth being reminded that the ear flower (*Cymopetalum penduliflorum*), which Hernández alleged to "inebriate like the mushrooms" when added to Cacao-based drinks, was also known by the *nahuatl* name *teonacaztli* or "divine ear".[874] I have not personally noted any marked psychedelic effects from the use of small qaunitites of *C. penduliflorum* in Cacao-based beverages, and there is insufficient information about the pharmacology of the whole plant to speculate about its effects on consciousness in combination with Cacao in anything but the most general ways. But it's curious that the name *teonacaztli* is, superficially, not very dissimilar from *teonanacatl* or "god-flesh", the *nahuatl* name for the divine mushroom itself; Mexica poetic symbolism being what it was, the name "divine ear" may have been applied not only because of its "divine" smell and flavour when mixed with Cacao, but also because the plant helped one obtain the ear of—or to hear—the gods when Cacao was consumed with *Psilocybe* mushrooms.

The other plant which may have been used with Cacao in the fearsome Mexica brew called *itzpacalatl*—the one made with actual human blood, which caused human sacrifices to happily lose their head, in more ways than one is *toloaxihuitl*, *Datura innoxia*. As described in Chapter 2, the characteristic effects of *Datura* intoxication—which may accurately be referred to as intoxication, because the plant is very poisonous, and overdosage can be fatal—are due to the presence of the tropane alkaloids hyoscyamine, hyoscine, and atropine.[875] These compounds block the release of the molecule called acetylcholine in the body and the brain.[876] Acetylcholine is the main messenger chemical of the body's autonomic nervous system, the nerve pathways which control numerous automatic and non-conscious responses such as digestive secretions, sphincter tone, pupil size, airway dilation, heart rate, blood flow, and many others. The autonomic nervous system is categorised in two parts, the sympathetic—which is active and reactive, or "fight or flight" at an extreme; and the parasympathetic, which is quiescent, controlling "rest and digest" functions. Acetylcholine is the messenger for the whole parasympathetic branch, but only part of the sympathetic; the main effective chemical for the sympathetic branch is adrenaline. Broadly speaking, by inhibiting acetylcholine, the alkaloids in *Datura* effectively halt the parasympathetic responses, inhibiting digestion and urination, and they also hamstring the sympathetic division—no control signals come through, but a residual trickle of adrenaline continues, elevating heart rate, dilating the pupils of the eyes, and opening the airways.

On a mental level, the effects are even greater—acetylcholine is fundamental to normal cognition and memory formation, so disrupting it causes the amnestic and deliriant-hallucinogenic effects characteristic of the plant. One of the principal features of *Datura* ingestion is fear—a sense of oppression or dread may be experienced even before the effects of the drug fully take hold, and *Datura*-induced visions are often nightmarish in character; amongst other things, the plant was traditionally used to see ghosts or communicate with spirits.[877] These effects suggest that the plant's alkaloids affect the amygdala, the brain's fear response centre; and, as we saw in the last chapter, it seems that Cacao can affect the amygdala and may reduce conditioned fear responses, and it certainly lowers cortisol and adrenaline levels. So if *Datura* was used in *itzpacalatl* to render a person suggestible, delirious, and forgetful, then basing the drink on Cacao may have had more than ceremonial significance. I propose that, in addition to its sacramental significance (described further in Chapter 9), Cacao may have been highly suitable as a vehicle for administering *toloaxihuitl*: a stimulant with fear-reducing properties, with the useful property of disguising its nauseous taste.

Cacao's host of Mesoamerican botanical collaborators were used to enhance and augment its flavour, its medicinal benefits, its physical and psychoactive properties. As with most real-world things, outside the confines of the laboratory, the categories are intertwined: the flavours of many of these plants depend on their volatile constituents, which may be partly responsible for their medicinal effects (as with the essential oil of allspice), or their psychoactive ones (as with vanillin in vanilla). The froth of Cacao-based drinks, produced by foaming agents such as *Smilax spp.*, may also enhance the psychoactive effects of aromatic constituents when bubbles burst in the mouth, releasing the volatile elements and facilitating their delivery to the brain, and the saponins may also enhance gastric absorption of other pharmacologically active constituents.

The story of Cacao, as with any medicinal plant, is a tale of remarkable transformations, as *Homo sapiens'* ongoing dialogue with the tree inspired innovations in its use. Other plants such as *Cymbopetalum penduliflorum*, *Vanilla planifolia*, and *Piper auritum* were drawn into the conversation, and formed a botanical constellation around it. By association with the star, the supporting cast members underwent major makeovers and significantly appreciated in value.

The elaborate fermentation processes used to transform vanilla pods and *Theobroma bicolor* seeds into ingredients for use in Cacao-based beverages are specific examples from the asterism of arcane gastronomic pharmacy that surrounds Cacao. But many of these traditional combinations, and the elaborate beverage formulations they engendered, have been forfeit in deference to added milk, sugar, and fat in the factory-farming-favourable production of chocolate. Although Cacao itself was historically perceived as a beneficial indulgence, these New World additives are largely responsible for its reclassification (in the form of chocolate) as a "junk food". So, in the next chapter, we ask whether, and in what circumstances, Cacao itself may be harmful. Is Cacao or its modern by-product, chocolate, truly addictive; and what effects, if any, do the confectioner's additives have on the health of chocolate consumers?

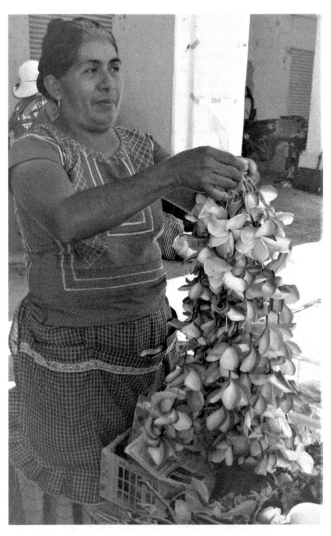

Woman selling Frangipani flower garlands, Juchitan, Guatemala, 2018

CHAPTER SEVEN

Chocolate, love, and bondage (Part II)

"Strength is the capacity to break a chocolate bar into four pieces with your bare hands—and then eat just one of the pieces."

(Judith Viorst, author, poet, and researcher)

"I don't think I have an obsession, however I do eat chocolate every day."

(Eric Ripert, chef)

It may be a far cry from opium, but chocolate's seductive appeal can't be ignored. Once a body has tasted real chocolate, the brain may select the flavour again for similar stimulating reasons that tea, coffee, or tobacco become preferred substances despite the first impression they make—and chocolate has the advantage of being delicious. Other foods with a similar flavour obtain some of Cacao's glamour and appeal; even carob, a cattle feed, has achieved international human food status mainly on the basis of its vague resemblance to chocolate, like a tribute act of dubious talents gaining employment owing to the popularity of the star they imitate. But is this appeal due to bitter brown Cacao, or the added sugar, fat, or milk that chocolate contains? What special magic makes chocolate so desirable—is it pharmacology or taste? And Cacao itself was a restricted drug for the Mexica, comparable to highly psychotropic *Psilocybe* mushrooms, not to be drunk "unthinkingly"[878]—were the Aztecs aware of some effects of the drug we are not attuned to, or of some potential for harm?

In fact many of the supposedly non-pharmacological attributes of chocolate which cause it to become a desirable and preferred flavour such as its fat content, its sweetness, and its complex flavour depend on the molecular structures of the chemicals themselves, because flavour is chemistry. As proposed in Chapter 5, traditionally processed Cacao beans and their by-products may be a kind of *hedonic modifier*: cocoa liquor appears to be a substance that increases its own desirability and the amount of pleasure one may feel by tickling the brain's reward circuitry and amplifying pleasure responses at a subtle background level. Cacao has always been associated with luxury, reward, and respite; and, given the great value that every culture exposed to Cacao has bestowed upon the bean, it seems likely that some pharmacological properties inherent to Cacao make it a suitable embodiment of these attributes. Yet no shadow of addiction, social harm, or health concerns besmirches the reputation of Cacao, despite its status as a sacred drug and restricted substance in pre-Colombian Mesoamerica. Could this psychoactive drug be so gentle and benign that no harm may arise from its use—or are the "nutritional" additives of sugar, milk, and extra fat altering the landscape?

Chocoholics: are they for real?

> It is now clear that cocoa and chocolate do not contain addictive substances in amounts high enough to cause cravings. Indeed, cravings are the result of an unhealthy relationship with the food ... the alleged craved-for chemicals are merely myths. (Paoletti et al., 2012)[879]

This quote by the editors of a scientific book about chocolate reflects the current consensus on chocolate cravings. Its wording also suggests that researchers are still looking for individual chemicals ("addictive substances") which may activate chocolate cravings; yet as we have seen, if chocolate does have any addictive potential, it's more likely that *combinations* of various chemicals in Cacao—the *whole drug*, not its separated parts—interact in complex ways with the chemistry of body and mind to modify pleasure and desire responses. Despite these scientists' views, throughout its history chocolate has been seen as a desirable and habit-forming food-drug; and as discussed in the previous chapter, the precise effects of chocolate on mood and cognition are far from settled, and are likely to be more complex and nuanced than the scant research into Cacao's psychoactivity has allowed for.

Reports of chocolate craving date back to the colonial era, when the Jesuit missionary José de Acosta noted that expatriate "Spanish men—and even more the Spanish women—are addicted to the black chocolate."[880] And in modern times chocolate is one of the most craved foods, accounting for "more than half" of all food cravings.[881] In addition to the cocktail of substances present in the bean, Cacao's nutritional qualities may play a role, too. For example, Cacao's magnesium content could subconsciously enhance its appeal to people whose diets are otherwise nutrient-poor, similar to the cravings of pregnant women for particular foods when the growing baby requires more of certain minerals or nutrients. Magnesium has notable stress-modulating effects, such that when oral magnesium was given to a group of triathletes in a placebo-controlled trial, the magnesium group had lower levels of pre- and post-exercise stress hormone, improved blood glucose control, and even enhanced performance (measured by greater reductions in running, swimming, and cycling times).[882] For self-identified "chocoholics" whose diet is otherwise low in vegetables, whole grains, and nuts (generally, good magnesium sources), chocolate could be their primary source of this essential mineral.

So is chocolate addiction ("chocoholism") really a thing? As one author put it, "Chocolate is probably the most common object of uncontrollable food cravings and food 'addictions' among women."[883] Research indicates that so-called "chocolate" craving (whether for dark or milk chocolate, or merely chocolate-flavoured foods) is *not* simply sugar or fat craving, because only the unique flavour of chocolate can satisfy it.[884] There are many more aspects to this question which will be addressed in this chapter, but let's proceed according to the established reality that whether or not chocolate addiction is accepted by mainstream science, chocolate cravings and psychological dependence on chocolate are real things. So the question then becomes: are these cravings the result of physical (pharmacological) or psychosocial (mental) causes? For now, let's set aside the issue of whether or not emotional, social, and chemical causes can really be fully separated, and take a closer look at the neurobiology of addiction.

Insatiable appetites and habitual needs

"Wanting" is a function of dopamine, the desire neurotransmitter, which—as we saw in Chapter 5—generates excitement and motivation, and is one of the main chemical messengers in the limbic system (the brain's "emotional response" area). Dopamine-releasing neurons are concentrated in the *ventral tegmental area* (VTA) and *nucleus accumbens*, the parts of the limbic system which generate desire (see Figure 8 in Chapter 5). The outer layer of the nucleus accumbens, referred to as its "shell", creates motivations and cravings which are necessary for survival, such as drives to seek food, water, sex, or new experiences in general. Habit formation is complex, so although the VTA/nucleus accumbens pathways are pre-eminent, several other regions of the brain are also involved in creating desire to repeat behaviours. These areas (the olfactory bulb, the frontal cortex in the rostral part of the brain, and the *nucleus tractus solitarii* in the caudal brain) are collectively referred to in science-speak as "operant reinforcers", meaning that they strengthen the desires and help to translate them into action.

The pathways linking these parts of the brain have been described as "incentive-forming brain circuits", and novel stimuli (such as an attractive person, or the smell of good food when hungry) light up the VTA/nucleus accumbens pathway, as do powerful stimulant drugs such as cocaine or amphetamine. Repeatedly activating this pathway causes a protein called *delta-Fos-B* (ΔFB) to be made in the whole *striatum* (an area of the brain of which the nucleus accumbens is part). ΔFB is the brain's habit-recording protein, a signal to turn behaviours into habits. Here, deep in the limbic system, ΔFB reinforces the desire to repeat an experience by creating long-term adaptive changes in brain cells.

It's possible to have habitual behaviours run entirely by "wanting" or anticipatory excitement (dopamine). We know that "liking" is transmitted by opioids (endorphins) in the brain, because these brain chemicals create feelings of pleasure and comfort. The VTA/nucleus accumbens pathway can be firing with dopamine without a high opiate level in the brain, generating a store of ΔFB which results in a powerful habit sustained by joyless craving, like a slot machine zombie in Las Vegas mindlessly feeding coins into a machine and pulling the lever, or a stressed-out chain smoker barely conscious of reaching for another cigarette. But "liking" is important for generating addictions, and the *initial* experience of consummating any sort of desire—eating the biscuit, shooting the heroin, having the orgasm—usually provides some sort of immediate feelings-based (endorphin) reward. So it's no surprise that when opiates are injected into the VTA of experimental animals, the drug increases the sensitivity of neurons to dopamine. In the language of neurology, the opiates "disinhibit" the dopamine-releasing brain cells, so that anticipatory excitement and cravings become even stronger.[885] In other words, *liking* increases *wanting*: pleasure invokes desire.

Another side to this story is the recent finding that cortisol, the stress hormone, affects the release of dopamine in the brain's reward pathways.[886] Short-term increases in cortisol, which may occur for example in a new social situation, or in training for a race, increase the turnover of dopamine in the reward pathways, helping to create useful motivation and excitement. But long-term increases in cortisol with chronic stress—as is commonly found in people with an emotionally troubled childhood—does the opposite, suppressing dopamine production here, and increasing depressive, demotivated, or *anhedonic* (joyless) states. Not only that, but cortisol makes these parts of the brain more sensitive to drugs of abuse such as cocaine and opiates.[887]

Presumably, cortisol increases sensitivity to pleasure-giving drugs because when the natural production of dopamine in the nucleus accumbens/VTA pathway is stunted by long-term stress, any substance which lights those pathways up becomes much more remarkable. People who have well-functioning pleasure pathways may not notice such a discrepancy between the drug-activated state and their natural state, whereas those who have their pleasure and desire circuits on a pilot light setting due to chronic stress may notice an enormous difference between a drug-activated state and their more depressed daily existence. This is one biological reason why a troubled past is more likely to lead to substance abuse, and corroborates the hypothesis discussed in Chapter 5, that a lack of stable Bonding in one's formative years contributes to addictive behaviours.

This mechanism of stress-related heightened narcotic reward sensitivity is consistent with the findings of former experimental psychologist Dr Bruce Alexander, who conducted the now-famous "Rat Park" study in 1979 with some colleagues.[888] Psychotropic drugs were—and still are—tested on animals confined in tiny cramped cages, and the drugs' addictiveness is measured in terms of how often the animals press a lever to self-administer the substance. Dr Alexander and his colleagues noted that these living conditions themselves are likely to be enormously stressful for rats, which by nature are free-roaming, so they designed a large open terrarium with many hiding spaces and easy access to food, water, and so-called addictive drugs such as morphine. The researchers named this habitat "Rat Park". The results of this set-up were that animals in Rat Park self-administered far fewer psychotropic drugs, and had markedly lower levels of addiction than those kept in ordinary cages. Dr Alexander hypothesised that in human social environments it is feeling "caged" or "trapped"—being isolated, under stress, or with few apparent options to improve or escape one's fate—that enhances addictive tendencies.[889]

Since Rat Park, several human population studies have confirmed that both short- and long-term stress increase the likelihood of "substance abuse", and demonstrated strong statistical links between psychotropic drug use in later life and childhood abandonment, neglect, emotional trauma, and physical or sexual abuse.[890] High cortisol also increases the activity of the excitatory neurotransmitter *glutamate* in the VTA, which allows dopamine levels to rise more quickly, reinforcing arousal in response to pleasurable stimuli, and encouraging habit formation.[891] Essentially, all addictions—whatever their specific forms and contents, determined no doubt by childhood conditioning and individual biochemical sensitivities and proclivities—are rooted in chronic stress.

Old World addictions? Sugar, fat, and milk

The "extras" in eating chocolate—fat, sugar, and sometimes milk—are often referred to as if they were pharmacologically inert, and any cravings for them are "psychological". Yet these substances markedly affect brain chemistry. "Palatability", or deliciousness, is partly an expression of the brain's response to eating nutrient-dense food: it makes us a little bit high. Endogenous opiates (endorphins) are released in the pleasure pathways when sugar or fat-rich foods are eaten,[892] rewarding us for refuelling; and as we have seen, opiates increase dopamine responses in the pleasure pathways and drive up reward-seeking behaviour. We are wired to seek out and consume such foods to ensure species survival; natural sources of sugars and fats usually contain other important nutrients together with the calories. Before the modern age of industrial farming, global transport, and food technology, which allow us to perennially and globally manufacture and distribute high-calorie, low-nutrient foods with a long shelf life, sweet, rich food wasn't so easily available to most people. Now that it is, we're all a little bit junky when it comes to diet.

The biggest elephant in the room when chocolate is discussed is *refined sugar*. The allegedly addicted colonial Spanish ladies were already accustomed to taking their chocolate with large amounts of added sugar, which the Europeans imported from their slave-powered sugar cane plantations. Research shows us that the human brain "lights up for sugar the same way it does for cocaine".[893] Rats given sugary foods overeat and get fat. When the sugar is taken away from animals accustomed to it they experience physical withdrawal symptoms, such as chattering teeth.[894] One study illustrates the compulsive appeal of sugars with lab rats, whose basic brain structure relating to emotional processing and drives (the limbic system) is very similar to our own. Rats given a 25% glucose solution mixed into their food for twelve hours every day were found to "binge" on the sweetened chow, and their consumption of the sugary mash *doubled* over ten days, as if they were chasing an initial "high". After the experiment, the rats' brains were compared to another group of sugar-free rats; lo and behold, the glucose-eaters' brains had increased dopamine receptor binding in the nucleus accumbens, and increased μ-opioid receptor binding in their brains' pleasure pathways (the cingulate cortex, hippocampus, locus coeruleus and nucleus accumbens shell), "much like [what happens with] some drugs of abuse".[895]

So what is refined sugar, and what about it makes it so compelling—addictive, even? Refined sugar usually refers to sugar that has been extracted from plant sources, such as sugar cane or sugar beet, or semi-synthesised from plant material, as in high-fructose corn syrup. Usually refined sugar means *sucrose*, or white table sugar. Sucrose is in fact made from two separate sugars, these being *glucose*—which cells use as fuel—and sweeter-tasting *fructose*, aka fruit sugar, which has to be transformed into glucose in the body before cells can use it. Fructose, which comprises 50% of sucrose and 55% of high-fructose corn syrup, is problematic if consumed too regularly as a food additive. When fructose is eaten, it must be transformed into glucose in the liver, which causes the production of fatty compounds called *triglycerides* that accumulate in the liver and are released into the bloodstream.

A regular excess of triglyceride production in the liver eventually results in non-alcoholic fatty liver disease, as the organ gets clogged up with the extra fats and starts to resemble a chronic alcoholic's liver. Blocking the liver's ability to make triglycerides can slow this down, but results in scarring the liver, or cirrhosis—an even worse outcome—so the body's excess triglyceride production is the safest way to dispose of the fructose.[896] The extra triglycerides in the blood magnify the release of insulin, the hormone which allows the body's cells to absorb glucose, fats, and proteins. High blood triglycerides also increase inflammation, and ultimately—after many years—result in a state of *insulin resistance*, whereby the cells' response to insulin becomes blunted.[897] This eventually leads to type 2 diabetes, when the cells stop responding to insulin completely.

The problem is that our biology is cued to the fact that our cells need glucose for fuel, but most naturally-occurring sweet foods also contain desirable compounds such as Vitamin C and other plant chemicals in whole plant foods such as antioxidant polyphenols which beneficially affect blood sugar, insulin, and other metabolic processes.[898] So there's an evolutionary impera-tive to eat sugars, which is why this drive is hard-wired into our biology. If sugars such as sucrose and fructose are consumed as integral parts of high-fibre plant foods like whole fruit, they appear to produce far less metabolic stress (predisposing to diabetes and liver problems) than when they're refined, and added to low-fibre foods.[899] Plant fibre (really just the cell walls and structural "filler" material in plants) is also a food for "good bacteria" in the gut, which generate and help us to absorb beneficial compounds and nutrients that we otherwise wouldn't get in the diet. Unfortunately, when sugars are stripped out of the food—specifically, when the fibre is removed—they're absorbed too fast, without many of the buffering compounds found in fruit or vegetables, and tax the system. Even fruit juices cause similar problems, despite their vitamin C content. Free sugars—unbound to fibre—also increase adrenaline levels, giving rise to the commonly observed "hyperactivation" of kids after eating high-sugar foods or drinking lots of juice, soda, or sugary cordial.[900]

The link between sugar intake, heart disease, and stroke[901] was mentioned in Chapter 4, but sugar's most well-known associations are with adult-onset (type 2) diabetes and tooth decay. It's well known that stress is a risk factor for physical and mental disease, and all forms of stress—particularly emotional stress—have been shown to increase the desire for fatty and sug-ary foods. It's one of life's ironies that precisely when we most need to look after ourselves by maintaining a healthy regime of good diet, rest, and exercise in order to be able to handle higher levels of stress, good intentions tend to evaporate in favour of cake, coffee, and procras-tination. When stressful situations arise, a hormone signalling cascade begins in the brain with corticotrophin releasing factor (CRF), which stimulates the anterior pituitary gland (which sits behind the front of the skull, just above the nose) to produce and release adrenocorticotrophic hormone (ACTH), which in turn causes the release of the principal stress hormone cortisol from the adrenal glands. Eating sugars stimulates the release of a hormone called cholecystokinin (CCK), which in turn stimulates the release of ACTH, which also enhances cortisol release from the adrenal glands.[902]

One study in rats found that injecting CRF directly into the nucleus accumbens increased the vigour of the rats' attempts to obtain sugar pellet rewards by responding to trained cues, as did amphetamine. This finding was interpreted to mean that stress could trigger bursts of "programmed compulsions" such as binge-eating, drug addiction relapses, or any "addiction" behaviour by intensifying dopamine-mediated drives.[903] Essentially, stress increased compulsive sugar consumption, at least in these tortured rats, and *refined sugar increases the stress response.*

So refined sugar not only raises the risk of disease over the longer term, but also increases the desire for more sugar. This hellish feedback loop contributes to obesity (due to the high circulating blood fats being stored), high blood pressure (due to inflammation damaging blood vessel walls and the body using fats to repair them, eventually narrowing the pipes, plus raised adrenaline levels causing blood vessels to constrict more), and eventually type 2 diabetes, when sugar-abused cells no longer respond to insulin at all.

The rise of added sugar in the diet, from sugary drinks to breakfast cereal to convenience foods, tracks well with the exploding incidence of the Western world's biggest killer diseases such as heart disease and stroke. But there are probable links to many other "diseases of affluence": high fructose intake causes increased levels of uric acid in the blood, giving rise to gout; increased levels of insulin correspond to higher incidences of cancer; and Alzheimer's disease corresponds to insulin resistance in the brain.[904] This is the end result of the excess refined sugar, protein, and saturated fat in the standard American diet, or SAD—comprising soda, burgers, fries, doughnuts, and ice cream—which has been successfully exported worldwide.

Carbohydrate craving is sometimes asserted to be a means of self-medicating depression by increasing the brain's level of serotonin. The theory goes something like this: carbohydrates increase the transport of the amino acid, tryptophan, into the brain, which is then turned into serotonin as required. But carbohydrate and fat cravings in general are associated with opioid systems in the brain, not serotonin pathways—bread and sugar "addicts" alike are seeking an opiate high.[905] Although fats also produce an endorphin "reward" for eating them, unlike sugars, they have no "taste threshold"—the more fat is added to a food, generally the more desirable it seems; yet consumers often can't tell if a food has extra fat in it or not. Sugar and fat, eaten in combination, have a synergistic effect on pleasure centres, and adding sugar to a food decreases the perception of its fat content.[906] Thus the European transformation of Cacao into extra-fatty, sugary eating chocolate made an already compelling substance into a truly habit-forming food.

Chocolate is now routinely prepared in Mexico and Guatemala with hot milk as well as added sugar. Cows were unknown in the Americas prior to the European invasion, but the Spanish brought their favourite foods—and their animal and plant sources—across the ocean with them. Cow's milk has had a fall from grace in the Western diet over the past decade or so, largely because many of its purported benefits have turned out to be over-hyped or attainable from other foods with less environmental impact and fewer potential health risks. While milk is a good source of calcium, over a certain threshold calcium intake provides no additional benefit for bone density, and calcium can be obtained from other foods such as green leafy vegetables. Because cow's milk is naturally low in Vitamin D, the vitamin required for proper absorption of calcium, it's often "fortified" by adding this vitamin, so fortified milk can help with calcium and vitamin D dietary requirements. But the "milk for strong bones" adage appears to be a myth: no benefits for bone density were found for dairy intake in children, and in adult women (72,000 of them, tracked over an eighteen-year period) there was no correlation between milk and dairy consumption and reduction in bone fracture risk. Milk intake also increases the risk of developing prostate cancer in men, and to a lesser extent, breast cancer in women; it may also increase the risk of developing ovarian cancer. Cow's milk consumption also raises the risk of type I diabetes in infants.[907]

But most intriguing, and relevant to its use in chocolate and the question of "chocolate addiction", is that cow's milk contains exorphins.[908] Exorphins (as in eXternal mORPHINe) are chemicals from foods or drugs which activate opiate receptors. The exorphins in cow's milk are "casomorphin peptides"—proteins which bind to opiate receptors, and encourage the baby cows to keep guzzling milk; human breast milk contains similar compounds. Milk casomorphins share this opiate-binding facility with constituents in some other foods, principally wheat gluten;[909] both of these highly craved foods—milk and wheat products, such as cheese and bread—are notoriously hard to give up, and the presence of the exorphins may explain the allure of pizza for dieters, and the recidivism of cheese-abjurers. Exorphins can be found in several plants: leaving aside the obvious one (*Papaver somniferum*, the opium poppy, which is the source of actual morphine), milder exorphins include cafestrol in coffee and epicatechin in Cacao and green tea.[910] So it's to be expected that the "comfort factor" of these foods or drugs would be high. Add to this the opiate-stimulating effect of sugar and fat, and you have a potently habituating cocktail in chocolate.

So fatty and sugary foods may intrinsically predispose us to overeat by stimulating our brains' pleasure centres to release endorphins, particularly via μ-opioid receptors, and other "habituating" neurotransmitters; and high-sugar foods also simulate a stress response in the brain, which may in turn increase compulsive or addictive dietary behaviours. Tragically, a large part of Cacao's homeland in Central America, Mexico, is now one of the fattest and most diabetic nations in the world: fully a quarter of Mexican men, and a third of the women are obese, and one in six Mexican adults is diabetic,[911] a legacy of the country's culinary love affair with refined sugar, cheese, meat, and rich high-protein, high-fat foods.

Meanwhile, research shows that, in common with many psychotropic drugs, when sugary chocolate is eaten to treat emotional problems—as a comfort food—it provides temporary satisfaction but actually *prolongs* any background low mood states.[912] This is very reminiscent of many drugs of abuse, which trade a short-term gain for long-term pain; but, as Rat Park demonstrated, the urge to take the drugs may be related to environmental stress and low mood in the first place. We don't yet know whether the prolongation of low mood applies only to confectionery chocolate, with its extra load of stress-inducing sugars, and the guilt often associated with disordered eating (on which subject, more shortly), or to all forms of Cacao.

Psychosocial chocoholism

A questionnaire given to 325 US university students asked which words people associated with chocolate. More women than men in the survey group self-identified as chocolate lovers, although only 6% of those surveyed claimed not to like chocolate. But while three quarters of respondents said chocolate was "attractive", only slightly fewer thought it was "addictive"; just over half associated the word "happy" with chocolate, but conversely a third of respondents thought chocolate was "harmful". Some of the other most commonly associated adjectives were "fattening", "energising", "good", "heavy", "unhealthy", "pleasant", and "exciting". Most interestingly—obviously, perhaps, but tellingly—91% of respondents agreed with the statement "chocolate is sweet".[913] Toasted Cacao beans and pre-Colombian Mesoamerican chocolate drinks are sour, bitter, and rich, but rarely—or barely—sweet. Chocolate's sometimes compulsive appeal is usually ascribed to its "high hedonic value" as a sweet, fatty, aromatically tantalising food. "Comfort eating" in general is a complex subject, but starchy or sugary foods are perennial choices, for all the reasons laid out earlier in this chapter.

And yet dietary habits and cravings aren't just chemical responses. Culture plays a big part: for example, British women experience more chocolate cravings than Spanish women. Thirty-seven women took part in a study comparing the effects of eating a chocolate bar or an apple on mood and satiation. Both apple and chocolate had the effect of abating hunger and improving mood and motivation, but the chocolate did so more effectively. Eating chocolate, but not apple, also caused joy—but for some of the women, the joy was followed by guilt. Predictably, the women who felt guilty also felt less joy after eating the chocolate.[914] While the latter study provides another reason for preferring traditional Cacao-based drinks to chocolate bars—less added fat and sugar!—both studies show that responses to chocolate are at least partially defined by the concept of it, one's cultural and personal beliefs and prejudices.

Fifty self-identified "chocoholics" who craved chocolate about six times and ate an average of twelve 60g chocolate bars each week credited their compulsion to the unique smell, taste, and texture of chocolate, rather than any pharmacological activity affecting their mood.[915] But humans are often exceptionally unreliable judges of their own addictions—note the centuries of collective denial that tobacco was in any way habituating or harmful, excluding a few voices in the wilderness. The previous survey's findings conflict with the online study described in Chapter 5, in which depressed chocophiles reported that their hankering for chocolate was more influenced by its mood-modifying poperties than its flavour.[916] Another interesting issue is why some women crave chocolate before or during their menstrual period. Although it's tempting to assume that chocolate's psychoactivity is being made use of here to self-medicate peri-menstrual low mood, this may not be the case. One study found that these "cravings" are also heavily culturally influenced, with American women being ten times more likely to spontaneously crave chocolate around their menstrual period than Spanish women. Subsets of American and Spanish men and women in the surveyed populations all reported chchocolate cravings after eating or while studying. The same proportion of men and women experienced such cravings.[917] So whilst it may be true that chocolate's pharmacological properties enhance its perceived value as a comfort food at stressful times or during emotional lows, there are currently no scientifically confirmed links between chocolate craving and menstruation other than food preferences and cultural beliefs.

One psychological theory about where chocolate cravings come from suggests that it's all about association. In childhood we receive chocolate during good times and festivities, the theory goes, so we come to associate the food with those emotions: "linked to memories of childhood, the maternal instinct and affection that comes with it"[918]—in other words, we seek out chocolate as a trigger of positive conditioned reward responses, as described in Chapter 5, wherein programmed unconscious reactions to chocolate may be invoked by its smell, or other triggers. In this scenario, chocolate recalls happy memories as easily as it absorbs odours.

As a complete explanation for chocolate cravings this "association theory" is hard to swallow. As far as we can tell, Cacao and its products have always been seen as desirable, and for a great deal of chocolate's three thousand year association with humankind, its ingestion by children was forbidden. And not all of Cacao's associations were positive, at least not in this sentimental way. A Classic Maya child, observing adults drinking *kakawa* at a funeral, or the Mexica youth seeing *itzpacalatl* administered to tomorrow's sacrificial captive so that he may dance in his cage with a smile on his face, may have found such a theory hard to comprehend, as well as questioning its necessity. A further flaw in this logic can easily be discovered by giving chocolate to a child who has never tasted it before. Many toddlers form an instant attachment to chocolate; when given a choice, preverbal children who appreciate chocolate have no difficulty in expressing a preference for chocolate over other foods after only one "exposure".

An alternative psychological explanation for chocolate cravings is what I call deprivation-attraction theory: by restricting a food (or anything else), it becomes more desirable. This supposes that when chocolate is used as a reward by parents, but access to it is limited, children naturally acquire a strong desire for the forbidden substance. This is in perfect accord with the historical restriction of Cacao consumption to Mexica and Maya nobility, and chocolate's perennial reputation as a luxury. With respect to chocolate, perhaps we can compare contemporary parents and children to pre-Colombian nobles and peasants. Cacao's value to the "little man" is enhanced by the glamour of limitation and celebration; access to the desired substance is permitted only at the discretion of those in authority, the keepers of the Cacao, or on special occasions. As with the former theory, there's more than a grain of truth here, but again the explanation is incomplete—it works on a social level, but not necessarily on the individual level: it doesn't explain why chocolate might be considered desirable enough to be a "treat" in the first place.

These psychological theories no more explain why some people self-identify as chocoholics than they explain the existence of alcoholism, or compulsive gambling, or "sex addiction". They go some way towards explaining why chocolate may be desired by some people, but not why these people claim they can't live for a single day without eating or drinking it.

A chemical addiction

As described in Chapter 5, Cacao contains chemicals that interact both directly and indirectly with opiate-releasing parts of the brain, including a few trace compounds which bind to cannabinoid receptors, and may increase sensitivity to opiates. The brain's own cannabinoid, anandamide (present in Cacao), also lowers desire and reward thresholds. Again, as we've seen, some substances in Cacao incline towards increased dopamine, serotonin, and phenethylamine turnover and sensitivity in the brain, and may raise the brain's level of anandamide too. By this logic alone we can deduce that Cacao and chocolate may generate cravings or even increase the potential for addiction. Cacao may also have unspecified and under-researched effects on the stimulating brain chemical glutamate, which has a poorly defined influence on many mood states; there's still a lot we don't know. But we can add another highly relevant finding—if Cacao (and chocolate) lowers blood cortisol levels, it may *reduce* addictive or habit-forming tendencies. So we have a conundrum: if Cacao might increase cravings through some mechanisms, and reduce them via others, what does it actually do?

Despite the scientific consensus that chocolate doesn't contain high enough levels of individual substances to cause chemical dependency, there are some compounds in Cacao which have been strongly linked to one form of addiction: alcoholism. The trace alkaloids *salsolinol* and the *tetra-hydro-beta-carbolines* (THβCs), produced during fermentation of the beans, are also spontaneously produced in the brains of alcoholics. When alcoholic drinks are consumed, the active ingredient, ethanol, is converted into acetaldehyde in the liver. Acetaldehyde can get through the blood-brain barrier and reach the brain, causing all the effects of drunkenness, where it also combines with dopamine to form salsolinol, and with serotonin or the related substances tryptophan and tryptamine, to make THβCs. The relevance of this finding is that when salsolinol and some THβCs are injected into the brains of monkeys or rats they have "reinforcing properties", meaning that they increase cravings and habit formation. Having salsolinol and THβCs in their system when they drink causes these animals to voluntarily increase their alcohol intake, and this effect lasts for a long time.[919] So while these compounds only account for a tiny percentage of the chemicals found in Cacao, their co-presence should make us sit up and take notice.

There's currently no proof that the level of salsolinol or THβCs in the bloodstream rises after eating chocolate, although of course absence of evidence isn't evidence of absence. And even though food preferences can be increased by the addition of caffeine, whole chocolate eaten in the normal way—with added fat and sugar providing the customary smell, taste, and feel of chocolate—is necessary to sate chocolate cravings, but cocoa powder given in capsules doesn't cause cravings.[920] So cravings may not be due solely to specific pharmacological constituents in Cacao, although as noted in Chapter 5, processed cocoa isn't an adequate substitute for whole Cacao, and as described earlier in this chapter, sugar alone has habituating properties. More likely, cravings are produced by a combination of psychological and pharmacological responses, as mood states affect brain and body chemistry, which is then influenced by the combined pharmacology of all the constituents in chocolate: Cacao, sugar, added fat, and/or milk—the whole package being greater than the sum of its parts.

Unfortunately there have been no studies of craving and satiation comparing unsweetened Cacao-based beverages to edible chocolate, which would allow a comparison between the more pharmacological aspects of *cacahuatl* (the traditional "whole drug") and the contemporary chocolate bar with its added fat, sugar, and—sometimes—milk. Having said that, the effects of white chocolate and dark chocolate on basic human brain chemistry *have* been tested. White chocolate is a perfect example of a food which is primarily composed of sugar, fat, and milk. It's referred to as "chocolate" on the basis that the fat it contains is cocoa butter, but it's not made with the "brown stuff"—the polyphenol, alkaloid, amine- and essential oil-rich cocoa liquor. Twenty-one younger adult males aged between twenty-five and thirty were each given 75g of dark or white chocolate to eat every day for twenty-eight days. The white chocolate contained 57g sucrose and 34g fat per 100g, and the dark chocolate contained 13g sucrose and 63g fat per 100g.[921] The volunteers' levels of dopamine (desire + motivation), serotonin (calmness), noradrenaline (excitement), and adrenaline (anxiety or excitement) were measured before, during, and after the trial.

There are three drawbacks with this experiment. First, it couldn't be "blinded"—in other words, all the participants knew what they were eating, and that could have affected the results, because belief can affect brain and body chemistry. Second, the chemicals were not measured in blood drawn from the brain, because it's much safer (and less unethical) to draw blood from arms than to drill holes in heads, but changes in chemistry of the general circulation may not accurately reflect changes in brain chemistry, because the blood-brain barrier effectively filters out many chemicals so they don't get carried into the brain. Third, there were very few volunteers involved—a small group size means the results are more likely to be skewed.

Nevertheless, the chocolate comparison trial gives us an idea, a "ball park" sense of what may be going on. The high-sugar white chocolate significantly elevated the volunteers' blood dopamine and serotonin levels, and caused noradrenaline to trend upwards, without raising it significantly. (We should note here that "significant" and "non-significant" are statistical terms; "significant" means the result suggests that something is mathematically likely to be linked to something else—it doesn't tell us whether the result is noticeable or not on a case-by-case basis.) As reported in Chapter 5, dark chocolate significantly reduced blood adrenaline levels, and caused a non-significant trend towards increased dopamine, while significantly elevating levels of the serotonin metabolite 5-HIAA.[922] The weaker effect of dark chocolate on dopamine levels is perhaps surprising, given the chemical compounds in Cacao which may affect dopamine turnover or production—but it appears that white chocolate pushed up dopamine levels very effectively, trumping the combined effects of Cacao, sugar, and fat in dark chocolate.

The authors of this paper suggested that the rise in dopamine with white chocolate could be due to fat-soluble compounds present in cocoa butter—possibly the biogenic amines themselves (dopamine, serotonin, etc.).[923] But this is illogical—the dark chocolate used in the experiment actually contained almost *double* the amount of cocoa butter, and the white chocolate had markedly more sugar and milk. The elevated dopamine response in the daily white chocolate consumers could be biological indicators of sugar habituation, perhaps reflecting increased craving or desire for the sugary, fatty food. This trial provides tangential support for the idea that while sugar, fat, and milk may be habituating, Cacao and dark chocolate could be less compulsion-forming, or that the stress-lowering effects of Cacao may actively counteract habituation. As we saw in Chapter 4, Cacao's polyphenols also blunt blood sugar spikes, which may inhibit the dopamine-releasing knock-on effect of high-sugar foods.

Experiments with rats accustomed to ingesting chocolate-flavoured beverages found that the drug Nepicastat suppressed chocolate-seeking behaviour following its withdrawal from their diet, but equally reduced hunger and flavour-driven food consumption.[924] Nepicastat is a dopamine β-hydroxylase inhibitor, a medication normally prescribed to cocaine addicts. The drug prevents dopamine conversion to the excitement-producing chemical noradrenaline in the brain, and reduces cravings for cocaine. Cocaine works partly on the basis of enhancing natural cravings by amplifying dopamine signals, but—most importantly for our purposes—chocolate showed no greater tendency to cause such cravings than other foods, at least in this animal trial. In other words, the mechanisms of comfort eating, at least in these rats, were similar to those which drove compulsive cocaine usage, and chocolate was being responded to by the rats only as a comfort food.[925]

The Nepicastat rats demonstrate that cravings can be biologically wired, dopamine and noradrenaline driven, and easily attached to palatable foods. But—is this the only interpretation of these results? One major problem with this (and many other) studies is the lack of attention paid to the quality of chocolate used—Cacao content relative to sugar and milk content, the origin and type of beans. In short, there wasn't enough focus on the potency and purity of Cacao, although to be fair, the researchers were mainly interested in the mechanisms of food cravings, rather than assessing the differences between different forms of Cacao! So, again, we can't tell if the results would have been different with high-Cacao chocolate. Also, these are stressed-out lab rats—as the Rat Park experiments showed, the environment in which the rats are kept strongly biases the inferences about addiction that may be drawn from such results.

The most interesting thing about the Nepicastat rat study is that it seems dopamine isn't the main brain chemical driving addictive behaviour—it's noradrenaline, a chemical which dopamine can be turned into in the brain. In the chocolate comparison trial, only white chocolate produced a trend towards rising noradrenaline. Dark chocolate *did* show a trend towards increasing dopamine in the bloodstream, even if the trend didn't reach a statistically significant level in the twenty-one-day trial period; but blood levels of noradrenaline rose initially, then fell back to baseline. On the other hand, there are several other significant compounds in the chemistry of addiction that weren't measured after consuming chocolate, notably cannabinoids such as anandamide, and the endorphins—specifically μ-opioid receptor stimulating endorphins like enkephalin.

Fortunately, there is one study which does assess the consumption of chocolate and the amount of enkephalin in the brain; unfortunately, again, it's a rat-based experiment, and enkephalin was injected directly into the rats' brains *before* the rats were given chocolate! After their brains were needled with drugs, the rats were given sugary chocolate to eat, which they did, to gross excess, while showing no signs of pleasure or enjoyment[926]—demonstrating behaviour similar to that of long-term gamblers, cokeheads, and unhappy addicts of all kinds. In another experiment, rats were trained to binge on chocolate, then given two opiate-blocking drugs. Both opiate blockers reduced bingeing behaviour, but the one which was more specific to μ-opioid receptors was more effective at evening out food consumption again.[927] This experiment showed that stimulating μ-opioid receptors enhanced specific dopamine pathway (wanting) activity in the brain, without increasing the general opiate-receptor or serotonin-mediated pleasure responses (liking).

The same issues remain with these experiments—what was the quality of the chocolate? How much real Cacao did it contain? How much were the effects due to the sugar in the chocolate, and how much to the Cacao? The first rat experiment shows that μ-opioid receptor stimulation is key to compulsive bingeing behaviour; and the second supports the hypothesis that eating chocolate triggers μ-opioid receptor activation. But neither experiment helps to answer the question of whether chocolate is any more addictive than other sweet, fatty foods, nor to define what role, if any, Cacao plays in these cravings. But as we saw in Chapter 5, Cacao may have a synergistic interaction with opiates by activating μ-opioid receptors and modulating endorphin turnover via nitric oxide; and, notably, the endorphin surges in rats' brains were *much stronger when the rats were eating chocolate than when they were eating other sweet foods*, which suggests that Cacao may have been amplifying the opiate response.

A study from the University of Hertfordshire recorded by author Julie Pech concluded that repression may be partly to blame for compulsive chocolate eating, where not vocalising thoughts of eating chocolate led to eating more chocolate, suggesting a more psychological mechanism for chocolate cravings.[928] But another experiment clearly demonstrated that chocolate does have a special relationship with food cravings: two groups of female undergraduate students were asked to avoid eating chocolate-flavoured sweet foods or vanilla-flavoured sweet foods for one week, and a third group was allowed to eat as normal. Once they were allowed to eat normally again, only the "chocolate flavoured" group ate a lot more chocolatey stuff than they used to; the "vanilla group" were content to eat the same amount of vanilla flavoured foods as they had before the trial. The chocolate group's deprivation had hit harder; their desire for chocolate had markedly increased with abstinence.[929]

But these foods were only flavoured with chocolate—they weren't high in polyphenols, caffeine, amines, or other constituents in Cacao. Even so, this result corroborates the results of the brain scans of rats eating chocolate, showing stronger enkephalin (endorphin) surges than rats eating other sweet foods *while they were eating*—before most of the chemicals in Cacao had a chance to be digested or absorbed into the bloodstream. In another human trial, just the *smell* of chocolate induced appetite suppression equivalent to actually eating it in a sample group of twelve women, even though the levels of a hunger-stimulating hormone called ghrelin remained high in their bloodstream.[930]

Two explanations spring to mind. The first possibility is that the reaction to chocolate-flavoured foods is a conditioned response, which triggers an immediate pharmacological effect—originally caused by the compounds in chocolate—when the same flavour cues are presented. The second interpretation is that Cacao's volatile constituents which comprise its unique aroma and much of its flavour (including PEA and other low-molecular-weight substances such as trimethylpyrazine) may trigger trace amine associated receptors (TAARs) in the limbic system, amplifying reward or motivation signalling there, as proposed in Chapter 5. Whether this results in appetite suppression or not perhaps depends on whether the subjects began eating; if they hold off, the effect of Cacao's scent on the brain's reward circuitry (whether conditioned or direct) may help restrain the appetite, but once the subjects began eating—particularly if the food has a high sugar and fat content—the endorphin-based reward system may take over, and, lubricated by Cacao's aromatic enticements, encourage more eating.

So, while chocolate may not be physically addictive—and the research so far seems to indicate that it isn't (see Table 6 below)—the evidence presented in this chapter does support the hypothesis that Cacao acts as an intention-reinforcing hedonic modifier. Just as Cacao appears to amplify good mood states according to the chocolate eater's intention, even to the extent the mere smell of it may enhance feelings of satiety and suppress appetite, conversely it may augment the pleasure response to sweet and fatty foods. Whether this translates into increasing their habit-forming potential, and may therefore contribute to physical and mental health problems such as obesity or eating disorders, will be discussed shortly.

Constructive dependency

It has been suggested, not unreasonably, that Cacao could be used as a "positive reinforcer" for desired behaviours to help achieve short-term goals,[931] because it's a substance which is currently thought of as physically non-addictive. Cacao's potential health benefits and apparent harmlessness when consumed in moderation may make it suitable for this kind of approach, as a reward food-drug. This is a valid suggestion, as short-term feelings of "joy" or elevated mood may be noted after chocolate consumption, but a longer-term antidepressant effect in humans hasn't yet been proven; in fact, as we've seen, the opposite association has been noted, as self-identified depressives eat more chocolate. So while "chronic chocolate intake" as a mood modifier remains unproven and controversial, short-term use as a reward is relatively easy to

Table 6. Evidence for chocolate and Cacao having addictive or non-addictive properties

Is chocolate addictive or not?

		Addictive	Direct evidence of addictive potential? If Yes, Score ×2	Non-addictive	Direct evidence of non-addictive properties? If Yes, Score ×2
Pharmacological effects	Non-human animal trials [Score: 1 point]	Salsolinol and THβCs have "reinforcing properties" in rat brains.	*Indirect* (isolated Cacao constituents) [Score: +1]	Rat trial: chocolate no greater tendency to cause cravings than other sweet foods.	*Direct* [Score: –2]
		Endorphin surges in rat brains increase when eating chocolate > other sweet foods.	*Direct* [Score: +2]	–	–
	Human trials [Score: 2 points]	Dark chocolate eaters score highly on Morphine-Benzedrine Group ARCI questionnaire.	*Direct* [Score: +4]	Cacao polyphenols reduce cortisol and adrenaline.	*Indirect* (isolated Cacao constituents) [Score: –2]
		Humans deprived of chocolate-flavoured sweets crave them and eat far more than other sweets when re-introduced into the diet.	*Indirect* (flavoured foods, not whole chocolate) [Score: +2]	Cacao polyphenols counter blood sugar spikes.	*Indirect* (isolated Cacao constituents) [Score: –2]
		–	–	Noradrenaline levels fell back to baseline after 21 days' dark chocolate consumption.	*Direct* [Score: –4]
Totals:			+9		–10
Result:		*–1. Evidence marginally favours non-addictive properties.*			

accept. Chocolate, in this sense, is a reinforcer and binder—using its desirability to "bind" its devotees to behaviours more conducive to achieving their goals:

> For many, chocolate is the most effective binding mechanism because even the promise of future chocolate is highly valued in the present … chocolate can become more successful as a positive reinforcer for long-term optimal behaviour if individuals are psychologically addicted to it. (Catherine S. Elliott, from Szogyi, 1997; ©Hofstra University)[932]

In other words, having a self-identified "addiction" or strong liking for chocolate makes it very suitable to use as an incentive for accomplishing onerous chores. A deliberate strategy making use of chocolate in this way could be therapeutically powerful in some circumstances, for example the depressed chocolate lover who keeps putting off the laundry—to use Cacao as a payment or self-administered reward either before or after the task.

This is symbolically in line with the traditional use of Cacao as money, and the folk use of chocolate in all its forms as both a consolation and a palliative for life's difficulties. It also agrees with the dopamine-elevating (and therefore motivating) effects of expectation, when "highly palatable foods" are anticipated. Chocolate's potential effectiveness and suitability as a reward or incentive is only limited by three possible factors: dislike of chocolate (which is rare), negative health effects produced by eating chocolate (which are uncommon), or feeling guilty after eating chocolate (which is, unfortunately, common). The latter is a negative effect particularly associated with dieting, or eating disorders.

"Chocolate" cravings and dysfunctional eating

> The literature tends to confound concepts of chocolate craving, carbohydrate craving and emotional eating and to a lesser degree obesity … it is probable that each phenomenon is driven by different motivations, [and] underpinned by different neurotransmitters. (Parker & Brotchie, in Paoletti et al., 2012)

Eating disorders are to be distinguished from simple chocolate cravings—bulimia nervosa, anorexia nervosa, orthorexia, and binge-eating are pathological, whereas chocolate cravings may be harmless. Similar neurochemistry applies though—it's been found that bulimics show increased activity in brain regions associated with food anticipation when their mood is low.[933] Cacao's effects on mood and cognition, brain chemistry, and food cravings have their own sets of chemical drivers, though in truth there may be overlap between all these categories simply because we regard chocolate as a food, not a drug, and components of food such as sugars and fats light up reward pathways in the brain in a similar way to many psychoactive substances. So it would be more surprising if these issues weren't a bit "confounded".

To investigate the effects of stress on eating patterns, a group of women aged forty-one to fifty-two were assessed and categorised as experiencing high or low levels of chronic stress, then put through a mock job interview designed to simulate a real-life stressful experience. The "chronically stressed" women ate less vegetables and more chocolate cake following their interview.[934] Interestingly, the chronically stressed women also had *lower* levels of cortisol in their bloodstream after the task than their more relaxed cohorts, which may suggest a kind of stress burnout factor, where chronic high demand for stress hormone reduces the adrenal capacity to produce it. This is a form of Selye's GAS. Hans Selye was a scientist, though not an unduly flatulent one (as far as we know): GAS is an acronym for general adaptation syndrome, whereby a continually stressed organism will adapt by blunting its stress response so that it's able to function, until—if the stress is maintained—collapse or breakdown eventually occurs.

One study recruited forty women, twenty of whom were self-identified "chocolate addicts", and monitored their eating habits over a week. The self-labelled "addicts" had more negative feelings like depression, guilt, and craving than non-"addicts", and after eating "chocolate" the "addicts" had higher levels of guilt than before.[935] We have no way of knowing whether these women really were addicted to chocolate—there were no objective assessments to show that this was or wasn't the case, we only know that they believed themselves to be addicts. There's also the recurrent issue of poor chocolate quality control assessment—we don't know whether the "chocolate" being consumed by these women was dark, milk, or even white chocolate. So this trial doesn't show that chocolate can't improve mood. But it does show that people who see themselves as having a problem with a particular food, in this case, chocolate-based products, experience negative emotional effects after eating that food.

A Dutch study with younger participants (eighteen to thirty-five years old) discovered that high-anxiety people found milk chocolate more effective for calming their nerves than dark chocolate.[936] This corroborates what we now know about the temporary endorphin-enhancing effects of added sugar, fat, and milk on brain chemistry. It may be that milk, and the higher sugar content, are the key to a more soothing chocolate bar—and, perhaps, one reason why binge-eaters often prefer sweet foods like high-sugar milk chocolate to more bitter dark chocolate. However, dark chocolate contains more Cacao, which has the property of reducing cortisol and adrenaline levels, whereas higher sugar intake elevates both. So we have the paradoxical situation where the more physically stress-relieving dark chocolate is perceived as less relaxing than milk chocolate, presumably because of dark chocolate's higher caffeine and lower sugar and milk content.

Binge-eaters given the opioid-blocking drug Naloxone ate less sweet and fatty foods during a brief tasting experiment, whereas there was no change in the amount consumed by people without this eating disorder.[937] This finding indicates that binge eaters may be using junk food like opiate drugs, to stimulate endorphin release, which would account for the variations on a theme of craving and bingeing which they experience. Other research emphasises the dopamine reward pathways, whereby excessive dopamine release in response to the anticipation of a reward causes the accumulation of delta-fos-B in the brain's reward circuitry. Because delta-fos-B causes physical changes to the circuitry of the brain, amplifying the response to that particular thing, eventually we become hard-wired so only that specific stimulus trips our reward switches—the desire for sex, money, or food becomes watching pornography every day, compulsive gambling, or overeating, to name only three possibilities.[938]

Ecstasy and agony: MDMA, chocolate, and binge eating

In Chapter 5 we saw that Cacao may enhance sensitivity to serotonin, dopamine, and noradrenaline signalling, and looked at some parallels between the effects of Cacao and MDMA. There's another recorded link between MDMA and Cacao: a published set of case studies of seven ex-MDMA users which revealed a pattern of symptoms and behaviours that developed after stopping regular MDMA use. Six of the seven people developed a very specific form of social paranoia—a fearful feeling of being ridiculed when in public, and in four cases this was intense enough to be labelled an "atypical psychosis". The authors noted that there were similarities to "the DSM-III-R description of social phobia" (Schifano & Magni, 1994).[939] Four of the cluster experienced appetite and weight loss, reduced concentration, and depression; three cases documented increased aggression, or outbursts of temper; and two of the group had symptoms of panic disorder (such as rapid heart rate, sweating, acute anxiety, breathlessness), and/or inverted sleep-wake patterns. All seven people developed chocolate and carbohydrate cravings, with binge-eating patterns involving chocolate and sugary, starchy foods up to thirty months after stopping regular MDMA use; the average length of time after stopping MDMA use for this behaviour pattern to develop was one year.[940] I can add one more individual to this roster, having myself had a similar experience a year after stopping regular weekend MDMA use in my early twenties.

As discussed in Chapter 5, the uniquely "empathogenic" effects of MDMA may be partly due to serotonin's secondary effects on neurohormones such as oxytocin. Serotonin also affects prolactin release in complex ways, and MDMA users released less of the hormone prolactin into the blood than non-users when they were intravenously dosed with the the serotonin precursor l-tryptophan.[941] We know that prolactin increases dopamine transmission in behavioural brain regions such as the nucleus accumbens and ventral tegmental area. Prolactin activation in these brain regions "does not prevent behavioural despair", but does seem to enhance the action of antidepressant drugs which combat it.[942] This property of prolactin is reminiscent of Cacao's observed effect of enhancing good mood states, but only if the subject wills it (with "intention"). Likewise, dosing opiate-addicted rats with prolactin decreases their self-administration of morphine, and prolactin is known to interact with opiate receptors; here, again, there is some tangential corroboration for a prolactin-enhancing effect of Cacao in the anecdotal potentiation of opiates by chocolate among recreational drug users. And as discussed in previous chapters, Cacao was traditionally used as a galactagogue, a drug to enhance breast milk production, which is a primary function of prolactin.

In bulimics and binge-eaters, binge frequency is "inversely correlated with serum prolactin response to D-fenfluramine" (a serotonin-releasing drug).[943] In other words, the less prolactin is produced in response to a serotonin-releasing drug—or presumably, by extension, a serotonin-releasing stimulus or a surge of tryptophan—the greater the likelihood of a binge. This suggests that bingeing may at least partly depend on abnormalities in serotonin levels or transmission in the brain, which correlates with the onset of bingeing behaviours in serotonin-depleted former MDMA users, and perhaps also their sudden appetite for chocolate. The authors of the paper on MDMA and chocolate craving speculated that chocolate's relatively high phenylalanine, tyrosine, and phenethylamine content may be responsible for its being craved in this case.[944]

As discussed in Chapter 4, phenylalanine and tyrosine are converted into dopamine and noradrenaline, and, like phenethylamine, these neurotransmitters increase positive mood states and motivation. In Chapter 5, we saw that former MDMA users and people who commit suicide tend to have lower levels of 5-HIAA in their brain and spinal cord, and higher blood levels of cortisol—effects which there is evidence to suggest Cacao may reverse or offset. Binge-eaters and bulimics also have higher blood levels of the stress hormone cortisol.[945] We also reviewed pharmacological, historical and anecdotal evidence that Cacao may affect blood levels of the hormone prolactin. So there are several possible links between MDMA use, binge-eating, elevated cortisol, altered serotonin and prolactin levels in the central nervous system, and unwitting impulses to self-medicate with Cacao.

In addition to the palatability and high content of the addictive sugar and fat combination in chocolate confectionery, Cacao's background-level effects on the brain's pleasure circuitry and perhaps secondary influence on prolactin suggest that chocolate may be implicated in binge-eating disorders. In the absence of significant amounts of Cacao's beneficial stress-modulating chemicals, chocolate flavouring may *reinforce* the drive to repeat a hedonic experience (i.e., to eat more chocolate, or over-consume junk foods); even when real chocolate is eaten, feelings of guilt may block and outweigh Cacao's intention-dependent mood-elevating effect. We may speculate that stressed-out binge-eaters are trying to medicate mood disorder with Cacao, but only succeeding in digging themselves in deeper by over-consuming sugary, fatty, nutritionally defective chocolate-flavoured junk foods. If we accept that Cacao can reinforce reward, then just as it may be consciously used to promote constructive behaviours, it could also amplify the appeal of negative ones. If Cacao could help to release us from our fears, when used "unthinkingly" it may also bind us more closely to our vices.

Chocolate toxicity?

So we know by now—and (if you've read the preceding chapters) you have some evidence to prove it—that Cacao has many beneficial pharmacological properties, and several interesting psychoactive ones. But anything with pharmacological activity, be it food, herb, or chemical, can have adverse effects. And just as Cacao has the potential to alleviate some mental health issues but may aggravate others, it may negatively affect some physical ailments. In gardening, a weed is just a plant in the wrong place, and so it is in medicine: side effects usually indicate a drug in the wrong place—the wrong person, dosage, or disease. Given that chocolate is consumed by many people on a daily basis, this issue deserves more attention than it has been given so far.

The internet, as ever, is a wonderful source of speculation, rumour, and hearsay. One website claims that "[a]ll grains, legumes, sugar, alcohol, caffeine and chocolate … cause inflammation in the gut and elsewhere in the body."[946] Ethanol is an irritant, and excessive consumption will cause a host of problems, and it's plausible that higher intakes of refined sugars may upset the balance of gut flora, and certainly contribute to non-alcoholic fatty liver disease, eventually causing health problems. But the entire statement is a fine example of *reductio ad absurdum*—making something so simple, it's a bit stupid. (The opposite of this is Occam's razor, a paraphrase of which is "the simplest explanation is the most likely one"; outside the artificial parameters of a laboratory experiment or theoretical construct, this is seldom true.) The website referenced above is a handy compilation of various allegations against Cacao's reputation as a healthy food. It asserts that Cacao contains "exceptionally high" levels of phytic acid, which inhibits digestive enzymes and reduces mineral absorption; that "some brands" of dark chocolate contain high levels of cadmium, lead, and *aflatoxin*, a carcinogenic poison produced by fungal contaminants; that Cacao's oxalic acid content can reduce mineral absorption and irritate the digestive tract; and that Cacao's theobromine and caffeine content can

> worsen anxiety, adrenal fatigue, chronic fatigue, depression, nervousness, insomnia, gastrointestinal disorders, nausea, nervous disorders, osteoporosis, oedema, heart and circulation disorders and many more ailments. [...] Chocolate … is actually a mind-altering, addictive drug … consequences include … anxiety, obesity, hyperactivity, elevation of chronic pain … and severe mood swings. (Miller, 2017)[947]

Fortunately, much of this catalogue of chocolate's crimes against human health can be disproved immediately. As we saw in Chapter 5, a clinical trial demonstrated that dark chocolate actually relieves symptoms of chronic fatigue syndrome, and, far from causing "adrenal fatigue", Cacao polyphenols lower the level of adrenaline and cortisol in the blood. "Heart and circulation disorders" is a risible allegation, given the wealth of experimental and clinical evidence of Cacao's beneficial effects on the circulatory system, detailed in Chapter 4. The claim of "addictive" properties has been dealt with in full earlier in this chapter. Some of the other accusations—osteoporosis, gastrointestinal disorders, depression, and problems caused by oxalic acid—may contain a crumb of truth, and will be considered in more detail shortly.

As to the assertions about anti-nutrients and toxins in Cacao, a brief survey of the research is illuminating. Cacao does contain phytic acid, a known mineral *chelator*—from the Latin *chelae*, meaning claws, because such compounds "grab" minerals. This can be good or bad, as chelators reduce absorption of both useful minerals and harmful heavy metals. Phytic acid is present at an upper limit of 0.75% dry weight in Cacao,[948] an amount comparable to many other beans and legumes, and most nuts contain higher levels. So this clearly isn't a major concern, unless you believe, as this website's author does, for reasons best known to himself, that beans are "inflammatory". Assuming the site's author has good intentions but poor fact-checking skills, this may be due to substances called lectins found in some uncooked beans, such as chickpeas (garbanzos) and kidney beans, which can trigger inflammatory responses. Most are removed by soaking and boiling, rendering their presence a non-issue (despite high-profile claims to the contrary, from doctors undeserving of the title). Some people may be lectin-sensitive, but as Cacao and chocolate contain negligible quantities of lectins, this is one tangent we shall not pursue.

Cacao's alleged heavy metal content may be more of a concern. Lead accumulation in the body is insidious, and can permanently damage the brain and nerves and other organs; excess cadmium intake may cause more rapid and obvious signs of poisoning such as digestive, respiratory, and kidney problems. Cadmium in chocolate doesn't seem to be an issue; high levels have not been reported, and cadmium assays of various cocoa-containing products in India revealed lower-than-certified values.[949] However, while lead levels in unprocessed, sun-dried Cacao bean samples taken from farms are very low, the lead content of *cocoa powder* can be among the highest found in all food types, most likely due to industrial contamination such as diesel fuels and lead-containing solder used in factory machines for processing the beans.[950]

But the story doesn't end there. Several compounds in Cacao and processed cocoa powder were found to bind "very firmly" to lead—so strongly that "the binding capacity exceeded about 1000 times the naturally present metal levels"[951] in laboratory conditions designed to mimic the chemical environment of the stomach and intestines. Once the cocoa powder had been mixed with fake digestive juices, only 5% of the lead present in the cocoa powder actually dissolved. In other words, the lead levels in cocoa powder would need to be several times higher for it to be a problem, and, far from potentially poisoning human consumers, Cacao products may actually chelate heavy metals and prevent them being absorbed from other foods in the stomach, or even remove them from the body of a person with high levels already present in their system.

The issue of fungal toxins in Cacao beans is also worthy of examination, as Cacao is a fermented food, and may be produced in imperfectly sanitised environments, although both traditional and industrial manufacturers take pains to sort the beans and discard any mouldy ones before processing them. The two kinds of poisons produced by moulds which are of most concern are excreted by *Aspergillus* and *Penicillium* species, namely *aflatoxins* and *ochratoxins*. Both of these fungal contaminants are resistant to heat, so will survive cooking if present in foods. Aflatoxins are the most potent and have been classified by the International Agency for Research on Cancer (IARC) as Class 1 carcinogens, in other words consuming them greatly increases the risk of cancer in humans, principally liver cancer; ochratoxins are also carcinogenic and may damage the kidneys, liver, and immune system, and ochratoxin A is classified by IARC as a group 2B carcinogen, a possible cause of cancer in humans.[952] Serious stuff.

In Europe, the EU sets an upper limit for the most dangerous aflatoxin, aflatoxin B1, of two to twelve micrograms per kilogram of produce ($2–12\mu g/kg$), and four to fifteen micrograms per kilogram ($4–15\mu g/kg$) for total aflatoxins;[953] maximum permitted ochratoxin content in foods ranges from two to ten micrograms per kilogram ($2–10 \mu g/kg$).[954] These limits are typically very conservative and err on the side of safety. So long as levels are below this, foods are safe for long-term consumption. A Canadian survey of eighty-five Cacao-containing products originating from all over the world in 2011–2012 found that all samples of cocoa liquor, drinking cocoa, cocoa butter, dark, milk, and baking chocolate were well below the EU minimum upper limit of both aflatoxin and ochratoxin. Only a couple of samples of "natural cocoa"—that is, raw and defatted Cacao powder—had a content of fungal toxins above the EU limits of $2.6\mu g/kg$ aflatoxin B1 and $4.72\mu g/kg$ total ochratoxins, but the average content of the samples was well below the safety margin.[955] The take-home message is that, for the most part, *Cacao and chocolate are well within safety margins for fungal contaminants*, but to be extra careful, if buying raw Cacao and natural cocoa powders, check their origins carefully and only buy from companies which screen their produce for contaminants.

Chocolate is, for many of us, one of life's few reliable pleasures. But here follows a list of possible chocolate-related "red flags".

1. Secret enemy of "man's best friend"

The alkaloid theobromine in Cacao and chocolate is toxic to many animals—surprisingly, much more so than caffeine or theophylline, which have a stronger stimulant effect in man. Dogs, foxes, horses, domestic fowl, and parrots are especially vulnerable; only 8mg/kg theobromine is sufficient to kill a dog. In other words, a small 25g bar of dark chocolate may be enough to endanger the life of a medium-sized 24kg dog. Moreover the combination of theobromine and caffeine in a 5:1 ratio (approximately that found in Cacao) was found to cause "optimal mortality" in research into coyote "pest control" in the USA.[956]

2. De-boning chocolate

Cacao has several benefits for the longer-term condition of skin and tooth enamel, but its ultimate effects on the skeleton may be less helpful. One small trial assessed bone density and chocolate intake in a random sample of 1001 older Australian women, aged seventy to eighty-five. Their diet was assessed by questionnaire, and greater chocolate consumption turned out to be linked to lower bone density: women who ate chocolate once a day or more had a 3.1% lower whole-body bone density than those who ate it less than once a week.[957] The authors speculated that Cacao's oxalic acid content may reduce calcium absorption, and noted that a single dose of 100g dark chocolate increased calcium excretion by 147%.

This was a preliminary study, with no control group, and the familiar methodological flaw: "chocolate" in the survey included all varieties, from drinking cocoa and low-Cacao milk chocolate to higher quality dark chocolate. So was the lower bone density due in part to higher sugar consumption or solely to Cacao intake, would the results be the same with traditional Cacao based drinks, and is this result reproducible, or a one-off? Only further research will tell. But until then, *older men and especially post-menopausal women at risk of osteoporosis may want to limit their chocolate intake*. Or at least weigh it up with their risk of heart disease and stroke, against which Cacao provides some protection.

3. Secret frenemy of men's "best friend"?

Possible benefits of Cacao for erectile dysfunction were discussed in the last chapter, but there may be a hidden dark side to Cacao's aphrodisiac mystique. Theobromine has been shown to cause testicular atrophy in rats,[958] decimating their fertility, and—more disturbingly—the same effect was found for cocoa powder as part of their diet. Acrylamide, too—produced during roasting—is a known mutagen (cancer-causer),[959] and its accumulation has been linked to testicular damage in rats.[960] It's not known whether cocoa would have the same effect in human males, but it's concerning that cocoa and chocolate consumption in eighteen different countries over a fifteen-year period (from 1965–1980) was strongly correlated with increased incidence of testicular cancer in men eighteen to thirty-seven years later in 1998–2002.[961] This may represent a delayed effect of chocolate and cocoa consumption causing testicular DNA damage in male infants and children, and perhaps even chocolate eaten or drunk by their mothers while pregnant or breastfeeding, because the effects of many mutagenic substances may only show up as cancer years or decades after the initial exposure. There was a similarly strong correlation between cocoa consumption during this period and next-generation male genital birth defects nineteen to thirty-eight years later (1999–2003).[962] So it's very possible that Cacao may cause DNA damage in male gonads and genitals which is passed down to the next generation, or shows up later in life as cancer.

By contrast, some animal research suggests that flavonoid-enriched cocoa powder may *reduce* DNA damage in the testes of adult male rats,[963] which suggests cancer-preventive effects. The polyphenols in Cacao also protect rats against prostate cancer development, and reduce the size of the prostate, which tends to increase in older animals and is a warning sign for prostate cancer.[964] But, again, human real-life data opposes this—there is a positive link between theobromine intake in the diet and prostate cancer in older men. Even 11–20mg of theobromine per day, the amount in a couple of squares of dark chocolate, has been shown to increase risk in a population survey.[965] This suggests that it may be the theobromine content of Cacao which is responsible for the observed anti-fertility properties in rats, and the possibility of carcinogenic effects in men. And chocolate is the major dietary source of theobromine—although theobromine can be produced from caffeine in the body, this study showed that of smoking, alcohol, *and caffeine intake*, none was associated with increased risk of prostate cancer[966]—so the issue wasn't coffee, tea, or other theobromine sources: it was most likely cocoa, or chocolate.

Given that the evidence of risks associated with Cacao in its most commonly consumed forms—cocoa and chocolate—on male fertility and reproductive cancers is stronger than the evidence against, it would be wise for *pregnant mums, young boys, and men with low sperm counts who are trying for a baby*, to limit their intake of shop-bought chocolate and especially cocoa. It's very likely that real Cacao drinks made from the whole bean with its much higher polyphenol content may counteract and outweigh any negative effects, and the risks shouldn't be overstated in any case; the population studies assessed relative risk, meaning that the real-life increase in the number of cases of testicular and prostate cancers which may be attributed to Cacao products if the link is confirmed by further research is very small. But it's there, and shouldn't be overlooked.

This may provide another retrospective justification for the Mexica prohibition of *cacahuatl* consumption by children and pregnant women, and their assertion that Cacao was "to be feared". It may be expected that cultures with a three-thousand-year intimate relationship with a plant would develop a sense of its true nature, even if its particular dangers and risks were not explicitly stated. Of course it may yet turn out that the risks to male reproductive health from early or late exposure to Cacao are insignificant; but, as the saying goes, better safe than sorry. My suspicion is that any negative health effects of Cacao may be completely context-dependent, speaking of which …

4. The Parkinson's controversy

Parkinson's disease is a condition wherein voluntary control of movement is gradually lost. Those afflicted by it incrementally acquire a shuffling gait, a resting tremor, mask-like facial features, and difficulty initiating and stopping movements. The movement disorder is associated with other symptoms such as mood swings, constipation, incontinence and sexual problems (wanting too much—usually a side effect of medication—or, more commonly, not being able to "perform"), and can lead to dementia in its advanced stages. Parkinson's is usually linked to aging, and is caused by the death of brain cells in a small region at the back of the brain called the *substantia nigra*, which is responsible for co-ordinating voluntary movements. The brain cells in this region use dopamine to signal, and once their numbers drop below 20%, symptoms of Parkinson's disease show up.

For years, there have been anecdotal reports by people living with Parkinson's that eating dark chocolate helps relieve their symptoms. This seemed to be confirmed by a 2009 study of 274 people living with Parkinson's, who were compared with a control group of 234 unaffected people. The Parkinson's group were found to consume much more chocolate than the non-Parkinson's people, regardless of their "depression scores"[967]—in other words, whatever else might be going on, it didn't look like they were eating chocolate just because they were unhappy. And the Kuna people of San Blas in Panama, who ingest an average of seventy-five grams of whole Cacao every day in beverage form, have 20% fewer cases of non-cardiovascular brain disorders (including Parkinson's disease) than city-dwelling Kuna émigrés, who don't regularly drink traditional Cacao-based beverages.[968] In laboratory tests, several of the polyphenols in Cacao have been found to protect brain cells from aging-related or inflammatory damage (see Appendix A for details), and rats fed very high doses of Cacao polyphenols as part of their normal diet had better brain function, lived longer, and much higher levels of dopamine were excreted in their urine.[969] So there's moderately strong real-world evidence that Cacao may help protect against Parkinson's disease.

In addition to providing general protection against oxidative damage in the brain and perhaps preserving dopamine levels, many of the individual polyphenolic compounds in Cacao may be anti-Parkinsonian; in laboratory experiments (*in vitro*), the flavanols quercetin, hesperetin, and caffeic acid prevented dopamine from being broken down into a toxic by-product,[970] and chlorogenic acid likewise prevented dopamine from oxidising and bonding to proteins in brain cells and causing damage,[971] while another by-product of Cacao's procyanidins, called protocatechuic acid, actually protects brain cells from damage and increases their rate of self-repair and adaptation in the laboratory.[972] Several other compounds in Cacao which are small enough to get into the brain—alkaloids such as tetramethylpyrazine and trigonelline, and the amino-acid based diketopiperazines—also have nerve cell protective properties in the petri dish,[973] and may well afford some protection against degenerative brain diseases such as Parkinson's.

So what's the issue? There are two. The first yellow flag is that more recent research hasn't shown any short-term benefit for dark chocolate on Parkinson's symptoms, which doesn't support the assertion of many people living with the disease that it helps them by providing noticeable improvement. In an experiment where two groups of Parkinson's disease patients ate single servings of either two hundred grams of dark chocolate or the same amount of white chocolate, the dark chocolate initially seemed to help symptoms one hour after eating it, in comparison with the symptoms recorded in the white chocolate control group; but on repeating the experiment twice, swapping the groups over each time, that initial positive result wasn't replicated.[974] Of course, this is only one experiment, using single doses of dark chocolate, and didn't measure the effects of regular consumption; further tests are needed. But the second and more concerning issue is that several compounds in Cacao have the potential to *accelerate* nerve damage to the dopamine-releasing neurons of the *substantia nigra*.

The true cause for concern is that, similar to depression, research has so far only confirmed *a link* between chocolate consumption and Parkinson's disease. As with depression, some people living with Parkinson's clearly feel that chocolate is beneficial to them, even if science has not yet confirmed that this is the case. A belief among consumers that it's doing them good isn't sufficient; the connection doesn't prove either benefit or harm. This is where evidence-based statistical medicine really comes into its own—because it's entirely possible for people to delude themselves about the benefits of a food, exercise, drug, or practice, particularly when it provides a noticeable short-term pleasure-based reward. It's important to objectively and statistically examine long-term health effects over whole populations, rather than rely on individual testimonies alone. There are reasons to be particularly vigilant about dietary concerns for Parkinson's disease, specifically. The Caribbean soursop fruit, *Annona muricata*, has been linked to outbreaks of an unusual form of Parkinson's disease on the island of Guadeloupe. Compounds in the fruit have been identified as cellular poisons, acting in similar ways to other chemicals that increase the risk of Parkinson's disease, and research has shown that these compounds are able to get into the brain following consumption of the fruits.[975]

So, what are the potentially risky compounds in chocolate or Cacao? Some research has focused on phenethylamine (PEA). PEA seems to be a good candidate for *enhancing* dopamine release, which should benefit Parkinson's sufferers, if anything; but its administration to rats actually *induces* a form of Parkinson's disease by depleting dopamine levels in the *substantia nigra*.[976] Of course the PEA in these experiments was injected directly into the rats' blood, in very high doses, quite unlike eating Cacao with its trace levels of the compound, so this isn't evidence that Cacao's small quantity of PEA could be harmful when Cacao or chocolate is eaten or drunk in normal amounts. But as we speculated in Chapter 5, the combination of PEA with other compounds in the bean is likely to magnify its effects to a significant extent—and why should all these effects be positive?

If the miniscule dose of PEA in an average serving of Cacao were the only risk factor, the evidence would still be in favour of a neutral-to-positive effect for Cacao in Parkinson's. But there are other compounds in Cacao and chocolate that could accelerate the death of dopamine-releasing brain cells. The alkaloid salsolinol, produced during fermentation of the bean, is present in small but pharmacologically significant quantities. Salsolinol is formed naturally in the human brain, and is not thought to be directly toxic to dopamine-producing brain cells; but under conditions of stress, such as high inflammation, salsolinol may contribute to brain cell injury.

When salsolinol is methylated—a chemical reaction which occurs naturally when dopamine mixes with acetaldehyde or formaldehyde in the brain—a toxic compound called n-methylI)-salsolinol (NMS) is formed. And NMS *does* directly kill dopamine-producing brain cells, by inhibiting the action of the damage-buffering antioxidant compound superoxide dismutase, or SOD. It also accelerates the breakdown of dopamine, thereby potentially increasing the rate at which dopamine-producing cells die off, while simultaneously reducing the levels of dopamine in the brain. You don't need to drink embalming fluid for this to happen: ordinary alcoholic beverages result in raised blood levels of acetaldehyde, as does fasting, starvation, diabetes, liver dysfunction, or a ketogenic (low-carbohydrate) diet. All these things accelerate production of salsolinol's more toxic chemical cousin in dopamine-releasing brain cells.[977] So Cacao or chocolate consumption in any of these situations may—theoretically—result in an increased production of the pro-Parkinsonian compound NMS in the brain.

Other compounds in Cacao and chocolate may also be toxic to some brain cells. Acrylamide, produced during roasting the beans, is a known carcinogen and nerve toxin, although the quantity of acrylamide in Cacao is also low. Rat experiments have shown that acrylamide exposure in young animals causes symptoms of neurological disease, and affects genes which provide blueprints for some of the dopamine pathways in the brain.[978] And another set of potentially psychoactive trace alkaloids in Cacao, the tetrahydro-beta-carbolines (THβCs), have an ambivalent role. While some of the THβCs protect nerve cells from damage in the laboratory,[979] their breakdown products, called β-carbolines—once they are absorbed and metabolised in the body and brain—may be "potent neurotoxins",[980] in addition to blocking the nerve-protecting enzyme MAO-A[981] and thereby raising the level of PEA in the brain.

One β-carboline alkaloid called harmane—a possible breakdown product of the THβCs in Cacao—is strongly implicated in the neurological disease called essential tremor,[982] a mostly benign age-related condition with continual shaking or tremor that affects different parts of the body. It's frequently misdiagnosed as Parkinson's disease, and often occurs together with it; and while the association of a β-carboline with this condition doesn't prove an association with Parkinson's disease, it demonstrates that this family of food-based compounds may cause symptomatic neurological disease. So some of the fairy dust compounds in Cacao which were discussed in Chapter 5 for their probable role in the pleasure-enhancing effects of Cacao and chocolate—PEA, salsolinol, and the THβCs—may also be risk factors for longer-term neurological problems in certain people.

As we saw in Chapter 4, Cacao is an especially rich dietary source of the essential trace mineral copper, such that a single decent-sized serving of 40g Cacao provides the entire recommended daily intake level of the mineral. Amongst other things, dietary copper is used to make copper-based enzymes which catalyse important chemical transformations, such as turning dopamine into noradrenaline in the brain—in a crude sense, turning "wanting" into "excitement". But high tissue levels of copper, and other minerals such as lead, iron, and manganese, have been linked to increased risk of developing Parkinson's disease, as defensive immune cells in the brain absorb these heavy metals and cause changes in the shape of some proteins these cells then manufacture, which accumulate and eventually cause malfunction and cell death. Copper also directly reacts with dopamine, causing production of hydrogen peroxide—a highly pro-oxidant substance, commonly known as bleach—as a waste product.[983] While hydrogen peroxide is produced naturally by some cells of the immune system as a means of chemically attacking invading organisms, if too much of this waste product is produced in dopamine-producing areas of the brain, exceeding the rate at which the body can comfortably get rid of it, brain damage may start to occur. More alarmingly, theobromine—the principal alkaloid in Cacao—is known to react with copper, also producing cell-damaging free radicals.[984]

Free radicals or reactive oxygen species (ROS) and the "antioxidant" phenomenon was discussed in Chapter 4, but to briefly recap, ROS are atoms with missing electrons which then steal electrons from neighbouring atoms and set off a chain reaction, eventually destabilising cellular structures. One way of visualising this is that when there are too many free radicals/ROS around, cells end up getting moth-eaten pretty fast, as oxidative damage occurs faster than the cells can "darn the holes", until the cells eventually disintegrate like rotten old carpets. NMS, PEA, and heavy metals all damage dopamine-releasing brain cells by "oxidative stress"—producing free radicals. Because older bodies can't buffer against free radical damage as efficiently as younger ones, NMS may build up in the brains of older people from a variety of dietary sources, and perhaps especially in those who go on ketogenic diets, drink alcohol, or are diabetic, giving rise to cumulative damage. Years of exposure to environmental pollutants such as heavy metals like lead from traffic fumes or old pipes, copper water pipes, or manganese from manufacturing or industrial pollution may cause these ROS-generating substances to accumulate in brain tissue; other compounds such as some pesticides have also been linked to a greatly increased risk of developing Parkinson's disease.[985]

While disease-related changes in the cells of the *substantia nigra* were accelerated by the presence of copper, at least in the laboratory,[986] a 2011 population study in Japan reassuringly found no link between dietary copper intake and the incidence of Parkinson's disease.[987] A 2013 meta-analysis of previous studies and a replication study corroborated this conclusion, finding no difference between the amount of copper in the brain and blood of people with Parkinson's and those without the disease.[988] But—Parkinson's disease patients were found to have higher-than-expected levels of *iron*, not copper, in the *subtantia nigra*, and low levels of the copper-transporting protein, ceruloplasmin.[989] This is because ceruloplasmin also transports iron out of organs and prevents toxic build-up. At least in rats, low copper intake has been found to cause excessive iron levels in the brain, whereas higher dietary levels of copper have no effect; and conversely, low iron intake is associated with copper accumulation.[990] So, perhaps, the high level of copper in Cacao may turn out to be helpful, especially because Cacao's probable metal-chelating effects may reduce absorption of metals in any case. But to make matters even more confusing, a Chinese population study in 2011 found that excessive dietary copper intake with low dietary vitamin E *was* associated with increased risk of developing Parkinson's disease.[991]

The solution to the problem of whether Cacao may be preventive, neutral, or causative for Parkinson's disease may reside in the last study. Cacao's anti-Parkinsonian compounds (the polyphenols) are principally antioxidants, and Cacao's pro-Parkinsonian compounds (PEA, salsolinol, copper + theobromine) may exert cumulative oxidative damage in the *substantia nigra*. Where polyphenol-rich, highly antioxidant real Cacao is being eaten or drunk, especially in the context of an antioxidant-rich diet, there is likely to be reduced risk of developing Parkinson's disease. But what about people exposed to nerve-damaging pesticides, industrial or airborne heavy metal contamination, and eating a nutrient-poor diet of processed foods? Especially those who are consuming high-theobromine, reduced-polyphenol forms of Cacao such as processed cocoa powder? They are liable to have a net excess of pro-oxidant compounds in their system, which the polyphenols in cocoa powder or low-quality chocolate are insufficient to counter. This finding may also explain the link between Cacao product consumption and testicular cancer, despite the apparently protective effects of whole Cacao in animal experiments. In real life, people often consume cheaper, more processed forms of Cacao, together with poor diet, cigarette smoking, and high environmental pollutant exposure—perhaps enough to tip the scale from Cacao's beneficial antioxidant polyphenols to minor but cumulative chemical insults from Cacao's potentially harmful copper, alkaloids, and trace compounds.

An interesting illustration of this possibility has been observed in fruit flies. Although fruit flies (*Drosophilia sp.*) may seem a bizarre object of study when investigating human biological possibilities, the advantage of studying them is that they have a very short lifespan, so the effects of a particular chemical or intervention can be observed over several generations in a matter of days. When the flies were given cocoa powder to eat, they lived longer—*except* when they were subjected to heavy oxidative stress, as when they were deficient in an enzyme that buffers against such stress. These flies died younger—their lives were *shortened* by cocoa consumption. This enzyme—called manganese-superoxide dismutase (Mn-SOD) just so happens to be the enzyme that NMS, the toxic by-product of salsolinol, deactivates. But the same study found that ingesting cocoa actually helped the flies to excrete excess heavy metals such as lead, iron, and copper, thereby providing some evidence to support the laboratory finding that Cacao may help prevent heavy metal poisoning.[992]

Hypothetically, an unholy combination of bad dietary habits such as inadequate food or nutrient consumption or low-carb (ketogenic) diets, high alcohol intake, poor blood sugar control, and contaminants such as some pesticides and heavy metals may lead to the onset of Parkinson's disease. All of these issues create oxidative stress and generate NMS in the brain, and all of them are reasonably common. In such conditions, regularly consuming more processed, low-polyphenol forms of Cacao such as cocoa powder could somewhat increase the risk of developing Parkinson's disease—even if, it appears, Cacao may help to reduce levels of heavy metals in the system. By analogy, rather like leaving the taps on with a half-blocked plughole, eventually the basin will fill up and overflow.

So, we know that people with Parkinson's tend to eat more chocolate; this small study needs confirming and replicating on a much larger scale, preferably with international epidemiological research to back it up. Consumption of different types of chocolate ought to be differentiated—cocoa powder vs. milk chocolate vs. dark chocolate vs. traditional roasted Cacao drinks, carefully checking for variations in subgroups who have greater or lesser antioxidant intakes, or pesticide and heavy metal exposure, also accounting for lifestyle factors such as diet, smoking, income, and occupation. Ideally, participants should have their mineral status assessed by means such as hair mineral analysis to detect systemic levels of heavy metals such as iron, copper, manganese, lead, and cadmium.

Given the preponderance of real-world evidence for benefit from high-quality Cacao (the Kuna study, anecdotal reports), it seems likely that *whole, unprocessed Cacao could be a helpful addition to the diet for people at risk of developing Parkinson's disease.* But given the known risk factors for developing Parkinson's, Cacao can only be recommended provided their dietary intake of Vitamin E and other antioxidant compounds (such as may be found in a great many pigmented fruits and vegetables) is adequate, and that they aren't diabetic, having liver problems, alcoholic, or on a high-protein and low-carb diet (all predisposing to form higher levels of NMS in the brain). In the meantime, those living with or at risk of developing Parkinson's disease should *avoid denatured forms of Cacao such as processed cocoa powder,* and moderate their intake of real, whole-bean Cacao drinks or dark chocolate.

5. "Allergies"

Genuine allergy to Cacao or chocolate is rare. Real allergic reactions, which range from mild itching to life-threatening anaphylactic shock, are so-called type 1 hypersensitivity responses caused by immune system components named type E immunoglobulins (IgE for short) reacting to a compound in the food and triggering the release of histamine from specialist defence cells called mast cells, which then sets off inflammation, the body's natural response to injury or invasion. Cacao contributes only 1.5% of allergic responses to the total range of documented food allergens. The usual suspects are fish, shellfish, and eggs, at 13% each, followed by dairy products, strawberries, and celery at 9.3% each; wheat flour and legumes such as haricot beans at 4.2% each; peanuts, fungi, and beef, at 2.3% each, then potatoes at 1.9%, with Cacao at the bottom of the list![993] Food "intolerances" are much more common, with diffuse and variable symptoms such as bloating, headaches, fatigue, joint pains, catarrh, and many more. Much of the time when people claim to be "allergic" to a particular food, they're referring to an intolerance. Intolerances are less severe than true allergies (which can be life-threatening). They're often secondary to the effect of a food on gut flora, or some pharmacological properties of compounds in the food to which that individual is especially sensitive, or simply a psychosomatic response to the food, not an immune response to the food itself.

Because of the trace amines produced during fermentation of the beans, Cacao does have a relatively high histamine content, and is on a list of high-histamine "trigger" foods for chronic urticaria (hives, an itchy skin rash like nettle stings), so it's recommended that Cacao be excluded from the diet of people with this condition.[994] It may be that long-term consumption of sugary foods, including eating chocolate (but perhaps not traditional unsweetened Cacao-based beverages) negatively alters the gut flora composition by providing an excess of simple sugars for less desirable microbes to feed on and multiply, contributing to the absorption of more inflammatory, histamine-releasing microbial by-products from the small intestine.[995] On the other hand, theobromine and theophylline, the principal alkaloids in Cacao, both reduce histamine release and protect against anaphylaxis.[996] More remarkably, feeding cocoa powder to rats has been shown to reduce IgE production in response to allergens, suggesting that Cacao overall may have mildly anti-allergenic effects[997] for people who aren't intrinsically allergic to the bean itself—which is to say, most of us.

Interestingly, lab tests suggest that raw Cacao beans may provoke more inflammatory immune reactions than toasted beans; in fact, the more processed the bean, the *less* likely are allergic skin reactions to it. So while 50% of subjects prone to dermatitis, eczema, asthma, or hayfever ("atopy", in medical lingo) had a skin reaction to raw whole beans applied as a paste directly to the skin, only 17% reacted to cocoa liquor made from toasted beans or cocoa powder, and none (0%) reacted to processed whole chocolate.[998] This is old data, and needs retesting; but if the findings hold up, this may be because molecular changes wrought by fermentation and toasting of Cacao beans causes the breakdown of many proteins present in the raw beans that could trigger immune responses in sensitive folk. Once these proteins are denatured into amino acids, glycoproteins, cyclotides, and the like, they become less inflammatory. It may also be because the antioxidant polyphenols are astringent—that's to say, they react with proteins in the skin, causing a tightening effect, which can irritate the skin; and perhaps the lower polyphenol levels in toasted Cacao beans may reduce their tendency to cause local skin irritation. Which is good news for everybody regularly applying melted dark chocolate to their skin.

But it's likely that the difference between processed chocolate bars, toasted cocoa liquor, or cocoa powder in this respect is due to the added cocoa butter in eating chocolate: cocoa butter on its own is considered an "emollient" or skin-soothing remedy. Its action here may depend on the anti-inflammatory properties of fat-soluble phytosterols or fatty acids, some of which may suppress the inflammatory response that could be provoked by proteins in the bean. But raw chocolate appears more likely to trigger allergic responses in some people, which is perhaps another reason for maintaining the traditional process of toasting Cacao beans before using them in food or drink.

In fact, recent research on toasted Cacao suggests that it may be *tolerogenic*, that is, inducing tolerance to certain substances, perhaps reducing food sensitivities. Cacao in the diet of lab rats suppresses the production of an intestinal immune system defence protein, or *antibody*, called IgA,[999] which can cause allergic reactions to some foods. In another experiment, young rats were made allergic to egg white protein, but adding Cacao to their diet reduced the production of IgE—typically associated with allergic responses—in the gut. At two weeks old, the rats were given a large dose of the egg protein to induce a massive allergic response, called *anaphylaxis*— the life-threatening sort of allergic response which some people have to bee stings or peanuts.

The rats which had been fed Cacao had faster recovery in the number of red blood cells, and a weaker immune system response to the allergen.[1000] Most notably, these effects were particularly noticeable in the rats fed whole Cacao, or "conventional Cacao"—*not* in the rats fed Cacao with added cocoa polyphenols, or raw Cacao. So here lies another small piece of evidence that compounds other than the polyphenols, some of which may only be found in fermented, toasted chocolate, have distinct pharmacological effects.

It looks like chocolate allergy is an overstated phenomenon, and Cacao may even have the opposite effect, helping to reduce food sensitivities. But there was one worrying finding in the "allergic rat" experiment: when the rats were killed and autopsied, it turned out that Cacao-fed rats also had more damage to the linings of their intestines. The damage didn't look to have been caused during the anaphylactic shock; instead, it appeared that the absorbent, finger-like filtering projections in the lining of the intestines called *villi* had atrophied, and the cells which produce mucus to lubricate and protect the guts were fewer in number in the rats who were regularly fed Cacao. These changes suggest that Cacao intake may have decreased the intestines' ability to filter out and absorb appropriate nutrients, and at the same time reduced their basic protective mechanisms. This implies that the tolerogenic effect of Cacao, produced by suppressing the IgA and IgE antibody response in the gut, may come at the expense of reducing the gut's basic defences, and perhaps increasing so-called "leaky gut", where more "undesirable" products of digestion are absorbed. In the laboratory, cocoa powder extracts inhibit several digestive enzymes produced by the pancreas, which help break down fat and carbohydrate;[1001] if this takes place in the gut, then perhaps these fats and starches travel down the gut less well-digested, and provide food for less desirable organisms, which may cause problems.

Fortunately, cocoa powder inhibits the growth of many disease-causing bacteria,[1002] which may be helpful in this case. And other immune defences—more typically used against viruses and fungal infections—were increased by Cacao over the long term, both in the gut and the whole system of the rats.[1003] Cacao also beneficially adjusts the gut flora—the balance of microbes in the intestine, otherwise known as the *microbiome*. In rats fed a 10% cocoa diet for four weeks, the balance of organisms in the animals' guts shifted substantially, reducing the growth of inflammation-promoting *Proteobacteria*.[1004] The researchers speculated that this change in the gut flora may be what affects the immune system in the gut, but not enough is known about it at this point. More significantly, beneficial effects on gut flora were shown in a human four-week trial, where twenty-two participants were given the equivalent of 41g Cacao every day. Researchers found significant decreases in the participants' unhealthy gut bacteria such as *Clostridium*, and increases in helpful *Lactobacilli* and *Bifidobacterium* (the bacteria found in "probiotic" yoghurts and supplements). As a consequence, the level of overall inflammation (measured in blood tests for an inflammatory marker called C-reactive protein) in the participants' systems decreased.[1005] This fits in nicely with the historical use of Cacao to treat diarrhoea and as a general tonic, as helpful gut bacteria will protect against gastrointestinal disease and improve overall health.

Traditional Chinese medicine suggests that chocolate is "warming, bittersweet and tonifying to the heart", but "too much will cause overheating, dampness, and overstimulation of the heart".[1006] Simplified, this translates as a substance which enhances positive emotions ("tonify ... the heart"), improves circulation ("warming"), helps recovery from illnesses and strengthens digestion ("bittersweet"), but—in excess—may produce anxiety, phlegm, and gut disturbances ("overheating and dampness"). The relevant conjecture here is that, because low IgA is linked to recurrent upper respiratory tract infections and increased risk of autoimmune disease, it's just possible that long-term excessive consumption of Cacao or chocolate may increase the risk of these things; and if the atrophic effects of Cacao on the gut lining of rats are replicated in humans, then the likelihood of such issues will be increased by greater absorption or reduced screening of potentially immune-triggering substances—known as *antigens* in the trade—such as digestive or microbial by-products from the intestines.

All in all, while true allergies to chocolate and Cacao do exist, *Cacao is less likely to trigger allergic responses than many other foods*. It *improves the microbial balance of the gut, reducing inflammation* throughout the whole body, and *increases tolerance to potentially allergenic foods*. On the other hand, *excessive consumption of Cacao may—hypothetically—thin the gut wall*, and its IgA damping effect may have other less positive ramifications, such as increasing the risk of catarrh or even autoimmune diseases, though this is speculation.

6. Migraine: chocolate-dependent headache?

Chocolate does have a bad reputation where migraine is concerned, but this reputation, too, may not be deserved. Only one in ten headaches are true migraines, marked by their severity, recurrence, and distinctive symptoms: "localised to half the head with pulsation, often accompanied by nausea and vomiting, more rarely with visual and mood disturbances".[1007] Migraine has been described as a "vascular storm", with two phases: the first, "prodromal" phase is accompanied by constriction of blood vessels in the brain; the second phase, the headache itself, is marked by blood vessel dilation with release of pain-inducing substances in the brain. However, more recent research has discovered that the blood flow changes are independent of pain in migraine: in other words, pain can occur before, during, after, or even without any change in the blood vessels.

What does happen is that there is a slow, spreading wave of electrical impulses in the brain, followed by reduced activity, in the painless so-called "aura" stage of some migraines (with alterations in smell, vision, movement, or other senses). Migraine pain itself seems to be accompanied by inflammation in the *dura mater* (Latin for "tough mother"), the protective lining of the brain filled with blood vessels just underneath the skull. The pain is due to "neurogenic inflammation", meaning inflammation triggered by nerve or brain cell activity, not by injury or other mechanisms—and some migraine pain may involve the trigeminal nerve (which has sensory branches covering the temples, cheeks, and jaw in the face, and roots at the top of the brain stem) and those connecting to it via the top of the neck, collectively called the *trigeminocervical complex*[1008]—so perhaps fixing neck problems may help. Several other brain areas are implicated. Some drugs which block serotonin receptors help to alleviate pain. The short version: the pain is something to do with wrong signals in the brain; it isn't caused by altered blood flow; blocking brain serotonin transmission helps; and we still don't know what really causes migraines.

Migraines aren't genetically determined for the most part, as they affect only 26% of identical twins. But high blood levels of the trace amine, tyramine—present in Cacao—are known to induce headaches. One study found that chronic migraine sufferers had very high blood levels of dopamine, noradrenaline and tyramine compared to people without migraines, and the longer the headaches' duration, the higher the blood level of tyramine.[1009] The study's authors suggested that anomalies in the metabolism of the amino acid tyrosine elevated levels of these three chemicals in the brain and blood, which could trigger the trace amine associated receptors (TAARs). Eventually, continually triggering the TAARs could lead to these receptors being "down-regulated", meaning that continuous activation causes the body to reduce the number of receptors to regulate the level of stimulation, rather like somebody eventually ignoring a continuously ringing doorbell. Unfortunately reducing the number of TAARs diminishes control over the dopamine, tyramine, and noradrenaline signalling, as one subtype of TAAR, called $TAAR_1$, acts like a brake—and this gets down-regulated too, leading to an upsurge in the release of these substances: like a persistent postman ringing the doorbell more frequently, and for longer.

Migraine sufferers thought to be sensitive to chocolate had the lowest blood levels of monoamine oxidase (MAO) following administration of 100mg of oral tyramine. MAO is the enzyme which breaks down tyramine, so this finding implies that migraine sufferers are naturally slow to break down amines such as tyramine, dopamine, and noradrenaline.[1010] Similarly, another small study found that people who had the lowest MAO release from platelets in the bloodstream after being given a tiny dose of oral phenethylamine (PEA)—suggesting that their ability to break down these naturally simulating, TAAR-triggering molecules was low—were the most migraine-prone and self-reportedly chocolate sensitive.[1011] PEA itself can trigger migraine in sensitive subjects at oral doses of 6–11mg, greater than the absolute level in Cacao; but given the "fairy dust" cocktail of MAO-inhibitors in Cacao, it's likely that the effects of both tyramine and PEA in Cacao are magnified—whether for pleasure or pain. The dose of PEA given to the migraine sufferers in this trial was 3mg, at least three to four times the amount in a strong serving of traditional Cacao beverage made with 40g Cacao—but recall that the presence of MAO-inhibitors can magnify the effects of PEA up to a thousand-fold. It could be that migraine-prone people with naturally low levels of MAO may be more sensitive to the migraine-triggering effects of the amines in Cacao, aided and abetted by Cacao's own minor MAO-inhibiting activity.

Yet Cacao's blood-flow-improving, inflammation- and pain-reducing effects should have the opposite net effect. One small study found 25g semi-sweet chocolate to be the equivalent of 81mg aspirin in the control of non-migraine headache.[1012] In fact Cacao is used in Central American folk medicine as a migraine preventive: a Mexican formula calls for the migraine sufferer to drink strong chocolate once a week, made with a turkey egg beaten into it.[1013] While this sounds fantastical, it may not be too far-fetched—Cacao improves pain tolerance, and has anodyne (mild pain relieving) properties; Cacao flavonoids have been shown to effectively reduce trigeminal nerve pain, and allay post-exercise muscle soreness and pain.[1014] The polyphenols in Cacao also increase nitric oxide release in the linings of blood vessels, improving blood flow to the brain, reducing inflammation and pain sensitivity, and should therefore have anti-migraine effects. Given the complex interactions that Cacao's fairy dust compounds appear to have with the xanthines and polyphenols in Cacao and brain chemistry, and the use of Cacao as an opiate and MDMA synergist, it seems plausible that a once-weekly dose of Cacao may reduce risk of migraine by modulating endorphin and serotonin metabolism. And the turkey egg? Perhaps it functions as a dietary source of tryptophan and choline, used to manufacture serotonin and various useful compounds, respectively.

While this doesn't rule out the possibility that chocolate may be a co-factor or secondary trigger for migraines in some people, larger trials of people claiming to experience chocolate-related migraines have shown no increase in migraine frequency with chocolate consumption,[1015] and the most recent rigorous trials and analysis demonstrate that chocolate is no more likely to cause headaches than placebo.[1016] So the consensus is that standard *eating and drinking chocolate or cocoa are not migraine trigger foods in the majority of cases.* Perhaps excessive consumption of stronger Cacao-based beverages or dark chocolate may be a risk factor for some individuals due to Cacao's tyramine content and mild MAO-inhibiting properties, but for such people occasional consumption of Cacao may even be preventive rather than harmful. It would be a useful experiment to see if once-weekly consumption of a good dose of real Cacao—say, 40–60g, perhaps taken with a low dose of the serotonin precursor 5-HTP—might prevent rather than trigger migrain

7. Fibromyalgia and gout

Gout in an excruciatingly painful condition, commonly affecting the big toe. It mostly occurs in later life as a result of a build-up of uric acid crystals in the joint, causing inflammation. Uric acid is a waste product normally excreted by the kidneys, so anything which results in abnormal accumulation of uric acid can cause this issue: kidney damage, some medications, genetic factors, lead poisoning, or over-consumption of foods which break down to produce uric acid, to name some of the more common causes. Because Cacao contains the xanthines—theobromine, caffeine, and theophylline—which break down to produce uric acid, it has been thought to predispose to gout. In fact, it doesn't[1017]—most likely, the opposite is true. Metabolic syndrome is a combination of high blood pressure, obesity, high cholesterol, and insulin resistance (or diabetes), and is known to predispose to gout.[1018] As Cacao tends to counteract metabolic syndrome to some degree, it may even prove to be helpful. So *Cacao and chocolate are neutral to beneficial for gout.*

Fibromyalgia is the name given to a condition with chronic pain in the muscles, "tender points" around the body, fatigue, and other physical or emotional issues. It's a diagnosis of exclusion, meaning that once other causes are ruled out, fibromyalgia is a possibility. The cause of the condition is unknown. Author Julie Pech notes that "Nearly 100% of the research advises against eating chocolate if you suffer from fibromyalgia."[1019] A search of medical databases online failed to turn up *any* research suggesting that Cacao was problematic in fibromyalgia, but several internet sites, such as the one cited at the beginning of this segment, claimed that chocolate was a problem.

Some researchers found that having a higher percentage of body fat, LDL cholesterol, and blood fats were linked to worse fibromyalgia symptoms.[1020] Others investigated oxidative stress and abnormal nitric oxide release in fibromyalgia, without drawing any firm conclusions[1021]—but if elevated cholesterol, oxidative stress, and inadequate nitric oxide release do play a part, Cacao ought to be helpful, not harmful. Another tantalising piece of evidence comes from research into the role of endocannabinoids like anandamide in fibromyalgia; the theory goes that endocannabinoids may be able to block cartilage destruction, reduce pain and inflammation, and help tissue rebuilding by modifying the activity of *fibroblasts*, cells that rebuild connective tissue.[1022] As we saw in Chapters 4 and 5, anandamide is found in trace amounts in Cacao together with compounds which retard its breakdown, but its role in the pharmacological action of Cacao is debatable.

Research on the effect of diet in fibromyalgia has focused on how some compounds in food can over-stimulate pain signals in the brain via the amino acid glutamate, which is used as a stimulatory signal. Glutamate release is triggered by the artificial sweetener aspartame, and glutamate is found in the food additive MSG (monosodium glutamate) and in natural sources such as soy sauce and parmesan cheese. Trial results have been mixed, but suggest that MSG is an aggravating factor for fibromyalgic pain, and excluding high-glutamate foods from the diet may help.[1023] Cacao contains unremarkable levels of glutamate. Salsolinol does enhance glutamate release,[1024] although the effect of whole Cacao or chocolate on glutamate levels in the brain isn't known. But Cacao's high magnesium and polyphenol content could be beneficial, as magnesium helps to muffle glutamate signals,[1025] and certain polyphenols (such as catechin) reduce oxidative damage caused by excessive glutamate signalling in the brain.[1026]

There's a theory circulating in the media and on the internet that oxalic acid found in many plant foods may set off inflammation and be the ultimate cause of fibromyalgia. A GP who wrote about it in a UK national newspaper did so in order to bring the benefits of the dietary changes she implemented for herself and many patients to the public. Like many other plant compounds such as caffeine, oxalic acid is produced by plants as an *antifeedant*, deterring insects who may feed on the plant by poisoning them. The theory connecting oxalic acid to fibromyalgia maintains that oxalic acid binds to calcium in the gut, forming calcium oxalate, which then precipitates out of the bloodstream into the tissues of people who eat the plants, causing pain and inflammation.[1027] This issue may be exacerbated by increased intestinal permeability or a deficit of good bacteria in the gut, such as may happen following antibiotic use, for example. Like many plant foods, Cacao contains oxalic acid, and several people claim that following a low-oxalate diet—which excludes chocolate and many other plant-based foods—completely relieved their fibromyalgia symptoms. The theory is plausible, but currently unsubstantiated.

Gut flora disturbance is also thought to contribute to fibromyalgia, as some organisms provoke inflammation, affect hormones, or stimulate the nervous system in the gut, all of which can initiate chains of events that increase fibromyalgia symptoms. Unhelpful gut microbes do this by secreting substances which affect the body once absorbed, or the immune system may attack the microbes themselves, triggering an inflammatory response directly.[1028] Cacao's beneficial effect on gut flora—retarding the growth of "bad" microbes, and encouraging the growth of helpful species such as *Lactobacillus*—could be useful here, as could the overall reduction in inflammation which follows regular Cacao consumption. This may be particularly relevant to the oxalic acid hypothesis of fibromyalgia, as *Lactobacillus* species are known to break down oxalic acid in the gut, making it harmless and preventing the formation of calcium oxalate kidney stones.[1029] This suggests that, rather similar to the heavy metal chelation situation, drinking Cacao may actually help to *reduce* net absorption of oxalates.

One hypothesis suggests that many chronic pain syndromes which are difficult to treat, including fibromyalgia, could be due to leakage of fluid from capillaries—small blood vessels—perhaps putting pressure on nerve endings. The cause of this could be a deficiency in adrenaline, dopamine, and noradrenaline signalling, which normally keep blood vessels constricted and reduce pain signals.[1030] If this theory is correct, Cacao may worsen fibromyalgia, as it lowers adrenaline levels; on the other hand, there is evidence to the contrary. Dietary polyphenols, including those in Cacao, appear to be helpful in fibromyalgia: a survey of seventy-three women, thirty-eight of whom had fibromyalgia, found that foods high in polyphenols tended to be associated with fewer tender points, and dark chocolate or red fruit intake was associated with better quality of life overall for fibromyalgia sufferers.[1031] In summary, extant evidence suggests that Cacao may be *neutral to beneficial in fibromyalgia*.

8. Digestive problems

While for most people *cacahuatl* improves digestion, for some, Cacao's high polyphenol content can cause constipation. Many people experience digestive discomfort or bowel disturbance after eating large quantities of sugary, fat-supplemented processed chocolate, particularly after meals. Very large quantities of even the best quality chocolate can lead to digestive problems owing to the toxicity of high doses of xanthines—as with overdosing on coffee or tea, side effects such as nausea, vomiting, headache, palpitations, and tremors can occur, the digestive component of which may be aggravated by chocolate's high fat content. Additionally, Cacao's caffeine content will increase digestive secretions but does also relax the cardiac sphincter, the valve at the top of the stomach[1032]—so if the stomach is very full, or the person is particularly active or stressed, *gastric reflux or "heartburn" can result*.

The effects of Cacao on the gut flora and food sensitivities have been discussed under "allergies", above. The short version is that *Cacao benefits the microbiome*—the organisms living in the gut—by encouraging the growth of bacterial populations beneficial to human health, such as *Lactobacilli*, and that Cacao also reduces hypersensitivity to "problem foods" by suppressing the immune response to them in the gut. In this way Cacao may benefit long-term gut health, and help problems such as chronic bloating or flatulence. The only caveat is that Cacao *may damage the absorbent surface in the small intestine* in the presence of food allergens and make it less efficient, if one rat experiment is anything to go by, and may *reduce digestion of some fats and starches*—and perhaps therefore reduce absorption of some fat-soluble vitamins, too.

The best time to consume chocolate—for maximum effect and minimal digestive disturbance—may be one to three hours after a meal; the lighter the meal, the sooner the Cacao can be taken. Thus a meal of fruit could be followed by drinking Cacao one hour later; a large cooked meal, three hours. Because the stomach isn't completely full, the Cacao will have a much stronger effect; it will still have positive effects on the microbiome, and any digestion-limiting or absorption-preventing effects it may have will be offset, as the food will have undergone some digestion, and has had time to pass out of the stomach into the small intestine (unless the meal was particularly high in fat, which delays gastric emptying). That said, the Mexica routinely rounded off their feasts with *cacahuatl*, although it may be that the *cacahuatl* was served some time after the last course. Recall that while Cacao may impede the digestion of fats and starches, nevertheless carbohydrate-based (starchy or sugary) foods assist the absorption of Cacao's beneficial polyphenols, so a starch- or fruit-based meal is best to maximise Cacao's pharmacological benefits—or a recipe combining Cacao with starch such as maize, as in *pozol* or other *atole*-type formulations.

9. Acne

It's common knowledge that chocolate "causes spots". This claim seemed to have been disproven in 1969, when a group of researchers showed that people with acne experienced no deterioration when eating highly concentrated dark chocolate bars in comparison to Cacao-free placebo or dummy bars, and a smaller group of acne-free subjects had no skin problems when eating extra chocolate either.[1033] But more recent work has validated the original claim, that chocolate—and dark chocolate in particular, which suggests that Cacao itself may share the same properties—may slightly increase acne symptoms.

A Turkish survey of 3826 people with acne (comparing them with 759 acne-free people) found a minor positive association between acne and chocolate consumption, as well as other foods, including bread, green tea, milk, white sugar, ripe banana, ice cream, apples, oranges, and red meat.[1034] A four-week study with seventeen young and sixteen middle-aged men given only 10g (2/5oz) of dark chocolate to eat every day found that all the participants had increased numbers of Gram-positive (spot-causing) bacteria on their faces at the end of the trial, particularly the younger men—who also had measurably more skin cell shedding,[1035] perhaps indicating the body's attempts to get rid of colonising bacteria a bit faster.

So, distressingly, it appears that *dark chocolate—and possibly Cacao—may exacerbate acne, particularly in young men*, although there's no evidence to suggest that chocolate causes acne (and, as we saw in Chapter 4, it appears to be otherwise very beneficial for skin health). It is entirely possible that only the combination of added fat and sugar with Cacao in ordinary chocolate may exacerbate acne, and plain Cacao or traditional Cacao-based beverages are not problematic—but more information is required to confirm or deny this.

* * *

In this chapter we saw that appetite and addiction are driven by dopamine signals in the nucleus accumbens of the brain, which in turn amplify noradrenaline signalling. Chronic stress, aggravated by isolation, confinement, or powerlessness, increases addictive tendencies—because the stress hormone cortisol eventually decreases dopamine release in the nucleus accumbens, so the dopamine-enhancing effects of many addictive substances become much more noticeable. Pleasure responses, caused by the release of endorphins or natural opiates in the brain, make the brain more sensitive to dopamine, so the urge to repeat the experience becomes stronger. Repeated behaviours get encoded in the brain by the protein delta-fos-B, creating powerful habits. Refined sugar and fat in chocolate temporarily increase brain dopamine and opiate responses and simultaneously elevate cortisol, and cow's milk proteins activate opiate receptors in the brain too, so many high-fat, added-sugar foods, especially those with added dairy products—like milk chocolate—are habit-forming. The phenomenon of chocolate dependency may be partly culturally conditioned, or linked to positive childhood associations, but Cacao's pharmacological properties of hedonic modification most likely also play a role, by modulating opiate responses via nitric oxide, and affecting serotonin and cortisol metabolism.

Pharmacological sensitivity to Cacao itself is likely to be state-dependent, so that those with higher-cortisol, lower-serotonin brain chemistry may notice its psychoactive effects more. This would explain chocolate's greater appeal to self-identified depressives, those with higher levels of neuroticism, former MDMA users, and people with hysteroid dysphoria. Other than a sample of former MDMA users who binged on chocolate, there appear to be no intrinsic links between chocolate and eating disorders. But chronically stressed compulsive eaters have lower cortisol and serotonin levels, and the observation that chocolate-flavoured foods are more craved than others in stressful situations is suggestive. Whether the latter finding is the result of a learned association between the pharmacological boost that Cacao adds to the opiate- and dopamine-releasing effects of high-fat, high-sugar foods, or something else, is unclear; but it's plausible that chocolate-seeking binge-eaters are subconsciously attempting to self-medicate mood disorders. Unfortunately, research shows that negative mood states following chocolate consumption tend to be aggravated by guilt. Even if binge-eaters weren't more likely to be eating poor quality chocolate to start with, Cacao's mood-enhancing properties may be eclipsed by powerful negative associations in eating disorders.

There are also many unanswered questions about Cacao and chocolate's long-term effects on health. It appears from the research that Cacao has many health-promoting properties (summarised in Chapter 4, and listed in full in Appendix A). Negative health effects on migraine and fibromyalgia appear to be myths, although it's feasible that Cacao may still be a problem for some people with these conditions; preliminary hearings have returned a verdict of not guilty, but rumours persist. High lead levels in some forms of processed cocoa and chocolate appear to be more than offset by Cacao's natural chelating properties, which reduce heavy metal absorption, and Cacao usually contains very low levels of fungal contaminants, well within safety margins.

On the other hand, while Cacao strengthens teeth and benefits the skin, it could also weaken bones in post-menopausal women. Cacao may reduce food sensitivity and benefit gut flora while—if animal research bears out—potentially weakening the gut wall in the presence of dietary allergens, and long-term Cacao intake may compromise primary immune defences in the gut (decreasing IgA). Hypothetically, too, Cacao may benefit male sexual function by improving blood flow and strengthening erections, but research has also linked its consumption by pregnant mothers and young boys to a slightly increased risk of later-life testicular cancer and next-generation newborn male genital defects. Likewise, Cacao's long-term effects on prostate cancer risk and Parkinson's disease risk appear to be beneficial or protective, but some evidence implies potential harm—perhaps under specific conditions of environmental stress, toxin exposure, or dietary deficiencies, or when consuming more denatured forms of Cacao such as sugary, highly processed drinking cocoa.

Overall, dark chocolate deserves its reappraisal as a beneficial substance, because the gifts of Cacao far outweigh its potential penalties. But it's naïve to assume that any drug, particularly one to which so many are emotionally attached, is universally beneficial and innocuous.

In plant-human relationships, *Theobroma cacao* has secured its pre-eminence through the provision of nutritional value to—and psychoactive persuasion of—its cultivators. Rather than eating the sweet fruit pulp, however, we perversely eat the bitter, stimulating seeds, the plant's precious next-generation genetic cargo. To do so, we render it edible and enhance its appeal by elaborate processes of fermentation and cooking. It shouldn't come as a surprise, then, that along with the benefits that the Cacao plant imparts, there may be a few stealth taxes on our health as well, as is the case with many cultivated plant foods. Traditional users of Cacao recognised its high value, but knew well that it was no panacea.

No doubt partly for this reason, in addition to more sybaritic motivations, pre- and post-Colombian Mesoamerican civilisations created their fantastic Cacao-based pharmacopoeia, combining prepared Cacao with native herbs and spices to modify flavour, texture, and effect. In the next chapter, fragments of this ancient formulary are reconstructed, and reformulations of ancient ingredients are suggested, in a compilation of reconstructed old-school and contemporary traditional recipes for the "food of the gods".

CHAPTER EIGHT

Chocolate formulary

"Tell us no more of Weapon-Salve,
But rather Doom us to a Grave;
For sure our Wounds will Ulcerate,
Unless they're wash'd with Chocolate.
[...]

There's ne'er a Common Council-Man,
Whose Life would Reach unto a Span,
Should he not Well-Affect the State,
And First and Last Drink Chocolate."

(From de Ledesma, 1631, translated by Wadsworth, 1652)

Authentic "Aztec chocolate" may not be possible to reproduce exactly, as there are no extant pre-Colombian recipes with precise quantities and measurements, nor are all the processes used by the Mexica, Maya, and other indigenous Mesoamerican people documented in detail. But many traditional ingredients and techniques are preserved in the living tradition of *atoles* and beverages incorporating Cacao in Central America, and detailed descriptions of the ingredients and tools used by the Mexica and Maya do exist, as do superficial descriptions of some of the different types of Cacao-based beverages prepared by the Mexica. So the procedure followed in this chapter will be to describe the optimal traditional processing methods for Cacao seeds, then fast-forward to the present day and recount contemporary Cacao-based recipes utilising indigenous ingredients, before attempting to reconstruct some Mexica high-class *tlaquetzalli cacahuatl* or Maya *kakawaa* formulas.

To begin with, which type of Cacao should be used? As described in Chapter 2, Hernández wrote that the Mexica distinguished four classes of indigenous *criollo* Cacao, and the seeds they used would most likely have been of the type nowadays referred to as *lavado*—very briefly fermented, for only twenty-four hours or even less. It makes more sense that Cacao wouldn't have been fermented for long, as a shorter fermentation produces less acids, and the traditional process of toasting Cacao on a *comal* and then grinding it on a *metate* yields a more complex flavour profile. The sour taste of fermented beans is mellowed by industrial conching

251

(the lengthy process of mechanically beating cocoa liquor for several days in large, open-air troughs), and/or offset by adding a larger quantity of sugar—which is both non-traditional and detracts from the medicinal value of the drinks. There are health benefits to a shorter fermentation period, too: while fermentation is necessary to produce several trace "fairy dust" compounds (see Chapter 4), it also breaks down the polyphenols which are arguably the most medicinally important constituents in Cacao, so a shorter fermentation is a useful compromise, generating both "fairy dust" and flavour without diminishing the polyphenol content. And it seems that in Alta Verapaz, Guatemala, one of the few locations in Central America where some locals still drink unsweetened, maize-free Cacao-based beverages (chocolate without sugar), the standard Cacao bean available for sale is only very lightly fermented.

The strongest argument for the ancient Mesoamericans not fermenting their beans for more than twenty-four hours is the lack of descriptions of fermentation in early post-conquest colonial accounts, such as the Codex Mendoza, which records only the Cacao beans being "removed from [their] pod, dried, roasted, and ground."[1036] Given that every stage of the processing was at least briefly described, why is fermentation not mentioned? Fermentation may have occurred almost inadvertently, when the fresh seeds and pulp were removed from newly-harvested pods and heaped up on a *petate* (a woven palm bedroll or mat); in tropical heat, piling the beans up in this way for only a few hours prior to washing them is sufficient to initiate fermentation. So for replicating traditional Mesoamerican Cacao beverages, I would recommend purchasing high-quality *criollo lavado*, grown in one of the historic Cacao-producing areas such as Chiapas or Tabasco in Mexico, or Suchitequepez in Gautemala.

One counterpoint to this "less is more" approach to Cacao fermentation in history comes from the seventeenth-century Italian doctor and chocolate enthusiast Antonio Colmero de Ledesma, who reported that Cacao produces foam "in greater quantity, when [it] is older, and more putrefied"[1037]—in other words, *fermentado* may produce more foam than *lavado* beans (and, as we will see in one variant of the drink known as *popo*, extra fermentation of moistened Cacao beans may further enhance their foam-producing properties). If this is true, it implies that recipes without added botanical foaming agents may work better with *fermentado* beans, so some traditional recipes likely called for them. In this chapter I've faithfully reproduced all recipes which name specific types of Cacao, but feel free to experiment, because unless or until more ancient sources of information arise, then as the maverick apothecary-astrologer Nicholas Culpeper counselled four centuries ago, "Every one, that desires to be called by the name of Artist, [should] have his wits in his Head, and not in his books."[1038]

Owing to the government-sponsored programmes of hybridisation and four centuries of uncontrolled experimentation, original Mesoamerican genetic stock of *criollo* Cacao is hard to find. For the same reason, dividing contemporary Central American Cacao into the four neat types distinguished by the Mexica is nigh-on impossible, as the morphological characteristics—such as bean size and shape—have been shuffled and modified many times since then, although a contemporary analogue of the high-quality *xochicacahuatl*, reputed to have a reddish seed coat, may be found in the "red Cacao" of Chiapas. Many of these farming initiatives were set up with the laudable aim of increasing farmers' profits, because growing Cacao is a tough gig: as recounted in Chapter 2, the plant is sensitive, with a minimum of six years before it is mature enough to produce fruits, and the whole cultivation and production process is highly special-ised and labour-intensive.

But some of the side effects of this hybridisation were also discussed in Chapter 2, including a possible deterioration in the chemical complexity of the stock. There are a few organisations attempting to protect and promote native *criollo* Cacao production, including AMCO (Agroin-dustrias unidas de MexiCO, sponsored by ECOM agro-industrial Corp. Ltd., and Hershey's) in Mexico, and APROCAV (Asociacion de PROductores y sembradores de Cacao en Alta Verapaz) in Guatemala. Such organisations attempt to conserve the genetic purity and quality of native *criollo* Cacao, but the conservation project is necessarily second to the primary goal of ensur-ing production and opening up new markets. This may prove to be an oversight, as the USP of *criollo* Cacao from Central America is its heritage, and preserving the original genotypes and—insofar as is practical—traditional methods of production for the highest grades of native Cacao should be a priority.

Señora Rocío Torres, an agronomist at the AMCO facility in Tapachula in south Chiapas, Mexico, explained that they grow and promote three varieties, two with "white" seeds from Tabasco (known as Echeverría and Marfil) and one with "red" (violet) seeds from Chiapas (the variety called Samuel), all from unmodified native *criollo* stock.[1039] The "white" varieties are more expen-sive and lower-yielding, as is traditional for *criollos*, with their higher alkaloid and lower polyphe-nol content; the "red" variety with its violet seeds will contain more polyphenols, and therefore have a more astringent or sour taste, but is still classified as a native *criollo*. These two Central American organisations that help to grow and supply quality Cacao are listed in Appendix E, in the hope that enterprising readers will support them by purchasing their wares, preferably in bulk!

Let food be your medicine

While the recipes in this chapter may be consumed for pleasure, they also have medicinal utility, particularly if added sugar is minimised. Diabetes is an epidemic, now the second leading cause of death in Mexico after coronary heart disease;[1040] arguably most of this death toll can be laid at the door of the European dietary imports of dairy—in the form of cheese—and, particularly, added sugar. It's true that most Cacao-based products taste better when sweetened, so where contemporary recipes call for large amounts of sugar, I've recorded this information but would strongly recommend that the sugar be reduced, omitted, or at least swapped for unrefined sug-ars such as *piloncillo* or *panela,* maple syrup, or raw honey. Milk, on the other hand, is unneces-sary, historically inauthentic, and detracts from the medicinal properties of Cacao's polyphenols by reducing their bioavailability (see Chapter 4).

Unrefined sugars such as *panela/piloncillo* still contain all the beneficial trace minerals and phytochemicals that are normally filtered out of white sugar,[1041] so they're better by a small margin. (Unless by some mischance you buy toxic honey, made from the nectar of poison-ous plant species such as nightshades, which has been known to happen. Nature loves her little jokes.) I also recommend using powdered whole green *Stevia rebaudiana* leaf alongside any sug-ary sweetener as a "sweetness booster", so you can cut the sugar in half; in some maize-based *atoles, Stevia* alone is enough to sweeten them, as it augments maize's natural sweetness. It's not historically authentic at all, but then neither is the use of sweetening (except for honey, and that seldom). Using whole *Stevia* leaf allows the production of sweet beverages (or foods) without adding grotesque amounts of sugar.

The isolated sweetening compounds from this plant are a collection of steviol glycosides called the steviosides, one of which—rebaudioside A—is now sold in various white, ersatz-sugar sweeteners. I'd recommend avoiding these isolated sweeteners, and using the powdered whole green leaf instead, because it may have beneficial effects on blood sugar control and blood pressure and even other diseases,[1042] so will augment any health benefits of the Cacao polyphenols in this respect. *Stevia* leaf works better as a sweetness extender rather than a stand-alone sweetener. As a rule of thumb, use the same amount of green *Stevia* leaf powder in a recipe as you would use cayenne (chilli) powder if you were trying to add heat: *Stevia* is as sweet as cayenne is hot, and just as too much cayenne can spoil a dish, too much *Stevia* will impart an unpleasant, almost bitter chemical sweetness—so, as with chilli powder, start with the motto "less is more", and taste-test before going crazy with the quantities!

Cacao's many potential health benefits (and its few potential hazards) have been described in the foregoing chapters. For those who are interested in exploring the medical uses of Cacao, a full monograph is available in Appendix A, with mini-monographs on many of the admixture plants and spices mentioned in this book in Appendix B. To use the recipes in this chapter for health benefits, effective doses of Cacao are necessary. For medium-term adjunctive treatment of active cardiovascular disease (CVD) or vascular complications of diabetes (VCD), where results may be required within weeks to months, higher intakes of cocoa polyphenols are recommended. Ideally 50–80g (1¾ < 3oz) Cacao should be ingested every day in traditional drinks, preferably with complex carbohydrates to facilitate polyphenol uptake—so some of the simpler Cacao-maize beverages such as *pozol*, *champurrado*, or *panecito* would be very useful, particularly as they don't require any fancy ingredients. In other words, traditional forms of chocolate are best, in order to ingest effective levels of polyphenols without surfeiting on added fat and sugar. Alternatively, 80–100g (3–3½oz) of manufactured high-flavanol dark chocolate *per* day may be substituted; in this case, I'd recommend going no lower than 85% cocoa solids—recall that the remaining 15% is all sucrose (white sugar), and a so-called "dark" 70% chocolate bar is almost ⅓ sugar.

Daily dosing is also recommended for prevention of CVD or VCD in high-risk groups, and preventive measures in pre-morbid groups such as the millions of people living with "metabolic syndrome", a combination of high blood pressure, abdominal obesity, high blood sugar, and high blood fats (triglycerides or LDL)—incidentally, whole Stevia leaf may be particularly useful in this condition.[1043] I'd recommend ingesting 30–40g (1–1½oz) whole Cacao daily as a medicinal dose for people living with such conditions, or at least five times a week for those seeking to prevent deterioration. Daily consumption of 20–25g (⅔–⅘oz) whole Cacao in the form of traditional beverages is advised for those in high-risk groups, such as having heart disease or diabetes in the family, smokers, etc. A minimum-intake disease-prevention chocolate protocol (for compliance) in high-risk groups could be eating 25g (⅘oz) dark chocolate (minimum 85% cocoa solids) four or five times weekly, or at least 20–40g (⅔–1½oz) whole Cacao (in traditional beverage form) three times a week.

All the forgoing dosages have been estimated for adults weighing between 10–12 stones (63–76kg). Those who are heavier may need to increase the dosages a bit; those who are lighter, reduce a bit. Elderly people and teenagers may need lower doses. Check with a physician or pharmacist before using chocolate regularly if you are taking heart medications (anti-arrhythmic drugs), migraine treatments, powerful anticoagulants, or antidepressants. Cacao will be safe in most cases, but some people are sensitive to it (although such people usually know when this is the case), and a handful of medications may interact with it, so caution is advisable.

Preparation is everything

Seed selection is very important for the flavour and effect of the final product, particularly when attempting to replicate traditional recipes. As above, the recommendation is that *criollo* Cacao *lavado* from Central America be used, and—if possible—acquired from an indigenous, non-hybridised variety grown in traditional Cacao-cultivating regions. But according to Cacao expert Juan-Pablo Porres Esquina, the final flavour profile and quality of Cacao is 20% dependent on genetics (hereditary characteristics), 15% on environment or microclimatic factors such as weather, soil type, carbon dioxide levels, and climate, 15% on cultivation methods and husbandry, and 50% on post-harvest processing such as fermentation method, sun- or fan-drying, cooking temperature and length, etc.[1044] As described in Chapter 4, the optimal temperature and duration for toasting Cacao is twenty to thirty minutes on a low heat (precisely: twenty-three minutes at 116°C or 241°F). So a relatively gentle flame under a heat-diffusing clay *comal* with a single layer of beans, constantly turned and moved with a wooden spoon or spatula for twenty-five minutes is ideal. A heatproof ceramic glass or stainless steel pan placed on top of a heat diffuser mat can also be used on a gas cooker to toast the seeds if you don't have a *comal* (or if you cook large quantities of seeds at one time, as I do, and have more than two cooking surfaces on the go at the same time).

The beans go through three subtle stages when cooking: first, they "ghost", acquiring a pale cast as fats start exuding through the shell; vinegary and sourer smells of fermentation become noticeable as residual moisture and organic acids start to evaporate. Then, they "spot", developing a vaguely mottled appearance as they begin to truly cook, usually around the five- to ten-minute mark with a medium-low flame; at this stage, wisps of smoke may begin to appear, and a delicious aroma of chocolate will start to develop. Finally, the seed coats begin to burn or develop blackened patches, they start to pop, and the chocolate aroma diffuses through the environment, drawing anyone else in the building into the kitchen; at this point, they're pretty much done. Many traditionalists roast the beans to within an inch of their life, whereas others whip them straight off the *comal* the moment they begin to pop. Ultimately the process, like all cooking, is organic and empirical—but let the scientific guidelines be of service, too: less may be more, in terms of a good balance of chemistry and flavour.

The seeds are then hand-shelled, which takes some time. They are best gently pinched and rubbed between thumb and fingers to loosen the shells before shucking off the skins. Acquiring the knack takes a while; many beans will simply fragment with the shell, or refuse to part with their charred endocarp. They're easier to flay while still warm, but I like to do them in batches, a few handfuls every morning as a sort of meditation, until the whole lot is naked (I cook and produce larger quantities in one go, two or three times a year). Use the charred shells as window-box mulch, or compost them; you can make tea out of them for a cocoa-flavoured infusion if you like, but you'll be maximising your acrylamide intake too, which isn't recommended. Prior to grinding, the shelled seeds should be stored in a glass container which is sealed or at least covered, and kept away from strong odours, because Cacao readily absorbs other smells.

To grind the seeds, a *metate* is required. Larger batches may be processed in a chocolate grinder or *melangeur*. But hand-grinding on the *metate* will produce a superior product, as explained in Chapters 2 and 4. In Mexico, the *metate* is often just placed in the sun for a while before working, and lit coals may be arranged underneath it to provide continual gentle heat and prevent it from cooling down completely. Putting the *metate* outside in the sun to heat it up works very well in tropical Mexico but is mostly counterproductive in England, so heating it in the oven becomes necessary. The *metate* and *mano* must first be warmed up in an oven heated to 175°C/347°F/Gas Mark 3, and left in there for an hour or so. Put the *mano* nearer the bottom of the oven as you will need this to cool down faster, because you hold it in your hands!

The toasted Cacao beans should be placed on the same shelf as the *mano* in a heatproof glass bowl, to warm them through for about twenty minutes—the idea is not to cook them further, just to heat them up; if a little further cooking does occur, so long as you've erred on the side of caution while toasting your beans, no harm done! Warming the beans isn't critical when working with a *metate*, as the grinding surface is hot, but is absolutely necessary when using a *melangeur*—cold Cacao seeds take a long time to liquefy, and may cause the machine to seize up if added in large quantities. Hervé Robert recommends not overheating the *metate* as it can spoil the flavour;[1045] conversely, I recommend heating it up a lot so the stone is baked through, then allowing it to cool sufficiently before you begin work, so the *metate* and *mano* should be taken out of the oven and left to cool for approximately twenty to thirty minutes before starting to grind. Tea lights (small candles) can be arranged underneath the *metate* on a trivet to provide steady warmth and prevent it cooling down while working. The upper surface of the *metate* should be just over blood-warm when beginning to work, not so hot that it further cooks the beans, but sufficiently hot that it liquefies the cocoa butter in the seeds and facilitates the work. The *metate* should be placed on a stable, heatproof and resilient surface so it doesn't slide around or damage the floor; a cushion or folded cloth may be placed at the foot of the *metate* to kneel on while working.

The toasted Cacao seeds may be added at the head of the *metate* a couple of handfuls at a time, and worked down the surface until liquid cocoa liquor starts to collect above the lip at the foot of the slope. Using a *metate* is highly labour-intensive, and there's a knack to it; professional athletes and weightlifters have nothing on the experienced señoras of Central America who can grind corn on a *metate* in a matter of minutes, while a *gringo* (such as I) may struggle for an hour or more to produce a sorry pile of mangled grains and the early warning signs of repetitive strain injury. Keep at it until a smooth, liquid consistency is achieved; scrape the liquid off into a ceramic or glass bowl, add more beans, and start again. When all the beans have been ground to liquid, pulverised spices may be mixed in; then the liquid with the spices is ground thoroughly a second time, and—if necessary—a third. The resulting liquid should be mirror-smooth, with no visible grains or (worse) lumps. By this time you will have been work-ing for anything from a couple of hours to a whole day, depending on the quantity of beans you're processing.

The spices must be properly prepared; some may need to be toasted, then all should be ground to a fine powder and sifted to remove lumps. Spices are best pulverised in a practical mortar and pestle or an electric mill, or using a combination of the two. The type of mortar and pestle I recommend are large granite ones, suitable for working hard materials, not the dinky, decorative ceramic types that are widely sold, and can just about handle small quantities of soft pastes. While spices can be reserved as dry powder and added to the Cacao immediately before making it into a beverage, this lazy method will produce inferior chocolate. All sources agree that adding the spices to freshly-ground cocoa liquor and grinding a second or third time produces a smoother drink with a better flavour—and no wonder, as the spices are being further pulverised and mixed with the warm liquid fats in the cocoa liquor, dispersing and mingling their flavour with the Cacao, which is a consummate odour-absorber. But I would recommend not adding any spices to any Cacao ground in a *melangeur*, a type of mechanical Cacao-grinder with granite grinding surfaces, unless you will be adding the same spice blend to your chocolate every time: the spice aromas will permeate the stone and flavour any future chocolate unless the *melangeur* is very well cleaned, and *melangeurs* are harder to clean than *metates*. Rather, grind a smaller quantity of beans separately on the *metate* and add an enormous quantity of spice to this; then, when grinding is complete, a small amount of the super-spiced hand-ground Cacao from the *metate* may be added to a larger quantity of plain Cacao from the *melangeur* to produce a beverage.

Once the Cacao has been ground, it may be poured into tablet moulds—or, far easier, directly onto sheets of greaseproof paper on a flat surface. Don't use ordinary paper, unless you enjoy papier-mâché-flavoured chocolate, and don't use wax paper, unless you want wax-flavoured chocolate, and don't use foil, unless you feel you need more aluminium in your diet. If you want a more environmentally friendly non-stick surface, de Ledesma recommends using evergreen or shiny-surfaced non-toxic leaves such as *pozole* leaves (*Calathea lutea*) here; banana leaves (*Musa spp.*) would do as well. If the ground Cacao is poured carefully, the little round puddles will set in the form of slim discs or wafers of chocolate, much easier to break up and make into drinks than chunky moulded tablets. These should be left to stand at room temperature for up to several days, depending on the ambient temperature. The Spanish chronicler Gonzalo Fernández de Oviedo y Valdés suggested that "The longer the cake was let stand, the higher the quality of the beverage product."[1046] In temperate latitudes such as the UK, this setting and proofing time is shorter; in winter, twenty-four hours is sufficient to allow complete hardening.

The opposite of what a confectioner wants to see often occurs: "bloom", or the appearance of white swirls, bubbles, or ripples of discolouration on the surface of the set cocoa liquor, formed as cocoa butter crystallises out from the cooling mass. There's no need for "tempering" to achieve a glossy texture when the Cacao tablets are going to be used to make drinks; besides, the designs produced by the precipitating swirls of lipids are beautiful and unique, being affected by temperature and small variations in the processing of the seeds. A matte appearance, an inflexible and brittle texture, and often some marbling or patterning on the surface show that the tablets are ready for storage. They may then be wrapped in non-coated greaseproof or prachment paper—I usually use the paper they are poured onto—wrapped again in foil, then stored in sealed, airtight, and odour-proof boxes, and refrigerated. In my experience the flavour of beverages produced from *fermentado* tablets seems to improve over several months' storage; the opposite appears to be true for tablets made from Cacao *lavado*.

The Maya were reputed to have drunk their *kakawa* hot, while the Mexica drank their *cacahuatl* cool.[1047] For making *kakawa*, hot water may be poured directly onto broken-up Cacao tablets or cocoa liquor fresh off the *metate* in a high-sided mixing vessel (a wide-necked jug or a bowl), then frothing it with a whisk or a *molinillo*. When making *cacahuatl*, it's worth remembering that "cool" in this context means "room temperature", and room temperature in Central America is often around 20–30°C (68–86°F). This is still below the average melting point of cocoa butter at 34°C (93°F), so the Cacao must either be in a liquid state already or, if dry tablets or discs of Cacao are being used, a smaller amount of hot water added first to melt the Cacao discs before adding the rest of the water. Very cold water should never be used, as this would further harden the fats in the Cacao and prevent it from dispersing in the liquid. If making the beverage from cocoa liquor, a little water at a time can be added and well mixed in to emulsify and incorporate it, and the process repeated until enough water has been added and the liquid is ready to be frothed (see later in this chapter for recipes).

Authentic atoles *and contemporary Cacao*

Before resuscitating some recipes for contemporary Cacao-based *atoles*, we first need a basic recipe. A white or yellow maize variety is normally used; Hernández calls for eight parts water, six parts maize, and one part lime. "Parts" means approximate volume, as in eight cupfuls of water to six cupfuls of fresh maize kernels to one cupful of lime.[1048] Lime, or *cal*, is available from Mexican and Guatemalan markets, and is sold on specialist online stores. It's cooked with maize to soften the grains—and, as recounted in Chapter 1, this improves the nutritional profile of maize as well as creating the characteristic "tortilla flavour" of nixtamalized corn. The water should be tasted when maize is being cooked with lime, and once it no longer tastes "spicy" and the corn develops a reddish tint, it's ready.[1049] The cooked corn is then rinsed well to get rid of any remaining lime or grit, then ground (with a little added water, if necessary) to produce a smooth dough or *masa* for making tortillas, tamales, or *atoles*. The cooked corn can also be dehydrated and ground to powder, making *masa harina*, a storable nixtamalized maize flour.

Many *atoles* are also made with non-nixtamalized maize, which is less nutritious but has a slightly sweeter taste, so for these recipes the lime should be omitted. Culinary researcher and author Diana Kennedy defines *atoles* as "a gruel ... traditionally prepared from dried corn that has been barely cooked, without lime, and ground to a fine masa".[1050] In fact fresh and dried, nixtamalized and non-nixtamalized corn are all used in the recipes below. In any case, maize should be cooked until soft, then drained, well-rinsed, and ground to a fine dough or tortilla *masa* by machine, or on the *metate*. This dough is then boiled with water in a clay jar; sometimes the resulting gruel is filtered to produce a kind of hot "corn milk" for some of the higher-grade *atoles*, but very often the boiled and unfiltered gruel is the finished product, known as *iztal atolli* to the Mexica, today's *atole blanco*. Several Mexica *atolli* recipes are recorded, including the sweet *nequatolli*, made by adding agave syrup; *iztac atolli*, with chilli, salt, and tomato; an *atolli* made with partly fermented dough and chilli, called *xocoatolli*; and *izquiatolli*, made by adding toasted ground maize and chilli,[1051] highly recommended for depressed dyspeptics.

1. Simple Cacao-based atoles

i) Pozol

Pozol is a cool and refreshing semi-ubiquitous *atole* in Mexico, especially popular on the hot and humid east coast. It's not to be confused with *pozole*, a hot Mexican soup or stew containing *hominy*, or toasted nixtamalized maize. *Pozol* was known as *posolli* by the Maya, and the pre-pared dough was often made into balls and packaged in the large, tough leaves of *Calathea lutea* for storage or fermentation. The same leaves are still used for wrapping tamales and other foods for cooking and preservation. There are several varieties of *pozol*, including a plain maize-based version, a "sourdough" fermented version, and the Cacao-based variety below, which can also be made with soured maize. Herbalist Tomas Villanueva from Puyucatengo outside Mexico City recounted drinking *pozol* made from fermented maize and Cacao "like water" while living in Tabasco.[1052] Claudia, the tour guide at the Haçienda La Luz Cacao plantation in Tabasco, said that many poor people eat only one meal a day, at midday, and use *pozol* as both breakfast and dinner[1053]—which, given the probable benefits of Cacao and caloric restriction for longevity, may help to partially offset the detrimental effects of poverty on life expectancy, depending on how much sugar is added to the beverage.

For most *atole* recipes, I don't insist on using a *metate y mano* to grind the Cacao—an electric or manual grinder is fine; and I would certainly suggest that maize be ground by machine rather than by hand if making *atole* from scratch. Grinding corn on a *metate* doesn't noticeably improve the flavour of the final product, so doing all the hard labour by hand just feels like masochism; and any *atole*, however elaborate, only features Cacao as one of many ingredients, and doesn't put it centre stage—the combination of ingredients means that the subtle flavour-refinement of *metate*-ground Cacao will be barely noticeable in most recipes, so why make life harder than it needs to be?

Note that quantities aren't given, because my source—a street vendor of *pozol* in Palenque who preferred to remain anonymous—said the ratios were *al gusto*—"to taste". Generally three or more parts maize to one part Cacao seems to be standard. This ratio is v/v, or "volume : vol-ume", rather than w/w (weight : weight, e.g., 30 grams : 10 grams) or w/v (weight : volume, e.g., 50 grams to one cup); in other words, three cups maize to one cup of Cacao. Versions made with soured maize have the additional benefit of being probiotic, containing various "friendly bacteria" including *Lactobacillus* and *Bifidobacterium* species,[1054] but only if made with cool or tepid water—because boiling water kills microbes. Consuming basic, unsweetened and unfermented *pozol* or tortillas reduced the negative impact of sugar-water on blood fats and pre-diabetic markers in a rat model of metabolic syndrome, and some of the bacteria in fermented *pozol* have additional blood sugar-lowering properties, so soured *pozol* may be even more beneficial.[1055]

Ingredients:
- Tortilla *masa* (see above for instructions on how to cook maize with lime: overcook the corn so it's very soft for this recipe), 3 parts (by volume)
- *Criollo* Cacao *fermentado* seeds, 1 part (by volume)
- Water
- Optional: *panela* or *piloncillo* sugar, to taste
- Ice cubes.

Equipment:
- Clay *comal*, for toasting Cacao
- *Metate* y *mano*, or manual or electric grinder for grinding Cacao (and maize, if preparing maize *masa* from scratch)
- Earthenware, glass, or china bowl, jar, or receptacle with a lid, for fermenting the *masa*, if desired
- Large earthenware, clay, or glass receptacle or tureen with a lid for mixing and serving the *pozol*.

Instructions:
The *pozol masa* can be made from scratch, by grinding the corn with a little water to make a damp but not sticky dough. Or, cheat: purchase *masa harina* (nixtamalized maize flour) and reconstitute it by making a dough with tepid water—just add a little water at a time and knead by hand. It should go without saying that hands and equipment must be scrupulously clean, especially if fermenting the *pozol*, as any organisms on your hands will be transferred to the dough and potentially be replicating in it. Keep adding tepid water and kneading until a soft, uniform, non-sticky dough is achieved. Good quality *masa harina* can be hard to find outside the Americas, though: most of the cheaper brands with international distribution are bleached, lack depth of flavour, and smoke when heated; and, for those who worry about such things, they're often made with genetically modified maize. Real, high-quality *masa harina* has a distinctive, "corny" smell, some natural speckling (not a uniform, sugary white appearance, which indicates a high degree of processing), gradually tans in the pan when dry-heated, and doesn't smoke until it's on the verge of burning. It has a vastly superior taste. Look for organic or at least unbleached whole *masa harina*, or make your own (it's easier to buy in bulk.)

For soured *atole*, cover the *masa* with a clean damp cloth to prevent it drying out and leave in a covered (but not airtight) earthenware, ceramic, or glass jar for one to three days. Even better, use a similar receptacle with some sort of airlock (so that air can escape, but not get in: a simple example is a crockpot for making *sauerkraut*, with a water-seal). After this time the dough should be checked: it should have a sour, somewhat vinegary smell but be free of mould or slime. If signs of decay or "off" smells are present, discard the *masa*, wash everything thoroughly with soapy water, sterilise the equipment by immersing in and rinsing well with boiling water, and begin again! Soured *atole* is often drunk to improve gut health and prevent diseases in Tabasco, with the caveat that people with very weak immune systems, such as those on chemotherapy, immunosuppressant drugs, or living with HIV should exercise caution, as ordinarily non-harmful microbes can cause a problem for such people. In these cases it may be best to stick to non-soured *pozol*. People with normal-functioning immune systems are more likely to benefit from the naturally fermented drink.

The Cacao is to be toasted, shelled, and ground. The liquid Cacao is then added to the maize *masa*—whether fermented or unfermented—and kneaded in very well. If your prepared Cacao is in the form of dried tablets, grind it to a homogenous paste or melt it first before mixing with the *masa*; the idea is to achieve a smooth, well-blended dough, not a gritty mess. Once the *pozol* dough is well mixed with the Cacao, the dough may be broken up, dropped into the mixing and serving receptacle. A little *panela/piloncillo* may be added just prior to mixing with water, if desired. If a little water is added at first and mixed in, then more water is added bit by bit as you mix, the dough will incrementally transition from a solid to a paste to a thick liquid to a lump-free beverage. Once the beverage is made, chill it in the fridge. Ice may be added to the finished *pozol*, if desired.

ii) *Champurrado*

Champurrado is a hot Cacao-based *atole* which has been Westernised with the addition of milk, sugar, cinnamon, and sometimes eggs and nuts. It has a thicker texture than *pozol* and is traditionally served as a breakfast drink, and is particularly welcome in mountainous regions where the nights and early mornings can be very cold, although the contemporary Mexican trend of sweetening everything until your teeth hurt is evident in most local variants of this semi-liquid chocolate porridge. The version given below is my standard breakfast version, which omits the additions of milk, eggs, and nuts, beefs up the Cacao content, and drastically reduces the sugar to produce a more savoury version of something approaching a pre-conquest Mesoamerican drink, but made from ingredients which are accessible to someone living outside the Americas! Champurrado is much more suitable for cooler climes than *pozol*, which is a great hot-weather drink.

Ingredients (serves one):
* 3–4 tablespoons good quality, unbleached yellow or white *masa harina*
* 20g (6–7 drams) prepared *criollo* Cacao *fermentado* (freshly made cocoa liquor, or pulverised/ grated tablets or discs)
* Ground spices, to taste (see below for ideas)
* One large mugful/½ litre of water (or, if desired, low-protein plant milk, e.g., almond, oat, or coconut)
* Sweetener: 1–3 teaspoons of *piloncillo* or *panela*, honey (or, if desired, maple syrup), to taste
* Optional: ⅕ teaspoon powdered stevia leaf, half a grated and toasted *mamey* seed.

Equipment:
* Enamelled or stainless steel pan
* Earthenware or ceramic jug for whisking
* Whisk.

Instructions:
Optionally—grate and quickly toast half a *mamey* seed, and set aside with ¼ of the *masa harina*. *Mamey* seed isn't a traditional ingredient of *champurrado* but it is a native Mesoamerican ingredient which adds a nice almondy undertone. Put ¾ of the *masa harina* in the pan, and toast it gently over a medium flame. When it achieves a light golden tan and smells like popcorn, add the rest of the *masa harina* (and toasted *mamey* seed powder, if using), pour in the water (or plant milk), whisk immediately and thoroughly to break up any lumps. If using milk, unsweetened oat or almond or coconut milk is recommended rather than soy milk because the higher protein content of the latter will reduce the health benefits of the Cacao—see Chapter 4 for the explanation.

Turn the heat up and bring it to a boil, whisking occasionally to prevent the *masa* from settling at the bottom of the pan, and sticking or burning. Meanwhile, grate or break up the Cacao and add to the jug—or just pour it in if freshly ground. Add spices, a pinch of powdered *Stevia* leaf, if using, and any sweeteners, such as a teaspoon or two of ground *panela*, honey, or maple syrup. Spices can include cinnamon, nutmeg, or aniseed, but I prefer indigenous Mesoamerican spices: I use my own blend of vanilla pods, chillies, toasted allspice berries, toasted *rosita de Cacao* flowers (see *tejate* recipe later in this chapter for instructions on how to toast the flowers), toasted magnolia flower petals and annatto seeds, ground to a fine powder.

Once the *masa harina* and water (or plant milk) comes to a boil, take it off the heat and pour it onto the Cacao, spices, and sweetener in the jug. Stir and whisk it well with a whisk or *molinillo*. It makes a moderately thick, soupy, barely sweet chocolate-cereal gruel which can be served in a bowl or wide-necked mug, on its own or accompanied by *tostadas* or other savoury biscuits for dipping (I favour home-made oatcakes—unsweetened biscuits made from rolled oats and water. I use flax and chia seeds as binding agents, so they contain no added oil).

iii) *Panecito* and *pinole*

These beverages are very common in Guatemala, particularly in the Suchitquepez region, although various forms of *pinole* may be found all over Central America. These are the "instant" *atoles* of the region, sold as bags of dried powder that may be stored for many months, and whisked into hot water to produce a quick meal replacement or accompaniment. Much like *pozol* in Tabasco, they serve as staple foods: *panecito* and *pinole* maker Señora Lopreto of San Antonio Suchitequepez in Guatemala, who gave me the recipes below, said that for herself and her daughter *panecito* is their daily breakfast, and *pinole* is usually drunk at lunchtime.[1056] This makes pharmacological sense, because *panecito* contains a higher proportion of caffeine-containing Cacao, whereas *pinole* is made with a lower proportion of *pataxtle* (*Theobroma bicolor*) instead of Cacao, which contains much lower levels of xanthine alkaloids—so the morning drink is more stimulating than the afternoon drink, providing a stepped dosage of stimulant-laced nutrition throughout the day. *Panecito* incorporates cinnamon, which isn't a native spice; but the recipe is so nearly fully native, so simple and delicious that I couldn't not include it! Besides, cinnamon has a number of medicinal properties, not least that it helps improve insulin sensitivity[1057] and is traditionally used to improve circulation, so it's likely to augment many of Cacao's health benefits if the beverage isn't over-sweetened.

The following recipes are instructions on how to make the powdered versions of *panecito* and *pinole*, for storage; details of how to make the powders into a drink are given after both recipes.

Panecito

Ingredients (bulk):
- Dried yellow maize kernels, 3lb/1.36kg
- *Criollo* Cacao *fermentado* seeds, 1lb/454g
- Whole dried cinnamon quills, 2oz/57g
- And, for making the *atole*:
  - Water
  - Optional: sweetener, such as dried powdered whole Stevia leaf, *panela*.

Equipment:
- Large *comal*, for toasting Cacao and corn
- Electric or manual mill or grinding machine, capable of handling larger quantities of coarse material, or a good food processor and/or hand-grinder for smaller quantities
- And, for making the *atole*:
  - Flour sifter or fine sieve
  - Bowl (for sifting powder into)
  - Mortar and pestle or smaller electric spice mill
  - Whisk or *molinillo*
  - High-sided jug or jar.

Instructions:
Toast the maize on the *comal* or in a pan until the grains tan and begin to caramelise. Keep the heat low and the process slow—popcorn isn't the goal! Then toast the Cacao, and shell the beans. Put the toasted corn, the toasted and shelled Cacao, and the cinnamon through the grinder. In Guatemala this is often done in bulk by taking the ingredients to a local mill; for kitchen cooks, scale down the quantities and grind them coarsely in a robust electric mill or food processor. For those who don't have fancy food processors, metal hand-cranked grinders may be purchased online, and the ingredients passed through these: two or three times should suffice. The result will be a fine, light brown dusty powder, with a delicious cereal-chocolate-cinnamon smell, which tends to clump a little on storage owing to the natural fat content of the Cacao.

Pinole

Ingredients (bulk):
- Dried yellow maize kernels, 3lb/1.36kg
- Raw *pataxtle (Theobroma bicolor)* seeds, ½lb/227g

- And, for making the *atole*:
  - Water
  - Optional: sweetener, such as dried powdered whole Stevia leaf, *panela*.

Equipment:
- Large *comal*, for toasting Cacao and *pataxtle*
- Electric or manual mill or grinding machine, capable of handling larger quantities of coarse material, or a good food processor and/or hand-grinder for smaller quantities
- And, for making the *atole*:
  - Whisk or *molinillo*
  - High-sided jug or jar.

Instructions:
As for *panecito*, toast the maize and the *pataxtle* seeds, then shell the *pataxtle*. Put the toasted corn and the toasted and shelled *pataxtle* through the grinder/food processor to make a fine powder with an appealing, cereal-like odour and pale beige colour.

To make one large serving of *panecito* or *pinole*, add two level tablespoons of either powder to a high-sided jar or jug. Sweetening such as *panela* may be added to taste, though I prefer to add just a pinch of dried *Stevia* whole leaf powder, and a pinch of chilli powder (the spice isn't traditional, but it goes well in both *atoles*). Note that Cacao is bitter, whereas *pataxtle* has a milder, more nutty taste, so slightly more Stevia or sweetener should be used to make *panecito*. Because *panecito* tends to clump on storage, you will need a flour sifter or sieve and a large bowl to sift out the lumps; then, re-grind the lumps to powder using a mortar and pestle or small mill, and sift them again. *Pinole* tends not to clump in this way owing to its lower fat content. Once you have a lump-free, optionally sweetened and spiced powder, pour on two mugfuls or one bowlful of boiling water—around ¾ of a pint/750ml. Froth the liquid very well using a *molinillo* or whisk. Allow it to stand and cool a bit—both beverages are usually drunk at room temperature in Guatemala, so you may wish to cover the jug and leave it for a while, although in colder climates they're best drunk hot. Whisk again to produce a significant froth; note that the froth on these beverages subsides rapidly, so don't expect a foamy drink. Pour into a bowl or wide-mouthed vessel to serve. Periodically stir or froth the beverage while drinking, as the maize flour tends to settle at the bottom.

iv) *Tiste*

Tiste is a popular Guatemalan cold drink, mainly consumed by *ladinos*—natives with mixed European and Mesoamerican heritage—and the list of ingredients reflects this origin, with its heinous sugar content. It's similar to *pozol* in its basic composition, as a powdered grain and Cacao mix which is dispersed in cold water, but it uses rice as the starchy base, and incorporates annatto seeds to colour the drink. I'd recommend omitting the sugar from the formula, and instead sweetening each drink to taste, in the manner of *panecito* or *pinole*, but I've replicated the original recipe here. The ingredients are used to make a powder which may be stored for several months.

Ingredients (bulk):
- Brown rice, ½lb/227g
- *Criollo* Cacao *fermentado* seeds, 1lb/454g
- Whole dried cinnamon quills, 2oz/57g
- Annatto (*Bixa orellana*) seeds, whole, 1oz/28g
- Vanilla pod, x1, chopped (optional)
- White sugar, 4lb/1.8kg (optional: preferably omitted, and substituted with a small quantity of powdered *Stevia rebaudiana* leaf, to taste).

Equipment:
- Large *comal*
- Electric or manual mill or grinding machine, capable of handling larger quantities of coarse material, or a good food processor and/or hand-grinder for smaller quantities
- Smaller spice mill or mortar and pestle
- Jug for mixing the drink
- *Molinillo* or whisk
- Cups or bowls, to serve.

Instructions:
Toast the rice to a golden-brown colour. Toast and shell the Cacao. Grind the annatto seeds in a spice mill or mortar and pestle. Then, grind the Cacao to a paste in the mill; grind again, with the toasted rice, cinnamon, powdered annatto seeds, and chopped vanilla pod added, to make a crumbly, powdery paste. If adding sugar, grind once more with the sugar to make a fine powder. Store in sealed glass jars, ideally with a desiccating pouch inside to prevent moisture-induced clumping.

To make one serving, put a tablespoon of the sugary powder—or a generous teaspoon of the unsweetened paste—in a jug. (Add a little sweetening, e.g., 1 tsp *panela* or honey at this point if you are using the sugar-free base.) Pour on a glassful of tepid water, a little at a time, mixing each time you add water. When a whole glassful of water has been added, whisk with the *molinillo*. It may be served immediately, or left to stand for fifteen to twenty minutes, then whisked again. Pour the beverage into a glass to serve—it should appear "as a brownish red liquid with half an inch of foam on the top".[1058]

2. Complex Cacao-based drinks

i) *Tejate* (a Zapotec recipe)

This famous Oaxacan *atole* is prepared in quantity in the early hours of the morning by women in villages outside town. Vendors stand at random street corners and intersections in the markets of Oaxaca city, easy to pass by if you don't know what you're looking for; they stand behind tables laden with large *cazuelas* or plastic tubs filled with nut-coloured liquid and a sudsy-looking beige blancmange; the "froth" on top are actually fluffy glaciers of aromatic fat that melt deliciously in the mouth. Such an elaborate drink made with indigenous ingredients is clearly of ancient origin. This recipe was donated and demonstrated by Señora Crispina

Navarro Gomez and her family, and like all the *atole* recipes in this section which were donated by vendors, makes a large quantity, enough to sell and serve many people; so scale it down for domestic use!

Ingredients (bulk):
- Fresh sweetcorn (maize) kernels, half a bucketful
- 15x *guacoyules*—Corozo Palm seeds (*Attalea cohune*)
- ~120 shelled *criollo* Cacao *fermentado* beans
- Handful *rosita de Cacao* (*Quararibea funebris*) dried flowers
- 1x *mamey sapote* seed (*Pouteria sapota*)
- 1x bucketful room temperature water.

Equipment:
- Wood ash, half a bucketful
- Large stockpot or clay *olla* (jar) for boiling
- Large metal colander
- Clay *comal*, for toasting
- *Metate* y *mano*
- Glazed earthenware, clay, glass, or china bowl
- Large earthenware *cazuela*, clay or china mixing bowl (holds 1–2 bucketfuls of liquid).

Instructions:
Mix the sweetcorn, wood ash, and *guacoyules* in the large stockpot; add water to cover, bring to a boil, and simmer for forty minutes or so. Strain the cooked corn through a large colander, rinsing thoroughly to disperse the wood ash. Next, pick out the *guacoyules*; they will have split during the cooking process. Select the ten best, with white insides—discard any with yellow insides. Any surplus "white inside" boiled *guacoyules* may be thrown away, or frozen and retained for use in a later batch.

Toast the Cacao beans for twenty to thirty minutes on a warm *comal*, moving them all the time (see instructions for preparation, above). Remove them from the *comal*, shell the beans, then set them aside. Next, pluck the stamens and styles (stringy central bits in the flower cones) from the dried *rosita* flowers, and set aside. Toast the flower cones for a couple of minutes, then add the stamens and styles and toast for a further minute. Remove from the *comal*, and set aside. Then, crush the *mamey* seed flat: put it in a plastic sandwich or zip-loc bag and pound it with the *mano* or a large pestle. Toast the flattened *mamey* seed on the *comal*, a minute or so each side.

Grind the ten cooked *guacoyules* to a paste on the *metate*; add the toasted *rosita de cacao* flowers and *mamey* seed and grind them altogether, to make an aromatic, yellow-white paste. Finally, add the Cacao beans, and grind to a homogenous mass. Add small palmfuls of warm water to the *metate* occasionally, so that it is well mixed in and helps form a loose, aromatic brown dough-like mass. Set aside in the small bowl, and cover. Next, purists may wish to grind the sweetcorn in batches on the *metate*; place the large bowl at the end of the metate to collect the ground corn and grind to a smooth consistency. As above, I would recommend mechanical grinding for the corn—it makes no difference to the flavour of the final product, and makes the job a lot easier! The other ingredients, however, should be ground on the *metate*, as this produces a superior product.

Knead the sweetcorn dough and the Cacao/*guacoyule* paste together by hand, then re-grind in batches on the *metate* to form an ultra-smooth pale brown mass. Place this mixture in the large bowl and add small cupfuls of room temperature water, one at a time, and mix each cupful in well before adding another. When it becomes liquid, stir with the flat of one hand (using the hand like a paddle), gently and consistently, while pouring water with the other; don't grip, squeeze, or beat the mixture. Continue adding water little by little until fats start to precipitate, then begin to pour the cups of water into the bowl from a height to aid production of the aromatic fatty froth which begins to form, and raise a good head of it.

When the bowl is full, it looks like a vaguely grey, yellow-brown to off-white liquid (depending on the proportion of Cacao relative to corn used in the recipe—the more sweetcorn, the paler it will be) with mounds of fatty scum floating in it like soft icebergs. The taste is savoury, earthy, vaguely granular, and creamy; the fatty topper dissolves deliciously on the tongue, releasing subtle flavours. Syrup (recommended: raw honey, maple syrup, or unrefined cane sugar) can be added to the drink to sweeten it before serving, if desired, but is unnecessary—it's pleasantly cereal-like without added sugar. Best served at room temperature, I recommend without ice—many outdoor vendors in Oaxaca city put ice cubes in the *tejate* in hot weather, which has the unfortunate side effect of congealing the floating fat to an unpleasantly hard consistency. This makes the drink rather like ingesting cold soup with lumps of suet, albeit more pleasant-tasting. On a hot day, I'd recommend seating the whole bowl in a larger bowl filled with crushed ice and water as a kind of insulating sleeve, rather than putting ice cubes into the *tejate* itself.

ii) *Chocolate atole*

This elaborate, foam-topped *atole* is prepared for *fiestas* and special occasions in Oaxaca, particularly in the famous textile-making town of Teotitlan del Valle. A highly labour-intensive production, the "magic ingredient" for making the foam is *cacao blanco*, the fermented seed of *Theobroma bicolor* or *pataxtle* (described and discussed in Chapters 2 and 6). Large quantities of *cacao blanco* are required to produce the foam, and it will only do so if carefully prepared—hands and utensils must be scrupulously clean and free from grease, as otherwise the finished product won't froth.[1059] If the *metate y mano* to be used for grinding *cacao blanco* has previously been used to process Cacao, and has a residual chocolatey smell, it may still have undetectable traces of cocoa butter on the surface, because granite is quite porous. To clean it, heat it well in the oven so that any fat "sweats" out of the surface, then blot the fat off with kitchen paper; wash well with a wire brush and plenty of soap in very hot water, being careful to rinse any suds off completely, and air-dry thoroughly before using.

A similar recipe is outlined in Diana Kennedy's wonderful culinary opus "Oaxaca *al gusto*" (©University of Texas Press, 2010), but this somewhat more detailed version was supplied by Doña Carina Santiago, owner of Tierra Antigua, a restaurant specialising in traditional and regional cuisine in Teotitlan del Valle.[1060] Because this is a very fine *atole*, not a meal replacement, the maize is not nixtamalized and is filtered to produce a very smooth, light *atole* base, a sort of hot "maize milk". This *atole* serves as the base of the beverage, and the cool Cacao-flavoured foam sits on top, a delightful contrast of flavour, texture, and temperature. Toasted corn was probably used instead of wheat before the Spanish conquest, but as discussed in Chapter 6, wheat was likely substituted because it assists foam formation more than maize; cinnamon is the other notable and ubiquitous post-conquest addition to the recipe. As with all the *atole* recipes in this chapter, the quantities here will serve many people, so scale it down considerably for domestic consumption! That said, the ingredients for making the foam are made into tablet form and may be stored for many months, or even longer if frozen, so it may be worth producing this quantity of "topper tablets" in one go and storing them.

Ingredients (bulk):
- For the foam topper:
  - *Cacao blanco* (fermented *pataxtle* seeds), 1kg/2lb 3oz
  - *Criollo* Cacao "*rojo*" *lavado*, 1kg/2lb 3oz
  - Brown rice, 2kg/4lb 7oz
  - Wheat grains, 1kg/2lb 3oz
  - Cinnamon quills, 1oz/28g
  - Dried yellow maize kernels, "one cup" (one mugful—not an exact measure)—for toasting
  - Optional: sweetener, to taste, e.g., *panela* or *piloncillo*.
- For the *atole*:
  - Yellow maize, 1kg/2lb 3oz—for making *masa*
  - 3L (5 pints) water
  - Optional: sweetener, to taste, e.g., *panela* or *piloncillo*.

Equipment:
- Large cheesecloth or muslin for straining
- Clay *comal*, for toasting
- Several bowls for holding and keeping ingredients separate during manufacture
- *Metate* y *mano,* and/or electric mill, grinder, or heavy-duty food processor
- Optional: high-powered blender
- Large earthenware *olla* (jar), enamelled, glass, or stainless steel pan for boiling the *atole*
- Large earthenware *cazuelas,* clay or china mixing bowls x2
- Coals or tea lights for keeping the *metate* warm
- Large *molinillo* without rings
- Calabash-bowls for scooping foam and serving.

Instructions:
To make the foam topper tablets, toast the wheat, rice, cinnamon, and one cupful of yellow maize separately on the *comal*, and set aside in two separate bowls: the rice and cinnamon are mixed in one bowl, and the maize and wheat are mixed together in another bowl. Toast the Cacao (but not the *cacao blanco*—this needs to be raw!). Peel the *cacao blanco* first—a fiddly job; be careful to remove all flaky dark skin from the seeds, and discard any that look greyish and

discoloured. Grind the *cacao blanco* seeds to a paste on a very clean room-temperature metate, and set aside. Then shell the toasted Cacao seeds, and set them aside too. Keep everything separate at this point! Heat the *metate* (outside, in tropical sun, or inside, in the oven), and place hot coals or tea lights arranged on a trivet beneath the *metate* to keep it warm—it should be just above blood-heat, but not too hot to touch or work on. First, grind the Cacao once on the *metate* to produce a coarse paste, then add the rice and cinnamon and grind them into the Cacao, then add the wheat and corn together and grind them as well, to make a homogenous chocolate-cereal mass. Finally, add the pre-ground *cacao blanco* to the *metate* and grind it in too, to make a greyish-brown paste. This order of grinding begins with the material which needs most work (Cacao) and ends with the softest (*cacao blanco*).

The ingredients may also be ground in a (very clean) electric grinder or mill: in this case, add all the grains and cinnamon together, and grind them twice or more to produce a fine powder; then add the Cacao and *cacao blanco* together, and run this through the machine once more to create the final product. This dough-like paste may now be shaped into little tablets or blocks, and set aside to dry for a few hours (in cooler climates, put them straight into the freezer or use a dehydrator to dry them out more thoroughly for storage). They may be kept for several months: put them in a paper bag to absorb excess moisture, and seal them in an odour-proof glass or non-reactive plastic airtight container and refrigerate or freeze.

To make the *atole*, soak 1kg (2lb 3oz) yellow maize overnight or for several hours. Grind the rehydrated maize twice or more to make a smooth *masa*, and mix well with 3L (5 pints) water, before straining through clean cheesecloth or muslin to make a cold "corn milk". Alternatively, blend the soaked maize and water in a high-powered blender (working in batches, making sure to portion out the corn and water evenly) before straining it. Decant the corn milk into a non-reactive enamelled, stainless steel, or clay pan or cooking jar, and place over a high heat to bring to a boil. Once boiling, turn the heat down to a simmer and skim any scum off the top; leave it to simmer for twenty minutes or so, then turn off the heat. Sweeten to taste—I prefer to leave the *atole* unsweetened, so its creamy blandness and warmth contrasts more with the sweet but dry coolness of the toasty-flavoured foam, but most people prefer the *atole* to be slightly sweetened.

Meanwhile, break up a foam-making tablet into a very clean mortar, add a little sugar or dry sweetener of choice, and grind to a fine powder to increase its surface area. Then put some of the powder into a glass, enamel, or earthenware bowl or *cazuela*, add any sweeteners (if using), and pour on a little warm water: the water should be around blood-warm, 40–60°C (104–140°F) to ensure the cocoa butter in the Cacao seeds melts. Froth briefly to break up any lumps and dissolve the sugar, then leave to sit for up to thirty minutes so that the powder infuses into the water. Then, taking a *molinillo* with no loose rings on it (as decorative rings will "cut" the foam, which we don't want) and holding it vertically above the centre of the bowl between two horizontal palms, rub the palms back and forth vigorously to raise a foam. This is hard work, as the *molinillo* needs to be rapidly rotated while not moving the head around (side-to-side) too much; foam making using *cacao blanco* is a delicate business. Raising a good head of foam may take some time. If foam isn't happening, you may need to adjust the ratio of foaming paste/tablet material to water: around two tablespoons per cup of water is approximately correct, but if the liquid looks very watery and tastes insipid, add more foaming paste, and if the mix looks very opaque or too soupy and thick, add more water. Start with a little less water, as it's better to add more water gradually than to use up more foaming tablets than you need! Build up a very large head of foam, at least twice as tall as the liquid is deep, before you allow yourself to stop.

Finally, pour the hot "corn milk" *atole* into bowls, filling them no more than halfway, and use another clean, non-greasy bowl or calabash to scoop a generous head of cool foam on top of the hot *atole*. The bowls should be served with a small spoon for eating the foam or stirring the *atole* if desired.

Alternative foam formula: I met Doña Antonia in Mercado Benito Juarez in Oaxaca city in 2008, where she was selling ready-made *chocolate atole* foaming powder. Her recipe is simpler than Doña Santiago's deluxe version, and the ratios are different:

Ingredients (bulk):
- For the foam topper:
  ○ *Cacao blanco* (fermented *pataxtle* seeds), ¼ kg (250g)/9oz
  ○ *Criollo* Cacao "*rojo*" *lavado*, ½ kg (500g)/1lb 2oz
  ○ *Masa harina* or whole-wheat flour, ½ kg (500g)/1lb 2oz.

Instructions:
Grind the *cacao blanco* first on a cool *metate*, using clean, grease-free utensils. Toast the Cacao, and shell it. Toast the *masa harina* or whole-wheat flour to a light golden colour. Grind the Cacao on a warmed *metate*, then mix with the flour and grind again; finally, grind in the *cacao blanco*. The result should be a greyish-brown, slightly clumpy powder, which may be stored as above in the fridge or freezer. To make the foam, re-pulverise the powder briefly to break up any lumps, and add one to two tablespoons to a jug or bowl, with approximately one cup of water. Whisk well, let stand for fifteen to twenty minutes, then whisk again to raise foam, as above.[1061] Also as above, adjust quantities and ratios as necessary. This basic "foam powder" is much simpler to make and contains a higher percentage of Cacao than the recipe above, but tastes less subtle and exquisite.

iii) *Chaw popox*

Chaw popox is a speciality of the humid Isthmus region in Oaxaca, some distance from the more arid and mountainous terrain of the Oaxacan heartland. Like *chocolate atole*, *chaw popox* is reserved for special occasions such as weddings and large *fiestas*, although it's also sold on market days by enterprising *señoras*, where it's popular with vendors and early morning shoppers. The following recipe was given by Señora Delfina Valverde of the little maritime town of San Mateo del Mar, but I've had to make some executive decisions about procedure in places, owing to issues of mutual comprehension as Spanish was also Señora Valverde's second language, after her native Huave (a Zapotec dialect).[1062] Sra Valverde had pre-prepared the *atole* before I arrived, so that I didn't get to see it being assembled, which would have eliminated many procedural questions. So any gaps have been filled in with Diana Kennedy's similarly sketchy account of the recipe (no disrespect intended, as without Ms Kennedy's groundbreaking research I wouldn't have known where to seek it out or what to look for—and I now fully appreciate the gaps in the recipe!)

Like *chocolate atole*, the finished beverage is a hot plain *atole* with a tepid chocolate-flavoured foam; and, also like *chocolate atole*, it's now customarily sweetened. The texture of the beverage is much less smooth than *chocolate atole*, because the *atole* isn't filtered, and the foam has a more pronounced chocolate-cinnamon taste. The dominant flavour of the beverage, unfortunately, was sugar, which rather spoiled my impression of it—so, once more, I recommend drastically reducing the added sugar. I'd also suggest barely sweetening the corn *atole* portion (if at all), to allow the natural sweetness of the corn to come through and contrast with the rich bitter-sweet Cacao-cinnamon flavour of the *panela*-sweetened foam.

Ingredients (bulk):
* *Criollo* Cacao *fermentado*, "one to four handfuls" (Diana Kennedy's source suggests "eight seeds", which seems far too little)
* Cinnamon quills, "a handful"
* Fresh outer stem bark of *n'ched (Gonolobus barbatus)*, "one handful", or a 50cm/19" strip of 1.5cm/⅔" diameter[1063]
* *Panela*, 500g/18oz or "a block"—in reality, to taste
* White sugar, 500g/18oz (optional)—to taste
* White corn, 2kg or two litres/4lb 7oz, or 3½ pints fresh or soaked (re-hydrated) corn
* Approximately 2L/3½ pints water.

Equipment:
* Clay *comal*, for toasting
* *Metate* y *mano*, and/or electric mill, grinder, or heavy-duty food processor
* Large earthenware *olla* (jar), enamelled, glass, or stainless steel pan for boiling the *atole*
* Large earthenware *cazuela*, clay or china mixing bowl for making foam
* Coals or tealights for keeping the *metate* warm
* Large *molinillo* without rings
* Calabash-bowls for scooping foam and serving.

Instructions:
Toast and peel the Cacao. Grind the fresh *n'ched* and dried cinnamon bark together once or twice on a *metate* or in an electric grinder, then add the Cacao and re-grind several times; once a smooth paste is achieved, *panela* (and, if desired—but not recommended—white sugar) may be added to taste and ground into the paste as well. Set aside; this foam-making paste may be refrigerated and stored for a week or so, or frozen and kept for longer.

To make the *atole*, soak approximately a litre or two pints (by volume) dried white corn overnight to make two litres of rehydrated corn, or weigh out approximately 2kg or 4lb 7oz of fresh white corn. Grind to a fine *masa*, adding a little water as necessary, then mix the prepared *masa* with two litres or three and a half pints of water in a clay *olla*, stainless steel or enamelled pan and bring to a boil, then turn the heat down and simmer for twenty minutes or so. The final *atole* should be slightly thicker than full-fat milk, a single cream or thin soupy consistency, but not completely smooth owing to the presence of fibre in the ground corn. If too thick, add more water!

Take a small handful of the prepared paste, break it up and drop it into the mixing bowl or *cazuela*. Pour in one or two cupfuls of tepid water, and whisk with the *molinillo* using the same technique as for *chocolate atole* above. Owing to the presence of the saponin-rich *n'ched*, it should foam more readily than the *chocolate atole* paste. Build up a large head of stable foam; if foaming isn't happening, adjust the ratios—add more paste, or more water, depending on whether the mixture is too thick or too thin. Finally, pour the hot *atole* into bowls, filling them no more than halfway, and use another bowl or calabash to serve a generous quantity of cool foam equal to the volume of *atole* on top. *Chaw popox* is normally served without any utensils, but being very similar in construction to the previous recipe, a small spoon for eating the foam would also be appropriate.

iv) *Bu'pu*

Bu'pu is a delight. Not as elaborate as *chocolate atole* yet just as refined and (in my opinion) even more delicious, this *atole* was the highlight of my time in the Isthmus region of Oaxaca. It's made and sold by ladies in the town square of Juchitan de Zaragoza from early evening, when enormous flocks of cawing birds congregate at dusk while live bands and performers strike up raucously festive Mexican tunes. The town square is surrounded by "Isthmus Jasmine" trees with white aromatic flowers releasing their subtle perfume—none other than *Bourreria huanita*, the popcorn flower, itself used in ancient Cacao-based drinks. Frangipani (*Plumeria rubra*) trees are dotted around the town centre too, with their day-glo yellow or pink five-petalled blooms, as symmetrical and perfect as artificial flowers, adding to the cocktail of scents that the warm breezes waft through the streets as the light fades, dispersing the lingering odours from the day-time street market as the last vendors pack up their stalls,leaving a shadowy warren of metal ribs and scraps of canvas.

Frangipani flowers are the special flavour ingredient and foaming agent in *bu'pu*, which, like the previous two recipes, features a hot plain *atole* with a cool and voluminous Cacao-flavoured foam on top. The foam of *bu'pu* is especially fine and fluffy, lacking the dry quality of the foam on *chocolate atole* or the slightly granular texture of *chaw popox*. Large quantities of fresh flowers are needed to produce the *atole*, so this recipe is something that can only be made in tropical regions where the frangipani grows—unless you happen to have a tropical plant greenhouse, or you're wealthy enough that you can arrange to have fresh cut tropical flowers delivered to you on demand. The flowers are sold in the market every morning, strung together in garlands or in loose mounds of petals. The red-pink blooms have a perfume a little like roses but less sweet and complex, and somehow richer; the yellow ones have a sweet smell with a lingering, rubbery pungency. Usually the two are mixed to produce *bu'pu*.

The recipe features ungodly amounts of *piloncillo* sugar, a post-colonial addition—most likely the traditional foam would have been unsweetened, made with just Cacao and frangipani flowers, bitter-tasting and much more aromatic. But I've left it as it is, because the complex caramel flavour of *piloncillo* is a large part of the appeal, quite unlike the shocking sweetness of refined sugar, and the *atole* is always served unsweetened, making a pleasant contrast between the sweet cool topping and the warm savoury beverage. Making the foaming layer without any *piloncillo* would be a worthy experiment, inverting the savoury-sweet layers of the drink while using only pre-Hispanic ingredients, although omitting all the *piloncillo* sugar would greatly increase the cost of making the drink—Cacao is expensive! The following recipe was given to me by Señora Anna Maria Vasquez Garcia, one of the vendors in the town square with the most regular customers;[1064] her daughter also makes and sells *bu'pu*.

Ingredients (bulk—serves 200!):
- For the foam topper:
  - *Piloncillo* sugar, 32kg/70lb 9oz
  - "Red" *criollo* Cacao *fermentado* from Chiapas, 2kg/4lb 7oz
  - Fresh *cacalosúchil* (frangipani flowers, *Plumeria rubra*), yellow and red, one full carrier bag
  - Sun-dried *cacalosúchil* (frangipani flowers, *Plumeria rubra*), yellow and red, crushed, approx. two tablespoonfuls
  - Approximately 1L/1¾ pints water.
- For the *atole*:
  - White corn, 6kg/13lb 4oz
  - *Cal*, or lime powder, a handful
  - Approximately 60L/106 pints water or more, for boiling and preparing the *atole*.

Equipment:
- Clay *comal*, for toasting
- Electric mill, grinder, or heavy-duty food processor
- Large earthenware *olla* (jar), enamelled, glass, or stainless steel pan for boiling the *atole*
- Large earthenware *cazuela*, clay or china mixing bowl or clean plastic bucket for making foam
- Large *molinillo* without rings
- Calabash-bowls for scooping foam and serving
- A large, insulated storage vessel for keeping the *atole* hot.

Instructions:
Toast and peel the Cacao. Crush the *piloncillo*: lay the blocks or tablets close together in a single layer in the centre of one half of a large, quadruple-layered clean linen or cotton sheet, then fold the other half over and tuck the edges under to trap the *piloncillo* between the layered cloths. Pound it with a heavy pole to pulverise, then open the sheet and scrape the pulverised sugars into a large bucket, breaking up any clumps by hand. Alternatively, run the *piloncillo* blocks through a powerful industrial mill—or, smaller quantities may be ground by hand with a large mortar and pestle (don't try to put whole blocks in a food processor—they're rock-hard and dense, and need breaking up a bit first). Grind the fresh frangipani flowers to a paste in the mill or food processor once; add the Cacao, and grind again; then, add the dried frangipani, and grind once more, to make a smooth paste. Add this paste to the pulverised *piloncillo* in the bucket, and stir well. Then add half a litre or up to a pint of water, and stir

to mix; keep mixing and adding a little water, up to a litre or one and three-quarter pints, to make a lumpy mush. This is then ground in the mill to produce a thick, syrupy paste. This may then be stored in the refrigerator for several weeks; according to Doña Garcia, the flavour improves with storage. It needs to be refrigerated briefly to thicken it, or it isn't so easy to make foam with it.[1065]

Take the white corn and boil it in water with the lime powder for around twenty to thirty minutes. Strain, rinse, and grind the corn in a mill, adding a little water if necessary, to produce a *masa*. Mix the *masa* well with sixty litres of water, then strain it in the manner of *chocolate atole* to produce a cold "corn milk", which is then boiled and simmered for twenty minutes to produce a smooth white *atole*. This may be decanted into an insulating tureen to keep it hot.

To make the foam, add two *jicaras* or scoops of the caramel-paste and an equal quantity of water to a mixing bowl or *cazuela*, stir well, then froth with a large *molinillo* (without rings, as usual). Raise a substantial amount of foam; serve the *atole* in the usual way, with a bowl or calabash half-full of hot *atole*, and use another *jicara* (calabash or gourd-bowl) to scoop an equivalent quantity of foam on top.

v) *Atole colorado*

This recipe is adapted from Diana Kennedy's excellent "Oaxaca *al gusto*" (©University of Texas Press, 2010). It's a foaming *atole*, made in the mountain village of Benito Juarez in Oaxaca, and the foam topper is made from a powder, referred to as *pinole*—a common name for various "instant" powdered beverages, (cf. the Guatemalan *pinole* recipe earlier in this chapter)—which, like the "topper tablets" or powder for *chocolate atole* can be made in bulk (as below) and stored until needed. *Atole colorado* relies on the relatively weak foam-promoting properties of a concentrated paste made from annatto seeds, called *pasta de achiote*, in conjunction with the usual emulsified fats from Cacao and dissolved grain starches. *Achiote* paste is prepared from annatto seeds by soaking and rubbing the fresh seeds in water to extract the dye, then flushing them through with boiling water until the colour is exhausted. The resulting bright red liquid is then cooked and evaporated gently in large pans over several days to concentrate it, stirring frequently.[1066] Salt and fat are often added to the thickening liquid; eventually a solid paste results, which is moulded into discs, balls, or logs, to be used as a red food colouring and spice.

You may make your own fat-free *achiote* concentrate by purchasing dried annatto seeds and soaking them in water overnight in a non-reactive (glass, ceramic, or stainless steel) cooking pan. Note that the seeds should be a vibrant red colour—old seeds are often duller or dark red, and may cause headache or stomach-ache when ingested. Bring the soaking seeds to a boil and strain out the water into another large, non-reactive stockpot set over a low heat to evaporate it slowly. Meanwhile, re-soak the seeds in fresh water, rubbing them with gloved hands (annatto is a dye—it stains!) to help extract the colour, then re-boiling them in a separate pan, and re-filtering this liquid into the stockpot. Repeat this until the seeds are colourless, and discard them. Evaporate the dye-infused liquid until it coats the back of a spoon, like a thin syrup, then pour this into moulds, such as ice cube trays, and freeze. Alternatively, add enough *masa harina* flour to thicken the concentrate and make a bright red dough, then roll this into balls and dehydrate until solid. Note that *achiote* balls made in the second way must be crushed before using and will not dissolve completely, but are suitable for use in *atoles* and solid foods.

Ingredients (bulk):
- For the foam topper:
  - Dry yellow corn or wheat grains, 4kg/8lb 13oz
  - "Red" *criollo* Cacao *fermentado* from Chiapas, 1kg/2lb 3oz
  - Cinnamon quills, 55g/2oz
  - *Achiote* paste, 55g/2oz
  - Optional: sweetener, to taste, e.g., *panela* or *piloncillo*.
- For the *atole*:
  - Yellow maize, 1kg/2lb 3oz—for making *masa*
  - 3L/5 pints water
  - Optional: sweetener, to taste, e.g., *panela* or *piloncillo*.

Equipment—as for chocolate atole:
- Large cheesecloth or muslin for straining
- Clay *comal*, for toasting
- Several bowls for holding and keeping ingredients separate during manufacture
- *Metate y mano*, and/or electric mill, grinder, or heavy-duty food processor
- Optional: high-powered blender
- Large earthenware *olla* (jar), enamelled, glass, or stainless steel pan for boiling the *atole*
- Large earthenware *cazuelas*, clay or china mixing bowls x2
- Coals or tea lights for keeping the *metate* warm, if using
- Large *molinillo* without rings
- Calabash-bowls for scooping foam and serving.

Instructions:
Toast and shell the Cacao. Toast the wheat or yellow corn grains, and toast the cinnamon. Grind all together on a pre-heated *metate* or in a grinder or mill, or heavy-duty food processor; again, if using a *metate*, grind the Cacao once first before adding the grains and cinnamon, but if machine-grinding run the grains and cinnamon through the machine first, then add the Cacao and process once more. Finally, grind in the *achiote*, which should give the resulting powder a vibrant red colour. This powder may be kept in a sealed glass jar for several months, or even longer if refrigerated; ideally add a desiccating agent, such as a silica pouch, to prevent the powder from clumping.

To make the *atole*, pre-soak 1kg or 2lb 3oz yellow maize, then grind twice or more to make a smooth *masa* and mix well with 3L water; or rinse the soaked maize, mix with three litres or five pints of water and blend the whole lot in a high-powered blender. Strain through clean cheesecloth or muslin, and place the strained *atole* over a high heat to bring to a boil; remove the scum and simmer for twenty minutes or so, then turn off the heat. Sweeten to taste.

To make the foam, take some of the red powder and put it into a bowl—locals use a clay bowl called an *apostle*[1067]—and add tepid water. One cup or 250ml (just under half a pint) of powder makes ten servings of foam, so scale accordingly. Add enough water to make a "thin paste", stir and leave to infuse for an hour. Then, add sweetening to taste, and froth with the *molinillo*. Serve in the usual way: scoop the cool red foam on top of the hot white *atole*.

vi) *Popo* (a Chinantecan recipe)

Popo is a tepid foaming drink sold in western Oaxaca and in the state of Veracruz on the south-west coast of Mexico. Or, rather, it's more than one drink—there are at least four (and probably many more) recipes for *popo*, all variants on the same theme. Unlike other very foamy *atoles*, *popo* doesn't separate the body of the drink and the foam—both are made together, as one homogenous liquid which is frothed up; moreover, the whole beverage is completely filtered, unlike the other recipes which tend to include at least some unfiltered plant material. All variants require one of three botanical foaming agents: the fresh root bark or fruit peel of *chupipe* (*Gonolobus niger*), *cocolmeca*, the fresh young stems of either *Smilax aristolochiifolia* or *Aristolochia laxiflora,* or *azquiote* (*Smilax aristolochiifolia*). Again, the foaming agents need to be fresh, making it difficult to acquire or use them outside the country unless you have the facilities for growing tropical plants.

All the recipes follow a similar protocol, having the foaming agent ground together with a sweet and starchy grain (corn or rice), toasted Cacao, cinnamon, and sugar to make a paste. This aromatic mass is then kneaded and strained in water through a straining bag, which—after multiple infusions—is discarded, and the resulting emulsion is then frothed. I've given two formulas for *popo*, one from Acuyacan in Veracruz on the west coast, and the other from Tuxtepec further inland in Oaxaca, representing the very different formulations which can exist for drinks of the same name and similar physical characteristics. As with other foaming beverages, my informants reiterated that utensils, bowls, and hands must be very clean and free from any traces of grease so that the foaming process works properly.

a) *Popo* from Acayucan: this is a composite of the same basic recipe, given by a street vendor who preferred to remain anonymous, and Doña Maria Matei and her mother in Heuyapan de Ocampo in Veracruz, Mexico.[1068]

Ingredients (bulk):
- White rice, 2–3kg/4lb 7oz—6lb 10oz (more rice produces a cheaper but milder beverage)
- "Red" *criollo* Cacao *fermentado* from Chiapas, 1kg/2lb 3oz
- Cinnamon quills, "ten pesos worth"—approx. 2–4 sticks or 25g/<1oz
- *Panela*, "a block" or to taste
- White sugar, same quantity as *panela*, to taste (omit if desired)
- Fresh *chupipe* root or fruit peel: the peel of two fruits, or decorticated ("peeled") root—a little more than the volume of cinnamon
- Water.

Equipment:
- Large cheesecloth or muslin for straining
- Clay *comal*, for toasting
- Dehydrator or low-temp oven, with baking parchment—or a *petate* and a sunny terrace
- Electric mill, grinder, or heavy-duty food processor
- Optional: high-powered blender
- Large earthenware *cazuelas*, clay or china mixing bowls
- Large *molinillo* without rings
- Calabash-bowls for serving.

Instructions:
Wash the rice in running water, then spread it out to dry—in Mexico, this can be done in the sun; in cooler climates, a dehydrator or low-temperature oven may be necessary. Toast the cinnamon and break it up. Toast and shell the Cacao. Crush the fresh *chupipe* root and discard outer bark (if the outer bark is retained, it will impart a bitter taste to the beverage); or, cut up the peel of two *chupipe* fruits. Grind the rice and cinnamon together in a high-powered or mechanical mill once; then re-grind, with the Cacao and either the crushed *chupipe* root or chopped fruit peel. If the paste which emerges is lumpy or granular, grind again to produce a homogeneous beige-brown dough. This dough can be frozen to preserve it until needed, or kept in the fridge for a few days.

To make the beverage, break off a good handful or two of the *popo* dough and drop into a mixing bowl or *cazuela*. Add tepid water to produce a thin soupy consistency and mix well, then strain the liquid through clean cheesecloth or muslin into another bowl, wringing it out very well to create a ball of strained-out material in the cloth. Squeeze the cloth-wrapped bolus of strained plant material around in the water to extract as much as possible, and then pour the liquid back through the squeezed-out plant material and wring out again. Repeat several times to maximally extract the flavours and constituents from the dough, and make the liquid as well-infused and concentrated as you can, then discard the exhausted plant material. Sweeten the expressed liquid to taste with crushed *panela* (and white sugar, if using), to taste—or omit. Finally, take a *molinillo* and froth to produce as much foam as possible, about twice the volume of the liquid. Decant some liquid and froth into bowls, calabashes, or cups to serve, with a ratio of one part liquid to two parts foam; scoop extra foam on top, as desired.

b) *Popo* from Tuxtepec: this version uses *pataxtle*, known locally as *cacao cimarrón* in place of Cacao, and replaces *chupipe* with *cocolmeca/azquiote*. It was given by *popo* vendor Doña Rosa Gregorio from Ojitlan, Oaxaca, Mexico.[1069]

Ingredients (bulk):
- Nixtamalized yellow corn *masa*, 2.5kg/5lb 8oz
- Raw *pataxtle* or *"cacao cimarrón"* (*Theobroma bicolor*) seeds, ½ kg/1lb 2oz
- Fresh *cocolmeca/azquiote* (*Sarsaparilla aristolochiifolia*) young shoots/tender stems, harvested before the leaves appear: "two carrier bags", or approximately three long stems (three separate young plants)

- Sweetening, to taste: *panela*, *piloncillo*, or white sugar, up to 1.5kg/3lb 5oz (may be omitted)
- Water.

Equipment:
- Large cheesecloth or muslin for straining
- Clay *comal*, for toasting
- Dehydrator or low-temp oven, with baking parchment—or a *petate* and a sunny terrace
- *Metate* y *mano*, and/or electric mill, grinder, or heavy-duty food processor
- Large earthenware *cazuelas*, clay or china mixing bowls
- Large *molinillo* without rings
- Calabash-bowls for serving.

Instructions:
Prepare the nixtamalized *masa*—soak yellow corn overnight, strain, boil with lime in the usual volumetric ratios (of 8 water : 6 corn : 1 lime) described earlier in this chapter, then rinse well and grind the corn to make the dough. Or, cheat: buy *masa harina* flour, reconstitute with sufficient water, and knead well to make a pliable, non-sticky dough. Let the dough rest for a while before making *popo* (thirty minutes to a few hours), leaving it in a cool place in a lidded glass or clay jar or pot, covered with a damp cloth to prevent it drying out.

Toast and shell the *pataxtle* seeds. They're toasted on a *comal* in the same way as Cacao, over a medium heat for approximately twenty to thirty minutes, and should be pale beige to light golden brown inside once toasted, not dark like Cacao—you're not making coffee! Then, lightly roast the whole fresh *cocolmeca* stems: place them on hot embers for thirty seconds to a minute each side, or very briefly pan-fry in a hot dry pan; the outside of the stems should be very lightly or barely charred, so that they're heated through but still look quite raw inside, like lightly cooked asparagus. Chop the *cocolmeca* into small chunks, then grind the shelled *pataxtle* and chopped *cocolmeca* twice on the *metate* or in the mill to make a smooth brown paste. This *pataxtle-cocolmeca* paste should then be kneaded well into the prepared corn *masa*, by hand, adding a little water if necessary. Once the dough is well-mixed—a uniform colour, with no marbling—the whole lot should be ground together once more. This dough can be frozen for several months, or stored for two to three days in the fridge before using.

Make the beverage in the same way as the previous version. Mix a handful or two of the *popo* dough with enough tepid water to produce a thin soupy consistency, then strain the liquid through clean cheesecloth or muslin into another bowl, wringing it out well and then kneading it in the liquid; pour the liquid back through the squeezed-out plant material and squeeze it again and again to make the extract as concentrated as possible. Discard the squeezed-out dry material. Sweeten the liquid to taste, froth with a *molinillo*, and serve.

vii) *Batido*

The last contemporary Cacao-based drink is a throwback to pre-Colombian *kakawa* or *cacahuatl*. Drunk in the Kek'chi Maya heartland of Alta Verapaz in Guatemala, *batido* is a starch-free Cacao-based drink made only from indigenous plants: Cacao, vanilla, annatto, ear flower, and mamey sapote seeds. These are made into a paste which is mixed with hot water to produce the beverage.[1070] The dried ear flowers (*Cymbopetalum penduliflorum*) are still sold in the marketplaces of Coban city as *muc'*, but I had a hard time tracking them down; and, while several informants told me that many locals still drink Cacao-based beverages unsweetened and flavoured with native spices, this tradition may be dying out as the Western lifestyle metastasises into rural Guatemala and soaks up indigenous traditions like a McDonald's napkin. My main source for this recipe is a hundred-year-old paper by the anthropologist Wilson Popenoe, who reported that in 1919 *bvatido* was "offered to visitors in the same manner as coffee is served by Europeans, and huge steaming pots of it are conspicuous features of all fiestas":[1071] no more.

Quantities have been estimated, based on Popenoe's description and my experience of other Cacao-based beverages; real ratios may vary, so please experiment!

Ingredients (bulk):
- *Criollo* Cacao *lavado* seeds, 1lb/454g
- *Muc'* or ear flower (*Cymbopetalum penduliflorum*), three dried petals
- Vanilla pods, ×2
- *Achiote* (*Bixa orellana*) paste, two teaspoonfuls (optional)
- *Mamey sapote* (*Pouteria sapota*) seeds, ×2
- Water.

Equipment:
- Clay *comal*, for toasting
- *Metate* y *mano,* and/or electric mill, grinder, or heavy-duty food processor
- Mortar and pestle, or spice mill
- Calabash-bowls for mixing and serving.

Instructions:
Toast the Cacao, and shell the beans. Crush the *mamey sapote* seeds and toast on the *comal*; cut up the vanilla pods into small segments. Lightly toast the *muc'*, then grind the toasted *muc'*, *mamey*, and vanilla to a paste, and set aside.

Grind half the Cacao beans to a coarse, gritty consistency, and set aside. Grind the rest of the Cacao to a smooth paste, then add the ground-up *mamey-muc'*-vanilla paste, and the *achiote* paste (if using), and re-grind. Mix the smooth, aromatic cocoa liquor with the coarsely ground Cacao to produce a gritty paste, and mould or pour into small blocks or roundels on grease-proof paper to cool. Store wrapped in greaseproof paper in airtight, odour-proof containers in a cool dry place or in the refrigerator.

To make the drink, take a teaspoonful or two of the freshly prepared paste (or pour a little boiling water on to pieces of the solid tablets to melt them) and add to a medium-sized bowl or calabash (breakfast cereal-size). Add a little warm water—must be warm enough to melt cocoa butter, so think "blood heat"—about a mugful. Stir until the paste is melted, then continue to beat gently with the hand until cocoa butter or globules of white fat start to separate and appear on top of the liquid. This manual method is also used to separate cocoa butter, and was described to me by Señora Aurelia Pop in San Luís, Peten, Guatemala; she attempted to demonstrate it using room-temperature water. But the weather was unusually cool that day (around

17°C/63°F), so the cocoa butter failed to materialise; it's important to make sure that the water is sufficiently warm. Once the paste is well mixed into the water and the fats have separated on top, the *Batido* is ready to drink. Popenoe says, "After drinking the liquid, the coarse fragments of Cacao which remain in the bottom of the *guacal* [calabash, or bowl] are tossed into the mouth and eaten … it is a murky, slightly oily liquid having a strong flavour … occasionally it is sweetened with cane sugar."[1072]

Back to the Old School

The pre-Colombian Mesoamericans were masters of Cacao-based drinks; the *atoles* above preserve only a handful of their techniques and ingredients. Bernardino de Sahagún listed a few of the Mexica Cacao preparations in the sixteenth-century "Florentine Codex".[1073]

* "Blue-green, made of tender Cacao"
* Chocolate made with wild honey
* Chocolate made with "flowers"
* Chocolate made with "blue-green" vanilla
* Chilli-red chocolate
* Pink chocolate
* Black chocolate, and
* White chocolate.

It's anyone's guess what some of these are. "Blue-green" (i.e., turquoise) doesn't mean literally blue-green, though—it's a Mexica metaphor meaning "highest quality", this being the colour of valuable jade or quetzal feathers. "Black chocolate" may simply be a plain Cacao beverage, and the "chocolate" made with wild honey, vanilla, or flowers will likely follow the basic procedure outlined below, being sweetened with honey or made with added vanilla or other floral enhancements such as *rosita de cacao* or ear flower. "Chilli-red chocolate" is likely made with chilli and *achiote* to give it a bright red colour. But pink or white chocolate are a mystery; for Westerners, "white chocolate" may conjure up images of some sort of sweet, creamy drink, like the candy, but the Mexica had neither dairy nor refined sugar. It may have been a fermented drink made from Cacao fruit pulp, or even a sort of unfermented pre-Hispanic *refresco*, produced by mixing the pale fruit pulp in water. Or maybe it was a filtered white corn *atole*, topped with Cacao-flavoured foam, like modern-day *chocolate atole*. Or perhaps it wasn't even white, and the name was metaphorical—maybe it referred to the white mould that grows on re-fermented Cacao, as in Diana Kennedy's *popo* recipe above. Perhaps "pink chocolate" was a white beverage, tinted with a little *achiote* or some chilli, giving it a pink hue.

When interviewing Señora Lopreto and her daughter, manufacturers of *panecito* and *pinole* from Suchitequepez in Guatemala, mention was made of an *atole* they called *pusum* or possibly *atole de ceniza* ("*atole* of ash"), made with whole immature Cacao pods.[1074] I went looking for this *atole*, but when I found someone who knew what it was, the recipe they gave me was rather different—a much more standard combination of toasted Cacao, toasted *pataxtle* and corn, made into a foamy drink.[1075] (I didn't recount this recipe in the previous section as my informant wasn't able to give enough detail about quantities, and I didn't have enough time in town to pursue it—if this book runs to a second edition, then perhaps.) I'm still intrigued by the idea of an *atole* made with stone-ground immature Cacao pods, as that may be behind the reference to "blue-green, tender" Cacao in Sahagún's list of Mexica Cacao-based beverages; such a drink would certainly be expensive, as it would use up entire pods like other recipes used up seeds! On the other hand, the only other reference to a drink made from "green Cacao" in the codex is where Sahagún states that too much of it "makes one drunk",[1076] so it may refer to an alcoholic beverage made from fermented and slightly caffeinated Cacao fruit (see Chapter 2).

A consistent feature of the surviving recipes for the highest quality pre-Colombian Cacao-based beverages is that foam was raised separately or set aside, and replaced on the finished beverage. Plain Cacao and water in the correct ratio can be frothed, and does produce a moderately stable foam, but a huge head of detachable bubbles imputes the use of foaming agents. Several contemporary *atole* formulas given earlier in this chapter include several such additives, so I've adapted these recipes using traditional ingredients to model possible procedures for making *kakawa* or *tlaquetzalli cacahuatl*. From Sahagún's accounts, water was "added sparingly" to ground Cacao—most likely little by little, and mixed in at each stage to emulsify it, much as *tejate* is made. Then the liquid was filtered, aerated, and poured "back and forth to make foam", following which the head was removed and set aside. The remaining liquid was "thickened", and more water was stirred in, before being served and topped with the foam.[1077]

So, putting Hernández's instructions together with processes used in making contemporary foaming *atoles*, one procedure (Template 1) for reconstructing the classiest ancient Cacao-based beverages might be:

1. Two batches of Cacao are prepared (toasted, shelled, and ground on the *metate*): one is plain, or made with the addition of whichever spices are required to make the body of the drink; this batch (A) is set aside.
2. The other batch (B) to be used for making the foam is ground with spices and foaming agents, so that they are fully incorporated into a paste, to which water is added.
3. This liquid can then be filtered through a fine sieve or even squeezed through muslin or linen cloth in the manner of *popo*, or simply well mixed and allowed to sit and infuse for a while. This liquid is then frothed to produce the foam.[1078]
4. Hot or tepid water is then incrementally mixed and stirred into the first batch (A), sweetening if desired. This is then frothed, and poured into individual gourd-cups or *jicaras*.
5. Finally, the voluminous froth from (B) is scooped out and dispensed on top of the individual servings of (A).

This method of keeping the two preparations separate—the body of the drink and the foam—is borrowed from the way that contemporary *chocolate atole*, *chaw popox*, and *bu'pu* are served, with a separate *atole* and foam topper. While it doesn't strictly follow the historical procedure outlined above, making the foam-producing portion of the drink separately allows us to incorporate more foam-facilitating additives so that foam may be generated more easily; and, using this two-batch process, we can create drinks with a cool head of foam and a hot body of liquid, or vice versa, as well as being able to serve the liquid and foam portions of the drinks more easily and evenly than if the drink is mixed in one vessel. Moreover, both batches can be set as tablets and stored separately, which is much more suitable for drinks using *cacao blanco* as a foaming agent, as larger volumes of these seeds are required (a 1:2 or 2:3 ratio of *cacao blanco* : Cacao), so it makes sense to make the foaming part of the drink separate from the non-foamy body of the drink. The only drawback of this method is that when using fresh plant material such as *n'ched (Gonolobus barbatus), chupipe (Gonolobus niger)*, or *cocolmeca (Smilax aristolochiifolia)* for the foaming agents in batch (B), the resulting foam-making paste must be frozen in order to keep it for anything more than a few days. But, for traditionalists, a more purist, one-batch approach (Template 2) might be:

1. Grind the toasted and shelled Cacao once, then re-grind with the spices and foaming agents to create a smooth liquid or paste.
2. Place or pour some of this into a jar or jug and add hot or tepid water little by little to produce an emulsion, mixing thoroughly every time water is added.
3. This liquid can then be filtered through a fine sieve or even squeezed through a muslin or linen cloth in the manner of *popo*. The filtered liquid is then frothed (with a *molinillo*, or by pouring back and forth from a height) to produce a head of foam.[1079]
4. The foam is skimmed off and placed in a separate bowl or high-sided jar, while the body of the drink may be thinned with the addition of more water, or thickened with the addition of more Cacao, and mixed again.
5. Pour the body of the drink in a thin continuous stream from on high into the middle of the foam. The final product should be a vessel filled with liquid, with a tall foam topper.

1. Basic drinks

These recipes are adapted from Hernández's accounts of Mexica Cacao-based drinks. The descriptions are sketchy, lacking precise quantities or clear instructions, so I've replicated the original quantities as far as possible and filled in the blanks with experimentation or educated guesswork where necessary.

i) Atextli

This is a pre-Hispanic *atole* recipe with a much higher Cacao-to-maize ratio than later *atoles*. Like contemporary *tiste* or *panecito*, it appears to rely solely on only Cacao's fats and emulsifiers in combination with maize starch to produce a foam, but contains too much fat to produce a dry powder, making a sticky and highly aromatic dough. It also utilises the three most popular Mexica Cacao spices, which Hernández claimed would "increase lust and excitation" when combined with Cacao, whereas plain Cacao "refrigerates"; he declared that this recipe "combats all poisons, and alleviates intestinal pains and colics".[1080] Hyperbole, but with a grain of truth: the spices are carminative (reduce flatulence) and as we saw in Chapter 4, Cacao may have some protective effects against snake venom, benefits the microbiome, and has some painkilling properties.

Ingredients:
- *Criollo* Cacao *lavado* seeds, x100
- Nixtamalized yellow maize *masa*, "an equal quantity" to the Cacao (by volume)

- *Tlilxochitl* (vanilla pods), x1–2
- *Xochinacaztli* (ear flower, *Cymbopetalum penduliforum*), x2 petals
- *Mecaxochitl* (holy leaf, *Piper sanctum*) dried flower spikes, x2
- Water.

Equipment:
- Clay *comal*, for toasting
- *Metate* y *mano*, and/or electric mill, grinder, or heavy-duty food processor
- Mortar and pestle, or spice mill
- A flour sifter or fine sieve and wide bowl
- Two large, high-sided clay or earthenware vessels, for frothing, or
- One large wide-necked jug and a *molinillo*
- Calabash-bowls for serving.

Instructions:
Prepare the maize *masa*: boil the maize with lime, rinse, and grind, or reconstitute *masa harina* flour with water. Set the *masa* aside in a cool dry place, covered with a damp cloth. Toast and shell the Cacao. Briefly toast the ear flower petals and the holy leaf flower spikes. Grind these with the finely chopped vanilla pods in a spice mill or mortar and pestle, periodically using the flour sifter or fine sieve over the bowl to separate out the well-ground material, and re-grind the coarse material until all the spices are finely powdered. Grind the Cacao once, then grind again with the spices; finally, mix well with the maize *masa*, combining them thoroughly, and grind the whole lot one more time.

To make the drink, place the finished dough in a large high-sided earthenware vessel or wide-necked jug, and add warm water little by little, stirring frequently to mix. When a milk-thin consistency is achieved, froth briefly with the *molinillo* or pour the liquid from a height into another tall-sided vessel. Cover the jug or vessel and allow the beverage to stand for twenty to thirty minutes, then pour back and forth repeatedly or whisk with the *molinillo* very well to raise a head of foam. Serve in the calabash-bowls.

ii) *Chocolatl*[1081]

The drink which may have given chocolate its name, even though it's nothing like it. Hernández described it as "fattening", so it may be a good recipe for convalescents or those who need to put on or maintain weight.

Ingredients:
- *Criollo* Cacao *lavado* seeds, "one handful" (or more)
- *Pochotl* (kapok or *Ceiba pentandra* seeds), the same volume as Cacao
- Water.

Equipment:
- Clay *comal*, for toasting
- *Metate* y *mano*, and/or electric mill, grinder, or heavy-duty food processor

- Mortar and pestle, or spice mill
- Two large, high-sided clay or earthenware vessels, for frothing, or
- One medium wide-necked jug and a *molinillo*
- Calabash-bowls for serving.

Instructions:
Hernández gives no quantities of Cacao and *Ceiba* seeds, saying only that an equal amount of each is used. Toast, shell, and grind the Cacao; toast the *Ceiba* seeds and grind them separately, then together with the Cacao to make a smooth paste. This paste may be set and stored in the same way as Cacao tablets. To serve one person, place approximately two tablespoons or 40g (1½oz) of the soft paste mixture into a jug; if the mix is hard, it should be broken up and a little boiling water added first to melt it. As with other fatty Cacao-based drinks, add a cupful of tepid water, stir well, then froth vigorously with the *molinillo* or by pouring the liquid back and forth between one high-sided vessel and another to produce the foam. Serve in the calabash-bowls.

2. Royal drinks, approximated

i) Basic *kakawa*

This recipe is my standard recipe for Mesoamerican chocolate. Because it lacks a botanical foaming agent or any added starch, it ordinarily produces only a small layer of foam, half an inch or so, though I suspect a more adept Mesoamerican *señora* could triple that amount. It's not based on any specific historical recipe, it's made using only the easier-to-find indigenous central American ingredients, and traditional processes. The spice blend is my own mish-mash of native spices, so feel free to extemporise.

Ingredients:
- *Criollo* Cacao *lavado* seeds, 500g/1lb 2oz
- Spices (adjust as desired):
    - Vanilla pods (*Vanilla planifolia*), x3
    - Dried allspice berries (*Pimienta dioica*), a small handful
    - Dried *rosita de Cacao* flowers (*Quararibea funebris*), a generous handful
    - Dried magnolia petals (*Magnolia dealbata*) and/or frangipani flowers (*Plumeria rubra*)
    - Dried annatto seeds (*Bixa orellana*), one teaspoonful
    - Chilli flakes (*Capsicum annuum*), one teaspoonful.
- Optional: sweetening, e.g., unrefined agave syrup, honey, maple syrup.

Equipment:
- Clay *comal*, for toasting
- *Metate* y *mano*
- Mortar and pestle, or spice mill
- A flour sifter or fine sieve and wide bowl
- Greaseproof paper
- Two large, high-sided clay or earthenware vessels, for frothing, or

- One medium wide-necked jug and a *molinillo*
- Calabash-bowls for serving.

Instructions:
Cut up the vanilla pods. Toast the allspice seeds, then the magnolia petals (if using), then toast the *rosita* flowers: detach the stamens, roast the flower cones briefly for a minute or so on a hot *comal*, then add the stamens and roast them for an additional thirty seconds. Don't toast the annatto, vanilla, or frangipani flowers (if using). Place all the spices in a large mortar and pestle and grind to powder; sift into a separate bowl and keep re-grinding the larger particles until the whole lot has been reduced to a reddish-brown sweet and spicy-smelling fine powder. Prepare the Cacao in the standard way: toast, shell, and grind once on a hot *metate*, then put the liquid in a bowl and stir in some spice: add about half to one teaspoon of spice blend for a cup-ful of cocoa liquor, and stir it in well. Re-grind the spiced cocoa liquor on the hot *metate* until a completely smooth, homogeneous liquid is formed. Drop this liquid onto sheets of greaseproof paper in the form of round puddles, and leave to cool. Wrap them individually in greaseproof paper, stack them, wrap the stacks in foil or seal in zip-loc bags, then store them in airtight, odourless glass or plastic containers in the fridge until ready to use.

To make the *kakawa*, weigh out 20g/¾ oz (small serving) or 40g/1½oz (large serving), and break up the disc in a jug or clay vessel. Sweeten if desired: for authenticity, use a teaspoon of unrefined agave syrup or Central American wildflower honey, although I prefer to use the less-authentic maple syrup, as the flavour combination works well. Pour 80–110ml/three to four fluid ounces of boiling water (for 20g/¾oz Cacao) or 160–220ml/⅓ to < ½ pint boiling water (for 40g Cacao) into each calabash-cup (to warm them), then pour this water onto the broken-up Cacao tablets and froth briefly with a *molinillo* or by pouring back and forth. Strain the liquid through a clean fine-mesh sieve or cheesecloth, then froth again very well. If making a large volume, skim off the foam with a clean calabash before serving, then replace it on each cup after pouring; if making only one or two cups, pour gently and directly into each serving cup so the foam comes out with the liquid (it's difficult to control how much comes out as you pour with this method, which is why the foam is traditionally removed then replaced, for accurate apportionment!)

ii) Devil's blood chocolate (chilli red: de Ledesma's recipe)

This recipe is taken from Antonio Colmero de Ledesma's seventeenth-century account of a very spicy Mexica chocolate drink coloured with annatto, following Template 2 above. I've rebranded it with a racy new name, appropriate for the post-colonial reconstruction of a fiery red "heathen" beverage made from ingredients produced in Catholic Central America.

Ingredients:
- *Criollo* Cacao *lavado* seeds, x100
- Dried chillies, x2
- Dried *mexasúchil/mecaxochitl (Piper sanctum)* fruits, x2
- *Pasta de achiote*, or *achiote* concentrate, 1–2 teaspoons
- Optional: sweetening, such as unrefined agave syrup, honey, or maple syrup.

Equipment:
- Clay *comal*, for toasting
- *Metate* y *mano*
- Mortar and pestle, or spice mill
- A flour sifter or fine sieve and wide bowl
- Greaseproof paper, banana leaves, or
- Two large, high-sided clay or earthenware vessels, for frothing, or
- A bowl and a *molinillo*
- Calabash-bowls for serving.

Instructions:

Toast and shell the Cacao. Toast the chillies and the *mecasúchil* on the *comal*. De Ledesma cautions against over-drying or burning the spices. When they're lightly toasted, grind and sift them to a fine powder. Grind the Cacao once, alone, on a hot *metate*; "But", de Ledesma cautions, "you must be very careful not to put more fire [under the *metate*] than will warm it, that the unctuous part do not dry away"[1082]—in other words, allow the *metate* to cool a little before working on it, and maintain a stable just-above-blood-temperature of the working surface, as suggested earlier in this chapter. Grind the cocoa liquor a second time, incorporating the spices and *achiote* paste, then pour the liquid aromatic chocolate onto sheets of greaseproof paper (or fresh banana or *pozole* leaves) in small round puddles, and leave to cool. He notes that Cacao will stick to hard surfaces, so it needs to be poured onto a smooth, flexible surface so the discs can be peeled off easily once they have dried. But greaseproof paper has longer keeping properties, and may also be used as wrapping paper to store the discs.

De Ledesma recommends the indigenous method for preparing the drink: pulverise or melt a "tablet", and pour on warm water (use above quantities: approximately 40g/1½oz Cacao to 220ml/⅓ to < ½ pint water). Sweeten, if desired. Mix well, and froth very well with a *molinillo* to raise a good head of foam, which should be separated into a serving bowl or larger calabash, and the drink poured from on high onto the foam—so that the head of foam ends up on top of the drink.

De Ledesma reported that this drink is very "Cold" and "agreeth not with all men's stom- achs", which I suspect may be caused by using old Annatto seeds or out-of-date *achiote* paste. He recommends making the drink with hot water, which is not traditional but certainly pleas- anter in cooler weather, and easier to prepare and froth.

iii) Motecuhzoma's chocolate (*yoloxochitl cacahutal*)

This recipe is a basic Mexica chocolate formula incorporating *yoloxochitl* (*Magnolia mexicana*), now known as *yolosúchil*, which was allegedly the favourite chocolate flavouring of the ill-fated emperor Motecuhzoma III (Montezuma).

Ingredients:
- *Criollo* Cacao *lavado* seeds, x100
- Dried *yoloxochitl*/*yolosúchil* (*Magnolia mexicana*) flowers, x3
- Optional: sweetening, such as unrefined agave syrup, honey, or maple syrup.

Equipment:
- Clay *comal*, for toasting
- *Metate* y *mano*
- Mortar and pestle, or spice mill
- A flour sifter or fine sieve and wide bowl
- Greaseproof paper
- Two large, high-sided clay or earthenware vessels, for frothing, or
- A bowl and a *molinillo*
- Calabash-bowls for serving.

Instructions:
Follow the procedure for the previous recipe, lightly toasting and pulverising the *yolosúchil* in place of the other spices. *Yolosúchil* is hard to obtain—it's a bright yellow, highly aromatic flower when dried. The herb sold as *magnolia* in Central American markets is the dried inflorescence or petals of *Magnolia dealbata*, and is a pale mango-orange colour with a much fainter smell; if using this as a substitute, double the quantity used in the recipe (use six whole dried flowers for the quantities given above).

iv) *Cacaloxochitl cacahuatl* (frangipani chocolate)

This recipe is based on *bu'pu*, using frangipani (aka *Plumeria spp.*: *cacaloxchitl*, or *cacalosúchil* in modern Mexico) as the foaming agent—essentially following the same procedure for making *bu'pu*, minus the huge quantity of added *piloncillo* sugar and the corn *atole*. Because this version maximises the flavours of Cacao and frangipani, without any "masking" or diluting flavours from sugar and the corn *atole*, I've suggested hand-grinding instead of machine-grinding to optimise flavour. I follow the second procedure (Template 2) for reconstructing pre-Colombian Cacao-based beverages, of making the drink in "one piece" rather than producing the foam separately, as the original recipe lends itself to this approach. Scale down quantities for domestic use—the following recipe could be used to cater a party!

Ingredients:
- *Criollo* Cacao *lavado* 500g/1lb 2oz
- Fresh *cacalosúchil* (frangipani flowers, *Plumeria rubra*), yellow and red, ¼ carrier bag full
- Sun-dried *cacalosúchil* (frangipani flowers, *Plumeria rubra*), yellow and red, crushed, approx. ½ tablespoonful
- Optional: sweetening, e.g., *piloncillo* sugar.

Equipment:
- Clay *comal*, for toasting
- Electric mill, grinder, or food processor
- *Metate* y *mano*
- A mortar and pestle, or spice mill
- A flour sifter or fine sieve and wide bowl
- Two large, high-sided clay or earthenware vessels, for frothing, or

- A *molinillo* without rings and a wide-mouthed jug or a clay, glass, or china mixing bowl for making foam
- Calabash-bowls for scooping foam and serving.

Instructions:

Toast and peel the Cacao. Grind the Cacao on the *metate*, then grind the fresh frangipani flowers to a paste on the *metate*. Grind and sift the dried flowers to make a fine powder, then stir the fresh flower paste and dried flower powder into the cocoa liquor, and grind again once or twice to make a smooth paste. This may then be dolloped onto greaseproof paper and allowed to set, or stored in the refrigerator for a few days.

To make the beverage, use 40g/1½oz of the paste per 220ml/⅓ to < ½ pint warm water. Warm the paste up first to blood-heat if it has been refrigerated, as the cocoa butter needs to be in a molten state for the process to work. Add a little sweetening, to taste, if desired. Add the water little by little to the paste, stir, and mix until well incorporated, then froth with the *molinillo* or by pouring back and forth from a height. Should produce a very large head of foam with small bubbles. Serve in calabash-cups.

v) Isthmus Jasmine chocolate

Sophie and Michael Coe recount a decadent post-Colonial European recipe for chocolate flavoured with jasmine flowers invented by the de Medici family physician Francisco Redi in their wonderful book on the history of chocolate.[1083] But it could be argued that this baroque delight was reinventing the wheel (ironic, since the wheel was barely used in Mesoamerica), because the native popcorn flower (*Bourreria huanita*), known to the Mexica as *izquixochitl*, has a rich sweet aroma so reminiscent of jasmine that its Spanish name is *jasmín del istmo*. Like Old World jasmine, the flowers of this tree are best used fresh, because they lose a lot of their fragrance when dried;[1084] so, as Sophie Coe suggests, "Perhaps [the] flowers were kept in a tightly closed vessel with the raw or roasted beans instead of being mixed with the liquid chocolate."[1085] But, as we've seen with *bu'pu*, it's entirely possible that fresh flowers may be ground into a paste and mixed directly with Cacao to flavour it. So I've incorporated both approaches in this admittedly made-up recipe—we do know that the Mexica used popcorn flower as a Cacao spice, so it's not entirely fanciful, although we don't know exactly how they used it. This recipe effectively incorporates its flavour.

Ingredients:

- *Criollo* Cacao *lavado*, whatever quantity
- Fresh *izquixochitl* (popcorn flowers, *Bourreria huanita*), twice the volume of the Cacao, freshly picked as required, in two batches (see Instructions below)
- Foaming agent: either fresh *chupipe* root, approx. 25g/≤1oz per kilo/2lb 3oz of Cacao; or *chupipe* fruit skin, approx. ½ peel of one fruit per kilo/2lb 3oz of Cacao; or fresh young *cocolmeca* stem, approx. one long stem (an arm's length) per kilo/2lb 3oz of Cacao
- Optional: sweetening, e.g., unrefined agave syrup, honey.

Equipment:

- Clay *comal*, for toasting
- Glass Kilner jar with an airtight seal, big enough to hold all the Cacao beans with a little room to spare; or a clay jar which can be made airtight
- Large cheesecloth or muslin for straining
- Electric mill, grinder, or food processor
- *Metate* y *mano*
- A mortar and pestle, or spice mill
- Two large, high-sided clay or earthenware vessels, for frothing, or
- A *molinillo* without rings and a wide-mouthed jug or a clay, glass, or china mixing bowl
- Calabash-bowls for serving.

Instructions:

Toast and peel the Cacao. Mix the toasted whole Cacao beans with an equal volume of fresh, aromatic *izquixochitl* flowers and put in a clean, dry, airtight glass or clay jar; close or stopper tightly, and keep in a cool, dry place for up to one week. The flowers may begin to brown and wilt slightly, but must not start to decay or liquefy! Refrigerate if necessary (i.e., in warm weather). Then, take out the Cacao, pick out all the flowers and discard them. Gather an equal amount of fresh *izquixochitl* flowers. Grind the Cacao into cocoa liquor on the *metate*. Meanwhile, prepare the foaming agent: for *chupipe* root, pulp it, pick out and discard the outer bark fragments, and grind to a paste; for *chupipe* fruit skin, chop the peel and grind well also. For *cocolmeca*, briefly toast the fresh stem, chop into small chunks, and grind to a paste. Grind the fresh *izquixochitl* flowers and foaming agent to a paste, then add the pulped fresh plant material to the cocoa liquor, and grind the whole lot once or twice on the *metate* to make a completely smooth, thick, and highly aromatic liquid. This may then be dolloped onto greaseproof paper and allowed to set, or stored in the refrigerator for a few days. Don't freeze it.

To make the beverage, follow the procedure for frangipani chocolate above. Use 40g/1½oz of the paste per 220ml/⅓ to < ½ pint tepid water. Warm the paste up first to blood-heat if it has been refrigerated; add a little sweetening, if desired; then add warm water little by little to the paste, stir, and mix until well incorporated, and froth with the *molinillo* or by pouring back and forth from a height, raising a huge head of foam. Serve in calabash-cups.

vi) Undead chocolate

This final recipe is also a personal invention, based on *chocolate atole* and its principal foaming agent, fermented *pataxtle* seeds, aka *cacao blanco*. I use my first method (Template 1) for producing facsimile Mesoamerican chocolate drinks here, creating separate mixtures for making foam and the body of the drink. The name comes from the fact that all the ingredients are—to some extent at least—fermented, and the controlled decay of fermentation is what gives them a new lease of posthumous life, with brand-new chemistry. The advantage of this recipe is that all ingredients are dry and may be stored for some time, so there's no issue of sourcing fresh tropical plants for those who live outside Central America! Because *cacao blanco* can easily be brought back to the UK, I've made this recipe at home, very successfully—it tastes wonderful, and produces an excellent head of foam.

Ingredients (bulk):
- For the foam topper:
  - *Cacao blanco* (fermented *pataxtle* seeds), 200g/7oz
  - *Criollo* Cacao "*rojo*" *fermentado*, 400g/14oz
  - Vanilla pods, x2
  - Optional: ear flower petals (*Cymbopetalum penduliflorum*), x2
  - Optional: holy leaf dried flower spikes (*Piper auritum*), x2–3
  - Optional: sweetener, to taste, e.g., *panela* or *piloncillo*, or coconut sugar.
- For the body of the drink:
  - *Criollo* Cacao "*rojo*" *lavado*, 600g/21oz
  - Optional: sweetener, to taste, e.g., *panela* or *piloncillo*, or maple syrup.

Equipment:
- Fine sieve for straining
- Clay *comal*, for toasting
- Wooden spoon
- Bowls for holding and keeping ingredients separate during manufacture
- *Metate* y *mano*
- Food processor (optional)
- Spice mill (optional)
- Mortar and pestle, fine sieve or flour sifter and bowl
- Greaseproof paper
- A *molinillo* without rings and a wide-mouthed jug
- A clay *cazuela*, or a clay, glass, or china mixing bowl
- Calabash-bowls for serving.

Instructions:
Ensure that all utensils and hands are free of any traces of fat or grease from previous work before beginning. To make the foam topper tablets, toast and shell the *Cacao fermentado*. Peel the *cacao blanco*, discarding any that look discoloured or mouldy. Crush the *cacao blanco* to a coarse powder with a clean mortar and pestle or on a *metate*, then grind to a fine powder in a very clean food processor, or continue to grind on the *metate* or in the mortar until finely powdered, and set aside. Finely chop the vanilla pods, and lightly toast the ear flower petals (if using—highly recommended, if you can get hold of them) then the holy leaf flower spikes on the *comal*. Then grind the spices to a coarse powder in the spice mill or mortar, sift them, and grind again until all the spices are finely powdered. Heat the *metate* and grind the Cacao once, then stir the powdered spices into the cocoa liquor and grind again. Then dump the powdered *cacao blanco* into the spiced cocoa liquor, and mix thoroughly with a wooden spoon. The mixture will look like a crumbly dough. Grind this once more, thoroughly incorporating the *cacao blanco* to produce a

highly aromatic chocolate-brown, thick and sticky semi-liquid paste. This aromatic paste may now be dropped onto greaseproof paper, patted into roundels, and left to set. The topper tablets may be stored for several months: wrap them in greaseproof paper, then foil, and seal them in an odour-proof glass or non-reactive plastic airtight container and refrigerate.

To make the main chocolate drink tablets, toast, shell, and grind the Cacao *lavado* twice or three times, to make a smooth liquid. Pour onto greaseproof paper in little puddles, allow the discs to set, and store as above. Label everything very clearly and keep the foaming tablets and *Cacao* lavado tablets separate!

To make the drink, break up a foam topper tablet straight from the fridge (still cool) in a very clean, non-greasy chilled mortar and pestle and grind quickly to a very fine powder. Put the powder in a clean, non-greasy glass or clay bowl or *cazuela*. Add sweetener (if using), and pour on warm water (warm enough to melt cocoa butter, 40–60°C [104–140°F]), then froth briefly with a *molinillo* to mix it up, then leave to sit for half an hour or more to cool. Then, froth the foaming mixture vigorously with the *molinillo*. You may need to adjust the ratio of foaming paste/tablet material to water if foam isn't happening; create lots of foam before you allow yourself to stop.

Meanwhile, take 40g/1½oz (per serving) of the Cacao *lavado* tablets (plain Cacao), break up, and drop into a jug. Add sweetening as desired. Add 210ml/⅓ to < ½ pint boiling water (per serving), and froth well with the *molinillo*. Strain the chocolate through a fine sieve, froth the liquid again, and pour into calabash-bowls to serve. Scoop the (relatively) cool foam on top of the already-served hot chocolate. Serving suggestion: add plenty of sweetening to the foam mixture, around 40–60% *piloncillo* or coconut sugar, but don't add sweetening to the body of the drink: chocolate made with Cacao *lavado*, if not over-toasted, has a milder flavour, so doesn't need much sweetening. Ensure that the volume of foam added to the drink is equal to the body of the liquid. That way there will be a pleasant contrast between the hot, relatively bitter liquid made from the Cacao *lavado* and the cool, sweet aromatic foam made from *fermentado*; the foam will serve to sweeten the body of the drink.

* * *

I wanted to close the chapter with a final recipe for drinking chocolate, representing one of the most decadent reinventions of Cacao-based beverages in Europe prior to the degrading (literally) of chocolate in the cocoa catastrophe, which has convinced millions that "hot chocolate" is an insipidly thin and overly-sweetened milky bedtime beverage made from a base of sugary powder. This baroque beverage is ambergris chocolate, described in Chapter 3, taken from the French gastronome Henri Brillat-Savarin's *Physiologie du Goût* (Physiology of Taste), written in 1826. This beverage, he assures us, is "marvellous for people before undertaking intellectual work" and good for people with chronic illnesses or "pyloric ailments", as well as general fatigue. He particularly remarked on its ability to dispel obsessiveness, claiming it will help "all men who are tormented by a fixed idea which kills freedom of thought".[1086]

The lowest quality, dark brown-black ambergris is expensive, and the highest quality white ambergris, astronomical—a lump of 83g (approx. 3 oz.) of brown ambergris was listed for sale on eBay for a mere £1375 (1799 USD, or $599.67 per ounce) as of February 2019, and 17.5g (approx. ⅗ oz., or 5 drachms) white ambergris was going for £1075 (1407 USD, or $2269.35 per oz.). Ambergris is that rare thing, an animal product which is acceptable for vegans and vegetarians, as no whales are harmed or exploited in its production. Ambrein, one of the main odour compounds in ambergris, has been determined to be an effective painkiller at relatively low doses in mice, and its effects were blocked by drugs affecting endorphin and noradrenaline release,[1087] suggesting that it works on opiate and trace amine pathways in the brain. Ambrein also increased sexual behaviour in male rats,[1088] while both ambrein and another ambergris compound, epicoprostanol, have been investigated for antioxidant and liver-protective activity, with mostly positive results.[1089] So the combination of Cacao and ambergris makes sense: a painkilling, neurotransmitter-modulating, antioxidant drug with an unforgettable, complex smell—this could be a description of either substance.

Brillat-Savarin's "Chocolate of the Afflicted":

- 1lb/454g prepared Cacao
- 60–72 grains (= 3.8–4.67g) high quality ambergris
- White sugar
- Boiling water.

Equipment:
- Porcelain *chocolatière*, or jug with *molinillo*
- Mortar and pestle
- Porcelain cups, for serving.

Instructions:
The "prepared Cacao" would have been made from toasted *criollo* Cacao *fermentado*, shelled and ground, then re-ground with up to 50% white sugar. I'd recommend cutting the sugar down to 20%, or preferably substituting it for unrefined *panela*, *piloncillo*, coconut sugar, or maple sugar. The ambergris is pulverised, then re-ground together with the chocolate paste, and allowed to set as tablets. These tablets are prepared in the usual way by grating or breaking them up, putting them into a *chocolatière* or jug, pouring on boiling water, and frothing with the *molinillo*. According the Brillat-Savarin, the beverage should be prepared the day before consumption, left to rest overnight at room temperature in a *chocolatière*, then re-warmed and frothed again immediately prior to consumption: "The night's rest will concentrate it and give it a velvety quality which will make it all the better."[1090]

Savarin also gives instructions for making it *ad hoc*, for those days when an immediate anti-depressant effect is required, by adding "the weight of a bean" of ambergris "pounded with sugar" to a cup of chocolate. So if one bean weighs approximately 0.3g (2½ grains), factoring in the cost of the Cacao, this drink sounds worth every penny of the £21.50 or 28 USD per cup this recipe would cost today. For anyone wishing to try this expensive chocolate tonic, without committing to making an entire batch and possibly turning to a life of crime to pay for it, I'd suggest using a stiff dose of 40–50g (1⅖–1⅘ oz) prepared Cacao in tablet form, breaking this up into the *chocolatière* with a little sweetening and the smashed ambergris, and using 400ml (slightly less than half a pint) of boiling water to make the drink

That ambergris is a fermented whale excretion, perhaps literally vomited up from the depths of the ocean, makes this European concoction especially remarkable: not only do these two substances appear to be gastronomically and pharmacologically compatible, but there's a symbolic syllogism, too. Like ambergris, Cacao is a fermented drug of great value, and had strong mythic ties to the watery Mesoamerican underworld. Savarin's combination of these two substances seems even more remarkable with a little knowledge of Cacao's metaphysics and its place in Mesoamerican mythology, to be explored in the next two chapters.

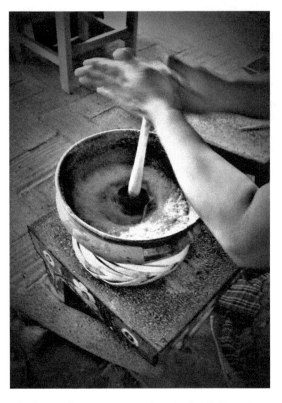

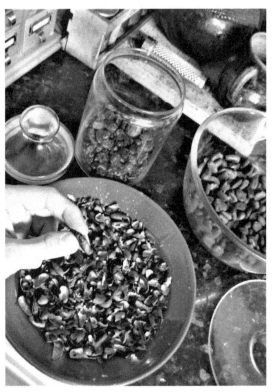

Chef Camilla Santiago makes froth of chocolate atole, Teotitlan del Valle, Oaxaca, Mexico, 2018

Peeling and sorting toasted Cacao seeds.

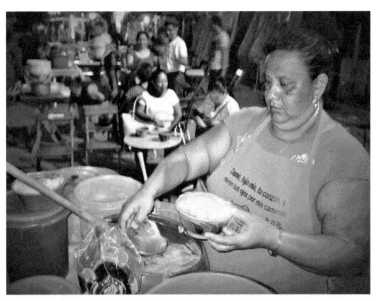

Señora Anna Maria Garcia Vasquez sells bu'pu, Juchitan, Oaxaca, Mexico, 2018

PART III

METAPHYSICAL CHOCOLATE

CHAPTER NINE

Death by chocolate

"This saying was said of Cacao, because it was precious … The common folk, the needy did not drink it. … it was said: *'The heart, the blood are to be feared.'"*

(Sahagún, quoted in Coe & Coe, 1996)

"What use are cartridges in battle. I always carry chocolate instead."

(Bluntschli, from George Bernard Shaw's play *Arms and the Man*, 1894)

Ceci n'est pas un pipe.

(Caption on the René Magritte painting, *La Trahison des Images*)

In the last chapter, traditional Mesoamerican recipes and formulae made with Cacao were described, and some reconstruction of ancient Cacao-based recipes was attempted. But you don't fully understand a subject unless you know where it's "coming from", belief-wise. Just like a person, it's not only what they've been through, but how these experiences are interpreted that matters: what myths surround them, and which rumours persist. After all, to consume a substance is to participate in its mythology, either because we believe contemporary myths in the form of advertising hype ("With these F****** ****** you are really spoiling us")[x] or because, in an ouroboric loop, we are drawn to use it in ways which reinforce its associations (I am sad because my partner has left me; I need chocolate ice cream; chocolate ice cream tastes good; when I am sad I will eat chocolate ice cream).

Even without the consumer knowing its heritage, the historical mythos of any substance informs its identity in both obvious and subtle ways. Superficial mythological impressions persist in Mesoamerican imagery or language used in branding speciality chocolates ("Maya Gold", "Montezuma's"), or the unquestioning beliefs people hold about chocolate's status as a luxury or comfort food. The notions which shaped Cacao's cachet in its previous incarnation as the most prestigious psychoactive substance in pre-Columbian Mesoamerica are less apparent today, but they bled into subsequent colonial concepts in more subtle ways. So to understand Cacao better, knowing what people believed about it is a necessary undertaking. A good place to start exploring the mythological matrix of Cacao is to look at how pre-Columbian

---

[x] This is a 1990s UK advertising reference. Apologies.

Mesoamerican peoples saw the world, and to attempt to see as they saw. It would be useful to examine their mythology, and look at why they worshipped as they did, and how they comprehended their universe: how they measured time, how they saw their place in it, and how they sought answers. After doing all that, it would be a good idea to look at Cacao's role in those myths and rituals. Let's begin by exhuming some old gods.

Theologia Mesoamericana

There were many indigenous cultures before the arrival of the Spanish. Even in contemporary Central America there are hundreds of different native languages and peoples with varying customs and beliefs—for example, "the Maya" actually consist of many different polities and peoples spanning more than two millennia. In many cases any surviving religious books were burned and their relics destroyed by zealous missionaries after the Spanish conquest, and adherents of the native religions were forcibly converted to Christianity, so that after half a millennium of missionary work, contemporary followers of the old pagan ways in Central America practise hybrid versions of the old beliefs with strong Christian liturgical influences. The paucity of written records, difficulties in translating Mayan hieroglyphs, and the lack of written language for many other Mesoamerican cultures make the theological landscape of older civilisations particularly difficult to decipher and comprehend. The already-strange nature of civilisations which didn't know the concept of total war yet widely practised human sacrifice, and which invented the wheel yet used it only for making toys, is made more alien by a lack of information.

But many legends and traditions survive in a culturally mutated form, so with ongoing excellent anthropological and archaeological work, and the post-conquest documentation of native religious practices by chroniclers like Bernardino de Sahagún, historians have begun to partially reconstruct the religious framework of many pre-Colombian civilisations. Their pantheons include overlapping characters, deities, and themes, but each nation had its own mythology and favoured patrons; just as a Martian more acquainted with London might feel when visiting Moscow, the cultural landscape is different, but familiar—there are differences, but the same basic structures and rules apply.

The Mesoamerican mindscape

Mesoamerican religion was polytheistic to an extreme degree, a consequence of their perception that spiritual powers inhabited and animated the world; almost everything had its own patron spirit or god. It may be more accurate to describe at least some of the later Mesoamerican theologies as *henotheistic*, meaning that all the gods and spirits were conceived of as aspects of one supreme power. The Mexica referred to this being as Ometeotl, "our Lord and Lady of duality", or Tloque Nahaque, "Lord of the Close and Near",[1091] the ultimate reality,[1092] compared to which everything else—gods included—was transient. It's thought that the Chichimecs, a nomadic group of tribes that may have migrated down into Mesoamerica from North America and perhaps overrun Toltec territory around the twelfth century CE, disseminated the concept of a dual-natured origin god/goddess, a pairing of Father Sky and Mother Earth.[1093]

The creation myths of the Maya and earlier cultures speak of similar all-from-one divine hierarchies, usually involving a sky deity and a water deity which call forth the land and the other gods. The dual nature of reality was a strong theme, too: day and night, fire and water, male and female, sun and moon are all paired dyads in Mesoamerican thought, being complementary opposites which can have positive or negative attributes;[1094] night had to exist for there to be day, shamans had to know how to inflict disease in order to cure illnesses, and so on. There is a striking similarity to ancient Old World "dual origin" gods or philosophical concepts such as the Hellenic Uranus-Gaia, Aristotelian fire/water and earth/air couplings, or Chinese yang-yin and Heaven-Earth polarities in Mesoamerican thought.

The Mesoamerican world view was essentially magical, and somewhat shamanic. These terms will be further unpacked in the next chapter; for now, this can be understood as a pan-cultural belief that the tangible world depended on invisible spiritual powers, and that these powers could be accessed and utilised through ritual, for the benefit of humans. The ritual relationship was reciprocal: the world existed because the gods had sacrificed themselves to create it, so it was the duty of humans not only to express gratitude, but to "feed" these forces with vitality so that the cosmos would continue to function; to insure against disaster and to ensure good outcomes in worldly actions.[1095] Humans had been created specifically to honour the gods, and the failure of the inhabitants of previous creations to do so resulted in their destruction.[1096]

There was a strong focus on earthly existence in Mesoamerican religious thought, and belief in some form of reincarnation or "perpetual cycle" was the norm. The emphasis was on securing health, fertility, and prosperity in this world, and predicting or finding the supernatural causes for natural disasters so that, where possible, they may be averted or neutralised.[1097] In return for sacrificial offerings, the gods sustained life and ensured success. The gods were "rich, happy, possessors of goods … always, forever, it germinates, it grows green, there in their house … Everywhere in the world, in various places they spread out their mat … They give to the people lordship, dominion, fire, [and] glory."[1098] So sacrifice was a core theological tenet in Mesoamerica; it was propitiatory, prophylactic, and pragmatic. The Mesoamericans believed sacrifices were fair trade for the provision of maize and water, which in some Maya legends were the ingredients of the dough from which the first humans of this creation were made—and, in the sense that maize and water were essential food and drink, this was an ongoing process, because the body alchemises whatever is eaten into new flesh.

All Mesoamerican theologies envisioned a tiered cosmos, broadly divisible into three "worlds": the underworld, this earthly material world, and the celestial world. The two "otherworlds"—that below, and that above—were immaterial, and inhabited by spirits and gods. In common with many other belief systems worldwide, the underworld was the place where the dead went, and the celestial world was where most of the gods resided. This three-layered world model was re-imagined by the twentieth-century surrealist and historian of magic, Kurt Seligmann, who submitted that all humans inhabit three realities from which our subjective universe is constructed: the imagined reality, the perceived reality, and the remembered reality.[1099] These could be said to loosely correspond to the Mesoamerican celestial, earthly, and underworld realms, respectively. A physical analogy could also be made: the celestial world being the brain or seat of higher intelligence, the middle world the heart, lungs, and stomach or seat of life, and the underworld the organs of elimination (bowels, kidneys, etc.) and generation (sex organs). These realms were in turn divided into separate "levels", although the division, naming, and function of these "levels" varied somewhat between cultures.

The Classic Maya civilisations believed there were thirteen "levels" of the celestial world, occupied by the gods, stars, planets, and luminaries;[1100] and that this celestial realm was mirrored by nine levels of the underworld, Xibalba, the "place of fear", inhabited by ancestor spirits, ghosts, and gods of death.[1101] The earthly realm of time and space was itself divided into "four skies" corresponding to the four principal directions, described below. The Mexica also divided Topan, the celestial realm, into thirteen levels, and concurred with the Mayan vision of nine levels in their underworld, Mictlan. Mexica poetry referred to the realm of the dead as Quenonamican, or "region-where-in-someway-one-exists."[1102] So there was some form of afterlife in Mesoamerican religious thought, which was entered by conscious remnants or aspects of the "soul" of the deceased individual.

Access to the various Mesoamerican afterlife options wasn't affected by morality in the human world at all, only by the manner of death;[1103] most people's souls went to the underworld. So, for example, in the Mexica cosmos, the souls of people who died by violence or misadventure ascended to one of the thirteen levels of Topan: warriors who died in combat, women who died in childbirth, those sacrificed to the gods, suicides, and people who drowned or were struck by lightning would automatically get a pass to the celestial realms, too.[1104] Lucky for them, as the underworld was no picnic: "souls" of the dead encountered delights such as clashing hills and obsidian-edged winds as they travelled through Mictlan, and they were whittled away until finally extinguished four years after death.[1105] So afterlife in the underworld sounds like a severe form of purgatory in most cases; and yet, this can't be the whole story, as ancestor-worship and a belief in reincarnation pervaded Mesoamerican culture.

For the Maya, as in Greek myth with the crossing of the river Styx, the dead entered Xibalba through a cave or the standing waters of a lake or ocean,[1106] and had to cross a body of water in a canoe before descending through eight levels of the underworld, which was "hot and steamy" (just as caves deep under the earth were hot, and decay is moist). The underworld was depicted in Mesoamerican art as a watery place, with seashells, fishes, and other aquatic symbolism, perhaps because the origins of the world were wet—the primordial sea from which the land arose. And, for those Mayan peoples who inhabited the Yucatan peninsula, which is like a giant calcified sponge, dotted with water-filled caves and sinkholes, going down into the earth meant getting wet. The entrance to the underworld lay in the west, where the sun sets. In Maya legends, the court of the Lords of Xibalba was on the ninth and lowest level, where the souls would be tested; they had to outwit the gods of death, in order to rise in the night sky as a star.[1107] The Mexica believed that dogs knew the way through Mictlan, so they often sacrificed dogs when a human died to act as guides for the deceased.[1108]

The Mayans also believed that ancestors affected the living, that rituals could empower objects by "ensouling" them with spiritual entities or forces, and that every human being had an animal aspect to their soul—called the *way* or *wayob* in some Mayan languages—into which some people (shamans and witches) could consciously transform. *Wayob* meant "to sleep" or "to dream", so they were primarily nocturnal avatars of a person's spirit, encountered in dreams. Planets or constellations were the *wayob* of the gods, uniquely visible and unchanging in the night sky. Every sentient being, both material and immaterial—humans, spirits and gods—had their own *wayob*;[1109] this is to be distinguished from the Mayan soul-stuff, *ch'ulel*, which suffused the world and was found in all things, animate and inanimate alike. The Mesoamerican world view was Animist: everything is somehow alive, and even inanimate objects are instilled with life and, in some sense, movement, which can be demonstrated over time in processes of erosion, decay, growth, and transformation. But, for the Maya, only gods, spirits, or humans had a *wayob*.

The Mexica believed in a tripartite soul. One aspect of consciousness was called *tonalli*, from the verb *tona* meaning warmth or sunshine. Like the sun, the source of life, it regulated growth and temperament. *Tonalli* resided in the head, and was reputed to stay with the body after death.[1110] It was linked to destiny,[1111] and the Mexica word *tonal* also means "spirit-familiar", an animal counterpart equivalent to the Maya *wayob*; the *tonalli* travelled in dreams or visionary experiences. *Tonalli* were thought to be sent from the "highest heaven" of Omeyocan and could be discovered after birth by contact with a particular animal, or divined from the day of birth using the 260-day divinatory calendar (described in the next chapter).[1112] The K'iche Maya also refer to the *nawal*, the "animal spirit of the soul" which is linked to the day of one's birth.[1113] So *tonal*, *wayob*, and *nawal* are metaphysically distinct but related concepts, roaming animal-shaped soul aspects which were linked to calendrical divination. *Teyolia*, the second Mexica "soul", was the power of reason which resides in the heart. The third aspect of the Mexica "soul" was *ihiyotl*, "breath", which resided in the liver and governed desires; a sort of miasma that endowed the ability to attract or influence others,[1114] halfway between pheromones and charisma.

The ascension of the successful "soul" as a star in Mayan theology suggests that the "souls" which were trialled in Xibalba could have been *wayob*—perhaps human *wayob* had a sporting chance to prove their worth, and join the *wayob* of the gods in the celestial realm. The "souls" which were erased in the Mexica underworld, Mictlan, may have been *teyolia*, which travelled to the otherworld after death.[1115] What is certain is that death was nothing to celebrate in Mesoamerican thought; spirits and gods queued up to be reborn, and death merely served to make life more poignant. Mexica songs consistently refer to distress at the fleeting nature of life on Earth, and are steeped with the bittersweet joy and nostalgic pain of transient earthly pleasures in the face of inevitable death.[1116] As one of Bernardino de Sahagún's native informants put it, "So that we would not die of sadness, our lord gave us laughter, sleep, and sustenance."[1117]

The pathways which allowed spirits to travel between levels and realms were conceptualised as a huge "world tree", most commonly the *Ceiba* (*C. pentandra*), and the gateways between realms functioned like valves in veins, or weirs in canals, so that the flow from spiritual to material was one-way only. The gods had placed barriers between the three realms through which the physical body cannot pass, but incorporeal mental or spiritual bodies can. The earthly realm and all material life was sustained by a constant flow of vivifying power from the celestial realm bearing both generative and destructive forces; every living thing was created as a celestial entity—god or spirit—that sacrificed itself to give life to something in the earthly realm. The material world, or world of the sun, was teeming with spiritual entities—invisible to humans—and ensouled beings, which included inanimate natural bodies such as rivers and rocks as well as living creatures, so that everything in the world of the sun possessed spiritual or divine power. In many Mesoamerican traditions, the sun itself was the middle-world body of a god who had sacrificed himself and been reborn. Changes in weather were thought to be the result of entities passing through our middle world, and the "heart" or life-force of every living creature was literally made from its patron-god:[1118] rabbit-gods, coyote-gods, human-gods … Yet the gods in this world, once embodied, became "passive and inert", especially during the day; but at night the gods could be contacted more readily, and their divine essences could separate from physical bodies and roam free.

Maya *ch'ulel* or *pixan*[1119] was immortal soul-stuff, present in everything; it generated identity, and mediated interactions amongst all things, and in humans was found primarily in blood—which is why bloodletting featured so strongly in sacrifices. Other things considered to be repositories of *ch'ulel* that were suitable offerings for the gods were selected on the basis of their aesthetic and symbolic value: maize, because it was humans' staple food and all its colours (red, blue, yellow) symbolically represented blood: arterial blood, blood in the veins, and blood as seen through the skin. Jade, because it is beautiful, the colour of water and plant life—symbolising life and death, verdancy and decay, water being associated with both—and is incredibly hard and durable, a permanent symbol of life-force, resilient and evergreen; and flowers,[1120] valued for their beauty, aroma, and transience. The Classic Maya described souls or spirit essences as being like flowers—perhaps because, like flowers, they cause life to bloom briefly in this world. But these spirit-essences are also described as "blooms on the world tree",[1121] and are therefore analogous to stars, which shine perpetually and revolve constantly with the sky, reflecting the immortal nature of some aspects of the "soul".

So the Mesoamerican religions contained a principle of replication, where all things on Earth originate in the celestial realm,[1122] like a god-haunted version of Plato's idea of timeless, transcendent Forms, and reminiscent of the Hermetic axiom "as above, so below". When the veil around the middle realm was disturbed by abnormal weather patterns or ritual action, entities were freed from their material bodies to move down into the underworld (presumably causing the death of their physical bodies), from where they could eventually return to the earthly realm. This endless process of god-animating and soul-cycling was tightly regulated, and could be monitored by spiritually blind humankind through divination.[1123] Under normal circumstances humans can only perceive "denser" material bodies, and our ability to affect or interact with the immaterial forces controlling the realm of the sun was limited, difficult, and risky.[1124] The risks were physical, and metaphysical: physical, because attaining the ability to see and interact with spiritual forces involved loosening and releasing a part of one's soul from the body; and metaphysical, because attempting to bargain with or command gods and spirits is a chancy business.

All the time in the world

Another key belief in Mesoamerican religious thought was the spiral nature of time: cycles within cycles—endings and beginnings were perceptible and present at every level, from day and night, or birth and death, up to immense loops of time involved in the recurrent genesis and abolition of the universe. Death and life were interdependent: the Classic Maya believed that after death, an individual's *ch'ulel* might hang around the burial site for a while, before returning to the underworld to be redistributed by ancestral gods as the soul of a newborn baby, so grandchildren possessed the *ch'ulel* of their great-grandparents.[1125] We ascribe the mechanics of familial traits and heritable characteristics today to genetics. The Maya name for corn kernels, their primary food and stuff of life, translated as "little skulls".[1126] The association is entirely logical, and obvious to an agricultural civilisation: death and decay are necessary to feed the soil, and permit the crops to grow. Life literally emerges from the underworld. Gardeners refer to this process as composting.

In the K'iche Maya creation myth, there was a primordial sea, and the dialogue between two gods (one in the water, the "Sovereign Feathered Serpent" and one in the sky, "Heart of Sky"[1127]) causes earth to rise up out of the water. There were three prior creations or "versions" of man: earth men, wood men, and maize men: the first were too stupid, the second too irreverent, and the third too perfect. The mud men were washed away, and the wood men were destroyed by a boiling deluge; those who escaped the inundation become monkeys. The maize men of the third creation had their sight "darkened" by the gods to limit their perceptions, creating the men of the current world. In Mixtec origin stories, the creator couple generate two sons, who transform into an eagle and a winged serpent; they create a huge garden, and restore humans to life from the "leftovers" of previous creations.[1128]

It may be more accurate to say that the Mayan view of time was coiled, rather than cyclical. Like a hosepipe—or a serpent. Themes recurred, but never precisely repeated. The past influenced the future, and perhaps vice versa; the universe was applied in layers, and the layers bled through, interacting with each other. Mesoamerican "cosmovision" was holistic and holographic—the small mirrored the large. Origin myths describe repeated creation and destruction of the cosmos, with "our" world, inhabited by humans, being only the latest in a series of creations. Every part of the world, too, nested within a greater analogous whole, and changes made to any smaller or larger structure could affect those further "up" or "down" the chain of scale and complexity; thus a single, small house was like a *milpa*, which resembled an entire community, which was part of the wider cosmos. In all cases, there were four directions and a centre, and every "tier" reciprocally supported and sustained the one above and below it.[1129]

The North American Hopi tribe share a common prehistoric ancestry with their southern kin, and have a fascinating cosmic set-up. They believe that each world eventually fails, and that people must then find a "hole in the sky" through which to pass into the next; the previous residence then becomes the world of the dead. For the Hopi, the celestial realm is the next human world, and the underworld is the previous one—humanity crawls "upwards" endlessly through time in a stacked universe like a hall of mirrors.[1130] The Mesoamerican view was less infinite; like the Maya, the Mexica believed there had been previous creations, but that there had been four worlds prior to this one, all of which were destroyed by the gods, each made primarily from one of the elements: water, earth, fire, and wind. This universe is the world of *ollintonatiuh*, the "sun of movement" or creation of the Fifth Sun, and is composed of a mixture of all four elements. The world of the Fifth Sun was imbued with *yoliliztli*, or "inside-movement", analogous to Mayan *ch'ulel*, Hellenic *pneuma*, Chinese *chi*, Egyptian *heka*, or Polynesian *mana*: life force.[1131] The Zapotecs had a similar concept: *pee*, which can be translated as "breath", "spirit", or "wind".[1132] The Nahuatl word *yollol* means "heart"; *yoliliztli* was concentrated in the heart, along with the *teyolia*, the rational part of the soul. Similarly, the Maya believed that spirits in the underworld required "seed-hearts" from previous generations of living beings in order to return to the world of the living.[1133]

Portals to power

The "divine right of kings" in Medieval Europe, where kings were also thought of as God's representative on Earth (below the pope, of course), was taken to the next level by the Olmecs and the Maya after them, who believed that their kings possessed "supra-human abilities"[1134] to contact the spirit realms. Auto-sacrifice, or bloodletting, was of central importance in Mesoamerica, and was a particular responsibility of the nobles and rulers. This duty was shared by commoners, too, but the onus for regular public shedding of blood fell on leaders because otherworldly power resulted in this-worldly outcomes and vice versa, so this-worldly power reflected otherworldly spiritual support. If commoners' blood was dial-up, noble blood was broadband. Maya noblemen used stingray spines and knotted cords with thorns to draw blood from the penis, or other parts of the body such as the lips, and noblewomen did the same with their tongues or other body parts during rituals. Blood was the necessary tithe to open a gateway to the celestial realm of the gods or the underworld of the ancestors, thereby gaining access to otherworldly power and counsel.

So what was the "vivifying power" which flowed from the celestial realms? And what constituted a "gateway"? The Maya conceived of an invisible force or immaterial magical substance they called *itz*, and a creator-god called Itzamna, the master shaman who made the starry sky, and who had "four bodies": the two "sides" of the Milky Way and the two "sides" of the zodiac[1135] (the band of constellations which form the backdrop through which the Sun appears to travel each year). *Itz* was the "blessed substance of the sky" which flowed out of gateways to the otherworld opened by the *itzam* or shaman. *Itz* was ritually invoked by resins, blood, sap, rubber, milk, sweat, tears, or semen—substances that change state or are produced by living tissues, and which congeal or leave residues. *Itz* was an invisible substance that caused change and generated new possibilities; the stuff of magical action, growth, and transformation in the world. *Ch'ulel* was a more fundamental and ethereal force, less dense than *itz*, often visualised as residing in clouds: in space, as nebulae among the stars; in the sky, as clouds; or above the altar, in the smoke of burning incense and offerings. In a sense, *itz* was the product of concentrated, focused *ch'ulel*: *ch'ulel* was to *itz* as clouds are to rain.

Blood sacrifice was performed to feed the gods with *ch'ulel*, and generate *itz*: *ch'ulel* in, *itz* out. *Itz* was generated in the ritual from the *ch'ulel* of the participants and offerings, or material representations of *itz* contained in resinous oblations such as rubber and copal could be exchanged for the much more powerful and dangerous otherworldly *itz*. Dangerous, because misuse of this ritual power by taking too much pride in personal wealth or directing *itz* solely for personal gain was an affront to the gods, and would incur personal or communal penalties such as disease, famine, or "bad luck". Pride was a universal sin in Mesoamerican thought: there was great cultural sensitivity to hubris, rising above one's station, and transgressing against the gods[1136]—a point in common with Christian Europe (Proverbs 16:18: "Pride goeth before destruction, and an haughty spirit before a fall"). Obtaining otherworldly *itz* was like a business contract with the gods: it permitted certain work to be done, but terms and conditions applied.

The Mesoamericans in general—certainly from the Maya onwards—also used rituals to invoke "vision serpents", a kind of living path or spiritual connection to the otherworlds above and below. These vision serpents were summoned in rituals incorporating state-altering technologies such as fasting, bleeding, dancing, music, and psychoactive plants. The maw of the vision serpent represented a portal to the otherworld, and faces or figures of ancestors or gods are often shown emerging from the open jaws of a snake in Mayan art, to communicate with the participant—the king, noble, or priest-shaman—during a ritual, presumably after the vision serpent has been summoned with sufficient quantities of *ch'ulel* from the blood of the participants, and invoked with ritual actions in an appropriate location.

The energy exchange of sacrifice was referred to by the Maya as *ch'am*, or "harvest":[1137] feeding the gods with the fruits of life, in order to sustain it. The Yucatec Maya called the sacrificial rituals necessary to open a portal to the otherworlds *pa'chi*, "opening the mouth", wherein they would smear blood on the lips of the gods' statues to "feed" them. (Incidentally, the ancient Egyptians had a very similar ritual for consecrating statues that they called *opet-re*, "the opening of the mouth and eyes", wherein a ceremonial adze was held to a god-statue's lips to channel the spiritual force known as *ka*, "all that enlivens", into the effigy.)[1138] *Pa'chi* also meant to "discover, manifest, or declare" as feeding the gods with *ch'ulel* allowed the "lightning to flow"[1139]—the awareness of divine *itz* manifesting, perhaps. Consecrated offering pots and bowls, "ensouled" and alive, were used to transfer the virtues of such offerings to the gods; these vessels were themselves considered to be little portals.

Because *ch'ulel* was present in blood, it was said that both one's ancestors and the vision serpent resided in the blood, and could be accessed during auto-sacrificial ritual.[1140] There is some material truth to this: some of our ancestors' DNA sequences are physically present in almost every cell of the body—ironically, with the exception of mature red blood cells, which have no DNA-containing nucleus; but white blood cells, also found in the blood, do contain genetic material. So the Maya would literally spend their souls to communicate with their supernatural patrons,[1141] summoning up vision serpents whose mouths opened into the celestial realm or the underworld.

All the Mesoamerican cultures used a fivefold division of space-time to map out the cosmos, based on the relationship to celestial events. As with Old World east and west, sunrise and sunset comprised the principal two directions for orientation in space. North—the "wind entering place"—was symbolically linked to the zenith, the sky, and the celestial world; south, the "wind leaving place", was linked to the nadir, the earth, and the underworld.[1142] The fifth direction was the centre, the place where one stood, and each of the four cardinal directions was supported by the "world tree", with its roots in the underworld and branches in the celestial realms,[1143] represented in the heavens by the Milky Way, named *wakah-chan* ("raised-up sky") by the Maya.[1144] The Maya referred to the centre of the sky as *yol*, the "heart of", *ek-wayob*, the "black transformer" or "white-bone-snake's mouth", a heavenly portal to the otherworld; these names explicitly reference the dark, starless void at the zenith when the Milky Way lies parallel to the horizon.

But the word *yol* also referred to earthly portals in sacred spaces.[1145] The Maya often rendered the "world tree" as a foliated cross,[1146] which marked shrines and holy places. The cross was a representation of the four directions and a central axis, the trunk of the world tree, with the addition of leaves, suggesting life and vitality, and each representation of a cross, as a magical object, had its own *ch'ulel*.[1147] Natural *yol* included mountaintops, springs, lakes, and "mouths" of the underworld such as caves, ravines, and the *cenotes* or *dzonots* of the Yucatan peninsula. A portal could be any place where shamans or sensitive folk felt the otherworld exhaling into the world of the sun. Unlike our own compass directions, Maya directions were alive, and always relative to sun, stars, and subject. In Maya territories, almost every mountain had (and often still has, to this day) a shrine with a foliated "doorway" cross where shamans can speak to the spirits which dwell "within" the mountain;[1148] the symbolism of the cross links the earthly portal to the celestial version, the white-bone-snake's mouth in the heart of the sky.

Like many Celtic sacred sites or places inhabited by Middle Eastern *djinn*, Mesoamerican sacred sites were often wild and abandoned, sometimes surrounded by thick brambles, best visited by shamans or priests trained to conduct ceremonies; it was commonly believed that the unwary could be harmed by venturing into one of these liminal locations, sometimes naïvely intending to strike Faustian bargains with otherworldly beings.[1149] These places exuded transformative power, visiting spirits or gods, or noxious "winds". This belief has many Old World equivalents too, such as the Celtic tradition of "thin places"; for example, in Europe, mushroom circles or "fairy rings" were thought to be similar gateways (which raises the interesting possibility that despite the lack of any historical record of *Psilocybe* mushroom use in Europe, perhaps this reputation arose from a vestigial cultural memory of magic mushrooms' potential to open a door into fairyland).

Mountains were especially important in Mesoamerica, because they represented a joining of earth and sky; the tips of mountains often pierce the clouds, while caves were mouths of the underworld. Moreover springs and streams sometimes emerge from them, and some mountains (volcanos) belch smoke and fire. Volcanos were, and are, most sacred, uniting all the elements and containing enormous generative and destructive forces. They were associated with a mythical "mountain of plenty" which features in one form or another in Mesoamerican myths, a hollow mountain from which staple foods and all human sustenance originate. In many places where the old ways are still practised, volcanos are thought to be "inhabited" by ancestors, deities, monsters, and spirits, and by interacting with them through ritual, dreams, and shamanic techniques, shaman-priests and other skilled, trained spiritual intercessors could meet and negotiate with the powers that controlled the world.[1150]

Portals could be constructed as well as found, which was useful for religious purposes: these were the temples, ballcourts, and sacred structures of Mesoamerican religion, and archaeological fame. The Olmecs and subsequent civilisations constructed their temples in the form of "stepped mountains" with a shrine at the top in order to replicate the conditions which made mountains sacred places, construing them as portals to the underworld via caves, and access points to the celestial world, towards which they pointed.[1151] Some Classic Maya referred to their temples as *uitz*, "mountains"; the Mexica's twin temples in the centre of Tenochtitlan mimicked the two volcanoes which flank the valley of Mexico, Popocatepetl ("po·po·ka·teh·peh·tul") and

Iztaccihuatl ("is·tack·see·wah·tul"). Broad plazas filled with dancing people represented the primordial sea and the exploits of the gods, while ballcourts evoked the underworld and the "game of life".[1152]

Ballcourts were sacred spaces, and ballgames were symbolic confrontations with death, evil, and disease, and may have culminated in a ritual human sacrifice.[1153] Some ballgame teams may have been comprised of prisoners of war, and others were members of the royal family (the "home team", perhaps). After important games captives would be sacrificed on the courtside steps. Ballcourt markers were shaped like quadrifoils, or foliated crosses, denoting their status as portals to the otherworld, and if a ballcourt is viewed in cross-section it forms a stepped V-shape, like the open jaws of a serpent.[1154] Ballcourts were decorated with mythic scenes relating to underworld themes. The K'iche name for the ballcourt, *hom*, is now the word for "grave",[1155] and *quic'*, "ball", means "blood".[1156] The emotional fervour of crowds and the celebrity status assumed by players at large football games today provide some insight into why the ballgame acquired such ritual significance: teams were playing the role of gods, and losing a game might result in sacrifice; literally, "heads will roll". How fortunate for sports team managers that the stakes aren't quite as high today.

War was a sacred duty for the Maya, necessary for acquiring captives to offer to the gods in sacrifice. War was also a battle between the *wayob* of the gods of the nations or tribes who were fighting, and victory was a sure sign that the *wayob* of one group's deities were stronger than their adversary's. Thus a victory in battle was the defeat of one god by another; humans were the willing participants in a celestial drama, and its purpose was the acquisition of sacrifices to feed the gods and perpetuate the world. Dead Maya kings were buried with their worldly goods—including, sometimes, their living wives, in sealed tombs. The *ch'ulel* of these objects (or people) would accompany the king into the underworld, so he would be properly provisioned and equipped for the arduous journey to the lowest level of Mictlan. These burial caches often included pots of prepared, foaming *kakawa*[1157]—along with other foods and beverages. But Cacao would have been an extraordinarily appropriate funeral offering, as we shall see.

Just So stories: origins

Page one of the pre-conquest "Borgia Codex", produced by a vassal nation of the Aztec empire under Mexica rule, illustrates the Mesoamerican equivalent of the "big bang": an explosion of stars and serpents pouring out of the top of a large turquoise bowl, presided over by a black, skeletonised being with clawed hands and feet. The serpents regurgitate beaked and taloned monkey-like homunculi, representing anthropomorphised wind or movement. The star-studded snakes have been interpreted as outflows of power, evoked by the Nahuatl couplet *yohualli ehectal*, "night-wind", imputing unfathomable, transformative, and dynamic forces. Serpents on either side of the bowl-face vomit up a bolus of obsidian on the left and what could be a bonsai-like copal tree (*Bursera jorullensis*) on the right, representing two of the necessary products for sacrifice—copal resin for incense, and obsidian for knife blades.[1158] This ophidian eruption resembles a dark head of foam effervescing out of a skull-faced bowl, from which one might consume a traditional Cacao beverage: are the origins of the universe depicted here as a bowl of frothy *cacahuatl*?

Mesoamerican creator deities included sky gods such as the ineffable Mexica dual god Ometeotl, or the Mayan Itzamna. In Mexica mythology, the world of the Fifth Sun came into being when the diseased god Nanahuatzin bravely threw himself into a fire to become the sun.[1159] Some of the oldest identifiable gods in Mesoamerican religious art are the rain gods,[1160] such as the hook-nosed Mayan Chac or the goggle-eyed Tlaloc of Teotihuacan and the Mexica. It may seem odd to modern people that rain gods could be so high up a spiritual hierarchy, but rain is crucial for agriculture and therefore survival, especially in regions which can be very arid. Meanwhile the rulers of the underworld, such as the Mayan "Earth Lords" or Lords of Xibalba, were often malevolent, inimical to life in the human world, and brought disease and affliction.[1161] They were objects of fear and derision, and were given names associated with contagion, afflictions, or putrefaction; one Mayan death god was named Cizin, the "flatulent one".[1162]

These lords of Xibalba play a key role in the K'iche Maya creation myth, written in their famous mythological history, the Popol Vuh. The story begins with two divine twins called Hun Hunahpu and Vucub Hunahpu, sons of the "divine midwife" goddess of humankind, Xmucane, and her husband Xpiyacoc. Xmucane and Xpiyacoc are the original Mayan "daykeepers", diviners and arbiters of social order.[1163] It was on their advice that the gods created the people of wood,[1164] which didn't work out so well but provided the necessary precursor to the current creation. Their sons live on Earth and like to play the native Mesoamerican ballgame. Their playing disturbed the Lords of Xibalba, who resented all the noise coming through their ceiling, so they requested that the twins come and pay them a visit. The twins went to the underworld, but the Lords of Xibalba tricked them, put them through several trials, because, we're told, "Xibalba is packed with tests, heaps and piles of tests".[1165] Tests and uncanny, impossible trickery: the ball in the ballcourt of Xibalba is a "spherical knife … surfaced with crushed bone",[1166] guaranteeing that the lords of death will win the game.

The twins fail the tests, and the Lords of Xibalba kill them; the twins' bodies are buried beneath the ballcourt, but Hun Hunahpu's severed head is placed in the fork of a tree by the main road in the land of the dead. Eventually, the underworld tree in which Hun Hunahpu's head was placed begins to bear fruits, which gain a reputation for being sweet and tasty, so much so that Xquic' ("Blood Moon"), the daughter of one of the Lords of Xibalba, comes to see what all the fuss is about. But one of the "fruits" in the tree is in fact the living head of Hun Hunahpu, inhabited by the spirits of both brothers; it spits in Xquic's palm when she reaches up to pick it, and impregnates her. She is then forced to flee the underworld and finds her way to the twins' mother, Xmucane. Perhaps unsurprisingly, Xmucane doesn't trust the pregnant stranger from hell—all she knows is that her sons went to Xibalba and never came back. So Xmucane tests her: she asks Xquic' to go into the garden and pick food for herself and her grandchildren, Hun Hunahpu's sons One Monkey and One Artisan. But the garden only has one exhausted clump of corn in it, so Xquic' beseeches the assistance of the goddess of corn and Cacao, who helps her fill her net with food, which she brings back to the house. Xmucane is then convinced that Xquic' really is her daughter-in-law, so she takes her in. Xquic' finally gives birth to a second generation of twins, named Hunahpu and Xbalanque.[1167]

When the twins grow up and discover their father and uncle's ballgame equipment, they also manage to irritate the Lords of Xibalba by playing a noisy ballgame, and are summoned to the court of Xibalba by the gods of death, where they, too, must undergo trials. Before they leave, the twins plant maize in Xmucane's house, telling her that if the maize dies, then they are dead too. During the trials in Xibalba, Hunahpu the younger is decapitated just as his father was, but the twins "fake it til they make it" by replacing his head with a squash. They have to play a ball-game against the gods of death, who replace the ball with Hunahpu's severed head as a comic wheeze; the twins retrieve it with the assistance of a rabbit which distracts the Lords of Xibalba by imitating the ball bouncing out of court, so that they have time to reattach Hunahpu's real head while the death gods are off-pitch, chasing the rabbit-ball. Having won the game, the twins realise that the gods of death are planning to burn them alive, so they voluntarily throw themselves into the fire; but before they do, they secretly instruct two diviners, Xulu and Pacan, to advise the Lords of Xibalba to scatter their ashes in a river in the underworld. Meanwhile the maize they planted on earth dies, and Xmucane mourns the death of her grandsons. The lords of Xibalba scatter their ashes in the river on the diviners' advice, and the twins are subse-quently reborn in the river as two fish, so the corn in Xmucane's house begins to sprout again, and she rejoices.

Having learned to defeat death, the reborn fish-twins emerge from the water in the under-world and become human again, presenting themselves as entertainers showing off a miracu-lous trick of sacrificing and resurrecting the denizens of the underworld. The Lords of Xibalba are amazed and delighted by this entertainment, and order the twins to perform for them, without realising their true identity. The gods of death willingly offer to participate and be reanimated—so the twins kill them but don't revive them, before unmasking themselves and holding the Lords of Xibalba to account. They visit their father's tree in Xibalba, and attempt to reanimate him, too, but can only do so partially, so they must leave him behind—although in earlier Maya legends, their father Hun Hunahpu is reborn as the maize god, emerging from the underworld through the back of a turtle. The Hero Twins finally exit the underworld as the sun and moon.[1168] (The relevance of the rabbit's appearance as a stand-in for the severed head of one of the twins in the ballgame becomes evident here, as the Maya saw a rabbit in the face of the moon.)

This creation myth embodies the Mesoamerican view of time as cyclical. The Hero Twins' underworld odyssey is a conditional triumph over death, disease, and decay, and rebirth as a result of sacrifice;[1169] challenges must be faced with ingenuity, and death must be bravely accepted so that life can go on. Natural cycles allow for a sort of reincarnation, where wisdom, trials, and gifts can all be passed down through generations. The twins must leave their father's and uncle's bodies in the underworld, and can't fully restore them, but can promise that "You will be prayed to ... you will be the first to have your day kept by those who will be born in the light ... Your name will not be lost."[1170] While the dead can't be brought back to life, their spirits can be honoured in the underworld. It's clear from the myth that, unlike the powers of death, the living can learn from the past and outwit the chthonian forces of destruction, and the next generation can surpass the previous one—if one is prepared to undergo the necessary trials, and survive them. The price of triumph is labour, sorrow, losing one's head, and a fearless willing-ness to immolate one's entire identity.

The decapitated father-twin Hun Hunahpu is one version of the Maya maize god, who is killed by the gods of death and reborn in the underworld as a plant, just as maize is "decapitated" every year when the ripe cobs are harvested, then reborn from the "heads" when the seeds are sown into the soil (compost being the "black gold" of the underworld). The other maize origin story features Yax-Hal-Witz, the "First True Mountain", sitting on the primordial sea at a location called "at the split [place], at the bitter water"[1171] in which maize and other essential food crops are found, including Cacao and *pataxtle*. Xmucane, the "first mother", ground this maize nine times with water to make a dough from which the bodies of the first humans of the third creation were made; the First Father then created their souls, and gave them life.[1172] The Mexica version of the "mountain of plenty" story features their cultural patron-god Quetzalcoatl, who transformed himself into a black ant to enter the mountain and stole corn kernels of all four colours (white, yellow, blue, and red), bringing them to the gods. They clearly appreciated it, because he went back and tried to steal the entire mountain, but couldn't carry it; so the sun god Nanahuatzin smote the mountain and broke it open, and the rain gods came and carried away the food,[1173] including Cacao, so that mankind could also have access to it: the gods of ingenuity, sun and rain made agriculture possible.

A Mayan deity labelled "God K" or K'awil by archaeologists is asserted to have rescued the seeds of edible plants from the great flood that obliterated the first creation, taking them to the thirteenth level of heaven. God K has been linked to the "Black Tezcatlipoca" in the Mexica pantheon, an aspect of one of their principal creator-gods, Tezcatlipoca and Quetzalcoatl (the latter is also sometimes known as the "White Tezcatlipoca"). Tezcatlipoca ("Smoking Mirror") was a god of rulers, fate, punitive justice, and sorcery, whose name evokes obsidian, or volcanic glass, from which mirrors and exceptionally sharp sacrificial blades were made. Tezcatlipoca was depicted with a "serpent foot" and wearing a smoking mirror on his forehead; the Mayan God K also had a serpent foot, and was depicted with a burning celt on his brow. God K, too, was also a patron of rulership, represented in the Maya kings' staff of office, a serpent-footed manikin sceptre. But the two gods weren't entirely identical: God K was associated with agriculture, which Tezcatlipoca was not, and God K seems to have had a more benign or human-friendly character. By contrast, Tezcatlipoca had a sinister, Voldemort-ish personality; his essence appears to be power, discord, and cathartic change. He had many names, including "the enemy", "night wind", "he whose slaves we are", and "possessor of the sky and earth".[1174]

Another important Mayan underworld deity was "God L", an elderly merchant god, associated with the planet venus.[1175] He is dark-skinned and wears jaguar pelts and a large owl headdress,[1176] owls and jaguars being underworld creatures, as befits nocturnal apex predators of land and air. God L appears to be a prototype of the later Mayan deity named Ek'chuah ("Black Scorpion"); he is at some point stripped of his wealth by the other gods, in a fit of vengeful envy.[1177]

The Mexica human origin myth involves Quetzalcoatl, the "feathered serpent". In Nahuatl, *quetz* means "spirit" or "wind"; the *quetzal* is a native bird with blue-green plumage which was prized more highly than gold in Mesoamerica, and *coatl* means snake.[1178] So Quetzalcoatl's name could be translated as "luxuriously feathered wind-spirit snake", and he also appears in Mexica myths as Ehecatl-Quetzalcoatl, wearing a beak-like mask commonly associated with depictions of wind gods. He was an important creator-god of the Toltecs and the Mexica, a principal deity of culture, invention, and ingenuity, and, like a composite of the Maya gods K'awil and Ek'chuah, he was a patron of rulers, priests, and merchants. The prototypes of Quetzalcoatl are the Teotihuacan-Mayan feathered serpent god Kukulcan, and the Mayan "war serpent" deity known as *waxak-lahun-ubah-kan*. The "feathered serpent" deity Kukulcan appeared at Teotihuacan and to a lesser extent in Mayan cultures which had trade connections with Teotihuacan, and was probably originally a water deity—perhaps one of the original creators of the world, as in the K'iche origin myth involving the feathered serpent creator-god in the primordial sea. *Waxak-lahun-ubah-kan* was a deified version of the vision serpent, intimately associated with the seasonal venus-Tlaloc ritual "star wars" imported from Teotihuacan.[1179]

The later, humanoid "feathered serpent" deity appears to have incorporated an actual historical figure: Ce Acatli Topiltzin, second king and son of the founding father of the post-Classic Toltec city of Tula, who was given the name Quetzalcoatl. He may have been a priest-king who didn't favour human sacrifice, but he was deposed in a military coup and banished by the warrior caste, whose patron god Tezcatlipoca demanded more sacrifices.[1180] The Toltec King Quetzalcoatl was reputed to have died in the year One Reed in "the land of writing", in other words somewhere in Maya territories.[1181] In Mexica myth, Quetzalcoatl descended into the underworld with his dog-boy sidekick Xolotl to retrieve the bones of the people from the previous world of the Fourth Sun which he had ruled, and had ultimately been destroyed by flood. Quetzalcoatl then gives the bones to the old goddess Cihuacoatl, who grinds them "like cornmeal" on a *metate*, adding blood from his penis to create a kind of living clay from which the first humans of the Fifth Sun were made.[1182] This occurred in the human origin-place called Tamoanchan, which is represented in codices as a flowering tree cut in half and gouting blood.[1183]

As with all Mesoamerican gods, Quetzalcoatl's worship included auto-sacrifice and offerings, but—unusually for a Mesoamerican deity—his preferred oblations were fresh flowers and butterflies, in contrast to his brother, Tezcatlipoca, who demanded living human hearts.[1184] Quetzalcoatl and Tezcatlipoca are best described as collaborating rivals, or frenemies with a case of mafia-level sibling rivalry. An origin myth of stunning violence reveals how the Mexica viewed suffering and bloodshed as intrinsic and essential aspects of reality. The two gods abducted the goddess Tlaltecuhtli, and, turning themselves into serpents, they wound themselves around her. One gripped her right hand and foot, and the other gripped her left hand and foot, and they tore her in two. Half the goddess became the sky, and the other half became the earth; her hair became vegetation, her eyes became lakes and waters, her nose became mountains, and her mouth became caves; in her ceaseless agony she cried during the night, begging for the hearts of men to eat, and would only consume food if it was first sprinkled with human blood. In return, as the gods ordained, her body brought forth food for men in the form of edible plants.[1185]

Decadence was taboo in Mesoamerica, as, like hubris, it could lead to spiritual delinquency and dereliction of one's proper duties, such as the human obligation to honour and worship the gods. The Mexica had five deities of pleasure and excess, the Ahuiateo; each governed a form of potentially excessive behaviour or vice such as gambling, drunkenness, or sexual misconduct, and associated diseases or misfortunes.[1186] Xochipilli, the "prince of flowers", god of feasting, dancing, painting, games, the midnight sun, and psychoactive plants—he whose statue is carved with representations of tobacco, *Psilocybe* mushrooms, and possibly funeral tree flowers—had an alter ego called Macuilxochitl, one of the Ahuiateo, who gave STDs, haemorrhoids, or boils to those who had sexual intercourse during periods of religious fasting.[1187]

One Mexica myth reveals how much they believed themselves to be negatively affected by the comforts of civilisation. The emperor sent sixty shaman-priests to find Aztlan, the historical Mexica homeland. They found a hill with spry, inexhaustible people living there who could control their physical age at will, growing younger as they climbed towards the top, where the serpent-skirted goddess Coatlicue lived. She told the magicians, "You have become old, you have become tired because of the chocolate you drink and … the foods you eat. They have harmed and weakened you. You have been spoiled by those mantles, feathers and riches that you wear and that you have brought here. All of that has ruined you."[1188]

Gods in the stars

Like all other ancient civilisations, the Mesoamericans perceived their gods in the heavenly bodies. At the tropical latitude of the Mayan civilisations, the Pole Star lay almost due north, and was "the navel around which the constellations rotate", and the ecliptic—the apparent path of the Sun around the Earth (which, as we now know, is in fact the opposite) is almost overhead.[1189] The stars were conduits of power, and the ecliptic was represented in Maya iconography as a double-headed serpent threading through the branches of the "world tree".[1190] The places where the ecliptic intersects with the Milky Way is represented in Mesoamerican carvings and illustrations as "sky bands", graphic representations of the sky and stars as a strip at the top or on the borders of illustrations. Certain constellations also feature as characters in myths and creation stories: Scorpio appears as a scorpion at the foot of the world tree in Maya art. The Maya saw the belt of Orion and the whole constellation of Gemini as a turtle, which explains why the reborn maize-sun god is often depicted emerging from the underworld from a turtle's back: on the Mayan "creation date", the sun was in Gemini, and rose with these stars. Orion's belt was also named the "three hearthstones", which appear in many Maya creation stories.[1191] In the K'iche myth of the Hero Twins and their fathers, Hunahpu the younger has been identified with the midnight sun, that is the sun in the underworld—the sun that can no longer be seen, whose Mexica equivalent is Xochipilli,[1192] the "prince of flowers".

The sun was often represented as a malevolent, aged deity in Maya art; by the post-Classic era, sun gods typically required offerings of live human hearts. The fierce nature of the deified sun makes sense in the tropics, where he burns and brings drought quite as much as he supports life.[1193] The Hero Twins and their father-uncle in the *Popol Vuh* are different aspects of the same (or at least connected) soli-lunar deities, while Xmucane and Xquic' represent the waning-new ("older") and waxing-full ("younger") phases of the moon, respectively. The Classic Maya moon goddess has been linked with the earth and with maize: likewise, Xmucane and Xquic' grow and harvest maize in the garden in the *Popol Vuh*, and the interweaving of the moon's phases with the solar year is an integral part of Mesoamerican calendrical time and the basis of the agricultural calendar, described in the next chapter. The moon is often rendered as a young or old woman in Maya religious art, although there are male moon deities—such as the Hero Twins—linked to the full moon,[1194] which makes sense as only the full moon rises at night and sets during the day; it culminates as the midnight sun anti-culminates beneath the Earth, so the full moon is the sun's night-time equivalent, its "twin". As in Europe, the moon was symbolically linked to water, plants, rain, and the sea.[1195]

The decapitation of one of the two twins in both generations of the Popol Vuh's "Hero Twins" saga is equated with eclipses,[1196] omens of upheaval. The moon maiden Xquic', the mother of the Hero Twins, may herself be an eclipse deity: "blood moons" are what happens when the moon's face is darkened by a partial lunar eclipse. Hunahpu the elder and Hunahpu the younger—a maize god and a Sun god—are different aspects of a single deity or metaphysical theme, as maize is a solar plant: it's yellow, needs much sunlight, and regularly dies and needs to be re-sown, just as the sun sets every night and rises every morning. The Tzotzil Maya, too, linked maize to their sun god, identifying it as "a hot food that came from his groin".[1197] The Maya wrote the word for sun using a pictogram of a frangipani (*Plumeria rubra*) flower,[1198] an important medicinal plant and *kakaw* spice, so this plant, like maize, was solar. As in the Old World, celestial bodies were associated with particular gods and specific earthly plants, people, and things; the stars became a magical meta-language for mapping the whole of creation.

The Popol Vuh tells of the fall of Itzam-Yeh, a gaudy macaw who sets himself up as the false sun of the world, before the real sun is made, and who is defeated and deposed by the Hero Twins, acting on the orders of the great creator-god, called Heart of Sky or Hurricane. Itzam-Yeh is possibly the *wayob* of the shaman-god Itzamna, and has been identified with the Big Dipper constellation: he "falls" from his perch on the "world tree" every night, as the Milky Way rotates from a vertical to a horizontal position in the sky and the Big Dipper descends towards the horizon.[1199] At the start of the hurricane season, in mid-October, the Big Dipper appears close to the "top of the tree" before dawn as the Milky Way is oriented perpendicular to the horizon at that time; but by the end of the hurricane season in mid-July, the Big Dipper is found "falling" from the tree in the small hours of the night: during the hurricane season, he topples from his perch.

Itzam-Yeh had two monstrous sons who also suffered from hubris: the monstrous crocodilian Zipacna, who believed himself to be the Earth, and his brother, Earthquake. Zipacna killed the "four hundred boys" who tried to trap him, crushing them under him when they were drunkenly (and prematurely) celebrating their victory; they became the stars known as the Pleiades, and represented the gods of drunkenness to the Maya.[1200] In one of the looping, multi-level associations which are so common in Mesoamerican myth, the same stars were also known as the "four hundred rabbits" and affiliated with the goddess of *pulque*, the Mesoamerican "beer" made from fermented *Agave* sap;[1201] the Maya saw a rabbit in the Moon's face, so rabbits, drunkenness, the moon, and pulque were all symbolically linked.

Zipacna and Earthquake were both killed by the Hero Twins, who lured each of them into a trap then buried them under the earth—providing a mythological explanation for earthquakes. For the K'iche Maya, the "world tree"—the Milky Way—was said to grow out of the abdominal wound of a human sacrificial victim lying on the back of an "earth monster". This image works on two levels, as the crocodilian "earth monster" Zipacna is the Milky Way in a horizontal position in the sky, whereas the "world tree" is the Milky Way perpendicular to the horizon; the crocodile "jaws" may be drawn by playing join-the-dots with the stars at the "base" of the "tree", which is why the "world tree" is sometimes rendered as a "crocodile tree".[1202] It's also been pointed out that crocodiles often bury their eggs on riverbanks, and trees frequently take root in these nitrogen-rich earthworks.[1203]

For the Mexica, the Milky Way was represented by two deities, Ilamatecuhtli ("She of the Star Skirt") and Mixcoatl ("Star Serpent"); and, like the Maya, they conceived of the Milky Way as a road or pathway to the otherworlds. The Milky Way is also represented as a goddess who gives birth to many gods, including Quetzalcoatl, who is born from her abdomen where the two-headed ecliptic serpent intersects with the Milky Way.[1204] Just as the Hero Twins walk the road on their way to and from Xibalba in the *Popol Vuh*, the Mexica gods Quetzalcoatl and Tezcatlipoca were said to have travelled along the Milky Way after they created the Earth (by brutally bisecting the goddess Tlaltecuhtli).[1205] The Classic Maya believed that the souls of the dead travelled down the world tree on the road to Xibalba, following in the footsteps of the maize-sun God.[1206] So the Milky Way was a sentient pathway to the otherworld; for the Maya, it may have been the "white-bone-snake", a celestial version of the "vision snake" summoned during sacrifice, although the white-bone-snake has also been tentatively identified as the constellation Scorpio, the "rift branch" of the Milky Way pointing to the *ek wayob*, the starless void in the middle of the night sky when the Milky Way rims the horizon.[1207]

The planet venus is the brightest star in the evening or morning sky, and periodically disappears and reappears on the other side of the sun, switching from a morning star to an evening star. To the Mesoamericans, venus was malevolent, and symbolised warfare. The principal venus god of the Mexica was Tlahuizcalpantecuhtli, a skeletal god of obsidian and coldness. The Maya, too, envisioned venus as an underworld-themed skeletal god, and timed the onset of their "star wars" to the first appearanc of venus in the sky after its conjunction with the sun as a morning star in the dry season.[1208] Likewise, for the Mexica the reappearance of Venus in the night sky (its heliacal rising) was a "baleful" omen.[1209] Like the luminaries, no one deity had a monopoly on venus—several gods appear to have been associated with the planet in different phases, and perhaps also in different seasons.[1210] For the Maya, venus is generally pernicious, as the Lacandon association with scorpions and poisonous ants, and the Yucatec name "wasp star" suggest.[1211]

Despite its malefic reputation, the benign creator-god Quetzalcoatl is one of the deities associated with venus. On his apotheosis, the Toltec-Mexica god-king Quetzalcoatl rose as the morning-star; venus is sometimes depicted as a "twin feathered serpent", showing the planet's "dual nature" in his different phases relative to the sun, as a morning and evening star. For some contemporary Maya, venus as morning star is the "white lord of the earth", whereas venus as evening star is the "false sun", or "he who makes the sun enter [the underworld]". Venus makes five stations in the sky every eighteen months, tracing out an approximately repeating pentacle-shaped pattern in an eight-year cycle. A "station" is a time when a planet appears to stand still in the sky for a night or two, before ostensibly reversing its previous direction of motion against the backdrop of the stars; this period of "retrograde motion" and the stations which bookend it are optical illusions.

The Hero Twins myth also alludes to venus's phases relative to the sun. During their trials in the underworld, the twins spend five nights in five infernal houses: the houses of Darkness, Cold, Jaguars, Bats, and Knives. Each house has been proposed to indicate a station of venus in the night sky, particularly as Jaguar and Bat are thought to be Mayan names for two constellations.[1212] The Hero Twins' visit to their father Hun Hunahpu's grave in the underworld after they have defeated the Lords of Xibalba is the start of a new venus cycle,[1213] when venus joins the sun and is therefore under the Earth and invisible for the whole night. Some skeletal or scorpion-tailed venus deities may have been associated with eclipses, as the interlocking of the venus cycle and the eclipse (metonic) cycles were used to time religious festivals, for example in the post-Classic Dresden Codex produced by eleventh- or twelfth-century Yucatec Maya from Chichen Itza, where venus periods are "rounded off" to interlock more precisely with the lunation cycle.[1214]

The wealthy Mayan underworld deity known as God K appears to be linked to the planet jupiter, particularly when jupiter is in retrograde—when it appears to be moving backwards against the constellations in the sky, relative to its normal direction. God K is shown being "speared" by a venus god in the Dresden Codex. Venus "spearing" other gods usually refers to a date when venus is opposite the planet or constellation represented by his "victim" in the sky, and on this date, as with other dates when God K is represented in codices, the planet we call jupiter was retrograde.[1215] God K and K'awil have also been identified with a late post-Classic deity named Bolon Dzacab or "Nine Generations"—linked to the nine levels of the underworld—a wealthy god who was petitioned to avert calamity in ceremonies which may have been calendrically associated with the planet jupiter.[1216] For the Mesoamericans, the sky was alive, and teeming with gods and their works.

Serpents and flowers

Before we move on to discuss Cacao's place in native Mesoamerican myth, a brief digression into two hugely important native symbols is necessary. Serpents feature heavily in Mesoamerican religion, probably because they combine several uncanny traits. Many snakes in Mesoamerica are highly venomous—the bushmaster (*Lachesis spp.*), fer de lance (*Bothrops asper*), and rattle-snake (*Crotalus spp.*) being the most deadly—and snakes slough their skins and swallow their prey whole, which is why they became emblematic of powerful spiritual forces in Mesoamerica: they could bring death or suffering, shed their "old selves" and regenerate, and entirely consume and absorb other creatures. The Mesoamerican practice of flaying some human sacrifices and wearing their skins to impersonate—or, perhaps more accurately, channel—a deity, is paralleled by the skin-sloughing of snakes: the human is "reborn" as a god by wearing the skin, until the decaying, deteriorating skin was discarded a few days later, and the human is "reborn" again as himself. The symbolism of shedding skin in order to grow corresponds with the notion of rebirth and transformation, which snakes symbolise,[1217] and which is a central theme of Mesoamerican religious thought.

Being striped, curved, multicoloured, and often living in or near water, snakes were the "companions of rainbows".[1218] They also symbolised lightning, perhaps because of the serpent-like coils and casts produced when lightning strikes sand and vitrifies it, or because of the rapid, dangerous nature of a lightning strike, reminiscent of a snake attack. While serpents are bound to earth and water, they also symbolised the sky: the Mayan word *can* or *caan* meant "sky", "serpent", or "four"[1219] (as in four directions, or the four Pauahtuns and Bacabs). The feathered serpent creator deity of the Popol Vuh dwells in the primordial sea, while his counterpart Heart of Sky rules the air; but clouds precipitate water, and sometimes produce lightning, so—as the feathers in the name "feathered serpent" suggest—snake-deities could be airborne. The circular or elliptical paths of the luminaries and wandering stars (planets) across the sky also suggested serpentine curvature to the Mesoamericans. Because of these associations with the airy celestial world and the watery underworld respectively, serpents were a symbol of rulership and authority in Mesoamerica. Mayan rulers were depicted as having a serpent-headed foot[1220] (a "lightning leg"), like the god K'awil and his dark Mexica descendant, Tezcatlipoca.[1221] The Mexica sun-war god Huitzilopochtli also wielded a living "fiery serpent" weapon, Xiuhcoatl, with all the power of a lightning strike. Mexica serpent-gods included Coatlicue (mentioned below), the beneficent Quetzalcoatl and his father Mixcoatl, "cloud serpent", a deity of the sky, the Milky Way, and hunting.[1222] These ophidian deities embodied the devastating power of lightning that granted authority, but also necessary transformative change, whether benign (K'awil, Quetzalcoatl) or terrifying (Tezcatlipoca).

Contemporary K'iche Maya speak of the "snake illness", one of six types of infirmity which call someone to the practice of divination. This illness may be accompanied by dreams of snakes, and features intense, recurrent, and painful cramps, as if the joints are "dislocated". The symptoms are only permanently relieved when the person begins to study to become a daykeeper (community spiritual leader and diviner) with a teacher, otherwise he keeps relapsing until the vocation is accepted. The diviner who accepts an apprentice may treat a new pupil by rubbing marigold flowers over his body and discarding them in the street, so that the next person who happens along "will take the snake illness with him".[1223] This kind of apparently callous attitude to the magical transference of misfortune seems typical of Mesoamerican thought, and is anathema to values shaped by Judaeo-Christian morality. But it typifies a strong fatalistic mindset that suggests the "right" person will happen along—what happens to anybody is their fate, or the will of the gods. If somebody walks into an invisible puddle of discarded illness, or if a person is cursed, that was meant to happen; similarly, if they are cured, or misfortune doesn't stick to them, then that, too, was meant to be.

As we shall see in Chapter 10, Mesoamerican divination means experiencing the "lightning in the blood", a kind of electric sensation, a somatic intuition which helps answer questions. This divine gift may be connected to the title *ahuacan* or "serpent", given to the chief priest and advisor to the throne in Classic Maya times, whose job was to draw up laws, divine, teach, and supervise the construction of sacred sites.[1224] Judaeo-Christian snakes symbolise dangerous knowledge which induces separation from God, and predisposes to sin; Mesoamerican snakes also symbolise knowledge, but this knowledge is desirable, bringing transformation and divine awareness. Either way, the process is never painless, or without consequences. Snakes could be said to symbolise the maxim "truth hurts".

There are the "vision snakes" depicted in Mayan art, showing deceased rulers and deities emerging from the mouths of serpents summoned during ritual; K'awil was often depicted standing in the mouth of a double-headed serpent. The ecliptic was often rendered as a double-headed sky serpent, winding through the "branches" of the celestial projection of the world tree, the Milky Way. The snake's maw was the *yol*, an open portal between realms.[1225] Snakes have been used as descriptors for the "living umbilical cord" or conscious pathways between the realms.[1226] Vision snakes were both snakes and ladders, the supernatural highways which conveyed non-material entities (spirits, gods, ancestors, *wayob*, or *tonal*) upwards or downwards, and were the means by which human "souls" were siphoned into their bodies, down an otherworldly saurian gullet into the womb.[1227]

Just as snakes symbolised life entering the body, they could also symbolise its departure: arterial blood spray—as after decapitation, or fatal injury—was often rendered as snakes streaming from wounds. The goddess Coatlicue, "she of the serpent skirt", was murdered by her other children at the very moment she gave birth to the Mexica's patron sun-war god Huitziopochtli, who sprung from her womb fully armoured and cut down his matricidal siblings. Statues of Coatlicue have serpents in place of head and hands, showing that these body parts have just been severed.[1228] Pain, hallucinatory delirium and death can accompany a snake bite; in Mesoamerica, snakes represented liminal moments between life and death, and all states of transition between this world and the otherworld: the moment when new life streams into the womb, or when living blood pours from the body, or when an ancestor or deity emerges from a portal during a religious ceremony.

Flowers, too, symbolise blood in Mesoamerican imagery. But in this case, they don't denote spectacular siphoning of life force in the blood to or from the otherworld via the living channels represented by serpents. The flower-blood metonym existed because blood carried *ch'ulel* or "soul", and, for the Maya, flowers were metaphors for stars, the "blooms on the world tree", which were thought to be individual souls.[1229] Flowers were an allegory for the spiritual essences of human beings, animals, or ritual objects, and a land of the dead known as the "flower world"—presumably one of the celestial realms, as it was beautiful, and filled with birds, butterflies, flowers, and rainbows.[1230] Flowers were also depicted as quatrefoils—literally, "four-leafs"—on Classic Mayan art, which connects them to the iconography of the foliated cross, the world tree, and implies they function as portals to the otherworld. This may be functionally true in the case of entheogenic plants (see below), or, to a lesser degree, the effects of seeing and smelling a beautiful flower: the word "transported" may be used to describe a powerful emotional response to beauty, or a pleasant aroma.

Maya kings wore flower-like ear flares,[1231] as flowers also symbolised the divine[1232]—perhaps because, in addition to resembling stars (the *wayob* of ancestors and gods), they were beautiful, underwent transformation into fruit or seeds which generated entire new plants, and sometimes possessed medicinal properties. They were also associated with the sun[1233]—they bloom in sunlight, and some flowers are heliotropic (they turn during the day to follow the sun), while most are phototropic (they grow towards the sun). Similarly, flowers are often brilliantly coloured, and some close their petals at night; others—those pollinated by moths, for example—open at night, and have lunar associations. Such soli-lunar links also made them royal symbols because, as in the Old World, sun and moon gods and goddesses were associated with rulership, as they govern life in the earthly realm, providing light, warmth, and energy, and manifestly affecting life on Earth.

Also like many other cultures worldwide, the symmetry, colour, fragrance, and overall aesthetic of flowers affiliated them with beauty, pleasure, and the arts. They were used as sacrificial offerings, particularly to Quetzalcoatl, patron of culture. Flowers were also metaphors for artistry, poetry, and song: "flowery" words indicated poetical recitation or formal, ballad-like speech, which is understandable—in contemporary English, to say someone's speech is "flowery" is to imply that it's unnecessarily embellished. In both cultural contexts, flowers as a figure of speech imply decorative modes of expression, but in Mesoamerican thought, "flowery" implied profundity, not frivolousness.

According to the Mexica, Quetzalcoatl created flowers—sort of. A bat (an underworld creature) emerged from his semen and bit a chunk out of the young flower goddess Xochiquetzal's vulva while she was sleeping. The other gods washed the bat-bitten genital flesh, and the bloody water produced malodourous flowers; but when the death god Mictlantecuhtli washed the same pudendal portion, the water spontaneously produced fragrant, beautiful blooms.[1234] This is a myth that could have turned Freud on. First, there's an act of sexual violence against a young goddess; but the violence is impersonal, carried out by a flying rodent and nocturnal pollinator, the bat, which emerged from the reproductive secretions of a creator-god. The goddess is unconscious when she is violated; and when the gods of life—the celestial beings—try to clean things up, they produce "malodorous flowers", but when the god of death does the same, he produces "fragrant flowers".

Nature, as symbolised by the bat, is a violator, with no regard for civilised mores; what spontaneously emerges from sexual urges can be dark and injurious (from the initial rupturing of the hymen, to the existence of STDs). Many natural and invisible by-products of sex, both physical and psychological, are potentially painful and destructive. When the higher gods attempt to sanitise things, the results are aesthetically displeasing; only the god of death is able to do a decent clean-up job, creating beauty from the mutilation. One interpretation might be that attempting to rationally rectify sexual crime or misadventure without acknowledging the chthonian powers which are inherent in the sexual domain at the level of nature produces "malodorous flowers". But the objects we call flowers are only produced due to fierce competition in the natural world, all of which occurs at the silent level of botanical struggles for survival and reproductive supremacy. The beautiful flowers which make us smile are literally a product of sexual warfare in the plant kingdom. As the reproductive organs of plants, flowers are assaulted by their pollinators, insects, birds, and bats seeking nectar, and then quickly disappear, turning into seeds or fruit. Fruit must be eaten, and its seeds excreted or buried: underworld processes are necessary to produce the next generation. Flowers embody the emergence of the exquisite from the intolerable; for the Mesoamericans, they symbolised all that was sacred and precious in life.

The style of warfare referred to as "flowery war"[1235] or *xochiyaoyotl* by the Mexica denoted recurrent, calendrically timed battles with the objective of acquiring prisoners for sacrifice, and many of the Aztec empire's bitterest enemies, such as the Tlaxcalans, resulted from it. The annual requirement to fight, the inevitable defeat by the superior forces of the Aztec empire, and the consequences—the "flower of their youth" (an interesting phrase) enslaved and fed to the heart-hungry gods of Tenochtitlan, every year—arguably produced more acrimony than a single, all-out war and conquest would have done.[1236] When the Spanish arrived, the Tlaxcalans allied themselves with the aliens, rather than unite with their Mexica neighbours. So the formal rules and ritualistic rationale of flowery war may have contributed to the destruction of the Mexica empire, no less than it seems to have done for the Classic Maya just over half a millennium earlier, as we saw in Chapter 1, when ongoing warfare abrogated the possibility of agricultural co-operation and trade in the Yucatan, incrementally tipping the whole region into a state of unsustainable conflict.

In formal Mexica poetry, war is alluded to as "intoxication"—the same descriptor for the effects of smelling beautiful flowers, drinking alcoholic beverages or *cacahuatl*; blood is described as "flowery nectar", and death in war was "flowery death". Flowers were associated with war because they were a constant reminder of the cycle of "souls", the brevity of mortal existence, and all that was worth fighting for in human life. Flowers were also associated with sexuality, particularly the seductive aspects of it, which correlates with the idea of being "intoxicated"—or, as the phrase goes, "under the influence". These forces could be weaponised: Aquiauhtzin, the ruler of Apayanco, a small village which was conquered by the Mexica in the fifteenth century, wrote a song in the character of a fictional woman from the conquered territory. She sings an erotic song to her new ruler, Axayacatl, submitting to him and taunting him at the same time:

> I weave my song with flowers […]
> You, with whom I do it, you, little Axayacatl,
> I weave flowers into you,
> I put flowers around you,
> I lift you up to join us together,
> I awaken you
> […]
> The boy calls me, the lord, little man,
> Axayacatl,
> He wants to have his pleasure with me.

She vows vengeance against the soldiers who have destroyed her homeland:

> I approach with my skirt of prickly fruit,
> With my blouse of prickly fruit.
> I will see them all dead.

(Aquiauhtzin, from León-Portilla, 1992.
© University of Oklahoma Press. Reprinted by permission)

The poem goes on to speak in various metaphors about becoming a vassal-state of Mexico-Tenochtitlan: prostitution, growing old and infirm, defeat, and the necessity to take pleasure in life where one can. These poems were typically sung in courts and noble houses; clearly Axayacatl had a well-developed sense of *schadenfreude*, as this was allegedly one of his favourite songs. The flower imagery implies seduction, influence, and being "lifted up"—although the implication is that Axayacatl is small and weak compared to the Amazon-woman of the poem. The implicitation is that he may have bitten off more than he can chew, and should be careful what he wishes for, although the poem ends on a note of resignation. So flowers also symbolise a state of being removed from one's normal subjective state of experience, inebriated by passion and powerful survival drives such as those which instigate sex or conflict. The flowers of seduction enable the protagonist to envision controlling Axayacatl, and those flowers become fruit: clothing made of "prickly fruit" which torments the wearer, like grief and the desire for vengeance. Mesoamerican flowers can be deadly.

This is literally true, too. Many native plants are toxic, but because of the symbolic association of flowers with "intoxication", they are also linked to entheogenic plants, some of which were certainly consumed with—or in—*kakaw* or *cacahuatl*. The psychoactive *Psilocybe* mushrooms were referred to as "little flowers", and several actual plant-kingdom Mesoamerican inflorescences are psychotropic, such as the darkly deliriant *toloaxihuitl* (*Datura inoxia*), the euphoriant-sedative water lily (*Nymphaea ampla*), or the unidentified aromatic Mexica floral smoking mixture called *poyomatli*, and many others (see Chapters 2 and 7). Murals at Tepanitla in Teotihuacan show flowers dripping with chimerical disembodied-eye droplets. Another surviving mural fragment from Techinantitla in Teotihuacan depicts several plants, some with eyes producing tear-like water globules, others festooned with dewdrops attached to eyes, while a giant feathered serpent hovers above them.[1237] The watery eyeballs may signify psychoactivity, imputing altered awareness or consciousness (as in "eye-opening"), being watched by the gods, being able to see the gods, or being enabled to see as they do, or all of the above. The link to water is perhaps through dew which gathers on plants, the rain which nourishes them and causes them to grow, the way that water reflects one's gaze like a mirror (a type of otherworldly portal), or even the tears associated with this brief mortal life—itself signified by the all-too-short blooming of a flower. It's also plausible that the melty eyeballs are associated with a specific sort of hallucination that occurs under the influence of some sacramental plant-based psychoactive brew—the native language of the otherworlds is, after all, the symbolism of dreams, which speak in a chorus of overwhelming totalities that resist rational comprehension. (Such as plants with drippy water-eyes.)

Serpent and flower imagery come together in Classic Maya depictions of vision serpents with beards of *Datura* flowers.[1238] *Datura* intoxication is notorious for producing hallucinations of snakes, spiders, and other phobia-inducing nightmarish creatures, as well as dead relatives; Datura flowers are often depicted on the head of cosmic war-serpents, such as the *waxak-lahun-ubah-kan*.[1239] Here is a flower which is a certain portal to the underworld, and will reliably produce vision snakes, or at least visions *of* snakes, and ancestors. The Yucatec Maya word for *Datura* is *tok'hu*, "true god"; the word *tok'* means "pierce", "let blood", or "flint".[1240] (This is another, minor testimony for *Datura innoxia* or *toloaxihuitl* being the principal psychoactive additive to *itzpacalatl*, the deliriant Cacao-based drink made from the "washing of obsidian knives" referred to in previous chapters.)

Flowers were like stars, and stars were also likened to eyes in the sky[1241]—clouds form in the sky, and rain comes from clouds, so water, eyes, flowers, and stars are connected. Flowers represented artistry, poetic speech, beauty, seduction and influence, states of fervour or ecstasy such as may be experienced in sexual intercourse or altered states of consciousness, as well as the divine aspects of being, and the gifts of life which arise from the necessity of death and processes of decay. Flowers also came to represent the poignant spiritual necessity of "flowery war". With their transformation into fruits and seeds, their aroma, and their medicinal or psychoactive properties, flowers were little portals to the otherworld, while serpents symbolised the living paths between the realms along which spirits and deities could travel. Snakes were transition-symbols, evoking states of movement or contact between this world and the otherworld, and the awesome power or life-shattering events this can entail, while flowers were symbolic of the divinity present in the human world, souls of otherworldly origin temporarily inhabiting the solar realm, and those states of "intoxication" to which humans are suscepti- ble, which recall our spiritual origins by transporting us into an extraordinary frame of mind. Flowers and snakes are symbols of transformation, so it should be no surprise that they feature in the mythology of Cacao.

Theobroma *theology*

There are many different Mesoamerican origin myths for Cacao, and the oldest are lost in the mists of time. The most generic Cacao origin story is that of the mountain of plenty, where Mesoamerican staple foods such as maize, Cacao, *pataxtle*, squash, black beans, and chillies are first produced, or—in the Mexica version—hidden, until they're discovered by the enterprising Quetzalcoatl and broken out by his celestial cronies like goodies from a *piñata*. In these legends, Cacao is lumped in with basic botanical foodstuffs and delivered from an otherworldly ware- house with the other groceries, after the divine equivalent of a ram-raid on the store. But these aren't the only origin stories for Cacao. When Hun Hunahpu is decapitated in the Popol Vuh, his head becomes the miraculous fruit in the underworld tree which impregnates Xquic', the death god's daughter. This tree is named as a calabash or gourd tree (*Crescentia cujete*), which correlates with the Aztec-era Borgia Codex depiction of the tree of the south, the direction of the underworld, as a calabash.[1242] But there are several post-Classic Maya ceramics which depict the tree with Hun Hunahpu's head in it as a Cacao tree.[1243]

In the Mexica Fejérváry-Mayer Codex, Cacao—not calabash—is the tree associated with the south cardinal direction, the "wind leaving place", and the underworld.[1244] Both Cacao and gourd trees flower and fruit cauliflorously (directly from the trunk), yet the tree into which Hun Hunahpu's head is placed is described as having sweet-tasting fruit. Gourd fruits are inedible; Cacao fruit pulp, however, is delicious. Perhaps the reason that the gourd tree is associated with the underworld in Mesoamerican mythology is its connection to Cacao, not the other way around. The apparently interchangeable nature of the two trees in folklore may be linked to *kakawa* being drunk from calabash-cups. Hemispherical, sawn-off-cranium-like dried gourds were the standard receptacles for frothy Cacao-based beverages, and imbibing from these vessels was likened to drinking from the maize-sun god Hun Hunahpu's skull[1245]—which is interestingly reminiscent of the Borgia Codex illustration of the birth of the universe, with the forces of creation exploding out of an effervescent death's head, a skull-shaped vessel contain- ing a dark, foaming liquid.

One Mexica legend says that Quetzalcoatl, patron god of kings, priest-magicians, and mer- chants, ruled the Toltecs during the last sun (as we saw earlier, this was probably a real-life king of Tula called Ce Acatli Topiltzin). He taught his people all the arts and sciences, cultivation and harvesting, astronomy, astrology, and how to measure time with the calendar. He also stole a bush from the gods—*Theobroma cacao*—and taught his people how to prepare it and make Cacao-based beverages.[1246] The gods grew jealous of Quetzalcoatl's people, and then angry, on discovering the theft of Cacao. So Quetzalcoatl's fraternal nemesis Tezcatlipoca came down to Earth on the thread of a spider, disguised himself as a merchant, and visited the Toltec king.

He convinced Quetzalcoatl to drink *pulque*, assuring him it was "the drink of happiness". Quetzalcoatl got drunk and made a fool of himself, so he had to abdicate, because public drunkenness was a great sin in Mesoamerican culture. Quetzalcoatl went into exile in the east, and as he walked, he wept as he saw that all the Cacao bushes he'd planted had become spiny maguey plants (the succulent from which *pulque* is made); this is why maguey, and not Cacao, grows in the arid Mexican heartlands. He planted his last Cacao seeds on the coast in present-day Tabasco, which is still a Cacao-growing region, and departed into the sea.[1247] This myth reveals that the Mexica thought of their humanoid feathered serpent god as the patron of Cacao and *cachuatl*, and Tezcatlipoca—the darker descendant of K'awil—as a patron of maguey and *pulque*; but Tezcatlipoca appears as a merchant here, recalling both the Maya underworld merchant god, "god L", who becomes a keeper of Cacao, and the Mexica *pochteca*, the traders for whom Cacao was both currency and merchandise.

There is another, bleaker Mexica origin story for Cacao. A princess stewards her warrior husband's estate and hides his treasure while he is away on a military campaign. In his absence, her husband's enemies, envious of his wealth, kidnap and torture her to extract the location of the treasure, but she keeps his secret. When she finally succumbs to death, Quetzalcoatl causes the Cacao tree to emerge from her blood. The fruit "hides the real treasure of the seeds", which are pink-tinted, strong, and bitter—representing blood, virtue, and "the suffering of love".[1248]

The gods of chocolate

Cacao is linked to various deities, both male and female, represented on Mayan bowls, statues, and figurines as fertile women and old or young men with Cacao pods growing out of their bodies.[1249] Little is known about any of these Cacao deities, although the Mayan underworld God K, or K'awil—he of the snake foot, physiognomic prototype of Tezcatlipoca—is shown emerging from the mouth of a serpent in a *dzonot*, a living portal between worlds, carrying Cacao seeds. K'awil's name means "sustenance",[1250] perhaps because of his mythical role rescuing plant life from the flood which destroyed a previous creation, and he is typically depicted with Cacao pods.[1251] While K'awil resembles Tezcatlipoca, his mythic persona seems closer to the Toltec-Mexica god Quetzalcoatl, the benefactor-god of rulership, culture, and merchandise who discovered maize, Cacao, and other crops in the Mountain of Sustenance.

The other Mayan deity often depicted with Cacao is the elderly merchant God L/Ek'chuah. When the other gods dispossess him, much of his hoarded wealth is in the form of Cacao, with which he is often depicted.[1252] The fifteenth month of the solar year was the month of Cacao planting, dedicated to Ek'chuah and the rain god, Chac; the festivities included the usual animal sacrifices, and offerings of precious substances, including Cacao. Cacao tree branches were handed to officials during the ceremonies, and the chosen animal sacrifice was a "chocolate dog"—a small dog with Cacao-brown spots.[1253] God K/K'awil is associated with leadership and divination, whereas God L/Ek'chuah is a merchant whose story is one of wealth, age, and loss. Ek'chuah is the predecessor of the Mexica merchant god Yacatecuhtli,[1254] who naturally had an association with Cacao, too, because of the merchants' primary task of locating and obtaining supplies of goods including Cacao, the coin of the realm.

Two unidentified deities in the Madrid Codex, a post-classic Yucatec Maya book, have blue-black skin and scorpion tails,[1255] and a scorpion-tailed, blue-skinned god is depicted standing next to a Cacao tree with a bird perched in its branches in a mural from Cacaxtla, a late Classic Maya site—which reminds us that Ek'chuah's name means "black scorpion". In this mural, the god also has jaguar-claw hands and feathered arms, wears a venus-symbol skirt, and is standing in a starry sky atop a watery underworld. He is flanked by a turtle, on his right, and a toad, on his left. Past the turtle on his right grows the Cacao tree, and to his left, grows a maize plant. Four dots and a stylised animal head next to the Cacao tree may represent the date "Four Deer" in the 260 day ritual calendar. The Cacao tree may represent the Milky Way—the world tree—with the Big Dipper constellation (Itzam-Yeh, "Seven Macaw") perching at the top, with the venus-god in the centre, standing between two constellations represented by the turtle (Orion) and the frog; the maize plant, we may speculate, represents the sun.

In older Maya myths, Cacao and other plants sprouted from the corpse of the maize god,[1256] as in Hun Hunahpu's death and rebirth as a fruiting tree—possibly Cacao—in the underworld. Mesoamerican maize god myths have common themes, beginning with the sacrificial death of the maize god at harvest time, leading to his burial in a mountain, at which point his spirit body ascends to the celestial world and his physical body in some way becomes food. This is where Cacao comes in: Cacao emerges from the maize god's body in the underworld and temporarily enriches the underworld god, such as god L/Ek'chuah, the elderly merchant-farmer deity. In other narratives, the serpent-footed "lightning bolt" god K'awil rescues Cacao and other foods from the underworld;[1257] this "agricultural avatar" role is later taken over by Quetzalcoatl. Finally, the maize god is reborn, which corresponds with the sprouting of maize grains to generate a new crop. The maize god's death allows Cacao to live, and the appearance of Cacao precedes the rebirth of the maize god.

In the post-Classic Mayan Dresden Codex, the text by an inscription of K'awil holding a handful of Cacao seeds reads "first or honoured maize's sustenance is Cacao", suggesting that maize—the staple food of humans, symbolically linked to the sun god—is in turn dependent on Cacao, whose supernatural sponsor is K'awil, god of agriculture, divination, magic, lightning, and rulership. Cacao is harvested at the end of the dry season, when maize is planted;[1258] one "begins" when the other "ends". These two primary food plants of Mesoamerica lend themselves to dualistic opposition: Cacao likes shade, maize likes sun; maize is annual, Cacao is perennial; Cacao pods grow down, maize cobs grow up. Both maize and Cacao seeds grow in a similar way, in a circular pattern around a central axis, producing a "cob"—only Cacao seeds are hidden inside pods with a leathery outer shell, but maize seeds grow outwardly, with a pithy central husk.[1259]

In the Popol Vuh, Xquic' calls for help from the spirits who guard the food crops in Xmucane's garden, the first of which is "Xkakaw, Ix Tziya"—"Cacao woman, Maize woman" or "Thunder Woman, Maize Woman".[1260] This is interesting on several levels—first, because this is not just the only female Cacao spirit to be explicitly named in surviving myths, it's the *only* specifically-named Cacao deity on record. Second, it exemplifies the dual-aspect nature of Cacao and maize. Third, the mention of thunder: both Quetzalcoatl and K'awil, the male deities credited with gifting or restoring Cacao to humankind, were also weather-gods—K'awil of lightning, and

Quetzalcoatl of wind. Quetzalcoatl in particular was the "road-sweeper" for the rain gods, ushering in the rain clouds to make the land fertile.[1261]

Cacao finds its way into contemporary Latin American myths as the *rilaj mam*, "ancient grandfather" in highland Guatemala. The *rilaj mam* is a sort of patron spirit of merchants, who "presides over the death of Christ" and "rules in his place for five days of holy week",[1262] before Christ (in a rather unconventional display of violence) engages him in battle on Easter Sunday and defeats him. During holy week, the idol of the *rilaj mam* is brought to the chapel and offerings of food, money, tobacco, liquor—and Cacao—are brought to the statue as offerings. It seems that the *rilaj mam* is a vestigial God L/Ek'chuah, Trojan-horsed into Christian ceremonies as a Satan-substitute, but the tributes paid to him during holy week bespeak a more complex relationship; habits of appeasement die hard, as do ancestral memories, or myths of a sun-maize god who is temporarily defeated by a powerful underworld deity before resurrecting. In another post-conquest K'iche Maya myth, Cacao is a keeper of the light, not a hostage of the dark: Cacao hides Jesus Christ from his pursuers by covering him with a blanket of white flowers, so Jesus promises that the tree will "ascend into heaven, and the clouds and mists of the sky will descend upon you in this world".[1263] He also decreed that Cacao was never to be used as firewood, and that chocolate should be served at all important ceremonies.[1264]

Theobroma *Logos: the mythical symbolism of Cacao*

There are several recurring tropes in the mythology and ritual usage of Cacao. Here are a few of the main affiliations:

1. **The World Tree.** The Mesoamerican Axis Mundi was sometimes referred to as the "crocodile tree", because when the *wakah-chan* (Milky Way) lay parallel to the horizon at night it became the "cosmic crocodile", like Zipacna in the Popol Vuh myth cycle. Cacao trees are sometimes depicted as crocodile-trees on Maya pottery,[1265] and some indigenous Mesoamerican groups explicitly designate Cacao as their world tree, not the more usual *Ceiba* or Kapok tree (*Ceiba pentandra*). Cacao is often represented emerging from of the jaws of an underworld serpent, a manifest *yol*, which is appropriate for a tree that grows on the edges of *dzonots*, those natural portals to the underworld. As we have seen, the Tzotzil Maya described the souls of the dead as "blossoms on the world tree". They also conceived of the Axis Mundi as a sky-tree "of many breasts" which suckle the souls of unweaned babies who died in infancy, now transformed into "flowers tied to the celestial cross";[1266] these descriptions are reminiscent of the flowers and pods which sprout directly from Cacao's trunk, as they do not from the *Ceiba*. Given the existence of Cacao-woman figurines sprouting Cacao pods, and the fertility symbolism associated with Cacao (see below) as well as its traditional medicinal use for promoting lactation (see Chapter 3), this suggests a strong symbolic overlap between Cacao and the Classic Maya *wakah-chan*.

2. **The Underworld.** The Mayan glyph for *kakawa* was two fish, because the word *ka* meant "fish"[1267]—so *ka-ka* is a poetic pun ("fish-fish")—and the underworld was a watery place. In Mesoamerican symbolism, birth was equivalent to emerging from water, like the feathered serpent calling forth the land from the sea, or the "waters breaking", and death was re-submergence; the "two fishes" reborn in the waters of the underworld evoke both entry and exit, rebirth and

death. Cacao's inclusion in the "food hoard" inside the mythic mountain of plenty, symbolic of the emergence of all plants from the earth, is made more explicitly chthonic by the under-world merchant god, God L or Ek'chuah, who sequesters and trades Cacao. In contemporary Belize, food and drinking chocolate are left in caves as offerings to underworld deities;[1268] and in Guatemala, cave offerings to the "earth gods and angels" consist of animal blood, Cacao, and fermented beverages,[1269] demonstrating old associations between earth, food, fermentation, the underworld, and Cacao. One of the more "civilised" portals to the underworld, the ballcourt—the mythic site of the twin generations' call to the underworld in the Popol Vuh, and the literal site of many sacrificial captives' dispatch to the underworld—were often decorated with carv-ings depicting Cacao trees and pods. The Cacao pods may symbolise decapitated heads, such as the mythic head of Hun Hunahpu, or the literal beheading of gameplayers, or sacrificial hearts, made as offerings to the gods.[1270]

3. **The maize god reborn; the eclipsed or midnight sun**. There is compelling evidence that the entire tale of the Hero Twins in the underworld—and presumably, therefore, older ver-sions of the Sun-maize god's underworld reincarnation myth, too—can be read as a complex allegory for Cacao production and processing: fermentation, roasting, grinding, and mixing with water. The twins' entrance to the underworld and the trials they undergo are equivalent to fermentation; they jump into the fire, and are roasted; their bones are ground, just as Cacao is ground on the *metate*; then their ashes are scattered into the water of an underworld river so that they can reincarnate as two fishes, just as Cacao is mixed with water to produce *ka-ka-wa*.[1271] While the Maya may or may not have extensively fermented their Cacao beans—this is dis-puted (see Chapter 2)—all the steps of the saga reflect the processing of Cacao. The Hero Twins are the future sun and moon, linked to both maize and Cacao—of the elder twins, one dies and one is decapitated and reborn as a Cacao tree in the underworld; of the younger, again one is decapitated, both die as a maize plant dies, and both are reborn in the underworld as "two fish": Cacao. Cacao is linked to trial, decapitation, and spiritual rebirth, and we know that eclipses were a sort of "decapitation" of the sun or moon, that Hun Hunahpu's Cacao-head impregnated an eclipse goddess, and that at night the sun visited the underworld to be reborn at dawn. So Cacao is symbolically linked to eclipses and the night-time sun on its journey through the underworld.

On a Classic-era Mayan *kakaw* pot, the maize god is shown seated in a canoe with two other deities—likely symbolising other planets or celestial bodies, as the Milky Way may also have been symbolised by a canoe with planets or constellations as "paddlers".[1272] The canoe is sail-ing out of the mouth of a *chihil-chan*, a "deer-serpent" with a fish body shaped like the Mayan glyph for Cacao, and the chimerical fish is itself emerging through a portal-like ring of brown foam: this may literally show the sun being reborn from a chocolate-rimmed doorway to the underworld (which sounds like a euphemism for some kinky sexual practice, but isn't). The Tz'utujil Maya of Atitlan still make a blood-red *atole* with Cacao and annatto which they refer to as "bones and blood", recalling the Mexica legend about blood from Quetzalcoatl's penis being ground with human bones to make the first people. Maize and Cacao make life; they are even grown together in some *milpas*, where Cacao is said to "protect" maize.[1273]

4. **Reincarnation, resurrection, and invoking ancestors**. This category is an offshoot of Cacao's role as an underworld plant. With its rapid growth and short life cycle, and its endless

renewal as each generation seeds the next and passes away, maize symbolises human life, our brief existence in the solar realm; whereas the perennial shade-loving Cacao represents rebirth, or the capacity for reincarnation and ceremonial contact with the ancestors, just as its seeds are killed, soured, darkened and utterly transformed—far more than maize—by fermenting and roasting and grinding. Maize and Cacao are the short life cycle and the long life cycle, respectively—the earthly avatars of life and death in the solar world, and death and rebirth from the underworld. Practically, maize is Mesoamerica's daily bread—its staff of life and staple food—and Cacao is a complementary life-enricher and life-extender, helping humans to bear trouble and grief. They are the bones and the blood, the sweet and the bitter, the visible and the occult sun.

The Hero Twins saga links the gods of the sun, moon and possibly venus to Cacao, and explicitly to their rebirth in the underworld—which occurs beneath the earth, just after new moons, eclipses, or venus's inferior conjunction with the sun, all preceding their visible reappearance in the sky (e.g., at dawn) when they rise from the sea in the east. The sun-maize-Cacao association in Mesoamerican thought has been extended to a sun-maize-Cacao-Christ overlap in contemporary Mayan mythology: modern day K'iche even say a blessing over Cacao seeds in Christian ceremonies, dedicating them to "the resuscitation of our Lord"[1274]—in this case, the persecuted, sacrificed, and resurrected Christ. For the pre-conquest K'iche, Cacao and maize beverages doubled down on Christian communion wafers and wine: such *atoles* were the body *and* the blood of the resurrected *twin* sons of god.

But the theology of Mesoamerican soul-recycling—the shuffling of human "souls" from the world of the Sun, to the underworld, or to the celestial world, and back again, is incompletely understood; it seems that some aspects of the soul could be reincarnated in different forms, appearing in the solar realm as plants or animals as well as humans. Especially important and venerated ancestors were often shown returning as Cacao trees, or their spirits being somehow accessible through them; Cacao trees were depicted growing right out of the ancestors' graves.[1275] Censers have been found at the late Classic Maya site Copan in the shape of Cacao trees with "floating faces" reminiscent of Hun Hunahpu's head in the underworld tree; these censers are thought to represent ancestors reborn as Cacao trees,[1276] though they just as likely represent some magical facility attributed to Cacao for helping to contact the ancestors.

This perceived ancestor-evoking property of Cacao may be one reason for its representation as the world tree, and its use as a sacramental substitute for blood: perhaps Cacao, like blood itself, was rich in *ch'ulel*, the Maya soul-stuff which facilitated contact with the otherworld. In the contemporary K'iche myth where Jesus blesses the Cacao tree for its protection, he declares that "clouds and mists"—synonyms for *ch'ulel*—will "descend upon you in this world". Or Cacao may have been a source of *itz*, the magic-stuff which caused things to happen: in the post-Classic Mayan Dresden Codex, the creator-god Itzamna is shown holding a Cacao glyph in a circle of dotted lines, perhaps a representation of Cacao as a vehicle of *itz*.[1277] On the other hand, the affiliation of Cacao trees with ancestor spirits could be allegorical, as grandchildren were often referred to as "sprouts",[1278] the process of reincarnation being analogous to vegetative reproduction.

Deceased Classic Maya rulers are sometimes depicted as Cacao trees on sarcophagi. In one scene on a late Classic Mayan vase, a person is shown emerging from the base of a Cacao tree, rising up towards a man with a resplendent headdress. Perhaps the man with the headgear is a king invoking a royal ancestor, as he stands welcoming the revenant with open arms; another man with chocolate-stained lips sits on the ground, looking up at the seated god K'awil, who gestures towards the Cacao tree, while a servant grinds Cacao seeds on a *metate* at his feet. Here, Cacao is explicitly linked to resurrection and royal power.[1279] Relief carvings of Cacao flank the entrance to the Temple of the Owls, messenger birds of the underworld, on two standing stones at Chichen Itza. The graven trees are dotted with representations of jade disks, which denote preciousness; fully three-dimensional carved figures emerge from the base of the trees, prone torsos and heads with arms crossed around their chests, and facial motifs indicating that they are breathing and speaking or singing. Serpentine, umbilical "tails" connect them to the trunk of the Cacao trees.[1280] Given their location, it seems likely that these are representations of ancestor-spirits being brought to life through Cacao. So Cacao may embody death and rebirth as an ancestor-spirit in the underworld, and may have been thought to facilitate summoning ancestor-spirits, the transformation of aspects of the soul into spiritual beings, or their reincarnation.

5. **Sacrifice and supplication**. In many Maya codices, gods are depicted piercing their earlobes and sprinkling Cacao pods with their blood.[1281] Why? In the myths, gods shed their blood to create physical beings, as when Quetzalcoatl creates the humans of the Fifth Sun. It could be that the figures bleeding over Cacao aren't deities at all, but costumed ritual participants auto-sacrifically honouring the gods. Sprinkling Cacao pods with blood becomes less bizarre if one considers blood as a magical fluid, replete with *ch'ulel*, and sacrifice as both reparation and down-payment: the gods (or human actors) auto-sacrificing to Cacao are doing so to "activate" some desired property of Cacao's, or to prepay or repay Cacao for a service. Perhaps the service is sustenance, and the magical power is something to do with Cacao's underworld affiliations; or maybe they're making a further security deposit on Cacao's *Ceiba*-substitute role as that living interdimensional scaffolding, the world tree. Although the tale of the Hero Twins is a myth of the K'iche Maya, there's another possible symbolic connection between Cacao and Mexica sacrificial practices: the *tzompantli* or skull-rack, used to display the heads of human sacrifices, was likened to a tree laden with fruit.[1282]

The Pipil of El Salvador were reported to hang "strings of Cacao pods" around the necks of young male captives to be sacrificed, and a Classic-era Mayan clay whistle depicts a kneeling man, with his hands tied behind his back, flaccid genitals exposed, with two Cacao pods hanging from a cord around his neck.[1283] The pods hang at chest level, like ridiculous fake breasts, as if to parody his uncovered testicles. Cacao may denote those marked for sacrifice by heart extraction, referencing the sacrificial victim's hermaphroditic ritual role: his sacrifice will combine an archetypally female element as he is penetrated by the blade, and a male function as he spurts blood, "fertilising" the ritual. The living heart and blood of the hapless captive will be a source of *ch'ulel* to open a portal and engender heavenly *itz* or magical, creative power; his death "gives birth" to new potential, the implication being that Cacao itself, like human hearts and blood, was also a source of such power.

Cacao itself was frequently used as an oblation, and many offering pots were decorated with Cacao pods.[1284] The Maya sometimes used non-perishable analogues of blood, such as ground hematite or cinnabar,[1285] and prepared *kakawa*—perhaps coloured blood-red with annatto—may have constituted an offering of this type. Contemporary Yucatec Maya still place prepared Cacao beverages on an altar so that the spirits can drink their "essence"[1286]—their *ch'ulel*, perhaps, or its equivalent. Cacao's association with rebirth and reanimation links it to "life" in the broader sense of summoning spirits or deities into objects or statues in rituals, and "ensouling" them. Lacandon Maya traditionally placed five Cacao beans, symbolising the heart, lungs, liver, stomach, and diaphragm into their "god pots", which were subsequently "ensouled" in a ritual to house their gods;[1287] the Cacao beans are the "vital organs" of the idols, without which the gods cannot inhabit them.

6. **Wealth, power, and ruin**. Cacao has mythic links with rulership and privilege. It was a very bad omen for a Mexica commoner to drink *cacahuatl*,[1288] perhaps signifying the destabilisation of society: to have their god-food consumed by plebeians may have been akin to seeing the pope's mitre or the crown jewels worn by a tramp. Ek'chuah, the aged Mayan merchant god, is stripped of his hoarded wealth by the other gods, who covet it; and in the Mexica myth of the sorcerers seeking their homeland, Aztlan, the goddess Coatlicue tells them how their riches and the Cacao they drink and food they eat has weakened and "ruined" them, so that they are at the mercy of old age and death. These myths can be read as morality tales cautioning against extravagance and presumption, or a warning to guard and moderate one's wealth, health, and fortune so as not to take them for granted; but Cacao, a symbol of abundance and authority, is explicitly associated with the enervating effects of indolent affluence, when avarice or complacency cause a dereliction of spiritual responsibilities.

The five Ahuiateo, the Mexica gods of vice and its consequences, were assigned to the southern compass point[1289]—the direction of the underworld. The potential syllogism between Cacao, wealth, and disaster can also be clearly seen in its Mexica origin stories. Quetzalcoatl loses his throne as a consequence of stealing Cacao from the gods to give to humanity, inspiring the other gods—in particular his dark brother Tezcatlipoca—to take revenge by inducing him to an act of public dissipation, forcing him to abdicate his throne and go into exile; the first Cacao tree is born from the blood of a princess who dies loyally guarding her absent husband's hidden wealth. Cacao is a magnet for envious retribution. It's a divine compensation for suffering, available in a buy-now-pay-later deal, or with one simple—fatal—prepayment.

7. **Fertility, sexuality, and reproduction**. Classic Maya artworks often depicted women and goddesses sprouting Cacao pods, or covered in Cacao seeds. The plant was strongly associated with femaleness and fertility,[1290] and this tradition continues with its folk medical use by Guatemalan *comadronas* (midwives) (see Chapter 3). The pendulous pods growing directly from the tree trunk also resemble testicles or breasts, and a late Classic Maya male figurine has a split Cacao pod on a stalk emerging from the top of his loincloth, like a penis (though one museum catalogue describes it, tactfully, as emerging from his "navel").[1291] In the Hero Twins myth, Hunahpu's pod-head impregnates the maiden Xquic', who later bears the Hero Twins, living embodiments of Cacao, so Cacao is a mythological symbol of both male and female fertility. A scene from the post-Classic Maya Madrid Codex shows a young moon goddess exchanging Cacao beans and sharing a pot of foaming *kakawa* with the elderly rain god Chac.[1292] *Kakawa* was

drunk when making alliances and important agreements, and this scene symbolises fertility in the wider sense of agricultural fecundity, dependent on the rains and—according to Mayan beliefs—the moon's cycles. Cacao has ancient use in rain and fertility rituals, both as an offering and a sacrament, and is strongly associated with water,[1293] the element which is paradoxically evocative of both the underworld and fecundity, because moisture is a precondition for growth and decay.

8. **Divination**. Cacao seeds were sometimes used in divination, as a substitute for maize kernels in sortilege (see Chapter 10 for more details of Mesoamerican divinatory practices).[1294] But Cacao's utility in divination and native magico-religious practice runs far deeper. Cacao's traditional consumption with psychedelic *Psilocybe* mushrooms in pre-Colombian Mesoamerica has been described and pharmacologically interpreted in Chapters 2 and 6, and it's highly plausible that Cacao facilitated altered states induced by the compounds in magic mushrooms, as well as being a beneficial modulator of the psychoactive effects of other native entheogens. Its ubiquitous consumption at both religious and secular ceremonies may be due, at least in part, to its psychoactivity—as postulated in Chapters 5 and 7, Cacao could act as a preparatory stabiliser and accelerant for revelatory, "portal-opening" entheogens.

There's also the anecdotally observed effect of central American chocolate or Cacao causing high-resolution technicolour dreams (see Chapter 5). *Sinicuichi* (*Calea zacatechichi*), one of the plants carved on the statue of Xochipilli, was used to induce lucid dreaming,[1295] the process of becoming aware while dreaming so one can consciously direct the actions of one's dream-self. This is considered to be an essential shamanic technique, as dreams are the travels of the *wayob* or *tonal* in the otherworld. So Mesoamerican shaman-priests could (and still do) seek answers from gods, spirits, and ancestors in their dreams,[1296] and perhaps Cacao was used ritually to facilitate this, which may be one reason it's so strongly associated with the underworld and communication with the ancestors in native Mesoamerican religion. More mundanely, when a contemporary K'iche diviner is accepted into his or her apprenticeship, the novice's family provides a ritual feast to which the teacher is invited, and which is traditionally rounded off by serving chocolate.[1297] While this may simply be a ceremonial gesture and a pleasant way of ending a meal, analogous to a cup of coffee or a champagne toast, Cacao's metaphysical signification of rebirth suggests that its use in this context may additionally symbolise the apprentice crossing a threshold into new spiritual awareness.

9. **Serpents and venom**. As laid out in this chapter, Cacao appears to have been a botanical representative of the theme of resurrection, or life-after-death, so it would be surprising if it wasn't associated with serpents. Even though you can't see the midnight sun, it still travels along the ecliptic—the snake in the branches of the Milky Way, aka the world tree, which is sometimes also depicted as Cacao. Cacao was traditionally used as an anti-envenomation elixir (as described in Chapters 3 and 4), and was gifted to humanity by the serpent-footed god K'awil, or the "feathered serpent" Quetzalcoatl. As we saw in Chapter 1, Cacao's affiliation with venom didn't just extend to prophylaxis, for which it has an ancient reputation; it could also be used to administer poisons. The post-colonial poisoning of the bishop who tried to ban chocolate's use in church by means of a cup of poisoned chocolate, causing "his skin to break and cast out white matter, which had corrupted and overflown his whole body"[1298] is particularly memorable.

Animistic spirits of water called "water serpents" are said to desire Cacao,[1299] which makes perfect sense given the mythological associations between water, fertility, and the underworld. I've also noticed that when Cacao beverages are made without added maize, the head of foam isn't dulled by added starches and particles. When these *tlaquetzalli*-class *cacahuatl* beverages are properly frothed, and the foam catches the light, the film of natural oils refracts it; every bubble contains a tiny swirling rainbow. In Mesoamerican terms, the foam on *kakawa* or *cacahuatl* is inhabited by thousands of tiny rainbow-serpents, reminiscent of the creation-drawing in the Borgia Codex, with snakes streaming out from the dark froth in the cosmic skull-bowl.

10. **The heart, the blood**. One of the Mexica poetic metaphors for Cacao was *yollol eztli*, or "heart, blood": as Bernardino de Sahagún relates, Cacao was "the heart, the blood … to be feared".[1300] *Yoliliztli*, the animating force of the world, which resided in the human heart, was analogous to Cacao, the blood of the heart torn out in sacrifice. The Mexica allegedly served those about to be sacrificed via heart extraction blood-red chocolate, presumably coloured with *achiotl* (*Bixa orellana*);[1301] this could have been intended to fortify the soon-to-be-late sacrificial candidate's spirit for its ascension to Topan. The post-Classic Toltec, Maya, and Mexica cultures, especially, seem to have used Cacao-based beverages as a ritual substitute for blood,[1302] but a carving on a Classic Maya stela in present-day Guatemala shows a whole Cacao pod being "sacrificed", spouting arterial blood as if it were a living human organ.[1303]

Mesoamerican ritual cannibalism may also provide a clue to the religious and ceremonial role of Cacao: prepared Cacao-based beverages were correlated with blood, Cacao pods with the heart or head (the receptacles for some parts of the "soul"), and Cacao beans served as the "organs" of gods in the Lacandon Maya "god pots". A belief that Cacao is a vehicle for vital power of divine origin is implicit in these correspondences. As described above, some post-Classic Mayan codices depict gods or human god-impersonators shedding their blood onto Cacao pods, and some figurines of sacrificial victims wear necklaces of miniature Cacao pods.[1304] Mixtec codices illustrate temples with bleeding Cacao pods growing from the roof and inside the doorway, so Cacao is intimately associated with these artificial portals to the otherworld, much as Cacao trees are known to grow naturally in the humid mouths of *dzonots* in the Yucatan peninsula.

The life cycle of Cacao is also used to time bloodletting rituals: contemporary Xeoj Maya of San Bartolomé offer blood from their ears and arms to the earth deities to ensure good weather when the Cacao trees bloom.[1305] These explicit connections between Cacao and blood, the liquid medium of life force and the gateway to the ancestors via sacrifice, support the hypothesis that Cacao itself was perceived to possess the very same life force—*ch'ulel* or *yoliliztli* or whatever local word for "identity-giving immortal spirit" was appropriate—and was revered for this reason. To drink beverages made with Cacao was to absorb and perhaps to replenish some of this life-giving force; to fortify the spiritual connection to the ancestors by invigorating the hereditary soul-force that resided in the blood.

Cacao's association with the heart is also metaphorically tied to its property of instilling courage. This can be seen in its historical use as a libation for sacrificial victims, warriors, and merchants—those who have faced, or are about to face death—and in its mythical associations with valorous acts, such as the Mexica princess's bravery, the daring of the selfless and ingenious benefactor-god Quetzalcoatl, and the courage of the Hero Twins. The heart is the first of the five vital organs symbolised by Cacao beans in the "god pots" of the Lacandon Maya. To remove a heart is to extract life-force; Cacao's synonymity with the heart and the blood identify it as a roborant at the level of the soul.

11. **Flowers and foam**. The Maya used *kakawa* as a baptismal liquid, mixing water taken from hollows in trees or rocks in the forest—natural fonts, or miniature portals—with Cacao and "certain flowers" to make a special anointing chocolate,[1306] which was painted onto the forehead, face, and spaces between the fingers and toes with a bone.[1307] Here, chocolate symbolises new life, and its use in baptism symbolically connects the infant to his or her ancestors in the underworld, and the cycle of life. The pairing with fragrant flowers and rainwater occurs because flowers denote the soul, joy, mortality, and the incarnation of divine powers into the solar realm, while water is both fertile and destructive, the element of the watery underworld and life-giving rain.

Contemporary Mexican folklore holds that while chocolate is good for the body, the foam is good for the soul.[1308] Restaurateur and *Chocolate Atole* maker Carmen Santiago of Teotitlan del Valle in Oaxaca refers to the foam as the best part of the drink—"*el lujo de la bebida es la espuma*" ("the high quality/abundance/wealth of the drink is its foam").[1309] The Lacandon Maya sing a special "frothing song" using "flowery words" of worshipful, poetic, and musical speech while making their sacred Cacao drink for the gods.[1310] Foam was taken to signify "divine presence",[1311] an immanent accumulation of *ch'ulel, yoliliztli,* or *pee*. This may be inferred from the "living" nature of bubbles, which move, pop, and subside, or burst in the mouth with little explosions of air. The combination of wind and water in foam merge the elemental media of sky and sea which the first gods inhabited and from which all creation arose.

Foams also arise as a result of fermentation, as in *pulque*,[1312] Tezcatlipoca's alcoholic gift. Fermentation is a living process, but also an underworld process, as it involves controlled decay. Cacao seeds, too, are partly fermented, but in contrast to *pulque*, the foam in Quetzalcoatl's beverages made from Cacao must be raised by frothing—a process of actively aerating the beverage, transferring "life energy" into it from outside. Contemporary Chatinos in south-eastern Oaxaca whip air into their remedies, so that "One's intentions, and the gods, [are] well-placed into the remedy."[1313] This belief that foams represent and absorb vivifying power is discernible today in the Oaxacan preparation of *Chocolate Atole*: if a woman can't make *atole* foam, a pregnant lady is brought in to beat it:[1314] two lives are better than one, and the vitality of the ripening foetus helps to invigorate the drink.

For the Mexica, *xochicacahuatl* or "flowery chocolate", made with aromatic flowers or spices and a generous head of foam, denoted luxury and sensuality.[1315] A cup of foaming chocolate tied the complex metaphor of flowers to Cacao's sacramental potency. Just as only the death god was able to make fragrant flowers from bloody water, so Cacao, the underworld plant replete with the same life-giving forces as blood itself, could be combined with fragrant flowers to produce a drink that evoked the joy, the sorrow, and the bittersweet triumph of life; it was a symbol of celebrating the present while accepting the inevitable. "Flowery chocolate" was the ultimate Mexica metonym for enjoying the best parts of life, while acknowledging the necessity of death. It mythically represented and pharmacologically evoked the pleasures of mortal existence and the need to give thanks to the gods for human life, bought by the sacrifices (literally) and struggles of the current generation. It invoked the presence of the ancestors in the blood, assisting the consumer to temporarily ward off death and inevitable rebirth as an ancestor oneself. A poem by Tlaltecatzin, the noble Mexica governor of Cuauhchinanco, sums it up:

> I alone, I sing
> To him, one who is my lord;
> In this place where the gods command,
> The flowering chocolate drink is foaming,
> The one which intoxicates men with its flowers.
> I yearn, oh yes!
> For my heart has tasted it:
> It intoxicated my heart –
> Songs, dreams, yearnings.
> My heart has tasted it.
> [...]
> The flowering chocolate drink is foaming,
> The flower of tobacco is passed around.
> [...]
> I only suffer and say
> May I not go
> To the place of the fleshless.[1316]

12. Celebrations, ceremonies, and contracts. Cacao was and is used by indigenous peoples in the ceremonies of all religions, past and present, in Central America.[1317] Anthropologist Dennis Tedlock points out that the K'iche Maya term *chokola* refers to the process of gathering food for a banquet, and the *nim chokoj* is a master of ceremonies at weddings and banquets where chocolate is drunk. Cacao is an essential pre-wedding gift from K'iche grooms to the families of their intended spouse,[1318] and Cacao-based beverages have been served at feasts, weddings, and funerals since ancient times. Cacao appears to feature in all celebrations, but particularly—as befits a drug bequeathed by serpent-gods (K'awil or Quetzalcoatl)—it is used to mark thresholds, important moments of transition from one state to another in life. The contemporary Catholic-influenced stamp of approval from Jesus for chocolate's ceremonial use is just the latest iteration of a long history of supernatural endorsements for this purpose. Cacao is also used to "attract good" in shamanic ceremonies, while chillies are used to "repel bad";[1319] it is a facilitator of positive change. In this sense, foaming chocolate is truly a substance of flowers and serpents: symbolising a new lease of life, honouring the past while shedding or letting go of it.

* * *

So Cacao has symbolic links to blood, rulership, women, the underworld, fertility, water, the heart, the head, and the "rebirth" of gods and ancestors as underworld spirits; it's mythically paired with maize and the maize god; it sometimes plays the part of the world tree.[1320] Cacao is the midnight maize, the eclipsed sun. Maize symbolises life-before-death, and Cacao designates life-after-death; their relationship is reciprocal, just as they support each other in the *milpa*, and one blooms as the other ripens. Cacao is a goddess of plenty, "Thunder Woman, Maize Woman", and Hun Hunahpu's chthonian alter ego. Cacao is the wealth of the aged ruler of the underworld, "Black Scorpion", the merchant hoarder who is later stripped of all his possessions, or the self-replenishing gift of the celestial diviner-kings, the serpent-footed K'awil and the feathered serpent Quetzalcoatl, who pilfer Cacao for the benefit of humankind. Cacao is the posthumous reward for valiant self-sacrifice, a product of transformation wrought from living blood; it's a magnet for wealth, envy, and vengeance, and a living vessel of ancestral wisdom.

Drinking *kakawa* or *cacahuatl* is to proclaim that one is alive, privileged, and grateful. To drink *kakawa* is to replenish *ch'ulel*, recharging one's ability to acquire *itz* and generate magical change in the world. Drinking *kakawa* is an implicit invitation to receive the wisdom and the burdens of ancestry, to make the scarifices which are necessary to effect change, to discard skins that no longer fit, to cross thresholds courageously and willingly. Drinking *kakawa* emboldens one to move forward, knowing that every step one takes is a step closer to the grave, when we, too, will become ancestors. In the next and final chapter we'll further explore Mesoamerican metaphysics, and the mutations which occurred in Cacao's mythological persona as the feathered serpent's gift took root in Old World culture.

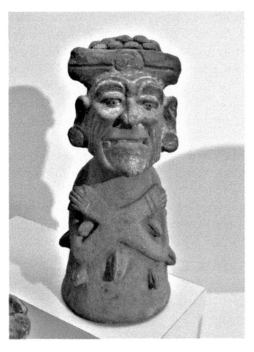

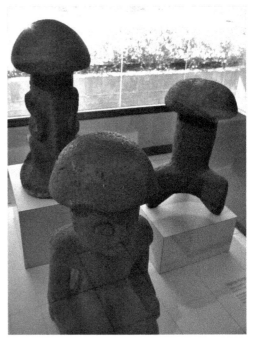

Classic-era Cacao god statue (elderly male, like God L), Popol Vuh museum, Guatemala city, 2011

Pre-Classic mushroom stones at the Popol Vuh museum in Guatemala city, 2011

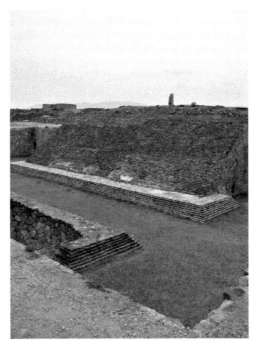

Ruined ballcourt at Monte Alban, Oaxaca, Mexico, 2008

CHAPTER TEN

The dark side of Venus

Morals have given rise to charity and pity, two suet balls that have grown like elephants, planets, which people call good. There is nothing good about them. Goodness is lucid, clear and resolute, and ruthless towards compromise and politics. Morality infuses chocolate into every man's veins.

(Translated from the DADA MANIFESTO by Tristan Tzara, 1918)

The distinction between "scientific" and "unscientific" knowledge is question-begging, the only valid question about knowledge being that of its truth.

(From E. F. Schumacher, *A Guide for the Perplexed*, 1977. Reprinted by permission)

"Una sopa de su propio chocolate."
"A soup of their own chocolate", meaning—"a taste of their own medicine".

(Contemporary Mexican phrase)

Let's assume that science as we know it in the early twenty-first century potentially has all the answers. Despite the imponderables fizzing at the borders of experiment and theory, stuffed with all manner of strangeness like fractals and zero-point fields and parallel universes, despite millennia of anecdote-not-data reports of mystical experiences and prophecies of variable accuracy and vast mutating tides of religious or ideological fervour, let's imagine that we can explain all of it with our current evidence-based rulebook. By these lights, our pre-Enlightenment ancestors were deluded, misguided, and ignorant. Religious beliefs and protocols often provide negative examples of "how not to do rational"—for example, by being ethically reprehensible, as in the case of human sacrifice, or religious war.

In the Mesoamerican paradigm, nothing could be more coldly logical than the systematic and carefully selected slaughter of a small percentage of the population (or even better, in the case of "flowery wars", someone else's population) for the reciprocal benefit of the gods, or willingly accepting ritual murder, so that the rest of the world may survive and prosper. But even discarding all religious belief as delusion, we can perhaps allow that there may be significant psychological truths embedded in the old myths; they're never one-dimensional, and demonstrate the remarkable power of ideology to motivate behaviour, to both horrific and transcendent effect.

Incredible works of art and entire civilisations coalesced around, and emerged from religious movements. Historical ideologies and protocols may show us new potentials: if we start by assuming that our ancestors weren't all idiots, that maybe there is *something* utilitarian in their beliefs and practices, then what could these older paradigms teach us?

To go even further: it may yet turn out that our whole universe is somehow conscious, or guided by consciousness other than our own. It may yet transpire that God, or gods, spirit, spirits, intention, soul, and magic really do exist in some form, even if that form is rather different than traditional conceptions allow. Perhaps the medieval alchemists were correct in asserting that matter really is the lowest and grossest manifestation of "spirit", whatever that is; if this is the case, then trying to explain our reality with contemporary science may be rather like a colour-blind man who doesn't know he's colour-blind drawing a rainbow for the benefit of children who have never seen the sky. But we can start our search for utility in traditional myths by looking at Mesoamerican spiritual technology: exploring divination, shamanism, and magic, and asking what even *is* magical thinking, or consciousness, for that matter? Then we could look at how Cacao's identity changed as it was removed from its native hydroponic myth-bath, enrobed in Christian ideology, and repackaged as a venereal substance in Europe, and what that may mean. Only then may we prise the sticky empty box out of Pandora's fingers, and talk some more about chocolate.

The calendrical cosmos

All human civilisations appear to have used divination. A dictionary definition of divination is "the art or practice of discovering future events or unknown things, as though by supernatural powers".[1321] In an uncertain world, knowing something of the future can be an asset; and, as the word "divination" implies, the existence of some form of divinity or universal intelligence is a precondition for accurate, non-probabilistic prediction. If the world is governed by conscious invisible entities, it makes sense to seek answers from these powers about what the future holds.

One way to do this is to open a direct line, using dreams, rituals, or shamanistic technologies to communicate with these intelligences. But these "immersive" methods are time-consuming, risky, and often require innate gifts; more accessible, rapid, and teachable means of acquiring such information was required, which is where divination using "external" signs comes in, either through spontaneous observation and interpretation of ambient phenomena, such as astrology or *augury* (divination by interpreting the flight of birds), or through the use of secondary devices like casting lots or reading Tarot cards. The basic premise of all divination is that because the world is alive, god-haunted, and fundamentally interconnected, reality inherently and constantly reflects the intentions and motions of the spiritual forces which govern it. In a divinatory landscape, divine will is legible in everything, like writing in the centre of a stick of rock, and may be perceived in various ways, by using appropriate tools and skills.

Astrology itself, in one form or another, has been used by all human civilisations, and this, too, is logical: the sky is the natural dwelling of gods and spirits, being an enormous, open, incomprehensibly vast and distant vault of heaven from which light and water spontaneously descend, and on which earthly life depends. The stars are a reliable, consistent feature of the environment, yet their configurations in relation to the Earth, sun, and moon constantly change, so as never to be exactly the same, even though—crucially—their courses and movements are, for the most part, predictable. So the night sky lends itself very well to the construction of systems of divination, because the arrangement of the heavenly bodies entails both inherent structure in the cyclical repetition of its components and their relationships to one another, and chaos in the ever-changing face of the whole. The chaotic element is critical, as this simulates the subjective randomness of life, but the predictable nature of these cycles is what makes astrology so ubiquitous: the night sky can be plotted as far into the past or future as a culture's astronomical acumen permits.

In Mesoamerica, as in the Old World, the principal divinatory technology was loosely based on astrology. But while Old World astrology was more "live"—charts were based on tables of the real-time movements of planets in the sky, and interpretations of their placements relative to each other—Mesoamericans utilised complex calendrical systems. The divinatory calendars of the Mexica were the *tonalamatl*, or "books of destiny"—based on a composite of the words *tonalli* (vitality/sunlight/life) and *amatl* (book). The K'iche Maya still refer to their calendrical books as *ilb'al*, or "seeing instrument",[1322] and the Mexica *tonalamatl* were used to "see time", bringing order out of the chaos of life and "perceiving" structure and meaning. But very few pre-Colombian divinatory codices and tables—other than those graven in stone—still exist, due partly to the passage of time and mostly to effective missionary work after the conquest. Only nine codices survive, dating from the late post-Classic era just before the conquest. Some of these are what the Mexica referred to as *tonalpohualli*, codices laying out the 260-day ritual calendar and its divinatory associations.

These painted screenfold codices detailed the meanings of each day, based on a cyclical calendar derived from astronomical observations: principally, the solar year, the lunar month, and the time that venus took to return to the same position in the sky in relation to the sun and the Earth.[1323] The Mesoamerican calendrical-divinatory systems are analogous to Chinese astrology in this respect, which uses a similarly "tidied" and more orderly and periodic calendrical abstraction of astronomical phenomena. But because these calendars were "rounded off" and cyclical, they diminished the chaotic, organic element which is necessary in divination; the gods don't speak in stock phrases. So the calendars were used with other "external" methods, including a type of sortilege (casting or drawing lots for the purposes of divination) using maize kernels or dried seeds, in conjunction with employing the innate gifts of certain individuals who could interpret physical sensations felt during a divinatory session. The layering of such techniques allowed for nuanced, multi-level "readings" that didn't rely simply on the rather rigid calendrical format.

The 260-day ritual calendar or *tzolkin* was used for divination and agriculture. It originates from 900–500 BCE,[1324] and approximates the human gestation cycle in length, as well as corresponding with astronomical lunar cycles and the venus cycle: nine lunar months, or the approximate duration of Venus's time as a morning or evening star (263 days).[1325] The *tzolkin* consisted of twenty months of thirteen days each, which are referred to as *trecenas* in contemporary scholarship (from the Spanish *trece*, or thirteen). Each *trecena* had some good and bad qualities, though some were generally more or less fortunate than others. There were twenty day signs or *uinal*, each represented by a specific glyph or pictogram with specific divinatory meanings.[1326] The numbers one to thirteen were combined with the twenty *uinal* to create an endless cycle of 260 days. The *uinal* which began each count of one to thirteen was the "lord of the *trecena*" and coloured the whole interpretation for that bundle of days.[1327]

One's date of birth in the *tzolkin* revealed certain aptitudes and vices, determined which days would be more beneficial for that person, and various other details; and it could be used for many other purposes, too, such as assisting with medical diagnosis, choosing the best days to initiate an action, to plant, or to harvest. Many almanacs detailed ritual protocols for ameliorating negative prognostications or capitalising on good ones, or to produce specific outcomes. One such ritual is performed for curing the pain caused by biting or stinging animals such as scorpions or snakes; instructions include such things as the placing of a specific number of offerings on a particular god's altar on certain days, or even the sacrifice of a precise number of people. One horrific example suggests that forty-eight infants be sacrificed to the rain god on the appropriate day.[1328] Babies in, water out.

The Mexica used the 260-day *tzolkin* in conjunction with the 365-day solar year calendar or *xihuitl*,[1329] which consisted of eighteen twenty-day months and an ill-omened "leftover" five-day period at the end of the year, known as the five *nemontemi* days.[1330] The months of the *xihuitl* were naturally twenty days long, this being the number of human fingers and toes. Some versions of both these calendars appear to have been in use in Oaxaca by 500 BCE, although the earliest definitive archaeological examples are from 100 BC. The calendars were used together to form a greater, fifty-two-year cycle, as fifty-two years is the common denominator of 260 and 365 days; so every fifty-two years, the cycles reverted, and the Mexica celebrated their "New Fire" festival on the last five days of the solar year. During this period people discarded old possessions, such as clothing, pots, and cooking utensils, and all fires were put out. Then, at the start of the new solar year, a priest sacrificed a high-born captive by cutting out his heart, and drilled a new fire in the chest cavity. This fire was taken to the major temples, and distributed from there to the minor temples, and then to the houses of the people,[1331] designating a rekindling and renewal of life and a fresh start.

Local rites were pinned to specific days of the 260-day ritual calendar, and would therefore fall at different times of the 365-day solar year every year, so the Spanish referred to such ritual observances as "moveable feasts". Personal rites were dependent on the birthday of any individual in the 260-day ritual calendar cycle too, so specific prayers and offerings were made to ameliorate any bad fortune and increase the good promised by their birth date.[1332] Sowing and harvesting of maize occurred between two annual zenith passages of the Sun at 15°N latitude, approximately 260 days apart: the first, in May, occurs at the onset of the rainy season, and corresponds with maize planting; harvesting precedes the second, in July–August, and is followed immediately by a second sowing of maize. Whatever day the sowing fell on, when the same day came around again in the 260-day calendar, it would be time to harvest. So while the agricultural cycles were naturally fixed to the 365-day solar calendar, which corresponded with the seasons, the 260-day calendar was a useful timing device for crop sowing and harvesting.

The Mesoamericans also used two major constellations, which we know as Scorpio and the Pleiades, to time the agricultural cycle: the Pleiades, which the Maya called the "four hundred boys", rose at dawn in May, heralding the onset of the rainy season, whereas Scorpio was associated with the beginning of the dry season,[1333] which was also the "star wars" season, from November to May. For the Classic Maya, May coincided with the month of *muan* and the merchant-god festival, during which traders returned from their long trading expeditions prior to the onset of the rains.[1334] The wet and dry seasons were linked to the Milky Way, the stellar backdrop to the sun's progression through the sky during the year. Many Classic Maya temples are adorned with sculptures of a two-headed cosmic monster—the ecliptic—with a fully-fleshed reptilian "front" head, linked to the onset of rains in May to June, when the sun was in the constellation we know as Taurus; but the "rear" head of the serpent is skeletal, representing the onset of the dry season in October to November when the sun was in Scorpio.[1335]

The Classic Maya had an extraordinarily sophisticated time-tabling system, which ran parallel to the 260-day and 365-day calendars, but which had been largely forgotten by the time of the Spanish conquest. This was the Long Count, used to keep track of vast cycles of time, from the creation of the world onwards. A Long Count date may be written 9.9.0.0.0., where each number represents a successively smaller unit: *calabtun, piktun, baktun, katun, tun, uinal, kin*. A *kin* is one day, twenty *kin* is a *uinal*, thirteen *uinal* (360 *kin*—just less than a solar year) is a *tun*, twenty *tun* is a *katun*, and twenty *katun* is a *baktun*, approximately 394 solar years. A *piktun* consists of twenty *baktun*, and a *calabtun* is twenty *piktun*,[1336] approximately 157,808 solar years. Because the Long Count "year" or *tun* was standardised to 360 days it gradually slid out of phase with the solar year calendar by five days every year. The Long Count was used to record dates on monuments such as stelae commemorating royal accessions or funerals, linking them to astronomical and mythical events.

The Long Count unit for one day, *kin*, was written with a solar glyph, explicitly tying the sun to a one-day period, and the measurement of time. In a temple at Copan, the door jambs cast no shadows at the winter solstice, indicating that the temple is aligned to the sun at that time. The doorframe is carved with a representation of the sun on one side, and a crocodile on the other; the sun sets perfectly framed by the doorway on the solstice, and captures the "crocodile jaws" of the Milky Way at night.[1337] The temples of some Maya sites are oriented towards the positions of the lunar apogee and perigee (when it is furthest away from or closest to the Earth, respectively), so were likely used for helping to predict eclipses.[1338] Mayan eclipse calculations were accurate to within twenty days, which was no mean feat for more than 400 years of eclipse tables, although more mistakes started to appear by the early post-Classic, Chichen Itza period, as the means of calculating the connections between the Long Count and the ordinary fifty-two-year calendar round were forgotten.[1339]

Venus' cycles in relation to the sun and moon were enormously important to the Mesoamericans, especially venus's phase, or position relative to the sun and Earth, which determines whether venus appears pre-dawn, as a morning star, or after sunset, as an evening star.[1340] For instance, the round, observatory-like structure known as the Caracol at Chichen Itza has windows obliquely angled towards the north and south horizon where venus's maximum elongation (its greatest distance from the sun, when it appears brightest) as the morning star would be visible.[1341] The onset of "star wars" during the dry season would be timed to coincide with venus's first appearance as an evening or morning star, or, much less commonly, with the inferior conjunction of venus with the sun—when venus, moving retrograde, lines up with the sun in the sky and is therefore completely invisible. But 96% of recorded "star wars" campaigns began when venus was visible in the sky, and of these, 70% were in the evening star phase: so the evening star venus was associated with more bellicose deities.[1342]

Although we're unsure which gods the Maya associated with the planet we call saturn, it seems likely that the merchant-underworld deity known as "god K" or K'awil was associated with jupiter. And it's certain that the Maya tracked the cycles of jupiter's and saturn's conjunctions, which occur every twenty years—approximately every *katun*, in the Long Count. The Maya appear to have used an 819 *kin* count to subdivide the jupiter-saturn cycles, and used the planet jupiter to time major dynastic ceremonies such as accession rituals and the apotheosis or deification of dead kings.[1343] Interregnum periods in Classic Maya times could be months long due to the wait for astrologically auspicious times to perform a ceremony,[1344] as the date of the previous king's death was often inconveniently out of sync with the optimal celestial timing for such purposes.

Magica Mesoamericana

A cereal-box definition of "magical" world views is that they imply non-material connections between things, in which human consciousness and our capacity for analogy and metaphorical thinking is accurately representative of the structure of reality. For example, the moon, water, silver, and pregnancy were somehow related in both European and Mesoamerican belief systems for various reasons: the moon affects the tides and appears to swell, expand, and diminish every month, while pregnancy often causes swelling of the breasts and sometimes "water retention"; the moon has a silvery appearance, and silver readily tarnishes and goes black when un-polished, just as the moon regularly loses light when it wanes. These sorts of associations were common to all mankind until the Enlightenment, the birth of experimental science, and the concept of "scientific objectivity". This presumes that thinking-by-analogy constitutes a reasoning error, as there is no substantive link between such dissimilar things, the only connection being one of "meaning", which is subjective and imaginal. Post-Enlightenment experimental science declares that non-causal connections between things are highly unlikely, so they bear a "burden of proof" requirement in replicable experimental conditions.

A general principle of traditional or pre-modern magical belief systems is that all naturally occurring beings and phenomena are the product of divine creation, and therefore contain some essence of divinity. One definition of magical techniques is that they are methods of accessing and communicating with this essence in oneself and other created things. Where associated with traditional religions, magical thinking may also involve belief in non-material forms of consciousness which inhabit or somehow exist within or in parallel to the physical world (spirits, djinns, angels, demons, gods, fairies, elementals, etc.). It's the divine or non-material part of the practitioner—whether layperson, shaman, or priest—which interacts with and influences, by fair means or foul, by force or persuasion, immaterial entities which may be autonomous (such as a spirit or deity) or immanent (such as a soul, or the divine essence in a being or object, like *ch'ulel*).

But there is a key difference between magical and religious practice: the primary focus of magic is on directly affecting—or commanding—non-material intelligences or forces in order to obtain a particular result, often with the aim of facilitating material changes. Religions, on the other hand, for the most part seek only to acknowledge, worship, and collude with whatever is perceived to be the agenda of these intelligences—the gods, or God, and associated entities. As in Mesoamerica and many ancient cultures, magic can be annexed to religious belief and practices, but need not be associated with a single religious orthodoxy. Magic is best thought of as a set of techniques based on common principles used in some religious or mystical belief systems.

To use the "moon" example, if pregnancy is associated with the moon and with silver, a non-denominational magical approach to enhance fertility and the possibility of conception may be to carry a plant associated with the moon for a month as a talisman; a magico-religious approach ("deific magic") could be to pray to or invoke a specific moon deity using silver instruments or offerings in a specially timed ceremony, perhaps on a particular day during the waxing (growing) phase of the moon, and specifically request or command their assistance; and a purely religious approach would be to pray and possibly make offerings to a lunar deity with reverent obeisance in the hope that they would assist. In practice, these categories often overlap or merge, but the main monotheistic religions of the Old World—Judaism, Islam, and Christianity—take a dim view of magical practices, because of the lack of faith implied by impious attempts to influence divine will; but as with many other "pagan" (polytheistic) religions, Mesoamerican religions were saturated with magical practices.

In Mexica legends, the "first couple" of divine beings following the creation of the world of the Fifth Sun were an elderly pair of diviners named Oxomoco and Cipactonal, whose equivalent in the K'iche legends of the Popol Vuh were Xmucane and Xpiyacoc, grandparents of the sun and moon. Oxomoco and Cipactonal were the Mexica patrons of divination via maize kernels and the calendar, and their early appearance in the creation myths and the pantheon shows the importance of the act of divination in Mesoamerican thought.[1345] The Mexica creator-god and cultural patron Quetzalcoatl was reputed to be the "ultimate soothsayer and sorcerer",[1346] equivalent in many respects to the Mayan creator-shaman god Itzamna. Divinities themselves practised divination, which is interesting, suggesting that even the gods weren't exempt from the vagaries of fate. Divination wasn't passive, it was a godlike, magical act of creation, because it sought to identify the root causes and probable outcomes of any given situation so that the most appropriate response could be taken to resolve any current issues or neutralise potential problems.

Divination may be divided into "external" and "immersive" categories. "External" methods are procedural, device or object-based, and included measuring the hand—the Mesoamerican equivalent of palmistry—and using representations or stand-ins for the person being asked about, such as maize grains or a model made from string. If maize grains sank in water or a string model could be disentangled easily, a sick person could be cured. But divination using the 260-day calendar combined an "immersive" (subjective and experiential) divinatory method with the "external" technologies of the calendar and a sortilege technique utilsing maize kernels. This skill was a divine gift from the subterranean dwarf deity known by the contemporary

Momostecan Maya as C'oxol or Tzitzimit, a volcano spirit who appears as a small boy or a red dwarf with a stone axe, which he uses to strike "lightning into the blood" of diviners.[1347]

Contemporary K'iche *ajq'ij*, or "daykeepers", possess this ability to hear the "lightning" in their blood. First, the diviner performs a ritual invocation of *pee* (life force), summoning "the breath, the cold, the wind, the cloud, the mist at the rising of the Sun"—descriptions very reminiscent of the smoke-like Classic Maya life force, *ch'ulel*—and acknowledges the "four corners of the sky and of the earth".[1348] Then the "face of the day" or *nawal* is determined by the calendar, and a whole 260-day cycle is counted out using maize kernels, seeds, or crystals. This count, called *ch'obonic*, "to understand",[1349] is used to generate more divinatory information; the seeds and crystals are lined up in little heaps, in a specific order, and interpreted. The diviner may seek more information by re-casting the seeds a second and even a third time. Throughout, the diviner "listens" for the blood "speaking" during a divination to confirm or deny an intuition, or add extra information.[1350]

The ability to "question the blood", called *coyopa*, is surely a cognate derivative of the Classic Maya *ch'ulel*. The "jumping" or "twitching" in the blood or muscles that occurs in response to subjects which come up during the divination, or direct questions that the diviner asks, is thought to be caused by the ancestors responding to the diviner via the "lightning in the blood". The pattern of sensations is interpreted according to a strict schema, based on polarities such as front/back, left/right, and distal/proximal.[1351] By combining the calendar reading with sortilege and listening to the "speaking of the blood" while questioning the querent, contemporary diviners produce very detailed and context-dependent responses. Given the greater sophistication of the Classic Maya calendar, ancient Mesoamerican divinatory processes may have been even more layered.

Like divinatory methods, magical techniques can be loosely grouped into "external" and "immersive" categories. Two major and universal principles of "external" magic are those of sympathy and contagion. Sympathetic magic is based on similarity or likeness, whereby the magical object resembles the thing to be influenced. This could be an allegorical likeness, intended to induce a desired effect, such as giving roses—a symbol of love and passion—on Valentine's Day to evoke similar feelings in their recipient. The Mexica used sympathetic magic in medicines made from centipedes and snakes to treat joint problems because they are extremely flexible, or applied semi-precious jasper to staunch bleeding because the stone is hard and blood-coloured.[1352] Another common example of sympathetic magic is the construction of a model or image of a person or objective, so that anything done to the model will affect the intended target, or vice versa—the form may be used to absorb or take on attributes of the living person. A variant of this method, known as "poppet" or doll magic is found all over the world, and has become infamous in popular cultural depictions of "voodoo" magical practices. It could be used to heal or harm;[1353] contemporary folk healers use this method to cure *susto*, by constructing a doll which can take on or absorb the illness from the child and may then be discarded, accompanied by ritual methods such as censing the child's bed with smoke.[1354]

Contagion is the notion that an effect may be transmitted by physical contact, so that wearing an amulet—such as the magico-medicinal Mexica amulet to protect travellers made from magnolia flowers and other ingredients, described in Chapter 3—will directly affect the wearer.[1355] In contemporary Guatemala, I was told how a scorpion sting may be treated by applying the entrails of the scorpion that stung you, wrapped in a handkerchief, to the wound; likewise, a harpoon injury sustained during fishing was treated by applying the entrails of a fish caught by harpoon. In the first instance, the "hair of the dog that bit you" is the principle: using the essence of the scorpion to neutralise its sting, so that it sympathetically draws out the poison, or renders the person immune to it. In the second case, there is a sympathy between the nature of the injury and a fish that has been caught in the same manner and at the same time, but the pain is transferred by "contagion" from the wounded man to the fish guts.[1356]

External magic can also be "deific"—that is, seeking the assistance of spirits or deities. Most performative Mesoamerican magic was deific: persuading, bribing, or coercing gods or spirits to perform or undo particular actions. Almost no magical activity in pre-conquest Mesoamerica was separate from worship. Deific magic could also be bound up with sympathetic magic, as with the Mexica recommendation to eat hummingbird meat to treat pustular diseases: the hummingbird was symbolically linked to the Sun, and one of the Mexica Sun gods was Nanahuatzin, the creator-god who was covered in pustules; so, eating hummingbird meat was a way of treating the illness by implicitly invoking a deity who might be quite literally sympathetic to the condition.[1357]

The contemporary Huichol and Cora view the world and all its life as a singular body, which requires vital force (*a xuturi*) to sustain it. Like the Classic Maya a millennium before, they have a reciprocal view of reality: human life depends on "father sun", and the life of the gods depends on sacrifice and magical ritual. They believe that the proper level of concentration necessary to effect magical actions can only be achieved during sacrifice; it requires the practitioner-priest to enter a flow state, and they say that only shamans and ancestors know how to "think correctly" to achieve this. Potent magic, they say, comes from thinking in this "correct" way.[1358] This is a very important point: without the correct state of mind, magical actions become merely artistic or performative. The beliefs, mental state, and focus of the ritual participants are what animate and empower ritual.

Ritual speech, chanting, or singing using "flowery words" or special phrases were commonplace in Mesoamerican worship—and, more particularly, in the performance of deific magic, which combined "external" elements like incense and offerings with "immersive" methods, such as the "ecstatic voyage" (summoning the vision serpent).[1359] This method was the most risky because it involves altering consciousness through the induction of trance states or the use of entheogenic plants, which can be physically or mentally hazardous. But "altering consciousness" is a modern, ethnographic-psychological-clinical turn of phrase; in most traditional magical systems, the "ecstatic voyage" would be thought of as literally entering another dimension, or perceiving and communing with other levels of reality, not merely a change in perception.[1360]

Ritual speech was highly metaphorical, as symbols are a means of condensing a great deal of potential outcomes into one thing; a "known unknown" can be expressed pithily, but without over-defining its potential range of expression. Ritual speech had its own particular jargon and cadences, and was referred to as "maize gruel tree speech" by the Maya, and *nahualatolli* or "speech of the sorcerers"[1361] to the Mexica—here, again, the word *atolli* signifies maize gruel. Maize gruel is a form of liquid nourishment which symbolically unites the four elements and the three realms, symbolising natural magical power. Sunlight from the breezy celestial world, plus earth, symbolising the underworld below, together yield this-worldly maize, which is mixed with water and cooked with fire to produce *atole*, a staple food-drink and the basic sustenance of humans on Earth.

Ancient Mayan doctor-priests or *ah menoob* used "the word" (*u t'an*), a divine gift received in a dream or during an ecstatic voyage. The *u t'an* technique used rhythmic speech patterns, distorted pronunciation, symbols, and metaphors, and applied this surreal manner of address in a structured way to rebuke the disease-causing entities. This technique is exemplified in the curative "ritual of the Bacabs", during which the *ah menoob* utilised singing and dancing, with the aid of psychotropic plants, to send spirit (his *wayob*, perhaps) via the world tree in a spiral journey, as if through a snake's body, entering the underworld or the celestial world to find the disease-causing spirit. He would then use the *u'tan* to address, bamboozle and defeat it. The final part of the ceremony consisted of applying medicines to the patient and singing curative songs, before the spirit of the *ah menoob* returned to his body. He then ritually closed the portal, and expressed gratitude to the Bacabs and gods of medicine.[1362]

The purpose of such "ecstatic voyages" was to to enter the otherworld in order to change conditions in the solar world; in such rituals the sorcerer or priest could direct the entity he or she contacted to enter the dreams of their patient or intended victim and heal or attack them there—dreams being the experience of the *tonalli* or *wayob* traversing the otherworld, so this was thought to seriously affect the target.[1363] Mexica *tlacatecolotl* or "owl men" were sorcerers who could both curse and cure; when cursed by one, only another *tlacatecolotl* could extract the hex, usually by removing pieces of bone or obsidian from their flesh that had been implanted with it; this sleight of hand provided impressive physical evidence which no doubt enhanced the cure.[1364] These traditions survive today in Central America in the form of *curanderos* and *brujos*, aka healers and witches: the first will only cure, usually for free, and are frequently paid in donations, gifts, or IOUs; the second will cure or curse—for a price.

Shaman tech

Mesoamerican magical actions varied from simple lay practices such as placing a *tejolote* (a pestle or grinding instrument) in a field to protect the crop from harm, to the most elaborate ceremonial magic, performed by "professionals" who experienced some sort of shamanic "call" to their vocation as sorcerers or priests.[1365] The word "shaman" originates from Siberia, but the term is applied to magico-religious practitioners worldwide, whose belief systems and techniques share many common elements. Shamans are intercessors between the human and spiritual domains, like priests but more hands-on: they cure or sometimes curse, they divine, and a key feature of shamanism is that it involves ecstatic journeying, the direct and immersive experience of the spirit world. The "call" to a shamanic vocation may include being struck by lightning, fainting during important rituals, a serious illness or life-shattering event, or visions in dreams or supernatural events which give the individual a spiritual mandate to practise.[1366] To refuse a call to shamanic practice, in the form of illness or dreams, may mean death.[1367] They minister to the tribe or social group, but they also work with individuals, mostly in a curing or problem-solving capacity.

The dream world is of central importance in all shamanic traditions, because the dream world is the spirit world. For Mesoamerican shamanic and magical practices, the technique of lucid dreaming was (and remains) part of the core curriculum, as only once a practitioner can control their dreams can they interact with, interrogate, and possibly control spirits.[1368] Once called by dreams, near-death experiences, or illnesses, or if a sorcerous vocation was endorsed by their birthdate, Aztec boys could be enrolled at the *calmecac* ("house of tears"), the extra-strict school for priests-in-training. Non-priestly magical practitioners could be apprenticed to practitioners, the most powerful of which were known as *nahualli*, or *nagual* in contemporary Mexico, who had the ability to transform into animals such as pumas, dogs, skunks, owls, snakes, or other animals.[1369]

The use of music to assist "altered states"—or to help open a portal—with and without entheogenic plants is ancient. More than 200 Guatemalan stone and ceramic effigies featuring mushrooms have been discovered dating from the first millennium BCE, including a seated figure beating a mushroom-shaped drum, and a ring of celebrants dancing around a giant mushroom.[1370] Singing and dancing contributed to the induction of altered states, and musical instruments included drums, bells, trumpets, flutes, rattles, and shells. Mexica music was often percussive, atonal, or in a minor key, such that the Spanish conquistadors described it as "doleful and tuneless" but nevertheless moving.[1371] The music must have been uncannily powerful in accompaniment to major ritual proceedings, with singing, dancing, and the ingestion of entheogens—such as the accession rites of the emperor Motecuhzoma III (mentioned in Chapter 1).

In the Mexica Codex Vindobonensis, Quetzalcoatl instructs nine deities on the ritual use of mushrooms;[1372] the feathered serpent who gave Cacao to humankind is also the original sponsor of the *Psilocybe* superhighway between humankind and the gods. The ritual use of *Psilocybe* mushrooms was exemplified by the twentieth-century Mazatec shaman Maria Sabina, who used them in ceremonies with chanting, singing, and percussive, rhythmic movements such as clapping or slapping the thighs. These were primarily curative sessions in which both shaman and patients participated, intended to help patients resolve illnesses and life dilemmas. Sabina described the mushrooms' purpose:

> There is a world beyond ours, a world that is far away, nearby, and invisible [...] a world where everything has already happened and everything is already known. That world talks, it has a language of its own [...] The sacred mushroom takes me by the hand and brings me to the world where everything is known [...] they [...] speak in a way I can understand. I ask them and they answer me. (Maria Sabina, quoted in Schultes & Hofmann, 1992)

The deities or spirits associated with entheogenic plants (or fungi, in this case) reveal themselves to those who ingest them, and communicate with them. The mushroom deities were "little men", and *ololiouhqui* (*Turbina corymbosa*) and *peyote* (*Lophphora williamsii*) were "venerable elders".[1373] This isn't to be taken lightly, and while the recreational use of entheogens wasn't unknown—such as the Mexica use of *Psilocybe* mushrooms at feasts—they were always treated with reverence. The Mazatec believe that inappropriate use of entheogens leads to insanity, so their use is ritually circumscribed.[1374] "Hallucinations" induced by ritual or entheogenic plants are the result of accessing non-ordinary reality, or "other dimensions of consciousness" from the contemporary anthropologist's perspective, which can be dangerous, or illuminating, or both.

The ingestion of sacred plants allows shamans or ritual participants to "see ... the essential structure of the world, where spirit and matter are one".[1375]

təˈmeltoʊ, təˈmɑːtəʊ: New World magic, Old World magic

The Perennial Philosophy can be defined as a magical world view that prevailed in all ancient cultures. The common elements consist of a cosmic order to which the gods themselves are beholden, and which is holistic, in that all beings and things share the same divine or life-giving essence. Central to this understanding were the notions of maintenance and reciprocity, with the gods and humanity engaged in a mutually beneficial relationship: the gods provide the world, and humans sustain the gods. Animal and sometimes human sacrifice was common, and ritual was of central importance—reinforcing the world-as-it-is through ceremony was a matter of survival. Actions and objects were animated or ensouled through ritual and sacrifice, and performative ceremonies in which participants re-enacted mythical events and embodied deities were a means of acquiring numinous potency, of "infusing mortal actions with divine strength".[1376] Every earthly thing was a replica of something in the divine or non-earthly world, which was invisible and eternal, in contrast to the tangible, temporal, and transient realm which humans inhabit.

So Mesoamerican beliefs clearly fit the Perennial Philosophy mould. In contrast to the Old World, there was no Axial Age in Mesoamerica: no emergence of groundbreaking philosophies, personalities, or semi-legendary figureheads like Buddha, Jesus, Lao Tzu, or Plato, who questioned the existing dogmas in Asia, Europe, and the Middle East from 900 BCE onward. It's possible that some of the parallels in pre-Axial Old World and Mesoamerican beliefs arose from shared prehistoric religious notions carried across the Bering strait ice sheets fourteen thousand years ago; or, perhaps, human minds and genetic tendencies are sufficiently similar to produce congruent religious notions in disparate regions, unconnected by anything other than ancestry and similar evolutionary challenges. A materialistically prosaic explanation: similar brains, similar beliefs. Alternatively, as Carl Jung proposed, certain commonalities exist in the human "collective unconscious", like disembodied entities which take analogous forms in many places and times. There is a fourth, currently unfashionable possibility, that such beliefs may reflect some objective truth, and have utilitarian value.

Several Mexica medical prescriptions from the Codex Badianus, described in Chapter 3, employed sympathetic magic—for instance, using the blood of jaguars in an unguent to transmit power and courage.[1377] Similar formulae can be found in pagan Old World medicine, such as the Greek *Kyranides* text from the second to the fourth centuries CE, which suggest using the brain of a peacock to create a love-potion, or making an ointment out of mouse-heads to cure hair loss.[1378] Such interventions combined the magical principles of sympathy and contagion. As in medieval Old World medicine, creating basic medicines didn't require the invocation of deity, but would invariably have been accompanied by prayer, or a specific chant to empower them, so deific magic was involved as well. The medieval European "doctrine of signatures" exemplified sympathetic magical principles—the idea that certain plants or animal parts resembled or were reminiscent of certain body parts, organs, or diseases, and that this indicated their medical usage. The Mesoamericans held similar views, for example their use of a seaweed called *tapachpatli* which they said resembled "crushed liver" to treat liver diseases, or *yoloxochitl* (*Magnolia mexicana*) to treat heart problems, because the mature flower is "shaped like a heart".[1379]

The universal magical principle of the importance of physical or temporal thresholds—boundaries or crossing-over points between different kinds of spaces or experiences—is well represented in Mesoamerican beliefs and practices, such as the concept of natural and artificial portals or *yol*, the use of *dzonots*, caves, and trees as access points to the otherworld, and the customary rituals associated with baptism, coming-of-age, marriage, and funerals. The astrological timing and location of rituals and sacred sites also echoes Old World practices such as the construction of the Egyptian pyramids and Celtic stone circles to line up with astronomical events, or the customary performance of religious rituals and festivals at particular times. Such notions survive in vestigial form in the calendrical approximation of major monotheistic religious festivals to events in the solar or lunar calendar, such as Christmas and Easter being adjacent to the winter and summer solstices in the northern hemisphere, or the occurrence of Ramadan in the ninth month of the Islamic lunar calendar.

The concept of "ensouling" objects or statues, or using them to house conscious, invisible spirit entities is also a global phenomenon. Old World versions of these beliefs and practices were common in pre-Christian pagan religions, and survived in monotheistic religion until the eleventh century with the Middle Eastern Harranian Sabians, before going underground with Gnostic and Hermetic mysticism or other forms of esoteric monotheism such as Kabbalah. For the Classic Maya, idols were imbued with *k'ul*, "holy spirits" or "gods", and priestly agents or *chilan* ("translators") would "channel" these spirits, voicing their responses and desires.[1380] A similar religious phenomenon can still be seen in the occurrence of crying or bleeding statues in Catholicism, which may be accompanied by visions of the Virgin Mary or angels "speaking" to people in dreams; although in Catholicism the statue is not considered to be alive or ensouled, but is a tangible "miracle" evidencing God's universal presence, whereas the Maya sought to routinely and deliberately house discrete spiritual entities in statues and communicate with them.

In common with other ancient cultures, the Mesoamericans believed that naturally produced objects and locations were already "ensouled", but that man-made objects and buildings needed to be consecrated, to have *ch'ulel*—or its equivalent—funnelled into them through rituals.[1381] European Hermeticists also used astrologically timed rituals to "ensoul" talismans cast in the image of men or beasts, and referred to the time in ancient Egypt when such things were common:

> statues ensouled or conscious … that foreknow the future and predict it by lots, by prophecy, by dreams and many other means; statues that make people ill and cure them, bringing them pain and pleasure as each deserves. (Ibn Qurra, ninth century CE, translated by Warnock, 2005)[1382]

Mayan rituals to invest objects or places with *ch'ulel* could include simpler ceremonies and bloodletting or animal sacrifices for smaller objects, all the way up the scale to ballgames, pageants, and feasts with human sacrifices for larger buildings or statues.

Once empowered or animated in this way, the magical efficacy—or ability of these objects or locations to attract specific types of fate—grew through ritual human use. If they were abandoned, however, they could become dangerous, as the event-attracting force or entity inhabiting them was no longer fed or steered by conscious human action, so the power contained had to be exorcised through a special "termination ritual".[1383] The Classic Maya used rituals to invest war standards or paraphernalia with the *wayob* of patron deities such as the *waxak-lahun-ubah-kan*, the feathered serpent of war, or the sun-jaguar, *K'in Balam*. Post-conquest Mayan accounts of their defeat by the Spanish describe the armies clashing as an almost incidental feature of an aetheric battle between the *wayob* of the Spanish forces, the "fair maiden" or Virgin Mary, the "footless birds" or angels, and hosts of saints, and the eagle, serpent, jaguar, and lightning *wayob* of the indigenous Maya, which were routed by the spiritual sponsors of the Christian forces.[1384]

The concept of serpents as representatives of otherworldly knowledge is also widespread. There's the ancient Chinese belief in dragons as powerful entities associated with rainfall, water, rulership, and supernatural wisdom, the south-east Asian *naga* or dragon-snake linked to the creator-deity Vishnu and Shiva, god of destruction, and the rainbow serpent of the Australian Aborigines which dwells in waterholes, shaped the land, and is associated with magical ability.[1385] The use of serpent and toad imagery, as well as the entheogenic use of mushrooms, toads, and plants in the nightshade family such as *Datura* are also reminiscent of European witchcraft. The image of witches riding broomsticks, for example, is thought to be connected to the production of hallucinogenic "flying ointments" made with nightshade-family herbs such as mandrake (*Mandragora officinarum*) or henbane (*Hyoscyamus niger*) which have a similar chemistry to *Datura*, replete with anti-cholinergic tropane alkaloids. These ointments were applied to broom handles, which could then be "ridden", in the x-rated sense—not something you'll find in Harry Potter.[1386]

The use of such ointments enabled a witch's spirit to fly from her body and commune with other disembodied entities; and the Mesoamericans used transformative unguents for similar purposes, regarding *Datura* and some of its botanical relatives as potent power plants with a dark side. For the Huichol, the sorcerer who chose to work with *kieri* (*Solandra brevicalyx*), the "Tree of Winds"—another tropane-containing nightshade—was capable of inflicting or reversing curses in a way that those who worked only with the more benign, mescaline-containing *peyote* (*Lophophora williamsii*) couldn't; it was a dangerous and solitary path to be a student of the plant's spirit, who was a "capricious patron", but could reward his acolytes with gifts of art and music and worldly wealth.[1387] So an entirely different religious tradition on a different continent came to similar conclusions about the nature and uses of this class of plants.

Belief in the importance of "cleans[ing], prepar[ing], and propitiat[ing]" before rituals is found in magical traditions worldwide. This has been described as a "removing of spiritual residues";[1388] in practical terms this may mean fasting, sexual abstinence, regular prayer and preparation to reduce material distractions and attachments and focus the mind, in addition to literally cleaning and consecrating the ritual space. Many Mesoamerican ritual actions, such as the creation of new god-statues, required strict protocols like celibacy, prayer, and seclusion on the part of sculptors and priests in order to maintain a "pristine" spiritual state before the statues were inaugurated or ensouled. The infamous Old World medieval magical grimoire *Picatrix* states that, among many other stipulations, effective magical action requires that you "make many suffumigations, have perfect faith, fast often, utter many prayers, choose a place appropriate to the work, and observe the … planets. These are the foundations of magical workings."[1389] No Mesoamerican priest would have disagreed.

Another remarkable parallel to Old World metaphysics can be found in the Mexica anatomy of the soul, with the animating *tonalli*, *teyolia*, and *ihiyotl* housed in the brain, heart, and liver, respectively. After Aristotle and Galen, Old World humoral medicine described the soul as having three parts, those being vegetative, sensitive, and rational, associated with the natural, animal, and vital spirits, housed in the liver, the brain, and the heart, respectively. (Natural spirits governed basic bodily functions such as nutrition and reproduction, animal spirits gave motion, sensation and cognition, and vital spirits gave life). The systems differ in the details, for example the vital spirits and the heart were metaphorically represented by the sun in the Old World system,[1390] but the sun was linked to the *tonalli* and the brain by the Mexica. But the overlap is remarkable for continents that had no regular or established means of physical contact or communication for millennia, even to the extent that the liver was thought to "house the passions" of the soul in the Aristotlean system,[1391] exactly like the seat of the Mexica *ihiyotl*. In both systems, the heart was the repository of life-force, will, and rationality (*yolliliztli* or vital spirits), and the capacity for imagination and motion were housed in the brain.

Behind the wizard's curtain: divination, magic, and consciousness

The eighteenth-century scientific world view that prevails in intellectual circles is *Materialist*, meaning that it focuses on *matter*: presuming that the universe is made up from "dead" or non-conscious material, and consequently—logically—prescribes that we can measure it, and find out how it all fits together. The *Vitalist* world view of traditional societies such a pre-Colombian Mesoamerica regards the universe and all living things as being perfused and animated by a vital force, which suggests that consciousness underlies reality: everything in the material world is, in a sense, either part of one large "spiritual organism" or under the aegis of non-physical conscious forces. This is the bedrock of a magical world view: in a Vitalist universe, things don't need to be in contact to affect each other. The other essential ingredient of a magical world is the belief in the oft-quoted "as above, so below"—that smaller "versions" of consciousness, such as our individuated awareness, mirror the larger universal god-consciousness in some tiny, particulate, but essentially similar way, and the two are continually in dialogue, just as a single cell, embedded in the matrix of a human body, retains its own separate micro-existence while being a dependent part of the whole.

Mesoamerican divination exemplifies these concepts, and was more nuanced than the calendars make it seem at first. As with astrology in Europe, Mesoamerican calendar divination was used for a variety of purposes, such as medicine, weather forecasting, predicting the outcome of battles and the fate of kings, finding lost objects or missing persons, or identifying thieves.[1392] Our understanding of Mesoamerican divination and religious beliefs is hampered by imprecise translations, too; most pictograms in the codices, such as "monkey", were complex symbols, relating not only to their literal representation but to a number of other social actions or associated meanings.[1393] "Water" in Mexica ritual speech was often referred to as "she of the jade skirt", "the dark green woman", or "the white priest",[1394] simultaneously describing the physical medium of water and a whole range of linked mythological associations and possibilities. This trait survives in modern Zapotec, where the name for the traditional Cacao spice *Bourreria huanita* is *guie xoba*, "sky flower"; the same phrase also means "de-husked corn"—which refers to its common name, "popcorn flower", as the flower's appearance is supposed to be reminiscent of popcorn; but the phrase also means "to swim".[1395]

As in Mesoamerican ritual speech, the use of symbol systems are an essential component of divinatory and magical lexicons worldwide, because symbols pithily express and conceptually unite a great number of possibilities and meanings, some literal, some poetic and allegorical. A sceptic may say this lack of specificity is because there is a need to generate unfalsifiability, or to maximise the probability that at least one divinatory interpretation is correct in hindsight. A magical practitioner may say this is because this is how the world actually works—that conceptual connections *are* real connections, because the universe is a product of Mind (with a capital M), and consciousness is the bedrock of reality; and/or because the meaning we impose shapes the reality we experience, that our perceptual filters are largely a product of subconscious programming, and the language of the subconscious is the symbolic language of dreams. The Mesoamericans may have put it differently: the gods manifest in all their works, and humans, as the gods' creations, must learn to speak their languages. Symbols are a language of the gods, or at least an approximate rendering of one.

Sceptics assert that divination is chicanery, and may be convincingly imitated by utilising techniques which make use of basic reasoning errors, good communication skills, and psychological tricks. But a sceptical accusation of "cold reading"—obtaining information from someone about their thoughts, desires, and hopes by "reading between the lines" of their speech and body language in order to dazzle and dupe them—would be confusing (or irritating) to a traditional diviner. Information was modified according to the querent's needs and circumstances, and addressing these needs by paying attention to their responses and "tells" was just an additional way of gleaning relevant information. Mesoamerican divination, like all divinatory systems, depended on an abstraction of real-world data into codifiable and interpretable forms; for example, the Maya seem to have modified or "rounded off" the length of venus's phases to make them more symmetrical so that they locked into the lunar cycles more exactly, to fit into their precise calendars. Venus spends an average of 236 days as a morning star and 250 days as an evening star, but these periods were considered to be of equal length in Meosamerican calendrical reckonings.[1396] This wasn't cheating: it was a matter of constructing a viable, symmetrically cyclical thought-mechanism abstracted from reality, which necessitated a little editorial discretion.

For Materialists—leaving aside the obvious issue of how dead matter and causally unrelated phenomena could speak to humans on the subjective details of their lives—this disregard for precision diminishes any claim to utility, as the data being used to obtain information from the natural world is non-representative and inaccurate. But for those of a magical mindset, including most ancient civilisations, human perceptions of reality, and the systems created to translate and interpret our perceptions, were as much a part of reality as the external phenomena which comprise it. In other words, in a magical universe, our thought processes are inseparable from—and reflective of—an underlying, divine reality. As the Old World "Emerald Tablet" has it, "That which is Below corresponds to that which is Above, and that which is Above, corresponds to that

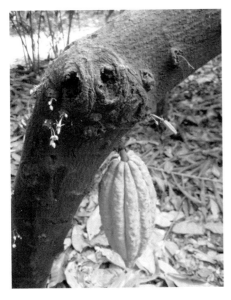

Above: *criollo* Cacao pod, San Antonio
Suchitequepez, Guatemala, 2011

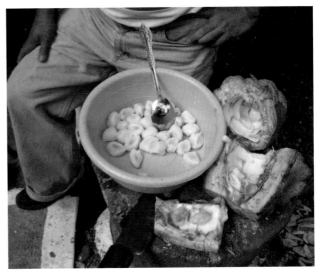

Above: cacao expert Jaun-Pablo Porres Esquina standing
with split *criollo* Cacao pod with fresh fruit and seeds,
San Antonio Suchitequepez, Guatemala, 2011

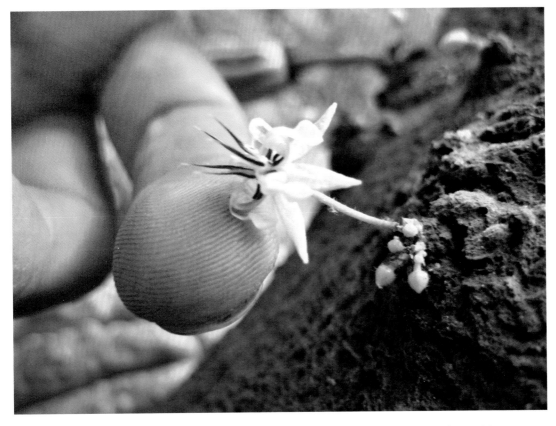

Above: *Trinitario* Cacao flower to scale, San Antonio Suchitequepez, Guatemala, 2011

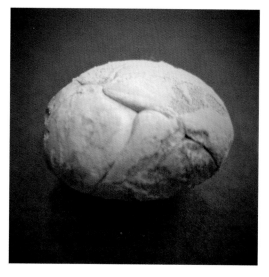

Above: peeled *cacao blanco*, an anaerobically fermented seed of *Theobroma bicolor*.

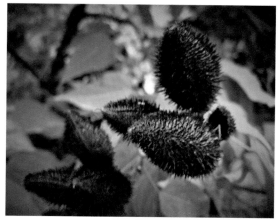

Above: *Bixa orellana* seed pods, Lanquin, Guatemala, 2011

Right: dried petals of *Cymbopetalum penduliflorum* or *muc'*, purchased from a marketplace in Coban, Guatemala, 2018

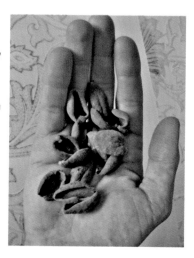

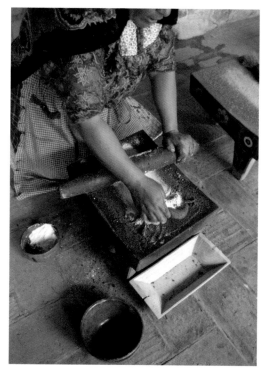

Above: one of the cooks at chef Carina Santiago's restaurant, *Tierra Antigua* in Teotitlán del Valle, Oaxaca, grinds *cacao blanco* with toasted Cacao seeds to prepare *chocolate atole*.

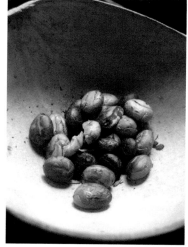

Left: toasted *cacao címarron* (*Theobroma bicolor*) seeds, for making *popo*, Tuxtepec-style.

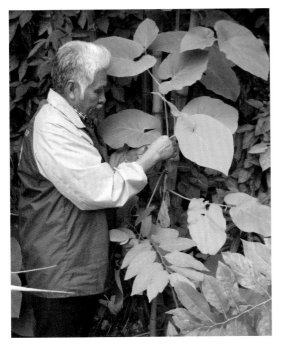

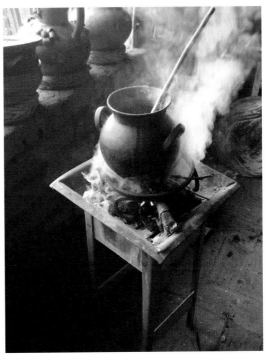

Above: herbalist Señor Reginaldo Huex with *hoja santa* (*Piper auritum*), San Jose, Peten, Guatemala, 2011

Above: boiling *atole blanco*, Teotitlan del Valle, Oaxaca, Mexico, 2018

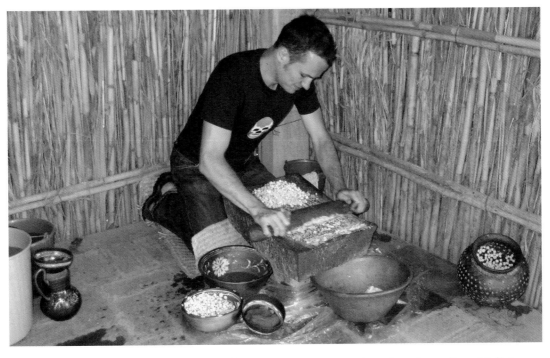

Above: the author grinding nixtamalized corn (*Zea mays*) to make *tejate*, Santo Tomal Julietza, Oaxaca, Mexico, 2008

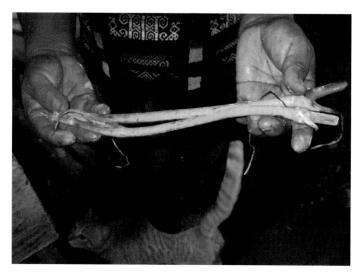

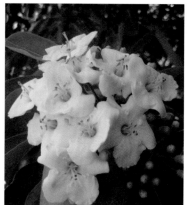

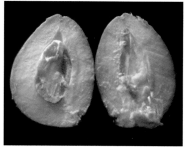

Above: Doña Rosa Gregorio holding toasted fresh *cocolmeca* (*Smilax aristolochiifolia*) she uses to make *popo*, Ojitlan, Oaxaca, Mexico, 2018
Top right: *Bourreria huanita* in bloom, Juchitan de Zaragoza, Oaxaca, 2018
Right: halved *chupipe* (*Gonolobus niger*) fruit.

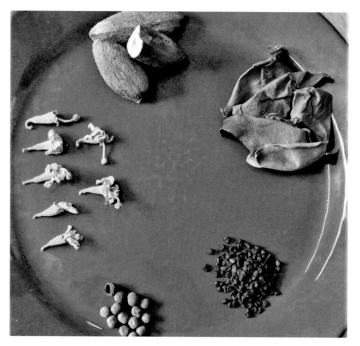

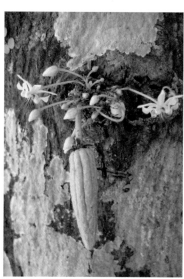

Above: immature *criollo* Cacao pod and flowers, San Antonio Suchitequepez, Guatemala, 2011

Above: some traditional Cacao-affiliated dried spices still used in Mexico. Clockwise from top: *mamey sapote* seeds (*Pouteria sapota*); *magnolia* petals (*Magnolia dealbata*); *achiote* seeds (*Bixa orellana*); allspice seeds (*Pimienta dioica*); *Rosita de cacao* (*Quararibea funebris*).

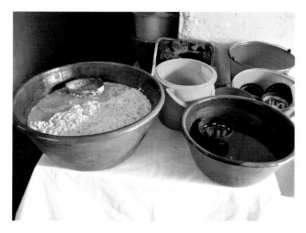

Above: *tejate* vendor's table, Oaxaca city, Mexico, 2008

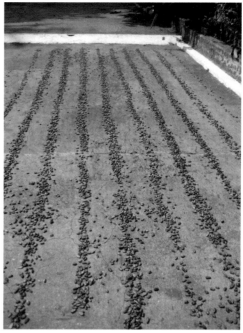

Above: *criollo* Cacao drying in the sun after fermentation, San Antonio Suchitequepez, Guatemala, 2011

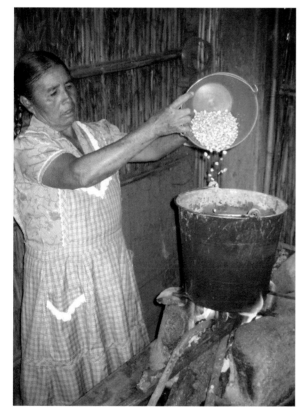

Above: Señora Crispina Navarro Gomez boiling corn (*Zea mays*) and *guacoyules* (*Attalea cohune*) seeds with lime to make *tejate*, Santo Tomal Julietza, Oaxaca, Mexico, 2008

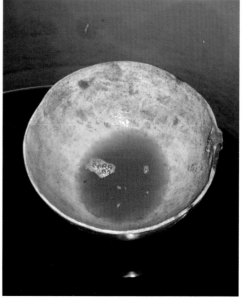

Above: a *jicara* of cocoa butter, extracted by boiling (wet method) cooling in a tub of water, Rex'hua, Guatemala, 2011

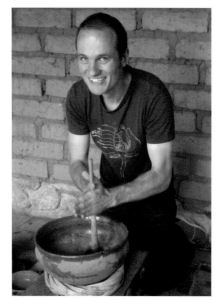

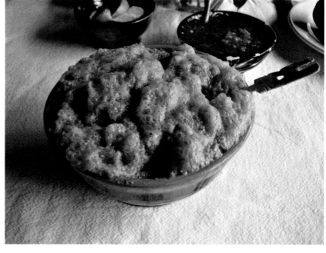

Above: *chocolate atole*, Teotitlan del Valle, Oaxaca, Mexico, 2018

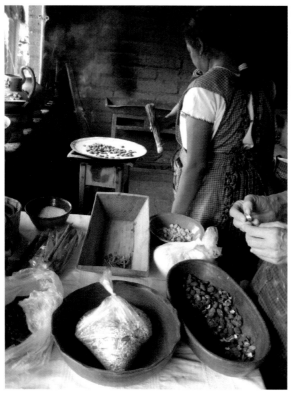

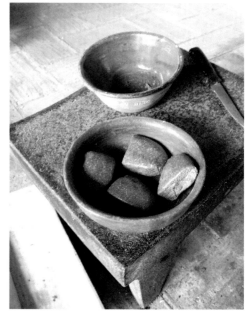

Top left: the author making foam for *chocolate atole*.
Above: the completed foam-making tablets for *chocolate atole*.

Above: chef Carina Santiago overseeing the toasting of Cacao beans (background), while an assistant peels *cacao blanco* (foreground) for making *chocolate atole*. Other ingredients on the table include rice, toasted dried maize, and *canela* (*Cinnamomum zeylanicum*). Teotitlan del Valle, Oaxaca, Mexico, 2018

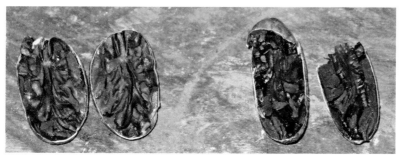

Left: side-by-side comparison of fermented (left) and Unfermented (right) *criollo* Cacao seeds. San Antonio Suchitequepez, Guatemala, 2011

Below, clockwise from top left:
Top left, "Undead chocolate" (recipe in Chapter Eight); top right, "Basic *kakawa*" (recipe in Chapter Eight); bottom right, breakfast *champurrado* (recipe in Chapter Eight); bottom left, grinding and sifting spices for "Basic *kakawa*".

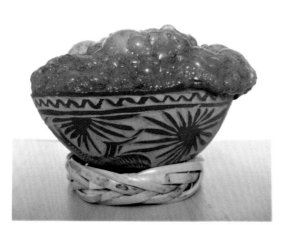

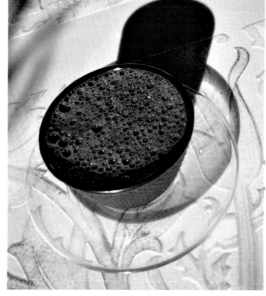

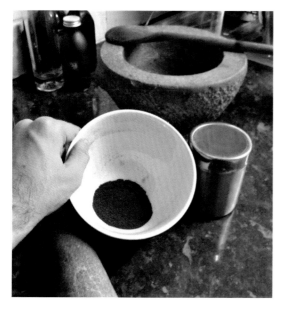

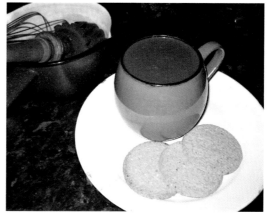

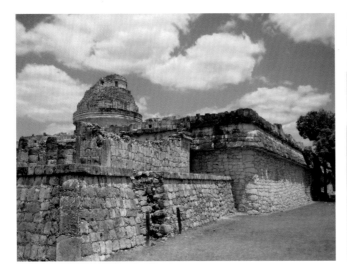

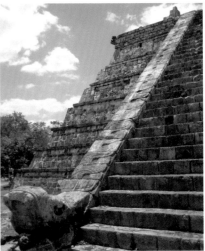

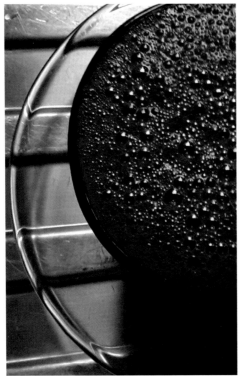

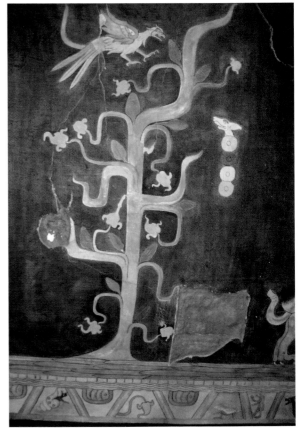

Top left: *el caracol*, the observatory at Chichen Itza, a temple for viewing the phases of venus.

Top right: serpent stairway, Chichen Itza.

Above: close up of the foam on "Basic *kakawa*" recipe, showing "rainbow serpents" in the bubbles.

Above: detail from the mural at Cacaxtla showing a Cacao tree with a bird, possibly representing the Big Dipper, in its branches. The tree stands to the right of a scorpion-tailed venus god (not shown).

which is Below, to accomplish the miracle of the One Thing."[1397] From this perspective, the process of weaving observed natural patterns into systematic forms from which narratives could be made, was entirely valid; the human mind and imagination was like a smaller reflection of the divine mind. Divination was as much an act of creation as of prognostication. To divine was to call forth spiritual powers; divination was a respected science, to the extent that events beheld by seers in dreams or visions could be used as evidence in Mesoamerican courts.[1398]

The discrediting of divination and magical thinking in the post-Enlightenment era occurred as a consequence of the rise of Materialism, in particular the insidious metaplasia of cause-and-effect mechanics from methodology to ideology. This can be clearly seen in the work of philosophical and scientific luminaries such as Karl Popper, Bertrand Russell, and Carl Sagan, who were opposed to the "irrationalism" of superstition and religion. Russell famously compared religious belief to a claim that a small teapot, far too tiny to be detected by the most powerful telescopes, is orbiting the sun, somewhere between Earth and mars; he argued that the unfalsifiability of this statement doesn't make it more likely to be true, or valid, and the burden of proof falls on those making similarly extraordinary claims. The weakness of Russell's analogy lies in the facile comparison of a teapot to religious belief, which reflects his prejudices, in addition to the question of who gets to define an "extraordinary claim". The assertion that God exists may be a hard case to prove for a fundamentalist, but for those who concede that religious myths may be allegorical rather than factual, the case against the existence of God seems as "extraordinary" as the case for it: in the words of Terry Pratchett, the current scientific paradigm asserts that "in the beginning there was nothing, which exploded".[1399]

But there are powerful arguments for the burden of proof: if something is to be relied upon, it must be seen to work on all levels, including, and perhaps especially, in the practical and physical domain; results can't be assumed, and should be demonstrable. Most divinatory techniques fail basic tests of scientific replicability, although not always, and not completely; there is often a consistent and highly significant just-above-chance level of success in trials of such techniques (including a famous "disproof" of astrology that has subsequently been called into question).[1400] A full discussion of the findings of "parapsychology" and scientific investigation into the practical efficacy of religious ritual, belief, and the occult would be a book in its own right, and certainly merits further investigation. The root of the matter, though, in terms of whether magic and deific religion are even *hypothetically* possible, is consciousness. This can be defined as our awareness of such things as pain, pleasure, love, and mortality—the qualities of life, or *qualia*,[1401] whose existence has been described as the "hard problem". Put simply, the "hard problem" is: why does the correct arrangement of brain matter produce what we call "consciousness"? "Because it does" is a parental response, not a scientific one.

The issue is that Mind seems so much greater than the physical structures that enable thought would suggest. Mind is an embodied, relational, self-organising, and open system, mathematically definable as "chaos capable" and non-linear; in other words, tiny inputs can generate disproportionately and often unpredictably large and variable outputs. Mind is defined as relational, yet it can still exist for those unfortunate people who are "shut-in", being blind, deaf, dumb, and immobile but with conserved higher cortical functioning following serious brain injury.[1402] Thought and sensory processing are clearly dependent on the physical matter of the brain, but the brain's structure doesn't explain why or how consciousness arises.

Broadly speaking, there are two schools of thought which seek to answer this question: Monism and Dualism. Time for some brief definitions of these hypotheses: Monism, as the name implies, suggests that reality is made from just one type of Stuff. If that Stuff is physical, and consciousness is produced—somehow—by the physical Stuff, then that is referred to as Physicalism: consciousness is a by-product of physical matter, like a computer program or projection. If the Stuff is Mental, and the "physical" is just an illusory, subjective by-product of the mental realm, as if the entire universe is a hologram, then that is Idealism.[1403]

There are two Physicalist schools of thought: Identity Theorists and Functionalists. Identity Theorists hold that the arrangement of physical matter in the brain automatically produces mental processes which give rise to consciousness, like a computer, although there are serious doubts about the viability of this proposal: under this definition, if we were able to grow a living brain in a vat in a laboratory, it would be expected to automatically develop consciousness. Functionalists adopt a more sophisticated version of the same concept, believing that mental states arise in the physical structure of the brain as a result of other mental states[1404]—so just cloning a brain and giving it an oxygenated blood supply would be inadequate; consciousness could only arise as a result of a chain reaction of networked and interdependent thoughts stimulated by responses to experience in the growing brain. Simply put, Functionalism suggests that given the right arrangement of matter, sufficient interconnectedness and complexity of mental signalling will eventually—with time and experience—give rise to consciousness. Both theories are Physicalist because they hold that consciousness arises from physical processes, and specifically from the cortical matter of the brains of higher mammals (and, speculatively, in alternative arrangements of physical matter in aliens, or other sentient beings in the universe) without any sort of "haunting" of the material realm.

Dualists, on the other hand, believe that consciousness doesn't reside solely in the brain. Substance Dualism, sometimes called Cartesian Dualism, is distinctly Vitalist and postulates "supernatural" or external causes of Consciousness, as it argues for the existence of separate and immaterial Stuff,[1405] such as the soul, which gives rise to life and thought. It's named after the philosopher René Descartes ("I think, therefore I am"), and is a philosophical box into which most world religions can be placed, including the monotheistic faiths and the ancient Mesoamerican belief systems, although the strong dividing line between "physical" and "non-physical" aspects of reality may have seemed bizarre to them. The philosopher and psychologist William James argued against Substance Dualism on the basis that brain injury or drugs are sufficient to destroy individual consciousness: so, he argued, the brain clearly produces consciousness.[1406] But there's a difference between functionality and causation—a brain may express or facilitate consciousness, yet not be its source, just as immersing a radio in water or smashing it may shut it down, but doesn't eliminate the radio waves carrying the programmes.

Property Dualism, on the other hand, is really more like a type of Materialism, but sneaks Dualist concepts in through the back door: Property Dualism recognises only one main type of physical Stuff, but regards Mind as a kind of non-physical stuff (small s) associated with it. Fundamental Property Dualism has a lot in common with Physicalism, asserting that consciousness is a non-physical property arising from physical matter, but posits a less linear relationship between matter and Mind, in the same way that electromagnetism or gravity are forces which arise from, or are linked to matter in some way; state changes must be detectable in physical matter for consciousness to change,[1407] but changes in consciousness may also cause alterations in physical states. In other words, alterations in blood flow, brain chemistry, and electromagnetic activity in the brain reflect and affect consciousness—but, in distinction to Identity Theory or Functionalism, don't necessarily correlate with it in a linear way.

Panpsychist Property Dualism—more usually referred to as Panpsychism—suggests that consciousness is an integral property of matter, which is latent in all physical Stuff.[1408] It can be biologically expressed as life by the proper arrangement of molecules into organisms displaying the characteristics of living beings such as nutrition, sensitivity, growth, reproduction, movement, excretion, and respiration (although viruses, which appear to be crucial players in evolution through their cut-and-paste interactions with DNA, are technically not alive by this definition). William James's argument that the brain must be the seat of consciousness can also be addressed from a Panpsychist perspective: if brains are a good arrangement for matter to express innate consciousness in perceptible ways, then destroying or shutting down the brain merely destroys the integrity of that individual human's consciousness. Brain damage reduces the coherence of an individual's consciousness without affecting the ubiquitous latent consciousness present in all matter.

Panpsychism is usually equated with panexperimentalism—the belief that everything has a form of consciousness, or "what-it-is-to-be-like"-ness, however basic—rather than pancognitivism, the belief that everything has *thoughts*, which would imply that they have an organic brain. Although Panpsychism isn't strictly Vitalist—as this would require belief in a Substance Dualist-type "vital force"—nevertheless Panpsychism has a kind of non-Dualist Vitalist perspective, and is compatible with several religious and non-religious (or not conventionally religious) metaphysical systems such as early Taoism or Zen Buddhism. To sum up these positions, the nature or origin of the universe can be described as Mind not Matter (Idealist), Matter not Mind (Physicalist), Mind before Matter (Substance Dualist), or Mind = Matter (Panpsychist).

The Physicalists are hoping to be able to demonstrate the material origin of qualia through neuronal correlates of consciousness (NCC): physical brain structures which are linked to the signals that accompany lived experience, and which particularly occur in the posterior cortex of the human brain. The elephant in the room: even the most sceptical scientist knows that on a subatomic level our perceptions and expectations affect the results we get. As the quantum physicist Werner Heisenberg famously noted, by observing something at the smallest discernible unit of reality, we change it. And as various other experiments such as the much-maligned work of Rupert Sheldrake or the investigative journalism of Lynne McTaggart have shown, this may well apply further up the scale, right up to the point of affecting how matter or living systems behave over time.[1409]

The "law of attraction", espoused in the popular film "The Secret", is an example of "magical thinking", currently used as a pathological term by psychologists to describe delusional associations between apparently coincidental things. But magical thinking is ancient and culturally universal, and may be compatible with some of the findings of modern physics; at the smallest discernible level of being, most matter turns out to be empty space, invested with particles which appear to wink in and out of being, and which are influenced by human thought.[1410] Strange things happen on close observation of our physical world, and the further down the rabbit hole we go, the stranger things get. But the truth of the "reality" of magic ultimately lies in the mind. This isn't a cop-out: as the Huichol say, magical action depends on "correct thinking"—in particular, the mode of thinking. Whether you believe magic is a matter of psychology or metaphysics, in either case the mind is the real portal between the human world and the otherworlds. When expectations and perception are altered, strange things happen; at the very least, magic and ritual can effect startling psychosomatic change. The bundled "reasoning errors" of magic add up synergistically; they constitute a totally different way of perceiving the world. And if it turns out that consciousness is universal, and not housed in individual brains as the Physicalists aver, then there will be no reason to dismiss the notion that perception, expectation, and directing one's consciousness towards a goal may produce an "objective" effect.

The catch-22 is that, in any model of consciousness, belief affects outcomes to some extent; the kind of results we expect to get in the real world are, largely, what we do get. But the "results" of magic, prayer, or ritual are wholly experiential and subjective, and proving or disproving any material outcomes from them is difficult, because they're variable and multifactorial. If a ritual performed to heal an illness is followed by a successful medical treatment, was the ritual responsible? If the person remains ill, did the ritual fail, did the medicine counteract the ritual, or has another malevolent magic-wielder annulled its effect? A shaman might say yes; or no, it's something else—a spirit, perhaps, or the fault of the patient, or some procedural or moral lapse in the shaman themselves. If we are to assume the perspective of the magician, then magic resists attempts at "objective" testing, because thoughts, intentions, or invisible entities influence outcomes.

The notion of "objectivity" in scientific experiment—the basis of the entire Enlightenment world view—may be less robust than was initially supposed. Being human may turn out to be the ultimate "confounding variable": in a non-causally interconnected and conscious Idealist, Substance Dualist, or even Panpsychist universe, scientific attempts to create a "sterile field" of objectivity would always be subject to the influence of the beliefs around which experiments are constructed. Over time, perhaps, statistical tests could be devised to evaluate the effects of different beliefs and practices on real-world outcomes, or perhaps tests designed by sceptics and true believers could be compared and run in parallel, or "crossed over" in different groups. Researchers such as Dr Dean Radin have begun to make inroads into such territory.[1411] But as the *Picatrix* stated almost a thousand years ago:

> The properties that are proposed and the examples that are given in the books of the prophets concerning this science [magic], if you were to try and deduce them by experiment, would seem to be of a fraudulent nature, nor would you be able to deduce the effects promised by them in eternity. If you understand them, however, in the manner we have said (that is, with the right attitude and a steady faith and an understanding of the causes of effects), then they will seem to be noble, high, and precious, and of a nature remote from the merely animal in man. (*Picatrix, Book III*, Ch. 12, trans. Greer & Warnock, 2011)

At the risk of straw-manning the argument, the standard ethnographic reasoning for the occurrence of identical principles and overlapping techniques in magico-religious practices occurring on several continents separated by millennia is that they arose due to similarity of human minds and thought-patterns, and the necessity to invent a pseudo-technology to give a "sense of control" of the world in the face of mortality. This may be true, but it's a condescending explanation, which takes as its starting point the notion that magical practices are ineffective; it's an interpretation built on an assumption. It also seems remarkably flimsy given the astonishing correlations which may be found in indigenous magical practices and beliefs from cultures geographically and temporally dispersed across the globe and throughout history, many of which endured in various forms for thousands of years.

However morally atrocious our ancestors' religious practices may have been, let's start with a different premise—we could concede that if their beliefs seem irrational and bizarre to us, the fault may reside, at least in part, in our comprehension. It may not be too much of a stretch to invert Arthur C. Clarke's famous line, that any sufficiently advanced technology is indistinguishable from magic: perhaps magic may not be distinguished until our technology is sufficiently advanced.

* * *

In occult circles, there's a theory that religion itself may have been an answer to the problem of the death of instinctual knowledge of what we now call "God". In other words, the development of organised religion may have been precipitated by a prehistoric erosion of collective consciousness, a poly-generational atrophy of awareness. Our ancestors inhabited a psychedelic, magical landscape; the development of the technologies of civilisation paralleled an incremental human separation from direct contact with nature, so that on the most basic level, the awareness of our dependence on natural drives and processes became attenuated. The biblical Eden, may, in a sense, be a collective dream-memory of a time when we were all amoeboid lifeforms floating in a soup of singular consciousness, before evolution kicked in.

What we call culture and technology may be the thick end of a wedge of clever human inventions, driven between us and "nature". Human cognitive development and inventions facilitate the development of our individuated consciousness, but artificially overcompensate for what we may have incrementally lost with the growth of the cerebral cortex: a direct line to what we may call "the divine", an immersive unity of being. From this perspective, even the rituals of the Perennial Philosophy were postlapsarian reactions. Of course, it's quite possible that all this speculation may be a manifestation of the human tendency to imagine we have lost something profound, because life is harder than we feel it should be. But what does any of this have to do with chocolate? To answer this, we must first take a detour to venus.

Venereal chocolate

Chocolate is a balm for life's slings and arrows; along the way, it's become symbolically associated with love, sex, romance, and the things of Venus's domain. Chocolates are a Valentine's Day gift, paired with roses; chocolates are a guilty snack, or a compulsive one; chocolate is synonymous with comfort, pleasure, and solace, as well as a Puritan awareness of the dangers of the primrose path—"moderation" is the keyword. Rubens's Venus would have disagreed: she advertises a capitalist's approach to expansion. In a consumerist economy, chocolate is a growth industry—it's big business. And contemporary Big Chocolate employs more slaves than the Mesoamerican Cacao-lords ever did. Like the Mexica and their steady supply of Cacao and captives for heart-sacrifice being cultivated or culled from remote regions by the *pochteca* and the armed forces, vassals and serfs in distant lands labour to supply today's lucrative chocolate and beauty industries with their raw materials, often in extreme poverty or joyless indenture.

As recounted in the last chapter, both the midnight sun and the "wandering star" we call venus were mythologically linked to Cacao in Mesoamerica. But while Cacao's traditional associations with luxury and celebration were retained when it was brought to Europe, its folkloric and ceremonial links with death and rebirth, blood sacrifice, and the ancestors were replaced by a reputation as an aphrodisiac. Chocolate became an exotic New World potion that cured melancholy and provoked venery. A dash of sugar, a drop of milk, and by some sleight of mind the Mesoamerican war gods were replaced by the Roman goddess of love and pleasure. Yet the scorpion-tailed and spear-wielding skeleton gods of the Mesoamerican venus never fully disappeared; Cacao's reputation has always had a darker edge. The voluptuary heathen drug, the disguiser of poisons, the insidious harm of excess—as if, when assuming symbolic ownership of Cacao, Venus surreptitiously appropriated some attributes from her astrological alter egos across the Atlantic. So how did this symbolic shift happen? And what do these transformations imply about the cultures that use Cacao, or the nature of the drug itself?

The death star

A *criollo* Cacao tree can live for between 100 and 150 years,[1412] or two to three fifty-two-year calendar cycles, two of which (102 years) neatly synchronise the cycles of the moon, sun, and venus in relation to the Earth. Cacao pods have a pentacle-like cross-section, a five-lobed star reminiscent of the pentagram which venus traces in the night sky over an eight-year period. In contemporary Guatemalan folk medicine, *curandero* Diego's uses of Cacao leaves and flowers (described in Chapter 3) in prescriptions for menstrual and urinary tract issues prompted me to ask him if he used Cacao to treat ailments of the throat, breasts, urinary tract, and reproductive system specifically, as these were all body parts affiliated with the planet venus in Old World medical astrology. He replied "exactly"[1413]—which may indicate either a coincidental local tradition of using Cacao to treat these parts of the body, or that his classification system has been influenced by Old World astrological thinking. Perhaps Diego or one of his predecessors categorised Cacao as a tree ruled by the Old World venus, and therefore appropriate for tonifying "venereal" parts of the anatomy. But this use may be ancient, as it's also congruent with some Mesoamerican personifications of Cacao as a female deity, and its associations with fertility, sexuality, and reproduction (see last chapter).

The mythical links between Cacao and several deitieswere also described in Chapter 9. The Mayan underworld deity God L, the prototype of Ek' Chuah ("Black Scorpion"), was a venus god,[1414] depicted with black face paint and carrying a war shield. In calendar divination, as we've seen, the first appearance of venus as a morning star in the dry season was used to time the onset of the "star wars" season, and God L was calendrically associated with this event.[1415] Such wars were intimately linked to the activity of merchants—of which God L and Ek' Chuah were patrons—who not only acted as unofficial spies and recon parties for their polities, but whose trading activity was a secular incentive for military campaigns,[1416] because the defeated state had to pay tribute, particularly in the form of Cacao or other valuables.

The Mexica associated the astronomical venus with the serious crime of adultery, and dangerous biting or stinging animals.[1417] The mural at Cacaxtla described in Chapter 9 depicts a blue-skinned scorpion-tailed venus deity standing between a Cacao tree and a maize plant, and the Mexica associated the evening star venus with their fearsome spear-hurling warrior god Tlahuizcalpantecuhtli, a god of coldness, stone, and punishment; the first appearance of venus as an evening star in the sky promised "stabbings and destruction", disease, and death.[1418] In short, there is an almost complete inversion in the Old and New World astro-mythological venus attributes, with New World venus deities depicted as spear-wielding or poison-bearing war gods. Even Quetzalcoatl, the Mexica's "patron saint of Cacao", is a post-Classic reinvention of the Classic era Teotihuacan-Mayan *waxak-lahun-ubah-kan*, or feathered serpent of war.[1419]

Temples of the post-Classic wind god Ehecatl-Quetzalcoatl in the Yucatan face west, the direction of the evening star venus and the setting sun.[1420] A variant of the myth of Quetzalcoatl's deposition in Tula had a different explanation for his public disgrace: in this account, instead of getting drunk, Quetzalcoatl had sex with Xochiquetzal, the young flower-goddess, who is also, it turns out, the patron of prostitution. Evidently this was a misstep, as he was punished by being burned alive, at which point his heart (his *teyolia*, perhaps) ascended to the celestial realm and appeared in the pre-dawn sky as the morning star.[1421] The more conventional tale of Quetzalcoatl's self-imposed exile into the east, when he departs into the sea, is also consistent with rebirth as the morning star venus, which rises from the ocean in the east before the sun.[1422] The creation account in the Popol Vuh has their feathered serpent creator-god floating in the primordial sea with "shining and brilliant" feathers before the first dawn—much like the morning star venus emerging from the sea and heralding the sunrise.[1423] So Quetzalcoatl, Cacao's patron deity, was consistently associated with venus in the post-Classic era.

In the K'iche Hero Twins myth, the cycles of death and rebirth of the twins have been interpreted as the phases of venus; the decapitation of Hun Hunahpu the elder and Hunahpu the younger may represent venus's direct and retrograde conjunctions with the sun. Hun Hunahpu's head being placed in "a tree in the west" may signify the appearance of venus as an evening star,[1424] an ill omen in Mesoamerican astrology, whereas venus's morning star appearance signifies the younger twins' rebirth and emergence from the underworld.[1425] In Mesoamerican lore, venus was sometimes described as an underworld god who "carried the sun on his shoulders" overnight through the underworld,[1426] much as the merchant god Ek' Chuah would have borne his bundle of Cacao beans.

The Yucatec Maya associated venus with the constellation of the Pleiades, which they called *Tzab*, or "the rattlesnake's rattle".[1427] The Ki'che later referred to the same asterism as the "four hundred boys", the gods of alcoholic intoxication, who attempted to save the Earth by capturing the giant crocodile Zipacna but were later crushed by him while drunkenly celebrating. The Yucatec Maya referred to the evening star venus as the "fire" of the Pleiades, which they used to time the onset of the coming rains for tending their crops, as for more than a thousand years venus's appearance as an evening star here heralded the onset of the rainy season. By contrast, venus's appearance in Scorpio preceded the dry season, and the season of war[1428]—perhaps one reason for the depiction of scorpion-tailed venus gods? Coinciden-tally, the Pleiades are placed in the venus-ruled zodiac sign of Taurus in Old World astrology, where they signified ambition, wanton behaviour, peacefulness, "success in agriculture … [with] disgrace and violent death".[1429]

While such metaphysical overlaps may not infer any links between the Old and New World versions of venus, they do suggest an interesting duality in the nature of Cacao's mythological links with the astronomical venus. Venus's appearance as a morning star or preceding the wet season was linked to gain from agriculture, trading, and tribute, in the manner of Ek' Chuah or the armed *pochteca* who fought for their wealth and status, or Quetzalcoatl's theft of Cacao from the gods or the Mountain of Sustenance. By contrast, it seems that the evening star or dry-season venus—the Mexica death god, the Mayan scorpion-tailed venus-god at Cacaxtla, or Hun Hunahpu's severed head in the fork of a tree—was inimical to human happiness, an omen of misfortune, war and pestilence. So it may be that the Mesoamerican venus as a planetary sym-bol had some affiliation to Cacao, and that Cacao, in turn, embodied some themes which over-lap with the European astrological venus such as luxury, value, acquisition and esteem when associated with the morning star, but inverted these meanings when appearing as an evening star. The overall complex of Cacao's symbolic meanings in Mesoamerica and its associations with planetary deities is most accurately reflected by an Old World version of venus with an additional retributive or acquisitive agenda; in astrological terms, venus with grim saturn, the lord of Karma, or venus ruled by furious mars, perhaps.

So Cacao's Mesoamerican venus-deities could be heroic benefactors, or harbingers of doom. But it's in the post-conquest culture clash that we find many of the most interesting seams and abutments in the reshaping of Cacao's cultural identity. Almost as if *Theobroma cacao*, hav-ing found its hosts overrun by an alien tribe whose ideology threatened to literally demonise everything of value in the native culture, including—and perhaps especially—its sacramental currency, seized the opportunity to expand its territory. In a few scant decades, Cacao had been insinuated into the new dominant culture; a new thought-chrysalis was spun from the threads of imported Judaeo-Christian mythology, and the old, heathen "bitter water" emerged trans-formed, as chocolate: palatable, fashionable, and—as ever—highly desirable.

Post-colonial venus

After the conquest of Mexico, chocolate became especially popular among women and monks in the colonies of New Spain.[1430] This connection is intriguing: perhaps, in an age when women's freedom to choose sexual partners was often severely curtailed, both groups appreciated the strong, evocative flavour of thick sweetened chocolate for their own reasons. Nothing amplifies sensuality more than its curtailment—hunger is the best sauce, as the saying goes, and choco-late is a classic love-substitute (the possible pharmacological reasons for this were discussed in Chapter 5). This was also an era in which chocolate was made more widely available in the colonies, and as it was sugared, it became more popular, and gained a reputation as a vehicle for women's sexual witchcraft. This was a spin-off from Cacao-based beverages' traditional functions as flavour-disguisers and medicaments, often with distinctly magical attributes (see Chapter 3); a few drops of menstrual blood, regarded in European witchcraft as a powerful magical fluid, could be discreetly added to chocolate without any perceptible alteration of fla-vour, as could other sorcerous ingredients of a botanical or anatomical nature.[1431]

Chocolate was used as a base for administering potions of seduction, compulsion, and repul-sion, or poisons. These potions were sometimes one-off, sometimes repeated prescriptions; a pretext for administering them was easy enough to find, as chocolate was drunk as a daily article of diet, and served to guests as a hospitable gesture. The reports of such use of chocolate exist because many potions failed to work, and those who made use of them dutifully "con-fessed" to local authorities—in contrition, or in spite.[1432] There were reports of colonial women in the West Indies feeding menstrually adulterated chocolate to their slaves to keep them from running away[1433]—not the first time that Cacao-based beverages had been mixed with human blood for similar purposes (such as the pre-sacrificial Mexica beverage *itzpacalatl*, discussed in Chapters 1, 2, and 6).

On a less sinister note, contemporary K'iche grooms traditionally give Cacao as a wedding gift, to be made into a drink for a banquet at the bride's house. In most Mayan marriage negotia-tions, Cacao is always a gift from the suitor; if the bride-to-be accepts, this signals that his pro-posal is accepted.[1434] Here Cacao and chocolate fulfil other traditional functions, as a celebratory substance marking the transition to another phase of life, or as a token of good-willed acqui-escence. But other interpretations apply: the gift of Cacao is a reproductive contract. Chocolate drunk in the matrimonial context symbolises another kind of binding spell, the sexual compact of husband and wife "til death do us part", and their intention to honour the ancestors by con-tinuing the bloodline. The historical use of chocolate as a vehicle for the more notorious forms of witchcraft shouldn't blind us to commonplace instances of ceremonial magic, for good or ill. A Mexican matriarch may have no use for covertly adding bodily fluids to chocolate to bind a lover, when she can more usefully and openly add chocolate to a wedding and bind a daughter to a well-descended son-in-law, or vice versa.

As with the offerings of Cacao beans to the *rilaj mam* during Easter week (see last chapter), Cacao still features in both pagan and Christian ceremonies in Central America. But while its reputation as an aphrodisiac and venereal substance never really took off until the Europeans took over, there were many traditional associations of Cacao in Mesoamerica that citizens of the Old World would have recognised as belonging to Venus's domain of sexuality, fertility, beauty, and relationships. In post-colonial Yucatan, Cacao seeds and chilli peppers are used in ritu-als and medicine to enhance sexuality and fertility, and "Cooling" Cacao's perceived property of "attracting good" versus fiery *Capsicum*'s role of "repelling bad" suggests an archetypally feminine role for Cacao.[1435] The San Blas people of Panama burn Cacao seeds over burial sites or graves during puberty rites,[1436] recalling the pre-Colombian ritual use of Cacao to contact ancestor spirits, but with the added dimension of a symbolic role in sexual maturity, which—as the onset of reproductive capacity—is an integral part of the process of life and death, affording the ancestors an opportunity to be reborn. The exchange of Cacao-based beverages in betrothal and marriage ceremonies, and its use in rain and fertility rituals in both post- and pre-colonial Mesoamerica also impute Old World Venusian attributes to Cacao.[1437]

The Bribri of Costa Rica have a legend that their creator-god Sibö visited the homes of four women in the celestial realm, asking for food and drink. Three beautiful women rejected his request, but the fourth woman, Tsura, described as "plainer" and more "homely", took the old man in and fed him. Then he bathed, became handsome, and asked her to marry him. When the four women came to Earth, the three formerly beautiful ladies became bitter, foul-smelling plants, but Tsura incarnated as a Cacao tree.[1438] There's a clear connection here between Cacao and "inner beauty", as well as the notion of being rewarded for morally right action. As in the antonymous Mexica myth of the princess who dies out of loyalty for her husband, Cacao is the personification—and the reincarnated reward—of a virtuous and loyal woman. The myth also displays a deep understanding of beauty as a powerful currency of social esteem, without which the final metamorphosis of beautiful ladies into disparaged plants, and the "plain" woman into the most esteemed and literally valuable plant of all (in a culture which used the seeds as money), would lack any sense of poetic justice. It would be interesting to find out whether people with body dysmorphia were more or less inclined to eat chocolate, because of Cacao's mythic associations as an embodiment of "true worth", and the social studies which link greater chocolate consumption with hysteroid dysphoria, depression, and pre-menstrual cravings (see Chapters 5 and 7), all of which may correspond to poor body image.

The convoluted Mexica legend of the birth of flowers from the flower-goddess Xochiquetzal's bat-bitten vulval wound-water (recounted in Chapter 9) tangentially links Cacao to Venusian themes, as Xochiquetzal is a young goddess of flowers, beauty, and sexuality. *Xochicacahuatl* or "flowery Cacao beverage" denotes foaming Cacao-based beverages of high quality that literally contain flowers as spices; only the god of death can cause beautiful flowers to bloom, recalling Cacao's underworld connections and the literal translation of the Mexica name for one of *xochicacahuatl*'s primary spices, vanilla: *tlilxochitl*, or "black flower". Vanilla is a pod, not a flower—*tlilxochitl* is an allegory for its sublime scent, produced only when the pod blackens during fermentation. The god of death "washes" the severed sexual organs of the green plant in the juices of decay as the vanilla pods wither and sweat, transforming the unprepossessing raw vanilla bean into an aromatic epiphany.

The legend of Coatlicue's mountain was recounted in the last chapter, wherein the serpent-skirted goddess chides the questing Mexica sorcerers for their extravagance and excessive Cacao-consumption, which has caused them to grow old. This myth is also replete with venereal themes, in this case the love of pleasure and luxury, and their debilitating consequences. This is personified by Macuilxochitl, the dark alter ego of Xochipilli, "prince of flowers", the god of psychoactive plants; as recounted in the last chapter, Macuilxochitl was the god of STDs and a member of the five Ahuiateo, or gods of excess, who—by virtue of their assignation to the southern compass direction in Mexica codices—were linked to the underworld, and to Cacao.

The Mexica poet Tlaltecatzin compared *xochicacahuatl*, the drink that "gives delight to all" to his favourite *ahuiani*, or "public woman"—the Mexica equivalent of the Japanese *geisha*, who host, entertain, play games, dance, and flirt with male patrons. Tlaltecatzin goes on to lament, in the inimitable Mexica style, how she, he, and all else he knows must pass away:

> You only lend yourself,
> Soon you must be abandoned,
> You will have to go away,
> There will be a defleshing.

(Tlaltecatzin, from León-Portilla, 1992. © University of Oklahoma Press. Reprinted by permission)

By implication, the pleasures of Cacao are compared to the beauty and sophistication of a high-class escort, and the inevitable separation after the sexual act; the mortal flesh that's sloughed at death like snakeskin, and the transactional nature of life itself, which is, like the beautiful *ahuiani*, only on loan. Cacao is mythically linked to flowers, joy, and luxury, but also to the enervating consequences of overindulgence, and ultimate death. This is the dark side of Venus, with which the Old World was familiar: consider the Galenic belief that excess venery (sex) caused Melancholy, or the French idiom for orgasm, *le petit mort*. Even the Mexica association of flowers with beauty, blood and battle is not so alien when viewed in the obsidian mirror of myth: after all, it was the beautiful Helen of Troy whose coveted face "launched a thousand ships" in the *Iliad*, and ignited the epic Trojan War.

Christianised Cacao

The Spanish conquistadors were horrified by native Mesoamerican religion, with its copious live human sacrifices, idolatry, cannibalism, and worship of "demons". They were also, one suspects, secretly gratified by the "barbarity" which gave them a mandate—a Christian duty, in fact—to conquer and reform the land by any means necessary. It would have been helpful to have their mission validated in this way, as they were so manifestly impressed by the cleanliness, orderliness, and civility of the culture in other respects. Conquistador Bernal Diaz del Castillo recounts his first impressions of the inner sanctum at the top of the 114 steps of the great pyramid temple of Huitzilopochtli and Tezcatlipoca in Tenochtitlan:

> There were some braziers with incense which they call *copal*, and in them they were burning the hearts of the three Indians whom they had sacrificed that day … All the walls were so splashed and encrusted with blood that they were black, the floor was the same and the whole place stank vilely.

"Half laughing", Cortés proceeds to suggest to Motecuhzoma, via the interpreter, that the gods he is worshipping are truly all devils, and would the king and his priests mind terribly if they erected a cross and a small shrine to the Virgin Mary at the top of the steps instead? Unsurprisingly, the *tlatoani*'s response is negative:

> Montezuma replied half angrily (and the two priests who were with him showed great annoyance), and said: "Señor Malinche, if I had known that you would have said such defamatory things I would not have shown you my gods, we consider them to be very good for they give us health and rains and good seed times and seasons and as many victories as we desire, and we are obliged to worship them and make sacrifices, and I pray you not to say another word to their dishonour". (Diaz del Castillo, trans. Maudslay, 1928)

It's tempting to ascribe only venal motives to the conquistadors, who had travelled with Cortés in search of fortune; but that would be to overlook their genuine bravery, and their equally authentic revulsion at native religious practices. Their conviction that the "Indians" were literally worshipping devils was as real as their desire for gold and glory.

The Spanish insistence that indigenous New World spirituality was satanic wasn't baseless, from their point of view. There are many unsettling affinities between Old World witchcraft or devil-worship and Mesoamerican religion, from the existence of shape-shifting sorcerers who used hallucinatory plants to the plethora of snake imagery, fanged gargoyle-like idols, and the consumption of human flesh in worship. The Maya even shed blood to summon a giant snake-spirit during their rituals, which then vomited up terrifying gods and ghosts. The "feathered serpent" Quetzalcoatl was venus as morning star—the same planetary body identified as Lucifer in the Roman tradition, later conflated with the Judaeo-Christian Satan because of its regular "falls" from heaven into the underworld as the planet moves towards conjunction with the sun.

In addition to being a god of knowledge who gave technologies such as astrology and magic to humankind—just as the fallen angels did in the non-canonical Book of Enoch—Quetzalcoatl could be associated with the serpent in the garden of Eden, which illicitly gave the "knowledge of good and evil" to mankind. This serpent, in turn, more than incidentally resembles the two-headed ecliptic serpent in the "branches" of the cosmic tree, the Milky Way. Perhaps, then, as the world tree can be *Theobroma cacao*, and Quetzalcoatl stole Cacao from the celestial realm to give to humankind, Cacao seeds could be said to be the Mesoamerican equivalent of the apple in Genesis. Indeed, after the conquest, the K'iche referred to Cacao as "the tree of sin and knowledge".[1439]

Despite the ideological aversion of the Spaniards and native Mesoamericans to each other's religions, there were several features of Mesoamerican thought which made the colonial Catholicisation of the country—at least superficially—somewhat easier. First, the pragmatic nature of the native religious contract with their deities meant that if they were defeated in battle, then the gods had either abandoned them or were weaker than the *wayob* or *nawal* of the tripartite Christian God and His retinue of angels and saints. Second, and more important in the long run, there were several theological overlaps between Christian and native theology and ritual. Like Jesus, the Mexica Quetzalcoatl was the result of an immaculate conception: his mother, Chimalman, was a human who conceived him after swallowing a precious stone—or being visited in her dreams by a god, or being shot in the womb by a divine arrow, depending on which local myth was told.[1440] The Mayan maize god suffered, died, and was reborn from the underworld,[1441] and maize was his flesh, water or Cacao-based beverages his blood in rituals—so the transubstantiation of bread and wine into the body and blood of the Lord at the Catholic Eucharist was a familiar concept.

Likewise, the most revered native sacrament translated almost seamlessly into Christian liturgical practice, as Cacao became identified with Christianity. The Hero Twins' rebirth in the underworld even took the form of two fish, an early Christian symbol. Contemporary K'iche say a blessing "to the resuscitation of our lord" over Cacao: a sleight-of-sacrament that makes sense once the native Cacao-lore is understood. It's not the first time in history that Christ has been symbolically linked to the morning star or the sun, either. From this perspective, it makes sense that Cacao and Christ have become liturgically linked in Central American lore.

As with most other ancient faiths, the native religions commemorated a great flood, which had destroyed a previous civilisation for their failure to behave and worship properly. Crosses were already in place at every shrine, although their purpose (designating the world tree, the four directions, and signposting a potential *yol*) was not the same as the Christian symbol. Indigenous Maya priests performed baptisms, anointing with *kakawa* rather than holy water. They also practised confession of sins, although in a rather more gory fashion: the penance was not a rosary, but bloodletting; or an old woman could be chosen as a scapegoat to hear the confessions of the entire community, then stoned to death.[1442]

Details and deities changed, but there was much conceptual and ritual architecture that the Christian faith could make use of. Such correspondences cut both ways, though. Just as they facilitated the conversion of many natives to Catholicism, they also enabled many indigenous people to continue practising their pagan ways under the guise of Christianity; as in many conquered territories, retaining the local religion became a means of passive resistance. Catholicism has been incorporated into native beliefs and pantheons in much of Latin America, with apparent success but questionable doctrinal probity; like the tips of icebergs, saints are now all that is visible of the old gods in many places. Over the centuries, the local and foreign deities and beliefs have diffused into each other, so that the K'iche Maya have taken the "fierce and wrathful" Spanish saint Santiago as their own; he speaks only Mayan now, and his local name means "venus morning star".[1443]

Theobroma thaumaturgy

As the archaeological and mythological evidence presented in the last chapter suggests, Cacao augmented the ability of participants to open portals, and to direct *itz*; ingesting *kakawa* or *cacahuatl* may facilitate ritual focus and relax internal barriers which prevent the spirit from accessing the otherworld. It can be used to make potions that amplify the effects of intention, and therefore help magic happen—which is perhaps another reason why the Mexica said, "The heart, the blood [*cacahuatl*] are to be feared."[1444]

Pharmacologically, there is some evidence that Cacao may modify fear and stress responses (see Chapters 4 and 5). In modern-day Santeria, a voodoo-like religion from South America, Cacao beans are burned with various herbs for the purpose of removing fear,[1445] and contemporary Guatemalan *curanderos* use Cacao to neutralise the folk illnesses known as *espanto* or *susto* ("fright", described in Chapter 3), a form of "soul loss" syndrome encountered in shamanic practices. This folk malady has pre-Colombian origins: the Mexica believed that a shock could cause the *tonalli*—the soul-aspect which resided in the head and journeyed in dreams or visionary experiences in animal form, like the Maya *wayob*—to depart, causing illness. To cure *susto*, a ritual may be performed wherein Cacao beans are buried or "planted" in the place where the initial shock occurred, as a form of "payment" to "distract" the evil that caused the fright.[1446] This method harks back to Cacao's mythological underworld connections, and its association with wealth. It seems the terrifying and disease-causing underworld spirits desire Cacao, so bail money is in order to secure the return of the soul-fragment.

The post-Colonial Mayan "ritual of the Bacabs" (deities of the four directions), described earlier in this chapter, was performed to cure ailments such as skin eruptions and fevers, and rounded off by administering a Cacao-based drink to the patient, such as *chacah*, a beverage made with Cacao, two chillies, honey, and tobacco juice.[1447] Cacao here combines its physical properties as a tonic and vehicle for other drugs with its magical attributes, perhaps animating ancestor-essences in the blood to assist with the ritual, helping to expel the disease-causing entity which the *ah menoob* is trance-chanting out of the patient's body. The pharmacological properties of Cacao aren't separate from its magical actions; using one to explain the other, we run the risk of annulling the mystery. Using psychoactive or medicinally active substances may be viewed as a form of spirit possession, where the consumer of the drug is temporarily taken over by the *daimon* or *deva* of the drug: consider the phrase "under the influence", referring to intoxication.

The spirit of the highly intoxicating *Datura innoxia* or *toloache* was conceived of as a young girl in one Mesoamerican legend. The story goes that she woke the king up by crying incessantly in the night; he took pity on her and invited her into the palace, but her unearthly beauty caused his five sons to quarrel, even to the point of threatening to duel each other to the death. So, like the evil queen in *Snow White*, the king ordered a servant to put her to death in the forest; but, also like the huntsman in *Snow White*, the servant couldn't do it—she was too beautiful, "like a flower after the rain", so he killed a rabbit instead to use its blood as proof that the deed was done. The girl wandered about looking for lodgings, but no one would take her in; in her anxiety her pupils dilated, and her eyes grew dark, becoming "filled with the light of fear". Eventually she saw a light at the bottom of an abyss, and ran towards it, finding a hut in which there resided a dwarf tending a garden with a marvellous flower in it. She climbed into the flower and hid, spending many nights fearfully awaiting pursuit, "without sleeping". The lovelorn princes, meanwhile, had turned into fire beetles, and came looking for her, but couldn't get near to the flower because of its "poisonous aroma". The girl hid in the flower for so long that eventually she merged with it. The girl is said to be able to leave the flower after the rains, "when the maize is green", and goes searching for her princes in the bodies of fallen fire bugs.[1448]

Photophobia or light sensitivity is a known effect of the tropane alkaloids in *D. innoxia*, as is mydriasis or pupil-dilation, which can last for days, accompanied by delirium and hallucinations, and often profound fear. The girl in the myth heads towards the underworld, and finds the plant in the garden of a dwarf-deity, a version of C'oxol or Tzitzimit, whose Old World equivalents would be the earth-spirits or dwarves known as gnomes or sylphs, similarly reputed to hoard and bestow wealth, and cause death to unwary trespassers.[1449] The myth of *toloache* describes the effects of the plant from the inside—what it feels like to be influenced by it, and what the spirit of the plant bestows on its consumers, both physically and psychologically. It's associated with archetypally female seductive power that can be dangerous to oneself and to others; with hidden things, and the ability to hide; the power of the victim; access to the underworld; and the ability to cause transformation and death, as well as to escape them.

This Animistic concept of a presiding entity, spirit, or governing personality may be applied to other altered states of mind, induced not by substances or trances but by special categories of stimulus, which were traditionally allotted deities of their own. Witness the liberal use of the phrase "intoxication" (*ihuinti*) by Mexica poets,[1450] referring to the effects of *xochicacahuatl*, war, or love, each of which had its affiliated gods or spirits. If the association of Cacao with the idea of being possessed or intoxicated seems bizarre, it's only because we're used to chocolate confectionery, which is much weaker than traditional *cachuatl*, and served without the attendant rituals and profound, placebo-enhancing theological reinforcement, or indeed the addition of other potent psychoactive substances. Besides, we live in a caffeine-steeped society, and have become numb to the miraculous effects of this class of stimulating alkaloids; more generally, we've forgotten how to *listen* for the effects of drugs and subtler influences on our moods and perceptions which are operating all the time. As Alan Watts said, the fish doesn't know water.

Alchemical chocolate

When Cacao was brought to Europe the medical establishment seized on it as a novel geriatric tonic and aphrodisiac, but a few industrious doctors were determined to explain its actions and reveal its true nature with experimental science. The enterprising Dr Stubbe detailed his alchemical experiments with Cacao in the 1662 publication of *The Indian Nectar, or … chocolate*, wherein he fractionally distilled a decoction of toasted, unshelled Cacao seeds. Old World alchemical taxonomy recognised three principal Kingdoms, the Animal, Vegetable, and Mineral, and distinguished three categories of substance: "Sulfur" was the purified vehicle of the soul or immaterial identity, "Mercury" was the receptacle for the vitalising principle, and "Salt" was the essence of the physical or material body. Sulfur was often piercing in smell and unique to the entity; Salts were less distinctive, but differed somewhat between entities, and were usually crystalline; and Mercury was usually liquid, and common to all entities in the same Kingdom. So alchemists sought to separate out these three principles in any substance, purify them, and then reunite them, to produce more powerful medicines and substances. Their motto was *solve et coagula*, "separate and reunite".[1451]

In plant alchemy, Sulfur is equivalent to the solid extract and essential oil of a plant, the Salt to its soluble mineral salts, and Mercury is ethanol ("alcohol"), the flammable solvent and preservative produced during fermentation of vegetable matter.[1452] Stubbe recounts again and again the similarity of many of his distillates of Cacao seeds to the alchemical products of human blood or flesh. His Spirits of Cacao—most likely what we would now consider an aqueous distillate or impure aromatic water—was initially white, but after a second distillation to separate out any oils, became "as red as blood … exceeding penetrative, and not unpleasant as to smell or taste, as other Spirits drawn from blood, or flesh". He also produced an "Oil" by distilling the infusion with a very hot fire, "such as I never put to any Vegetable", which was also "red as blood, but clear", and cooled to a waxy consistency—no doubt an impure cocoa butter, coloured with procyanidins.

These two extracts are both varieties of alchemical Sulfur, which was divided into Volatile and Fixed components; his "Spirits" containing more of the Volatile, and the Oil containing more of the Fixed Sulfur. The *caput mortuum* or "death's head" were the insoluble salts produced after burning the plant residue to ash and washing the ashes with distilled water, and were usually discarded, as they represented the "Salt of the Salt", the grossest parts of physical matter. Stubbe's Cacao *caput* had "no taste, [and was] exceeding light", with a smell reminiscent of "fat flesh, when boiled".[1453] Stubbe noted that his "Spirits of Cacao" soon became "turbid and sour", which indicates that he hadn't distilled it sufficiently—had he fractionated off the essential oil and evaporated the residue, this wouldn't have happened. He noted that the Oil, or un-purified Fixed Sulfur, was "exceeding piercing" in taste, and had an "inexpressible aromaticalness on the tongue; and seemed to delight and refresh the Heart, and Stomach: but with a great resemblance still of flesh".[1454]

Although these experiments seem to modern pharmacists like a child playing with a chemistry set, there was a great deal of magic in alchemy; it was inextricably bound up with theology, informed by the notions of body, soul, and spirit, and the Galenic concept of the four elements. So alchemy wasn't just the precursor of chemistry, it was (and is) its own thing, and the parts into which it divided substances were qualitative rather than elemental in the modern sense. The subjectivity of its categories and the reliance on intuition and organoleptic properties—taste, smell, and appearance—in alchemical procedures should allow us to recognise that alchemy wasn't only proto-pharmacological tinkering, but also an art. Stubbe's testimony reveals how he was struck by the "blood"—or "flesh"-like products of his efforts to dismantle Cacao, and how their quality was pleasanter than similar meaty by-products, like a more refined, elevated Vegetable facsimile of alchemical extracts from the Animal kingdom. It reminds us of the Mesoamerican comparison of Cacao with human blood and organs, and their belief that the seeds contained the same life-giving invisible properties, to the extent that they used Cacao-based beverages as a sacramental substitute for the products of human sacrifice.

Complementary chocolate

Homœopathy is a three-hundred-year-old alternative medical system with a controversial public image. It was invented by the German physician Dr Samuel Hahnemann, and is based on the principle of *similia similibus curantur*, or "like cures like". Hahnemann was an empiricist, meaning that he tried things out to see if they worked or not, and based his philosophy on real-world experience. The homœopathic system is derived from his observation that highly diluted substances (drugs, foods, minerals, animal parts, bodily fluids, or even pathological products such as pus) produced reactions in the body which cured the same set of symptoms they would produce when taken in full doses. For example, a homœopathic medicine originally made from coffee could be used to treat some forms of insomnia. Homœopaths also "succuss" their remedies at every stage of dilution, which means they vigorously shake them, as they believe this maximises the efficacy of the remedy—a process highly reminiscent of the indigenous Mesoamerican Chatino practice of whipping air into their remedies to make them sacred and place "one's intentions … into the remedy".[1455]

Homœopathy isn't herbal medicine, and is distinct from traditional medicine systems the world over in two main ways. First, homœopathy uses miniscule doses—often so small that no chemical trace of the original substance remains, in contrast to systems utilising traditional herbal drugs, which usually employ large and pharmacologically active doses, particularly in acute diseases. Hahnemann's original medicines would have contained minute, but detectable quantities of the original substance, but since then homœopathy has evolved to include more and more dilute medicines, as it holds the interesting position that the more dilute, the more potent the remedy—and the more specific its indications. Second, traditional medical systems practise allopathy, meaning "contrary cures", whereby a fever can be lowered by administering fever-reducing, Cooling remedies, whereas homœopathy may employ a remedy made from a substance which in full doses produces a fever for the same purpose.

But these are oversimplifications; traditional herbal medicine may use Hot drugs to treat a fever, by assisting the body to break a sweat and lower its own temperature; and the homœopathic system also includes remedies that have a "symptom picture" which contrast with the effects produced by a full dose of the substance they're made from. This is because the "like cures like" theory isn't applied dogmatically. Instead, the indications for administering a homœopathic preparation are created by observing the symptoms produced by that medicine in a real live group of healthy people, a process called "proving" the remedy. These people take the remedy for a period of time and note any unusual physical or emotional "reactions" in minute detail. These "reactions" then became the indications for administering that remedy. This procedure has been highly criticised by the scientific and medical communities because it prioritises uncontrolled subjectivity in small, self-selected groups of people over replicable experimental conditions.

Like magical systems in general, the objective truth of homœopathy may depend on whether the universe we inhabit is Materialist or Vitalist, or—in terms of consciousness—Physicalist or Dualist. In a Physicalist universe, it would require a whole new mechanism of medicinal action to be revealed—not an impossible proposition, but rather less promising. So homœopathy is controversial for several reasons, principally because it has more in common with magical than with scientific thinking; there is currently no known way for a substance so diluted that no trace of it remains to produce any biological effects, and the process of "proving" isn't "blinded"—in other words all the people taking the remedy know what the remedy was made from, and this knowledge may affect the things they experience when taking it.

Nevertheless many people experience subjective benefit from taking homœopathic remedies. It is, essentially, an esoteric system, which often performs poorly in one-size-fits-all clinical trials and has no discernible pharmacological mechanism, which has led some people who call themselves rational to describe it as a pseudo-science. That's rather unfair; it would be equally logical to call science pseudo-magic, for its failure to capitalise on the great power of meaning and ritual revealed by first-hand experience or study of shamanism, traditional medicine, and contemporary scientific investigations into the tip of the "placebo effect" iceberg.

Discussing the classification and uses of chocolate in homœopathy reveals some of the meanings attached to the substance, if nothing else. Believers may conclude that the "proving" of *chocolatum* reveals essential truths about chocolate, while Materialist sceptics can still infer some of the cultural preconceptions or subconscious notions which have accreted around chocolate, at least in a small group of homœopaths. Admittedly, that's a less impressive proposition than the possibility of discerning a grand narrative like the "personality" or spirit of chocolate, but in both cases the cultural identity of chocolate informs—or is revealed by—the resulting testimonies, at least to some extent. The remedy was first prepared in 1989, made from a tincture (a water and ethanol extract) of "best quality Belgian dark chocolate",[1456] diluted to 3c, which means one drop was added to a hundred drops of water, then one drop of that was added to another hundred drops of water, and a drop of *that* was added to a hundred more drops of water, producing a dilution of more than 10^{-6}. This solution was then further diluted to produce higher "potencies" (dilutions), many of which exceed the Avogadro constant, the level beyond which there is no detectable molecular trace of the original substance.

The decision was made to turn confectioner's chocolate into a remedy rather than Cacao because processed chocolate is the substance that's craved, and more commonly used in the Old World societies where homœopathy is practised (although homœopathy also has a growing following in other countries such as India). A group of eight female and four male provers took part, who noted the following "reactions":

- Irritability with loved ones, and the world in general, with a tendency to swear, and a desire to flee from and abandon one's nearest and dearest
- Difficulty connecting with people, with feelings of isolation and vulnerability, more able to live alone
- A strong desire to hide, with a feeling of "not belonging", yet—paradoxically—feeling better in company
- Many anxieties, some paranoia, as if being watched or observed, with health fears
- Changeable and extreme emotional highs and lows
- A need to see the horizon, with a desire for freedom, and sometimes dreams of flying
- A feeling of lack of nurture, particularly in infancy—sometimes accompanied by breast sensitivity, food cravings, or weight issues
- A strong, urgent need to tell the truth, with confidence in one's own opinions, and feeling more able to communicate at a deeper level
- Feeling as if they have been lied to and deceived, with a need to react against that
- Congestive headache
- Tiredness and restlessness, with difficult sleep
- Strong awareness of the heartbeat (almost palpitations)
- Difficulty getting and staying warm
- High and low energy on alternating days, with all symptoms strongly aggravated in the evening
- And, a strong desire for short and bristly hair, either one's own or with the impulse to touch other people's hair or beards.[1457]

The provers considered that *chocolatum* exhibited many features of "the drug remedies", uniquely combining the restlessness and sensitivity associated with homœopathic preparations of stimulants such as cocaine with the feelings of isolation, dullness, and floating that were more typical of remedies made from narcotics such as morphine. This correlates with the anecdotal observations and lab work described in Chapter 5, which suggested that Cacao may augment the effects of both monoamine (stimulant) and endorphin (opiate) brain chemicals, and drugs which activate these pathways. By far the majority of physical sensations experienced with the remedy were in the head. Hun Hunahpu would have understood.

Many of the issues which came up in the proving could be linked to some of the sociological findings described in Chapters 5 and 7: the higher neuroticism of self-confessed chocoholics, for example, with their tendency to irritability and rejection sensitivity (hysteroid dysphoria), as well as the use of chocolate by elderly persons, more happily correlated with lower levels of social isolation. I hypothesised that Cacao may modify the circuitry of attraction in the brain, specifically accelerating Infatuation and possibly modifying Bonding in social and sexual relationships; and that Cacao may benefit certain people such as those with PTSD, but on the negative side may also enhance compulsive behaviours or addictions in subjects with susceptible brain chemistry, such as people who have experienced a lack of well-bonded or stable caregiving relationships in infancy. In this regard, some of the results of the proving are particularly striking—feelings of isolation, difficulty connecting, and problems with nurture, as well as irritability with loved ones are all issues which may be encountered with a history of insecure or unpredictable caregiver relationships. Also, it does look like the provers have written a personality profile of me. Although that could just be paranoia.

Homœopaths regard *chocolatum* as a key remedy for "sex hormone imbalances" in women, specifically those which give rise to emotional issues, and note that many patients appear to be "seriously addicted to [chocolate]". They compare it to two other remedies with similar indications: *Sepia*, made from cuttlefish ink, used for more delicate constitutions who are drawn to dance, are sexually excitable or excessive, and often experience despair, with feelings of domination or dependency; and *Lachesis*, made from snake venom, linked to jealous, sexually powerful, competitive, but slightly "poisonous" personality types, the *femme fatale* of the repertory.[1458] The strong awareness of the heartbeat coupled with loneliness experienced by the provers of *chocolatum* also correlates with the public use of chocolate as the "heartache food" or Valentine's Day gift, as much as it does with the Mesoamerican association of Cacao with heart extraction. Being a prisoner of war given a final drink of *cacahuatl* before lying back on the *chacmool* to have one's heart cut out must have been a lonely experience; some people in that scenario may have wanted to swear, or felt a bit concerned about their health.

The provers' perception of increased desire to tell the truth, feeling confident in their opinions, and the facilitation of deeper communication reminds us of Cacao's traditional associations with courage, removal of fear, and communing with ancestors. The compulsion towards short hair and bristly beards experienced by the provers, unless merely a quirk of all twelve participants—it's recorded as a "characteristic peculiarity of the remedy"—seems oddly anomalous. It may perhaps represent a childlike fascination with adult stubble, a vague, semi-eroticised desire for protection or comfort such as may be sought from sweet, milky foods like chocolate. Curiously, Quetzalocatl was the only Mexica deity explicitly described as "bearded" by Sahagún's native informants.[1459]

Chocolate has also been linked to the heart in traditional Chinese medicine (TCM), where it's named *qiaokeli*—a phonetic rendering of "chocolate" with Mandarin pronunciation. The traditional Chinese medical system is analogous to the Galenic-humoral system outlined in Chapter 3, only with a different structure (five elements, not four; *chi*, not *pneuma*, and many other variables). Like the Galenic system, its postulates may be physiologically inaccurate in terms of anatomy and pathophysiology—there is no literal organ called the "triple burner", for example—but as an empirical medical system which records, observes, and adjusts patterns of symptoms and physiological reactions it is exceptionally subtle and precise. *Qioakeli* is said to enter the Heart, Liver, and Kidney meridians,[1460] which broadly means it influences emotional balance and appropriate action (Heart), digestive function, self-respect, and bodily repair and maintenance (Liver), and fluid balance and ageing (Kidneys). The translations of the Chinese so-called "organs" are misleading, as they really refer to groups of *functions* which we may ascribe to several physiological organs, including quite separate ones; many of the processes ascribed to the Heart, for example, are clearly mediated by the brain and central nervous system, but are described as residing in the Heart because the clearest physical symptoms are often felt in that region of the body (palpitations, physiological awareness of emotional states).

Qiaokeli is classified as a substance which tonifies the Heart and Kidney Yang. "Tonifying the Heart" means it assists "consciousness, intention, volition, thought, reflection and self-awareness",[1461] and may remediate Heart disturbances such as situational anxiety, inappropriate responses, palpitations, and insomnia. In TCM, the heart is the repository of *shen*, or Spirit, defined as

> the domain of human life that defies the limitations of time and space. It is the human capacity for relationships that are not restricted by physical or temporal contact. [...] Spirit allows a person to worship an ancestor [...] Spirit recognizes and pursues ultimate goals such as "self-transformation", [...] Spirit is felt whenever human consciousness forges compelling bonds and special relationships. Spirit is invoked by imagination, intention, awe, enchantment, and wonder. (Kaptchuk, 2000)

Tonifying the Kidney Yang means that *Qiaokeli* also replenishes the ability of the Kidneys—which functionally include the actual kidneys, the thyroid gland, the adrenals, and the hypothalamus, the part of the brain which regulates hormonal functions—to energise the body and prevent collapse. From Bensky and Gamble's *Chinese Herbal Medicine Materia Medica*:

> From a modern biomedical standpoint, the pathophysiology of deficient Kidney Yang is exceedingly complex and is far from being completely understood. Based on clinical observations and experimental results, one part of its aetiology seems to be related to disorders of the endocrine system. Patients with decreased Kidney Yang very often have decrease in plasma thyroid hormone-binding proteins, 24-hour urinary 17-ketosteroids, and rate of glycolysis. When treated with herbs that tonify the Kidney Yang, these measurements can increase into the normal ranges [...] In general, it is thought that from a biomedical standpoint the functions of this class of herbs include:
>
> • Regulation of the functions of the adrenal cortex
> • Regulation of energy metabolism
> • Promotion of sexual functions
> • Promotion of growth
> • Strengthening of resistance. (Bensky & Gamble, 1993)

As research into Cacao and chocolate have shown, several of these functions appear to be borne out in the case of *qiaokeli*—Cacao lowers plasma levels of adrenaline and cortisol, may reduce symptoms of chronic fatigue syndrome over several weeks, alters the microbiome so as to affect metabolism, and appears to have complex effects on the immune system—in addition to its traditional reputation as an aphrodisiac, which remains unproven but is supported by anecdotal and pharmacological testimonies (see Chapters 4 and 5 and the Cacao monograph in Appendix A for full details).

Chocolate may also be recommended in TCM to assist recuperation after long illness, to lower blood pressure, to "move blood" (assist circulation), and to slow down aging, although as a very Western foodstuff it's doubtful that many classical Chinese medicine practitioners actually prescribe it. But these indications are supported by scientific evidence (Chapter 4) and by Cacao's traditional use as a tonic, particularly suitable for older people. It's also indicated in TCM for clearing phlegm from the chest, for lowering fevers with colds, and for helping recover appetite. This dovetails nicely with the Mesoamerican and Galenic classification of Cacao as a Cooling, fattening remedy which is useful in fevers, and was particularly recommended for use in chronic lung ailments (Chapter 3). Cacao's use as a Heart tonic also highlights the overlap between the metaphorical Heart as the seat of the emotions, which stores *shen* in TCM and the Vital Spirits in Galenic medicine, and the physiological heart: Cacao appears to benefit both. Another interesting side-note: like other psychostimulants, MDMA or ecstasy is said to deplete the heart's *shen*,[1462] and Cacao may support or help to restore it. This is noteworthy, given the craving for chocolate recorded in a small sample of former regular MDMA users within a year of giving up, and the parallels between some of the subjective and objective effects of MDMA and Cacao ingestion described in Chapter 5.

So the remedy picture for homœopathic *chocolatum* has an affinity with venomous serpents and the defensive excrescence of frightened sea creatures, with drugs, neuroticism, and an enhanced sense of personal mission. The desire for freedom and dreams of flying experienced by the test group are also said to be typical of the "bird remedies" in homœopathy. It's as if the myths were extruding into the provers' unconscious, so that even with a ballast of sugar and fat, the feathered serpent Quetzalcoatl came flying out of the watery underworld on a truth-telling quest to elevate mankind, bearing his stolen gift that ultimately resulted in public disgrace, and its attendant sorrows. TCM's classification of chocolate also fits neatly with the Mesoamerican symbolic association of Cacao with the heart and the blood; *Qiaokeli* as a Heart and Kidney Yang tonic corresponds with the Mesoamerican use of Cacao as a bravery-enhancing and vitalising substance that amplifies spiritual force and power. Many of the symptoms experienced by the provers of *chocolatum* would be classified by TCM practitioners as "Heart Blood deficiency", or "Heart and Kidney Yang deficiency".[1463] Whether or not you have any faith in these therapeutic systems, their classification of chocolate apparently endorses many of the traditional medicinal and metaphysical affiliations of Cacao—and does so in the absence of any direct transmission of the indigenous Mesoamerican myths and uses of the plant.

Cacao culture

When a cohort of more than 300 undergraduates at New York's Hofstra University were asked for their opinions about chocolate in the 1990s, 91% said "sweet". "Attractive" slightly out-weighed "addictive" at 75% and 70%, respectively, but "heavy" topped "happy" at 57% and 56%. A third of the students believed chocolate to be "harmful". More women than men took part, and more women reported liking chocolate; the chocolate-consumers went on more diets, ate more junk food, and smoked more.[1464] The preponderance of females may be partly cultural, given the findings described in Chapter 5 that men showed a stronger desire for chocolate in the Addiction Research Center survey, but as described in Chapter 7, women's pre-menstrual cravings for chocolate appear to be culturally determined. Similarly, there's no reason to assume that the "feminine" image of chocolate in Europe—hearts, flowers, and all—wouldn't skew the responses, although the Mesoamerican personification of Cacao as a female deity, and its association with pregnancy, breastfeeding and fertility suggests there may be a deeper historical connection with female sexuality.

The survey results are exactly what one might expect from the hypothesis advanced in Chapters 5 and 7 that Cacao is a hedonic modifier which has the potential to reinforce either good or bad habits in a state-dependent or situation-dependent manner. But there's no saying what type of "chocolate" was being consumed by the students—as the rat experiment in Chapter 7 showed, chocolate *flavour* may dramatically enhance the reward response following consumption of sugary junk food. But a survey of sixty-five psychology students at Villanova University in Philadelphia found that most chocolate-consumers identified as more self-reliant, believing that success comes with personal effort, and isn't dependent on fate.[1465] This seems out of step with the finding described in Chapter 5 that self-identified chocolate-eaters may be more neurotic, but while susceptibility to negative emotion and an internal locus of control may not vary independently, they aren't the same thing. More to the point, both survey groups were self-selected from a specific demographic, a relatively narrow age range of university attendees—which suggests that these student samples may not be representative of Joe Public. But taking both these findings at face value, a tentative conclusion may be that chocolate is favoured by those who seek to master their internal terrain; the self-medicating neurotic and the non-determinist chocophile may share an inclination to augment their locus of control.

In the twentieth-century Russian novel *Chocolate* by Tarasov-Rodianov, a reformed prostitute bribes the chief of the military police's family with chocolate taken from a former lover, then uses this knowledge to take him down with her when she is arrested.[1466] Shades of homœopathic *Lachesis*, or Aquiauhtzin's vengeful seductress with her skirt and blouse of prickly fruit (see Chapter 9). Cacao's mythic function as a magnet for envy, vengeance, and downfall brought about by treachery is a perceptible story arc in many traditional legends; arguably, too, in the historical fate of the Mexica empire at the hands of the Spanish and their native collaborators. But in Europe, Cacao's affiliation with femininity and female sexuality has been emphasised since the twentieth century. Even though Spanish colonists noted the enthusiasm with which women took to drinking chocolate, men also drank chocolate in the courts, stately homes, and coffeehouses of Europe throughout the seventeenth and eighteenth centuries. The Meosamerican correlation of Cacao with courtship, with the formal gifting of Cacao beans to new brides, and drinking chocolate at engagement ceremonies and weddings has been diffused, amplified, and effeminised in the Old World by the marketing of chocolate confectionery as a romantic gift:

> Chocolate symbolised the impending breaking down of sexual resistance ... a woman could re-enact Eve's role by tempting [a man] with just one or two out of her own box, or ... by offering a discreet after-dinner mint that does not threaten his masculinity with any suggestion of need, want, or unseemly desire ... As the [box] designs suggest, chocolates are associated with flowers ... flowers also symbolise the female ... both put on a colourful show to attract fertilization. (Barthel-Bouchier, in Szogyi, 1997; © Hofstra University, New York)

Here, chocolate is the domain of the Old World Venus, but the association of woman with chocolate and the Biblical Eve is revealing—like Xquic' in the Hero Twins saga, Eve plucked her father's forbidden fruit from a magical tree and was expelled from her domain. Flowery Cacao has been transformed from a theocratic sacrament into a weapon of seduction, but the same archetypal mycelium nourishes the roots of Cacao's identity in both Old and New World cultures.

In the 1908 operetta *The Chocolate Soldier*, Oscar Straus's version of George Bernard Shaw's play *Arms and the Man*, two characters sing a duet to a moulded chocolate soldier on the stage:

> Oh you little chocolate soldier man,
> You're far too sweet and pretty,
> Oh you funny chocolate soldier man,
> For you I feel great pity.
> Oh you silly chocolate soldier man
> Just made to please young misses,
> So sweet you'd melt, if e'er you felt
> A full grown maiden's kisses.

(Straus, quoted by Kaler, in Szogyi, 1997.
© Josef Weinberger Limited, London. Reprinted by permission)

These lines are reminiscent of Aquiauhtzin's female character simultaneously seducing and belittling the warrior-king Axayacatl, but here chocolate is used to symbolise immaturity, ineffectuality, and the orgasmic neutralisation of Mars by Venus, like the Botticelli painting where Mars sprawls unconscious while Venus sits upright, wide awake and serene, and satyric cupids play with Mars's war-gear. With the addition of milk and sugar, Cacao has done a 180 from its Mesoamerican role as the soldier-fortifier and become emasculating, symbolising the triumph of female sensuality over masculine will. But chocolate is still cast as a soldier; and in the original play, it's chocolate stolen from a boudoir which allows the starving trooper Bluntschli to survive. Bitter *cacahuatl*'s mutation into sweet chocolate enhanced its feminine associations, but the ancient correlation of Cacao with soldiery, the "flowers" of youth and the altered states induced by love and war are preserved in the inversion.

The apogee—or nadir—of Cacao's Old World association with sexuality is surely found in the eighteenth-century stories of the chocophilic Marquis de Sade, who famously wrote a letter to his wife from a prison cell in the Bastille requesting that she bring him a cake "as black inside from chocolate as the devil's ass is black from smoke".[1467] De Sade noted the coprophagic symbolism of chocolate, declaring that chocolate was an appropriately "abundant, delicate, soft food"[1468] to fatten participants for gory, feculent orgies. De Sade wasn't the only person to have made the connection between chocolate and excrement; he just liked his characters to play with their food. Twentieth-century author Dale Pendell noted that *Theobroma cacao* belongs to the *Sterculiaceae* plant family, named after Sterculius, the Roman god of manure,[1469] and there is a theory (mentioned in Chapter 1) that the name "chocolate" was adopted instead of *cacahuatl* because, de Sade apart, drinking a brown liquid called *caca*-anything may not have gone down so well in Europe. But two contemporary Mexican *atoles* made with Cacao have scatologically adjacent names: *popo* and *bu'pu*—amusingly close to *pupú*, an infantile Spanish colloquialism for faeces, like poo-poo in English. It shouldn't be a surprise that Cacao retains etymological ties to the underworld: manure is just fertiliser, after all, and the god of death produces the most fragrant flowers.

Tristan Tzara's scathing quote from the Dada manifesto at the top of this chapter affiliates chocolate with stultifying conventional values: "Morality infuses chocolate into every man's veins." For Tzara, chocolate represents vacuous virtue-signalling that dulls sensibilities and perverts right action. Here we see an echo of the Mexica anxiety over Cacao's potentially enervating effects as a luxurious substance which may induce decadence; but, unlike the Mexica and their fatalistic preoccupations, there are no intimations of hubris with Tzara's critique. Twentieth-century chocolate has been transmuted into a low-grade dependency so that, for Tzara at least, it becomes synonymous with defective purpose. Cacao is once more a state-sanctioned drug, but this time around it's not a sacred drink empowering a grand narrative of sacrifice, but an item of confectionery acting as a budget anaesthetic for the soul. In either scenario, it could be said that Cacao is an agent of imperialism. In Mesoamerica, bitter Cacao beverages were a sacrament consumed by warriors after battle, couples before marriage, and sacrificial victims before death; in the twentieth century, sweet chocolate became a daily reward, a rationed treat in two world wars, a palliative coating on the break-time biscuits of office workers everywhere.

Europe absorbed the foods and substances of the Americas into Old World culture like a hungry amoeba, profaning and destroying local rituals and traditions in the process. The *devas* of tobacco (*Nicotiana tabacum*) and coca (*Erythroxylum coca*) have exacted their retribution for such sacrilege through the agency of their alkaloids, nicotine and cocaine. It may be said that the pillaging of the conquistadors and early European settlers who enslaved, abused, and decimated the native population of the Americas has been paid back in kind over several generations through the agency of their sacred plants. Looked at in the clear light of history, the various tobacco-associated health problems and cocaine or crack addiction are simply consequences of our distribution of these drugs, our competitive and expansionist cultures, and the growing number of disaffected people who have the financial means and leisure time to perpetrate self-destructive addictions. But contemplated in the torch-lit twilight of magical thinking, these scourges are the chemical warfare of angry spirits: two sides of the same coin, perhaps.

Cacao, by contrast, appears to be entirely benign; but as the myths show, Cacao's *leitmotif* is survival through death and rebirth. The history of civilisations closely associated with Cacao in any form suggests that the drug has an affinity for hierarchical and fatalistic social structures and conditions. Cacao was the lifeblood of commerce in Mesoamerica, literally being used as currency, and contemporary chocolate is big business. Like many psychoactive drugs (such as tea, opium, or coca leaves), Cacao's pleasures have always been paid for by conquest and drudgery, but for the most part it has had a consistently socially acceptable and glamorous image, tainted only with accusations of decadence or indulgence (which, if anything, add to chocolate's popular appeal). Cacao's predominantly benign—or, at most, softcore controversial—public relations is at odds with the stark discrepancy between impoverished farmers and affluent consumers which has been a consistent theme in the history of *Theobroma cacao*'s interactions with *Homo sapiens*.

At the turn of the twenty-first century, a shocking documentary aired on the UK's Channel 4 television network exposed the child slavery and abuse inherent in the international cocoa trade, particularly on the Ivory Coast of West Africa, where 90% of plantations used slave labour; the researchers estimated that 40% of the world's chocolate was "contaminated by slavery". Slaves were malnourished, physically and psychologically intimidated, and viciously beaten if they tried to run away. One boy interviewed on a plantation said, "Tell them, when they are eating chocolate, they are eating my flesh."[1470] *Theobroma cacao*'s partnership with humankind isn't always symbiotic; it seems to have an affinity for inequity, though perhaps it's unfair to blame the plant for the way we humans organise ourselves around it.

From an Animist perspective, the god of Cacao appears to be loyal to power, and, cat-like, will reward those who feed it, on its own terms. If aliens invaded the Earth tomorrow and took the population hostage, a new Cacao-based product would probably become a valued part of their culture within a few decades; or perhaps the aliens, having a different awareness of consciousness, would take a few Cacao trees and other valued plants with them to learn from and ignore the upright monkeys, leaving baffled *Homo sapiens* to indignantly protest their superior cortical development.

For the Mexica, it was taboo for women and children to consume Cacao. Now, chocolate has become women's favourite sweet, and is widely eaten by children. But Cacao is still associated with the resurrection of a deity, being sold as the Easter drug for kids: the festival of Jesus Christ's resurrection is commercially commemorated with an egg made of chocolate. The pagan custom of exchanging painted eggs after the spring equinox, symbolising new life, was annexed to Easter. Chocolate eggs became popular in the nineteenth century, and have remained so. These eggs are typically made with Cacao and maternal bovine secretions, combining an ancestor-summoning resurrection-drug with the fattening, soporific milk produced by a mother cow for a baby that has been stolen at birth in order to usurp her milk supply. They are bizarre, unlikely gifts, but seen from the perspective of Cacao's mythological history, this is less true. Even wearing its new guise as chocolate, Cacao naturally ends up signifying new life emerging from death, as an egg—a hard-shelled birthing pod, the type from which snakes or birds hatch. Cacao, the feathered serpent's gift to humankind, the Hero Twins reborn, in the form of little hollow mountains filled with tasty treasure.

The infantile and mammary symbolism of adults consuming sweetened milk products shouldn't be overlooked. One contemporary theory proposes that preferences for sweet or salty tastes are linked to different personality types. "Salties" are allegedly energetic, assertive, dynamic, decisive, self-confident, and honest, whereas "sweets" apparently look for protection, and are introverted, self-absorbed, and conciliatory.[1471] If this is true, the increasing tendency to sweeten foods, knowing that added sugars are habituating, may parallel a societal trend towards greater solipsism, dependency, narcissism, and enforcement of normative social values (groupthink).

But Cacao and chocolate can also be associated with social conscience and virtuous enterprise. John Cadbury, a Quaker, established his chocolate manufacturing company in the UK in 1824, and as the company expanded his sons George and Richard Cadbury built Bournville, an "ethical factory" outside the city centre in pleasant rural surroundings, with excellent amenities and accommodation for its workers, including detached houses with their own gardens.[1472] As Quakers, the Cadburys were teetotallers, and regarded chocolate and cocoa as a superior substitute for alcohol;[1473] their religious beliefs informed their ethics, and morning prayers for the whole workforce were held at the factory for many years. The wholesomeness of their vision and of their perception of Cacao informed the results of their enterprise. As ever, Cacao was bound into a hierarchical belief system which endorsed expansion and effort in return for pleasure, but the sacrifices demanded were in labour and dedication, not human blood and suffering. The Cadburys' chocolate business came together successfully because they were guided by a set of shared principles and a coherent family identity that they expanded on to create a community.

* * *

As Krishnamurti wrote, "It is no measure of health to be well adjusted to a profoundly sick society."[1474] Is modern society sick? On the "no" side, many human populations live longer, have more material wealth, and a lower percentage of infant mortality than ever before. On the "yes" side, global inequity is greater than ever, wars are more destructive and potentially geno- cidal, the average human lifespan still doesn't far exceed the Biblical "three score years and ten", and the negative environmental impact of humanity on the planet threatens our species' survival and that of many others. Despite the rise of globalism, a paradoxical feeling of "dis- integration" is pervasive.

Assisting *integration* may be the optimal response to our carcinogenic culture of greed, solip- sism, and endless growth. But this can't come at the expense of stifling individuality through compulsory adherence to dogma, or reducing the problem to small, controllable, atomised parts. Religion, that ancient provider of meaning and social coherence, can become a monstrous dragon when leashed to humanity's unconscious fears, as the horrific scale of human sacrifice in Mesoamerica shows, or for that matter the tendency of healthy human beings infected with sick doctrines to commit acts of terrorism or war. Fundamentalism constitutes an abdication of personal responsibility, by eliminating the "anxiety of doubt".[1475]

But post-Enlightenment creeds also have their own share of pathology: prominent atheist critics of religion conveniently forget that the greatest acts of state-sanctioned mass murder have occurred in societies where religion was disapproved of or outlawed, and were justified on the basis of entirely secular ideologies. In the absence of religious faith there is a desperate and dangerously unconsciously-directed search for solutions, a polarization of secular ideolo- gies and political movements, as religious drives—lacking a philosophical outlet—get siphoned into political allegiances, to incendiary effect. Nietzsche, the philosopher-genius who famously wrote "that which does not kill us, makes us stronger" (which is demonstrably false; Nietzsche himself had a catastrophic mental breakdown at the age of forty-four from which he never recovered), predicted this state of affairs—the "death of God" producing increasing nihilism.

The solution requires a multi-level holistic approach. If the Mesoamericans used Cacao to help catalyse change in accordance with the will, then perhaps it can play a part. As a tree of the underworld, Cacao was intimately connected to the blood, the ancestors, and the poten- tial to receive ancestral guidance. The mythology and pharmacology of Cacao indicate that it may help to bring dreams (or nightmares) into reality—either as a Materialist's crutch, or as a Vitalist's magic potion. Consciousness is key: if the Physicalists are correct, then all the myths and ritual uses of Cacao reflect the values and mores of the societies which produce and con- sume it; but if the Idealists or the Substance Dualists or the Panpsychists are correct, the myths may reveal underlying truths about Cacao, its secret life, and its purpose. In any case, Cacao's history suggests that as a remedy for heartache, this drug may assist societies to tolerate—or endorse—the intolerable.

Quetzalacoatl is the logical Mexica patron of foamy *cacahuatl*, a mixture of air and water with a rainbow serpent in every bubble. Quetzalcoatl was also a patron of Mexica priests, those arbiters of magical technologies such as the ritual calendar, divinatory techniques, and deific magic. Cacao's exalted status in Mesoamerica may depend on its integral role at all levels of Mesoamerican ritual: as a substance which can provide pleasure, augment the effects of entheogens, and provide a measure of protection against snakebite, Cacao was a worthy addition to the Mesoamerican pharmacopoeia. Cacao's particular value may have resided in an ability to enhance the efficacy of "immersive" divinatory and magical techniques such as listening to the "lightning in the blood", dream travel, or the visionary "ecstatic voyage". This conclusion be inferred from Cacao's regular use as an oblation, its underworld affiliation, and its connection with the living blood of sacrifice, the heart and the ancestors; it has some measure of corroboration in Cacao's vivifying, fear-allaying, monoamine-modifying potentials; and it is endorsed by Cacao's consistent mythological association with transformation and resurrection.

Even after the conquest of Mexico, chocolate's medicinal and cultural associations in the Old World reveal the underlying influence of the Mesoamerican myths. Cacao continued to be associated with protection and dangerous knowledge: the tree that sheltered Jesus was also a stand-in for the Biblical forbidden fruit. An early alchemical experiment declared Cacao's essential similarity to flesh and blood. Confectioner's chocolate became a repository for female sexual power, enticing but potentially emasculating—like the male captive given Cacao-pod breasts, to "impregnate" the ritual through his death. As if possessed by Quetzalcoatl, *chocolatum*'s homœopathic provers dreamt of flying, felt deceived or lied to, and were attracted to beards, and noted its similarity to a remedy made from Bushmaster (*Lachesis*) venom, one of the most poisonous snakes native to Central America. Traditional Chinese medicine classes *qiaokeli* as a remedy to tonify the Heart Yang, augmenting consciousness and intention. Meanwhile Cacao's involvement with slavery continued unabated through the industrial revolution, merely changing its form and location. And chocolate has become alloyed to two popular festivals: commemorating sexual pair-bonding with edible hearts on Valentine's day, and ostensibly celebrating the resurrection with a pagan egg at Easter.

There are worse spirits to trade one's soul with than Cacao, a substance which belongs to the dark side of Venus. Cacao's intoxicating effect, which was so clear to the Mesoamericans, isn't recognised as such in our sybaritically saturated culture. To be under the influence of Cacao is to feel temporarily more contented and competent, but greasing the wheels of pleasure in a person or culture with no firm bedrock of familial and social ties can inadvertently exacerbate melancholy by intensifying the awareness of how transient and fleeting mortal joys are. The societies which held it in the highest regard have been the wealthiest and most successful within the bounds of their known worlds, but such empires cast long shadows: acquisitive expansion, oppression, enslavement, perpetual border warfare, and escalating structural unsustainability precede their inevitable collapse.

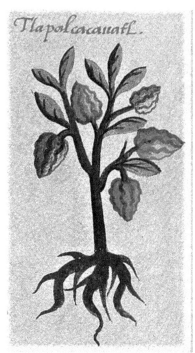

Cacahuatl drawing from
Codex Badianus.

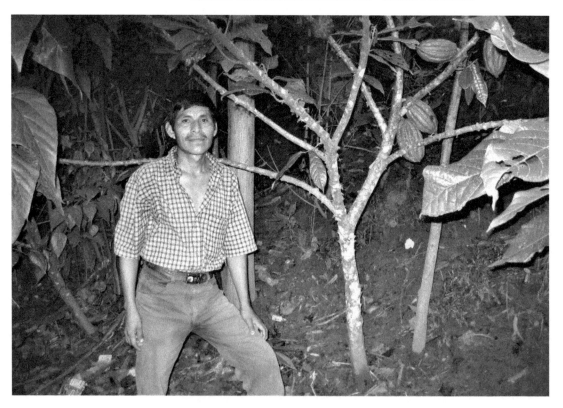

Don Juan Francisco of APROCAV with one of his grafted Cacao trees, Lanquin, ALta Verapaz,
Guatemala.

Conclusion

"Hearts live by being wounded. Pleasure may turn a heart to stone, riches may make it callous, but sorrow—oh, sorrow cannot break it."

(Oscar Wilde, *A Woman of No Importance*, 1893)

Toma chocolate, paga lo que debes.
(Drink your chocolate, pay what you owe.)

(Cuban proverb, from Grivetti & Shapiro, 2009)

Every drug is a doorway. Where it leads depends not only on the drug, but on the disposition of the person receiving it, the context in which it is taken or administered, and the attitudes or intentions of those who control it. This book has told the story of the premodern development and use of *Theobroma cacao* seeds as a drug, and built a case from historical, pharmacological, and mythological perspectives that they are entheogenic: a word which ethnopharmacologist Jonathan Ott defined as meaning

"realizing the divine within", the term used by the ancient Greeks to determine states of poetic or prophetic inspiration, to describe the entheogenic state which can be induced by sacred plant drugs. (Ott, 1996)[1476]

It may seem strange to class Cacao alongside powerful mind-altering organisms such as *Psilocybe* mushrooms, *peyote*, or tropane-alkaloid-containing botanicals such as *Datura* species, but Cacao's historical uses in ritual and ceremony, the tree's mythic association with death and rebirth, and the pharmacology of the seeds all suggest that Cacao is a subtle modifier of consciousness and perception. It's possibly more accurate to call Cacao a proto-entheogen, or an entheogen-enabler, as the evidence presented in Chapter 5 shows that it may act as a poly-drug potentiator, and an amplifier of intention.

A central hypothesis of this book is that Cacao is a *hedonic modifier*, and an *anti-phobic*, stress-modulating agent which facilitates and stabilises positive changes in mood and perception. But as with any psychoactive substance, its widespread consumption may be expected to both reflect and affect the cultures which consume it, and not all those interactions need be for the good. As Dale Pendell wrote in his wonderful chapter on chocolate,

> If we accept the world as a playground, sometimes a battlefield, of poisons [psychoactive substances], history becomes a story of shamanic alliance and conflict, a story of magic spells and their dissolution by new spells. We can say that all governments are in the business of enchantment, to keep the sacrificial victims from rising up and overthrowing those who sacrifice and eat them.[1477]

Class cannibalism isn't generally regarded as desirable (unless you're a Marxist who takes the slogan "eat the rich" at face value), but it's possible that Cacao may amplify the desire nature, which in imbalanced persons or societies—those who have a dearth of stable Bonding in their individual or cultural background—could aggravate habits of destructive consumption. On a personal level, this could just be an increased proclivity to gorge on chocolate-flavoured junk food; but on a societal level, there may be an association with affluenza, an obsession with material possessions. This expansionism may arguably be seen in ancient Mesoamerican societies and our own, although a case may be made that this is simply a sign of cultural dominance and success, with which Cacao has always been associated. The word "spoil" springs to mind: to the victor the spoils, you're spoiling us with these chocolates, a spoilt child.

But Cacao's pre-Colombian patrons Quetzalcoatl and K'awil were benefactor-gods, and, similarly, Cacao has been identified with Christ in Central America. Chocolate consumption seems to be predominantly associated with beneficial epidemiological and social outcomes such as significantly reduced risk of heart attack or stroke, more well-adjusted elderly people, and happier babies, so this "spoiling" may be imaginary—or simply displaced onto impoverished workers in distant lands, toiling to grow Cacao for the international market. Just like Cacao's effect on mood, its interactions with individuals and cultures may be partially state- and intention-dependent: the health-conscious person may benefit from good quality chocolate, but the binge-eater may eat even more if the biscuits are flavoured with cocoa. As the Cadbury family demonstrated, the business of chocolate need not be intemperate or unethical.

It makes sense that K'awil was a "god of spiritual force in material objects",[1478] because Cacao's venerated status in Mesoamerica may have depended on precisely this property: its embodiment of spiritual power, enhancing processes of self-transformation and manifestation. Metaphysically, Cacao was used to augment magical and ritual action, and to communicate with the ancestors. How different from the sticky-fingered, compulsive consumer of cake, biscuits, truffles, and confections: the palliative "chocolate" of today, the mass-market methadone of a purpose-starved society. Contemporary Cacao is so heavily sugared that the real thing tastes too complex, too bitter, too sour; like mortality, like hard work, like responsibility. But this is slander: surely chocolate's current identity is a more suitably sweetened persona for a modern age, where "ancestral responsibilities" such as ritual murder and theocratic magic are, thankfully, things of the past?

Cacao still sings its flowery song in the blood of those individuals and societies who consume it, but we live in such a stimulant-saturated world that its heady "intoxication" could almost be missed, even if it weren't attenuated and transformed and bound to that other magical slave-farming substance, sugar. As it is, we see evidence of its nature in the scientific literature, such as the effects on the heart, the blood. We may perceive its cultural associations, as a "treat" and

a pleasure, rarely consumed by those who toil at the base of an economic hierarchy to produce it, where the revenue streams run mostly uphill. Canvassing opinions from its devotees,
the self-identified "chocoholics", we find that it is a guilty pleasure, highly regarded for mood
adjustment, yet oddly strongly correlated with depression; consumed by the privileged and
well-adjusted, yet regarded as an addiction by the neurotic.

If Cacao had a motto, it would be "every pleasure has its price". Buy a chocolate bar, indulge
yourself, you're worth it; the slave child starves in Africa, the waistline expands. When one
speaks of "the heart's desire", Cacao may be used to assuage its absence or, perhaps, to attain it;
Cacao mitigates fears and soothes the heart, so the ills of old age and the terrors of death may be
staved off and reduced, but the nature of any drug used to palliate existential angst is the danger
that the issues underlying the troublesome appetites and anxieties it allays remain unassuaged.
Cacao's nature seems to be truly benign, but if the myths have any truth then the spirit of
Cacao will benefit only those who are willing to visit the underworld; as a desirable substance,
it speaks to unvoiced emotional, survival-level cravings for appreciation, for safety, for dominance. If our hungers and horrors are unacknowledged, Cacao may assist us to displace them,
by projecting them onto the world, and the "other". Like the venus-gods of Mesoamerica, Cacao
represents not Rousseauian, chocolate-box love, but "flowery war": it demands sacrifice; and,
as the myths show, true rewards only follow when the hero or heroine is prepared to sacrifice
themselves.

* * *

The history of human belief systems can be imagined as a long road from Vitalist animism to
Materialist atheism. The immersive shamanic and magical beliefs of ancient cultures, which
have survived for millennia in challenging environments such as the Amazon jungle or the
wilds of Siberia, mutated with agriculture into the more ornate and abstracted forms of religion:
people didn't speak with and see the gods anymore, and the ineffable became increasingly
tied up with the hierarchies of state, rather than curated by esteemed outsiders like shaman.
External magical methods such as astrology, calendrical divination, object-based magic became
more commonplace, and religion became an indoor experience. Latterly, religion itself has
been greatly challenged by a further move towards philosophical abstraction, with the post-
Enlightenment atheism moving from the position that the spiritual doesn't exist to postmodern
relativism, where no innate value exists in anything. This sequence can be seen as an inevitable
and progressive consequence of the development of technology and increased networking, or
as a kind of devolution or fall from direct experience of the spiritual to mediated and prescriptive experience to no experience at all.

It's likely that both perspectives are inaccurate and incomplete, but we certainly don't see the
world as our ancestors did. One remedy for this might be to detach ourselves from value judge-
ments before parsing historical beliefs and practices from multiple angles in order to examine
the utilitarian pros and cons of their perspective. We tend to assume that our view is superior,
being most recent, "higher up the mountain of history"; but much of the path below is blan-
keted in the mists of time, and our memory of the ascent is imperfect. We look at the things our

ancestors believed and discard most of them as rubbish, not troubling ourselves with the fact that our descendants are as likely to do the same thing with most of our dearest doctrines—contemporary culture, and perhaps most materially successful cultures, suffers from a bad case of hubris and "chronic general ingratitude".[1479] Every age has something to teach.

"Objective truth" (if there is such a thing—idealists and postmodernists may say not) could be conceived as a courtyard, a vast circular atrium with overlooking windows set into the upper storey. Behind every window is a room, and each room has a different view of the courtyard. Each room, and its view, is one paradigm: one philosophical or metaphysical reality model. Some have better views of the courtyard than others; some have tiny grubby windows, or the view is partially blocked, but no single room shows the entire view. Humanity has lived in only a few of the rooms; there are—impossibly, yet truthfully—an infinite number. Different technologies, techniques, and insights are required to unlock the doors and pass between the rooms. We spend time arguing through the walls about whether this bit of that statue in the courtyard we can see is really a woman's elbow or a dolphin's nose, because people in different rooms, looking out of different windows, have different views. Of course some of the interpretations may be right, and others wrong; but none encompasses the whole.

With any luck, we may be entering what the German polymath and chocolate enthusiast Goethe imagined as the fourth epoch of the sciences: the first is childlike, poetic, and superstitious; the second is empirical, investigative, and curious; the third, dogmatic, didactic, and pedantic; and the last is ideal, methodical, and mystical.[1480] If the extraordinary placebo effect rabbit hole is any guide to the immense possibilities of the effects of meaning on well-being, then by making a concerted collective effort to anatomise, customise, and utilise religious, shamanic, and magical rituals in the way they were originally intended, as means of curing humanity of the ills consequent to our limited perspective, perhaps we could open up new possibilities to change ourselves. The pharmacology and mythology of Cacao suggest that it may be a valuable facilitator of de-traumatisation and transformation. At the very least, it is a mostly beneficial, low-toxicity substance with potentially vast public health benefits in the prevention of cardio-metabolic and age-related diseases.

Re-familiarising ourselves with the old, powerful, unsweetened Cacao-based drinks may therefore be helpful. They can be drunk secularly but mindfully, using intention and meaning to harness the "placebo effect"—with ritual purpose, binding us to small personal goals with the intent of improving ourselves, and, ultimately, humanity. Or they may be employed therapeutically, to assist in overcoming fears, and for strengthening *shen*—the pursuit of self-transformation by augmenting "imagination, intention ... enchantment and wonder".[1481] Maybe Cacao could help us save the world, if we let it. If not, at the very least, it's a pleasant medicine to try.

ENDNOTES

Introduction

1. Yuker, in Szogyi, 1997 [Book].
2. Williams, 2003 [Book].
3. Takahashi *et al.*, 2000 [Journal].
4. Kurek *et al.*, 1996 [Journal].
5. Lopresti, 2017 [Journal].
6. Norling, Ly & Dally, 2017 [Journal].
7. Yanovski, 2003 [Journal].
8. Davinelli *et al.*, 2018 [Journal].
9. Wolfe & Holdstock, 2005 [Book].
10. Schifano & Magni, 1994 [Journal].

Chapter One

11. Miller & Taube, 1993 [Book].
12. Rudgley, 1998 [Book].
13. Takahashi, 2000 [Journal].
14. Ji, 2012a [Internet].
15. Young, 1994 [Book].
16. Miller & Taube, 1993 [Book].
17. *Ibid*.
18. Tedlock, 1992 [Book].
19. Miller & Taube, 1993 [Book].
20. Reents-Budet, in McNeil, 2006 [Book].
21. *Ibid*.
22. Miller & Taube, 1993 [Book].
23. Dreiss & Greenhill, 2008 [Book].
24. Young, 1994 [Book].
25. Miller & Taube, 1993 [Book].

26. Tedlock, 1992 [Book].
27. Miller & Taube, 1993 [Book].
28. Reston, 2003 [Book].
29. Miller & Taube, 1993 [Book].
30. *Ibid.*
31. Freidel, Schele, & Parker, 1993 [Book].
32. Dreiss & Greenhill, 2008 [Book].
33. Mann, 2005 [Book].
34. *Ibid.*
35. Reston, 2003 [Book].
36. Miller & Taube, 1993 [Book].
37. *Ibid.*
38. Coe, 1994 [Book].
39. *Ibid.*
40. Mann, 2005 [Book].
41. Milbrath, 1999 [Book].
42. Reston, 2003 [Book].
43. Freidel, Schele, & Parker, 1993 [Book].
44. Miller & Taube, 1993 [Book].
45. *Ibid.*
46. Freidel, Schele, & Parker, 1993 [Book].
47. Miller & Taube, 1993 [Book].
48. Freidel, Schele, & Parker, 1993 [Book].
49. *Ibid.*
50. Miller & Taube, 1993 [Book].
51. *Ibid.*
52. Coe, 1994 [Book].
53. Miller & Taube, 1993 [Book].
54. León-Portilla, 1992 [Book].
55. Graulich, 2004 [Journal].
56. Coe, 1994 [Book].
57. Boone, 2007 [Book].
58. Pendell, 2010 [Book].
59. Coe & Coe, 1996 [Book].
60. Hamnett, 1999 [Book].
61. Boone, 2007 [Book].
62. Persoone, 2008 [Book]; Dreiss & Greenhill, 2008 [Book].
63. Young, 1994 [Book].
64. *Ibid.*
65. Miller & Taube, 1993 [Book].
66. Coe & Coe, 1996 [Book].
67. Miller & Taube, 1993 [Book].

68. Glockner, 2017 [Periodical].
69. Miller & Taube, 1993 [Book].
70. *Ibid.*
71. *Ibid.*
72. *Ibid.*
73. Coe & Coe, 1996 [Book].
74. Ott, 1985 [Book].
75. Diego Durán, quoted in Coe & Coe, 1996 [Book].
76. Coe & Coe, 1996 [Book].
77. Young, 1994 [Book].
78. Sampeck, 2016 [Journal].
79. Sahagún, 1950–82, 9: 48; *quoted in* Coe, 1996 [Book].
80. (2013), en.m.wiktionary.org/wiki/caco#Latin [Internet].
81. Briggs, 2008 [Book].
82. Coe & Coe, 1996 [Book].
83. Ullmann, in Szogyi, 1997 [Book].
84. Aguilar-Monero, in McNeil, 2006 [Book].
85. Coe & Coe, 1996 [Book].
86. Young, 1994 [Book].
87. Ullmann, in Szogyi, 1997 [Book].
88. McGee, 1984 [Book].
89. *Ibid.*
90. Duran, quoted in Coe, 1994 [Book].
91. Wagner, 2001 [Book].

Chapter Two

92. Coe & Coe, 1996 [Book].
93. Colombo, Pinorini-Godly, & Conti, in Paoletti *et al.*, 2012 [Book].
94. Beckett, 2000 [Book].
95. Young, 1994 [Book].
96. *Ibid.*
97. Aguilar-Moreno, in McNeil, 2006 [Book].
98. Dreiss & Greenhill, 2008 [Book].
99. Kew Science, http://powo.science.kew.org/taxon/urn:lsid:ipni.org:names:320783-2 [accessed 9 August 2018].
100. Young, 1994 [Book].
101. 20 April 2008: Interview with tour guide Claudia at Hacienda La Luz, Tabasco, Mexico.
102. Young, 1994 [Book].
103. *Ibid.*
104. *Ibid.*
105. De Schawe *et al.*, 2018 [Journal].

106. http://faculty.ucr.edu/~legneref/medical/ceratopogonidaemed.htm;   https://extension.entm.purdue.edu/publichealth/insects/bitingmidge.html [accessed 13 August 2018].

107. Shelley & Coscaron, 2001 [Journal].

108. 20 April 2008: Interview with tour guide Claudia at Hacienda La Luz, Tabasco, Mexico.

109. Young, 1994 [Book].

110. *Ibid.*

111. *Ibid.*

112. *Ibid.*

113. *Ibid.*

114. Source: Mexico travel notebook 2011, Juan-Pablo Porres Esquina.

115. Persoone, 2008 [Book].

116. Young, 1994 [Book].

117. 20 April 2008: Interview with tour guide Claudia at Hacienda La Luz, Tabasco, Mexico.

118. Persoone, 2008 [Book].

119. Young, 1994; 26 January 2011: Interview with Cacao farming expert Juan Pablo Porres Esquina at Don Ramiro's finca in San Antonio Suchitequepez, Guatemala.

120. 29 January 2011: Interview with Cacao farmer and APROCAV technical advisor Don Juan Francisco, Cohoban, Alta Verapaz, North Guatemala.

121. Young, 1994 [Book].

122. Persoone, 2008 [Book]; and Young, 1994 [Book].

123. Young, 1994 [Book].

124. https://www.barry-callebaut.com/about-us/media/press-kit/history-chocolate/theobroma-cacao-food-gods [accessed 16 August 2018].

125. Source: Mexico travel notebook 2011, Juan-Pablo Porres Esquina.

126. Persoone, 2008 [Book].

127. Young, 1994 [Book].

128. *Ibid.*

129. *Ibid.*

130. 20 April 2008: Interview with tour guide Claudia at Hacienda La Luz, Tabasco, Mexico.

131. Bertazzo *et al.*, 2013 [Book].

132. 29 January 2011: Interview with Cacao farmer and APROCAV technical advisor Don Juan Francisco, Cohoban, Alta Verapaz, North Guatemala.

133. Young & Severson, 1994 [Journal].

134. Young, 1994 [Book].

135. Teixeira, Thomazella, & Pereira, 2015 [Journal].

136. Meinhardt *et al.*, 2008 [Journal].

137. Henderson & Joyce, in McNeil, 2006 [Book].

138. Ogata, Gomez-Pompa, & Taube, in McNeil, 2006 [Book].

139. Montamayor *et al.*, 2008 [Journal].

140. Cornejo *et al.*, 2017 [Internet].

141. Coe, 1994 [Book].

142. *Ibid.*

143. Stubbe, 1662 [Book].
144. Kennedy, 2010 [Book]; 21 September 2018: Interview with restauranteur and chef Carmen Santiago, Teotitlan del Valle, Oaxaca, Mexico.
145. McNeil, in McNeil, 2006b [Book].
146. Telly, from Szogyi, 1997 [Book].
147. Soto, 2005 [Internet].
148. Beckett, 2000 [Book].
149. Ziegleder, from Beckett, 2009 [Book].
150. *Ibid.*
151. Source: Mexico travel notebook 2011, Keith Wilson—orders beans from ladies who toast them on metal trays, then remove them from the heat "as soon as the first bean pops". [See Appendix C, Interview 3.]
152. *Ibid.*
153. Source: Mexico travel notebook 2018, observed and photographed Sra Anna Maria Garcia Vasquez, maker and vendor of Bu'pu in Juchitan de Zaragoza, Oaxaca, Mexico, using this method to process Cacao.
154. De Gortari, 2012 [Internet].
155. Source: Mexico travel notebook 2011, "cold method" demonstrated by Sra Aurelia Pop, Rex'hua, Alta Verapaz, Guatemala.
156. Source: Mexico travel notebook 2011, "hot method" demonstrated by Sra Juana Ca'al, midwife, Alta Verapaz, Guatemala.
157. Source: Mexico recordings 2008, tour guide Claudia at Hacienda La Luz, 2008; Beckett, 2000.
158. Beckett, 2000 [Book].
159. Source: 29 Jan 2011: Interview with Sr Ignacio Cac Sacul, president of the Cacao grower's association, Alta Verapaz, Guatemala.
160. Source: Mexico recordings 2008, tour guide Claudia at Hacienda La Luz, 2008.
161. Young, 1994 [Book].
162. Fredholm *et al.*, 1999 [Journal].
163. Pech, 2010 [Book].
164. Briggs, 2008 [Book].
165. Beckett, 2000 [Book].
166. Fredholm *et al.*, 1999 [Journal].
167. *Ibid.*
168. Beckett, 2000 [Book].
169. https://ghirardelli.com/about-ghirardelli?storeId=11003&langId=-1 [accessed 20 August 2018].
170. Briggs, 2008 [Book].
171. Coe & Coe, 1996 [Book].
172. Fredholm *et al.*, 1999 [Journal].
173. Beckett, 2000 [Book].
174. *Ibid.*
175. Persoone, 2008 [Book].

176. Briggs, 2008 [Book].
177. Persoone, 2008 [Book].
178. Beckett, 2000 [Book].
179. Pech, 2010 [Book].
180. Coe, 1994 [Book].
181. Pech, 2010 [Book].
182. https://webmd.com/vitamins/ai/ingredientmono-893/bloodroot [accessed 22 August n2018]; *Ibid.*
183. Gay & Clark, in Grivetti & Shapiro, 2009 [Book].
184. Stubbe, 1662 [Book].
185. Badiano, 1552 [Book].
186. Hernández, 1615 [Internet].
187. Coe & Coe, 1996 [Book].
188. Robert, 1957 [Book].
189. De Ledesma, 1631 [Book].
190. Robert, 1957 [Book].
191. Stubbe, 1662 [Book].
192. Hughes, 1672 [Book].
193. *Ibid.*
194. Hughes, quoted in Paoletti *et al.*, 2012 [Book].
195. Steinbrenner, in McNeil, 2006 [Book].
196. 20 Jan 2011: Interview with Señora Leon, chocolate tablet maker, San Antonio Suchitequepez, Guatemala.
197. Persoone, 2008 [Book].
198. Henderson & Joyce, in McNeil, 2006 [Book].
199. Trilling, 1999 [Book].
200. Source: Mexico travel notebook 2008, tour guide Claudia at Hacienda La Luz, 2008; Beckett, 2000 [Book].
201. Aguilar-Moreno, in McNeil, 2006 [Book].
202. Coe, 1994 [Book].
203. Faust & Lopez, in McNeil, 2006 [Book].
204. Popenoe, 1919 [Journal].
205. Soto, 2005 [Internet].
206. Popenoe, 1919 [Journal].
207. Kennedy, 2010 [Book].
208. *Ibid.*
209. Stross, 2011 [Journal].
210. McNeil, in McNeil, 2006b [Book].
211. *Ibid.*
212. Kennedy, 2010 [Book].
213. Source: Mexico travel notebook 6 May 2008, info provided by *Tejate*-maker Señora Crispina Navarro-Gomez, Santo Tomal Julietza, Oaxaca, Mexico.
214. Trilling, 1999 [Book].

215. Kennedy, 2010 [Book].

216. *Ibid.*

217. https://laroussecocina.mx/diccionario/definicion/cocolmeca [accessed 23 July 2017].

218. Dharmananda, 2001 [Internet].

219. 22 February 2011: Interview with *Popo* vendor, Acuyacan, Veracruz, Mexico.

220. Source: Mexico travel notebook 12 September 2018, info provided by Veronica Juarez, technician at the MEXU herbarium, UNAM, Mexico City.

221. 2 October 2018: Interview with *Popo* vendor Doña Rosa Gregorio, Ojitlan, Oaxaca, Mexico.

222. 18 October 2018: Interview with stallholder Sra Claudia Maribel Ya'teni, Coban, Alta Verapaz, Guatemala.

223. Popenoe, 1919 [Journal].

224. 29 January 2011: Interviews with Ignacio Cac Sacul, president of the Cacao Grower's Association, and Don Juan Francisco, Cohoban Cacao Grower's Association technical advisor and Cacao farmer, Alta Verapaz, North Guatemala.

225. 14 February 2011: Interview with Don Mateo Poptchu, Mopan Maya spiritual guide and diviner, San Luis, Peten, West Guatemala. [Appendix C, Interview 6.]

226. Coe & Coe, 1996 [Book].

227. Kennedy, 2010 [Book].

228. Stross, 2011 [Internet].

229. Dunning & Fox, in Grivetti & Shapiro, 2009 [Book].

230. Kennedy, 2010 [Book].

231. 21 September 2018: Interview with Doña Carmen Santiago, chef and owner of Tierra Antigua restaurant, with her student, Kalisa Wells, Teotilan del Valle, Oaxaca, Mexico.

232. Kennedy, 2010 [Book].

233. 26 September 2018: Interview with Sra Delfina Valverde, maker of *chaw popox*, San Mateo del Mar, Oaxaca, Mexico.

234. Kennedy, 2010 [Book].

235. Coe & Coe, 1996 [Book].

236. *Ibid.*

237. Persoone, 2008 [Book].

238. Source: Mexico travel notebook 2011, tour guide Boris at Tikal, Guatemala.

239. 11 February 2011: Interview with Sr Reginaldo Huex, herbalist and director of the Asociacion Bio-Itza, San Jose, Peten, West Guatemala. [Appendix C, Interview 4.]

240. Coe & Coe, 1996 [Book]; Coe, 1994 [Book].

241. Persoone, 2008 [Book].

242. Source: Mexico travel notebook 2018, Notes from MUCHO, the *Museo de Chocolate* in Mexico City.

243. Field notes, Coban, Alta Verapaz, October 2018.

244. *Ibid.*

245. McNeil, in McNeil 2006a [Book].

246. Coe & Coe, 1996 [Book].

247. McNeil, in McNeil 2006a [Book].

248. McNeil, in McNeil 2006a [Book].

249. Coe & Coe, 1996 [Book].
250. *Ibid.*
251. Young, 1994 [Book].
252. Henderson & Joyce, in McNeil, 2006 [Book].
253. McNeil, in McNeil, 2006b [Book].
254. Henderson & Joyce in McNeil, 2006 [Book].
255. Coe, 1994 [Book].
256. Schultes & Hofmann, 1992 [Book].
257. Coe, 1994 [Book].
258. Ott, 1996 [Book].
259. Stubbe, 1662 [Book].
260. Safford, 1910 [Internet].
261. Coe & Coe, 1996 [Book].
262. Coe, 1994 [Book].
263. Mills, 1991 [Book].
264. Coe, 1994 [Book].
265. http://maya-ethnobotany.org/mayan-ethno-botany-tropical-agriculture-edible-flowers-medicinal-plants-flavoring-guatemala-mexico-belize/plumeria-rubia-flor-de-mayo-frangipani-cacao-balche-aphrodisiac-fragrance.php [accessed 18 December 2017].
266. Hernández, 1615, translated by Ximenez. [Internet.]
267. www.maya-ethnobotany.org [accessed 18 December 2017].
268. Da Silva & Alba, 2004 [Internet].
269. Coe & Coe, 1996 [Book].
270. *Ibid.*
271. 23 September 2018: Interview with Señora Teresa Olivera, stallholder in mercado Benito Juarez, Oaxaca city, Oaxaca, Mexico.
272. Coe, 1994 [Book].
273. de Ledesma, quoted in Grivetti & Shapiro, 2009 [Book].
274. Raffauf & Zennie, 1993 [Journal]; Ott, 1996 [Book]; https://toptropicals.com/html/toptropicals/plant_wk/quararibea.htm [accessed 5 January 2018].
275. Ott, 1996 [Book].
276. *Ibid.*
277. Pendell, 2010 [Book].
278. Fagetti, 2017 [Periodical].
279. Wasson, 1980 [Book].
280. *Ibid.*
281. Carod-Artal, 2015 [Journal].
282. de la Garza, 2017 [Periodical].
283. *Ibid.*
284. Schultes & Hofmann, 1992 [Book]; Carod-Artal, 2011 [Journal].
285. de Sahagún, book 6, p. 256, quoted in Coe & Coe, 1996 [Book].
286. Shulgin & Shulgin, 2013 [Book].

287. *Ibid.*
288. De la Garza, 2017 [Periodical].
289. Schultes & Hofmann, 1992 [Book]; Carod-Artal, 2015 [Journal]; Hernández, translated by Ximenez, 1615 [Internet].
290. Schultes & Hofmann, 1992 [Book].
291. Carod-Artal, 2015 [Journal].
292. Personal experimental notes, 2013.
293. Carod-Artal, 2015 [Journal].
294. Wasson, quoted in Ott, 1996 [Book].
295. De la Garza, 2017 [Periodical].
296. Franciotti, 2016 [Internet].
297. Spiegel, 2016 [Journal].
298. Torquemada, quoted in Coe & Coe, 1996 [Book].
299. Carod-Artal, 2015 [Journal].
300. Schultes & Hofmann, 1992 [Book].
301. *Ibid.*
302. *Ibid.*
303. http://expat-chronicles.com/2009/10/scopolamine-in-colombia/ [accessed 16 September 2018]

Chapter Three

304. Tilburt & Kaptchuk, 2008 [Internet].
305. Tobyn, 1997 [Book].
306. Stanhope *et al.*, 2009 [Journal]; Lim *et al.*, 2010 [Journal].
307. Wojcicki & Heyman, 2012 [Journal]; Zelber-Sagi, Ratizu, & Oren, 2011 [Journal].
308. Bray & Bellanger, 2006 [Journal].
309. https://nottingham.ac.uk/news/pressreleases/2015/march/ancientbiotics---a-medieval-remedy-for-modern-day-superbugs.aspx [Accessed 26 February 2019].
310. Withering, 1785 [Book].
311. Bifulco *et al.*, 2014 [Journal].
312. Parkinson, 1640 [Book].
313. Williams, E. (2003) [Book]; and Szabo *et al.*, 2009 [Journal].
314. Three sample papers among thousands: the first, on the potential utility of herbal medicine in cancer treatment (Tavakoli *et al.*, 2012 [Journal]), and the second two on the efficacy of the much-maligned Kava Kava (*Piper methysticum*) as an anxiolytic (Thompson, Ruch, & Hasenöhrl, 2004; Sarris *et al.*, 2013 [Journals]).
315. https://goodreads.com/author/quotes/248774.Hippocrates [accessed 13 March 2019].
316. https://poetryfoundation.org/poems/46565/ozymandias [accessed 13 March 2019].
317. Bletter & Daly, in McNeil, 2006 [Book]; Paoletti *et al.*, 2012 [Book].
318. Grivetti, in Grivetti & Shapiro, 2009 [Book].
319. Hernández, 1615 [Internet].
320. Bletter & Daly, in McNeil, 2006 [Book].

321. Dreiss & Greenhill, 2008 [Book].
322. Grivetti, in Grivetti & Shapiro, 2009 [Book].
323. *Ibid.*
324. Interview with Señor Mario Euan, senior teacher at U-Yits-Ka'an school of Agriculture and Ecology in Mani, Yucatan, Mexico, 18 April 2008 [Appendix C, Interview 1].
325. 4 February 2011: Interview with Doña Juana Ca'al, Rex'hua, Alta Verapaz, Guatemala; also taken from field notes in conversation with Señora Aurelia Pop, Lanquin, Peten, Guatemala, in 2011.
326. 4 February 2011: Interview with Doña Juana Ca'al, Rex'hua, Alta Verapaz, Guatemala.
327. Eggleston & White, *from* Watson *et al.*, 2013 [Book].
328. Monroy-Ortiz & Castillo-España, 2007 [Book].
329. *Ibid.*
330. Noriega & González, in Grivetti & Shapiro, 2009 [Book].
331. Field notes in conversation with Señor Juan Gomez, a Cacao worker in San Antonio Suchitquepez, Guatemala, 2011.
332. Field notes in conversation with Doña Juana Ca'al, Rex'hua, Alta Verapaz, Guatemala, in 2011.
333. *Ibid.*
334. 3 February 2011: Interview with Don Antonio Xoc, Ya'al Pemech, Alta Verapaz, Guatemala.
335. Field notes, Guatemala, 2011.
336. Grivetti, in Grivetti & Shapiro, 2009 [Book].
337. Bletter & Daly, in McNeil, 2006 [Book].
338. Field notes, Guatemala, 2011.
339. *Ibid.*
340. 3 February 2011: Interview with Don Antonio Xoc, Ya'al Pemech, Alta Verapaz, Guatemala.
341. Field notes, Guatemala, 2011.
342. *Ibid.*
343. Grivetti, in Grivetti & Shapiro, 2009 [Book].
344. Bletter & Daly, in McNeil, 2006 [Book].
345. *Ibid.*
346. Grivetti, in Grivetti & Shapiro, 2009 [Book].
347. *Ibid.*
348. Falade *et al.*, 2005 [Journal].
349. https://goodreads.com/author/quotes/248774.Hippocrates [accessed 13 March 2019].
350. Hernández, 1615 [Internet].
351. Dreiss & Greenhill, 2008 [Book].
352. Coe & Coe, 1996 [Book].
353. Robert, 1957 [Book].
354. Robert, 1957 [Book].
355. de Ledesma, 1631 [Book].
356. *Ibid.*
357. Hughes, 1672 [Book].
358. *Ibid.*

ENDNOTES 393

359. *Ibid.*

360. *Ibid.*

361. De Ledesma, 1631 [Book].

362. Grivetti, in Grivetti & Shapiro, 2009 [Book].

363. *Ibid.*

364. Stubbe, 1662 [Book].

365. Wilson, in Paoletti *et al.*, 2012 [Book].

366. Wang *et al.*, 2018 [Journal].

367. Hughes, 1672 [Book].

368. Robert, 1957 [Book].

369. *Ibid.*

370. Murphy *et al.*, 2003 [Journal].

371. Hughes, 1672 [Book].

372. Kennedy, 2008 [Book].

373. Bone, *from* Brice-Ytsma & Watkins, 2014 [Book].

374. de Ledesma, 1631 [Book].

375. Robert, 1957 [Book].

376. *Ibid.*

377. *Ibid.*

378. Hughes, 1672 [Book].

379. Robert, 1957 [Book].

380. de Ledesma, 1631 [Book].

381. Steinbrenner, in McNeil, 2006.

382. *Ibid.*

383. Hosseinzadeh *et al.*, 2011 [Journal].

384. Evrensel & Ceylan, 2015 [Journal].

385. Robert, 1957 [Book].

386. *Ibid.*

387. *Ibid.*

388. Moore, 2017 [Book].

389. *Ibid.*

390. Culpeper, 1653 [Book].

391. Tobyn, 1997 [Book].

392. Robert, 1957 [Book].

393. Coe & Coe, 1996 [Book].

394. Robert, 1957 [Book].

395. *Ibid.*

396. Stubbe, 1662 [Book].

397. *Ibid.*

398. Hughes, quoted in Wilson, in Paoletti *et al.*, 2012 [Book].

399. de Ledesma, 1631 [Book].

400. See Appendix A: *Theobroma cacao* monograph.

401. Robert, 1957 [Book].

402. Hughes, 1672 [Book].

403. *Ibid*.

404. Akatsu, 1917 [Journal].

405. Robert, 1957 [Book].

406. Byrne, 2013 [Internet].

407. Culpeper, 1653 [Book].

408. Hernández, 1615 [Internet].

409. Philomath, quoted by Grivetti, in Grivetti & Shapiro, 2009 [Book].

410. de Ledesma, 1631 [Book].

411. Stubbe, 1662 [Book].

412. Hecquet, quoted by Robert, 1957 [Book].

413. Stubbe, 1662 [Book].

414. *Ibid*.

415. Kennedy, 2010 [Book].

416. *Ibid*.

417. Robert, 1957 [Book].

418. *Ibid*.

419. Chevalier & Bain, 2002 [Book].

420. De Montellano, 2004 [Periodical].

421. Tedlock, 1992 [Book].

422. Tobyn, 1997 [Book].

423. Miller & Taube, 1993 [Book].

424. Trotter & Chavira, 1997 [Book].

425. Miller & Taube, 1993 [Book].

426. de Montellano, 2004 [Periodical].

427. Miller & Taube, 1993 [Book].

428. Miller & Taube, 1993 [Book].

429. Tedlock, 1992 [Book].

430. *Ibid*.

431. Hernández, 1615 [Book].

432. León-Portilla, 1992 [Book].

433. Hernández & Sahagún quoted in Barrera & Aliphat, in McNeil, 2006 [Periodical].

434. Dreiss & Greenhill, 2008 [Book]; Wilson, in Paoletti *et al.*, 2012 [Book].

435. Dreiss & Greenhill, 2008 [Book].

436. Badiano, 1552 [Book].

437. *Ibid*.

438. *Ibid*.

439. Linares, Bye, & Flores, 2000 [Book].

440. *Ibid*.

441. Miller & Taube, 1993 [Book].

442. Hernández, 1615 [Book].

443. Bucay, 2002 [Journal].

444. Trotter & Chavira, 1997 [Book].
445. 2 May 2008: Interview with stallholder in *Mercado Benito Juarez*, Oaxaca City, Oaxaca, Mexico.
446. Hernández, 1615 [Book].
447. Badiano, 1552 [Book].
448. *Ibid.*
449. Safford, 1910 [Internet].
450. Glockner, 2017 [Periodical].
451. Hobbs, 1986 [Book].
452. Culpeper, 1653 [Book].
453. *Ibid.*
454. Hernández, quoted in Schultes & Hofmann, 1992 [Book].
455. *Ibid.*
456. Monroy-Ortiz & Castillo-España, 2007 [Book].
457. Robert, 1957 [Book].
458. *Ibid.*
459. Hernández, 1615 [Internet]; Holzmann *et al.*, 2014 [Journal].
460. Stubbe, 1662 [Book]; Hernández, 1615 [Internet].
461. Hernández, 1615 [Internet].
462. Da Silva & Alba, 2004 [Internet].
463. Hernández, 1615 [Internet].
464. Monroy-Ortiz & Castillo-España, 2007 [Book].
465. Da Silva & Alba, 2004 [Internet].
466. Monroy-Ortiz & Castillo-España, 2007 [Book].
467. Culpeper, 1653 [Book].
468. Hernández, 1615 [Book].
469. Stubbe, 1662 [Book]; and personal notes from chocolate-making, 2016.
470. Hernández, 1615 [Internet].
471. *Ibid.*
472. *Ibid.*
473. Montalvo & Parra, 1999 [Journal]; Estrada-Reyes *et al.*, 2013 [Journal].
474. Hernández, 1615 [Internet].
475. 18 April 2008: Interview with Sr Mario Euan, herbalist and teacher at U-Yits-Ka'an school of Agriculture and Ecology, Mani, Yucatan peninsula, Mexico. [Appendix C, Interview 1].
476. Hernández, 1615 [Internet].
477. Field notes, Guatemala, 2011; and 13 February 2011: interview with Don Angel Chiac, San Luis, Peten, Guatemala.
478. 11 February 2011: Interview with Sr Reginaldo Chayax Huex, San Jose, Peten, Guatemala, [Appendix C, Interview 4].
479. Hernández, 1615 [Internet].
480. University of California and Los Angeles, 2002 [Internet].
481. Zhang & Lokeshwar, 2012 [Journal].
482. *Ibid.*
483. Linares, Bye & Flores, 1999 [Book]; (2017), *Canak* [...], www.maya-ethnobotany.org [Internet].

484. Badiano, 1552 [Book].
485. (2017), *Canak* […], www.maya-ethnobotany.org [Internet].
486. Monroy-Ortiz & Castillo-España, 2007 [Book].
487. (2017), Neglected crops […], www.fao.org [Internet].
488. (2018), *Pouteria sapota: Plants for a Future.* http://pfaf.org [Internet].
489. (2017), Neglected crops […], www.fao.org [Internet].
490. (2018), *Pouteria sapota: Plants for a Future.* http://pfaf.org [Internet].
491. Monroy-Ortiz & Castillo-España, 2007 [Book].
492. *Anonymous, 1975 [Journal].*
493. Hernández, 1615 [Internet].
494. Rudgley, 1998 [Book].
495. Griggs, 1997 [Book].
496. Linares, Bye & Flores, 1999 [Book]; Bown, 2002 [Book].
497. Bone, 2003 [Book].
498. Bensky & Gamble, 1986 [Book].
499. Bucay, 2002 [Journal].

Chapter Four

500. Carper, 1988 [Book]; Pizzorno & Murray, 2006 [Book].
501. Moerman, 2002 [Book].
502. *Ibid.*
503. *Ibid.*
504. Khan & Nicod, in Paoletti *et al.*, 2012 [Book].
505. Khalil *et al.*, 2000 [Journal].
506. Berges *et al.*, 1995.
507. Awad *et al.*, 2003 & 1996 [Journals]; Bouic *et al.*, 1999 [Journal].
508. Singh *et al.*, 2012 [Journal]; Murugan *et al.*, 2009 [Journal].
509. Colombo, Pinori-Godly & Conti, in Paoletti *et al.*, 2012 [Book].
510. Pech, 2010 [Book].
511. Ristow & Schmeisser, 2014 [Journal].
512. Castell *et al.*, from Watson *et al.*, 2013 [Book].
513. Sudano *et al.*, in Paoletti *et al.*, 2012 [Book].
514. Panneerselvam, 2010 [Journal].
515. Castell *et al.*, from Watson *et al.*, 2013 [Book].
516. Sakagami *et al.*, 2008 [Journal].
517. Elwers *et al.*, 2009 [Journal].
518. Bisson *et al.*, 2008 [Journal].
519. Sokolov *et al.*, 2013 [Journal]; Mastroiacovo *et al.*, 2014 [Journal].
520. Mao *et al.*, 2003 [Journal]; Verstraeten *et al.*, 2004 [Journal]; Wollgast, 2004 [Acacdemic Paper: doctoral dissertation].
521. Mao *et al.*, 2002 [Journal]; Kenny *et al.*, 2007 [Journal]; Heptinstall *et al.*, 2006 [Journal]; Panneerselvam *et al.*, 2010 [Journal].

522. Zhu *et al.*, 2005 [Journal].

523. Roura *et al.*, 2008 & 2007 [Journals]; Schramm *et al.*, 2003 [Journal].

524. Sanchez *et al.*, 1973 [Journal].

525. Pang *et al.*, 2016 [Journal]; Migliori *et al.*, 2015 [Journal]; Huang *et al.*, 2013 [Journal].

526. Li *et al.*, 2015 [Journal]; Mansour & Tawfik, 2012 [Journal]; Jayanthi & Subash, 2010 [Journal]; Oktar *et al.*, 2010 [Journal]; Coban *et al.*, 2010 [Journal]; Kart *et al.*, 2010 [Journal]; Pari & Karthikesan, 2007 [Journal]; Ciftci *et al.*, 2012 [Journal]; Tsai & Yin, 2012 [Journal].

527. Cinkilic *et al.*, 2013 [Journal]; Oboh *et al.*, 2013 [Journal]; Teraoka *et al.*, 2012 [Journal].

528. Horman, Brambilla & Stalder, 1981 [Journal].

529. Fallarini *et al.*, 2009 [Journal]; Bardelli *et al.*, 2011 [Internet]; Park, 2007 & 2005 [Journals].

530. Stark *et al.*, 2008 [Journal].

531. Poulsen *et al.*, 2013 [medium not given].

532. Tome-Carneiro *et al.*, 2013 [Journal].

533. Nakano *et al.*, 2012 [Journal].

534. Extrapolated from Zoumas, Kreiser & Martin, 1980 [Journal].

535. Briggs, 2008 [Book].

536. Smit, in Fredholm, 2011 [Book].

537. *Ibid*.

538. Fredholm *et al.*, 1999 [Journal].

539. Smit, in Fredholm, 2011 [Book].

540. Baggot *et al.*, 2013 [Journal].

541. Smit, in Fredholm, 2011 [Book].

542. Sugimoto *et al.*, 2014 [Journal].

543. Smit, in Fredholm, 2011 [Book].

544. Slattery & West, 1993 [Journal].

545. Smit, in Fredholm, 2011 [Book]; Giannandrea, 2009 [Journal].

546. Smit, in Fredholm, 2011 [Book].

547. Barnes, 2013 [Journal].

548. Barnes, 2013 [Journal]; Dubuis *et al.*, 2014 [Journal].

549. Motegi *et al.*, 2013 [Journal].

550. Ebadi *et al.*, 2005 [Book].

551. Hipólito *et al.*, 2011 [Journal].

552. Airaksinen *et al.*, 1984 [Journal].

553. Carr & Lovering, 2000 [Journal]; Mravec, 2006 [Journal].

554. Misztal *et al.*, 2010 [Journal].

555. Kang, 2007 [Journal].

556. Quertemont & Didone, 2006 [Journal]; Polache & Granero, 2013 [Journal].

557. Airaksinen & Kari, 1981 [Journal].

558. Preza *et al.*, 2010 [Journal].

559. (2013), http://urticaria.thunderworksinc.com [Internet].

560. Berry, 2004 [Journal].

561. Zucchi *et al.*, 2006 [Journal].

562. Berry, 2004 [Journal].

563. Marseglia, Palla, & Caligiani, 2014 [Journal].

564. De Laurentiis *et al.*, 2010 [Journal]; Luce *et al.*, 2014 [Journal].

565. (2012) lipidlibrary.aocs.org [Internet].

566. di Tomaso, Beltramo & Piomelli, 1996 [Journal]; Beltramo & Piomelli, 1998 [Journal].

567. Cornacchia *et al.*, 2012 [Journal].

568. Prasad, 2005 [Book].

569. Hoenicke & Gatermann, 2005 [Journal].

570. Borawska, in Sikorski, 2007 [Book].

571. Gröber, Schmidt, & Kisters, 2015 [Journal].

572. Eby & Eby, 2010 [Journal].

573. *Ibid.*

574. Bertazzo *et al.*, in Watson, 2013 [Book].

575. Nakamura *et al.*, 1999 [Journal]; Reddy *et al.*, 2009 [Journal].

576. Beckett, 2009 [Book].

577. Bertazzo *et al.*, in Watson, 2013 [Book].

578. *Ibid.*

579. Ziegleder, Stojacic & Stumpf, 1992 [Journal].

580. Beckett, 2000 [Book].

581. Bertazzo *et al.*, in Watson, 2013 [Journal].

582. Copetti *et al.*, 2012 [Journal].

583. do Nascimento *et al.*, 2013 [Journal].

584. Bertazzo *et al.*, in Watson, 2013 [Book].

585. Beckett, 2009 [Book].

586. Bertazzo *et al.*, in Watson, 2013 [Book].

587. Beckett, 2009 [Book].

588. *Ibid.*

589. Bernaert *et al.*, in Paoletti *et al.*, 2012 [Book].

590. *Ibid.*

591. Abecia-Soria, Pezoa-García, & Amaya-Farfan, 2006 [Journal].

592. Beckett, 2000 [Book].

593. Farah, Zaibunnisa, & Misnawi, 2012 [Journal].

594. Beckett, 2000 [Book].

595. *Ibid.*

596. *Ibid.*

597. *Ibid.*

598. *Ibid.*

599. *Ibid.*

600. *Ibid.*

601. *Ibid.*

602. Visioli *et al.*, in Paoletti *et al.*, 2012 [Book].

603. *Ibid.*

604. Buijsse *et al.*, 2010 [Journal].

605. Castell *et al.*, from Watson *et al.*, 2013 [Book].

606. Buitrago-Lopez *et al.*, 2011 [Journal].
607. Djoussé *et al.*, 2010 (Dec.) [Journal].
608. Djoussé *et al.*, 2010 (Sept.) [Journal].
609. Buijsse *et al.*, 2010 [Journal].
610. (2013), http://extras.bhf.org/heartstats [Internet].
611. (2018), https://giftshop.bhf.org.uk/dechox [Internet].
612. Matsumura *et al.*, 2014 [Journal].
613. Grassi *et al.*, 2008 & 2005 [Journals]; Muniyappa *et al.*, 2008 [Journal]; Davison *et al.*, 2008 [Journal]; Faridi *et al.*, 2008 [Journal].
614. Mellor & Nuamovski, 2016 [Journal].
615. Modell & Darlison, 2008 [Journal].
616. Drake *et al.*, 2007 [Journal].
617. Crichton, Elias, & Alkerwi, 2016 [Journal].
618. Moreira *et al.*, 2016 [Journal].
619. Visioli *et al.*, in Paoletti *et al.*, 2012 [Book].
620. Wang *et al.*, 2014 [Journal].
621. Loffredo & Violi, in Paoletti *et al.*, 2012 [Book].
622. Francis *et al.*, 2006 [Journal].
623. Mastroiacovo *et al.*, 2014 [Journal].
624. Visioli *et al.*, in Paoletti *et al.*, 2012 [Book].
625. Bisson *et al.*, 2008 [Journal]; Matsumura *et al.*, 2014 [Journal].
626. Grassi *et al.*, 2016 [Journal].
627. Messerli, 2012 [Journal].
628. Becker *et al.*, 2013 [Internet].
629. Stark *et al.*, 2008 [Journal].
630. Usmani *et al.*, 2005 [Journal].
631. Barnes, 2013 [Journal].
632. Simons *et al.*, 1985 [Journal].
633. Erkkola *et al.*, 2012.
634. Triche *et al.*, 2008 [Journal]; Saftlas *et al.*, 2010 [Journal].
635. (2019), https://forums.horseandhound.co.uk [Internet].
636. Misztal *et al.*, 2010 [Journal].
637. *Ibid.*
638. Eggleston & White, from Watson *et al.*, 2013 [Book].
639. *Ibid.*
640. *Ibid.*
641. Reiche, Nunes, & Marimoto, 2004 [Journal].
642. Reuter *et al.*, 2010 [Journal].
643. Shacter & Weitzman, 2002 [Journal].
644. Wirtz *et al.*, 2014 [Journal].
645. Osakabe *et al.*, 2009 [Journal].
646. Goya *et al.*, 2016 [Journal].
647. Ohno *et al.*, 2009 [Journal]; Yamagishi *et al.*, 2002 [Journal].

648.   Loffredo & Violi, in Paoletti *et al.*, 2012 [Book].
649.   Ramiro-Puig & Castell, 2009 [Journal].
650.   Nakamura *et al.*, 1999 [Journal].
651.   Silva, Simeoni & Silveira, 2009 [Journal].
652.   Carnésecchi *et al.*, 2002 [Journal].
653.   Baharum *et al.*, 2014 [Journal].
654.   Fredholm *et al.*, 1999 [Journal].
655.   Barnes, 2013 [Journal].
656.   Copeland *et al.*, 2005 [Journal].
657.   Girish *et al.*, 2009 [Journal].
658.   Wahby *et al.*, 2012 [Journal]; Kemparaju *et al.*, 2006 [Journal].
659.   Neukam *et al.*, 2007 [Journal].
660.   Heinrich *et al.*, 2006 [Journal].
661.   Williams, Tamburic, & Lally, 2009 [Journals].
662.   Buijsse *et al.*, 2006 [Journal].
663.   Eggleston & White, from Watson *et al.*, 2013 [Book].
664.   Epel *et al.*, 2004 [Journal].
665.   Martin *et al.*, 2009 [Journal].
666.   Farhat *et al.*, 2014 [Journal].
667.   *Ibid.*

Chapter Five

668.   Coe & Coe, 1996 [Book].
669.   9 April 2008: Interview with stallholders at Santeria stall "El Elefante", Mercado de Sonora, D.F., Mexico.
670.   Castell *et al.*, in Watson *et al.*, 2013 [Book].
671.   Scholey & Owen, 2013 [Journal].
672.   Fredholm *et al.*, 1999 [Journal].
673.   Smit, 2011 [Book].
674.   Smit, Gaffan & Rogers, 2004 [Journal].
675.   Baggot *et al.*, 2013 [Journal].
676.   Smit, in Fredholm, 2011 [Book].
677.   *Ibid.*
678.   Haertzen & Hickey, in Bozarth, 1987 [Book].
679.   Nasser *et al.*, 2011 [Journal].
680.   Haertzen & Hickey, in Bozarth, 1987 [Book].
681.   Nasser *et al.*, 2011 [Journal].
682.   van Ree, in Niesink *et al.*, 1999 [Book].
683.   Scholey & Owen, 2013 [Journal].
684.   Castell *et al.*, in Watson *et al.*, 2013 [Book].
685.   Meier, Noll & Molokwu, 2017 [Journal].
686.   Massee *et al.*, 2015 [Journal].

687. Pase *et al.*, 2013 [Journal].

688. Rose, Koperski & Golomb, 2010 [Journal].

689. Parker & Brotchie, in Paoletti *et al.*, 2012 [Book].

690. *Ibid.*

691. Borawska, from Sikorski, 2006 [Book].

692. Schuman, Gitlin and Fairbanks, 1987 [Journal].

693. Yu *et al.*, 2012 [Journal].

694. Yamada *et al.*, 2009 [Journal].

695. Rusconi *et al.*, in Paoletti *et al.*, 2012 [Book].

696. Wirtz *et al.*, 2014 [Journal].

697. Martin *et al.*, 2009 [Journal].

698. Becker *et al.*, 2013 [Journal].

699. Parker & Brotchie, in Paoletti *et al.*, 2012 [Book].

700. Yamada *et al.*, 2009 [Journal].

701. Graeff, Netto, & Zangrossi, 1998 [Journal].

702. Smeets *et al.*, 2006 [Journal].

703. Drexler *et al.*, 2015 [Journal].

704. Thomson, 2012 [Internet].

705. 26 January 2011: Interview with "Cacao shaman" Keith Wilson, San Marcos La Laguna, Lake Atitlan, Guatemala [Appendix C, Interview 3].

706. Sathyapalan *et al.*, 2010 [Journal].

707. Chatzitoffis *et al.*, 2013 [Journal].

708. Räikkönen *et al.*, 2004 [Journal].

709. *Ibid.*

710. McIntosh, Kubena, & Landmann, in Szogyi, 1997 [Book].

711. Strandberg *et al.*, 2008 [Journal].

712. *Ibid.*

713. Galli, in Paoletti *et al.*, 2012 [Book].

714. Møller, 1992 [Journal].

715. Morrison & Tweedy, in Morrison, 2000 [Book].

716. Willeit *et al.*, 2003 [Journal].

717. "Chris", 2006 [Internet].

718. Airaksinen, Ho, An, & Taylor, 1978 [Journal].

719. Trilling, 1999 [Book].

720. Fredholm *et al.*, 1999 [Journal].

721. Xie, Krnjević, & Ye, 2013 [Journal]; Airaksinen *et al.*, 1984 [Journal].

722. Stone, 2011 [Journal].

723. Rusconi *et al.*, in Paoletti *et al.*, 2012 [Book].

724. Duke, 1983 [Internet].

725. Shulgin & Shulgin, 2013 [Book].

726. Bodor & Farag, 1983 [Journal].

727. Sabelli *et al.*, 1978 [Journal].

728. Berry, 2004 [Journal].

729. di Tomaso, Beltramo & Piomelli, 1996 [Journal].
730. (2012), lipidlibrary.aocs.org [Internet].
731. (2017), https://chronichives.com [Internet].
732. Panneerselvam *et al.*, 2010 [Journal].
733. Stefano & Kream, 2011 [Journal].
734. Bershad *et al.*, 2016 [Book].
735. Parrott, 2001 [Journal].
736. Parrott *et al.*, 2014 [Journal].
737. Zucchi *et al.*, 2006 [Journal].
738. Amoroso & Workman, 2016 [Journal].
739. Saunders, 1996 [Book].
740. McGuire, 2000 [Journal]; Morgan *et al.*, 2002 [Journal].
741. Robledo *et al.*, 2004 [Journal].
742. Battaglia *et al.*, 1988 [Journal].
743. Rodríguez-Arias *et al.*, 2013 [Journal].
744. Diaz del Castillo, 1982 ex. Coe, 1994 [Book].
745. Robert, 1957 [Book].
746. *Ibid.*
747. *Ibid.*
748. Rosen *et al.*, 2000 [Journal].
749. Salonia *et al.*, 2006 [Journal].
750. Smit, in Fredholm, 2011.
751. (2016), https://pubchem.ncbi.nlm.nih.gov [Internet]; Stammel *et al.*, 1991 [Journal].
752. Smit, in Fredholm, 2011 [Book].
753. Schiavi *et al.*, 1990 [Journal].
754. Miner *et al.*, 2012 [Journal].
755. Asprey, 2016 [Internet].
756. Kamatenesi-Mugisha & Oryem-Origa, 2005 [Journal].
757. 18 April 2008: Interview with Señor Mario Euan, senior teacher at U-Yits-Ka'an school of Agriculture and Ecology in Mani, Yucatan, Mexico. [Appendix C, Interview 1].
758. Rawson, 2013 [Journal].
759. Kohl & Francoeur, 1995 [Book].
760. Fisher, Aron, & Brown, 2005 [Journal].
761. McManamy, 2011 [Internet].
762. Fisher, 1998 [Journal].
763. Ott *et al.*, 2013 [Journal].
764. Sims, 2010 [Internet].
765. (2014), www.cdc.gov/violenceprevention/acestudy [Internet].
766. Esch & Stefano, 2005 [Journal].
767. *Ibid.*
768. *Ibid.*
769. Baskerville & Douglas, 2010 [Journal].
770. Winick-Ng, Leri, & Kalisch, 2012 [Journal].

771. Heinzen, Booth, & Pollack, 2005 [Journal].

772. Hervera *et al.*, 2011 [Journal].

773. Winick-Ng, Leri, & Kalisch, 2012 [Journal].

774. Barnes, 2013 [Journal].

775. Esch & Stefano, 2005 [Journal].

776. Luce *et al.*, 2014 [Journal].

777. di Feliceantonio *et al.*, 2012 [Journal].

778. Sathe *et al.*, 2001 [Journal].

779. Hawkes, 1992 [Journal].

780. Kruger *et al.*, 1998 [Journal], & Exton *et al.*, 1999 [Journal].

781. Soaje & Dreis, 2004 [Journal]; Bowen *et al.*, 2002 [Journal].

782. Gordon *et al.*, 2010 [Journal].

783. Larsen & Grattan, 2012 [Journal].

784. Misztal *et al.*, 2010 [Journal].

785. Carlson *et al.*, 1985 [Journal].

786. Farah, Zaibunnisa, & Misnawi, 2012 [Journal].

787. Esch & Stefano, 2005 [Journal].

788. Dreiss & Greenhill, 2008 [Book].

789. Coe & Coe, 1996 [Book].

Chapter Six

790. Holzmann *et al.*, 2014 [Journal].

791. Bucay, 2002 [Journal].

792. Coe & Coe, 1996 [Book].

793. Xu & Kong, 2017 [Journal].

794. Vilar *et al.*, 2014 [Journal]; 18 April 2008: Interview with Sr Mario Euan, herbalist and teacher at U-Yits-Ka'an school of Agriculture and Ecology; Mani, Yucatan Peninsula, Mexico. [Appendix C, Interview 1.]

795. Chen *et al.*, 2013 [Journal].

796. Bucay, 2002 [Journal].

797. Dzib-Guerra *et al.*, 2016 [Journal], Gutierrez *et al.*, 2010 [Journal]; Gonzalez, Gutierrez, & Cotera, 2014 [Internet].

798. Gonzalez, Gutierrez, & Cotera, 2014 [Internet].

799. Hänsel & Leuschke, 1975 [Journal].

800. Abbey *et al.*, 2008 [Journal].

801. Zhang & Lokeshwar, 2012 [Journal].

802. Badiano, 1552 [Book]; Holzmann *et al.*, 2014 [Journal].

803. Da Silva & Alba, 2004 [Internet].

804. Shinde, Patil, & Bairagi, 2014 [Journal].

805. Alencar *et al.*, 2015 [Internet]; Shinde, Patil, & Bairagi, 2014 [Journal].

806. Shinde, Patil, & Bairagi, 2014 [Journal].

807. Das *et al.*, 2013 [Journal]; Alencar *et al.*, 2015 [Internet]; Mondal *et al.*, 2016 [Journal].

808. Badiano, 1552 [Book].
809. Shinde, Patil, & Bairagi, 2014 [Journal].
810. (2017), Flor de Mayo, http://maya-ethnobotany.org [Internet].
811. Nishino *et al.*, 2015 [Journal].
812. Ezekiel & Oluwole, 2014 [Journal].
813. Hernández, 1615 [Book].
814. Fernandez Garcia *et al.*, 2005 [Journal].
815. Zhang & Mueller, 2012 [Journal]; Shanmugavalli, Umashankar, & Raheem, 2009 [Journal].
816. Xu *et al.*, 2015 [Journal].
817. Chen *et al.*, 2013 [Journal].
818. Raffauf & Zennie, 1993 [Journal].
819. Ho *et al.*, 2011 [Journal].
820. Yan *et al.*, 2017 [Journal].
821. Menon & Nayeem, 2013 [Journal]; Srinual, Chanvorachote, & Pongrakhananon, 2017 [Journal].
822. Zhang & Lokeshwar, 2012 [Journal].
823. Zhang *et al.*, 2015 [Journal]; Shamaladevi *et al.*, 2013 [Journal].
824. Shinde, Patil, & Bairagi, 2014 [Journal].
825. Clark & Lee, 2016 [Journal].
826. Núñez *et al.*, 2004 [Journal].
827. Chen *et al.*, 2013 [Journal].
828. Silva, Simeoni, & Silveira, 2009 [Journal]; (2018), *Pouteria sapota*, http://pfaf.org [Internet].
829. 18 April 2008: Interview with Sr Mario Euan, herbalist and teacher at U-Yits-Ka'an school of Agriculture and Ecology, Mani, Yucatan Peninsula, Mexico. [Appendix C, Interview 1.]
830. Vilar *et al.*, 2014 [Journal]; Ferreira *et al.*, 2013 [Journal].
831. McCarty, DiNicolantonio, & O'Keefe, 2015 [Journal].
832. Shinde, Patil, & Bairagi, 2014 [Journal].
833. Tzounis *et al.*, 2010 [Journal].
834. Alanis *et al.*, 2005 [Journal].
835. Calzada, Yepez-Mulia, & Aguilar, 2006.
836. *Ibid.*
837. Gonzalez *et al.*, 2014 [Journal].
838. Velazquez *et al.*, 2009 [Journal]; Calzada *et al.*, 2017 [Journal].
839. Calzada *et al.*, 2017 [Journal].
840. Stubbe, 1662 [Book]; Hernández, 1615 [Book].
841. Hernández, 1615 [Book]; Williams, 2003 [Book]; Marzouk *et al.*, 2007 [Journal].
842. Fontaine *et al.*, 2016 [Journal].
843. Tsuruma *et al.*, 2012 [Journal].
844. (2016), European Food Safety Authority [Internet].
845. Chopan & Littenberg, 2017 [Journal].
846. Buijsse *et al.*, 2006 [Journal].
847. Pepling, 2003 [Internet].
848. Chiarini, 2013 [Internet].
849. Kennedy, 2010 [Book].

ENDNOTES 405

850. Shinde, Patil, & Bairagi, 2014 [Journal].

850. Shinde, Patil, & Bairagi, 2014 [Journal].
851. Monroy-Ortiz & Castillo-Espana, 2007 [Book]; Badiano, 1552 [Book]; Bone, 2003 [Book].
852. Ban *et al.*, 2008 [Journal]; Ban, Jeon *et al.*, 2006 [Journal]; Ban, Cho *et al.*, 2006 [Journal]; Shao *et al.*, 2007 [Journal]; She, Zhao *et al.*, 2015 [Journal]; She *et al.*, 2015 [Journal]; Sa *et al.*, 2008 [Journal]; Li *et al.*, 2007 [Journal].
853. Jiang & Xu, 2003 [Journal]; Williams, 2003 [Book]; Bone, 2003 [Book]; She *et al.*, 2015 [Journal].
854. Bone, 2003 [Book].
855. Trilling, 1999 [Book].
856. Kennedy, 2010 [Book].
857. Trilling, 1999 [Book].
858. 8 October 2018: Interview with *Popo* maker Doña Matei and her mother, Hueyapan de Ocampo, Veracruz, Mexico.
859. Trilling, 1999 [Book]; 22 February 2011: Interview with *Popo* vendor, Acuyacan, Veracruz, Mexico.
860. Lam *et al.*, 2014 [Journal].
861. Coe & Coe, 1996 [Book].
862. (2009), http://bpi.da.gov.ph [Internet].
863. Shulgin & Shulgin, 2013 [Book].
864. Bletter & Daly, in McNeil, 2006 [Book].
865. *Ibid.*
866. Passie *et al.*, 2002 [Journal].
867. *Ibid.*
868. *Ibid.*
869. Curran, Nut, & DeWit, 2018 [Journal].
870. Francis *et al.*, 2006 [Journal].
871. Raffauf & Zennie, 1993 [Journal].
872. Ott, 1996 [Book].
873. De La Garza, *ex*. Lacy & Orellana, 2017 [Periodical].
874. Ott, 1996 [Book].
875. Williams, 2003 [Book].
876. Spinella, 2001 [Book].
877. Schultes & Hofmann, 1992 [Book].

Chapter Seven

878. Coe & Coe, 1996 [Book].
879. Paoletti *et al.*, 2012 [Book].
880. Coe & Coe, 1996 [Book].
881. Pech, 2010 [Book].
882. Golf, Bender, & Grüttner, 1998 [Journal].
883. Drewnowski, 1992 [Journal].
884. Parker & Brotchie, in Paoletti *et al.*, 2012 [Book].
885. Fredholm *et al.*, 1999 [Journal].

886. Sinha, 2008 [Journal].
887. *Ibid.*
888. Hadaway *et al.*, 1979 [Journal].
889. Alexander, 2010 [Internet].
890. Van der Kolk, 2014 [Journal].
891. *Ibid.*
892. Yanovski, 2003 [Journal].
893. Moss, 2013 [Book].
894. *Ibid.*
895. Colantuoni *et al.*, 2001 [Journal].
896. Choi & Diehl, 2008 [Journal].
897. Taubes, 2017 [Book].
898. Hanhineva *et al.*, 2010 [Journal].
899. Petta, Marchesini, & Craxi, 2014 [Journal].
900. *Ibid.*
901. Djoussé *et al.*, 2010 [Sept.]
902. Parker & Brotchie, in Paoletti *et al.*, 2012 [Book].
903. Peciña, Schulkin, & Berridge, 2006 [Journal].
904. Djoussé *et al.*, 2010 [Sept.]
905. Castell *et al.*, from Watson *et al.*, 2013 [Book].
906. Moss, 2013 [Book].
907. (2016), http://pcrm.org [Internet].
908. Kurek *et al.*, 1996 [Journal].
909. Takahashi, 2000 [Journal].
910. Ji, 2012b [Internet].
911. H.T., 2013 [Internet].
912. Parker, Parker, & Brotchie, 2006 [Journal].
913. Yuker, in Szogyi, 1997 [Book].
914. Macht & Dettmer, 2006 [Journal].
915. Hetherington & MacDiarmid, 1993 [Journal].
916. Parker & Brotchie, in Paoletti *et al.*, 2012 [Book].
917. Zellner *et al.*, 2004 [Journal].
918. Molinari & Callus, in Paoletti *et al.*, 2012 [Book].
919. Quertemont & Didone, 2013 [Journal].
920. Smit, 2011 [Book].
921. Rusconi *et al.*, in Paoletti *et al.*, 2012 [Book].
922. *Ibid.*
923. Fredholm *et al.*, 1999 [Journal].
924. Zaru *et al.*, 2013 [Journal].
925. *Ibid.*
926. Thomson, 2012 [Internet].
927. Giuliano *et al.*, 2012 [Journal].
928. Pech, 2010 [Book].

929. Molinari & Callus, in Paoletti *et al.*, 2012 [Book].
930. Massolt *et al.*, 2010 [Journal].
931. Elliott, in Szogyi, 1997 [Book].
932. *Ibid.*
933. Bohon & Stice, 2012 [Journal].
934. Tryon, LeCant & Laugero, 2013 [Journal].
935. Parker & Brotchie in Paoletti *et al.*, 2012 [Book].
936. Martin *et al.*, 2012 [Journal].
937. Drewnowski *et al.*, 1992 [Journal].
938. Wilson, 2012 [Internet].
939. Schifano & Magni, 1994 [Journal].
940. *Ibid.*
941. Price *et al.*, 1989 [Journal].
942. Drago, 1990 [Journal].
943. Monteleone *et al.*, 1998 [Journal].
944. Schifano & Magni, 1994 [Journal].
945. Gluck *et al.*, 2004 [Journal].
946. Miller, 2017.
947. *Ibid.*
948. Aremu & Abara, 1992 [Journal].
949. Dahiya *et al.*, 2005 [Journal].
950. Rankin *et al.*, 2005 [Journal].
951. Mounicou *et al.*, 2002 [Journal].
952. (1997), http://inchem.org [Internet].
953. Lawley, 2013 [Internet].
954. *Ibid.*
955. Turcotte, Scott, & Tague, 2013 [Journal].
956. Smit, 2011 [Book].
957. Hodgson *et al.*, 2008 [Journal].
958. Smit, 2011 [Book].
959. Fuhr *et al.*, 2006 [Journal].
960. Wang *et al.*, 2010 [Journal].
961. Giannandrea, 2009 [Journal].
962. *Ibid.*
963. Orozco, Wang, & Keen, 2003 [Journal].
964. Bisson *et al.*, 2008 [Journal].
965. Slattery & West, 1993 [Journal].
966. *Ibid.*
967. Wolz *et al.*, 2009 [Journal].
968. Visioli *et al.*, in Paoletti *et al.*, 2102 [Book].
969. Bisson *et al.*, 2008 [Journal].
970. Vauzour *et al.*, 2008 [Journal].
971. Teraoka *et al.*, 2012 [Journal].

972. Xue *et al.*, 2011 [Journal]; Guan *et al.*, 2011 [Journal].

973. Kao *et al.*, 2006 [Journal]; Tohda *et al.*, 1999 [Journal]; Cornacchia *et al.*, 2012 [Journal].

974. Wolz *et al.*, 2012 [Journal].

975. Lannuzel *et al.*, 2006 [Journal].

976. Borah *et al.*, 2013 [Journal].

977. Kang, 2007 [Journal].

978. Seale *et al.*, 2012 [Journal].

979. Ichikawa *et al.*, 2006 [Journal].

980. Cao *et al.*, 2007 [Journal].

981. Airaksinen & Kari, 1981 [Journal].

982. Louis & Zeng, 2010 [Journal].

983. Nishino *et al.*, 2011 [Journal].

984. Smit, 2011 [Book].

985. Ascherio *et al.*, 2006 [Internet].

986. Rose, Hodak, & Bernholc, 2011 [Journal].

987. Miyake, 2011 [Journal].

988. Mariani *et al.*, 2013 [Journal].

989. Kristinsson, 2012 [Journal].

990. Collins, Prohaska, & Knutson, 2010 [Journal].

991. Fukushima *et al.*, 2011 [Journal].

992. Bahadorani & Hilliker, 2008 [Journal].

993. Robert, 1957 [Book].

994. (2017), https://chronichives.com [Internet].

995. *Ibid.*

996. Firth & Smith, 1964 [Journal].

997. Abril-Gil *et al.*, 2012 [Journal].

998. Robert, 1957 [Book].

999. Ramiro-Puig *et al.*, 2008 [Journal].

1000. Abri-Gil *et al.*, 2016 [Journal].

1001. Farhat *et al.*, 2014 [Journal].

1002. Park *et al.*, 1979 [Journal].

1003. Ramiro-Puig & Castell, 2009 [Journal]; Pérez-Berezo *et al.*, 2009 [Journal].

1004. Camps-Bossacoma *et al.*, 2017 [Journal].

1005. Tzounis *et al.*, 2010 [Journal].

1006. Leggett, 2017 [Internet].

1007. Robert, 1957 [Book].

1008. Goadsby, 2012 [Journal].

1009. D'Andrea *et al.*, 2013 [Journal].

1010. Hanington, 1967 [Journal].

1011. Robert, 1957 [Book].

1012. Pech, 2010 [Book].

1013. 9 April 2008: Interview with stallholders at *Esperancita* herb stall, Mercado de Sonora, Mexico City.

1014. Eggleston & White, in Watson, Preedy, & Zibadi, 2013 [Book].

1015. Robert, 1957 [Book].

1016. Lippi, Mattuzzi, & Cervellin, 2014 [Journal].

1017. Singh, Reddy, & Kundukulam, 2011 [Journal].

1018. Schlesinger, 2010 [Journal].

1019. Pech, 2010 [Book].

1020. Cordero *et al.*, 2013 [Journal].

1021. Ozgocmen *et al.*, 2006 [Journal].

1022. McPartland, 2008 [Journal].

1023. Holton, 2016 [Internet].

1024. Xie, Krnjević & Ye, 2013 [Journal].

1025. Okiyama *et al.*, 1995 [Journal].

1026. Yazawa *et al.*, 2006 [Journal].

1027. Morrison, 2012 [Internet].

1028. Galland, 2014 [Journal].

1029. Sadaf, Raza, & Hassan, 2017 [Journal].

1030. Check *et al.*, 2008 [Journal].

1031. Costa de Miranda *et al.*, 2016 [Journal].

1032. Lohsiriwat, Puengna, & Leelakusolvong, 2006 [Journal].

1033. Fulton, Plewig, & Kilgman, 1969 [Journal].

1034. Karadağ *et al.*, 2017 [Journal].

1035. Chalyk *et al.*, 2018 [Journal].

Chapter Eight

1036. Berdan & Anawalt, 1997 [Book].

1037. De Ledesma, 1631 [Book].

1038. Culpeper, 1655 [Book].

1039. 12 October 2018: Interview with Sra Rocío Torres Torres, agronomist-technician at AMCO, Tapachula, Chiapas, Mexico.

1040. (2019), https://worldlifeexpectancy.com [Internet].

1041. Jaffé, 2015 [Journal].

1042. Momtazi-Borojeni *et al.*, 2017 [Journal].

1043. Carrera-Lanestosa, Moguel-Ordoóñez, & Segura-Campos, 2017 [Journal].

1044. Field notes, J-P, October 2018, Tapachula, Chiapas, Mexico; and personal correspondence, March 2019.

1045. Robert, 1957 [Book].

1046. Steinbrenner, in McNeil, 2006 [Book].

1047. Coe & Coe, 1996 [Book].

1048. Hernández, trans. Ximenez, 1615 [Internet].

1049. 18 February 2011: Interview with lime vendor in Ocotlan market, Oaxaca, Mexico.

1050. Kennedy, 2010 [Book].

1051. Coe, 1994 [Book].

1052.   12 April 2008: Interview with herbalist Tomas Villanueva, Puyucatengo, Mexico.

1053.   20 April 2008: Interview with tour guide Claudia at Hacienda La Luz, Comalcalco, Tabasco, Mexico.

1054.   Romero-Luna, Hernández-Sánchez, & Dávila-Ortiz, 2017 [Journal].

1055.   Cano, Aguilar, & Hernández, 2013 [Journal].

1056.   26 January 2011: Interview with Señora Lopreto, *Panecito* and *Pinole* maker, San Antonio Suchitequepez, Guatemala.

1057.   Santos & DaSIlva, 2018 [Journal].

1058.   Popenoe, 1919 [Journal].

1059.   Kennedy, 2010 [Book]; and 21 September 2018: Interview with Doña Carina Santiago, restaurateur, chef and owner of *Tierra Antigua* restaurant, Teotitlan del Valle, Oaxaca, Mexico.

1060.   21 September 2018: Interview with Carina Santiago, chef and owner of Tierra Antigua restaurant, with her student, Kalisa Wells. Teotitlán del Valle, Oaxaca, Mexico.

1061.   Field notes, Oaxaca, Mexico, 2008.

1062.   28 September 2018: Interview with Sra. Delfina Valverde, msker of Chaw Popox, San Mateo del Mar, Oaxaca, Mexico.

1063.   Kennedy, 2010 [Book].

1064.   26 September 2018: Interview with Señora Anna Maria Garcia Vasquez, market vendor and maker of *Bu'pu*, Juchitan de Zaragoza, Oaxaca, Mexico.

1065.   *Ibid.*

1066.   Trilling, 1999 [Book].

1067.   Kennedy, 2010 [Book].

1068.   22 Feb 2011: Interview with vendor of Popo in Acayucan, Veracruz, Mexico; and 8 October 2018: Interview with Doña Maria Eugenia Navarrete Matei, Heyapan de Ocampo, Veracruz, Mexico.

1069.   2 October 2018: Interview with Doña Rosa Gregorio, vendor of Popo, Tuxtepec and Ojitlan, Oaxaca, Mexico.

1070.   Coe & Coe, 1996 [Book].

1071.   Popenoe, 1919 [Journal].

1072.   *Ibid.*

1073.   Sahagún, quoted by Coe, in Szogyi, 1997 [Book].

1074.   26 January 2011: Interview with Señora Lopreto, Panecito and Pinole maker, San Antonio Suchitequepez, Guatemala (with my guide and Cacao expert, Juan-Pablo Porres Esquina).

1075.   14 October 2018: Interview with Señora Ernestina Tawal, market vendor, San Antonio Suchitequepez, Suchitequepez, Guatemala.

1076.   Sahagún, quoted in Grivetti, from Grivetti & Shapiro, 2009 [Book].

1077.   Coe & Coe, 1996 [Book].

1078.   Robert, 1957 [Book].

1079.   *Ibid.*

1080.   Hernández, *trans.* Ximenez, 1615 [Internet].

1081.   Coe, 1994 [Book]; Coe & Coe, 1996 [Book].

1082.   De Ledesma, 1631 [Book].

1083.   Coe & Coe, 1996 [Book].

1084. Verified by personal experiment from *Bourreria huanita* flowers picked in Juchitan de Zaragoza, October 2019.

1085. Coe, 1994 [Book].

1086. Brillat-Savarin, quoted in Robert, 1957 [Book].

1087. Taha, 1992 [Journal].

1088. Taha, Islam, & Ageel, 1995 [Journal].

1089. Raza, Alorainy, & Algasham, 2007 [Journal].

1090. Brillat-Savarin, *quoted by* Szogyi, in Szogyi, 1997.

Chapter Nine

1091. Léon-Portilla, 1992 [Book].

1092. Coe & Coe, 1996 [Book].

1093. Chevalier & Bain, 2002 [Book].

1094. Tedlock, B., 1992 [Book].

1095. Chevalier & Bain, 2002 [Book].

1096. Boone, 2007 [Book].

1097. Miller & Taube, 1993 [Book].

1098. Chevalier & Bain, 2002 [Book].

1099. Mach, hosted by White, 2018 [Podcast].

1100. Tedlock, B., 1992 [Book].

1101. Freidel, Schele, & Parker, 1993 [Book].

1102. Léon-Portilla, 1992 [Book].

1103. Miller & Taube, 1993 [Book].

1104. *Ibid*.

1105. *Ibid*.

1106. Tedlock, B., 1992 [Book].

1107. Miller & Taube, 1993 [Book].

1108. *Ibid*.

1109. *Ibid*.

1110. Bassett, 2008 [Internet].

1111. Chevalier & Bain, 2002 [Book].

1112. Miller & Taube, 1993 [Book].

1113. Freidel, Schele, & Parker, 1993 [Book].

1114. Bassett, 2008 [Internet].

1115. Bassett, 2008 [Internet].

1116. Léon-Portilla, 1992 [Book].

1117. Coe, 1994 [Book].

1118. Austin, 2004 [Journal].

1119. de la Graza, in Orellana & Sanchez Lacy, 2017 [Periodical].

1120. Miller & Taube, 1993 [Book].

1121. *Ibid*.

1122. Miller & Taube, 1993 [Book].

1123.   Austin, 2004 [Journal].

1124.   *Ibid.*

1125.   Freidel, Schele, & Parker, 1993 [Book].

1126.   *Ibid.*

1127.   *Ibid.*

1128.   Miller & Taube, 1993 [Book].

1129.   *Ibid.*

1130.   Hays-Gilpin & Hill, 1999 [Journal].

1131.   *Ibid.*

1132.   Miller & Taube, 1993 [Book].

1133.   Austin, 2004 [Journal].

1134.   Hamnett, 1999 [Book].

1135.   Milbrath, 1999 [Book].

1136.   Graulich, 2004 [Journal].

1137.   *Ibid.*

1138.   Cheak, in Coppock & Schulke, 2018 [Book].

1139.   Freidel, Schele, & Parker, 1993 [Book].

1140.   Sterger, 2010 [Thesis].

1141.   Freidel, Schele, & Parker, 1993 [Book].

1142.   Tedlock, B., 1992 [Book].

1143.   Austin, 2004 [Journal].

1144.   *Ibid.*

1145.   Freidel, Schele, & Parker, 1993 [Book].

1146.   *Ibid.*

1147.   *Ibid.*

1148.   *Ibid.*

1149.   Austin, 2004 [Journal].

1150.   Glockner, 2004 [Periodical].

1151.   Freidel, Schele, & Parker, 1993 [Book].

1152.   Freidel, Schele, & Parker, 1993 [Book].

1153.   Freidel, Schele, & Parker, 1993 [Book].

1154.   Dreiss & Greenhill, 2008 [Book].

1155.   Freidel, Schele, & Parker, 1993 [Book].

1156.   Dreiss & Greenhill, 2008 [Book].

1157.   Miller & Taube, 1993 [Book].

1158.   Boone, 2007 [Book].

1159.   Boone, 2007 [Book].

1160.   *Ibid.*

1161.   Freidel, Schele, & Parker, 1993 [Book].

1162.   Miller & Taube, 1993 [Book].

1163.   Tedlock, D., 1996 [Book].

1164.   *Ibid.*

1165.   *Ibid.*

1166.   *Ibid.*
1167.   Coe & Coe, 1996 [Book].
1168.   Tedlock, D., 1996 [Book]; Freidel, Schele, & Parker, 1993 [Book].
1169.   Freidel, Schele, & Parker, 1993 [Book].
1170.   Tedlock, D., 1996 [Book].
1171.   Freidel, Schele, & Parker, 1993 [Book].
1172.   *Ibid.*
1173.   Boone, 2007 [Book].
1174.   Miller & Taube, 1993 [Book].
1175.   Vail, in Grivetti & Shapiro, 2009 [Book].
1176.   Miller & Taube, 1993 [Book].
1177.   Dreiss & Greenhill, 2008 [Book].
1178.   Miller & Taube, 1993 [Book].
1179.   Freidel, Schele, & Parker, 1993 [Book].
1180.   Hamnett, 1999 [Book].
1181.   Milbrath, 1999 [Book].
1182.   Chevalier & Bain, 2002 [Book]; Grofe, 2007 [Thesis].
1183.   Miller & Taube, 1993 [Book].
1184.   Miller & Taube, 1993 [Book].
1185.   Miller & Taube, 1993 [Book].
1186.   *Ibid.*
1187.   *Ibid.*
1188.   Coe & Coe, 1996 [Book].
1189.   Freidel, Schele, & Parker, 1993 [Book].
1190.   *Ibid.*
1191.   Freidel, Schele, & Parker, 1993 [Book].
1192.   Milbrath, 1999 [Book].
1193.   *Ibid.*
1194.   *Ibid.*
1195.   *Ibid.*
1196.   *Ibid.*
1197.   Milbrath, 1999 [Book].
1198.   *Ibid.*
1199.   Freidel, Schele, & Parker, 1993 [Book].
1200.   *Ibid.*
1201.   Miller & Taube, 1993 [Book].
1202.   Freidel, Schele, & Parker, 1993 [Book].
1203.   Milbrath, 1999 [Book].
1204.   *Ibid.*
1205.   Miller & Taube, 1993 [Book].
1206.   Freidel, Schele, & Parker, 1993 [Book].
1207.   Milbrath, 1999 [Book].
1208.   *Ibid.*

1209. Miller & Taube, 1993 [Book].
1210. Milbrath, 1999 [Book].
1211. *Ibid.*
1212. *Ibid.*
1213. Tedlock, D., 1996 [Book].
1214. Milbrath, 1999 [Book].
1215. *Ibid.*
1216. *Ibid.*
1217. Miller & Taube, 1993 [Book].
1218. Milbrath, 1999 [Book].
1219. Miller & Taube, 1993 [Book].
1220. Freidel, Schele, & Parker, 1993 [Book].
1221. Miller & Taube, 1993 [Book].
1222. *Ibid.*
1223. Tedlock, B., 1992 [Book].
1224. Reston, 2003 [Book].
1225. Freidel, Schele, & Parker, 1993 [Book].
1226. Sterger, 2010 [Thesis].
1227. Freidel, Schele, & Parker, 1993 [Book].
1228. Miller & Taube, 1993 [Book].
1229. Milbrath, 1999 [Book].
1230. Hays-Gilpin & Hill, 1999 [Journal].
1231. Freidel, Schele, & Parker, 1993 [Book].
1232. Miller & Taube, 1993 [Book].
1233. Sterger, 2010 [Thesis].
1234. Boone, 2007 [Book].
1235. Coe, 1994 [Book].
1236. Graulich, 2004 [Journal].
1237. Ott, 1996 [Book].
1238. Sterger, 2010 [Thesis].
1239. *Ibid.*
1240. *Ibid.*
1241. Milbrath, 1999 [Book].
1242. Boone, 2007 [Book].
1243. Grofe, 2007 [Thesis].
1244. Dreiss & Greenhill, 2008 [Book].
1245. Tedlock, D., 1996 [Book].
1246. Grivetti & Cabezon, in Grivetti & Shapiro, 2009 [Book].
1247. Cano, 2009 [Internet].
1248. Grivetti & Cabezon, in Grivetti & Shapiro, 2009 [Book].
1249. Dreiss & Greenhill, 2008 [Book].
1250. *Ibid.*
1251. Martin, *from* McNeil, 2006.

1252.   Dreiss & Greenhill, 2008 [Book].
1253.   Grivetti & Cabezon, in Grivetti & Shapiro, 2009 [Book].
1254.   *Ibid.*
1255.   Martin, in McNeil, 2006 [Book].
1256.   *Ibid.*
1257.   *Ibid.*
1258.   Dreiss & Greenhill, 2008 [Book].
1259.   Kufer & Heinrich, in McNeil, 2006 [Book].
1260.   Tedlock, D., 1996 [Book].
1261.   Miller & Taube, 1993 [Book].
1262.   Henderson & Joyce, in McNeil, 2006 [Book].
1263.   Reents-Budet, in McNeil, 2006 [Book].
1264.   Dreiss & Greenhill, 2008 [Book].
1265.   Martin, in McNeil, 2006 [Book].
1266.   Freidel, Schele & Parker, 1993 [Book].
1267.   Coe & Coe, 1996 [Book].
1268.   Dreiss & Greenhill, 2008 [Book].
1269.   McNeil, in McNeil, 2006b.
1270.   Dreiss & Greenhill, 2008 [Book].
1271.   Grofe, 2007 [Thesis].
1272.   Freidel, Schele, & Parker, 1993 [Book].
1273.   McNeil, in McNeil, 2006b.
1274.   Grofe, 2007 [Thesis].
1275.   Dreiss & Greenhill, 2008 [Book].
1276.   McNeil, in McNeil, 2006a.
1277.   Dreiss & Greenhill, 2008 [Book].
1278.   Martin, in McNeil, 2006.
1279.   Dreiss & Greenhill, 2008 [Book].
1280.   *Ibid.*
1281.   *Ibid.*
1282.   Miller & Taube, 1993 [Book].
1283.   Mazariegos, 2006 [Booklet].
1284.   Freidel, Schele, & Parker, 1993 [Book].
1285.   *Ibid.*
1286.   Faust & López, in McNeil, 2006 [Book].
1287.   Dreiss & Greenhill, 2008 [Book].
1288.   Coe & Coe, 1996 [Book].
1289.   Miller & Taube, 1993 [Book].
1290.   Reents-Budet, *from* McNeil, 2006.
1291.   Dreiss & Greenhill, 2008 [Book].
1292.   *Ibid.*
1293.   McNeil, in McNeil, 2006b.
1294.   McNeil, in McNeil, 2006b.

1295. Schultes & Hofmann, 1979 [Book].
1296. Glockner, 2004 [Periodical].
1297. Tedlock, B., 1992 [Book].
1298. Stubbe, 1662 [Book].
1299. McNeil, in McNeil, 2006b.
1300. Coe & Coe, 1996 [Book].
1301. Dreiss & Greenhill, 2008 [Book].
1302. Coe & Coe, 1996 [Book].
1303. McNeil, in McNeil, 2006a.
1304. *Ibid.*
1305. Dreiss & Greenhill, 2008 [Book].
1306. *Ibid.*
1307. Coe & Coe, 1996 [Book].
1308. Dreiss & Greenhill, 2008 [Book].
1309. 21 September 2018: Interview with Señora Carmen Olivera, chef and owner of Tierra Antigua restaurant, Teotitlan del Valle, Oaxaca, Mexico.
1310. Dreiss & Greenhill, 2008 [Book].
1311. Stross, 2011 [Journal].
1312. *Ibid.*
1313. Stross, 2011 [Journal].
1314. Kennedy, 2010 [Book].
1315. Coe & Coe, 1996 [Book].
1316. Tlaltecatzin's poem, quoted in Pendell, 2002 [Book]; Léon-Portilla, 1992 [Book].
1317. Grivetti & Cabezon, in Grivetti & Shapiro, 2009 [Book].
1318. Tedlock, D., 1996 [Book].
1319. Faust & López, in McNeil, 2006 [Book].
1320. Martin, in McNeil, 2006.

Chapter Ten

1321. Hanks, 1989 [Book].
1322. Tedlock, 1985 [Book].
1323. Boone, 2007 [Book].
1324. Milbrath, 1999 [Book].
1325. Boone, 2007 [Book].
1326. Miller & Taube, 1993 [Book].
1327. Boone, 2007 [Book].
1328. *Ibid.*
1329. *Ibid.*
1330. *Ibid.*
1331. *Ibid.*
1332. *Ibid.*
1333. Milbrath, 1999 [Book].

1334. *Ibid.*

1335. *Ibid.*

1336. Miller & Taube, 1993 [Book].

1337. Freidel, Schele, & Parker, 1993 [Book].

1338. Milbrath, 1999 [Book].

1339. *Ibid.*

1340. Milbrath, 1999 [Book].

1341. *Ibid.*

1342. *Ibid.*

1343. *Ibid.*

1344. Miller & Taube, 1993 [Book].

1345. Boone, 2007 [Book].

1346. *Ibid.*

1347. Tedlock, B., 1992 [Book].

1348. Tedlock, 1992 [Book].

1349. *Ibid.*

1350. *Ibid.*

1351. Tedlock, 1992 [Book].

1352. de Montellano, 2004 [Journal].

1353. Austin, 2004 [Journal].

1354. 13 February 2011: Interview with Señor Ca 'al, San Luís, Peten, Guatemala [Appendix C, Interview 5].

1355. *Ibid.*

1356. 13 February 2011: Interview with Señor Ca 'al, San Luís, Peten, Guatemala [Appendix C, Interview 5].

1357. *Ibid.*

1358. Alcocer & Neurath, 2004 [Journal].

1359. Austin, 2004 [Journal].

1360. Schultes & Hofmann, 1992 [Book].

1361. Boone, 2007 [Book].

1362. Cortés, 2004 [Journal].

1363. *Ibid.*

1364. Austin, 2004 [Journal].

1365. Austin, 2004 [Journal].

1366. Glockner, 2004 [Periodical].

1367. Tedlock, 1992 [Book].

1368. Glockner, 2004 [Periodical].

1369. Austin, 2004 [Journal].

1370. Schultes & Hofmann, 1992 [Book].

1371. Miller & Taube, 1993 [Book].

1372. Schultes & Hofmann, 1992 [Book].

1373. de la Graza, 2017 [Periodical].

1374. de Orellana, 2017 [Periodical].

1375. Glockner, 2004 [Periodical].

1376. Armstrong, 2006 [Book].

1377. Badiano, 1552 [Book].

1378. Warnock, 2005 [Book].

1379. de Montellano, 2004 [Journal].

1380. Freidel, Schele, & Parker, 1993 [Book].

1381. *Ibid.*

1382. Ibn Qurra, *ed. & trans.* Warnock, 2005 [Book].

1383. Freidel, Schele, & Parker, 1993 [Book].

1384. *Ibid.*

1385. Cotterell, 1999 [Book].

1386. Rudgley, 1998 [Book].

1387. Alcocer & Neurath, 2004 [Journal].

1388. Illes, 2004 [Book].

1389. *Trans.* Greer & Warnock, 2010 [Book].

1390. Tobyn, 1997 [Book].

1391. Cummins, in Coppock & Schulke, 2018 [Book].

1392. Austin, 2004 [Journal].

1393. Tedlock, 1992 [Book].

1394. *Ibid.*

1395. Field notes, on the road from Juchitan de Zaragoza to San Mateo del Mar, October 2018: thanks to Hector, my Zapotec taxi driver.

1396. Milbrath, 1999 [Book].

1397. Moe, 2014 [Internet].

1398. Miller & Taube, 1993 [Book].

1399. Pratchett, 1992 [Book].

1400. Ertel, 2009 [Journal].

1401. Koch, 2018 [Periodical].

1402. Goldhill, 2016 [Internet].

1403. Blackmore & Troscianko, 2018 [Book].

1404. Marlow, 2013 [Internet].

1405. *Ibid.*

1406. Blackmore & Troscianko, 2018 [Book].

1407. Marlow, 2013 [Internet].

1408. *Ibid.*

1409. McTaggart, 2001 [Book]; Sheldrake, 2009 [Book].

1410. McTaggart, 2001 [Book].

1411. Radin, 2018 [Book].

1412. 29 January 2011: Interview with Ignacio Cac Sacul, President of the Cacao Grower's Association, Alta Verapaz, North Guatemala.

1413. Field notes, 2011.

1414. Vail, in Grivetti & Shapiro, 2009 [Book].

1415. Milbrath, 1999 [Book].

1416. Miller & Taube, 1993 [Book].

1417. Milbrath, 1999 [Book].

1418. Miller & Taube, 1993 [Book].

1419. Milbrath, 1999 [Book].

1420. *Ibid.*

1421. Hamnett, 1999 [Book].

1422. Milbrath, 1999 [Book].

1423. Milbrath, 1999 [Book].

1424. Tedlock, 1992 [Book].

1425. Cano, 2009 [Internet]; Grofe, 2007 [Thesis].

1426. *Ibid.*

1427. Milbrath, 1999 [Book].

1428. *Ibid.*

1429. Robson, 1923 [Book].

1430. Szogyi, in Szogyi, 1997 [Book].

1431. Briggs, 2008 [Book].

1432. Cabezon, Barriga, & Grivetti, in Grivetti & Shapiro, 2009 [Book].

1433. Briggs, 2008 [Book].

1434. Dreiss & Greenhill, 2008 [Book].

1435. Faust & Lopez, in McNeil, 2006 [Book].

1436. Bletter & Daly, in McNeil, 2006 [Book].

1437. Henderson & Joyce, & Aguilar-Moreno, in McNeil, 2006 [Book].

1438. Grivetti & Cabezon, in Grivetti & Shapiro, 2009 [Book].

1439. Grivetti & Cabezon, in Grivetti & Shapiro, 2009 [Book].

1440. Hamnett, 1999 [Book]; supplemented by Wikipedia https://en.wikipedia.org/wiki/Quetzalcoatl#cite_ref-21, accessed 30 January 2019.

1441. Freidel, Schele, & Parker, 1993 [Book].

1442. Miller & Taube, 1993 [Book].

1443. Freidel, Schele, & Parker, 1993 [Book].

1444. Sahagún, quoted in Coe & Coe, 1996 [Book].

1445. 9 April 2008: Interview with stallholders at *El Elefante*, a *Santeria* supply store in the Mercado de Sonora, D.F., Mexico.

1446. Grivetti, in Grivetti & Shapiro, 2009 [Book].

1447. Dreiss & Greenhill, 2008 [Book].

1448. Valle, 2017 [Periodical].

1449. Paracelsus, 1656 [Book].

1450. León-Portilla, 1992 [Book].

1451. Junius, 1979 [Book].

1452. *Ibid.*

1453. Stubbe, 1662 [Book].

1454. *Ibid.*

1455. Stross, 2011 [Journal].

1456. Fraser, 2018 [Internet].

1457. *Ibid.*
1458. *Ibid.*
1459. Sahagún, 1829 [Book].
1460. 2017, www.whiterabbitinstituteofhealing.com [Internet].
1461. Kaptchuk, 2000 [Book].
1462. Saunders, 1997; Berry, 2009 [Internet].
1463. 2019, www.sacredlotus.com [Internet].
1464. Yuker, in Szogyi, 1997 [Book].
1465. Starr & Starr, in Szogyi, 1997 [Book].
1466. Fyne, in Szogyi, 1997 [Book].
1467. Coe & Coe, 1996 [Book].
1468. Lekatsas, in Szogyi, 1997 [Book].
1469. Pendell, 2002 [Book].
1470. Bales, 2000 [Booklet].
1471. Molinari & Callus, in Paoletti *et al.*, 2012 [Book].
1472. 2019, www.cadbury.co.uk [Internet].
1473. Briggs, 2008 [Book].
1474. Bodhipaksa, 2007 [Internet].
1475. Foley, 2010 [Book].

Conclusion

1476. Ott, 1996 [Book].
1477. Pendell, 2010 [Book].
1478. Freidel, Schele, & Parker, 1993 [Book].
1479. *Ibid.*
1480. Pendell, 2010 [Book].
1481. Kaptchuk, 2000 [Book].

APPENDICES

Expanded monograph

Theobroma cacao L.

FAMILY: Malvaceae [Juss.] (formerly Sterculiaceae)

COMMON NAMES: Cacao, Cocoa Tree

HABITAT: Cacao is an equatorial understorey tree, 12–15m tall, growing in evergreen rainforests from 20°N to 20°S. It requires temperatures of 27°C/80.6°F and above, not lower than 16°C/60.8°F, in regions where annual rainfall averages between 1500 and 3000mm.[1] It prefers lower elevations, growing at less than 700m above sea level in rich soil.[2] Indigenous to Central America, Cacao often grows in *cenotes* (sinkholes) in the Yucatan peninsula of Mexico due to their humid and sheltered microclimate, which also benefits Cacao's insect pollinators (see below), whose larvae often require damp conditions to thrive. Silt in the water of *cenotes* helps to sustain the humid microclimate, which Cacao favours, and their scattered locations reduce disease transmission and spread.[3]

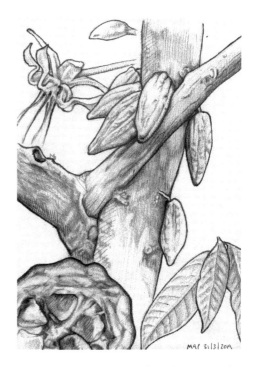

CULTIVATION: Requires deep, fertile soil, partial shade, high humidity, and high annual rainfall.[4] Cacao cannot tolerate more than four months of continuous dry weather.[5] Likes shelter; high winds and low temperatures easily damage the tree.[6] Traditional "shade trees" are taken from the nitrogen-fixing Leguminosae family, and include "Madre de Cacao", *Gliciridia sepium*, as well as species of *Inga* and *Erythrina*. Food crops were traditionally grown alongside Cacao in Mesoamerica, a mutually beneficial "companion planting" system reminiscent of the *milpa* ("maize field") agricultural method devised in the same location.[7] Cacao flowers at the start of the rainy season; the flowers are pollinated by "chocolate midges" of various families, such as haemovores in the *Ceratopogonidae* family, including *Forcipomyia* species,[8] *Cecidomyiidae*, and stingless bees (*Meliponinae*). Wild Cacao flowers appear to have a narrower range of pollinators but a higher volume of insect visitors than *Theobroma* cultivars,[9] and wild ancestral *T. cacao* phenotypes have a more complex essential oil with a higher molecular weight profile, mimicking the exocrine secretions of some insect pollinators.[10]

Cacao trees begin fruiting at about two or three years old, but only attain maximum yields from six or seven years. The trees are highly susceptible to diseases and pests such as capsids, cocoa borer moth, or fungal infections like black pod disease and witches' broom disease (*Moniliophthora perniciosa*).[11] *Criollo* (*Theobroma cacao ssp. cacao*), the type of Cacao cultivar indigenous to Central America, is most valued for its seeds, but is also more susceptible to disease and lower-yielding than the Amazonian cultivar known as *forastero* (*Theobroma cacao ssp. sphaerocarpum*). These subtypes have been variously hybridised to form a third variant, known as *trinitario* (owing to its origins in Trinidad) or *mestizo*, combining the milder flavour of *criollo* with the hardiness and higher yields of *forastero*.

PARTS USED: <u>Seeds</u>, variably fermented and dried, toasted, roasted or raw, shelled, ground and mixed with water and other plant-based (edible or medicinal) additives, to make traditional Cacao-based beverages. Ground seeds are mixed with various combinations of added fat and sugar, with or without dehydrated milk and emulsifying agents to make chocolate for eating or drinking. De-fatted, pulverised, and alkali-treated seed, known as "cocoa powder", used in beverages and baking. <u>Fat</u> extracted from the seeds is known as cocoa butter, and used in food and medicine. <u>Seed husks/shells</u> are sometimes used in infusions. <u>Inner stem bark</u>, as decoction; <u>leaves</u>, as infusion, juice, or in decoction; <u>flowers</u>, in infusion; <u>root bark</u>, as decoction.

TRADITIONAL VIEW OF MEDICINAL EFFECTS: Cacao is generally regarded as a Cooling plant, both in Renaissance Europe and in Mesoamerican folk medicine, past and present. In Europe, it developed a reputation as an aphrodisiac and geriatric tonic.[12] The old-school European Galenic-humoral system classified prepared chocolate—the seeds made into a drink with some sugar and hot water—as slightly warming or temperate, particularly useful for Phlegmatic persons, or to be drunk in winter and old age.[13] The pre-Colombian Mesoamericans utilised Cacao seeds in prescriptions to treat agitation, vision-quest hangovers, insanity, to encourage or prohibit sleep, and to increase courage or reduce fear. It was also combined with other remedies to provide relief for physical ailments such as fevers, "skin eruptions" (unspecified), diarrhoea and bloody dysentery, indigestion and flatulence, "lung problems" (also unspecified), exhaustion, impotence, to delay hair growth, to clean the teeth, and as a prophylactic against snakebite.[14]

Cacao seeds are used in traditional folk medicine for stimulant and anti-fatigue properties, to assist weight gain and convalescence, as a prophylactic and disease preventative, and as a pre-medication to protect against envenomation such as snakebite and wasp, bee, or scorpion stings.[15] The seeds are also used to assist in chronic cough or lung ailments, to improve diges-tion and counter dysentery or diarrhoea, and—conversely—to assist elimination of wastes via bowels and kidneys.[16] They have also been used as a febrifuge, a parturient and galactagogue,[17] and to relieve pain.[18]

Cocoa butter is used externally to help heal and prevent damage to the skin, as a hair tonic, and as an abdominal massage oil by midwives, who use it in a special manipulative technique to turn a breach baby.[19] Cocoa butter is also internally administered to treat coughs, and pro-mote bowel movements.[20] Cacao flower infusions have been used to treat urinary tract prob-lems and "apathy",[21] and applied topically to heal cuts and scratches on the feet[22] or to treat "screw-worm of the eye".[23] A decoction of Cacao seed husks or "shells" with indigo dye is used to treat body lice in Cuba.[24] Cacao leaf infusions are used in the treatment of diabetes, heart pain, menorrhagia, and dysmenorrhoea;[25] externally, as a poultice, to treat headaches, cuts, and abrasions.[26] Cacao root bark has been used in the treatment of anaemia in Nigerian folk medicine.[27]

Technical data

BOTANY:

The tree is a tropical evergreen with a deep taproot,[28] dark grey-brown bark, and glabrous, ellip-tic-obovate to ovate leaves, with a shallowly cordate base. Leaves grow in two or three annual "flushes", increased by water stress or direct sunlight from unsheltered conditions.[29] Small, five-petalled cymose flowers grow directly from the trunk (cauliflorously), and are pollinated by midges (see above); most do not develop into fruit. The flowers measure 18mm in diameter, with 12mm pedicels; they have a pink calyx, with narrowly lanceolate lobes and hairy margins, 5-angled and 5-celled obovoid ovaries, with 14–16 ovules per locule in two rows; the style is cylindrical.[30] Fertilised ovaries take about five to six months to develop into large, slim rugby-ball-shaped pods—an ellipsoid, longitudinally 10-grooved drupe, with a thick endocarp. Pods weigh from two hundred grams to over a kilogram each.[31] Pods are filled with a mucilaginous white pulp containing 30–45 seeds; each seed has an outer shell coat, or testa, two cotyledons or "nibs", and a small embryo plant germ.[32]

CONSTITUENTS:

SEE TABLES on FOLLOWING PAGES

Class	Amount in Cacao seed	mg/40g Cacao	Bio availability	Pharmacological mechanism + effects (general)
ALKALOIDS—total: Of which:		≤ 1,600 [~ 762]		
Xanthines, total:	Approx. 4% dry weight	≤ 762		
	≤ 19mg/g		Clearance rates & sensitivity vary widely; Tobacco smokers clear caffeine more rapidly.	CNS stimulants (phosphodiesterase inhibitors = raise intracellular cAMP + adenosine antagonism), sympathomimetic: positively ino- & chrono-tropic, increase respiratory rate, bronchodilators; paradoxically also increase GIT acid & pepsin secretion. Inhibit TNF-α & leukotrine synthesis: vs. inflammation, reduce innate immunity. CNS: enhance dopamine sensitivity via adenosine A2 receptor antagonism.
Of which:				
Theobromine	1.22%[33]	488	*Theobromine:* Peak absorption 2h; *Caffeine:* Peak absorption 0.5h; metabolised to Paraxanthine (84%), Theobromine (12%) & Theophylline (4%).	Vasodilator, diuretic, cardiac stimulant (positively ino- & chrono-tropic), vagal parasympatholytic & antitussive; hypotensive? Lower affinity for adenosine receptors = **weak CNS stimulant**. PARP-1 inhibitor: vs. vascular inflammation. Anticariogenic. Thymolytic, spermatolytic, genotoxic to testicular & prostate tissue, angiogenesis inhibitor.
Theophylline	3,254–4,739ppm[34]	130–190		Bronchodilator, cardiac stimulant (positively ino- & chrono-tropic, coronary vasodilator), hypertensive, diuretic, respiratory stimulant. Restores histone deacetylase sensitivity in smokers' lungs—improves sensitivity to steroids in COPD, asthma etc. High affinity for adenosine receptors.
Caffeine	0.21%[35]	84		**Most potent CNS stimulant in Cacao.** Moderate affinity for adenosine receptors; hypertensive, diuretic, GIT peristalsis stimulant, cardiac & respiratory stimulant. **Weak MAO-A & MAO-B inhibitor.**
Tetrahydroisoquinolines[36]				
Salsolinol (1-methyl-1,2,3,4-tetrahydroisoquinoline-6,7-diol)	25µg/g	≥ 1[37]	Crosses BBB; also formed endogenously in presence of aldehydes or ketones.	CNS opiate agonist, **dopamine modulator** (region-specific effects), **habituating/reinforcing; reversible MAO-A inhibitor** (increases Tyrosine → Tyramine, L-DOPA, NA, adrenaline, 5-HT levels). **CNS stimulant.** Neurotoxin precursor: methylated product, N-methyl-R-salsolinol is neurotoxic to dopaminergic neurons (pro-Parkinsonian). Thrombogenic.

Pyrazines, total:		1.4mg/kg	0.056		
Of which:	Tetramethylpyrazine[38]	Approx. 0.525mg/kg	0.021	Rapid absorption & excretion; ≥ 100mg t.d.s. necessary for oral activity.	Calcium channel antagonist & vasodilator, vascular anti-inflammatory, nephroprotective, neuroprotective, antioxidant, lowers fibrinogen = antifibrotic, antithrombotic.
	Trimethylpyrazine	Approx. 0.875mg/kg	0.035		Unknown
Indoles:					
Of which:	Tetrahydro-beta-carbolines [THBC's]—total:	0.87–7.86µg/g	0.03–0.72[39]	Produced in fermentation.	A variety of β-carboline alkaloids with an extra hydrogen atom instead of a double carbon bond. β-carboline effects: • Reversible inhibition of **MAO-A & 5-HT uptake** • **Benzodiazepine, opiate & dopamine receptor binding** • Inhibition of Na+ dependent transports.[40] MTCA = mutagenic n-nitrosamine precursors.
Of which:	6OHMTHβC[41]	0.16–3.92µg/g	0.006–0.3	Human CNS pK unknown.	
	TCHA[42]	0.01–0.85µg/g	0.0004–0.1	Suspected to partly metabolise by oxidation to β-carbolines *in vivo*.	
	1S, 3S-MTCA[43]	0.35–2µg/g	0.014–0.2		
	1R, 3S-MTCA[44]	0.14–0.88µg/g	0.006–0.1		
	MTHβC[45]	0–0.21µg/g	0–0.02		
Pyridine					
	Trigonelline	14–124nmol/g^{-1} in fresh material[46]	0.002–0.02 [?][47]	"Specific drug delivery system" for PEA to CNS[48], a metabolite of Niacin.	Smooth muscle spasmolytic, anti-histamine, neurotropic, dopamine & phenylethylamine conveyance to CNS (?), bacteriostatic, **CNS stimulant** & GABA antagonist.

Class		Amount in Cacao seed	mg/40g Cacao	Bio availability	Pharmacological mechanism + effects (general)
POLYPHENOLS—total: Of which:		12g/kg[49] = 12mg/g; Estimated ≤ 4% dry weight after traditional processing.	~ 480–1600	Oxidised during fermentation & roasting. Milk reduces absorption. Flavan-3-ol & Procyanidin absorption facilitated by ascorbate.	In vitro inhibitors of: xanthine oxidase activity, ACE (angiotensin-renin), prostate cancer cell growth, lymphocyte production & B-cell Ig production; in vitro stimulators of macrophage CSF production from PBMCs. Decrease colonic epithelial fluid secretion & cellular proliferation (vs. polyamine synthesis). In vitro (animal): **antidepressant and dopaminergic effects with high doses**; enhanced lifespan & cognition, nootropic; anti-atherosclerotic; higher doses = decreased tumorigenesis in prostate, lung, thyroid & pancreatic cancer models; vs. ethanol-induced gastric ulceration; vs. testicular carcinogenesis. In vitro (human): vs. platelet function; **increase circulating nitric oxide (NO) levels.**
Proanthocyanidins:				Flavan-3-ol "prodrugs".	**MAO-A & MAO-B inhibitors**; inhibit endothelin-1 production; stabilise elastin & collagen; anti-oedema. In vitro (animal): analgesic & sedative effects at very high doses.
Procyanidins, total:		0.6–1.35%[50]	≤ 240[51]	Stable in gastric milieu. B2 & other dimers	"Dominant antioxidants in ... chocolates"[52]
Including:[54]	Dimer B1	≤ 112mg/100g	≤ 44.8		In vitro: vs. H_2O_2-induced apoptosis, antimutagenic & anti-angiogenic; stabilised T-cell membranes, decrease lipoxygenases;
	Dimer B2	≤ 72mg/100g	≤ 28.8		• Cinnamatannin A2 = Hyaluronidase inhibitor, E. coli anti-adhesion[53]
	Trimer C1	≤ 24mg/100g	≤ 9.6		In vitro (human): modulated TGF-B production.
	Cinnamatannin A2	≤ 33mg/100g	≤ 13.2		
Flavan-3-ol monomers, total: x7, including:		0.37%	≥ 146	Carbs increase plasma levels of catechin & epicatechin, unaffected by fats or proteins; plasma levels peak 1–2h after ingestion. 18.3% ingested dose found in urine.	Intake inversely correlated with CHD mortality in the elderly.[55]
	(-)-epicatechin	0.35–1.68%	63		In vitro 5-lipoxygenase inhibition; reduce LDL peroxidation; stimulate IgA production; increase PBMC reactivity; inhibit platelet aggregation/ activation, vs. monocyte & neutrophil activation.
	(+)-catechin	0.31–0.49%[56]	43		• Epicatechin & Catechin = **MAO-B inhibitors** [L-dopa, PEA]
	Epicatechin gallate	18mg/100g	7.2		• Epicatechin in vitro: inhibits xanthine & NADPH oxidase, reduces plasma levels of endothelin-1, increases cortical neuron CREB activation
	Epigallocatechin	4.95mg/100g	1.98		
	Epigallocatechin Gallate (EGCG)	76.5mg/100g	30.6		
[57]	Glucopyranosides: Quercetin, hesperetin, luteolin, naringenin, apigenin, etc.	?	?		

	mg	%	Bioavailability	Effects
Hydroxycinnamic acids		0.12%		
Caffeic acid (& derivatives)	1220mg/kg	≤ 49[58]	Found in human plasma following ingestion of polyphenol-containing foods.[59]	• Epicatechin & Catechin have cardioprotective effects vs. ischaemia-reperfusion injury via δ-opioid receptor binding • Catechin & 3-O-methyl epicatechin: protection vs. free-radical induced haemolysis • Catechin inhibits polysaccharide hydrolysis via α-glucosidase • Quercetin, Hesperetin and Caffeic acid **reduce production of neurotoxin dihydrobenzothiazine (product of dopamine metabolism).**
Chlorogenic acid	8.8–17.5mg/kg[60]	0.35–0.7	Levels decrease with roasting. Well absorbed orally.	• Hypoglycaemic: retards intestinal glucose uptake; hypotensive • Anti-thrombotic: suppresses thromboxane A2 • Neuroprotective, inhibits acetylcholinesterase and butyrylcholinesterase • Hepatoprtotective, gastroprotective, anti-ulcerogenic • Thiamine antagonist.
Phenolic Acids[61]		0.16%		
Gallic acid	97.5mg/100g	39	Protocatechuic acid = metabolite of anthocyanins & pro-anthocyanidins. Low levels detectable in plasma after ingestion.	*In vitro*: Antifungal, antiviral, cytotoxic to cancer cells; vs. human rheumatoid arthritis inflammatory gene expression, pro-apoptotic. *In vivo* (animal): vs. gastric cancer cell metastasis; high doses vs. oxidative kidney damage.
Protocatechuic acid	60mg/100g	24		*In vitro*: anti-inflammatory; pro-apoptotic to leukaemia cell lines; increases neural stem cell proliferation, neuroprotective; antithrombotic vs. shear stress induced clotting; insulin-like action on adipocytes. *In vivo* (animal): huge doses = anti-inflammatory, analgesic; vs. intestinal ischaemia-reperfusion injury.

(Continued)

Class	Amount in Cacao seed	mg/40g Cacao	Bio availability	Pharmacological mechanism + effects (general)
N-phenylpropanoyl-l-amino acids x9, including:				
Clovamide (N-caffeoyl-3-hydroxytyrosine), N-Caffeoyldopamine or Caffedymine	Up to 1.26mg/kg[62], or 30mg/100g[63]	0.05–12	Roasting = < 60% decrease in clovamide content. Bioavailable: levels peak in plasma & urine 2h after oral ingestion.	Antioxidant, possibly neuroprotective,[64] possible p-selectin inhibitors.[65] may therefore reduce cancer metastasis & inflammatory responses.\n\n*In vitro* β-2 adrenoreceptor agonists.
Dideoxyclovamide (N-*trans*-p-coumaroyl-L-tyrosine), N-Coumaroyldopamine	4.3mg/100g	≤ 1.7		• Clovamide: *in vitro* neuroprotective; regulates monocyte activity, anti-inflammatory; β2 adrenoreceptor agonist, COX-1 & -1 inhibitor, anti-thrombogenic.\n• Dideoxyclovamide: vs. platelet-leukocyte interaction, anti-thrombogenic.
N-*trans*-caffeoyl-L-tyrosine)	?	?		
Stilbenoids:	0.018%			
Resveratrol (3,4,5-trihydroxystilbene) & derivatives:	8.99μg/g	0.37–0.74	Resveratrol absorption = high, but rapidly metabolised so poor bioavailability; highly variable metabolism by gut flora.	Resveratrol: Neurotrophic, neuroprotective to dopaminergic neurons; **MAO-A inhibitor.**\n\n*In vitro*: reduced lipogenesis; increased cellular vulnerability to EBV; cytotoxic to bone-marrow derived macrophages; inhibits malignant NK cells; vs. NO production; pro-apoptotic in pancreatic & naso-pharyngeal cancer cells; vs. VEGF production by osteosarcoma; inhibits non-androgen dependent prostate cancer cells; telomerase inhibitor; vs. vascular endothelial oxidative injury.\n\n*In vivo* (animal): huge doses (= 5g in a 10st human) = antidepressant, increasing 5-HT, NA & DA turnover due to MAO-A inhibition.\n\n*In vivo* (human): 8mg + grape phenolics = anti-inflammatory effects over 1 year; resveratrol on its own, no change in glucose production/sensitivity in obese subjects.
Of which: Trans-piecid	7.14μg/g	0.3–0.6[66]		
Trans-resveratrol	1.85μg/g	0.07–0.14		
Quinones	0.0008%			
Pyrryloquinoline quinone	0.34–0.76μg/g[67]	0.01–0.03	Very stable molecule. Human Equivalent minimum dose for animal trial effects = ≥ 1.4mg/day.	Stimulate mitochondrial repair & regeneration (as exercise & caloric restriction do); neuroprotective, antiparkinsonian.\n\n*In vivo* (animal): reduced myocardial damage following infarction.\n\n*In vivo* (human): 20mg/day = improved memory (2000× cacao 40g dose).
Lignin [Husk]	?	Trace (?)	Uncertain. Large molecule, so effects probably limited to GIT; alkalinity & heat may be required for systemic absorption, so limited intestinal absorption may be possible.	Astringent & anti-diarrhoeal; *in vitro* antiviral activity (influenza & HIV)[68]

Class		Amount in Cacao seed	mg/40g Cacao	Bio availability	Pharmacological mechanism + effects (general)
FATTY ACIDS		57% (nibs)	22800 (22.8g)		
Saturated:	Stearic acid = Octadecanoic acid [$CH_3(CH_2)_{16}CO_2H$]	~19%	~7600 (7.6g)	Stearic: Part-metabolised to Oleic acid; less likely than PA to form cholesterol esters.	In vitro neuroprotection vs. oxidative & excitotoxicity; vs. lymphoma cell proliferation; increased neuronal apoptosis.
				Palmitic: Excess dietary carbohydrate converted to PA; incorporated into cholesterol esters; desaturates to Palmitoleic acid.	In vitro (mouse): Topically vs. burns.
	Palmitic acid = Hexadecanoic acid [$CH_3(CH_2)_{14}CO_2H$]	~15%	~6000 (6g)		In vitro (human): increases post-prandial fibrinogen & factor VII coagulant activity.
					Vs. insulin & leptin appetite suppression; possible increased CHD risk
					In vitro pro-apoptotic in breast cancer; HIV CD4 fusion inhibitor.
					In vitro (human): no elevation in LDL cholesterol if mono- & polyunsaturated fats also high.
mono-unsaturated	Oleic acid = cis-9-Octadecenoic acid, oleate [$C_{18}H_{34}O_2$]	~20%	~8000 (8g)	Linoleic: converted to GLA, thence to AA's, pro-inflammatory eicosanoids, but GLA forms DGLA in the body, which inhibits AA-derived leukotrines' pro-inflammatory properties. However, the transformation to GLA blocks production of EPA, so has net pro-inflammatory effects. Moreover oxidised LA metabolites activate capsaicin receptors and may increase pain sensitivity.	Vs. Adrenoleukodystrophy; hypotensive; high dietary intake assoc. increased breast & possibly also prostate, colon & rectal cancer risk.
					In vitro: reduces ESR, blood viscosity; improves erythrocyte flexibility; negates pro-apoptotic effects of palmitate on breast cancer.
					In vitro (human): increases post-prandial fibrinogen & factor VII coagulant activity > saturated fats; inhibits elastase.
Poly-unsaturated	Linoleic acid = cis-9,cis-12-Octadecadienoic acid, [$C_{18}H_{32}O_2$]	~2%	~800 (0.8g)		In vitro (human): inhibits gastric & colon cancer cells.
					In vivo (animal): increased breast, prostate & colon carcinogenesis.
					In vitro (human): Italian population: high intake correlated with higher melanoma incidence; but low intake associated with relapse in recovering cocaine addicts; lowers BP, platelet aggregation, improves erythrocyte flexibility; higher intakes may protect vs. pneumonia, pre-eclampsia, and reduce keratoconjunctivitis sicca symptoms.
Phytosterols		276mg/100g	110.2		Competitively inhibit GIT cholesterol absorption. Possibly protect vs. lung, ovarian, breast & colon cancers.

(Continued)

Class	Amount in Cacao seed	mg/40g Cacao	Bio availability	Pharmacological mechanism + effects (general)
4-desmethylsterols				
Including:				
Sitosteryl	216mg/100g	86.4	Insoluble in water, poorly soluble in fat, soluble in alcohol; poorly absorbed from intestine, with faster hepatic metabolism than cholesterol. Metabolised to bile acids in the liver.	• B-sitosterol: *in vitro* pro-apoptotic in breast cancer cells, vs. colon cancer cell growth; *in vivo* (human) reduced post-exercise inflammation & immunosuppression; improved urinary flow in BPH.
Stigmasteryl	123.3mg/100g	49.3		• Stigmasterol: hypoglycaemic, thyroid-inhibiting; vs. breast, prostate & colon cancer risk; vs. cartilage deterioration.
	60.1mg/100g	24		• *In vivo* (mice): vs. scopolamine-induced memory loss.
Campesteryl	18.7mg/100g	7.5		• Campesterol: vs. cartilage deterioration.
Triterpenes (4,4'-dimethylsterols)				*In vitro* & *in vivo* (animal): cancer chemopreventive;
Including:				
Cycloartenyl	44mg/100g	17.6		• Cycloartane *in vivo* (animal): vs. UV-B tumour promotion.
	18.9mg/100g	7.6mg		
4,4',14-Trimethyl-24-methylene-5α-cholest-7-en-3β-yl	10mg/100g	4		
24-Methylene-cycloartanyl	5.8mg/100g	2.3		
4-methylsterols				
Including:				
Citrostadienyl	15.56mg/100g	6.2		• Obtusifoliol *in vitro*: inhibits EBV activation.
Obtusifoliol	5.56mg/100g	2.2		
	2.07mg/100g	0.8		
Lophenyl	1.39mg/100g	0.6		
Phospholipids	"30% of 2% of 98% of cacao lipids"[769] (= 0.3352%)	13.4		Animal cell membrane constituents;
Including:				• Phosphatidylcholine: surfactant (emulsifier) & major component of lecithin
Phosphatidylcholine	35-41%	≤ 5.5		• Phosphatidylinositol: abundant in brain tissue; primary source of arachidonic acid; used to manufacture diacylglycerol signalling molecules which regulate cellular metabolism and life cycle via protein kinase C
Phosphatidylinositol	24-30%	≤ 4		• Phosphatidylethanolamine: **anandamide precursor**; crucial roles in cellular fusion + fission, autophagy, & protein synthesis
Phosphatidyl-ethanolamine	11-20%	≤ 2.7		• Lysophosphatidylcholine: a hydrolysed product of phosphatidylcholine with demyelinating properties
Lyso-phosphatidylcholine	4-10%	≤ 1.3		• Phosphatidylserine: facilitates animal cell phagocytosis following apoptosis.
Phosphatidylserine	2-4%	≤ 0.5		• Phosphatidic acid: lipid precursor, and intracellular signalling lipid.
Phosphatidic acid	0.3-4%	≤ 0.5		
-Unidentified x 4	5-14%	≤ 1.9		

Class	Amount in Cacao seed	mg/40g Cacao	Bio availability	Pharmacological mechanism + effects (general)
ORGANIC ACIDS	14.8–33.3g/kg [1.5–3.3%]	592–1332		
Lactic acid	1.2–23g/kg	48–920		Minor antibacterial properties; primary brain "fuel" in humans (more than glucose).
Acetic acid	3–8.3g/kg	120–332		Major taste compound. Minor food-preservative and antibacterial properties.
Citric acid	3–7.2g/kg	120–288		Minor food-preservative properties; alkalinises urine.
Oxalic acid	1,520–5000ppm, 0.2–0.5g/100g, 3.5–5.9g/kg	60.8–236		Moderately toxic; inhibits dietary calcium absorption; causes calcium oxalate formation, can lead to kidney stones & kidney failure and/or joint pain in excess. Also possibly anticarcinogenic/antimetastatic.[70]
Phytic acid	0.59–0.75%[71]	236–300		Indigestible mineral chelator; trypsin inhibitor; reduced during fermentation.

Class	Amount in Cacao seed	mg/40g Cacao	Bio availability	Pharmacological mechanism + effects (general)
PROTEINS	12.00–28,570ppm 0.12–2.9%	≤ 4,400		Functional & structural molecules.
Albumins	52% total protein[72]	2288	Undetermined; possibly low or limited to upper GIT.	Albumin fraction from semi-fermented, but not unfermented cacao: in vitro anti-tumour & antioxidant.
Globulins	43% total protein[73]	1892		
Glutelins	5%	220		
Prolamines	1%	44		
Amino Acids				Precursors required for protein manufacture.
Aspartic acid (= asparaginic acid)	?	?	Aspartic acid: Forms acrylamide with dicarbonyl compounds during roasting.	Non-essential.
Glutamic acid	10,200ppm	≤ 408	Glutamic acid: crosses BBB via specific transport receptors.	Non-essential. Excitatory neurotransmitter, helps learning & memory; facilitates synaptic plasticity. Precursor for GABA. Key metabolic agent; used to remove excess nitrogen via the liver.
Glycine	900ppm	36	**Phenylalanine: Competes with Tryptophan to cross BBB.**	Non-essential. Inhibitory neurotransmitter in brain stem, spinal cord & retina; also NMDA receptor co-agonist, with glutamate.
Isoleucine	5,600ppm	224	**Tryptophan: CNS uptake increased by insulin release, especially following carbohydrate ingestion.** Competes with other AAs to cross BBB so levels must be very high to influence mood.	Essential. Branched-chain. Requires Biotin for metabolism.
Lysine	800ppm	32		Essential. A serotonin antagonist: dulls overactivation of 5-HT4 receptors in the gut. Deficiency can be anxiogenic. Dietary intake may prevent cold sores & modulate blood pressure.
Phenylalanine	5,600ppm	224	Tyrosine: Crosses BBB via specific transporters.	Essential. Tyrosine [→L-DOPA] & PEA precursor. Larger quantities can interfere with serotonin production.
Threonine	1,400ppm	56		Essential.
Tryptophan	6.39–17.26mg/100g[74]	2.6–6.9		Essential. **Precursor for serotonin, melatonin & niacin.** May augment antidepressant effects, but may also increase insulin resistance and CNS senescence in excess.
Tyrosine	5,700ppm	228		Non-essential. Can be synthesised from phenylalanine. Precursor of tyramine & **catecholamines: → L-Dopa** (→ dopamine, adrenaline, noradrenaline) & thyroid hormones.
Valine	5,700ppm	228		Essential. Branched-chain.
Non-protein Amino Acids:				
γ-aminobutyric acid (GABA)	31.7–101.2mg/100g[75]	12.9–40.5	Crosses BBB via high-affinity transporters.	Inhibitory: anxiolytic, antispasmodic, regulates muscle tone. Excitatory in developing brain; regulates neuronal development. Increases HGH.
β-aminoisobutyric acid	?	?		Unknown. Increases hepatic fat oxidation.

Compound	Concentration	Value	Pharmacokinetics	Activity / Function
Amino Alcohols		0.02–5.9		
Arachidonoylethanolamide (Anandamide)	0.05–57 μg/g⁻¹[76]	0.002–2.28	Oral bioavailability not >5%; lipophilic; transported by reversible serum albumin binding. Active at nanomolar concentrations.	Binds to cannabinoid & vanilloid receptors; attenuates pain, anxiety & fear; modulates body temperature & appetite. Promotes food intake & lipid storage (anabolic). Decreases heart rate & b.p., anti-inflammatory. **Modulates neurohypophyseal oxytocin and vasopressin release.**
N-acyl-ethanolamines[77]		0.02–3.6		
N-oleyl-ethanolamine (OEA)	0.5–90μg/g⁻¹[78]	?	?	OEA: Produced in small intestine after food; binds to cannabinoid receptor. Anorectic, promotes fat breakdown;
N-linoleoylethanolamine (LEA)	?	?	Inhibit Anandamide degradation by fatty acid amide hydroxylase, causing anandamide to accumulate at sites of action in gut & CNS. 5μM LEA causes 50% inhibition of anandamide breakdown.	CNS: facilitates memory consolidation through enhancement of noradrenergic transmission; ceramidase inhibitor, i.e. pro-apoptotic; assists cardiac glucose metabolism under endotoxic stress.
Biogenic Amines		0.92–4.9		
Tyramine	9.56–71.68μg/g	0.4–2.9	Low—except in the presence of MAOIs. Biogenic Amines cannot cross BBB, only their precursors can.	Peripheral sympathomimetic; no CNS activity. Increases systolic b.p. with high intake; possibly pro-migraine; increases gut activity.
Dopamine*	5.3–25.85μg/g	0.2–1	PEA orally inactive up to 1600mg p.o.[79] 5–10 minutes half-life; but **MAO-B** inhibitors increase CNS PEA levels by ≤1000-fold. *Tyramine* causes mild hypertensive response with **MAO-A** inhibitors at	Classical monoamine neurotransmitter in the CNS, associated with motivation, memory, reward-seeking behaviour, attention & problem-solving in CNS, as well as movement control and suppression of nausea. Activates β-adrenergic cardiac receptors, dilates renal arteries.
PEA [Phenylethylamine]	2.79–14.95μg/g	0.1–0.88[80]	6–10mg p.o.; 10–25mg p.o. + MAO-I's = hypertensive crisis.	Trace amine neurotransmitter in the CNS. Centrally antidepressant; CNS dopamine & noradrenaline agonist; increases gut activity.
Serotonin*	2mg/kg	0.08*	*Dopamine*: **MAO-A & MAO-B** degrade it. Ingested *Serotonin* has no effect on CNS serotonin levels.	Found in GIT, platelets & a classical tryptamine neurotransmitter in the CNS. Regulates peristalsis: secreted in gut, stored in platelets; vasoconstrictor; in CNS, regulates mood, appetite & sleep; role in bone density regulation, tonic control of insulin release.
Histamine*	1mg/kg	0.04*[81]		Pro-inflammatory mediator. Classical monoamine neurotransmitter in CNS, suppresses sleep & appetite, increases arousal / attention in CNS; mediates T-cell differentiation; pro-erectile activity in male corpus cavernosum; Type I hypersensitivity & inflammatory mediator released from mast cells.

*CNS neurotransmitters.

(Continued)

Class	Amount in Cacao seed	mg/40g Cacao	Bio availability	Pharmacological mechanism + effects (general)
Heterocyclic Compounds				
2,5-diketopiperazines x25:	62.4–84.1mg/kg[-1] [82]	2.5–3.4	Highly stable, resistant to proteolysis, small molecules; cross BBB.	Diverse activities: antimicrobial (antiviral, antifungal, antibacterial), antileukaemic, radioprotective, immunomodulatory, hypoglycaemic, neuroprotective.[83]
Including: cis-cyclo [Pro-Val], cis-cyclo [Ille-Pro], cis-cyclo [Val-Leu], cis-cyclo [Ala-Ile], cis-cyclo [Ala-Leu].				
Cyclo [Val-Pro]	1724ppm[84]	69.7mg		Weakly antimicrobial *in vitro*.[85]
Cyclo [Vala-Pro]	228ppm[86]	9.1mg		Cytotoxic to cancer cell lines, modulates cytokine activity in macrophages *in vitro*.[87]
Acrylamide	≤909μg/kg	≤0.036	Originates from baking, frying or combustion of starchy foods: asparagine + reducing sugars or carbonyl compounds; also cigarette smoke. Most ingested acrylamide is absorbed, but well metabolised.[88]	Neurotoxin, carcinogen; **accumulation linked to testicular damage**; mucous membrane irritant.

Class	Amount in Cacao seed[90]	mg/40g Cacao	Odour[89]	Pharmacological effects (general)
VOLATILE COMPOUNDS (principal)[90]				
2- & 3-Methylbutanoic Acid (isovaleric acid)	Trace: up to 1mg/kg of each	Trace: up to 0.04mg of each	Sweaty, cheesy	Possible anticonvulsant & sedative, oestrogen competitive inhibitor, EBV-inducing.
3-Methylbutanal			Malty	**Sympathomimetic** & mucous membrane irritant at low doses, sympatholytic in high doses.
Ethyl 2-methylbutanoate			Fruity / "Peasy"	None yet found.
2-Methoxy-isopropylpyrazine			Earthy, beany	None yet found.
Hexanal			Green	Antifungal, bacteriostatic, possibly **CNS dopaminergic**, weak carcinogen, possibly hepatotoxic and anti-spermatogenic, pro-haemolytic.
2-Methyl-3-(methyldithio) furan			Cooked meat	None yet found.
2-Octenal			Fatty, waxy	Possibly neurotoxic to dopaminergic neurons.
2-Noenal			Green, fatty	Antimalarial *in vitro* (*Plasmodium falciparum*).
Phenylacetaldehyde			Honey-like	*In vitro* **Dopamine beta-monooxygenase inhibitor**: interrupts tyrosine metabolism, preventing the conversion of dopamine to noradrenaline.
4-Heptanal			Biscuit-like	None yet found.
δ-Octenolactone			Coconut-like	Fly repellent *vs.* Tsetse flies!
γ-Decalactone			Peach-like	Inhibit human CYP2A6 enzymes *in vitro*.
Dimethyl trisulphide			Sulphurous	Inhibits yeast > bacterial growth *in vitro*.
Nonanal			Soapy	Anti-diarrhoeal in mice, with no effect on normal bowel transit; *in vitro* inhibition of AA metabolism to TXB2, HHT & 12-HETE at 0.25μm.
2-Ethyl-3,6-dimethylpyrazine			Nutty, earthy	None yet found.

(Continued)

Class	Amount in Cacao seed	mg/40g Cacao	Odour[89]	Pharmacological effects (general)
2-Phenylethanol			Sweet, yeasty	Antimicrobial, esp. vs. *E. coli*; inhibits platelet aggregation *in vitro*.
Ethyl 2-methylpropanoate			Fruity	None yet found.
2-Decanal			Fatty, green	None yet found.
2,4-Nonadienal			Fatty, waxy	*In vitro* toxicity to human fibroblasts & endothelial cells; vs. UV-induced mutagenesis in *E. coli*.
Ethyl cinnamate			Cinnamon	*In vitro* cytotoxicity vs. human melanoma & leukaemia cell lines, and antimicrobial vs. Gram –ve organisms, esp. *E. coli* & *C. albicans*; absorbs UV light, weak xenoestrogen.
3-Hydroxy-4,5-dimethyl-2(5H)-furanone			Spicy seasoning	None yet found.
3-Hydroxy-5-ethyl-4-methyl-2(5H)-furanone			Spicy seasoning	None yet found.
Tetramethylpyrazine[91] (Ligustrazine)	Approx. 0.525mg/kg	0.021	Nutty, musty, chocolatey[92]	Neuroprotective, nephroprotective, vascular anti-inflammatory, Ca^{2+} channel inhibitor (vasodilator), anti-fibrotic.
Trimethylpyrazine	Approx. 0.875mg/kg	0.035	Baked potato, peanut, burnt notes	None yet found.

Class	Amount in Cacao seed[93]	mg/40g Cacao as drink [est.]	RDI	Pharmacological mechanism + effects (general)
VITAMINS, MINERALS, etc.				
Ascorbic acid (Vitamin C)	31ppm	1.2	75mg [f]; 90mg [m] (+35mg if smoking)	Used to make collagen & repair tissue; protects against oxidative tissue damage. Enhances iron absorption. Reduced by cigarettes. Low levels reduce endothelial and connective tissue repair and increase CV disease & osteoarthritis risk.
Calcium	800–1,100ppm; 106mg/100g	32–44	1000mg	Assists bone density; used in neurotransmission, muscle contraction, regulating heartbeat. Requires Vitamin D for absorption.
Copper	24ppm	0.96	0.9 mg	Bacteriostatic, fungicidal; facilitates iron absorption; essential component of many enzymes; high levels in liver, muscle & bone. Cuproenzymes involved in cellular energy production, cross-linking collagen & elastin, myelin maintenance, neurotransmitter metabolism, anti-oxidation, melanin production. Free copper ions = strong free radical inducer. Prevents iron-deficiency anaemia. High serum copper associated with increased CHD risk; may be linked to PD.
Iron	36–37ppm, 0.01%	**1.4–5.56**	8mg	Crucial component of haemoglobin & myoglobin, cytochrome p450 & many other redox enzymes. Accumulates in SN in Parkinson's, and hippocampus in Alzheimer's.
Magnesium	0.014%; 429mg/86g cocoa powder[94]	40[95]–200[8]	400–420 [m]; 300–320 [f]	Essential mineral; used for ATP synthesis. Variably affects calcium absorption, reduces vascular calcification & atherosclerosis. Preventive of metabolic syndrome, hypertension, type 2 diabetes; reduces asthma, osteoporosis severity/occurrence.

(Continued)

Class	Amount in Cacao seed[93]	mg/40g Cacao as drink [est.]	RDI	Pharmacological mechanism + effects (general)
Manganese	0.002%	0.8	N/D; est. 2–5mg	Used to manufacture many important enzymes such as Mn-SOD. Dietary excess produces neurotoxic effects.
Niacin (Vitamin B3)	17–18ppm	0.7	14mg [f] 16mg [m]	Essential nutrient. Precursor of critical metabolic enzymes, necessary for energy production, DNA repair, and steroid hormone manufacture. Dietary deficiency leads to depressive and anxious symptoms. Manufactured from Tryptophan. Lowers cholesterol, may cause flushing.
Nicotinamide	21ppm	0.8		Amide of niacin, a metabolite of it; lacks cholesterol-lowering or flush-inducing properties. Anxiolytic, and reduces skin inflammation; nootropic activity through sirtuin activation (Sirtuins = proteins that mediate apoptosis, stress resistance, energy efficiency and DNA transcription).
Pantothenic acid	13ppm	0.5	5mg	Essential nutrient used in protein, fat & carbohydrate synthesis, and to manufacture Coenzyme-A used in cellular respiration & to make other compounds e.g. cholesterol, ACh.
Phosphatidylcholine	96–1,328ppm	3.8–53.1	550mg [m], 425mg [f][96]	Component of cell membranes. Higher intakes found helpful for liver cell & bowel lining repair, e.g. in hepatitis & inflammatory bowel disease.
Phosphorus	3,600–5571ppm; 0.04%	144–223	700mg	Essential mineral, used in DNA, RNA & ATP and all cell membranes. Approx 1–3g consumed and excreted daily; principally found in protein-rich foods.
Potassium	0.29%	116–610	4700mg	Necessary ion for cellular function, together with sodium. Prevents muscle contraction, regulates nerve function & osmotic balance. Higher intakes may reduce risk of hypertension, cerebrovascular and cardiac disease.

Pyridoxine (Vitamin B6)	1ppm	0.04	2mg	Helps RBC production, required for monamine manufacture (used to make decarboxylase for conversion of 5-HTP & L-DOPA into neurotransmitters). Excess can cause peripheral neuropathy.
Riboflavin (Vitamin B2)	1–4ppm	0.04–0.16	1.3mg [m], 1.1mg [f]	Essential to proper energy metabolism, component of FAD & FMN which are cofactors for several redox reaction enzymes involved in cellular respiration and the metabolism of fatty acids, carbohydrates, proteins, vitamins and other functional molecules e.g. glutathione.
Selenium	14µg/100g	0.0056	0.075 [m]; 0.06 [f]	Essential micronutrient; used to manufacture the detoxification enzyme glutathione peroxidise, and as a cofactor for thyroid hormone metabolism and mercury detoxification.
Sodium	0.14%	56	2400mg	Necessary ion for cellular function, together with potassium. Regulates nerve function and maintains osmotic balance, etc. High intakes reduce NO production, increasing tendencies to vasoconstriction, platelet aggregation and atherosclerogenic processes.
Zinc	0.005%	2	11mg [m], 8mg [f]	Essential mineral; commonly deficient. Benefits immune system, retards aging, speeds tissue healing. Necessary for synaptic plasticity, i.e. learning and adaptability of brain function. Used to make enzymes essential for CO_2 regulation and protein digestion. Both deficiency and excess (> 100mg/day) can be harmful.

Pharmacodynamics and pharmacokinetics

Alkaloids: *Theobromine, theophylline* and *caffeine* (collectively known as the xanthine alkaloids) are the main stimulant compounds in Cacao, at least in terms of quantity and documented CNS stimulant properties. Unfortunately, to date there are no large studies comparing the stimulating effects of the three alkaloids. So far there are a handful of very small human trials which indicate non-synergistic effects, and a weaker caffeine-like stimulation from theobromine alone, with anecdotal reports of a theobromine withdrawal syndrome similar to the symptoms of caffeine withdrawal[97] (headaches, muscle tension, fatigue, and low mood). Doses as low as 12.5mg caffeine have behavioural effects in humans; all three xanthine alkaloids can act as positive reinforcers, increasing taste preferences for foods when administered concomitantly in lower doses, becoming aversive (negatively reinforcing) at high doses.[98] The CNS stimulation ranking for the three alkaloids is considered to be caffeine > theophylline > theobromine.

Adenosine, the neurotransmitter inhibited by xanthines, is a breakdown product of intracellular ATP metabolism; it appears to have a "signal-damping" role, predominantly inhibiting neurotransmission, thereby acting as a natural "decelerator" of neuronal activity. Adenosine acts at various CNS cell receptor sites, and caffeine chiefly blockades adenosine A1 and A2a receptor subtypes, present in all areas of the brain, but most prevalent in the *hippocampus* (part of the limbic system involved in emotionally-driven and instinctive behaviours), *cerebral* and *cerebellar cortexes* (processing consciousness, perception, intellect, and voluntary activity [cerebral cortex]; co-ordination and muscle tone [cerebellar cortex]), and some *thalamic nuclei* (sensory relays). A1 receptors are found throughout the CNS, linked to D1 (dopamine) receptors; A2a receptors are found on GABAergic neurons concentrated in dopaminergic regions such as the substantia nigra. A2a receptor activation decreases dopamine binding affinity to D2 receptors, but only at very high doses. So blockade of adenosine receptors largely results in local dopamine-mediated signal amplification by removing the damping effect of ATP metabolite accumulation, giving rise to caffeine's characteristic stimulating effects.

Theobromine comprises approximately 1.2% of the dry weight of Cacao. Like caffeine, it exerts stimulant activity via adenosine receptor blockade, having a higher affinity for A1 than A2 receptors; it binds to all adenosine receptor subtypes more weakly than caffeine, probably accounting for its milder CNS stimulant effects. Theobromine levels peak in the blood 2.5h after oral ingestion—but theobromine absorbed from whole chocolate or Cacao peaks slightly faster, at around two hours, and caffeine also peaks slightly faster than it normally would at under thirty minutes post-ingestion (see below). In mice, oral theobromine produced stimulatory behavioural effects (increased movement at the higher dose, and faster avoidance response to negative stimuli at the lower dose) only two to three hours after ingestion in doses equivalent to that contained in 15–49g of pure Cacao for a 10st human; curiously though, theobromine prevented many of the stimulating effects of caffeine.[99] Orally administered theobromine did not increase sleep latency in human subjects on its own, whereas caffeine alone or in combination with theobromine did. Theobromine decreased calmness three hours after ingestion, and lowered blood pressure one hour after ingestion; caffeine increased alertness and contentedness more rapidly and markedly one to three hours after ingestion, but also increased blood pressure one hour after ingestion. The differing effects on blood pressure suggest that there are differences in their mechanism of action. A combination of theobromine and caffeine (T:C = 700:120mg, i.e. the same ratio as in Cacao, at high dosage) had a similar effect to caffeine alone on mood, with no net effect on blood pressure. There is a wide range of individual sensitivity to theobromine's stimulant effects if it is administered alone: increased "energy", "motivation to work", and decreased "sleep(iness)" have been reported in comparison to placebo, but these responses are highly variable. Oral doses of 250–500mg isolated theobromine had "limited subjective effects" and "dose-dependently increased heart rate", producing anxiety and discomfort at the higher doses.[100]

Physiologically, theobromine is a PARP-1 inhibitor,[i] modifying DNA repair and intra-nuclear cell protein manufacture: it may therefore increase some cancer cells' mortality, inhibit vascular dysfunction and inflammation, and be of use for lowering risk of stroke or heart attack, and treating ischemia-reperfusion injury, diabetes, and COPD. Theobromine also has anti-angiogenic effects in tumours via inhibition of carcinoma adenosine receptors; recent research has also revealed that theobromine specifically inhibits malignant glioblastoma proliferation by inhibiting phosphodiesterase-4 expression in tumour cells,[101] which the researchers speculate could lead to Cacao's use as a preventative "nutraceutical" agent for this type of cancer. However theobromine also has some reproductive toxicity: in male rats, seven weeks' dietary intake of 0.6% theobromine or cocoa powder at 5% of the diet caused irreversible testicular atrophy, decreased spermatogenesis, and reduced thymus gland weight, indicating an anti-fertility and anti-spermatogenic effect as well as possible immunosuppressive effects at high doses.[102] Similarly, very high intakes of theobromine (not achievable with normal dietary ingestion) were teratogenic in animals. Theobromine reduces copper, generating free radicals, and may share caffeine's property of impairing DNA strand repair, which may account for an observed association between *in utero* and developmental (childhood and pubertal) theobromine exposure and both adult testicular cancer and next-generation neonatal hypospadias.[103] There is some evidence of association between theobromine exposure and prostate cancer, especially for older men consuming more than 11–20mg theobromine per day[104]—a level of intake easily achieved with Cacao consumption. Theobromine has mild diuretic activity weaker than or equivalent to caffeine through adenosine inhibition resulting in renal vasodilation, and possesses cariostatic activity, increasing dental enamel hardness and repair.[105] In common with theophylline, theobromine has anti-tussive properties (it suppresses the cough reflex), and also has some bronchodilatory activity: the mechanisms are still unclear, but may be somewhat similar to theophylline's PDE-3 mediated effects (see below). Theobromine is more efficacious than codeine for reducing persistent coughing, for example, lingering after viral infections.[106]

At around 0.4% of Cacao's dry weight, **theophylline** is a less potent CNS stimulant than caffeine,[107] but has a very high affinity for adenosine receptors. It also has notable cardiac stimulant activity, exerting positively inotropic, chronotropic, and hypertensive effects. Theophylline is a coronary vasodilator, strongly inhibits bronchospasm, and possesses diuretic and respiratory stimulant activities. It is bronchodilatory via phosphodiesterase-3 (PDE-3) inhibition,

---

[i] PARP-1 = Poly [ADP-ribose] polymerase-1, a DNA-modifying enzyme. PARP-1 inhibitors protect against some cancers by stopping PARP-1 enzyme from repairing DNA strand breaks in rapidly dividing cancer cells, therefore leading to cell death; they protect against oxidative damage by activating 'survival pathways' in cells.

anti-inflammatory via PDE-4 inhibition and histone deacetylase-2 (HDAC-2) activation,[108] and anti-tussive by reducing excitability of vagal afferent nerves via calcium-activated potassium channels.[109] Deficiency or congenital lack of this subtype of HDAC causes cardiac defects and vascular repair deficiency syndromes. HDAC2 expression is inhibited by tobacco smoke and is the target of corticosteroids' anti-inflammatory effects; theophylline restores its normal activity and therefore increases the anti-inflammatory potency of corticosteroids, even at low doses,[110] so dietary Cacao intake may therefore be of service in corticosteroid-resistant COPD or asthma. In animal models, 100mg/kg i.p. theophylline prevented priapism-induced corpus cavernosum cell apoptosis;[111] this finding appears to be of little direct use or relevance to chocolate pharmacology owing to the non-oral mode of administration and the colossal dose used (equivalent to 6.4g theophylline in a 10st/64kg human, vastly exceeding a toxic dose)! However, it may imply that the more modest dose of theophylline in chocolate may have beneficial effects in tandem with the cell-membrane-stabilising polyphenolic components, if used in the medium- to long-term treatment of erectile dysfunction of vascular origin or disorders such as Peyronie's disease (see below for the polyphenols' vascular endothelium-protective effects).

Theophylline also inhibits histamine release from human skin mast cells *in vitro* via non-specific phosphodiesterase receptor inhibition.[112] Bitter taste receptors in general (tripped by the xanthine alkaloids), particularly the TAS2R subtype, have been found to induce bronchial relaxation independently of known bronchodilatory pathways.[113] High doses of theophylline are known to increase seizure risk and occasionally cause acute encephalopathy; it may cause these effects by triggering excess astrocytic NO release in the presence of Gram-negative bacterial exotoxins.[114] Both theophylline and caffeine induce *in vitro* apoptosis of canine hemangiosarcoma cells and enhance the chemotherapy drug Doxorubicin's cytotoxicity via inhibition of ATM/ATR kinases (enzymes which repair DNA damage, or mediate apoptosis if the damage is too extensive).[115] This may have implications for complementary use of theophylline- and caffeine-containing drugs such as tea and chocolate in Doxorubicin chemotherapy.

Approximately 0.2% of Cacao's dehydrated mass is **caffeine**, "the most widely used of all psychoactive drugs".[116] At normal human intakes, caffeine decreased striatal mRNA expression for Neuronal Growth Factors 1-A & -B, suggesting that caffeine alone may decrease neuronal growth, neuron and myelin repair, and could hypothetically aggravate bipolar disorder, and reduce pain sensitivity. It should be noted that this caveat would likely not apply to polyphenol-rich natural caffeine sources such as coffee, tea, chocolate, kola, guarana, or maté, but may be relevant for caffeine tablets or "energy drinks" with added caffeine. Unlike cocaine or amphetamines, caffeine doesn't increase motor activity by dopaminergic mechanisms, but its effects "are synergistic with actions of dopamine or dopaminergic drugs [in] the nucleus accumbens".[117] Unlike other psychostimulants, caffeine alone doesn't increase dopamine D1 receptor neurotransmission in the nucleus accumbens, but does increase D2 receptor activation; overall it *decreases* nucleus accumbens activity (again, in contrast to cocaine or amphetamine). Despite this, caffeine has weak reinforcing properties, presumably as a result of the D2 receptor activation. caffeine increases hippocampal serotonin, and high doses increase dopamine and noradrenaline (norepinephrine) release; it activates glutaminergic neurons and mesocortical cholinergic neurons—in short, its CNS stimulant activity involves secondary catecholaminergic, glutaminergic, and cholinergic effects.

Counter-intuitively, isolated caffeine decreases cerebral blood flow up to 30%, but simultaneously increases brain metabolism and glucose uptake, and has been found to benefit memory consolidation. (Theobromine has minimal effects on cerebral blood flow and glucose utilisation, whereas theophylline has similar effects to caffeine in this regard.[118]) Higher doses provoke a "stress-like response", increasing blood levels of cortisol, growth hormone, and thyroid stimulating hormone at oral doses in excess of 500mg. Lower doses (up to 250mg) increase feelings of energy, good mood, sociability, self-confidence, and alertness. Excessive intake of more than 1000mg/day can give rise to "caffeinism", a dependency syndrome associated with generalised anxiety, but there are considerable individual differences in sensitivity. Caffeine also exerts minor analgesic effects due to A2 receptor blockade on hyperalgesic sensory nerve endings, and has additive effects with other CNS analgesics such as Paracetamol. Caffeine has weak anorectic effects, reducing frequency of meals. In general, women are more sensitive to caffeine than men, with some sex-linked differences in psychoactivity: caffeinated men experience decreased perception of effort in complex tasks, whereas for women the opposite is true.[119] It's possible that at least part of chocolate's statistically greater popularity among women may depend on the relatively lower level of caffeine in the drug, as opposed to coffee, for example.

Caffeine has biphasic effects on acetylcholine (ACh) in most regions of the brain: in general, low doses of caffeine inhibit ACh while high doses increase ACh activity, but caffeine dose-dependently increases cortical ACh without inhibiting it at lower levels. Higher caffeine doses also increase CNS Serotonin (5-HT), muscarinic, and δ-opioid receptor activation, which begs the question (as yet unanswered), does theobromine also do this, despite its lower CNS-stimulant activity? Low doses of caffeine give "a cue that resembles a weak dopaminergic stimulus",[120] so they are more readily generalised to cocaine and amphetamine in animal experiments, with an inverse relationship between caffeine dose and predilection for cocaine. Only very modest euphoria was noted at oral doses of 200–800mg in human experiments with isolated caffeine. But the presence of the xanthines in Cacao account for a substantial amount of its psychoactivity, and of chocolate's popular appeal. One double-blind, placebo-controlled clinical trial compared a group of thirty-two people given a drink without alkaloids to another group of thirty-two drinking an identical beverage spiked with 19mg caffeine and 250mg theobromine (similar quantities to those found in cocoa) over six separate, non-consecutive mornings, and found that participants' liking for the xanthine-adulterated drink increased.[121]

It's common knowledge that caffeine reduces sleep quality and sleepiness, and is relied on for its sleep-retarding effects, but there is huge variation in individual sensitivity and caffeine metabolism which strongly affect this characteristic property of the drug. Caffeine primarily increases activity in brain regions related to motor activity and the sleep-wake cycle, which persist for five to six hours after caffeine ingestion. Most strikingly, there is no tolerance to caffeine's effects on cerebral energy metabolism: the same regions of the brain are stimulated to some degree after chronic administration. Caffeine increases anxiety in previously anxious people, but doesn't do so in depressed people. Interestingly though, depressed populations have lower caffeine intakes; this result may mean that caffeine intake reduces depression, or that depressive people choose to take less caffeine! [122] Notably, despite the lack of tolerance to caffeine's effects on brain metabolism and the drug's stimulating effects, adaptations to long-term caffeine ingestion result in *decreased* locomotor activity, *reduced* susceptibility to seizures, and *reduced* ischaemic brain damage, in absolute contrast to acute doses. Likewise many negative effects of initial high-dose caffeine ingestion such as anxiety are decreased on continued use, but once such adaptation has taken place a withdrawal syndrome on caffeine cessation is more likely to ensue (headache, lethargy, depressed mood, anxiety, etc.).

The addition of caffeine and milk to beverages independently improved mood and reduced anxiety in sixteen *caffeine-withdrawn* subjects thirty to sixty minutes post consumption in a cross-over study; hot beverages in general were found to increase skin conductance and temperature, with peak effects ten to thirty minutes post consumption (owing to vasodilation), but added caffeine reduced the increase in skin temperature and slightly increased blood pressure due to its pressor effects.[123]

Ninety-nine per cent of ingested caffeine is absorbed forty-five minutes after ingestion, and in contrast to theobromine, plasma levels peak relatively quickly at thirty minutes. Caffeine is highly bioavailable, readily crossing the blood-brain barrier and the placenta, and has a two and a half to four hour half-life in adults, which doesn't alter significantly with age, being similar for young (over six months old) and elderly persons. Caffeine is mostly metabolised to the equally active paraxanthine (84%), in addition to some theobromine (12%) and theophylline.[124] It's been noted that sucrose (as found in eating chocolate, or Cacao beverages sweetened with table sugar, coconut sugar, or maple syrup, for example) decreases caffeine's CNS stimulation. While caffeine is metabolised to the still-active paraxanthine and theobromine, theobromine is immediately converted to inactive metabolites. However, there are "substantial individual differences" in theobromine and caffeine clearance rates; smokers, for example, have been noted to clear xanthines 30–50% more quickly, but conversely caffeine metabolism takes four to six times longer in the last trimester of pregnancy. Paradoxically, increased xanthine consumption (as in heavy coffee drinkers) results in decreased clearance speed. In non-human animals, theobromine causes little increase in locomotion when administered on its own, but displays stimulant synergy with caffeine, although no such amplification of effect has been noted in humans. Theobromine's half-life exceeds theophylline's, which in turn exceeds caffeine's; the intermediary metabolite paraxanthine is metabolised most rapidly of all.[125]

Present at up to 25µg/g or 0.0025% of Cacao's dry weight, **salsolinol (SAL)**, aka 1-methyl-1,2,3,4-tetrahydroisoquinoline-6,7-diol is a relatively minor constituent in Cacao, but may contribute to the psychoactivity of Cacao given that the alkaloid readily crosses the blood-brain barrier. It should be noted that tetrahydroisoquinolines (TIQs) such as SAL are also found in whisky, wine, cheese, bananas, broiled sardines, flour, eggs, beer, and milk. In some of these foods the concentrations of other TIQs are far higher than in chocolate, for example, 1-methyl-TIQ at 354ng/g in white wine vs. ≤ 12ng/g (= 0.012µg/g) in cocoa, 15ng/g TIQ in Emmenthal, vs. approximately 1 ng/g in cocoa (= 0.001µg/g).[126] SAL is produced endogenously in the CNS as a natural by-product of dopamine metabolism, in reactions where catecholamines are co-present with aldehydes or α-keto acids from such variables as fasting, diabetes, following a ketogenic diet, or hepatic dysfunction. SAL is most commonly produced as a condensation product of dopamine and acetaldehyde following ethanol intake. It is thought to be responsible for alcohol's activation of dopaminergic neurons in the ventral tegmental area (VTA) of the brain,[127] which plays a role in habit formation, craving, and addiction. SAL can also be synthesised from dopamine and pyruvic acid.

In the VTA of experimental rats, SAL increases nucleus accumbens dopamine release, and "induces a strong conditional place preference"; also rats readily self-administered SAL by injection directly into the VTA and nucleus accumbens, indicating "addictive" or reinforcing properties[128] (q.v. caffeine's synergy with dopaminergic drugs in the nucleus accumbens). SAL has positive effects on heart rate and muscle contractions through β-adrenoreceptor stimulation (dose and quantity not stated),[129] and increases locomotor activity,[130] yet it also decreases plasma levels of adrenaline and noradrenaline during episodes of acute stress by decreasing sympatho-adrenal stimulation[131] (q.v. Whole Chocolate—clinical trial in Chronic Fatigue).

SAL is a reversible inhibitor of monoamine oxidase type A [MAOI-(A)] and tyrosine hydroxylase, thereby retarding both the production and the breakdown of dopamine, and elevating levels of other catecholamines. MAOIs in general are antidepressant, especially indicated for atypical depression such as "hysteroid dysphoria" (rejection sensitivity, sweet food cravings). *In vitro* work indicates that SAL accelerates dopaminergic (DA) neuron firing by three mechanisms: (1) by direct depolarisation, (2) by activating GABA-inhibiting μ-opioid receptors on GABA-ergic DA neuron inputs, and (3) by activating D1 receptors on presynaptic glutaminergic terminals, thereby enhancing presynaptic glutaminergic neurotransmission. D1R glutamatergic effects are shared with ethanol, but salsolinol's glutamatergic effects are 1–2 *million* times greater than ethanol.[132] Opioid-mediated effects are also significant: some opiate-blocking drugs (Naltrexone and Gabazine) reduce the dopaminergic response to SAL. However, salsolinol's affinity for opiate receptors in rat synaptosomal membranes was not particularly high, suggesting that μ-opioid receptors are not salsolinol's principal site of action.[133] SAL also evinced biphasic dopaminergic effects, with peak activity at 0.1μM, diminishing at higher doses.[134]

SAL may accumulate in dopaminergic neurons, and has been linked to the development of Parkinson's disease: SAL methylation produces the neurotoxic compound N-methyl(R) salsolinol (formed from dopamine + acetaldehyde, or dopamine + formaldehyde), which accumulates in the nigrostriatum and accelerates the senescence of dopaminergic neurons.[135] Methylation may be induced by concomitant presence of heavy metals such as copper, magnesium, iron, or aluminium. It has also been noted that Parkinsonian patients have elevated N-methyltrans-ferase activity in lymphocytes compared to non-Parkinsonian research participants, indicating increased production of neurotoxic N-methyl-salsolinol.[136] SAL is also an *in vitro* inhibitor of hydroxysteroid (17-beta) dehydrogenase 4.[137] SAL also competitively inhibits substrate binding to cytochrome p450 XVII, a principal enzyme in the biosynthesis of androgens.[138] If these actions are confirmed *in vivo*, then exogenous SAL consumption may turn out to affect steroidogenesis (especially testosterone) and sexual behaviour or development.

SAL also decreases pro-opiomelanocortin [POMC] gene expression. Given that μ-opioid receptor activation is known to increase the release of POMC products such as β-endorphin and α-MSH,[139] this could represent a down-regulatory effect of SAL on endogenous opioids, or possibly a consequence of competitive inhibition between SAL and other compounds with higher affinity for μ-opioid receptors leading to a net reduction in signals calling for POMC products and a consequent reduction in POMC gene expression. It has been speculated that this effect may account for the central opioid deficiency encountered in chronic alcoholism, wherein SAL levels are increased by the presence of central acetaldehyde from ethanol metabolism.[140] In sheep, SAL increases prolactin (PRL) secretion, but "[T]he secretion of PRL is under the inhibitory control of DA, and SAL does not antagonize the [pituitary?] DA receptor's action";[141] and "[Oral] administration of a solution of SAL or cocoa (another salsolinol-containing beverage) did not stimulate PRL secretion in normal women."[142] However, more recent research in nursing sheep found that SAL levels rise in tandem with PRL during suckling in response to endogenous opioid stimulation (particularly at μ-opioid receptors) in the mediobasal hypothalamus, and that this response (elevated SAL and PRL) was blocked by opiate receptor antagonists.[143] This research, taken alongside the moderate binding affinity of SAL for mu-opioid receptors, suggests that SAL may enhance PRL release in the presence of endogenous opiates.

Cacao also contains very low levels (0.0014%) of **pyrazines**, aromatic alkaloids present in the essential oil of the toasted or roasted beans. One of these, **tetramethylpyrazine (TMP)**, is the major active constituent in the Chinese medicinal herb Chuanxiong (*Ligusticum wallichii*), which is used in cardiovascular disease, headaches, and vertigo. TMP also happens to be a major flavour ingredient in maple syrup. TMP possesses the following properties in isolation, *in vitro* or in animal testing: antioxidant, protective against renal failure, pulmonary vasodilator and protective against pulmonary fibrosis. High doses of TMP lower fibrinogen, suggesting possible use as a preventive against stroke.[144] Animal studies go some way to confirming this: TMP provided *in vitro* (spinal) and *in vivo* (cerebral) protection against neuronal ischaemia-reperfusion injury.[145] TMP also produced vascular protection against the endothelial destruction caused by hypoxia in rats,[146] and *in vitro* calcium channel antagonist activity has been identified, suggesting vasodilatory action.[147]

TMP is rapidly absorbed following oral ingestion, and excreted via urine. But the amount of TMP in Cacao is far lower than could be expected to produce measurable haemodynamic effects: oral doses of at least 100mg repeated three or more times daily would be required to elicit measurable physiological responses.[148] However, the low levels of pyrazines present in Cacao contribute to the flavour and aroma of the roasted bean, and may exert additive effects with other antioxidant compounds in Cacao which influence circulation, such as the polyphenols. Lower-temperature roasting (~116°C) of Cacao beans for twenty to twenty-five minutes produced an optimal balance in terms of the best compromise between flavour and toxicity as represented by the ratio of beneficial pyrazines to carcinogenic acrylamide in the roasted beans. Pyrazines and polyphenols are somewhat mutually incompatible, in that higher polyphenol contents reduce pyrazine concentration as polyphenols bind to pyrazine precursors such as amino acids;[149] moreover, pyrazines are formed during roasting, which reduces polyphenol levels.

Trace amounts of several **tetrahydro-beta-carboline (THβC)** alkaloids are present in fermented Cacao (a maximum of 7.9μg/g, or up to 0.0008% of the dry weight of Cacao). Like salsolinol, low levels of compounds in this class of alkaloid also occur in many other fermented foods and drugs, and in some fruit juices, where they appear to contribute to free-radical scavenging (antioxidant) activity.[150] Also like SAL, THβCs are produced endogenously in the human brain following ethanol consumption. Both SAL and THβCs have been implicated in the development of alcoholism, as the endogenous formation of both involves acetaldehyde, the principal psychoactive metabolite of ethanol. Acetaldehyde combines with dopamine to form SAL, and with indeolamines (serotonin, tryptophan, tryptamine) to form THβCs, and administration of salsolinol and some THβCs have been found to reinforce alcohol or heroin dependency in lab rats and primates.[151]

Larger amounts of related β-carboline compounds constitute the main psychoactive constituents of the principal plant used in the famous Amazonian entheogenic purgative drug, Ayahuasca (*Banisteriopsis caapi*). THβCs may oxidize to form psychoactive β-carbolines in vitro, although the details of their human pharmacokinetics are currently unknown. β-carbolines have been observed to inhibit MAO-A and serotonin reuptake at low concentrations, and (like SAL) are known to bind to opiate and dopamine receptors.[152] β-carbolines may exert profound effects at low dosages:

> [they] have been shown to intercalate into DNA, to inhibit CDK, topoisomerase, and monoamine oxidase, and to interact with benzodiazepine […] and 5-hydroxy serotonin receptors. Furthermore, these chemicals also demonstrated a broad spectrum of pharmacological properties including sedative, anxiolytic, hypnotic, anticonvulsant, antitumor, antiviral, antiparasitic as well as antimicrobial activities. (Cao et al., 2007)[153]

(Note: CDK = Cyclin-Dependent Kinase, an enzyme that mediates the cell cycle, so blocking CDK halts mitosis (cell division); topoisomerases are enzymes regulating DNA winding, so topoisomerase inhibitors are also anti-mitotic, pro-apoptotic, possibly antimicrobial and/or anti-neoplastic or mutagenic, depending on the situation.)

More specifically, several THβCs have been found to bind to serotonin receptor subtypes 1A and 2A. Central nervous system 5HT-1A receptor activation is associated with antidepressant, anxiolytic, nootropic (cognition-enhancing) and endorphin-releasing analgesic effects, while type 2A agonists are typically "psychedelic" (having LSD or psilocybin-like effects). Clearly the dosage and specific molecular structure of THβC compounds are very important here, as people don't generally "trip" on fruit juices, but Cacao's content of several THβCs together with other MAO-inhibitory compounds is worthy of note, especially in light of the historical use of chocolate beverages as a base for *Psilocybe* mushroom ingestion, and modern "user reports" claiming that Cacao intensifies the effects of various psychoactive compounds including opiates and MDMA (see Chapter 5). However, plasma levels of salsolinol and THβCs following chocolate consumption are currently undetermined.

At an estimated 0.00005% of the fresh, undried whole Cacao plant, the alkaloid **trigonelline** is a trace presence, although it hasn't yet been quantified in dried Cacao beans. Trigonelline is also found in coffee (≤ 1.3%) and fenugreek seeds (0.13%), in addition to various other foods such as soy, onions, tomatoes, and shellfish. In addition, 5% of ingested dietary niacin (vitamin B3) is converted into trigonelline, so the actual *in vivo*, post-metabolism content of trigonelline in Cacao is likely to be higher than the absolute content would suggest.[154] Being bacteriostatic against *Streptococcus mutans*, trigonelline has anti-cariogenic activity, in addition to possessing apparent hypocholesterolaemic, hypoglycaemic, anti-migraine, and sedative activity in animal and *in vitro* work.[155] Trigonelline has also been found to elevate seizure thresholds in rats,[156] and possesses *in vivo* CNS stimulant activity, which is corroborated to some extent by *in vitro* work suggesting GABA antagonist and neurotropic properties.[157] *In vitro*, trigonelline is spasmolytic to ileal smooth muscle, but has uterotonic activity.[158] Based on *in vivo* experiments, trigonelline may serve as a specific drug delivery mechanism for PEA to the CNS[159]—which is interesting given the small but measurable content of PEA in Cacao, and the co-presence of MAO-A inhibitory compounds in the bean.

Polyphenols

The antioxidants in Cacao prevent rancidity, so prepared drinking chocolate can remain potable at room temperature for several days, and even with added milk the liquid won't sour for a surprising amount of time.[160] Cacao has a very high ORAC (oxygen radical absorbance capacity) value, though this has only been measured *in vitro* and it remains unclear what value the ORAC "score" has as a predictor of Cacao's *in vivo* pharmacological activity, other than being an approximate measure of the polyphenol content. The flavonoids and other so-called "antioxidants" may exert physiological activity via different and specific mechanisms unrelated to free radical production; for example, increased serum antioxidant levels following chocolate consumption may be due to elevated uric acid production consequent to polyphenol or xanthine metabolism, rather than the presence of phenolic constituents in the bloodstream. The "free radical" theory of aging (whereby antioxidants may reduce the aging process by inhibiting oxidative damage on a cellular level) is unproven, and while it's accepted that degenerative processes involve free radical production, it doesn't follow that free radicals are the cause of aging. In fact "free radicals" are essential components of immune defences and apoptosis. While free radical activity contributes to DNA cross-linking, metaplasia, connective tissue breakdown (e.g., wrinkles) and LDL oxidation predisposing to atherosclerosis, it's also suspected that highly radical-inducing practices such as caloric restriction or intermittent fasting can reduce the net effects of oxidative damage by inducing repair (and have other effects), decreasing overall mortality.[161] Ergo, exogenous "antioxidants" need not be beneficial *per se*, and indiscriminate supplementation with such products has in some cases been associated with *increased* morbidity.[162] For example, both uric acid and glutathione are endogenous antioxidants; the former is a metabolic waste product which can give rise to an inflammatory condition (gout), the latter protects liver cells from chemical injury.

The apparent health benefits and effects of Cacao polyphenols depend on mechanisms specific to each compound's physiological actions, which may be linked to their radical-neutralising activity, but not necessarily so. There are two molecular mechanisms of the Cacao polyphenols' radical-reducing capabilities which may have positive ramifications for human health. The two mechanisms are ROS (reactive oxygen species) scavenging, and inhibition of NADPH (Nicotinamide Adenine Dinucleotide Phosphate) oxidase, a major enzymatic generator of ROS used in immunological respiratory burst responses to pathogens, but also elevated in atherosclerosis, diabetes, cancer, Alzheimer's disease, and primary immunodeficiency. Inhibiting this enzyme might be expected to reduce platelet aggregation and modulate inflammation, neurotransmission, and cytotoxicity.[163]

Nitric oxide (NO) is also known as "endothelium-derived relaxing factor" for its vasodilatory effects. NO inhibits endothelial proliferation, platelet aggregation, and leukocyte adherence, and its vasoprotective role is underscored by research revealing that the endothelial production of NO is impaired in atherosclerosis, diabetes mellitus, or hypertension. Although the vasodilatory effects of NO release afford some protection against tissue ischaemia, very high levels are known to cause direct tissue toxicity. Cacao polyphenols increase levels of circulating NO by several mechanisms, thereby exerting vasodilatory and vascular-endothelium protective effects. The specific mechanisms by which Cacao polyphenols achieve these effects are *inhibition* of reactive oxygen species formation, Angiotensin Converting Enzyme (ACE), and l-arginine oxidation; and *promotion* of calcium ion release, protein kinase C activity, the COX prostacyclin pathway, and endothelium-derived hyperpolarizing factor activation.[164]

The polyphenols comprise up to 4% of the dried weight of raw sun-dried criollo Cacao beans, and up to 6% of the dry weight of forastero beans; once fermented, these quantities decrease to 3% of fermented criollo, and 5% of fermented forastero beans.[165] Interestingly, despite the current flurry of interest in polyphenols' health benefits, the *criollo* variety is more esteemed, mostly due to their less astringent/sour "polyphenol" flavour, but perhaps also due to their higher caffeine content: *criollo* Cacao typically contains 0.4–0.8% caffeine, while *forastero* Cacao contains only a quarter of this, at 0.1–0.2% caffeine.[166] *Criollo* also contains higher amounts of particular polyphenols such as caffeic acid derivatives, while *forastero* subtypes generally contain more proanthocyanidins, which are sometimes completely absent from *criollo* varieties.[167] A dietary whole polyphenol extract of Cacao reduced obesity in mice fed a high-fat diet, without affecting fasting blood glucose; the *in vitro* mechanism for this effect was found to be a reduction of mitotic clonal expansion of preadipocytes and inhibition of insulin receptor kinase by binding directly to the enzyme.[168] While it can't be assumed that this effect would be replicated in humans eating or drinking chocolate, particularly given Cacao's traditional usage to help gain weight, recent research on Cacao's effect on diabetes and cardiovascular health does bear this out (q.v. "Whole chocolate research" later in this monograph).

The polyphenols in Cacao may be classified in the following molecular hierarchy, giving the largest "parent compounds" first, and smaller, metabolically downstream categories later:

- Polyphenols > condensed tannins: proanthocyanidins > procyanidins
- Polyphenols > flavonoids > flavan-3-ols (flavanols) > catechins.

Cacao polyphenols (CP), and the proanthocyanidins in particular, have been screened for preliminary *in vitro* anti-neoplastic or cytotoxic activity. Speculation about the chemopreventive potentials of these compounds has led to the identification of several possible mechanisms of action:

> "Other proposed mechanisms by which polyphenols may prevent, delay or alleviate the progression of cancer that, however, have not yet been studied particularly with chocolate, cocoa or polyphenols isolated from cocoa include: complexation (chelates) of divalent cations, inhibition of the activity of enzymes including telomerase, xanthine oxidase, lipoxygenase, protein kinase C and protein tyrosine kinases, inhibition of MAP kinase as well as growth factor signalling, induction of hepatic electrophile-processing (Phase II) enzymes, modulation of the activity of enzymes such as cytochrome P-450 isozyme, induction of apoptosis, and inhibition of angiogenesis" (Wollgast, 2004).[169]

Laboratory (*in vitro*) work with CP demonstrated total inhibition of prostate cancer cell line growth at 0.2% concentrations, with no effect on normal prostate cells,[170] but the polyphenols also inhibited lymphocyte proliferation and B-cell immunoglobulin production "in a dose-dependent manner",[171] indicating possible Th-2 immunosuppressive activity. But the procyanidins also appeared to stimulate innate immunity *in vitro* by enhancing peripheral blood mononuclear cell (PBMC) production of granulocyte macrophage colony-stimulating factor and B-cell markers CD69 and CD83.[172] The procyanidins also had dose-dependent xanthine oxidase inhibitory activity.[173] If this also occurs *in vivo*, it may indicate some anti-plasmodial (antimalarial?) activity, as many microorganisms—including the various *Plasmodium* species responsible for malaria—require hypoxanthine (one of the enzyme's products) to survive. This property may also benefit other conditions in which xanthine oxidation is implicated, such as corneal degeneration and gout.

Rats with drug-induced prostate cancer also benefited from CP. Doses of 24 or 48mg/kg administered orally every day for nine months reduced tumour size and appearance as compared to carcinogen-treated but polyphenol-deprived rats. Notably, however, the group receiving the lower dose of polyphenols fared better than the higher intake group, with no tumours in any of the lower dose rats after nine months, whereas *the higher dose group still developed tumours*.[174] The low dose group was still ingesting a high dose of polyphenols in terms of the quantity of Cacao which would have to be consumed (24mg/kg in a 10st or 63.5kg human adult = 1524mg polyphenols per day = 120g whole Cacao per day), but the greater therapeutic response in the lower dose group suggests that there may be an optimum "dosage window" for CP. The optimum therapeutic dosage may correspond to or overlap intake levels which are achievable by consumption of non-toxic quantities of whole Cacao, if the type of cancer induced in these rats proves to be similarly responsive to orally administered polyphenolic chemoprevention in humans.

CP dose-dependently reduced weight gain and ingestion rates of testosterone-treated rats, and reduced the rats' serum DHT levels and prostate size ratio—in this case, the higher dose was more effective.[175] Huge doses of oral polyphenols in mice (40 or 200mg/kg, equivalent to 240g–1kg whole Cacao in a 10st human) reduced dermal markers of inflammation and carcinogenesis after topical mutagen/toxin was applied.[176] In another experiment, male rats were poisoned with several carcinogens over thirty-six weeks, but CP at 0.025–0.25% of their diet had chemopreventive effects at the higher dosage for lung and thyroid cancers, but didn't protect against cancers of the kidneys, colon, or small intestine. CP at 0.025–0.25% of the diet in female rats similarly poisoned by a carcinogen over forty-eight weeks had protective effects at the higher dosage against pancreatic, but not mammary carcinogenesis.[177] It should be noted however that this dosage (0.25% of the diet as pure polyphenols) is equivalent to an excessive daily intake of Cacao for the average human, at the upper limits of tolerance—not only would this level of intake take time to work up to, it would be extremely costly, and is up to four times greater than the maximum tolerable daily intake of Cacao for many people: if the average daily human food intake is 1277g, then 0.025–0.25% = 319–3190mg polyphenols = 266g whole Cacao per day. Most people experience side effects such as nausea, headaches, digestive distress, or vomiting after consuming over 80–100g whole Cacao in one sitting. Dividing this dosage over twelve hours or more would be tolerable for most adults, but >200g would likely still produce symptoms of toxicity such as headaches or nausea unless a high tolerance had been acquired. At the very least, such dosages would be aversive.

However, as noted earlier, other constituents in the whole Cacao bean may increase or oppose the potency of the polyphenols with regard to specific activities. For example, in this case we may speculate that theobromine may antagonise CP's chemopreventive effects on prostate cancer, but the THβCs may enhance the anti-neoplastic activity of CP in some cell lines. In any case it should be recalled that the activity of a chemical extract such as isolated polyphenols isn't always reflected in the efficacy of the whole plant, or *vice versa*.

Cocoa liquor polyphenols also dose-dependently inhibited lipid accumulation in preadipocytes derived from mice, suppressing mitotic clonal expansion in fat cells and decreasing mRNA expression of fatty acid synthase,[178] suggesting that Cacao may help prevent weight gain if these results are borne out by animal and human studies.

Cocoa extract or isolated flavanols applied directly to colonic epithelia caused a partial inhibition of chloride ion secretion from the mucosa, thereby decreasing fluid secretion, which may be a relevant mechanism of action in controlling secretory diarrhoea, one condition for which Cacao was traditionally prescribed.[179] CP from unroasted beans administered orally also exhibited "antidepressant-like effects" in rats (forced swimming test) at dosages of 24mg/kg and 48mg/kg, equivalent to 1524mg or 3048mg polyphenols in a 10st adult human, which could only be achieved by ingestion of a minimum of 120–240g whole Cacao, in excess of the upper dosage limit, although 120g total daily consumption is feasible in divided doses—this is close to the approximate daily intake of Cacao for the Kuna people in San Blas, Panama. However, there may be synergy or additive effects between the polyphenols and other constituents in the beans such as the alkaloids, and/or cumulative effects; of course it should also be noted that there can be huge variations in inter-species pharmacokinetics. Tests would need to be conducted in humans ingesting higher doses equivalent to 80g (an upper tolerable single-dose limit for many people, perhaps divided into two smaller doses of 40g) whole Cacao daily. A similar daily dose of 24mg/kg polyphenols improved cognitive performance and increased the lifespan of lab rats, also preserving urinary free dopamine levels.[180]

Rabbits bred to develop atherosclerosis given cocoa polyphenols as 1% of the dry weight of their daily diet for six months had lower blood pressure and resting heart rate and significantly reduced aortic atherosclerosis, without significant change in blood lipid levels as compared to the comparison group of rabbits fed a polyphenol-free but otherwise identical diet. The polyphenol group also maintained better cardiac output under stressful conditions and retained "parasympathetic tone" as they aged.[181]

CP administered to rats before intra-gastric ethanol poisoning reduced damage to stomach mucosa equivalent to the protection attained from the use of standard anti-ulcer drugs Cimetidine and Sucralfate. The orthodox drugs achieve this either by completely suppressing hydrochloric acid production, which impairs primary protein digestion and the "sterilisation" of food in the stomach, or by binding to the ulcer's surface and sealing it, which can produce constipation or other digestive disturbances further down the alimentary canal. On the other hand CP worked by reducing free-radical damage in cells affected by inflammation, but also modified leukocyte activity to decrease pro-inflammatory activity in gastric muscosa via xanthine oxidase inhibition (most likely effected by the procyanidins, as described above).[182] These mechanisms suggest there may be complementary applications of CP in peptic ulceration. In other animal torture experiments, mice were fed a diet with added CP (human equivalent = approximately 12.77g polyphenols per day, equivalent to 106g whole Cacao/day). Some of those mice were then poisoned with diesel exhaust, and those with CP in their diet had greatly reduced metabolic indicators of oxidative stress in their lungs, and reduced signs of lung injury overall on autopsy.[183] Purified CP administered to streptozotocin-induced diabetic rats as 0.5% of their daily diet reduced cataract formation over ten weeks. Unfortunately, while this may lead to future research or drug development, this level of intake represents an absurd quantity of Cacao in humans: if 1277g is assumed to be the weight of an average Briton's daily food intake,[184] then 0.5% diet = 6.39g polyphenols, representing a ludicrous 532g whole Cacao/day!

One human double-blind placebo-controlled clinical trial, involving thirty-two subjects given a daily dose of either 6mg (designated "placebo") or 234mg CP over twenty-eight days, found significant reduction in platelet function in the high-polyphenol group, together with elevated plasma levels of ascorbic acid.[185] These results suggest that Cacao may be useful to decrease the risk of thrombus formation, for example in people with a higher risk of stroke, heart attack, DVT, or similar. Interestingly, there was no change in oxidation markers or overall antioxidant status in either group, again underscoring the likelihood of specific pharmacodynamic mechanisms for the cardiovascular effects of CP independent of their "antioxidant" status.

Higher levels of CP give beans a sourer or more bitter taste, so more highly prized bean varieties tend to have relatively lower CP content. CP levels in Cacao also fall during fermentation as they are oxidised when exposed to air due to dissolution of the parenchyma (plant cell walls), so the CP are dissipated into the fermentation liquid. Longer fermentation and drying times, and longer, higher roasting temperatures also reduce CP content. However in all these processes the beans' high saturated fat content protects many CP from oxidation, so by far the most destructive process is alkalisation of defatted cocoa mass, or "Dutching", the process used to increase the water-dispersive properties of cocoa powder, which results in loss of up to 80% of the polyphenols. CP comprise approximately 6–8% of the dry weight of unfermented and unroasted Cacao beans.[186] Natural (simple roasted and defatted) cocoa contains 34.6mg/g flavanols, whereas processed alkalised cocoa contains almost ten times less than this, 3.9mg/g flavanols, and dark chocolate is little better, with 1.7–8.4mg/kg CP,[187] due to its added fat and sugar content diluting the CP percentage.

The **proanthocyanidins** are procyanidin "prodrugs", just as the flavonoids are flavan-3-ol (flavanol) prodrugs: their downstream procyanidin metabolites exert the principal pharmacodynamic effects. Cacao has the highest concentration of proanthocyanidins of any natural food or drug, more than some of its closest "competitors" such as bilberry, tea, red wine, or acai berries. The "antioxidant" or ORAC ranking of these foods, indicating only "antioxidant" properties (and, as discussed earlier, not necessarily indicative of intrinsic health merit) is cocoa > red wine > green tea > black tea.[188] Cacao's proanthocyanidins cause vasodilation *in vitro* by inhibiting production of the protein endothelin-1 which constricts blood vessels, they stabilise collagen and elastin, and have *in vivo* anti-oedema activity. Cacao's proanthocyanidins give fresh beans a purple colour; *criollo* beans are a lighter mauve, as they contain higher levels of caffeine but up to two-thirds less anthocyanins than the less esteemed *forastero* varieties.[189] *In vitro*, anthocyanins reduce lipoxygenase[ii] production and may therefore exert anti-inflammatory effects *in vivo*, depending on their bioavailability.[190] An enormous 80mg/kg dose of purified

---

[ii] Lipoxygenase = enzymes which catalyse the production of pro-inflammatory leukotrines derived from arachidonic acid, among other functions.

proanthocyanidins, equivalent to that found in a toxic dose of 400g Cacao given to a 10st/63.5kg human, when administered to heat-tortured mice caused a potentiation of their sleeping time, and "behaviour similar to those receiving morphine".[191]

Researchers aver that the concentration of highly antioxidant **flavanols** in Cacao isn't sufficient to explain the prevention of free-radical induced tissue damage:

> Other mechanisms compatible with the physiological levels reached by flavanols may explain the observed changes in cell or tissue oxidation levels after flavanol consumption. These mechanisms are *beyond the ability of flavanols and other flavonoids to directly prevent free radical-mediated tissue damage* [my italics]. Thus, the question remains of attributing beneficial effects to cocoa polyphenols vs. cocoa as a whole. Other compounds in cocoa are known to be bioactive. (Wollgast, 2004)[192]

Epidemiological data comparing flavanol intake and cancer incidence is inconsistent, but for coronary heart disease mortality in the elderly there is a strongly positive inverse association, even when confounding variables such as "antioxidant vitamin" intake and income status are excluded.[193] Cacao flavanols accumulate in the hippocampus and other areas of the brain linked to learning and memory following chronic ingestion, and have collectively been found to exert potentially profound effects on these faculties. The flavanols induce expression of neuropeptides which potentially improve brain repair, prevent neuronal damage, and increase neuroplasticity. They also improve blood flow and increase angiogenesis in the brain. One *in vitro* study modelling Alzheimer's disease found that Cacao polyphenols counteracted neurite dystrophy by activating the brain-derived neurotrophic factor (BDNF) survival pathway in cells affected by amyloid-β accumulation.[194] Real-life benefits of cocoa flavanols have been demonstrated in animal models and human observational studies of cognitive function in aging, dementia, and stroke.[195] However, there is currently no conclusive research demonstrating *acute* beneficial effects of cocoa flavanols on cognitive function.[196] One small-scale medium-term DBPC clinical trial found that a once-daily dose of chocolate containing 500mg polyphenols (equivalent to approx. 40g Cacao) over a period of one month significantly improved "self-rated calmness and contentedness" relative to placebo, with no acute effects on mood and none noted on cognition at any dose.[197]

Cacao flavanols (a mixture) were administered to older adults aged 61–85 years over an eight-week period in a double-blind, placebo-controlled, parallel-arm study testing the effects of three levels of Cacao flavanol intake on cognitive function, metabolic profile and blood pressure. The three dosage levels were 48mg ("low flavanol"), 520mg ("intermediate flavanol"), or 993mg ("high flavanol") per day, approximating to daily dosages of whole Cacao of 13g, 143g, and 272g, of which an upper dosage limit somewhere between the first and second group is feasible with whole Cacao. All dosage levels improved performance on the trail making and verbal fluency tests of cognitive function, with the intermediate and higher flavanol intakes showing the greatest improvements, and the two higher flavanol intake groups also showed the greatest improvements in insulin sensitivity, lipid peroxidation, and blood pressure.[198]

Polyphenols in general (from sources other than, but not excluding Cacao) also inhibit LDL biosynthesis, increase hepatic LDL receptors, and inhibit hepatic apolipoprotein B100, and may therefore lower plasma LDL. However, high doses of Cacao polyphenols are cytotoxic to hepatocytes; (-)EGCG in particular acts as a pro-oxidant in this environment.[199] Isolated cocoa flavanols at a high dose of 10mg/kg (equivalent to 108g whole Cacao for a 10st/63.5kg adult, likely to produce emesis if administered in a single dose) administered to mice caused an acute increase in plasma adrenaline and enhanced thermogenesis/anti-lipemic effects. Interestingly, epicatechin alone caused few of these effects, suggesting that the combination of flavanols was responsible for this activity.[200] These results indicate that high doses of the mixture of flavanols found in Cacao, equivalent to the upper end possible for human ingestion of Cacao (bordering on a toxic dose), may exert anti-obesity, thermogenic, and adrenergic effects. It should be noted, however, that whole Cacao extracts may *reduce* plasma levels of adrenaline and cortisol in adult humans.[201] These results from testing isolated cocoa flavanols indicate their therapeutic potential, but there is a need for further studies before extrapolating the effects of individual constituents or chemical groups to benefits of a whole plant product in a particular condition (e.g., Cacao in Alzheimer's disease or cardiovascular disease).

Cacao's **procyanidins**, especially **procyanidin B2**, retarded hydrogen peroxide-induced apoptosis *in vitro* by inhibiting kinase enzyme activity,[202] and displayed anti-mutagenic activity through a similar anti-kinase mechanism.[203] They are also anti-angiogenic, preventing cultured aortic endothelial cell proliferation.[204] Procyanidins administered to healthy human subjects (n=7) modulated TGF-β1 secretion (reduced when high, increased when low).[205] TGF-β is anti-proliferative, pro-apoptotic, and reduces T-lymphocyte activation and monocyte phagocytosis, yet this cytokine is typically overproduced by cancer cells, whereby the malignant cells' growth and spread are enhanced despite its anti-proliferative properties, as elevated TGF-β induces local immunosuppression and angiogenesis. So if the procyanidins' anti-kinase effects are also shown to be active following oral administration, Cacao may be a useful anti-metastatic agent in certain cancers. Moreover, TGF-β is usually elevated in the blood and CSF of Alzheimer's disease patients, although it's not yet clear whether this is a compensatory response to neurodegeneration or an element of the pathological process.

In vitro, the procyanidins stabilised T-cell membranes,[206] suggesting that—if bioavailable (see below), orally administered Cacao procyanidins may both modulate and conserve specific immune system components. There was a reduction in polyamine synthesis in Caco-2 cells (a cellular model of the intestinal epithelium) treated with 50microg/ml procyanidin extracts. Polyamines are cellular metabolites which play an essential role in growth and proliferation, so the implication is that Cacao's procyanidins may have anti-proliferative effects on intestinal epithelia.[207]

Some of the procyanidins are hyaluronidase inhibitors, suggesting multiple applications, including potential utility in bronchitis or COPD, and some bacterial infections such as cystitis, as they inhibit *E. coli* adhesion to urinary epithelium.[208] The hyaluronidase inhibitory activity of Cacao goes some way towards explaining Cacao's traditional use as a general or supportive tonic in many illnesses including pulmonary ailments, and possibly its use as a prophylactic antivenom against some types of snakebite, as many snake venoms contain hyaluronidases and inhibiting this enzyme with plant extracts significantly reduces their morbidity in experimental models.[209] And as is the case with the phenolic constituents in general, the whole bean is superior to processed cocoa: roasted and fermented Cacao beans or cocoa liquor contain four times as much total procyanidins as Dutched cocoa powder.[210]

While the larger condensed tannin proanthocyanidins have low bioavailability due to their high molecular weight, small intestinal and colonic microflora degrade some to bioactive phenolic acids, which are detectable in urine forty-eight hours after chocolate consumption.[211] However, their procyanidin by-products are very stable in the gastric milieu, and do reach the small intestine intact.[212] A rat study found that oral administration of whole cocoa extract, or procyanidin complexes isolated from hazelnuts (*Corylus avellana*) with or without whole Cacao extract, resulted in high renal concentrations of phase 2 procyanidin metabolites, indicating that the kidney may be the primary site of procyanidin metabolism. Phenolic acids were detected in all tissues, particularly the kidney, liver, lung, and brain.[213]

It's notable that *in vitro* ascorbic acid stabilised flavan-3-ols and procyanidins in alkaline media (comparable to the pH of pancreatic secretions), whereas these phenolics were otherwise degraded in a few hours at a similar pH,[214] suggesting that consuming procyanidins with fruits high in Vitamin C may increase their bioavailability. However procyanidins such as PB2 were detectable in human plasma thirty minutes after plain cocoa ingestion, peaking at two hours after consumption. So even though intestinal catechol-O-methyltransferase (COMT) activity would suggest degradation to (still-active) metabolites catechin and epicatechin, high concentrations of procyanidins reduce COMT activity (by saturation?) and may therefore permit rapid absorption of intact procyanidins, which would explain their presence in the bloodstream[215]— and may infer utility in Parkinson's disease treatment, if taken with l-dopa containing drugs or natural products such as Cowhage (*Mucuna pruriens*) or Broad Beans (*Vicia faba*).

Flavan-3-ols including **epicatechin** are found in whole Cacao, as well as being produced *in vivo* as flavonoid metabolites following hydrolysis by gut bacteria. They inhibit 5-lipoxygenase activity, thereby reducing leukotrine synthesis, and even millimolar concentrations in the blood have been found to reduce LDL peroxidation.[216] Flavan-3-ols may preferentially stimulate IgA production *in vivo*, and when applied orally have been found to reduce the risk of developing periodontal disease.[217] High flavan-3-ol and epicatechin-containing natural products such as Cacao could be useful for enhancing specific mucosal defences, which may imply adjunctive therapeutic roles in HIV, cancer patients undergoing chemotherapy, and many other conditions where mucosa may be compromised and opportunistic infections could take hold. *In vitro*, flavan-3-ols were also found to be "potent stimulators of both the innate immune system and early events in adaptive immunity" on the cellular level.[218] Yet they also evinced inhibition of monocyte and neutrophil activation, with 4-O-methyl-epicatechin being particularly active in this regard, and similar effects were noted *in vivo*, so their ultimate effect on immunity is yet to be determined.[219] *In vitro* flavanols and their metabolites also inhibited platelet aggregation, activation, and conjugation with monocytes or neutrophils, in a similar manner to aspirin, demonstrating anti-thrombotic activity.[220]

The flavan-3-ols epicatechin and **catechin** inhibit amyloid-β protein induced neuronal apoptosis and provide protection against oxidative stress in neurons *in vitro*, from which potential neuroprotective or anti-neurodegenerative activity may be inferred.[221] Both compounds are MAO-B inhibitors, possibly increasing central dopamine and phenylethylamine levels, suggesting antidepressant and perhaps antiparkinsonian effects. Other flavan-3-ols in Cacao such as **quercetin**, **hesperetin**, and **caffeic acid** inhibit *in vitro* production of the dopamine metabolite 5-S-cysteinyl-dopamine and its neurotoxic oxidised by-product, dihydrobenzothiazine,[222] again suggesting potential antiparkinsonian activity if these phenolics cross the blood-brain barrier. *In vitro*, epicatechin also inhibits xanthine oxidase, thereby reducing ROS ("free radical") formation, and increases extracellular cyclic AMP response element binding protein (CREB) in cortical neurons, which implies that this compound may increase capacity for long-term memory formation. Epicatechin also exerts cardioprotective activity via δ-opioid receptor stimulation[223] and reduces plasma endothelin-1, causing vasodilation.[224] In animal experiments, catechin and **3-O-methyl epicatechin** produced a dose-dependent inhibition of free radical-induced haemolysis,[225] which may infer a complementary role for Cacao in haemolytic anaemias.

The flavan-3-ols epicatechin and catechin are absorbed in significant amounts, with a twelvefold peak increase in the amounts in the bloodstream two hours after chocolate ingestion, and plasma ORAC increased by 31%, returning almost back to baseline six hours after ingestion. In eight human subjects given up to 0.50g Cacao per kg bodyweight (0.5g/kg), procyanidin B2, epicatechin, catechin, and 3-O-methyl epicatechin were all detected in plasma one hour after Cacao consumption.[226] So while the larger proanthocyandins weren't well absorbed, the procyanidin dimers, flavan-3-ols and smaller polyphenolic molecules and their metabolites are systemically bioavailable. Flavanol monomers are easily absorbed from the small intestine,[227] and polymeric procyanidins are metabolised by colon microbiota into various phenolic acids which may then be absorbed—so to some extent the procyanidins may be considered prodrugs as well as active constituents of Cacao in their own right. Two hours after human volunteers ingested procyanidin- and flavonoid-enriched cocoa, epicatechin was measurable in their blood plasma at 5.3mg/g, and their blood samples evinced decreased markers of oxidative stress.[228]

Milk reduces the absorption of flavan-3-ols from beverages and foods containing Cacao, as measured by metabolites in the urine of nine volunteers in a one-off trial. Flavan-3-ol absorption declines from 18.3% of the ingested dose in non-milk chocolate consumers to 10.5% when Cacao is taken with milk.[229] Milk didn't substantially affect the *in vivo* metabolism of flavan-3-ols in this smaller group, but in another two trials with twenty-one volunteers milk had less of an inhibitory effect on flavan-3-ol absorption, but some changes in metabolism of the compounds were recorded, possibly due to differences in the ratio of Cacao to milk in the tested foodstuffs.[230] It was observed that consuming 40g cocoa powder with 250ml whole milk instead of plain water did cause a reduction in the consequent plasma epicatechin metabolite level, even though this wasn't reflected in the urinary metabolite measurements.[231] A cautious conclusion may be that milk somewhat reduces the absorption of at least some of Cacao's flavanol components. The mechanism for this is unknown, but could be that the proteins in milk form complexes with the flavanols in Cacao, and the resultant molecules are then too large to be transported across the intestinal lumen unless first hydrolysed by intestinal microorganisms. Again, therefore, the degree to which milk (and perhaps other protein-containing foods or liquids) impacts the absorption of Cacao's flavanols may depend on the microbiome.

By contrast, sugars and starches (as in corn, bread, biscuits, etc.) increased the plasma content of catechin and epicatechin by 140% compared with controls when consumed with cocoa in twenty-four subjects, and significantly raised their plasma antioxidant capacity at 1.5 and 2.5h post-consumption compared to cocoa alone, indicating increased plasma flavanol content. Consuming protein, fat, or even antacids (proton pump antagonists such as Omeprazole) had negligible effects on flavanol absorption.[232] This implies that the traditional consumption of

Cacao beverages after meals, or with corn in *Atoles* or contemporary corn-based Mexican drinks such as *Tejate, Champurrado*, or *Pozol*, and even the European innovation of adding sugar to solid eating chocolate, may maximise the pharmacological effects of the flavan-3-ols in Cacao by increasing their bioavailability.

However, it should not be assumed that Cacao's polyphenols are necessarily the components responsible for the elevated plasma antioxidant capacity. In a double-blind crossover trial, eighteen volunteers ate chocolate containing either 200ml flavanols/day or a low-flavanol version containing <10ml/day every day for four weeks. All participants had a measurable reduction in faecal water free radical content with *both types of chocolate*, suggesting that other, non-polyphenolic components, may be responsible for measurable changes in antioxidant levels, at least in the gut.[233] The result in this case (the low faecal free radical content) may be a consequence of secondary effects, such as other components in Cacao affecting gut microflora. In another trial, an epicatechin metabolite was detected in plasma up to two hours after oral cocoa beverage consumption,[234] and plasma epicatechin levels also increased up to twelve times above baseline, peaking at two hours after cocoa ingestion, and returned to baseline after six hours.[235] Phenolic acid metabolites of the polyphenols in chocolate are produced in quantity by gut microflora and excreted in the urine. It is these metabolites which are hypothesised to be responsible for many of the observed effects of cocoa polyphenols *in vivo*, although the procyanidins were also found to be remarkably stable in the gut[236] and were detectable in plasma thirty minutes after ingestion.[237] It may therefore be speculated that at least some of the polyphenols' pharmacological activity in humans is dependent on a functional microbiome ("gut flora").

Cacao's **hydroxycinnamic acids** include **caffeic acid** and **caffeic acid derivatives**, which are found in Mexican/Central American criollo Cacao at higher levels than in other varieties, or those grown in other parts of the world—around 1.2mg/g (non-Mexican varieties contain 0.5–1.1mg/g).[238] Caffeic acid is an ubiquitous compound in plants, as it is a necessary intermediate in the formation of Lignin, but some herbs and spices contain exceptionally high amounts, and Cacao falls into this category; caffeic acid comprises around 0.122% of Cacao's dry weight. Caffeic acid is well absorbed from foods and can accumulate if such foods are consumed regularly, being detectable in human plasma following daily ingestion of fruits containing Caffeic acid over an eight-week period at levels significantly above baseline.[239] Caffeic acid prevented acetaminophen-induced hepatotoxicity, protected endothelial cells against ischaemia-reperfusion injury, and buffered neurons from acrolein[iii]-induced oxidative damage *in vitro*,[240] suggesting possible benefit for liver, cardiovascular, or renal disease, and Alzheimer's disease. In rat experiments (*in vivo*), the caffeic acid derivative, caffeic acid phenethyl ester reduced cholestatic and ethanol- or cisplatin-induced liver damage, normalising liver enzyme and bilirubin levels, and mitigated gamma radiation or isoprostenol-induced heart damage.[241] Caffeic acid phenethyl ester is found naturally in bee propolis, but it is currently not documented if this particular compound is present in Cacao.

The **phenolic acids** in Cacao include gallic and protocatechuic Acid. **Gallic acid** comprises almost 0.1% dry weight of the bean, and has topically anti-fungal, anti-viral, and antioxidant

---

[iii] A simple aldehyde, acrid and toxic, most commonly encountered/ingested by heating cooking oil beyond its smoke point.

properties, as well as being cytotoxic to several cancer cell lines. Plants containing high levels of gallic acid are often used ethnomedically as "astringents" to counter bleeding or haemorrhage, administered orally as anti-diabetic agents, and externally applied to treat psoriasis and haemorrhoids.[242] Many of these uses are clinically unconfirmed, but *in vitro* research notes that gallic acid inhibits pro-inflammatory gene expression in the synoviocytes of people with rheumatoid arthritis, and induced apoptosis in many of these cultured cells.[243] *In vivo* animal research does exist: applied topically, gallic acid had a de-pigmenting effect via inhibition of melanin production,[244] and orally administered gallic acid inhibited gastric cancer cell metastasis in mice.[245] High-dose i.v. gallic acid protected rats from ethanol-induced pancreatic injury,[246] and daily oral administration of gallic acid for one week (at a dose of 20mg/kg, equivalent to 1270mg per day for a 10st human) ameliorated sodium fluoride-induced oxidative damage to rat kidneys.[247]

0.06% of Cacao's dry weight is **protocatechuic acid** (**PCA**), which has *in vitro* anti-inflammatory, anti-hyperglycemic, neuroprotective, and anti-carcinogenic/anti-proliferative properties (the latter by inducing apoptosis of cultured human leukaemia cells).[248] Under laboratory conditions PCA induces neuronal maturation and neurite outgrowth, increases neural stem cell proliferation, and promotes survival of stressed cortical neurons.[249] It also reduces shear-stress induced platelet aggregation, but doesn't affect clotting induced by other factors such as collagen, thrombin, or ADP, and caused no reduction in bleeding time, which suggests that PCA intake may reduce the risk of post-traumatic thrombus formation without increasing bleeding, depending on its bioavailability.[250] PCA has insulin-like activity on adipocytes, increasing their glucose uptake, thereby demonstrating potential activity against insulin resistance.[251] Intraperitoneal administration of PCA to fifty mice over a three day period as a pre-treatment before induced intestinal ischaemia-reperfusion injury protected the phenolic acid-treated mice from collateral damage to lung tissue.[252] Orally administered PCA also protected rat heart tissue from oxidative damage at a dose of 100mg/kg,[253] equivalent to over 6g daily in a 10st human, a near-impossible dose to derive from food or natural sources. Similarly, PCA as 1–2% of the diet protected mice from brain injury associated with D-galactose, indicating a possible role in the prevention or alleviation of age-related cognitive decline.[254] In addition, PCA was deemed to have anti-inflammatory and analgesic activity in rats "comparable to standard drugs".[255]

PCA is one of the main metabolites of the anthocyanins and procyanidins in Cacao,[256] so its presence in the bloodstream following Cacao or chocolate ingestion and its contribution to Cacao's pharmacology may be more than expected from the quite low level of PCA in the whole bean. The only pharmacokinetic data on PCA specifically available to date are from an experiment using mice, which showed that a 50mg/kg oral dose of PCA[iv] gave a maximum plasma concentration at five minutes post-ingestion, and was detectable for eight hours post-ingestion. This result is of questionable relevance to Cacao research, because it would be necessary to consume over 5kg of beans or cocoa liquor in one sitting to achieve this level of PCA in the bloodstream. However, a small trial in which adult humans were given 60g black raspberry powder to eat showed that low quantities of PCA (ng/ml) were detectable in plasma following ingestion.[257] It's hard to know what to make of this information, other than that at least some

---

[iv] Equivalent to 3175mg in a 10st human. To achieve this level of intake with Cacao, it would be necessary to consume over 5kg of beans or cocoa liquor in one sitting.

of the PCA from Cacao or *in vivo* procyanidin metabolism would find its way into the general circulation, but as yet there is no indication whether or not the quantities absorbed from a given dose of Cacao could be pharmacologically significant.

The **N-phenylpropanoyl-l-amino acids (NPAs)** are present in Cacao at levels of up to 30mg/100g Cacao, or up to 0.03% dry weight. These compounds in Cacao are also "antioxidants", with ascorbic acid-like anti-radical activity. *In vitro*, **clovamide** prevents neuronal damage by oxidative stress, ischaemia-reperfusion injury, and excitotoxicity;[258] it exerts dose-dependent anti-inflammatory effects by modulating human monocyte activity, and by inhibiting respiratory burst, intracellular NF-kB activation, and release of pro-inflammatory cytokines;[259] it activates β-2 adrenoreceptors; and it also inhibits COX-1 and COX-2 inflammatory pathways.[260] If its *in vitro* actions prove to be systemically viable, then clovamide may have bronchodilatory activity as potent as (the adrenergic drug) Salbutamol, and it may decrease atherosclerotic inflammation and tendency to thrombus formation via COX-pathway inhibition of thromboxane B2 production and platelet p-selectin expression, and monocyte modulation. Clovamide is bioavailable following chocolate consumption, as it is detectable in the urine of human trial subjects after drinking cocoa, peaking at two hours post-ingestion.[261] **Dideoxyclovamide** also inhibits platelet p-selectin expression and platelet-leukocyte interactions *in vitro*, showing similar potential to clovamide for antithrombotic and anti-metastatic effects—also suggestive of additive or synergistic potential with Cacao's procyanidins as anti-metastatic, anti-thrombotic, and even as prophylactic snake anti-venom agents, as suggested by Cacao's traditional use.

The level of clovamide and its derivatives in Cacao is highly variable, depending on the bean's provenance. Like other phenolic constituents, roasting or pyrolysis degrades Cacao's NPA constituents, reducing clovamide content by up to 60%.[262] Cacao's NPAs such as clovamide were detected in urine after humans consumed Cacao beverages, peaking two hours after consumption, indicating systemic bioavailability.[263] It should be noted that other NPAs have been found to enhance mitochondrial activity (as does pyrryloquinoline quinone [PQQ], also found in Cacao), and to accelerate liver and skin cell proliferation.[264]

Chlorogenic acid (CA), the principal **hydroxycinnamic acid** found in Cacao, is an intermediate compound in lignin synthesis and is therefore a common secondary metabolite in plants. CA has antioxidant and hypoglycaemic activity, the latter by delaying glucose absorption, and protects human lymphocytes against X-ray DNA damage *in vitro*.[265] CA also has some direct cytotoxic activity, to which lung cancer cells are only marginally more sensitive than normal lung fibroblasts, so CA is only partially selectively cytotoxic at moderate concentrations of 0.5–5mM. However, CA has a relatively narrow therapeutic window in this regard, with some carcinogenic potential through causing DNA damage to healthy cells.[266] CA is neuroprotective *in vitro* by inhibiting acetylcholinesterase and butyrylcholinesterase activity and reducing oxidative damage to neurons.[267] CA may also exert antiparkinsonian effects—it inhibits oxidation of dopamine and the interaction of oxidised dopamine with alpha-synuclein, preventing Lewy body formation and acting as a cytoprotective agent in dopamine-producing neurons.[268]

CA suppressed production of thromboxane-A2 *in vitro*, and may therefore be anti-thrombogenic in vascular endothelial injury.[269] In animal experiments, huge intraperitoneal doses of CA had anti-hyperalgesic properties in rats. CA also attenuated induced chronic liver injury and hepatic fibrosis, and had anti-ulcerogenic and gastroprotective properties against ethanol damage in rats—all at higher doses than those which could reasonably be consumed in the form of Cacao or other foodstuffs.[270] In a randomised, double-blind, and placebo-controlled human clinical trial with twenty-three mixed-gender participants, an acute oral dose of 400mg CA significantly lowered both systolic and diastolic blood pressure, by approximately –2mm Hg.[271] CA also has some anti-nutrient properties in solution, reacting with quinines and proteins to form caffeic and quinic acids which limit thiamine (Vitamin B1) absorption.[272] Although CA is present at only low levels in Cacao, it is "well absorbed orally",[273] but levels decrease with roasting of the bean, so raw or lightly roasted beans have higher CA content.

Resveratrol is a naturally occurring phytoalexin: a compound that protects plants against pathogens. It's present in Cacao at very low levels, approximately 0.0009% of the beans' dried weight. There is about half as much resveratrol in Cacao as there is in red wine, weight for weight.[274] While a 175ml (medium) glass of wine contains 0.00175–2.5mg resveratrol, a 40g serving of whole Cacao contains 0.37–0.74mg. Resveratrol absorption is very high, but it has poor bioavailability as it is rapidly metabolised by gut microorganisms, with a high degree of variability.[275] In common with some of the proanthocyanidins in Cacao, resveratrol has monoamine oxidase inhibitory (MAOI-A) properties, preventing the breakdown of the peripheral catecholamine-releasing amino acid tyramine as well as the catecholamines themselves, the neurotransmitters dopamine, noradrenaline, and serotonin, and the neurohormone melatonin. Resveratrol is found in high concentrations (much higher than found in Cacao) in grape skins and in the Japanese Knotweed (*Polygonum cuspidatum*). *In vitro*, human adipocytes incubated with 100mM resveratrol became sensitised to β-adrenergic receptor-induced triacylglycerol breakdown and reduced lipogenesis, demonstrating potential anti-obesity or thermogenic ("fat-burning") properties.[276]

Resveratrol also exhibits a battery of anti-neoplastic effects *in vitro*. It decreased EBV-induced human B-Lymphocyte oncogene activation and inhibited infected cell survival;[277] it also induced cell cycle arrest in malignant natural killer cells, in a dose and concentration-dependent manner.[278] These data suggest that—if bioavailable following oral consumption—resveratrol, and perhaps dietary sources of resveratrol such as Cacao, may protect against post-mononucleosis health risks such as lymphoma. Resveratrol also inhibited nitric oxide production *in vitro* through non-antioxidant/free radical independent mechanisms, and was dose-dependently cytotoxic to bone-marrow derived macrophages,[279] again suggesting that it may be a useful adjunct in some leukaemias, but that its action may somewhat counterbalance the nitric oxide-releasing effects of other Cacao polyphenols. Resveratrol dose-dependently induced apoptosis of pancreatic cancer cells,[280] human naso-pharyngeal cancer cells,[281] and suppressed mTOR, a regulatory protein; mTOR deactivation counteracts cell growth and neoplasia.[282] Resveratrol also reduced "aggressive", non-androgen dependent prostate cancer cell viability and tendency to metastasis,[283] and inhibited VEGF (vascular endothelial growth factor) production by human osteosarcoma cells,[284] limiting their pro-anigiogenic capacity and viability. Again, depending on resveratrol's bioavailability, these data suggest that dietary resveratrol may protect against various cancers.

Resveratrol protects cultured dorsal root ganglia neurons from ethanol damage.[285] Resveratrol also has *in vitro* growth and repair-promoting properties in dopaminergic neurons by stimulating neurotrophic factor release from astroglia,[286] and protects astroglia from ammonia toxicity via principally anti-inflammatory and non-antioxidant mechanisms.[287] These properties of resveratrol suggest the possibility of additive or synergistic antiparkinsonian effects with the antioxidant, dopamine-sparing Cacao polyphenols. Resveratrol also prevented hydrogen peroxide-induced oxidative injury to vascular endothelium,[288] and protected cardiomyocytes from ischaemia-reperfusion injury via nitric oxide synthetase inhibition.[289] Resveratrol also shows potential for lifespan enhancement by inducing *in vitro* telomerase activity.[290] **Trans-resveratrol** has *in vitro* and *in vivo* (animal) anti-inflammatory, anti-cancer, cardioprotective, and oestrogenic effects.[291]

With regard to trans-resveratrol's bioavailability and *in vivo* efficacy, one study in which very high oral doses (80 mg/kg) were administered to rats demonstrated antidepressant activity. The test animals had a marked increase in brain serotonin turnover, with central noradrenaline and dopamine levels also rising, in accordance with resveratrol's MAOI-A activity.[292] However, the dosage used was equivalent to over 5g (5000mg) pure trans-resveratrol for a 10st/63.5kg human, a quantity all but impossible to achieve through dietary intake, especially considering that a reasonably high 40g dose of whole Cacao contains less than 1mg of resveratrol, and only 0.1mg trans-resveratrol. A more realistic oral dosage of 8mg, co-administered with grape phenolics, was used in a triple-blind, randomised placebo-controlled clinical trial with seventy-five human subjects. After one year, the active group showed a 9.6% increase in serum adiponectin (a marker of reduced inflammation) and an 18.6% decrease of serum Plasminogen Activator Inhibitor-1 (a thrombogenic compound), in addition to down-regulated expression of several pro-inflammatory genes as compared to the placebo and control groups.[293] However, in another double-blind placebo-controlled clinical trial, when 500mg trans-resveratrol was administered to twenty-four obese healthy male subjects over a four-week period, no changes in glucose production/turnover, blood pressure, lipid metabolism, or inflammatory biomarker levels relative to the placebo group were noted.[294] These results imply that resveratrol and trans-resveratrol may have different actions, that very high doses may be necessary for measurable effects, or that resveratrol may synergise with other polyphenols to produce measurable effects at lower levels of intake over longer periods of time.

Quinones are trace compounds in Cacao, with antioxidant and putative neuroprotective properties. They are very stable and highly bioavailable. *In vitro* research shows that quinones reduce mercury and oxydopamine damage to neurons, and prevent alpha-synuclein aggregation; they also stimulate mitochondrial repair and regeneration in old cells—a very unusual property, as only intense exercise, caloric restriction, and a handful of medications can otherwise induce this process. Animal trials demonstrate that quinones may have antiparkinsonian (preventive/protective) effects, and may be prophylactic against cortical ischaemia-reperfusion injury (stroke damage). Quinones also reduced damage to animal heart tissue in artificially induced myocardial infarction. The dosage used in animal trials is equivalent to human intake of ≥1.44mg/day, whereas the amount of quinones in 40g whole Cacao is only 0.01–0.03mg, so humans consuming Cacao would be ingesting up to 144 times less quinone than the amount which demonstrated pharmacological efficacy in clinical trials. Nevertheless, quinones may have an important role in mammalian nutrition as a trace nutrient/phytochemical, and additive or synergistic potentials with other Cacao compounds have not yet been assayed. Much larger doses of quinones than are normally present in foods may help to preserve memory and cognition in animals and humans, as measured by a very small open label (preliminary) clinical trial, in which 20mg quinones were orally administered every day to seventeen middle-aged adults, and marked improvements were found in measures of sleep quality, duration, mood, and waking cortisol response.[295] Again, it is unlikely that this result has much relevance with regard to Cacao, because the trial was not large or carefully controlled, and the dose used was 1000-fold greater than that found in a fairly high daily intake of Cacao; however, it is worth mentioning owing to the possibility of synergy or additive effects between the trace presence of **pyrryloquinoline quinone** and other compounds in Cacao.

Lignin is a common plant cell wall component, principally found in Cacao stem and root bark as well as in the discarded seed husks of Cacao. Cacao lignins show anti-HIV activity *in vitro*; they also enhanced the antioxidant activity of ascorbic acid, and "stimulated NO generation by mouse macrophage-like cells", demonstrating potential immunomodulatory properties. A complex of lignin and carbohydrate from Cacao mass, prepared from whole ground seed as opposed to cocoa husks, had higher *in vitro* anti-HIV activity than lignin alone.[296] Whether this has any relevance whatsoever to human consumption of Cacao is not yet known, but lignins are large molecules, so any anti-retroviral activity may be limited to the human gastrointestinal tract (they may perhaps act on HIV in the MALT—the mucosa-associated lymphatic tissue in the gut, the largest collection of lymphatic tissue in the human body). Lignins' solubility is increased by heat and by alkaline conditions, so certain preparations of Cacao—such as hot beverages incorporating nixtamalized (lime-treated, and therefore alkalised) corn or *masa harina*—may increase lignin bioavailability.

Fatty Acids and Phytosterols

Cacao beans are 50% fat, referred to as "cocoa butter", which has the useful property of being liquid at body temperature but solid at temperatures below 25°C;[297] this means the beans can be used to make chocolate which is solid at room temperature in cooler climates yet melts in the mouth (pleasant), and the isolated fat can be used to make suppositories which melt after insertion (useful).[298] The fat profile of the beans is as follows:

Saturated fats: **palmitic acid** (PA) is the most common fatty acid in animals and plants, and reduces the appetite-suppressing effects of insulin and leptin, which may account for Cacao's traditional reputation of having "fattening" properties. Excess carbohydrates in the diet are converted to palmitic acid, which is then used to produce longer fatty acids; high PA intake may increase the risk of developing cardiovascular diseases. PA desaturates to palmitoleic acid. PA is an *in vitro* CD4 fusion inhibitor for HIV,[299] which may have some relevance if cocoa butter is traditionally used on the hands and skin of those who may come into contact with HIV-infected body fluids, for example obstetricians (cocoa butter as a massage oil for trans-abdominal foetal manipulation, or cervical manipulation by traditional midwives) or use as a sexual lubricant. However PA also enhances glioma cell growth *in vitro*[300]—contrast theobromine (q.v.). *In vitro* palmitate dose-dependently inhibited breast cancer cell proliferation by inducing apoptosis.[301] Most importantly, human *in vivo* trials showed that PA intake does not elevate total or LDL cholesterol if mono- and poly-unsaturated fat intake is increased commensurately.[302]

Stearic Acid (SA) is usually more abundant in animal fats, cocoa butter being a rare vegetable exception. In common with most fats, SA is transported through the lymphatic vessels; it is partly metabolised to oleic acid, and actively lowers LDL production.[303] Dietary administration of SA to mice slightly increased their pancreatic insulin secretion, and potentiated glucose-induced insulin secretion. Chronic *in vitro* exposure of rat pancreatic beta-cells to stearate, palmitate, and oleate reduced insulin secretion in response to glucose, whereas acute exposure to these fatty acids increased insulin responses in human beta-cells. This data may suggest that chronic dietary intake of SA may induce insulin tolerance or a "blunting" of pancreatic insulin secretion.[304] SA also afforded dose-dependent neuroprotection against oxidative (H2O2) or glutamate-induced neurotoxicity *in vitro*; on the other hand, exposure of neurons to a mixture of stearic and palmitic acids increased apoptosis—however, this research may have little relevance to Cacao's pharmacology as palmitic, oleic, or stearic acid can not cross the blood-brain barrier.[305] Stearate also dose-dependently reduced prolactin-induced rat lymphoma cell proliferation *in vitro*.[306] Palmitate and stearate altered aortic smooth muscle metabolism *in vitro*, and increased post-prandial plasma factor VII coagulant activity and fibrinogen in humans,[307] suggesting possible thrombogenic effects of high dietary SA intake. Topical SA greatly assisted resolution of burns in mouse skin,[308] which accords with the traditional use of cocoa butter as an emollient for superficial burns.[309]

Monounsaturated Fats: **Oleic acid** (OA) is an $\Omega 9$ fatty acid, and the most abundant fatty acid in human adipose tissue. High OA intake may be hypotensive, and may hinder adrenoleukodystrophy (ALD[v]) progression. Higher concentrations of OA in red blood cells may be associated with increased breast cancer risk, and dietary supplementation with OA was found to have a mild co-carcinogenic effect on colon cancer development in rats,[310] but no promoting effect on skin tumours in mice was found.[311] *In vitro* oleate stimulated breast cancer cell proliferation, negating the pro-apoptotic effects of palmitate.[312] Patient studies suggest high dietary OA intakes may indeed increase risk for prostate, colon, and rectal cancers.[313] On the other hand, OA *in vitro* causes reversible alteration of erythrocyte shape, reduction of blood viscosity, and reduced ESR,[314] whereas *in vivo* OA increased post-prandial plasma factor VII coagulant activity and fibrinogen more than stearate and palmitate in humans[315]—this suggests both thrombogenicity and possible utility in conditions of erythrocyte deformation, such as sickle cell anaemia, if the *in vitro* findings are replicated *in vivo*. OA also inhibits *in vitro* and *in vivo* elastase activity.

Polyunsaturated Fats: **Linoleic acid** (LA), an $\Omega 6$ fatty acid, is converted to γ-linolenic acid (GLA) by delta-6-desaturase, and thence to arachidonic acid—but GLA is also converted to dihomo-γ-linolenic acid (DGLA) which is a precursor for anti-inflammatory series one thromboxanes and prostanoids, which inhibit the pro-inflammatory action of arachidonic acid metabolites. However, the production of GLA from LA blocks the endogenous production of the anti-inflammatory precursor compound eicosapentanoic acid (EPA), so LA intake has net pro-inflammatory effects. LA has some *in vitro* bacteriostatic activity against Gram-positive organisms,[316] which may have relevance to the topical usage of cocoa butter, and higher dietary

---

[v] ALD is a rare, genetically linked disorder of fatty acid metabolism, whereby very long chain fatty acids accumulate in the adrenal cortex, and leydig cells of the testes, and displace CNS myelin, resulting in severe and progressive neuro-endocrine disruption.

LA intake was found to protect against pneumonia in a study of 38,378 US health professionals aged forty-four to seventy-nine years.[317] Human gastric and colon cancer cell growth was dose-dependently inhibited by LA *in vitro*; however, LA enhanced *in vivo* rat and mouse breast and prostate carcinogenesis, and LA added to the diet of captive rats increased colon cancer incidence.[318] There was also a higher incidence of gastric tumours in mice fed linoleic and oleic acids in refined corn oil,[319] though it should be noted that the oil itself, and the artificial diet (lacking chemopreventive cofactors) may have been a significant predisposing cause, more than, or in addition to, the LA content of the diet. However, a case-control study in northern Italy also found higher human dietary LA intake increased the relative risk of melanoma, especially in women,[320] so excessive or relatively high levels of dietary LA may in fact *increase* the risk of developing certain cancers.

One study noted that low plasma LA in recovering cocaine addicts was "a better predictor of relapse than cocaine use, sociodemographic or clinical parameters",[321] suggesting that additional dietary LA may be of benefit in such cases. Unsaturated fatty acids added to the diet of lab rats significantly inhibited serum nitric oxide and endothelin-1 production, while saturated fats increased endothelin-1 production, so both types of dietary fat had a net effect of reducing endothelium-dependent vasorelaxation in lab rats.[322] Despite this finding, higher dietary LA intake in humans may protect against heart attack and stroke through lowering blood pressure, platelet aggregation, and enhancing erythrocyte flexibility, as assayed in a randomised case-control study.[323] A randomised, double-blind, placebo-controlled trial observing eighty-six women in the third trimester of pregnancy, supplementing 450mg LA and 600mg calcium every day observed a significant reduction in pre-eclampsia,[324] which suggests that whole Cacao may be of benefit. One placebo-controlled clinical trial in which 57mg of LA and 30mg of GLA were administered daily improved keratoconjunctivitis sicca symptoms in patients with rheumatoid arthritis.[325] A measure of 40g Cacao contains 800mg LA, but also contains other "competing" essential fatty acids and no GLA, so whether it would be beneficial in these cases is unknown. Oxidised LA metabolites are also known to activate capsaicin receptors and increase pain sensitivity. The pro-inflammatory properties of LA may account for some of the cancer-promoting effects observed in trials, but this observation, and the potentially hypertensive/thrombotic effects of dietary fat intake, may be more remarkable *in vitro* and in animal trials than in human dietary interventions, where other dietary factors can offset or alter outcomes completely.

Phytosterols have a chemical structure similar to cholesterol, and are found in many plants and plant-based foods. Owing to this structural similarity, they competitively inhibit gastrointestinal cholesterol absorption, so that if human daily dietary intake exceeds 1.3g, they can lower blood lipoprotein (especially LDL) and triglycerides, and daily intakes of over 2g lower LDL by 8–9%. Cacao seeds contain only 86–87mg phytosterols per 40g, around 0.2% dry weight, so Cacao only contributes to total dietary phytosterol intake and isn't a major source of such compounds. Regular dietary intake of phytosterols may provide some protection against lung, colon, ovarian, and breast cancers.[326] Phytosterols are barely soluble in fat, more readily dissolving in fatty or alcoholic media—however, they are present in beverages made from Cacao due to the nature of these beverages being a suspension (cocoa) or a suspension-emulsion (traditional Cacao drinks). They are poorly absorbed from the human intestine, and more rapidly metabolised in the liver than cholesterol, where they are transformed into C21 bile acids for excretion.[327]

The addition of emulsifying agents to Cacao beverages or chocolate is likely to enhance their bioavailability.

Of the **4-desmethylesterols** (**sitosterol**, **stigmasterol**, and **campesterol**), dietary stigmasterol intake, specifically, may reduce risk of ovarian, prostate, and colon cancers. Stigmasterol is hypoglycaemic and thyroid-inhibiting at high intakes. Stigmasterol and campesterol may also slow cartilage deterioration in osteoarthritis.[328] Stigmasterol also reduced scopolamine-induced memory impairment in mice by an unspecified mechanism.[329] **Beta-sitosterol** induces apoptosis in breast cancer cells, and reduces colon cancer cell growth *in vitro*; a small pilot clinical trial (double-blind and placebo-controlled) in human marathon runners showed that orally administered beta-sitosterol decreased athletes' post-marathon cortisol to DHEA ratio and elevated their CD3 and CD4 lymphocyte counts, indicating a reduced inflammatory response and less immunosuppression following intense physiological stress.[330] Another double-blind, placebo-controlled clinical trial in men with benign prostate hypertrophy using 20mg beta-sitosterol three times daily (60mg/day) produced improved symptoms and urinary flow.[331] These findings may be significant in the case of Cacao, as not only has whole Cacao been found to increase cortisol excretion (see "Experimental Data & Clinical Trials" section in this monograph), but a 40g serving of Cacao contains around 49mg of beta-sitosterol, a quantity not much less than that used in this trial. However, *in vitro* work has also found that cocoa polyphenols exert much stronger anti-proliferative effects against human prostate cancer cell lines, which eclipse the effects of the much weaker beta-sitosterol, with which they have no additive or synergistic properties.[332] So while beta-sitosterol may contribute to Cacao's pharmacology, any contribution to chemoprevention of prostate hypertrophy or cancer remains to be demonstrated.

The **4,4'-dimethylsterols (triterpenes)** in Cacao have demonstrated cancer chemopreventive properties *in vitro* and *in vivo* (animal trials only). **Cycloartane**, specifically, attenuates UV-B tumour-promoting effects in mice.[333] Of the **4-methylsterols** (**citrostadienyl**, **obtusifoliol**, and **lophenyl**), obtusifoliol inhibits Epstein-Barr virus activation *in vitro*.[334]

The various **phospholipid** compounds in Cacao, comprising around 0.03% of the beans' dry weight, were defined in 1969. The phospholipids are usually animal cell membrane constituents, less commonly found in plants. **Phosphatidylcholine** is a surfactant (natural emulsifier) and a major component of lecithin. **Phosphatidylinositol** is most abundant in brain tissue, and a primary source of arachidonic acid, required for eicosanoid synthesis. Phosphatidylinositol is also used to manufacture diacylglycerol signalling molecules which regulate cellular metabolism and the cellular life cycle via protein kinase C signalling. **Phosphatidylethanolamine**, found at 6.75mg/100g, or 0.0068% of Cacao's dry weight, is an anandamide precursor, and has crucial roles in cellular fusion and fission, autophagy, and protein synthesis. **Lysophosphatidylcholine** is a hydrolysed product of phosphatidylcholine, with demyelinating effects—high dietary intakes of this phospholipid compound have been linked to multiple sclerosis. However, it comprises a smaller proportion of Cacao's phospholipid cache, around 0.00325% of the beans' dry weight, and its demyelinating effects are most likely more than offset by neuroprotective effects of the polyphenols. The water solubility of one of Cacao's flavanol monomers, quercetin, was improved twelve-fold by phospholipids with no loss of antioxidant activity,[335] and the hepatoprotective properties and serum concentration of orally administered ellagic acid in rats were dramatically increased when co-administered with phospholipids.[336]

These bioavailability-enhancing properties are likely to be highly relevant in any consideration of the pharmacology of Cacao, particularly as *Theobroma*'s phenolic compounds are increasingly recognised as important mediators of the drug's physiological activity.

Organic Acids

The organic acids in Cacao are present in variable quantities depending on the seeds' processing, comprising up to 3.3% of the dried seeds' weight. They are produced by microorganisms during fermentation, and contribute sourness to the distinctive flavour of Cacao. Some are evaporated during toasting or roasting, and (in commercial chocolate) conching and Dutching. The acids facilitate oxidative reactions during fermentation by destroying the parenchyma of cotyledons (plant cell walls in the seeds) and allowing oxygen to mingle with cellular contents.[337] On ingestion, many organic acids are anti-nutrients, for example **phytic** and **acetic acid** reduce calcium absorption, and phytic acid also creates insoluble complexes with calcium in the intestinal lumen. Acetic acid is best known as the by-product of *Acetobacter spp.* in the fermentation of carbohydrate into vinegar, but this common bacterial waste product may exert hypotensive, hypoglycaemic, and hypercalacemic effects when ingested—when an acetic acid solution was fed to rats over a six day period their plasma renin and aldosterone levels fell. Acetic acid ingestion also enhanced the absorption of calcium from the distal colon in human subjects. This substance may therefore contribute to Cacao's weakly anti-hypertensive and anti-diabetic activities (q.v.). Similarly, ingestion of acetic acid solution before carbohydrate-based meals significantly reduced post-prandial blood sugar levels and increased subjective feelings of satiety, and taking vinegar before the morning meal was found to reduce total daily calorie consumption in a blinded, randomised, placebo-controlled trial. Acetate ions are formed intra-gastrically as acetic acid deprotonates, and have been found to increase colon cancer cell differentiation, and to reduce colon cancer cell division and motility *in vitro*; acetic acid may therefore exert some chemopreventive effects in the gastrointestinal tract.[338]

Oxalic acid forms oxalates which then chelate minerals such as calcium, inhibiting their absorption. Some oxalates are also naturally produced in the gut by bacterial action on carbohydrates. The resultant compounds may then precipitate as potentially kidney- and joint-damaging salts, mainly calcium oxalate. Cacao's oxalic acid content isn't high—by comparison, purslane (*Portulaca oleracea*) contains 1.31g/100g oxalic acid, carrots (*Daucus carota*) contain 0.5g/100g, while Cacao contains only 0.15–0.5mg/100g. *In vitro* studies suggest that oxalic acid may also have anti-carcinogenic and anti-metastatic effects; a novel hypothesis suggests that the calcium-salt forming properties of oxalic acid may increase apoptosis among some types of cancers, by preventing calcium from leaving the cell and causing a lethal intracellular build-up of calcium salts.[339] Oxalates also inhibit glycolysis, and as cancer cells are extremely sugar-hungry yet energy inefficient (the so-called Warburg effect), they inhibit cancer cell growth. [340]

Lactic acid is another common organic compound produced as a waste product of pyruvate metabolism, and is the most quantitatively variable acid in Cacao, ranging from the least to the greatest amount among all the acids present in the prepared bean. Its accumulation is partly responsible for the burning sensation in muscles experienced during exercise, and yet, when consumed orally, lactic acid retards the onset of exhaustion in high-intensity exertion, and its presence may play a small role in Cacao's efficacy in CFS (q.v.).[341] **Citric acid** salts are calcium and iron chelators, and possess anticoagulant and antioxidant activity; their presence in Cacao-based beverages may therefore enhance the "shelf life" of the prepared drinks. Citric acid also increased faecal excretion of aluminium in animal trials, so its presence in foods or Cacao-based beverages may be a useful aid to preventing aluminium toxicity.[342]

Proteins, Amino Acids, and Biological Amines

Cacao is approximately 11% **protein** by dry weight, mainly **albumin** > **globulin**. Cacao's globulin has a unique structure, resembling vicilin, the generic seed storage protein in legumes.[343] The albumin fraction from semi-fermented (but not unfermented) seeds has *in vitro* anti-tumour and antioxidant activity—both of these activities are "uncorrelated", so the anti-neoplastic effects are unrelated to the antioxidant properties of the protein.[344] What relevance this may have *in vivo* following Cacao or chocolate consumption, if any, is unclear—proteins, being larger molecules, often don't exert systemic effects following oral administration, though their metabolites may. Long roasting reduced the solubility of cocoa proteins, and roasting at 150°C caused some diminution of total protein content—13% of the protein had degraded after thirty-eight minutes' roasting, and after forty-two minutes' roasting, levels of protein began to decline more rapidly.[345] Traditional lower-temperature seed-toasting methods are therefore more likely to conserve Cacao's protein content and bioavailability, and although fermentation causes some diminution of Cacao's polyphenols, other bioactive compounds (such as the anti-neoplastic albumins) are generated.

Ten of the twenty-two basic **<u>amino acids</u>** used as precursor compounds for protein manufacture are found in Cacao. Amino acids may also be utilised in gluconeogenesis, with the nitrogenous portion of the molecules being oxidised to urea and CO_2 when energy requirements are exceptionally high, or carbohydrate intake is low. Nine amino acids are essential, as the body can't manufacture them. Amino acids are also used to make various neuroendocrine signalling compounds. **Glutamic acid**, for example, is a non-essential amino acid found in moderately high concentrations in Cacao, at up to 1.02% dry weight, or 10,200ppm. While containing far less than soy protein isolate, which at up to 17.5% glutamic acid is the richest (artificial) dietary source of this amino acid, Cacao's glutamic acid content is comparable to other legumes at the higher end of the plant-based glutamic acid percentile.[346] *In vivo*, glutamic acid is oxidised to glutamate, a γ-amino butyric acid (GABA) precursor and an excitatory neurotransmitter in its own right, used in learning and memory, and contributing to synaptic plasticity. Glutamate doesn't diffuse across the blood-brain barrier, but, akin to other amino acids utilised in the CNS, it is actively taken up into the CNS by specific transporters. Pathologically, excessive glutamate release is excitotoxic, and contributes to several CNS disorders such as post-stroke ischaemic damage (CVA), Alzheimer's disease, and ALS. Glutamate also has an important role in metabolism, being utilised in the process of transforming other amino acids into intermediary compounds, and excreting excess nitrogen via hepatic metabolism.

Tyrosine is another non-essential amino acid found in Cacao at just over half the concentration of glutamic acid, and is a precursor of tyramine, L-dopa, and thence the stimulating catecholamines dopamine, adrenaline, and noradrenaline; it's also a precursor for melanin, and thyroid hormones. Oral supplementation with 100mg/kg tyrosine (equivalent to 6500mg/day for a 10st adult human) had little effect on mood in non-stressed individuals, but improved apparent resistance to stress and grief, although it was less effective in this regard than the immediate dopamine precursor compound, l-dopa. This is presumably because l-dopa requires less intermediary conversion steps to form dopamine, whereas tyrosine can be "siphoned off" into other metabolic pathways to make thyroid hormones or melanin. Larger "doses" or intakes of tyrosine inhibit histamine degradation, and can therefore exacerbate allergic or anaphylactic responses, though this is unlikely to occur with normal food intake. **Phenylalanine** is an essential amino acid found at relatively high concentrations in Cacao, a startlingly high concentration for a relatively low protein plant product, around 0.9%, much higher than most other foods with the exception of soy protein isolate (at >4%) and some dairy products (>1%).[347] Phenylalanine can be converted into tyrosine *in vivo*, but is also a precursor compound for the biogenic amine, phenylethylamine or phenethylamine (PEA), which has a controversial and much-debated role in the psychopharmacology of Cacao (see below).

Phenylalanine competes with **tryptophan**, another essential ámino acid, to cross the blood-brain barrier. Tryptophan is a precursor compound for the manufacture of serotonin, melatonin, and niacin. Tryptophan intake needs to be quite high to positively influence mood due to competition for brain uptake with other amino acids. Although there is a high level of tryptophan in Cacao compared to other food sources, the level is low relative to Cacao's phenylalanine content, and, as noted above, where phenylalanine intake is high, tryptophan uptake will be low. Very high levels of tryptophan occur in egg white, cod, soya beans, and parmesan cheese, but uptake will be highest when low phenylalanine food sources of tryptophan are consumed with carbohydrates. This occurs because carbohydrate-induced insulin release causes larger branched chain amino acids to be absorbed into muscle, leaving smaller (less branched) tryptophan molecules in the bloodstream. The higher ratio of tryptophan in the blood relative to other amino acids leads to a net increase of tryptophan transport across the blood-brain barrier and into the CNS, predisposing to more serotonin and melatonin manufacture, and thereby to improved mood, and drowsiness. For this to occur, however, tryptophan intake must exceed that of other Amino Acids, and carbohydrates must also be ingested at the same time. Lower levels of tryptophan in the blood are linked to depression, which leads to the interesting speculation that regular intake of phenylalanine-rich foods may predispose to low mood or depression through a net decrease in tryptophan uptake and CNS serotonin manufacture. On the other hand, lower dietary tryptophan intakes in animals have been linked to longer lifespans, and it's known that there is an age-related increase in CNS serotonin levels.[vi] Additionally, excessive dietary tryptophan has been observed to exacerbate insulin resistance in pigs via an unidentified mechanism.

Cacao is a relatively poor source of the essential amino acid **lysine**, which inhibits serotonin activity in the gut and amygdala while potentiating CNS benzodiazepine receptor binding

---

[vi] This is an intriguing observation, as the highest measured tryptophan levels in food occur in the nutritional algae spirulina, and in egg white, both of which foods would have been designated "phlegmatic" in traditional humoral (Galenic) medicine. Phlegm was the humour naturally associated with old age, tranquillity, and sedation—all effects associated with elevated CNS serotonin levels. See Tobyn, 1997 [Book].

affinity, thereby reducing anxiety and stress-related diarrhoea. Adequate lysine intake is necessary for proper immune function, and possibly for blood pressure control. **Glycine** is a non-essential amino acid, also found at relatively low levels in Cacao. It can act as inhibitory CNS neurotransmitter, or an excitatory co-agonist at NMDA receptors. Cacao also contains a relatively high level of **histamine**, which has appetite-suppressing, sleep-retarding, and pro-inflammatory effects. Cacao not only contains histamine, like many other fermented foods, but is said to trigger histamine release directly from mast cells, though this allegation is currently unsupported by evidence. Several other foods can do this: alcohol, pineapple, tomatoes, strawberries, raw egg white, and shellfish are common triggers. Cacao is therefore listed as one of the foods most likely to cause urticaria, along with shellfish, fish, egg, nuts, berries, tomatoes, cheese, milk, and wheat, as Cacao both contains and—allegedly—may trigger the release of histamine.[348]

Non-protein amino acids found in Cacao include **γ-amino butyric acid (GABA)**, made from the amino acid glutamate. GABA is an anxiolytic, anticonvulsant, pro-amnestic neurotransmitter. GABA is critical for neuronal development, and, while sedative in adults, it has excitatory activity in immature brains, and has a role in regulating muscle tone. GABA's oral bioavailability is currently unknown, and thought to be low—however, orally administered GABA increased human growth hormone release following strenuous exercise, and it's known to cross the blood-brain barrier via high-affinity membrane transports. These findings suggest the possibility that supplementation or dietary intake of GABA may have some activity. The closely related **β-aminoisobutyric acid** is little researched at present. It's known to increase hepatic fat oxidation.

The so-called **amino alcohols** in Cacao are **N-acylethanolamines**, fatty acid amides present in trace amounts of debatable physiological relevance (in terms of quantities that may reasonably be consumed in Cacao). The most referenced of these—although not the most abundant—is **anandamide**, a compound formed from the union of arachidonic acid and ethanolamine. In Cacao, anandamide is found in concentrations not exceeding 57μg/g, or 2.3mg per 40g serving,[349] but may be present in far lower quantities (source estimates vary). Anandamide's oral bioavailability is less than 5%, as the compound is swiftly hydrolysed in the intestinal lumen by fatty acid amide hydrolase (FAAH) enzymes. Anandamide reversibly binds to serum albumin for transport, and is highly lipophilic. However, it should be noted that anandamide is also active at "nanomolar to sub-micromolar concentrations."[350] Physiologically, anandamide has a role as a neurotransmitter which attenuates pain sensation via cannabinoid and vanilloid receptor binding. The CB1 (cannabinoid-1) receptors to which it binds are found in the CNS, small intestine, heart, testes, and uterus.

Anandamide also affects perception of pain, anxiety and fear, regulation of body temperature, and appetite. It decreases heart rate and blood pressure, and is considered to be anabolic, increasing food intake and promoting lipid storage. Anandamide is also produced by macrophages, by which it is released on contact with bacterial endotoxin, and thereby mediates some anti-inflammatory and anti-cancer processes. Anandamide also appears to modulate central oxytocin and vasopressin release from the neurohypophysis, displaying a two-stage stimulatory-inhibitory action *in vitro*. Anandamide stimulates central oxytocin release from the hypothalamic neurons *in vitro* through activation of hypothalamic CB1 receptors, but it also activates neurohypophyseal CB2 and TRPV1 receptors, stimulating nitric oxide synthesis, which suppresses oxytocin and vasopressin release.[351] It's unclear at present whether anandamide has a role in the psychopharmacology of Cacao, but Cacao's traditional reputation as a drug to prevent fear, gain weight, and assist in lactation and breastfeeding is intriguing.

N-oleoylethanolamine (OEA) is an amino alcohol formed from oleic acid and ethanolamine. OEA is produced endogenously in the small intestine after feeding. It has anorectic activity, acting locally in the gut to induce satiety, and it stimulates fat breakdown, opposing anandamide's effects in this regard. OEA binds to a variety of cannabinoid receptors, and enhances memory consolidation through CNS noradrenergic mechanisms. OEA is also a ceramidase inhibitor: in other words, it increases accumulation of the lipid ceramide in cell membranes, activating apoptosis, and may help to maintain cardiac glucose metabolism under conditions of endotoxic stress.[352] Neither OEA nor its sister compound **LEA (N-linoleoylethanolamine)** activate brain cannabinoid receptors, but they do inhibit anandamide breakdown in rat brains (EC^{50} ~5µM).[353] A double-blind placebo-controlled clinical trial of the OEA precursor N-oleyl-phosphatidylethanolamine, given orally at a dosage of 85mg, was co-administered with 50mg epigallocatechin gallate (EGCG) as a daily supplement for 138 overweight men and women. The combination produced improvements in insulin resistance, post-prandial satiety, depressive symptoms, and severity of binge eating.[354] While levels of EGCG in a 40g serving or dose of unmixed Cacao approach the dosage used in this trial, the quantity of OEA in Cacao is infinitesimal by comparison. Nevertheless, these compounds are both present in measurable and potentially pharmacologically active quantities.

Both OEA and LEA retard anandamide breakdown, and only very low levels of OEA and LEA are necessary to effect this inhibition. OEA and LEA inhibit anandamide degradation by fatty acid amide hydroxylase, so, researchers have speculated,

> These compounds might contribute to the hedonic properties of chocolate by causing non-metabolized anandamide to accumulate at its sites of action ... elevated anandamide levels could cooperate with other pharmacological components of chocolate (for example caffeine, theobromine) to produce a transient feeling of well-being.[355]

Although this may seem unlikely given the very low quantities of these N-acylethanolamine compounds in Cacao, only miniscule quantities of LEA may be necessary to prevent anandamide's intragastric hydrolysis: 5µM of LEA caused 50% inhibition of anandamide breakdown. The N-acylethanolamines are lipophilic, so the very high fat content of Cacao favours their absorption.[356] The quantities of N-acylethanolamines present in traditional whole-bean Cacao beverages are very low (approximately 1mg Anandamide and 1.5mg total OEA and LEA in 40g Cacao), but cannot be dismissed as pharmacologically insignificant without human *in vivo* assessment of the combined pharmacokinetics of the amino alcohols within the matrix of compounds found in whole Cacao seeds. It should be noted that these compounds, like salsolinol, and unlike the tetrahydro-β-Carbolines and trigonelline, are not present in coffee.

Amines are smaller, nitrogenous components of amino acids. Amine levels in Cacao rise with fermentation, and may also increase with roasting as more amino acids are hydrolysed, but levels decrease with alkalisation during cocoa production. Amines are concentrated in the non-fat portion of the bean.[357] Some amines function as neurotransmitters, such as dopamine and noradrenaline, which belong to the so-called classical monoamine neurotransmitters, and serotonin, a tryptamine neurotransmitter. **Dopamine** is a CNS neurotransmitter, associated with extraversion and excitement and with the reward-driven learning system in the mesolimbic region of the brain, incentivising the initiation and learning of new behaviours. The Ventral Tegmental Area of the midbrain contains the highest number of dopamine receptors, the so-called "reward neurons", and dopamine-releasing neurons are also found in the *substantia nigra pars compacta* of the midbrain, where they play a role in the reward system and in movement control. Some dopaminergic neurons originate in the hypothalamic arcuate nucleus just above the brainstem, from where they project to the anterior pituitary and inhibit prolactin release. The dopaminergic neurons in the frontal lobes of the brain are involved in memory, attention, and problem-solving. Dopamine release also increases goal-directed behaviours.

Systemically, dopamine has a pressor effect, in other words it raises blood pressure and heart rate. D1 and D5 dopamine receptor activation effects increased intracellular cAMP, stimulating neuronal depolarisation, while D2–D4 receptor activation decreases intracellular cAMP by inhibiting adenylate cyclase, with inhibitory or signal-damping effects. D1 is the most prevalent CNS dopamine receptor subtype. Activation of D2 receptors in the "chemoreceptor trigger zone" of the medulla in the brainstem are associated with nausea and vomiting, while low cortical D2 binding is associated with social anxiety, and low *substantia nigra* dopamine levels with Parkinson's disease. Generally low dopamine levels result in anhedonia, tardive dyskinesia, diminished serum testosterone and DHEA in men, and hyperprolactinaemia in both men and women. Similarly, low CNS dopamine is positively associated with "burning mouth syndrome", fibromyalgia, attention deficit hyperactivity disorder (ADHD), and restless legs syndrome (RLS). Dopamine also activates resting T-cells, but inhibits them once activated. Having effected its role as a neurotransmitter, dopamine is reabsorbed presynaptically and degraded by monoamine oxidase type A and type B (MAO-A and MAO-B). Dopamine itself can't cross the blood-brain barrier, but its precursors L-phenylalanine, L-tyrosine, and L-dopa can, while the B-vitamins folic acid, pyridoxine, niacin, and nicotinamide are all necessary cofactors for dopamine metabolism, also required for the manufacture of the related catecholamines adrenaline and noradrenaline. While Cacao isn't a significant source of these nutritional cofactors, it does contain a relatively high level of the precursor compounds phenylalanine and tyrosine, in addition to several compounds with MAO-inhibitory activity, and the dopamine-amplifying xanthine alkaloids, which suggests that dopamine modulation may be an important aspect of Cacao's psychopharmacology.

Serotonin, aka **5-hydroxytryptamine (5-HT)**, is mainly found in the gastrointestinal tract, as a neurotransmitter in the CNS, and in platelets. Ninety per cent of the body's serotonin is manufactured in the gut, where it is released from enterochromaffin cells to regulate intestinal movements, and subsequently absorbed into the bloodstream and stored in platelets. Although Cacao is not a significant food source of serotonin, it does contain several compounds which may elevate central serotonin activity, and has been demonstrated to affect serotonin metabolism in humans (elevated serum and urinary levels of the serotonin metabolite, 5-HIAA, following chocolate consumption).[358] When released from platelets as they clump together during clotting, it functions as a vasoconstrictor. The serotonin precursors tryptophan and 5-HTP, but not serotonin itself, may cross the blood-brain barrier, so ingested serotonin has no effect on

CNS serotonin levels. In the CNS, serotonin regulates mood intensity, appetite, and sleep; it affects memory and learning; and it alters perceptions of resource availability and social dominance or rank.

Elevated extracellular serotonin leads to intensification of mood states, and most pharmaceutical antidepressants, anxiolytics, anti-psychotics, psychedelics, and empathogens target 5-HT receptors. Serotonin is made by tryptophan hydroxylase, and a deficiency of this enzyme in animals results in defective maternal care and increased aggression. 5-HT also suppresses appetite by switching off dopamine via 5-HT2C receptors on dopaminergic neurons. There is a diurnal rhythm in serotonin release and receptor expression, peaking in the morning; and in early aging, CNS serotonin levels increase, but they fall off again in later old age. Because serotonin modulates osteoblast activity, lower blood serotonin levels predict lower bone density. Serotonin also induces endothelial nitric oxide activation, enhancing vasomotor signalling. However, serotonin also has an inhibitory effect on insulin and insulin-like growth factor (IGF), suppressing pancreatic beta-cell insulin release, and can act as direct growth factor in fibrotic conditions such as liver cirrhosis, while defective brain serotonin signalling has been associated with sudden infant death syndrome (SIDS).

Phenylethylamine or **phenethylamine (PEA)** is a neurotransmitter in the mammalian CNS, made from phenylalanine. In common with several psychoactive drugs such as amphetamine or MDMA, phenylethylamine activates CNS trace amine associated receptors (TAARs) on dopaminergic neurons, effecting dopamine and noradrenaline release, so if PEA is administered centrally (at very high levels) it has "an amphetamine-like action".[359] However, lower, more physiologically typical CNS concentrations of PEA potentiate the effects of dopamine, serotonin, and other neurotransmitters, functioning as neuromodulators acting via central trace amine receptors, or TAARs.[360] PEA is metabolised by several enzymes: both types of monoamine oxidase (MAO-A, but principally by MAO-B); aldehyde dehydrogenase, a group of enzymes which break down ethanol and acetaldehyde, ethanol's chief toxic metabolite; and dopamine-beta-monooxygenase, the enzyme that transforms dopamine into noradrenaline. Endogenous PEA levels in the CNS are found to be low in ADHD and clinical depression, whereas high concentrations are associated with schizophrenia. Outside the CNS, both PEA and tyramine increased guinea pig and rat gut contractility *in vitro*, and relaxed the vasculature around the gut—so, depending on its metabolism, PEA may exert local digestion and peristalsis-enhancing effects.[361] PEA normally has a ten minute half-life following oral ingestion, but MAO inhibitors prevent PEA-based drugs being metabolised before reaching the CNS, although they may actually blunt PEA's stimulant/euphoriant properties.

There is only a trace quantity of up to 0.88mg PEA per 40g serving of Cacao, and when administered as a single drug, PEA is orally inactive at doses up to 1,600mg; even intravenously, doses of less than 50mg fail to produce any psychoactive effects.[362] Oral PEA is rapidly metabolised by MAOs in the small intestine—if it were not, local (gastrointestinal) increases in PEA would also necessarily lead to increased serum tyramine levels (see below) which would cause nausea, headaches, raised blood pressure, tachycardia, and other signs of sympathetic arousal. However, Cacao also contains some compounds which have been known to make PEA more available in the CNS, such as trigonelline, which ferries PEA across the blood-brain barrier into the CNS. The β-carboline alkaloid derivatives (THβCs) in Cacao have MAO-inhibitory properties, which have been known to affect CNS bioavailability of PEA-based drugs. However, β-carbolines in general are reversible, shorter-duration MAO-inhibitors, and probably too weak to block amine metabolism thoroughly enough to cause a hypertensive crisis, or to elevate serum PEA; also they block MAO-A but not MAO–B, so even if the THβCs in Cacao possess this property, they are unlikely to unlock the psychotropic potential of the very low level of PEA in Cacao, but may rather inhibit it through partial agonism at central 5-HT2 receptors, which inhibit PEA's psychoactivity.[363]

Nevertheless, low PEA levels in the CNS can be increased 1000-fold with MAO-B inhibitors, but only up to three or four times when levels are already high.[364] One uncontrolled clinical observation study noted that a daily oral dose of 10–60mg PEA, taken with Selegiline, an irreversible MAO-B inhibitor, improved mood in twelve of fourteen patients with major (clinical) depression over five months to a year;[365] the doses used in this trial can therefore be considered equivalent in terms of psychoactivity to oral doses of up to 10–60 *grams* of PEA (10,000–60,000mg). The dose of PEA used in this trial was at least fifteen times greater than that found in a 40g serving of Cacao, and taken with a much stronger MAO inhibitor than any of the other phytochemicals with MAO-B inhibitory properties found in Cacao, which include several polyphenols, such as the proanthocyanidins and the flavan 3-ols catechin and epicatechin, enhanced by the action of trigonelline. Even if a 1000-fold *in vivo* magnification of the psychotropic effects of Cacao's PEA content is assumed because of the co-presence of these compounds, a maximal "CNS equivalence" of 880mg PEA could be achieved from 40g Cacao, which suggests that Cacao's PEA content is unlikely to be a major contributor to its psychoactivity, although PEA may feasibly exert some slight psychotropic activity given higher intakes of Cacao with a higher PEA content, *if* the combined effect of the polyphenols and trigonelline is found to possess adequate PEA-enhancing efficacy in the CNS. It has been noted that PEA administered with MAO-B inhibitors in rats occasioned an additive decrease in CNS B-1 adrenoreceptors, and D1-like receptors in rat striatum,[366] which suggests that the PEA/ MAO-B inhibitor compound combination in Cacao, if sufficiently active, may cumulatively reduce neuronal excitability, possibly even altering cognition and neuronal growth; however, this can't be known without measuring the effects of whole chocolate on these variables in human subjects.

Tyramine is another common trace amine, produced during decay or fermentation of many foods, such as hard cheeses, smoked meats, alcoholic beverages, and chocolate. Tyramine levels are much higher in cheeses, and when ingested together with MAO-A inhibitor drugs cause hypertyraminaemia, the so-called "cheese reaction", giving rise to symptoms such as headache, flushing, nausea, and a hypertensive crisis. An amount of 6–10mg tyramine is sufficient to cause a mild reaction in the presence of MAO-A inhibitors. There is up to 3mg tyramine in a 40g serving of Cacao, or 4.35mg in 60g, a serving size of Cacao above which side effects such as nausea and headaches may occur. In other words, there are subcritical but pharmacologically active quantities of tyramine in Cacao, if combined with MAO-A inhibitors—such as several compounds co-present in Cacao, specifically salsolinol, THβCs, resveratrol, and (to a lesser degree) caffeine. It's interesting that single-dose servings of Cacao over 60–80g typically border on the level of tyramine intake necessary to produce side effects in the presence of MAO-A inhibitors, and that such side effects do occur (headache, anxiety, palpitations, tremor, nausea, and vomiting are prominent features of Cacao overdose). These adverse effects are often attributed to the xanthine alkaloids, but the tyramine content may play a significant role. There is a possible, though disputed link between dietary tyramine intake and migraine; although some studies have suggested no connection, it's noted that cluster headaches and migraines are accompanied by increased CNS tyramine turnover. However, no change in the EEGs of migrainous subjects after chocolate intake was noted,[367] although the dosage of Cacao may have been too low to properly assess this. High dietary tyramine intake (at cheese rather than chocolate levels) increases systolic blood pressure, although tolerance develops with repeated exposure, leading to a decreased pressor response.[368] In common with several psychoactive drugs such as amphetamine and MDMA, tyramine and phenethylamine act via trace-amine associated receptors in the brain—or, perhaps more accurately, the psychoactive drugs hijack these receptors, for which PEA and tyramine are endogenous ligands.[369]

Histamine is best known as a principal chemical messenger triggering allergic (type 1 hypersensitivity) and inflammatory responses. Cacao is naturally high in histamine relative to other foods, and has been reported to induce urticaria (a histamine-dependent condition) in some people, and may directly trigger the release of histamine from mast cells.[370] In common with many of the other amines in Cacao, it is produced by microbial activity during fermentation. Orally ingested histamine is sufficiently bioavailable to produce systemic effects, as in "scombroid food poisoning" from eating decayed fish, in which the principal toxin is high levels of histamine produced by microorganisms. In the human body histamine is stored in mast cells in mucosa, on internal surface-air interfaces (e.g., the respiratory tract), and in blood vessel linings. Histamine type H1 receptor activation is involved in hypersensitivity or inflammatory responses outside the CNS, and activation of H2 receptors in vascular smooth muscle is vasodilatory, in the gastric mucosa serving to stimulate parietal cells to secrete gastric acid. Within the CNS, histamine's principal function is as a neurotransmitter preventing sedation and appetite suppression, although activation of the histamine H3 receptor subtype has a suppressive or negative feedback-like effect, decreasing histamine, acetylcholine, noradrenaline, and serotonin release. Inhibiting CNS histamine receptor activation has the net effect of decreasing vigilance, and under normal circumstances CNS histamine-releasing cells or neurons fire only while awake. In common with dopamine and phenylethylamine, higher levels of histamine metabolites are found in the cerebrospinal fluid of schizophrenic subjects. Immunologically, histamine may also help with T-cell differentiation, at least according to animal experiments, as activation of histamine receptor subtypes[vii] on T-cells stimulates or suppresses different aspects of immunity.[371] Histamine also has a role in the male reproductive tract, helping to maintain erections through its vasodilatory activity.

* * *

The **diketopiperazines (DKPs)** are heterocyclic compounds biosynthesised from paired amino acids, and were until recently considered to be pharmacologically inert. In fact the group has

---

[vii] Histamine H1 receptor activation enhances Th1 immune responses, whereas H2 receptor activation appears to suppress both Th1 and Th2 type immune responses.

diverse activities. Some DKP derivatives are oxytocin antagonists,[372] but the ones in Cacao are not. The DKPs have a very bitter taste, and are therefore important flavour compounds in chocolate; they are produced during fermentation, and many DKPs are also found in other fermented foods such as coffee and beer.[373] Levels of DKPs in Cacao increase with roasting. DKPs are relatively small compounds and resistant to proteolysis, so probably survive the digestive process; they are also known to cross the blood-brain barrier.[374] DKP variants have diverse actions, and can exhibit anti-microbial, anti-tumour, anti-lukaemic, hypoglycaemic, radioprotective, immunomodulatory, neuroprotective, or nootropic activity via several mechanisms.[375] The major DKPs in Cacao have been identified, but their pharmacological properties haven't yet been fully defined. They include cis-cyclo (Pro-Val)—also found in roasted coffee and fungi; cis-cyclo (Ile-Pro)—also found in roasted coffee; cis-cyclo (Val-Leu), cis-cyclo (Ala-Ile), and cis-cyclo (Ala-Leu).[376] Two of the most abundant relative to other food sources are the weakly anti-microbial cyclo (L-Val-L-Pro) at 1742ppm, and cyclo (L-Vala-L-Pro) at 228ppm, which is cytotoxic to many cancer cell lines and has immunomodulatory activity, regulating cytokine signalling in macrophages.

* * *

Cacao's **acrylamide** content increases with roasting, or more precisely it increases proportional to roasting temperature, but acrylamide levels plateau then decrease with further heating. Acrylamide is formed from the amino acid asparagine and dicarbonyl compounds during roasting (a Maillard reaction). Acrylamide concentrations in toasted/roasted Cacao decrease with storage time, and this is speculated to be a result of degradation by ongoing reactions with sulfhydryl groups (thiols) from aromatic compounds formed from cysteine when Cacao is roasted.[377] Levels of acrylamide in cocoa powder are between seven and thirty times higher than in dark chocolate;[378] it's therefore to be expected that traditional Cacao beverages (made with Cacao beans toasted at low temperatures, not industrially roasted) may contain proportionally lower levels of acrylamide. Acrylamide is a proven carcinogen, and its dietary intake is possibly linked to endometrial and ovarian cancer in post-menopausal women,[379] but it hasn't been conclusively linked to other cancers in the human population. It has also been alleged to cause damage to the nervous system.[380] The chronic intake levels required for human carcinogenicity are up to 900x higher than carcinogenic doses in experimental rats, and human acrylamide detoxification systems are up to four times more effective than rats'.[381] However, the available *in vitro* and animal research suggests that higher dietary intakes may increase cancer risks, and a safe level of intake hasn't yet been determined for humans.

Vitamins and Minerals

Cacao contains very high levels of **copper**: one serving of traditional Cacao beverage made from 40g beans contains just over the RDA limit of copper (900mcg), which is very high compared to other high-copper food sources, for example 40g cashew nuts contains 888mcg copper. Copper is used to manufacture various important enzymes (cuproenzymes) involved in several processes, including but not limited to: mitochondrial energy production, connective tissue formation and repair, dopamine conversion to noradrenaline in the CNS, MAO production, myelin sheath repair, superoxide dismutase manufacture (redox balance), regulating gene expression, and melanin formation. Adequate copper intake is essential for iron absorption, because copper is a component of the proteins hephaestin and ceruloplasmin. Hephaestin transports iron from epithelial cells to plasma ("opens the gates"), and caeruloplasmin converts iron into a form in which it may be transported in plasma.[viii] Serum copper is usually elevated above control in subjects with depression,[382] although it's not known whether this finding reflects a cause or a consequence. Copper excretion and absorption is normally well-regulated, which prevents toxicity. However, copper accumulation has been implicated in Parkinson's disease aetiology.

There are also significant amounts of **iron** in Cacao; in greater absolute quantity than that found in beef or chicken liver (although being non-haem iron, it's less biologically active than iron from animal products—only 5–10% is absorbed *in vivo*).[383] Iron's main physiological use is as an oxygen-binding metal: it is an integral component of haemoglobin, myoglobin, and redox enzymes. Iron also accumulates in the *substantia nigra* of persons with Parkinson's disease, and in the hippocampus of Alzheimer's patients, and is thought to contribute to oxidative cell damage and disease progression in both cases.

Cacao is also relatively high in **magnesium**. A 40g serving contains up to 172mg, almost half the RDA for men and over half the RDA for women. Magnesium is an essential mineral, used in many enzymes, and is essential for the manufacture of all the enzymes used in ATP synthesis. Low levels of magnesium increase the severity of asthma, and predispose to diabetes and osteoporosis; hypomagnesia is also associated with hypertension and metabolic syndrome. Low levels of magnesium in the CSF are positively associated with treatment-resistant suicidal depression, but not with depression in general. Magnesium is a natural calcium antagonist: adequate dietary intake reduces vascular calcification and atherosclerosis, and has anti-thrombotic effects, attenuating collagen-induced platelet activation and reducing ADP-triggered platelet aggregation.[384] Magnesium allegedly competes with calcium for absorption at high levels of intake, causing a variable net decrease of calcium absorption via undetermined mechanisms,[385] but in one small study oral co-supplementation of magnesium and calcium showed no significant effect on each other's absorption;[386] it's mostly stored in the skeleton, and intracellularly. A four-week, double-blind, placebo-controlled clinical trial compared daily administration of 17 mmol/d magnesium orotate to placebo in a small group of twenty-three triathletes. At the end of the study, the magnesium group were found to have lower serum cortisol before and after exercise, a reduced post-exercise serum creatine kinase and leukocyte count (indicating lower levels of inflammation or tissue damage), and improved blood glucose control (higher levels during exercise with lower insulin); taken together, the results indicated a reduced stress response.[387] Cacao added to the diet of rats fed a low-magnesium diet was sufficient to prevent magnesium deficiency.[388]

Cacao also contains significant amounts of **manganese**. Manganese-containing enzymes are very prevalent in mammalian physiology, such as manganese-superoxide dismutase (Mn-SOD) used to buffer/prevent toxic superoxide effects. Manganese ions are cofactors for many enzymes. Manganese is less toxic than copper, but high amounts can be neurotoxic and give rise to a Parkinson's disease-like syndrome which is unresponsive to l-dopa, and has been

---

[viii] Ceruloplasmin oxidises ferrous iron (Fe^{2+}) to ferric iron (Fe^{3+}).

implicated in childhood behavioural problems and neurodegenerative diseases through oxidation, excitotoxicity, and protein aggregation.

There's also a relatively high potassium content in Cacao. Cacao's natural potassium (K) to sodium (Na) ratio is approximately 3:1, as compared with the reference daily intake ratio of approximately 5:2. Given the preponderance of high-sodium (salted) foods in contemporary diets, Cacao is considered a useful dietary potassium source, although it only marginally favours potassium in terms of recommended relative intake. Both electrolytes are necessary for maintaining osmotic balance and are essential for nerve function by maintaining proper electrical signal conduction along the nerves (hence the "electrolyte" label), and to maintain proper muscle function (including cardiac muscle). Higher intakes of dietary potassium may reduce risk of hypertension and stroke, although Cacao should not be considered an especially good source of this common dietary mineral.

Cacao also contains moderately high levels of **zinc**, such that a 40g serving contains a quarter of the female RDI for zinc and just under one fifth of the male RDI. Zinc is necessary for proper immune function, tissue repair, growth, reproductive function (especially spermatogenesis), gene expression, and regulation of cellular lifespan (apoptosis). Low levels have been associated with Parkinson's disease.[389] Zinc is a common dietary deficiency, but excess intakes (e.g., through supplementation) may cause iron and copper deficiency over time,[390] increasing the risk of anaemia. Conversely it has been noted that high iron intake can inhibit zinc absorption through competitive inhibition of the intestinal epithelial divalent transporter-1.[391]

Volatile compounds

Seeds

Pharmacolological research on all the volatile compounds that comprise Cacao's unique aroma is patchy and diverse. It's possible that, being volatile, these compounds may be inhaled and act rapidly via the olfactory-limbic pathway to exert some central effects, if they possess psychotropic activity. **Isovaleric acid** (3-methylbutanoic acid) is sedative, possibly anti-convulsant, and inhibits oestrogen-mediated oocyte maturation *in vitro*. It is barely water-soluble but dissolves easily in organic solvents, and is easily absorbed from the gastrointestinal tract. **3-methylbutanal** is sympathomimetic at low levels. **Hexanal**, a compound that also contributes to the smell of freshly mown grass, is anti-fungal and has concentration-dependent Dopaminergic effects in the CNS of laboratory rats.[392] Hexanal is produced during lipid peroxidation *in vivo*, and presumably likewise formed during fermentation or roasting of Cacao. *In vitro*, hexanal is carcinogenic, inducing DNA strand breakage; it is also pro-haemolytic and anti-spermatozoic. **Phenylacetaldehyde** inhibits dopamine beta-monooxygenase, so retards conversion of dihydroxyphenethylamine (dopamine) to noradrenaline; however, the alternative catechol-O-methyltransferase (COMT) pathway to convert dopamine to 3-methoxytyramine means it has only a weak dopamine-sparing effect.[393] It's entirely plausible, therefore, that these four compounds may contribute to Cacao's psychoactivity. However, **trans-2-octenal** increases oxidative damage to dopaminergic neurons in fruit flies.[394]

2-noenal inhibits *Plasmodium falciparum* replication in human red blood cells *in vitro*; as an *in vitro* effect of a trace aromatic compound in Cacao, this property is unlikely to confer significant anti-malarial activity on whole Cacao, but may provide support for Cacao's traditional use as a cooling febrifuge and tonic in the context of chronic malaria. **Gamma-decanolactone** inhibits the human enzyme responsible for nicotine metabolism; however, this likely pales in comparison with the inducing effects of the xanthines in Cacao on nicotine metabolism. **Dimethyl trisulphide** has an inhibitory effect on microorganism growth *in vitro*: yeast growth is inhibited at ≥20ppm, while ≥200ppm is required to inhibit bacterial growth.[395] **Nonanal** has an anti-diarrhoeal effect in rodents, with no effect on normal bowel function; additionally, micromolar concentrations of nonanal inhibited formation of thromboxane B2 and arachidonic acid metabolites *in vitro*, implying a modulating effect on inflammatory and blood clotting mechanisms.[396] Topically applied **2-phenylethanol** exerted anti-microbial effects on *E. coli* and other bacteria via membrane and DNA association disruption. 2-phenylethanol is metabolised by alcohol dehydrogenase, and inhibits platelet aggregation *in vitro*.[397] These aromatic compounds may therefore play a role in Cacao's traditional ethnomedical uses as a drug with anti-diarrhoeal and prophylactic anti-venom properties (some snakes and biotoxins have coagulant and pro-inflammatory activity).

2,4-nonadienal is toxic to human fibroblasts and endothelial cells *in vitro* at micromolar concentrations,[398] an effect which would be utterly reversed by Cacao polyphenols; however, it also has anti-mutagenic effects against UV-induced mutatagenesis in *E. coli*, enhanced by benzaldehyde[399]—which is of particular interest given Cacao's combination with Mamey seed (*Pouteria sapota* [q.v.], a source of benzaldehyde compounds) in the traditional beverage known as *Tejate*, and the potential for additive chemopreventive effects with the polyphenols on UV-induced mutagenesis in humans. **Ethyl cinnamate** has *in vitro* anti-microbial activity against Gram negative organisms, particularly *E. coli* and *Candida albicans*.[400] Ethyl cinnamate also absorbs UV light and has weak xenoestrogenic activity,[401] though it exhibited *in vitro* cytotoxicity against human melanoma and leukaemia cell lines.[402] These two compounds may therefore influence Cacao's effects on the skin (Cacao as an "internal cosmetic" agent) and carcinogenesis. (For information on the volatile compound tetramethylpyrazine, aka ligustrazine: see alkaloids, above.)

Flowers

Cacao's tiny flowers also produce a complex volatile oil, but this oil varies by phenotype; one Mexican *criollo* variety, which is closer to wild, ancestral-type Cacao, contained compounds of higher molecular weight and attracted many more Cacao-associated midges and stingless bees than other Cacao cultivars.[403] Steam-distillation of *T. cacao* flowers yielded seventy-eight compounds, 50% of which was **pentadecane**, with **pentadecene** a secondary component. Little is known about the pharmacology of these compounds, except that they are found in the essential oil of several medicinal plants. They are acyclic alkanes, and exist as colourless liquids in their natural state.[404] 1-pentadecene is a volatile component of beef and oak moss oleoresin, and acts as a surfactant, with some cytotoxic and genotoxic properties.[405] It was noted that Central American *criollo* flower oil attracted more midges than oils extracted from other varieties, owing to the greater complexity of its essential oil.[406] Bolivian wild and cultivated Cacao both attracted many insects of the genus *Hymenoptera*, but while cultivated Cacao drew a wider range of bug species, greater numbers of insects were enticed to the flower of the wild plant.[407]

Experimental data and clinical trials

In vitro *research*

Most *in vitro* research is necessarily preliminary, being a guideline for further investigation and experimentation, and must be confirmed by *in vivo* and clinical trial findings.

Cardiovascular and metabolic: Theobroma cacao root decoction had high membrane stabilising activity on erythrocytes,[408] suggesting potential therapeutic benefit in haemolytic anaemia, malaria, or other disorders characterised by haemolysis.

Nervous system: Mouse brain hippocampal slices were used for assessing the effects of different Cacao extracts on neurological changes predisposing to Alzheimer's disease, specifically oligomerisation of amyloid-β protein. Extracts from higher-polyphenol beans were found to exert the strongest prophylactic activity, restoring long-term neuronal potentiation response; short-fermentation *lavado* beans were more effective than the fully fermented and roasted "natural" beans. Lower-polyphenol Dutched cocoa extract had no effect.[409] Aqueous Cacao extracts have also been shown to inhibit the activity of indeolamine 2,3-dioxygenase which catalyses the breakdown of serotonin to kyneurine, and significantly suppressed tryptophan breakdown in human peripheral blood mononuclear cells; the experimenters hypothesised that this conservation may partly explain Cacao's beneficial effects on mood.[410]

Cacao polyphenols' inhibition of NADPH oxidase, and their modulation of other pathways mediating neuronal apoptosis,[411] suggests possible utility of Cacao as a dietary adjunct or supplementary treatment in neurodegenerative disease. Certainly amyotrophic lateral sclerosis (ALS), Parkinson's disease, and Alzheimer's disease all heavily involve oxidative stress as a pathogenic mechanism; the flavan-7-ol EGCG (found in Cacao and the tea plant, *Camellia sinensis*) alone has been found to halt ALS progression in mice—but so far there are no human studies to replicate this finding.[412] (See Chapters 4 and 6 for discussion.) Un-processed (un-Dutched, *lavado*, or natural) whole Cacao bean extracts prevent oligomerisation of amyloid-β *in vitro*,[413] suggesting anti-Alzheimer's activity.

Immune system and neoplasia: Crude Cacao extracts inhibited metabolic activation of the carcinogen benzo-α-pyrene[ix] by cytochrome P450 (CYP) 1A; however, Cacao extracts did not protect against another mutagen which worked by free radical generation,[414] confirming that not all Cacao's cytoprotective properties are dependent on antioxidant mechanisms. Cacao extract dose-dependently inhibits inflammatory cytokine and chemokine secretion from macrophages, and, when the macrophages were treated with Cacao extract before applying an inflammatory stimulus, there was greater inhibition of TNF-α.[415] If borne out by *in vivo* research, this finding may have relevance to Cacao's traditional usage as a prophylactic remedy for snakebite, as TNF-α is a principal cytokine in the inflammatory cascade triggered by some snake venoms.[416] The extract also down-regulates T-lymphocyte activation,[417] and high-procyanidin cocoa had

---

[ix] Benzo-α-pyrene is naturally found in coal tar, exhaust fumes—especially diesel, cigarette smoke, and charred food.

anti-proliferative effects in cultured human colon cancer cells by inhibiting biosynthesis of polyamines[x].[418] Both aqueous and ethanolic extracts of Cacao also suppressed pro-inflammatory pathways in activated T-cells.[419] Cacao extracts also caused inhibition of growth factors, and MAPK pathway[xi] modulation, and evinced variable effects on transcription factors, cellular proliferation, apoptosis, transformation, migration, and angiogenesis.[420] Aqueous extracts of Cacao inhibit the formation of neopterin in human peripheral blood monocytes, a biomarker of inflammatory processes and oxidative stress; this is often associated with Th-1 type hypersensitivity responses, which suggests that Cacao may help to quell overactive immune responses.[421]

Antimicrobial properties: Five per cent cocoa powder inhibited growth of 102 microorganisms belonging to thirteen genera; especially sensitive were *Shigella*, *Staphylococcus*, *Micrococcus*, and *Bacillus* species. Casein in milk greatly attenuated this effect.[422] Of these, *Staphylococcus* may be the most relevant due to the spread of MRSA; *Staphylococcus* species are common and usually harmless unless they penetrate the skin, but some varieties can produce toxins which can cause food poisoning. Likewise, *Bacillus* species can cause food poisoning, and *Shigella* species may be dysentery-causing. *Micrococcus* are only liable to be problematic in immunocompromised people, such as those living with HIV, leukaemia, or on immune-suppressing medications. These observations bear out traditional observations of the long keeping properties of chocolate drinks prepared with water, and the seventeenth-century rhyme by the Spanish surgeon, Antonio Colmenero de Ledesma, on washing wounds (physical or emotional) with chocolate to prevent them festering.[xii]

Digestive system: Cocoa extracts also dose-dependently inhibited the pancreatic digestive enzymes α-amylase, lipase, and phospholipase A2, and may thus interfere with fat and carbohydrate digestion and absorption.[423]

In vivo *research (animals)*

Author's note: I strongly object to animal research on the basis that it is atrocious to perform experiments causing suffering and premature death to sentient beings where consent is impossible owing to their lesser intellect. If we would object to carrying out similar research on humans with lower intellectual capacity, such as babies, brain damaged adults, or those with learning difficulties on the basis of their ability to feel pain and suffer, then—logically—the same should apply to non-human animals with the capacity to feel pain and fear, and to experience suffering in similar ways. I've included results from such research in this book because there's so much of it, and not to include it would be a gross omission of extant information; however, almost all the conclusions which may be drawn from such research could be made from human clinical trials, cleverly designed in vitro *or laboratory research using cultured human cell lines. This is particularly the case with herbal drugs and foods which are known to be safe for human consumption, where vivisection is even more gratuitous. Volunteer* in vivo *studies, functional assays, and clinical trials would be the more ethical choice. Often animals are tortured and killed to*

[x] Intracellular signalling molecules necessary for cell division: growth, maturation, and survival; levels are elevated in neoplasia.
[xi] Mitogen-activated protein kinase, an intracellular enzyme regulating cellular survival and replication processes.
[xii] See Chapter 8 epigraph.

obtain quite trivial information, because such studies are far cheaper and less difficult to organise than human trials—justification is assumed on the ethically dubious basis of intellectual hierarchy (might = right, or our right to acquire information supersedes the right of other species not to suffer), or historical religious mandate.

Nervous system: While eating chocolate, lab rats experienced enkaphalin surges of more than 150% over baseline levels in the anterior dorsomedial striatum, likely as a response to palatability (a natural response to foods high in fat and sugar) rather than pharmacological rewards.[424] However, several pharmacological actions not dependent on Cacao's fat, sugar, or xanthine content have been demonstrated in animal experiments: pre-treatment with Cacao extract by directly injecting it into the temporomandibular joint (TMJ) before injecting capsaicin caused suppression of sensory trigeminal nerve activation in rats,[425] demonstrating anti-nociceptive effects, although the real-life value of this research is questionable or negligible owing to the bizarre approach of injecting chocolate directly into the joint!

Acute oral doses of cocoa mass at 100mg per 100g bodyweight (equivalent to single or regular daily doses of 63.5g Cacao for a 10st human) altered conditioned fear responses in rats in the elevated t-maze test, an experiment designed to induce and evaluate anxiety. "Conditioned fear" in this model is a *learned* fear which causes the animal to stay in the "safe zone" (covered tunnels or "arms" in the maze), demonstrating an unwillingness to come out into the open and be exposed to greater risk; an excessive fear response is equated with generalised anxiety disorder in humans, or PTSD. Avoidance latency (time taken to venture from the enclosed, "safer" part of the maze, and explore) was significantly ($P < 0.5$) reduced in animals given these one-off doses of cocoa mass, suggesting that their conditioned fear response was diminished. This effect was stronger than the reduction of conditioned fear responses in animals given intraperitoneal injections of benzodiazepine at 0.1mg/kg. However, there was no change in escape latency (time taken for the animal to "unfreeze" and move away from the exposed arm of the maze, into the safer covered zone) in the Cacao group, suggesting that acute doses of Cacao reduced conditioned, but not unconditioned fear responses. ("Unconditioned fear" in this model is an *instinctual* fear which causes the animal to "freeze" in the "unsafe zone"—the open, elevated space—of the maze; an excess of it is equated to panic disorder, aka "panic attacks" unrelated to specific cues in humans.) There were no measurable effects on brain noradrenaline, serotonin, or dopamine concentration in these rats. When the rats were fed cocoa mass for two weeks at 1% of their diet, there was a slight, non-significant *increase* in avoidance latency, in other words in "conditioned fear-related behaviour", accompanied by a rise in brain serotonin concentration and turnover.

The authors concluded that acute doses of Cacao had anxiolytic activity, whereas "chronic" (two weeks') usage did not;[426] however, it should be noted that the elevated serotonin turnover and increased avoidance latency after two weeks' consumption suggest that the Cacao improved the rats' facility to learn by association, or slightly *increased* their generalised anxiety levels, which may suggest an amplified tendency to risk aversion. Caffeine and amphetamine produce no effect in the elevated T-maze model of anxiety,[427] which strongly suggests that the psychoactivity of Cacao does not depend wholly on caffeine—in rats, at least. It may also be worthy of consideration that Cacao's effects on monoamines were measured, but not on CNS levels of opioids, GABA, and cannabinoids; and the absolute level of monoamines measured may not reflect changes in sensitivity (i.e., brain monoamine levels may remain constant while intracellular metabolism or receptor affinity changes).

Cardiovascular and metabolic: Obese-diabetic rats orally dosed with cocoa extract at 600mg/kg body weight (equivalent to a daily intake of 38.1g cocoa mass in a 10st adult human) over four weeks produced no measurable change in plasma insulin or fasting glucose, but there was a significant acute reduction in plasma glucose sixty to ninety minutes post-ingestion.[428] However, an earlier trial using an 80% ethanolic 1:10 extract of cocoa in diabetic rats at 1–3% of their dietary intake found a dose-dependent reduction in total triglycerides as well as serum glucose levels.[429] A systematic review of short-term randomised feeding trials reveals that cocoa and chocolate lower blood pressure, reduce inflammation, have anti-platelet activity, increase HDL and reduce LDL oxidation, and may lower coronary heart disease mortality.[430] A 2014 review of research into Cacao and obesity found that rats and mice fed cocoa as part of a normal or high-fat diet showed less weight gain and mesenteric white adipose tissue accumulation than the control group or other animals eating a high-fat diet without added cocoa. Dietary cocoa intake also decreased the hepatic expression of genes involved in fatty acid synthesis and transport, and up-regulated uncoupling protein 2 expression, which may enhance thermogenesis or decrease fat accumulation.[431]

Whole Cacao at 0.5, 1, or 2% of rats' diet maintained erythrocyte glutathione levels.[432] This experiment was performed with whole Cacao, so the results are potentially more applicable to whole chocolate or Cacao products, although the precise constituents or combinations thereof which may be responsible for the observed effects necessarily remain obscure. 0.5, 1, or 2% of the diet represents an approximate human equivalent of 6, 13, or 26g Cacao per day, a very achievable level of intake. These findings suggest that dietary Cacao may protect against some types of anaemia dependent on damage to erythrocytes.

Immune system and neoplasia: Three weeks' "high-dose" dietary intake of cocoa in rats (at 4% and 10% of the diet) strongly reduced intestinal secretory Immunoglobulin A (sIgA), though sIgA levels were only slightly reduced in Peyer's patches.[433] Long-term Cacao intake augmented systemic Th1-dependent immune responses, elevating intestinal γδ T-lymphocyte counts (these being the most prevalent T-cell subtypes in gut mucosa), while Th2-dependent antibody-secreting response declined.[434] A subsequent study in which stool analysis was performed on Wistar rats fed a 10% Cacao diet found that the microbiome was substantially altered, with increased faecal counts of *Tenericutes* and *Cyanobacteria* and lower levels of *Firmicutes* and *Proteobacteria*.[435]

A food allergy to ovalbumin was induced in newly weaned rats, who were then fed conventional Cacao or non-fermented Cacao extract as part of their diet, or a cocoa-free diet. At fourteen days old they were exposed to ovalbumin to induce allergy, and at twenty-seven days old anaphylaxis was induced; the rats were then killed and autopsied. Conventional Cacao-fed rats had no increase in serum leptin or glucagon-like peptide following allergy induction, and conventional Cacao in the diet completely prevented increases in Th-2 dependent serum IgG1 and IgG2a. Total and anti-ovalbumin intestinal IgA was significantly decreased in the conventional Cacao group, but not in the non-fermented Cacao group, and intestinal anti-ovalbumin IgE production was also strongly suppressed. Following induction of anaphylaxis, the conventional Cacao diet partially prevented serum increase in mast cell protease, and promoted haematocrit recovery two hours following the event. However, acute anaphylactic effects such as a drop in body temperature and decreased movement may have been exacerbated by Cacao intake—possibly due to vasodilatation—and rats on a conventional Cacao diet also showed increased villous atrophy and a decreased number of goblet cells in the intestinal lumen.[436] That these effects were more pronounced in the lower-flavanol conventional Cacao group suggests that other compounds in the bean, perhaps produced during fermentation and roasting, may be responsible.

Cocoa liquor extract also reduced enzymatic markers of liver cell necrosis in rats with liver cancer.[437] There were measurable changes in the lymphoid tissue of rats regularly given cocoa in their diet, especially GALT (gut-associated lymphoid tissue), with a reduction in the proportion of T-helper lymphocytes in Peyer's patches, spleen, and mesenteric lymph nodes, and decreased GALT (gut-associated lymphatic tissue) IgA secretion.[438] Previous research by the same team had revealed that Cacao in rat food promoted T cell maturation and reduced intestinal IgM and IgA secretion. So regular cocoa intake caused a net reduction in antibody-mediated autoimmunity and gastrointestinal specific immune surveillance, and decreased antibody-mediated mucosal defences.

Reproductive system: Whole Cacao at 0.5, 1, or 2% of rats' diet also lowered the concentration of testicular 8-hydroxy-2'-deoxyguanosine (8-OHdG) over two weeks, but did not have the same effect in the rats' heart or liver tissues.[439] 8-OHdG is a pivotal marker for measuring the effect of endogenous oxidative damage to DNA and therefore of carcinogenesis,[440] and glutathione is an endogenous "antioxidant" which buffers cells from "free radical" damage. These findings suggest that dietary Cacao may protect against testicular cancer. On the other hand, it should be noted that the human epidemiological data currently available is in conflict with this finding, given that higher Cacao intakes have been correlated with higher incidences of testicular cancer eighteen to thirty-seven years later (described shortly).[441]

Oral health: There was a measurable reduction in gingival levels of oxidative stress markers in rats fed a diet containing 10% Cacao over a four-week period as compared to rats on a Cacao-free diet, although there was no difference between the two groups in the development of induced periodontitis.[442]

Metabolic effects: Moderate Cacao supplementation increased the lifespan of fruit flies, although higher dietary concentrations of Cacao did not. The experimenters also noted that Cacao supplementation caused earlier morbidity and death in the flies when manganese-superoxide (a primary antioxidant enzyme) was deficient, and concluded that Cacao could act as a pro-oxidant when oxidative stress levels were abnormally elevated. However, when excess heavy metals were present, Cacao extended lifespan, showing "metal-chelating effects".[443]

Human studies and results

Endocrine system: A 2012 meta-analysis of trials assessing the utility of chocolate and cocoa in blood sugar control demonstrated "consistent acute and chronic benefits of chocolate or cocoa" on circulation and insulin resistance, as assessed by FMD and HOMA-IR.[444] Nineteen hypertensive adults with impaired glucose tolerance participated in a fifteen-day trial, ingesting 100g of flavanol-rich dark chocolate daily: their mean systolic and diastolic blood pressure decreased by –4mm Hg, and all subjects had increased flow-mediated dilation and reduced total and LDL cholesterol, with significantly improved insulin sensitivity and pancreatic β-cell function.[445] A randomised crossover trial with twenty active male subjects consuming 40g dark choco- late every day for two weeks recorded improved fatty acid mobilisation during exercise, and decreased metabolic impact of exercise (reduced F2-isoprostanes and oxidised LDL), although no improvement in exercise performance was noted.[446]

A small study from 2010 found that when overweight and obese subjects consumed daily dark chocolate containing 500mg polyphenols (equivalent to 42g whole Cacao) over two weeks, there was a slight decrease in blood pressure and fasting blood glucose, with a trend towards reduction of urinary cortisone. Notably, chocolate containing a daily dose of 1000mg polyphenols was no more effective than 500mg/day.[447] Similarly, a functional assay assessing the acute effects of dark chocolate ingestion on blood clotting found that medium doses of high-flavonoid cocoa (0.375g chocolate per kg bodyweight, equivalent to 30–35g whole Cacao in a 10st subject) had a "faster and stronger … effect than either low or high doses" on reducing platelet reactivity and stabilising red blood cells.[448] It should be noted that an intake of 500mg Cacao polyphenols per day may be harder to achieve with eating chocolate and occasion some weight gain, requiring the consumption of 80–100g dark chocolate daily, but is much more pal- atable with traditional chocolate drinks, requiring only one or two cups of *cacahuatl* totalling 40g Cacao, or one or two mug-sized portions of a Cacao-based *atole* per day (see Formulary, Chapter 8).

A 2014 placebo-controlled clinical trial assessed the acute effects of 50g dark chocolate (72% cocoa solids) on the stress response in a cohort of sixty-five healthy non-smoking adult males by measuring their saliva and blood levels of adrenaline, noradrenaline, cortisol and ACTH before and after administering a standardised stress test (the Trier social stress test). Although there were no differences in ACTH or noradrenaline, all participants in the *verum* (dark chocolate) group "showed a significantly blunted cortisol and [adrenaline] … reactivity to psychosocial stress compared to the placebo group. Additional controlling for age, BMI, and MAP did not significantly change these results."[449] In a fourteen-day (medium-term) trial, thirty participants were classified into those having high or low anxiety traits, and all participants were given 40g dark chocolate every day. The chocolate reduced participants' urinary excretion of cortisol and catecholamines, indicating a decreased adrenal stress response (in other words, less cortisol and catecholamines were being released to be metabolised). Most interestingly, those with higher anxiety traits had a stronger response. Authors concluded that the chocolate modified the gut microbiome, and reduced the effects of stress on metabolism.[450] These trials demonstrate that Cacao modifies the adrenal and systemic stress response.

Nervous system: Single, acute doses of flavanol-rich cocoa (containing 450mg of flavanols, equivalent to a 40g dose of whole Cacao, a moderate-large dose) increased cerebral blood flow to grey matter, and five days' administration of cocoa containing 150mg flavanols/day (equivalent to twelve to thirteen grams whole Cacao/day) produced a measurable increase in oxygenated blood circulation through the cerebral cortex of sixteen healthy young volunteers, though no alterations in behavioural reaction times were noted.[451] Brain imaging revealing blood flow in six healthy adults given flavanol-rich chocolate also revealed increased signal intensity during a task requiring concentration compared to scans performed prior to chocolate consumption, although it isn't known whether this reflected increased nerve firing or just increased blood flow to the activated brain areas.[452] The assumption is that the chocolate enabled the brain to increase its blood and therefore oxygen supply as necessary—but as this was such a small trial with no placebo group it's not possible to be certain whether it was the chocolate or the participants' expectations which caused this response. Another study found that subjects who ate 85g chocolate fifteen minutes before a cognitive function test performed up to 20% better than the control group—but, interestingly, the milk chocolate group did better than the dark chocolate group.[453] This could reflect the greater placebo value of familiar and comforting milk chocolate, or the anti-anxiety effects of exorphin (sedating, opiate-like) compounds in milk pairing with the stimulants in chocolate, or poor quality of the chocolate used! It should be noted however that fifteen minutes isn't long enough for many of the compounds in chocolate to get into the bloodstream, so all this study shows is that being given chocolate before doing mental work may improve performance.

One study utilised a low dose (250mg) of cocoa powder, administered acutely and once daily to a group of forty subjects from twenty-one to twenty-eight years old. The subjects were assessed with repeated ten-minute cognitive demand battery tests, and a mental fatigue scale. The only notable result was an acute reduction in mental fatigue and improvement in a "serial sevens" (rapid mental arithmetic) task.[454] However, the exceptionally low dose of poor-quality Cacao should be noted, as this is likely to account for the unimpressive results of this trial. Most studies suggest a positive, nootropic effect of dark, high-flavanol chocolate on cognition. Nine hundred and sixty-eight residents of Maine and Syracuse in the United States, aged twenty-three to ninety-eight, were assessed using neuropsychological testing, and higher chocolate consumption was strongly associated with better overall cognition, and specific enhancements over baseline in visual-spatial memory and organisation, working memory, scanning and tracking, abstract reasoning, and in the mini-mental state exam (MMSE). All but the last were not mainly due to "cardiovascular, dietary and lifestyle factors"—the improvements were specifically the result of regular chocolate consumption.[455] Another study evaluated 531 senior citizens over the age of sixty-five for a period of four years, using the MMSE. Adjustments were made for risk factors such as age, smoking, obesity, diabetes, alcohol consumption, etc. Chocolate consumption was again found to be strongly associated with a reduced risk of cognitive decline, but only if daily caffeine consumption did not exceed 75mg.[456] One study assessed the effects of chocolate on sleep deprivation in thirty-two participants, who were administered either high- or low-flavanol chocolate two hours prior to assessment in both sleep-deprived and well-rested states. The high-flavanol chocolate preserved working memory accuracy in women following sleep deprivation, and improved circulatory parameters such as flow-mediated dilation and blood pressure in sleep-deprived men and women.[457]

Clinical studies on chocolate's effect on mood have produced varying results. In general, eating chocolate was found to improve negative moods but not "neutral and positive moods"; most interestingly, *intention* was found to enhance mood-raising properties of chocolate.[458] Another study corroborated this finding: 258 participants randomised into chocolate-eating or cracker-eating groups found that "mindfully" eating a small dose of seventy-five calories of chocolate (approximately thirteen grams) produced a greater increase in positive mood than those eating chocolate "unmindfully" or those eating crackers, "mindfully" or not.[459] A systematic review of research on chocolate's effect on mood and cognitive function found that eight studies met their inclusion criteria, and five of these showed either an improvement in negative mood or an attenuation of negative mood, while three showed evidence of cognitive enhancement. Two studies showed neither of these things but identified "significant alterations in brain activation patterns".[460]

In a sample of 1018 adults living in San Diego, California, depression (assessed by the Center for Epidemiologic Studies Depression Scale [CES-D] questionnaire) was positively correlated with higher chocolate intake for men and women, independent of general fat, carbohydrate, or calorie intake: respondents with low depression scores ate an average of 5.4 servings per month, higher scorers ate 8.4 servings, and the highest scores ate an average 11.8 servings/ month.[461] Another study used a standardised questionnaire comparing 72 regular chocolate eaters with 122 non-chocolate consumers and 22 recovering alcoholics found that people who "self-medicated" low mood with chocolate or other sweet foods were "more likely to have personality traits associated with hysteroid dysphoria, an atypical depressive syndrome".[462]

In an online survey with 3,000 respondents who self-identified as having suffered from clinical depression, 45% of respondents reported chocolate cravings (male : female = 51 : 31%). Respondents acknowledged "hedonistic effects" (*sic*), but referred to chocolate's "capacity to settle 'emotional dysregulation' ... and this aspect was ranked above aesthetic factors".[463] Apparent mood-altering effects of the chocolate were rated higher by cravers than its taste or appearance. Depressed chocolate cravers consistently evinced higher levels of neuroticism; in particular, they had higher levels of irritability and rejection sensitivity, the latter being a prominent feature of hysteroid dysphoria. In another online survey of 2,692 self-identified clinical depressives, 61% of chocolate cravers (by contrast, the women outnumbered the men in this survey) rated chocolate's mood-raising properties as moderate to very important, and chocolate was perceived by such users as a means of reducing anxiety and irritability.[464]

In another small medium-term (twenty-eight day) clinical trial exploring chocolate's effect on catecholamine levels, daily intake of 75g dark chocolate was compared to 75g white chocolate in twenty-one healthy adults. The daily chocolate rations were divided into three servings of 25g. It was estimated that the dark chocolate group were consuming 877mg of polyphenols and 694mg theobromine daily as compared to none in the white chocolate group (excepting those found in other foods, such as polyphenols from wine or theobromine from maté tea or post-caffeine metabolism, respectively). Added sugar consumption (from the chocolate) was 9.75g in the dark chocolate group vs. 42.75g in the white chocolate group. Plasma levels of dopamine, noradrenaline, adrenaline, serotonin, and its metabolite 5-HIAA taken from peripheral venous blood samples were monitored in both groups. There was a statistically significant increase in 5-HIAA and decrease in adrenaline in the dark chocolate group, with a consistent but not quite statistically significant trend towards increased serotonin. Surprisingly, there was a statistically significant increase in dopamine and serotonin levels in the white chocolate group, with no increase in 5-HIAA, and a trend towards increasing noradrenaline.

So this small trial assessing the effect of chocolate on central monoamines found that white chocolate "outperformed" the dark in terms of increased levels of the active "pleasurable/stimulating" catecholamines. It should be noted however that there was a linear trend towards dopamine increase in the dark chocolate group, and likewise towards a reduction in adrenaline, both of which—if sustained—may have achieved statistical significance over a longer period of time;

certainly serotonin metabolism was affected as evinced by elevated 5-HIAA, and these changes are in line with positive mood state effects noted by consumers. The authors speculated that "Some active compound, and/or combination … present in both dark and white chocolate could be responsible," and suggested that the lipophilic amino acid amides could be present in cocoa butter (the fat from Cacao), of which white chocolate has more, and may account for these effects.[465] However, as discussed in the main text of this book (Chapter 5), the dark chocolate in this trial actually contained more cocoa butter. Moreover, it should also be noted that the trial was of relatively short duration, and a longer, larger trial would be necessary to substantiate these results.

A very small double-blind, randomised, pilot crossover placebo-controlled study of ten patients with chronic fatigue syndrome (CFS) showed a significant decrease in chronic fatigue and subjective handicap, as well as a decrease in anxiety and depression after eight weeks of daily high polyphenol chocolate intake, in comparison with the placebo chocolate group, whose symptoms worsened. The Cacao was administered as 15g of chocolate containing 85% cocoa solids (including cocoa butter) three times daily: total 45g/day, containing 68.1% cocoa liquor with up to 4% polyphenols = 27.5g Cacao per day, containing up to 1096mg total polyphenols per day. The authors of the study speculated that the improvements may have been an effect of Cacao's putative serotonergic activity, and its content of anandamide and PEA.[466] However, improvements may also be due to increased excretion of cortisol and adrenaline, as well as improved vascular endothelial and circulatory function (see cardiovascular and endocrine studies below).

A 2013 study compared the cerebrospinal fluid (CSF) levels of 5-HIAA, cortisol, and the precursor hormone DHEA in twenty-eight un-medicated people who had recently attempted suicide, with nineteen control subjects. The result: "Suicide attempters had higher CSF and plasma cortisol levels compared to healthy volunteers … female suicide attempters had lower CSF 5-HIAA levels compared to male and female healthy volunteers respectively … Suicide victims [sic] tended to have low CSF 5-HIAA and high CSF cortisol."[467] Another study of rhesus macaque monkeys found that infants who experienced more maternal rejection had lower 5-HIAA levels, while those who were overprotected against perceived threats by their mothers had higher cortisol levels; the authors concluded: "Since exposure to high levels of maternal protectiveness and rejection is known to affect the offspring's behaviour and responsiveness to the environment later in life, our results are consistent with the hypothesis that these effects are mediated by long-term changes in the activity of the offspring's HPA axis and brain serotonergic system."[468] This research is relevant to human psychosocial adjustment, as exposure to stressful events and relationships during childhood strongly predicts mental, physical, and social health during adulthood.[469] Therefore, Cacao's ability to increase cortisol and catecholamine excretion, while raising CNS 5-HIAA—if borne out by larger trials and studies—may have very practical applications in developing treatment protocols for people living with social anxiety, suicidal ideation, or hysteroid dysphoria. Speculatively, there may be a role for *Theobroma* in the treatment of post-traumatic stress disorder, or other forms of conditioned fear, as the extinction of conditioned fear is mediated by the ventral prefrontal cortex and its neuronal projections to the nucleus accumbens and amygdalae,[470] brain regions which are strongly dependent on dopamine, cannabinoid, and nitric oxide signalling, all of which Theobroma's constituents may modify.

Cacao has analgesic properties. These are speculated to be partly due to fat- and sugar-associated endorphin release following chocolate consumption ("hedonic ingestion analgesia"), but this fails to adequately explain the traditional use of Cacao-based beverages against pain—such beverages being mostly unsweetened, and without added fat. Animal models demonstrated that expectation of macronutrient-rich food increased analgesia during consumption of such foods, so it seems that the high cultural cachet of Cacao as a nourishing food-beverage may have enhanced psychosomatic analgesia.[471] Cacao's phenylethylamine (PEA) and anandamide content are largely dismissed as relevant to this property due to their low level, although chocolate craving has been noted in MDMA users and those with low serum PEA,[472] and other compounds that conserve and potentiate anandamide and PEA[xiii] are co-present in Cacao. The greatest pharmacological contribution to chocolate analgesia comes from the flavonoids and methylxanthines. Methylxanthines have minor, centrally mediated analgesic effects, and the Cacao flavanols act as immuno-regulatory anti-inflammatories, decreasing local inflammatory mediator production and vascular inflammation, and increasing microcirculation. Cacao flavanols also attenuate trigeminal neuralgia by inhibiting neuronal calcitonin gene-related peptide (CGRP) production while up-regulating MAP kinase phosphatase enzyme expression, which has a net anti-nociceptive effect.[473]

Cardiovascular system

Atherosclerosis, wherein thickening of blood vessel walls leads to increased risk of clot formation, heart attack, and stroke, was formerly assumed to be a consequence of high intakes of saturated dietary fat, but is now thought to be primarily an inflammation-driven process. On a chemical level, there may be an imbalance between cellular production of antioxidant "buffers" such as SOD, and nitric oxide (NO). Platelets in the blood release inflammatory mediators once activated, which can induce atherosclerotic plaque rupture or vascular ischaemia.[474] It appears that NO is more significant in the pathogenesis of cardiovascular disease than LDL cholesterol, because reduced levels of NO are associated with hypercholesterolemia, increased platelet aggregation, and endothelial monocyte adhesion, indicative of atherogenesis and increased risk of thrombus formation.[475] Due primarily to the NO-inducing properties of its polyphenols, Cacao may play a significant role in the treatment or prevention of atherosclerotic pathologies.

Numerous clinical trials have demonstrated pharmaceutical utility of Cacao in the prevention or treatment of cardiovascular pathology. It is notable that the most carefully controlled trials produced outcomes demonstrating mild to moderate benefit in terms of reduced cardiovascular pathology risk factors, for example, blood pressure, endothelial function, serum cholesterol, and insulin sensitivity:

1. A double-blind placebo-controlled clinical trial with forty-nine participants assessed the effect of cocoa flavanols on blood pressure. Daily consumption of 360mg cocoa flavanols in

---

[xiii] Anandamide: the N-acylethanolamines OEA and LEA; Phenyltheylamine: Proanthocyanidins, Epicatechin, and Catechin.

chocolate bars was compared to the effect of low-flavanol placebo chocolate bars on systolic blood pressure over an eight-week period, and a mean systolic blood pressure decrease of 6mm Hg was observed in the *verum* (non-placebo) group. In a non-blinded extension of this trial, twenty-five participants were given 12g sugar with and without 26g cocoa powder per day for twelve weeks, and their serum lipoproteins were measured; the cocoa-consuming group had a 24% increase in HDL, with decreased LDL oxidation.[476]

2. Forty subjects with coronary artery disease participated in a double-blind placebo-controlled clinical trial, wherein daily consumption of 444mg isolated Cacao flavanols from cocoa/chocolate[xiv] were compared with the effect of taking isocaloric placebos over a six-week period as measured by brachial artery flow-mediated dilatation (FMD), systemic arterial compliance, and cellular adhesion molecules: no benefits were noted in the *verum* group, either acutely or over the six-week period.[477]

3. In another randomised double-blind placebo-controlled clinical trial, twenty-one partici-pants were given high-flavanol chocolate containing 213mg procyanidins and 46mg epi-catechin (approximately the amount found in 40g whole Cacao) daily, over a two-week period. There was a significant improvement in brachial artery FMD of +1.3% in the high-flavanol group, which coincided with an elevation in plasma epicatechin.[478] No changes in LDL oxidation, blood pressure, serum lipids, or the oxidative stress marker 8-isoprostane were observed.

4. Twenty un-medicated hypertensive subjects were given flavanol-rich cocoa twice daily for two weeks in a randomised, double-blind placebo-controlled crossover trial. (The fla-vanol intake was high, at 900mg per day, equivalent to 75g/day whole Cacao: a feasible intake, if given as three divided 25g doses or two high doses of 37.5g.) There were no sig-nificant changes in blood pressure, insulin resistance, or epithelial adhesion molecules, but increased insulin-stimulated changes in brachial artery diameter were noted. In view of the improvement in insulin-mediated vasodilation during the trial, it was concluded that two weeks was too short for other changes to become apparent.[479]

5. A single-blind, randomised placebo-controlled trial compared the effects of acute inges-tion of liquid cocoa (22g) to solid dark chocolate containing 22g cocoa powder, in sugared and unsweetened varieties, on vascular endothelial function and blood pressure in forty-five healthy overweight adults. The mean age of participants was fifty-three. The cocoa improved FMD and reduced blood pressure, and it was observed that the sugar-free cocoa had significantly stronger effects, with the liquid formulations being slightly more effective than solid chocolate.[480]

6. Forty-four unmedicated prehypertensive or mildly hypertensive adults aged between fifty-six and seventy-three participated in a randomised controlled trial comparing the effects of dark and white chocolate ingestion on blood pressure and serum oxidative stress markers over an eighteen-week period. A dose of 6.3g of dark chocolate containing 30mg polyphenols was administered daily, compared to an isocaloric dose of white chocolate. There was a slight reduction in blood pressure in the dark chocolate group after eighteen

---

[xiv] An equivalent dosage of whole Cacao would be 40g, which contains approximately 480mg total Polyphenols.

weeks (–2.9mmHg Systolic, –1.9mmHg Diastolic), and hypertension prevalence in the dark chocolate group fell from 86% to 68%. There was a sustained increase of s-nitrosogluta-thione (GSNO) in the plasma of the dark chocolate group, but no changes in the oxidative stress marker 8-isoprostane, indicating improved nitric oxide (NO) formation and vasodilation.[481]

7. Twenty-two heart transplant recipients participated in a double-blind, randomised trial with no placebo group to investigate the acute effects of ingesting 40g of high-flavanol dark chocolate with 70% cocoa solids. Each serving contained 0.27 and 0.9mg/g catechin and epicatechin, respectively, a quantity equivalent to 15–20g whole Cacao. The effects on coronary artery dilation and platelet adhesion were assessed, and two hours after ingesting the dark chocolate there was a significant increase in coronary artery dilation and a reduction in platelet adhesion, positively correlated with serum epicatechin concentration.[482]

8. The acute effects of ingesting high-flavonoid cocoa were assessed in a randomised double-blind crossover trial with twenty participants divided into two groups of ten individuals. High-flavonoid cocoa contained 187mg flavonoids per 100ml serving. No changes in plasma F(2)-isoprostane levels were noted unless the cocoa ingestion was combined with strenuous physical exercise—then a significant difference was noted, with lower F2-isoprostane levels in the high-flavanol group.[483] This suggests that the antioxidant effects of Cacao, and any physiological consequences, are more notable under conditions of physiological stress.

9. A small randomised double-blind crossover trial with ten participants assessed the acute effects of chocolate ingestion on plasma inflammatory markers. Each dose of low-polyphenol chocolate contained 3.33mg procyanidins, and the high polyphenol chocolate contained 148mg procyanidins (approximately equivalent to 25g of whole Cacao). Participants taking the higher polyphenol chocolate had altered serum eicosanoid synthesis, with a 32% elevation of plasma prostacyclin levels, and a 29% decrease in plasma leukotrienes, indicating anti-inflammatory, anti-thrombotic, vasodilatory, and anti-asthmatic effects.[484]

10. A double-blind trial with no placebo group tested the effects of drinking chocolate on haemodynamic factors in thirty-two post-menopausal hypercholesterolaemic women. The women were divided into two groups of sixteen, and given either a high-flavanol beverage containing 446mg flavanols/day, or a low-flavanol beverage containing 43mg flavanols/day over a six-week period. After six weeks, brachial artery hyperaemic blood flow increased by 76% in the high flavanol group and by 32% in the low flavanol group, and there was a significant reduction in plasma soluble vascular cell adhesion molecule-1 in the high flavanol group only.[485]

11. Eleven smokers participated in a small randomised, double-blind crossover trial with no placebo group, testing the effects of acute cocoa beverage ingestion on vasodilation. Once again, high flavanol cocoa (containing 176 to 185mg of flavanols) was compared with low flavanol cocoa (<11mg). Two hours after ingesting high-flavanol cocoa, there was a significant increase in plasma NO species and flow-mediated dilation, reversed by the NO inhibitor *n*-methylarginine. This is especially relevant, as vascular disease in smokers is caused by impaired NO synthesis.[486]

12. Thirty-six normotensive ("prehypertensive") subjects participated in a twelve-week randomised controlled trial, with a daily "dose" of 50g of dark chocolate containing 70% cocoa

solids. Difficulties with compliance were noted, and there were no recorded blood-pressure lowering effects.[487]

13. Twenty-seven adults participated in a five-day single-blind, placebo-controlled trial of the effects of very high flavanol Cacao on vasodilation. Participants ingested 821mg flavanols per day, equivalent to 80g whole Cacao. A marked and statistically significant (P = 0.009) increase in vasodilation was observed after the five-day period, particularly when ischaemia was induced. A comparison with flavanol-poor cocoa (such as may be found in standard processed cocoa) produced much weaker vasodilatory responses.[488]

14. A randomised, single-blind clinical trial assessed the effects of two weeks' daily high-flavanol chocolate intake in comparison with zero-flavanol white chocolate on cardiovascular and metabolic factors in thirty-nine healthy male participants aged between twenty-three and forty. The daily dose of high-flavanol chocolate contained 550mg flavanols, equivalent to approximately 46g of whole Cacao. Significant improvements in coronary flow velocity reserve (CFVR) were recorded for the high-flavanol chocolate group after two weeks, independent of changes in lipid profile, blood pressure, and oxidative stress.[489]

15. Forty-nine obese or overweight adults took part in an open trial comparing the effects of high-flavanol cocoa intake with and without exercise to the effects of ingesting low-flavanol cocoa with and without exercise on haemodynamic and metabolic factors (vasodilation and erythrocyte nitric oxide production, and blood glucose control, respectively). The high-flavanol cocoa contained 902mg of flavanols per day, equivalent to 70g whole Cacao (a very high dose), and the low-flavanol cocoa contained 36mg flavanols/day, equivalent to 9.5g whole Cacao. Independent of exercise, high-flavanol cocoa acutely increased participants' mean FMD by 2.4% (measurements taken 2h after ingestion) and increased baseline FMD by 1.6% after daily administration over a two-week period. The high-flavanol cocoa also induced a slight reduction in BP (1–2mm Hg), and reduced insulin resistance by 0.31%. The higher flavanol beverage also reduced erythrocyte arginase activity *in vivo*, causing vasodilation.[490]

16. Forty-two volunteers determined to be at high risk of developing cardiovascular disease took part in a four-week randomised crossover trial, testing the effects of milky cocoa on serum inflammatory markers. Daily ingestion of 40g cocoa powder taken with 500ml skimmed milk was compared with a daily intake of 500ml plain skimmed milk. The cocoa + milk significantly lowered serum markers of inflammation (-selectin and intercellular adhesion molecule-1) compared with the milk-only group.[491]

17. Twenty-three healthy subjects with a mean age of thirty-six participated in a randomised crossover study comparing the effects of the average American diet on serum cholesterol and lipid oxidation to the average American diet supplemented with 22g cocoa powder and 16g dark chocolate per day over a four-week period. The chocolate group was ingesting 466mg polyphenols per day, equivalent to 40g whole Cacao. Participants in the chocolate group had a significantly prolonged LDL oxidation time with raised HDL and increased serum antioxidant capacity at the end of the four-week study, but their HDL:LDL ratios remained unchanged.[492]

18. Thirty healthy adults took part in a functional assay comparing the acute haemodynamic effects of cocoa, water, or a caffeinated beverage after ingestion. Cocoa consumption

decreased clotting tendencies two to six hours after ingestion, and adrenaline-stimulated primary haemostasis was significantly attenuated at six hours post-ingestion; caffeine also decreased ADP-induced primary haemostasis two and six hours after ingestion. However, cocoa reversed adrenaline-induced platelet glycoprotein production caused by caffeine. Researchers concluded that cocoa had an "aspirin-like effect" on primary haemostasis.[493] This early result was confirmed by a crossover study with sixteen healthy participants, in which the ingestion of a cocoa beverage containing 897mg flavanols, equivalent to 75g whole Cacao per day, was compared with aspirin alone, and both cocoa and aspirin together. Taken with aspirin, the high-flavanol cocoa had short-term additive effects on platelet reactivity,[494] but there was no detectable change in eicosanoid synthesis over two weeks of concomitant administration, demonstrating limited anti-thrombotic efficacy.

19. Twenty people at risk of cardiovascular disease participated in a trial to assess the acute haemodynamic effects of high-flavanol cocoa. Increased plasma nitroso compounds and flow-mediated dilation of the brachial artery were recorded after ingestion, indicative of increased NO- mediated vasodilation.[495]

20. Eight people participated in a functional assay to test acute effects of cocoa on haemolysis. Single doses of cocoa preceded by a meal of bread and water were administered to participants at one-week intervals. Three doses of cocoa were tested: 0.25, 0.375, or 0.5g/kg cocoa, which equates to 15.9g, 23.8g, or 31.8g cocoa for a person weighing 10st/63.5kg. Blood was taken before consumption of cocoa, and following ingestion at intervals of one, two, four, and eight hours. Researchers noted that participants' erythrocytes showed reduced susceptibility to free-radical induced haemolysis, and the medium dosage of Cacao had more marked anti-haemolytic effects than either the low or high doses. They also claim that *unpublished* data shows the medium dosage to be more effective for *in vitro* inhibition of adrenaline- (epinephrine-) stimulated platelet activation (reducing stress-induced thrombosis); they speculate that the methylxanthines in cocoa could reduce erythrocytes' structural integrity by inhibiting phosphorylation-dependent cystoskeletal maintenance, accounting for the reduced anti-haemolytic effects observed with the higher dose.[496]

21. Ten medicated diabetic patients participated in a trial testing the effects of acute and medium-term (thirty days) consumption of flavanol-rich cocoa on brachial artery FMD. The acute dose of cocoa contained 963mg flavanols, equivalent to a large dose of 80.3g whole Cacao. There was a significant increase in FMD at two hours post-ingestion. If this dose of cocoa flavanols were administered in the form of a single dose of whole Cacao (not standardised to contain a higher level of flavanols) it would likely cause some side effects such as vomiting or headache from xanthine overdose and/or borderline hypertyraminemia, as 80g Cacao contains up to 6mg tyramine. However, a split-dosage trial was also performed in which the participants were given Cacao standardised to contain 321mg flavanols three times daily over thirty days, equivalent to a dosage of 28g whole Cacao taken three times daily, a high but feasible dose, similar to the level of consumption of Cacao by the Kuna of Panama. This thrice daily thirty-day regimen increased participants' baseline FMD by 30%, indicating a reversal of diabetic vascular dysfunction.[497]

22. Thirteen male subjects consumed 35g delipidated cocoa, equivalent to 70g whole Cacao. Blood drawn two hours post-consumption showed prolonged LDL oxidation.[498]

23. Fifteen younger people (under the age of fifty) and nineteen older people (over the age of fifty) participated in an uncontrolled short-term study to assess the effects of acute and short-term (four to six days) cocoa ingestion on haemodynamics. Acute FMD and short-term PWA (pulse wave amplitude) increased in both groups, but more markedly in the older group. L-NAME, a nitric oxide antagonist, reversed these changes.[499]

24. Forty-five healthy volunteers participated in a three-week trial, in which some participants consumed 75g dark chocolate per day, the same quantity of white chocolate, or 75g dark chocolate with added polyphenols. HDL rose in the groups consuming dark chocolate, and dark chocolate with extra polyphenols (+11.4 and +13.7%, respectively). There were no changes to serum lipid oxidation, fatty acids, or plasma inflammatory markers (F-2 isoprostanes) in any group. However, it was noted that lipid peroxidation decreased in *all three* groups, including the polyphenol-free white chocolate group. The authors speculated that the fatty acids in Cacao "may modify the fatty acid composition of LDL and make it more resistant to oxidative damage".[500]

25. Twenty-eight volunteers took part in a pilot study assessing the effects of one week's high-flavanol chocolate consumption on platelet reactivity and inflammation. The chocolate used contained a daily dose of 700mg flavanols, equivalent to 58g whole Cacao, a feasible intake. LDL decreased by 6% and HDL rose by 9%, with decreased platelet reactivity in blood drawn from the participants; notably, there was a reduction of high-sensitivity C-RP in female subjects only, indicating reduced inflammation (cf. women and perimenstrual chocolate consumption).[501]

26. Twenty-eight young male football players aged eighteen to twenty took part in a non-blinded, uncontrolled crossover trial comparing milk chocolate to white chocolate intake over one month, with a two-week crossover period. The milk chocolate dosage took the form of a daily dose of 105g of a brand-name chocolate containing a daily dose of 168mg flavanols. Several haemodynamic changes occurred in the milk chocolate group, with a mean reduction of –5mm Hg diastolic blood pressure, an average total cholesterol change of—11%, LDL cholesterol reduced by 15%, and urate levels declined by 11%. No changes in plasma epicatechin were recorded. It should be noted that these results are greater than those noted in later trials for such a low dose of flavanols, and that two of the authors work for Mars, Inc.[502]

27. Twenty-five subjects participated in a controlled twelve-week study, monitoring plasma cholesterol changes in participants ingesting either 12g sugar (sucrose) per day, or 12g sugar taken with 26g cocoa powder. Those taking cocoa with sugar had a 24% increase in plasma HDL and a 9% reduction in LDL oxidation from baseline, as compared to a 5% increase in HDL cholesterol in the sugar-only group.[503]

28. A small, five-day single-blind trial enlisted twenty-seven healthy subjects to consume cocoa containing 821mg flavanols per day, equivalent to a feasible intake of 68g whole Cacao. Subjects had marked peripheral vasodilation responses, and more rapid vasodilation following ischaemia due to nitric oxide activation.[504]

29. After six weeks on a diet supplemented with 36.9g dark chocolate and 30.95g cocoa powder every day, twenty-five healthy subjects' serum showed lower LDL oxidisability, but there were no measurable effects on urinary F2 isoprostane levels or inflammatory markers.[505]

30. Fifteen healthy participants were observed over fifteen days in a non-blinded crossover trial in which daily ingestion of 100g dark chocolate containing 500mg polyphenols (equivalent to 42g whole Cacao) was compared with a daily supplement of 90g white chocolate. The dark chocolate consumers had significantly increased insulin sensitivity, slightly decreased systolic blood pressure, and the HOMA-IR (homeostatic model assessment of insulin resistance, a standardised quantitative measure of insulin resistance and pancreatic beta-cell function based on fasting blood glucose and insulin levels) was also significantly lower after dark than white chocolate.[506]

31. Nineteen hypertensive subjects with impaired glucose tolerance took part in an uncontrolled and unblended crossover trial. All subjects ingested 100g dark chocolate containing 1008mg polyphenols [equivalent to 84g whole Cacao/day] for fifteen days, then did the same with isocaloric white chocolate (no polyphenol content). The subjects consuming dark chocolate noted increased beta-cell function and insulin sensitivity, decreased insulin resistance, decreased total and LDL cholesterol, increased FMD, and slightly decreased BP.[507]

32. Ten women took part in a crossover study comparing the acute haemodynamic effects of two varieties of 100ml cocoa drink. The first drink contained 329mg flavanols, including 61mg epicatechin, and the second drink contained 27mg total flavanols, including 6.6mg epicatechin. The higher flavanol beverage augmented O_2 saturation of haemoglobin by ×1.8 (i.e., an 80% increase) at two hours after ingestion.[508]

Overall, effects on blood pressure, cholesterol, and clotting seem to be replicable and reasonably robust, but mild. A 2007 **meta-analysis** of clinical trials assessing **cocoa's effect on blood pressure** included five eligible trials with a total of 173 subjects, a median two-week duration, and a mean BP reduction of –4.7mmHg Systolic and –2.88mmHg Diastolic pressure.[509] A more conservative 2012 meta-analysis concluded that the effect of chronic Cacao consumption on blood pressure was even less dramatic, at –1.6mm Hg Diastolic pressure.[510]

Cacao's effects on vasodilation and increasing insulin sensitivity also appear to be consistent, and, interestingly, may be more emphatic in post-ischaemic states (Trial 28) and older subjects (Trial 23). Other notable properties of Cacao in these trials are anti-haemolytic (Trial 20), anti-coagulant (Trials 7, 9, and 18), and coronary vasodilator (Trials 7 and 14). Of these, the anticoagulant effects, though mild, were acute, and replicated in three separate trials, and coronary vasodilation was observed both acutely and as a consistent effect following two weeks' dietary supplementation.

Three trials detected no cardiovascular benefit from Cacao. One was a randomised, double-blind placebo-controlled high quality trial assessing vasodilatory effects via brachial artery blood flow (Trial 2); another was testing for effects on blood pressure (Trial 12); and the third "null" trial was an open trial assessing serum fatty acid oxidation and inflammatory markers (Trial 24). The first was a well-designed trial, but it used only isolated polyphenols, not whole

Cacao—and this may be a problem, as some trials detected haemodynamic effects from Cacao independent of changes in serum oxidative status—such as Trial 14, where Cacao-induced changes in coronary blood flow were found to occur independently of changes in serum oxidation. Therefore the circulatory effects of Cacao may not be due to polyphenols alone, but to interactions with other constituents *in vivo*. The second trial assessed only normotensive subjects, and found no changes in blood pressure. But as noted above, Cacao's effects on circulation and blood chemistry may be at least partially state-dependent, and it's feasible that more hypertensive subjects could have had a stronger response. In the final trial, an open trial, it may be that the chocolate quality was poor; certainly this result conflicts with the results from other trials.

In summary, it appears that Cacao may be a vascular amphoteric, producing stronger responses in older subjects with compromised circulation, demonstrating clear vascular anti-inflammatory and endothelium-restoring effects. It is a feature of many drugs, and particularly natural products with complex chemistry, that they can induce different effects in different people (e.g., the cortisol- and adrenaline-lowering effects of Cacao being more pronounced in anxious subjects, or the greater increase in pulse wave amplitude and flow-mediated arterial dilation induced by Cacao in older subjects).

Skin

Twenty-four women participated in a randomised, double-blind, uncontrolled trial to assess the effect of Cacao flavanols on photoprotection and skin aging. There were two groups of participants, both drinking one daily cup of cocoa for twelve weeks, containing either 326mg flavanols (containing 61mg epicatechin and 20mg catechin), or 27mg flavanols (including 6.6mg epicatechin and 1.6mg catechin). UV-induced erythema was significantly reduced in the high-flavanol group only, with measurable increases in cutaneous blood flow and skin hydration and density, and reductions in transepidermal water loss, roughness, and scaling, with no perceptible change in wrinkles. Researchers concluded that overall skin appearance, skin repair, and health were improved, and "cosmetically relevant skin surface and hydration variables" were affected.[511] Thirty healthy people participated in another randomised, double-blind uncontrolled trial ingesting 20g of high or low flavanol chocolate for twelve weeks, and determined that the high-flavanol chocolate conferred "significant photoprotection", and that "ordinary chocolate had no such effect".[512] Another small crossover design study with ten female participants found that high flavanol cocoa (containing 329mg flavanols, equivalent to 27g whole Cacao) effected a significant (70%) increase in dermal blood flow two hours after ingestion.[513]

Dental

Cacao inhibits dental caries by a probable combination of two pharmacological mechanisms, polyphenolic cariostasis and xanthine-induced hardening of dental enamel, with accelerated surface recrystallisation.[514] Some compounds in Cacao, most likely the polyphenols, also inhibit the enzyme dextran sucrose, which cariogenic (cavity-causing) oral bacteria produce to help them break down sugars and acquire energy, and therefore reduce plaque formation and tooth decay.[515]

Gastrointestinal

A serving of 0.55g/kg dark chocolate (equivalent to 14–26g whole Cacao) acutely attenuated the postprandial increase in hepatic venous pressure gradient (HVPG) in patients with liver cirrhosis within thirty minutes after consumption, as compared with white chocolate, and there was a simultaneous fifteen- to fifty-fold increase in plasma flavonoids.[516] The medical implications of this are that Cacao may be incorporated in the diet of cirrhotic patients to reduce the risk of portal hypertension, which can cause severe and life-threatening complications such as damage to the kidneys and spleen, peritonitis, ruptures, and haemorrhages. Cacao could be administered in a traditional drink form (no added fat and minimal added sugar) together with carbohydrate—such as a traditional *atole* (see Chapter 8), as part of a reduced-protein, reduced-fat diet, to increase the absorption of the vasodilating and anti-inflammatory polyphenols. Although the authors correctly cite the flavonoids as the main compounds responsible for this effect, it should be noted that some NPAs (N-phenylpropanoyl l-amino acids) are known to increase hepatocyte proliferation and repair, so long-term administration of high quality Cacao may have additional benefits in attenuating progression or reducing complications of liver disease.

A small randomised double-blinded crossover study with twenty-two healthy participants found that daily intake of high-flavanol cocoa (containing 494mg flavanols, equivalent to 41g whole Cacao) over a four-week period significantly increased faecal counts of desirable gut flora (*Bifidobacterium* and *Lactobacilli*) and decreased pathogenic *Clostridium*, and decreases in plasma C-reactive protein levels were linked to enteric changes in populations of *Lactobacilli*.[517] This exemplifies secondary or indirect effects of plants or drugs, whereby systemic inflammation may be reduced as a consequence of altered intestinal microflora, and also provides another mechanism for Cacao's traditionally anti-diarrhoeal action. Cacao's effects in this regard are normally ascribed to astringent ("binding") effects of the polyphenols, and in a medical questionnaire filled in by 200 healthy people, 766 people with irritable bowel syndrome, and 122 people with chronic constipation, 48–64% of the respondents cited chocolate as a constipation-causing food, ahead of two other culprits, bananas and black tea.[518]

Respiratory

Forty-four un-medicated, pre-hypertensive, or mildly hypertensive adults aged between fifty-six and seventy-three participated in an eighteen-week double-blind randomised controlled trial with no placebo group. Participants were given daily doses of either 6.3g of dark chocolate containing 30mg polyphenols, or isocaloric white chocolate. Sustained increases of s-nitroso-glutathione (GSNO)[xv] were recorded in the plasma of the dark chocolate consumers, with no

---

[xv] Endogenous Nitric Oxide signalling mediator and precursor.

change of the oxidative stress marker 8-isoprostane. In common with the cardiovascular trial above, these results indicate improved nitric oxide formation and vasodilation.[519] As nitric oxide (NO) metabolism is involved in cardiovascular and respiratory disease, and in the development of immune tolerance following organ transplantation (see below), it is possible that Cacao intake may be supportive in these circumstances. Raised GSNO may also help in cystic fibrosis, as GSNO and NO modulate respiratory tract inflammation and bronchodilation. As tangential support for this hypothesis, maternal consumption of chocolate (dark or milk) during pregnancy was associated with a decrease in incidence of wheezing in their children up to five years of age, along with leafy vegetables, apples, and pears. Curiously, however, higher levels of fruit and berry *juice* consumption during pregnancy were positively associated with risk of allergic rhinitis in children.[520]

Musculoskeletal

A randomised controlled trial with no placebo group and 1,001 elderly female participants aged between seventy and eighty-five found that more regular chocolate consumption was associated with reduced bone density and strength. Women eating chocolate every day had 3.1% lower whole-body bone density than those consuming chocolate once a week.[521]

Urinary tract: Theobroma cacao is used to treat renal problems in Caribbean ethnomedicine; in Trinidad & Tobago the "core" (root?) is eaten for "urinary problems".[522] A study of the acute effects of dark chocolate (70% cocoa solids) ingestion on renal blood perfusion in ten healthy subjects found that the chocolate caused an increase in renal medullary oxygenation, which the authors speculated may indicate nephroprotective effects for Cacao, which would corroborate its Caribbean ethnomedical use.[523] On the other hand, ingestion of 50–100g 70% cocoa solids dark chocolate in six healthy male subjects caused greater than 200% increase in urinary oxalic acid excretion after two to four hours. The study authors pointed out that this hyperoxaluria may result in increased risk of calcium oxalate kidney stone formation with regular chocolate consumption.[524]

Reproductive and Gynae

Female: One small prospective cohort study found a reduced prevalence of pre-eclampsia and gestational hypertension among women who consumed chocolate during pregnancy: chocolate-eaters had a 45% risk reduction for pre-eclampsia in the first trimester, and a 44% risk reduction in the third trimester, with a 35% risk reduction for gestational hypertension in the first trimester only.[525] An earlier study found that women consuming chocolate five or more times every week had a 19% reduced risk of developing pre-eclampsia in the first trimester, and a 40% risk reduction in the last trimester.[526]

American women were up to ten times more likely to report peri-menstrual chocolate cravings than Spanish women, suggesting a cultural or psychological basis for peri-menstrual chocolate cravings.[527] Tangential support for this hypothesis comes from the observation that peri-menstrual chocolate cravings decreased after menopause by only 13.4%, showing that the craving is mostly non-hormonal in origin.[528] Interestingly, given the traditional use of Cacao for nursing mothers, chocolate has also been fed to cows to increase their milk supply[529]—though there is no evidence to show whether it is effective for this purpose.

Male: While erectile dysfunction (ED) is polycausal, the involvement of nitric oxide releasing parasympathetic pathways is essential for achieving erection by facilitating vasodilation and blood flow into the corpus cavernosum, and impaired endothelium-dependent vasodilatation is a major contributory factor to the pathogenesis of ED (aggravated by conditions such as diabetes, hypercholesterolaemia, and atherosclerosis). Oxytocin and vasopressin release in hypothalamic nuclei may also be involved in facilitating physiological arousal.[530] Cacao enhances endothelium-dependent vasodilation, protects vascular endothelium from oxidative or inflammatory injury, and may be helpful in the treatment, or attenuate the development, of vasculogenic ED. Dietary Cacao intake may even influence central oxytocin and vasopressin release over a period of time, or at higher levels of intake, via its content of weak MAOI compounds (affecting serotonin metabolism as measured by elevated serum levels of 5-HIAA, and thereby potentially enhancing oxytocin release), and trace amounts of anandamide and anandamide-potentiating N-acyl-ethanolamines (which inhibit the release of both neurohormones).

But animal feeding studies also found that high intakes of isolated Theobromine *or whole cocoa powder* are toxic to the testes, reducing sperm quality and causing testicular atrophy, and epidemiological evidence found a positive correlation between national per capita cocoa consumption and testicular cancer rates and hypospadias (developmental disorder in newborn males) in the same populations from eighteen to thirty-seven years later.[531] Average per capita consumption of cocoa and chocolate in eighteen different countries across five continents in the period 1965–1980 is positively correlated (p<0.001) with incidence of adult male testicular cancer in 1998–2002, the eighteen to thirty-seven year gap reflecting apparent delayed effects of chocolate exposure *in utero* and during childhood on the development of adult cancer. A similar positive correlation was found between cocoa consumption and the prevalence of male genital birth defects such as hypospadias or cryptorchidism in the period 1999–2003.[532]

These data strongly suggest that antenatal and childhood Cacao consumption may be a risk factor for development of testicular cancer later in life, and may cause DNA damage to spermatozoa in adulthood leading to next-generation infant male birth defects. Given the animal research data showing that two weeks' consumption of Cacao reduced a marker for testicular DNA damage,[533] these data may be the result of other coincidental factors (such as Cacao routinely being ingested with another food product which may be responsible for these findings in this part of the world), or that long-term Cacao consumption causes cumulative damage which overtakes an initial protective effect. But a scientific rationale for the traditional Mesoamerican taboo against children and (in some cultures) women consuming Cacao may be inferred from this data, if the correlation proves to be robust and causal.

Immune system and Cancer

A short (twenty-eight day) trial with twenty-one healthy adult participants was conducted to determine chocolate's effect on immunity. Daily intake of 75g dark chocolate was compared with 75g white chocolate, divided into three daily doses of 25g each. The researchers estimated that the dark chocolate group were consuming 877mg of polyphenols and 694mg theobromine daily as compared to none in the white chocolate group (except that found in other foods, such as polyphenols from wine or theobromine from maté tea or post-caffeine metabolism, respectively). The daily added sugar consumption was 9.75g for the dark chocolate group (13%) vs. 42.75g (57%) in the white chocolate group. Neither group noted any side effects. No statistically significant immunological differences in the dark chocolate group were noticed over the relatively short trial period, but there was a trend towards increasing levels of total leukocytes and eosinophils and reduction of TNF-α. In the white chocolate group there was a decline in monocyte levels with a statistically significant rise in IL-10 production and reduction of TNF-α.[534]

The fact that both groups' levels of TNF-α were lowered indicates a possible trend towards *reduction* of tumoricidal activity; this may be due to the added sugar intake, or simply an artefact of the experiment. Similarly the markedly different trends in both groups may also be experimental artefacts—a longer trial of several months' duration would be needed to ascertain that—but the expansion of eosinophil and leukocyte populations in the dark chocolate group suggest an immunomodulatory effect; conversely the trend towards monocyte decline and significantly increased IL-10 production in the white chocolate group suggests a more active suppression of specific immunity, possibly as a consequence of high sugar consumption (elevated IL-10 may be the causal factor for the observed trend towards monocyte decline in this group as it suppresses monocyte production).

* * *

Summary of actions

Confirmed: short-term stimulant; vascular endothelial anti-inflammatory; anti-ischaemic, vasodilatory; weak hypotensive; anti-thrombotic; increases insulin receptor sensitivity; anti-ulcerogenic; astringent; adrenaline-lowering, cortisol-reducing; anti-cariogenic; anti-tussive.

Inferred: coronary vasodilator; hedonic modifier—amplifies pleasure responses and attenuates conditioned fear (acute/short-term effect); anxiolytic (long-term effect); nootropic; weak bronchodilator; enteric microbial trophorestorative; tolerogenic; mild analgesic; nephroprotective; chemopreventive.

Indications

Based on **human clinical trials**, Cacao *is likely to be useful* as a <u>longer-term</u> complementary treatment or dietary supplement for the following applications:

Cardiovascular

- **Atherosclerosis**, as a component of **stroke and coronary heart disease prevention** strategies
- As a dietary adjunct to assist control of, and protection from adverse effects of **hypertension**
- Prophylactic use against CVD in **smokers**

- To assist **recovery following heart transplants** or **cardiovascular surgery**
- Adjunctive benefits in **diabetes**, e.g., **diabetic vasculopathies**, neuropathy, etc.

PNEI

- Subjective alleviation of **chronic fatigue syndrome** symptoms and associated anxiety and depression.

Endocrine

- To reduce **insulin resistance** and attenuate the development of **metabolic syndrome**.

Obstetric

- To reduce the risk of developing **pre-eclampsia** or **gestational hypertension**.

Gastrointestinal

- As a dietary supplement for patients with **cirrhosis** of the liver, to reduce risk of portal hypertension and organ damage.

Integumentary

- As an "internal sunscreen" to **reduce UV skin damage** and tendency to redden or burn
- As an "internal cosmetic" agent for **maintaining skin hydration and appearance** (although see contra-indication for acne, below).

Based on **human clinical trials**, short-term or acute administration of Cacao is *likely to be useful* for the following applications:

Neurological

- General **mood enhancement**
- To alleviate temporary **fatigue**, and improve cognitive function in **sleep deprivation**
- Symptomatic relief from **trigeminal neuralgia**
- To **potentiate Paracetamol's analgesic effects** (utilising the synergy between Paracetamol and Caffeine).

Cardiovascular

- To assist in **recovery from high-intensity exercise**.

Based on *in vitro* **and** *in vivo* **research** on individual phytochemicals in Cacao, whole Cacao extract, and Cacao's traditional medicinal uses, *longer-term* complementary treatment or dietary supplementation with Cacao *may be useful for* the following applications:

Neurological

- Alleviating some atypical depressive disorders such as **hysteroid dysphoria**
- **Vascular dementia,** and possibly also other forms of **dementia**, such as **Alzheimer's disease**
- To slow deterioration in progressive neurodegenerative conditions such as **ALS** (though see cautions re: Parkinson's disease, below)
- To assist with **post-ischaemic recovery in CVA ("stroke")**, including recovering neurocognitive functionality.

Cardiovascular

- To assist with **post-ischaemic recovery in CHD ("heart attack")**
- Diseases featuring reduced erythrocyte oxygen-carrying capacity, haemolysis, or coagulopathy, such as **sickle cell disease** or **thalassaemia**
- Treatment of **Reynaud's phenomenon** and **Buerger's disease**
- As a prophylactic drug or dietary supplement to **prevent or reduce angina attacks**
- **Erectile dysfunction**, where it is a consequence of atherosclerotic and/or diabetic circulatory impairment
- As a dietary supplement in **haemochromatosis** (with reference to its mineral-chelating effects in fruit flies).[535]

Endocrine

- For adjunctive benefits in **diabetes**, e.g., **diabetic vasculopathies**, neuropathy, etc.
- For **Cushing's disease**, to lower cortisol levels
- To reduce DHT formation and possibly prevent **benign prostate hypertrophy**.

Integumentary

- To slow the development and appearance of **varicose ulcers** in bed-bound or sedentary patients, or those with diabetes
- To reduce long-term skin damage from **tobacco smoking** (counteracting vasoconstrictor and pro-oxidant effects of tobacco smoke).

Dental

- Regular consumption of high cocoa content dark chocolate or *unsweetened* chocolate beverages to reduce **dental caries** ("cavities") and strengthen **weak tooth enamel**.

Gastrointestinal

- To correct **enteric dysbiosis**, resulting in diarrhoea or meteorism (bloating)
- To protect against **peptic ulceration**.

Respiratory

- To assist with symptomatic relief and retarding disease progression in **cystic fibrosis**
- To assist with **symptoms** of, and improving **long-term prognosis** in **COPD**, through mild bronchodilatory, cough suppressant, and hyaluronidase inhibitory effects, in addition to reducing cumulative lung tissue injury
- Reducing incidences of **asthma** in the offspring of pregnant women with a personal or family history of atopy.

Urinary

- To **protect the kidneys** by preserving renal blood perfusion.

Reproductive

- To help **prevent or alleviate vasculogenic erectile dysfunction**
- To help in treatment of **Peyronie's disease**.

Obstetric

- To reduce the risk of developing **gestational diabetes mellitus**
- As a **galactagogue** during breastfeeding.

Anti-neoplastic

- As a **chemopreventive** agent against **cancer** in general, and **prostate cancer** specifically
- As a dietary adjunct in **prostate cancer** or **colon cancer** (procyanidins and flavanols)
- As a dietary adjunct in **glioblastoma**, or to reduce the likelihood of an astrocytoma developing into a glioblastoma (theobromine)
- To **augment Doxorubicin cytotoxicity** (caffeine).

Miscellaneous

- To **enhance Th1 (cell-mediated specific) immunity** and suppress enteric **secretory IgA production** (conventional or *fermentado* Cacao only)
- As a dietary supplement for prophylaxis of, or recovery from ill effects of **snakebite**.

Based on *in vitro* **and** *in vivo* **research** on individual phytochemicals in Cacao, whole Cacao extract, and Cacao's traditional medicinal uses, short-term or <u>acute administration</u> of Cacao *may be useful* for the following applications, although there is currently a lack of clinical evidence:

PNEI

- As pharmacological adjunct in hypnotherapeutic or psychotherapeutic intervention strategies to treat panic syndromes associated with elevated cortisol such as **social anxiety disorder (SAD)** and **post-traumatic stress disorder (PTSD)**. Acute doses (40–60g) of Cacao have potential for use in conjunction with de-conditioning therapies as a pharmacological enhancer of conditioned stimulus extinction, to facilitate blockade of fear reconsolidation during and after fear memory retrieval or presentation of conditioned stimuli in PTSD, or recall of anxiety-provoking social contexts in SAD. (See Chapter 5 for discussion, and Appendix D for a clinical experiment.)

Cardiovascular

- As a **low-potency anti-thrombotic**, for example on long-haul flights, to **prevent DVT**
- As a vehicle for, or adjunct to the administration of other drugs for **acute angina**
- To aid **recovery from acute circulatory symptoms** such as **chilblains, intermittent claudication**, or simple **cramp**.

Respiratory

- Symptomatic relief from **cough**.

Gastrointestinal

- To treat mild **diarrhoea**
- To prevent or treat **portal hypertension** in liver disease.

Preparations and dosages

Although sugar and carbohydrates do increase the absorption of Cacao polyphenols, it has been demonstrated that the action of whole Cacao does not solely depend on the polyphenols,[536] and that simple sugars reduce pharmacological effects of the polyphenols on vascular endothelium.[537] However, consuming Cacao with milk or other proteins should be avoided, as this does reduce the flavan-3-ols' bioavailability.[538] In fact, **for maximum efficacy all internal formulations utilising Cacao should be low in sugar, in liquid form, and taken with a small amount of complex carbohydrate** (e.g., maize meal) **to maximise pharmacological potency**.[539] Suggested daily adult dosages of whole Cacao, lightly toasted/roasted and prepared as unadulterated chocolate (no added fat or sugar), are:

- <u>Longer-term supplementation</u> for cardiovascular, endocrine disorders, etc: **20g one to two times daily**, or **140–280g per week**. Lower doses for prevention/health maintenance in at-risk persons, higher end for treatment.
  - As commercial chocolate, this approximates to **25–30g dark chocolate with at least 80% cocoa content, up to three times daily**.
- <u>Acute doses</u> for rapid mood adjustment, cortisol and adrenaline reduction, or more noticeable physiological effects, for example, recovery from an angina attack, trigeminal neuralgia, or sickle cell crisis: **40–60g, followed 90–120 minutes later by a 20g supplementary dose, if required** or desired.
  - It's not recommended that commercial chocolate be used for reliable acute effects; traditionally prepared Cacao-based beverages containing the requisite dose of Cacao (see Chapter 8) are much more effective. However, if necessary a dose of **70–80g dark chocolate (minimum cocoa solids: 80%)** would approximate to this dosage, although the effect will be *considerably* weaker, and entails an unnecessary quantity of added sugar and fat.

Cautions and contraindications for use:

High-risk:

- **Allergy** to chocolate or Cacao.

Moderate risk:

- **Tyramine sensitivity**: people with known tyramine sensitivity or who are taking **some antidepressant drugs** (**MAOIs**, such as Moclobemide, Phenelzine, Isocarboxazid, or Tranylcypromine) should avoid higher doses of Cacao or dark chocolate.
- Renal calculi: patients with **calcium oxalate kidney stones** or hyperoxaluria should be wary of chocolate or Cacao products, as Cacao greatly increases renal Oxalic Acid excretion.[540]
- Due to its high copper content, high dietary Cacao or chocolate intake is contra-indicated for individuals with **Wilson's disease**.
- **Acne**, especially in adolescent males. A small four week study in men given 10g dark chocolate to eat every day found increased numbers of Gram-positive facial bacteria on all chocolate consumers.[541] However this result needs to be corroborated by other trials, and it is unclear whether this result is generalisable from chocolate to Cacao and traditional beverages with a lower content of added sugar and fat.
- **Urticaria**: due to its Histamine content, Cacao and chocolate are thought to exacerbate urticaria in some individuals.[542]
- Because Cacao appears to lower serum cortisol and adrenaline levels, it should not be used by individuals with **Addison's disease**. However, Cacao appears to be beneficial for many individuals with so-called "adrenal fatigue" or chronic fatigue syndrome, whose adrenals are functionally sound.

Low or uncertain risk:

- Male infertility: **men with low sperm counts** should avoid high daily intake of Cacao. In an animal study, cocoa powder at 5% of the daily diet caused decreased spermatogenesis and irreversible testicular atrophy due to its high theobromine content.[543]
- **Male infants and children with a family history of prostate and/or testicular cancer**: an epidemiological study indicated that high Cacao intakes during childhood were linked to mutagenic epigenetic changes in the immature reproductive system which may increase risk of testicular cancer in later life.[544]
- Similarly, pregnant or nursing mothers of male infants may wish to avoid regular consumption of chocolate, as it has also been significantly linked to **higher incidences of genital birth defects in newborn males** in the same epidemiological study.[545] However, these findings should be counterbalanced by the observed decrease in asthma incidence and apparently improved moods of infants of both sexes born to chocolate-consuming mothers in other studies.[546]
- **Post-menopausal women with low bone density**: preliminary research links regular chocolate consumption to lower bone density in this group.[547]
- **Parkinson's disease**: it is currently unclear whether chocolate is beneficial, neutral, or harmful for individuals living with Parkinson's disease. There is a statistical link between incidence of Parkinson's disease and higher chocolate consumption.[548] Recent clinical research using single doses of dark chocolate demonstrated no acute effect on movement disorder for individuals living with Parkinson's disease,[549] although no longer-term studies have yet been published. Cacao contains some substances which are neuroprotective (several polyphenolic compounds, including catechin and epicatechin, protocatechuic acid, chlorogenic acid, and quinones; and the diketopiperazines) and some substances which are neurotoxic to dopaminergic neurons (salsolinol, β-phenethylamine, tetra-hydro-β-carbolines, and copper, with copper-reducing theobromine). Therefore it would be prudent at this stage for Parkinsonian patients to avoid excessive chocolate consumption. See Chapter 7 for full discussion.

Note also that Cacao, particularly in combination with sugar, may have habituating effects in people with higher morphine-benzedrine sensitivity on the Addiction Research Center Inventory (ARCI) scales (used to assess reinforcing properties of abused drugs), who exhibit stronger preferences for dark chocolate.[550] There are currently no large-scale studies to support this speculation, although smaller epidemiological studies have established a tenuous link between chocolate intake, depression, and neuroticism.[551] Whether this link is robust, causal, or evidence of self-medication is currently unclear, and any longer-term health implications are currently speculative.

Consumers should also be aware that cocoa powder and some chocolate products may contain very high levels of lead from industrial contamination; several samples of Nigerian fermented and dried cocoa beans collected from farms following sun-drying showed very low levels, up to 0.5ng/g, but manufactured cocoa had a lead content "among the highest of all foods", up to 230ng/g, precisely 230% of the 1ng/g maximum permissible level of lead proposed by the

Codex Alimentarius Commission.[552] Although the absorption of lead from cocoa powder and chocolate appears to be very low,[553] the denuded polyphenol levels, higher acrylamide content, and reduced shelf stability of cocoa powder in addition to its higher lead content suggest that whole-bean Cacao products or low-sugar dark chocolate are far better choices than cocoa powder for those using Cacao as a health supplement or medicine.

Endnotes

1. Coe & Coe, 1996 [Book]; Colombo, Pinorini-Godly, & Conti, in Paoletti *et al.*, 2012 [Book].
2. Beckett, 2000 [Book].
3. Young, 1994 [Book].
4. McNeil, in McNeil, 2006a [Book].
5. Young, 1994 [Book].
6. Beckett, 2000 [Book].
7. Young, 1994 [Book].
8. Colombo, Pinorini-Godly, & Conti, in Paoletti *et al.*, 2012 [Book].
9. De Schawe *et al.*, 2018 [Journal].
10. Young & Severson, 1994 [Journal].
11. Young, 1994 [Book].
12. Wilson & Hurst, 2012 [Book].
13. Wilson, in Paoletti *et al.*, 2012 [Book].
14. Dreiss & Greenhill, 2008 [Book]; Wilson, in Paoletti *et al.*, 2012 [Book].
15. Grivetti, in Grivetti & Shapiro, 2009 [Book].
16. *Ibid.*
17. 4th February 2011, interview with Doña Juana Ca'al, Rex'hua, Alta Verapaz, Guatemala; also taken from field notes in conversation with Señora Aurelia Pop, Lanquin, Peten, Guatemala, in 2011.
18. Eggleston & White, in Watson, Preedy, & Zibadi, 2013 [Book].
19. Field notes in conversation with Doña Juana Ca'al, Rex'hua, Alta Verapaz, Guatemala, in 2011.
20. Field notes in conversation with Señor Juan Gomez, a Cacao worker in San Antonio Suchitquepez, Guatemala, 2011.
21. Field notes, Curandero Diego in San Antonio Suchitequepez, Guatemala, 2011; Grivetti, in Grivetti & Shapiro, 2009 [Book].
22. Grivetti, in Grivetti & Shapiro, 2009 [Book].
23. Bletter & Daly, in McNeil, 2006 [Book].
24. Noriega & González, in Grivetti & Shapiro, 2009 [Book].
25. Bletter & Daly, in McNeil, 2006 [Book]; Field notes, Curandero Diego in San Antonio Suchitequepez, Guatemala, 2011; 3 February 2011: Interview with Don Antonio Xoc, Ya'al Pemech, Alta Verapaz, Guatemala.
26. Field notes, Curandero Santiago A'echis of Lanquin in Peten, Guatemala, 2011; Grivetti, in Grivetti & Shapiro, 2009 [Book].
27. Falade *et al.*, 2005 [Journal].

28. 2018, http://powo.science.kew.org [Internet].

29. Young, 1994 [Book].

30. 2018, http://eol.org [Internet].

31. Beckett, 2000 [Book].

32. *Ibid.*

33. Values extrapolated from Zoumas, Kreiser, & Martin, 1980 [Journal].

34. Values taken from Dr Duke's Phytochemical and Ethnobotanical Database, http://ars-grin.gov/cgi-bin/duke/farmacy2.pl [Accessed 15 June 2012].

35. Values extrapolated from Zoumas, Kreiser, & Martin, 1980 [Journal].

36. THIQ alkaloids are "formed in the plant from two phenylethylamine units and a C9 terpenoid precursor": Evans, 2002 [Book].

37. Melzig *et al.*, 2000 [Journal].

38. Values extrapolated from approximate quantity of 1.4mg/kg Alkyl Pyrazines in Mexican Cacao, at a ratio of 1.5:2.5 for Tetramethypyrazine: Trimethylpyrazine in Cacao at normal roast levels. From Ziegleder, in Beckett, 2009 [Book].

39. Extrapolated from Herraiz, 2000 [Journal]. Only processed chocolate was tested (dark, milk, cocoa, & cocoa-containing cereals), so the given lower limit per 40g Cacao reflects the lower limit Herraiz found in processed chocolate, whereas the upper limit reflects his upper limit values multiplied by two to obtain something closer to the upper limit of what may be found in pure unadulterated Cacao. Even multiplying by two may give low values, given that most dark chocolate on the market is only 60–70% Cacao solids, of which perhaps 20–30% is added cocoa butter.

40. Airaksinen & Kari, 1981 [Journal].

41. 6-Hydroxy-1-methyl-1,2,3,4-tetrahydro-β-carboline.

42. 1,2,3,4-tetrahydro-β-carboline-3-carboxylic acid.

43. 1S,3S-1-methyl-1,2,3,4-tetrahydro-β-carboline-3-carboxylic acid.

44. 1R,3S-1-methyl-1,2,3,4-tetrahydro-β-carboline-3-carboxylic acid.

45. 1-methyl-1,2,3,4-tetrahydro-β-carboline.

46. Khan & Nicod, in Paoletti *et al.*, 2012 [Book].

47. I was unable to find a precise quantification for Trigonelline in Cacao seeds. The given value is highly speculative, as it is extrapolated from the wide $nmol/g^{-1}$ range given by Khan & Nicod (see previous endnote) for trigonelline in the fresh juice of leaves and fruits of *Theobroma cacao* specimens of undetermined age and provenance. Trigonelline is also denatured by roasting, so its level in traditional roasted Cacao bean-based beverages is likely to be very variable, but higher than in commercially available, factory-processed chocolate.

48. Bodor & Farag, 1983 [Journal].

49. Wollgast, 2004 [Journal].

50. Kosman *et al.*, 2007 [Journal].

51. Gu *et al.*, 2006 [Journal]: Procyanidins = 40.8mg/g in non-alkalised cocoa powders, i.e., defatted, roasted cocoa beans.

52. *Ibid.*

53. Wollgast, 2004 [Journal].

54. Procyanidin dimer refs from http://phenol-explorer.eu/reports/43 [Accessed 22 August 2012]; from cocoa powder.

55. Wollgast, 2004 [Journal].
56. Gu *et al.*, 2006 [Journal].
57. EG, EGC, & EGCG refs extrapolated from http://phenol-explorer.eu/reports/43 [Accessed 22 August 2012]; taken from dark chocolate, all values multiplied by 1.5 to reflect differences between factory processed eating chocolate & basic toasted beans.
58. Redovniković *et al.*, 2009 [Journal]; Elwers *et al.*, 2009 [Journal].
59. Koli *et al.*, 2010 [Koli].
60. Watson, Preedy, & Zibadi, 2012 [Book].
61. Phenolic acids values also extrapolated from http://phenol-explorer.eu/reports/43 [Accessed 22 August 2012]; taken from dark chocolate, all values multiplied by 1.5, as above.
62. Arlorio *et al.*, 2007 [Journal].
63. Values extrapolated from http://phenol-explorer.eu/reports/43 [Accessed 22 August 2012]; the website states 30mg clovamide/100g cocoa liquor; although this seems absurdly high given other estimates of N-phenylpropanoid contents. One analysis [Wollgast, 2004] quantifies Cacao NPAs between 20–24% of total polyphenol content.
64. Fallarini *et al.*, 2009 [Journal].
65. Park and Schoene, 2006 [Journal].
66. Extrapolated from Hurst *et al.*, 2008 [Journal]. Values detected in cocoa powder; higher level of the range in 40g Cacao = double the lower, to approximate the effects of processing (high temperature roasting, hydraulic pressing, and alkalisation) on the antioxidant content of the beans.
67. Kosman *et al.*, 2007 [Journal].
68. Sakagami *et al.*, 2008 [Journal].
69. Parsons, Keeney, & Patton, 1969 [Journal].
70. Embi *et al.*, 2012 [Journal].
71. Aremu & Abara, 1992 [Journal].
72. Voigt, Kamaruddin, & Wazir, 1993 [Journal].
73. *Ibid.*
74. Bertazzo *et al.*, in Watson, Preedy, & Zibadi, 2013 [Book].
75. Marseglia, Palla, & Caligiani, 2014 [Journal].
76. Di Tomaso, Beltramo, & Piomelli, 1996 [Journal]: values obtained from samples of cocoa powder and chocolate following solvent extraction and three different kinds of chromatography (column, gas + mass spectrometry, & HPLC).
77. Beltramo & Piomelli, 1998 [Journal].
78. Di Tomaso, Beltramo, & Piomelli, 1996 [Journal].
79. Shulgin & Shulgin, 1991 [Book].
80. Values extrapolated from Kosman *et al.*, 2007 [Journal] ("grated cocoa" [sic] used); and Bertazzo *et al.*, in Watson, Preedy, & Zibadi, 2013 [Book].
81. *These values from Pastore *et al.*, 2005 [Journal]. Likely to be lower than actually found in Cacao as processed chocolate was used.
82. Bonvehi & Coll, 2000 [Journal].
83. Borthwick & Da Costa, 2015 [Journal].
84. *Ibid.*
85. *Ibid.*

86. *Ibid.*
87. *Ibid.*
88. Fuhr *et al.*, 2006 [Journal].
89. List taken from Ziegleder, in Beckett, 2009 [Book].
90. *Ibid.*
91. Values extrapolated from approximate quantity of 1.4mg/kg Alkyl Pyrazines in Mexican Cacao, at a ratio of 1.5:2.5 for Tetramethypyrazine: Trimethylpyrazine in Cacao at normal roast levels. From Ziegleder, in Beckett, 2009 [Book].
92. Odour descriptions from http://leffingwell.com/pyrazine.htm [Accessed 2 September 2012].
93. % values for minerals from Aikpokpodion & Dongo, 2010 [Journal]—using Ghanaian Cacao beans; ppm values from Dr Duke's Phytochemical & Ethnobotanical Database online, http://ars-grin.gov/duke/
94. From nutritiondata.self.com/facts/sweets/5471/2 [Accessed 28 June 2013]. Based on 86g unsweetened cocoa powder, estimated to correspond with 100g whole Cacao bean.
95. Smit, in Fredholm, 2011 [Book]—based on upper limit of value for dark chocolate; may be slightly higher in pure bean beverages.
96. Adequate Intake data for Choline from the Linus Pauling institute, http://lpi.oregonstate.edu/infocenter/othernuts/choline/ [Accessed 26 July 2013].
97. Ott, 1985 [Book].
98. Smit, 2011 [Book].
99. *Ibid.*
100. Baggot *et al.*, 2013 [Journal].
101. Sugimoto *et al.*, 2014 [Journal].
102. Smit, 2011 [Book].
103. Smit, 2011 [Book]; Giannandrea, 2009 [Journal].
104. Slattery & West, 1993 [Journal].
105. Smit, 2011 [Book].
106. Briggs, 2008 [Book].
107. Yu *et al.*, 1991 [Journal].
108. Barnes, 2013 [Journal].
109. Dubuis *et al.*, 2014 [Journal].
110. Barnes, 2013 [Journal].
111. Karakeci *et al.*, 2013 [Journal].
112. Eskandari, Bastan, & Peachell, 2013 [Journal].
113. Grassin-Delyle *et al.*, 2013 [Journal].
114. Ogawa *et al.*, 2013 [Journal].
115. Motegi *et al.*, 2013 [Journal].
116. Fredholm *et al.*, 1999 [Journal].
117. *Ibid.*
118. Grome & Stefanovich, 1986 [Journal].
119. Spinella, 2001 [Book].
120. *Ibid.*
121. Smit & Blackburn, 2005 [Journal].

122. Fredholm *et al.*, 1999 [Journal].
123. Quinlan, Lane & Aspinall, 1997 [Journal].
124. *Ibid.*
125. Lelo *et al.*, 1986 [Journal].
126. Ebadi *et al.*, 2005 [Journal].
127. Polache and Granero, 2013 [Journal].
128. Xie, Krnjević, & Ye, 2013 [Journal].
129. Smit, 2011 [Book].
130. Hipólito *et al.*, 2010 [Journal].
131. Mravec, 2006 [Journal].
132. Xie, Krnjević, & Ye, 2013 [Journal].
133. Airaksinen *et al.*, 1984 [Journal].
134. *Ibid.*
135. Naoi, Muruyama, & Nagi, 2004 [Journal].
136. Mravec, 2006 [Journal].
137. 2016, https://pubchem.ncbi.nlm.nih.gov/compound/Salsolinol [Internet].
138. Stammel *et al.*, 1991 [Journal].
139. Carr & Lovering, 2000 [Journal].
140. Mravec, 2006 [Journal].
141. Hashizume *et al.*, 2009 [Journal].
142. Carlson *et al.*, 1985 [Journal].
143. Misztal *et al.*, 2010 [Journal].
144. Dharmananda, 2012 [Internet].
145. Fan *et al.*, 2006 [Journal]; Kao *et al.*, 2006 [Journal].
146. Zhang, Deng, & Zhou, 2011 [Journal].
147. Pang, Shan, & Chiu, 1996 [Journal].
148. Farah, Zaibunnisa, & Misnawi, 2012 [Journal].
149. Jati *et al.*, 2004 [Journal].
150. Herraiz & Galisteo, 2003 [Journal].
151. Quertemont & Didone, 2013 [Journal].
152. Airaksinen & Kari, 1981 [Journal].
153. Cao *et al.*, 2007 [Journal].
154. Tice, 1997 [Internet].
155. *Ibid.*
156. *Ibid.*
157. Hossain *et al.*, 2003 [Journal]; Tohda *et al.*, 1999 [Journal]; Tohda, Kuboyama, & Komatsu, 2005 [Journal].
158. Fung *et al.*, 1988 [Journal].
159. Bodor & Farag, 1983 [Journal].
160. Beckett, 2000 [Book].
161. Mattson & Wan, 2005 [Journal]; Tapia, 2006 [Journal].
162. Bjelakovic *et al.*, 2004 [Journal]; Miller *et al.*, 2005 [Journal].
163. Loffredo & Violi, in Paoletti *et al.*, 2012 [Book].

164. Sudano *et al.*, in Paoletti *et al.*, 2012 [Book].
165. Elwers *et al.*, 2009 [Journal].
166. Davrieux *et al.*, 2005 [Internet].
167. Radojcic *et al.*, 2009 [Journal].
168. Min *et al.*, 2013 [Journal].
169. Wollgast, 2004 [Journal].
170. Jourdain *et al.*, 2006 [Journal].
171. Sanbongi, Suzuki, & Sakane, 1997 [Journal].
172. Kenny *et al.*, 2007 [Journal].
173. Lee *et al.*, 2006 [Journal].
174. Bisson *et al.*, 2008 [Journal].
175. Bisson *et al.*, 2008 & 2007 [Journals].
176. Lee *et al.*, 2006 [Journal].
177. Yamagishi *et al.*, 2003 & 2002 [Journals].
178. Farhat *et al.*, 2014 [Journal].
179. Schuier *et al.*, 2005 [Journal].
180. Bisson *et al.*, 2008 [Journal].
181. Akita *et al.*, 2008 [Journal].
182. Osakabe *et al.*, 1998 [Journal].
183. Yasuda *et al.*, 2008 [Journal].
184. Bingham, McNeil, & Cummings, 1981 [Journal].
185. Murphy *et al.*, 2003 [Journal].
186. Zumbé, 1998 [Journal].
187. Miller *et al.*, 2008 [Journal]; Wollgast, 2004 [Journal].
188. Lee *et al.*, 2003 [Journal].
189. Wollgast, 2004 [Journal].
190. Knaup *et al.*, 2009 [Journal].
191. de Oliveira, Santos, & Côni, 1975 [Journal].
192. Wollgast, 2004 [Journal].
193. *Ibid.*
194. Cimini *et al.*, 2013 [Journal].
195. Sokolov *et al.*, 2013 [Journal]; Mastroiacovo *et al.*, 2014 [Journal].
196. *Ibid.*
197. Pase *et al.*, 2013 [Journal].
198. Mastroiacovo *et al.*, 2014 [Journal].
199. Galli, in Paoletti *et al.*, 2012 [Book].
200. Matsumura *et al.*, 2014 [Journal].
201. Martin *et al.*, 2009 [Journal]; Rusconi *et al.*, in Paoletti *et al.*, 2012 [Book].
202. Cho *et al.*, 2008 [Journal].
203. Kang *et al.*, 2008 [Journal].
204. Kenny *et al.*, 2004 [Journal].
205. Mao *et al.*, 2003 [Journal].
206. Verstraeten *et al.*, 2004 [Journal].

207. Carnésecchi *et al.*, 2002 [Journal].
208. Wollgast, 2004 [Journal].
209. Wahby *et al.*, 2012 [Journal]; Kemparaju *et al.*, 2006 [Journal].
210. Tomas-Barberan *et al.*, 2007 [Journal].
211. Rios *et al.*, 2003 [Journal].
212. Rios *et al.*, 2002 [Journal].
213. Serra *et al.*, 2013 [Journal].
214. Zhu *et al.*, 2003 [Journal].
215. Spencer *et al.*, 2001 [Journal].
216. Sies *et al.*, 2005 [Journal].
217. Mao *et al.*, 2002 [Journal].
218. Kenny *et al.*, 2007 [Journal].
219. Heptinstall *et al.*, 2006 [Journal].
220. *Ibid.*
221. Heo & Lee, 2005 [Journal]; Ramiro-Puig *et al.*, 2009 [Journal].
222. Vauzour *et al.*, 2008 [Journal].
223. Panneerselvam *et al.*, 2010 [Journal].
224. Visioli *et al.*, in Paoletti *et al.*, 2012 [Book].
225. Zhu *et al.*, 2005 [Journal].
226. *Ibid.*
227. Khan & Nicod, in Paoletti *et al.*, 2012 [Book].
228. Wang *et al.*, 2000 [Journal].
229. Mullen *et al.*, 2009 [Journal].
230. Roura *et al.*, 2008 & 2007 [Journals].
231. *Ibid.*
232. Schramm *et al.*, 2003 [Journal].
233. Record *et al.*, 2003 [Journal].
234. Roura *et al.*, 2005 [Journal].
235. Rein *et al.*, 2000 [Journal].
236. Rios *et al.*, 2003 & 2002 [Journals].
237. Holt *et al.*, 2002 [Journal].
238. Redovniković *et al.*, 2009 [Journal]; Elwers *et al.*, 2009 [Journal].
239. Koli *et al.*, 2010 [Journal].
240. Pang *et al.*, 2016 [Journal]; Migliori *et al.*, 2015 [Journal]; Huang *et al.*, 2013 [Journal].
241. Li *et al.*, 2015 [Journal]; Mansour & Tawfik, 2012 [Journal]; Jayanthi & Subash, 2010 [Journal]; Oktar *et al.*, 2010 [Journal]; Coban *et al.*, 2010 [Journal]; Kart *et al.*, 2010 [Journal]; Pari & Karthikesan, 2007 [Journal].
242. 2013, http://en.wikipedia.org/wiki/Gallic_acid [Internet]
243. Yoon *et al.*, 2012 [Journal].
244. Kumar *et al.*, 2013 [Journal].
245. Ho *et al.*, 2013 [Journal].
246. Kanbak *et al.*, 2012 [Journal].
247. Nabavi *et al.*, 2013 [Journal].

248. Masella *et al.*, 2012 [Journal].
249. Guan *et al.*, 2011 [Journal]; Xue *et al.*, 2011 [Journal].
250. Kim *et al.*, 2012 [Journal].
251. Scazzocchio *et al.*, 2011 [Journal].
252. Wang *et al.*, 2012 [Journal].
253. Ciftci *et al.*, 2012 [Journal].
254. Tsai & Yin, 2012 [Journal].
255. Lende *et al.*, 2011 [Journal].
256. Masella *et al.*, 2012 [Journal].
257. Chen *et al.*, 2012 [Journal].
258. Fallarini *et al.*, 2009 [Journal].
259. Bardelli *et al.*, 2011 [Journal].
260. Park, 2007 & 2005 [Journals].
261. Stark *et al.*, 2008 [Journal].
262. Arlorio *et al.*, 2007 [Journal].
263. Stark *et al.*, 2008 [Journal].
264. Hensel *et al.*, 2007 [Journal].
265. Cinkilic *et al.*, 2013 [Journal].
266. Burgos-Moron *et al.*, 2012 [Journal].
267. Oboh *et al.*, 2013 [Journal].
268. Teraoka *et al.*, 2012 [Journal].
269. Cho *et al.*, 2012 [Journal].
270. Bagdas *et al.*, 2012 [Journal]; Shi *et al.*, 2013 [Journal]; & Shimoyama *et al.*, 2013 [Journal].
271. Mubarak *et al.*, 2012 [Journal].
272. Bertazzo *et al.*, in Watson, Preedy, & Zibadi, 2013 [Book].
273. Shimoyama *et al.*, 2013 [Journal].
274. Hurst *et al.*, 2008 [Journal].
275. Gambini *et al.*, 2013 [Journal]; Bode *et al.*, 2013 [Journal].
276. Gomez-Zorita *et al.*, 2013 [Journal].
277. Espinoza *et al.*, 2012 [Journal].
278. Quoc Trung *et al.*, 2013 [Journal].
279. Lucas & Kolodziej, 2013 [Journal]; Sueishi & Hori, 2012 [Journal].
280. Liu *et al.*, 2013 [Journal].
281. Zhang, Zhou, & Zhou, 2013 [Journal].
282. Wu & Liu, 2012 [Journal].
283. Sheth *et al.*, 2012 [Journal], Li *et al.*, 2013 [Journal].
284. Liu, Li, & Yang, 2012 [Journal].
285. Yuan *et al.*, 2013 [Journal].
286. Zhang *et al.*, 2012 [Journal].
287. Bobermin *et al.*, 2012 [Journal].
288. Liu *et al.*, 2013 [Journal].
289. Shen *et al.*, 2012 [Journal].
290. Bollheimer *et al.*, 2012 [Journal].

291. Colombo, Pinorini-Godly, & Conti, in Paoletti *et al.*, 2012 [Book].
292. Yu *et al.*, 2012 [Journal].
293. Tome-Carneiro *et al.*, 2013 [Journal].
294. Poulsen *et al.*, 2013 [Journal].
295. Nakano *et al.*, 2012 [Journal].
296. Sakagami *et al.*, 2008 [Journal]; Sakagami *et al.*, 2011 [Journal].
297. Beckett, 2000 [Book].
298. *Ibid.*
299. 2019, https://en.wikipedia.org/wiki/Palmitic_acid [Internet]; Lee *et al.*, 2009 [Journal].
300. Yamashita *et al.*, 2000 [Journal].
301. Hardy, Langelier, & Prentki, 2000 [Journal].
302. Clandinin *et al.*, 2000 [Journal].
303. 2019, https://en.wikipedia.org/wiki/Stearic_acid [Internet].
304. Warnotte *et al.*, 1999 [Journal]; Ayvaz *et al.*, 2002 [Journal]; Itoh *et al.*, 2003 [Journal].
305. Ulloth *et al.*, 2003 [Journal]; Wang *et al.*, 2007 [Journal]; Edmond, 2001 [Journal].
306. Sylvester, Ip, & Briski, 1993 [Journal].
307. Yu *et al.*, 2001 [Journal]; Tholstrup, 2005 [Journal].
308. Khalil *et al.*, 2000 [Journal].
309. Bletter & Daily, in Mc.Neil, 2006 [Book].
310. 2019, https://en.wikipedia.org/wiki/Oleic_acid [Internet]; 2012, https://pubchem.ncbi.nlm.nih.gov/compound/445639 [Internet].
311. 2012, https://pubchem.ncbi.nlm.nih.gov/compound/445639 [Internet].
312. Hardy, Langelier, & Prentki, 2000 [Journal].
313. 2012, https://pubchem.ncbi.nlm.nih.gov/compound/445639 [Internet].
314. *Ibid.*
315. Yu *et al.*, 2001 [Journal]; Tholstrup, 2005 [Journal].
316. Kabara *et al.*, 1972 [Journal].
317. Merchant *et al.*, 2005 [Journal].
318. Sasaki *et al.*, 2006 [Journal]; Rose, 1997 [Journal]; Sakaguchi *et al.*, 1984 [Journal].
319. 2012, https://pubchem.ncbi.nlm.nih.gov/compound/445639 [Internet].
320. Vinceti *et al.*, 2003 [Journal].
321. Buydens-Branchey *et al.*, 2003 [Journal].
322. Song *et al.*, 2006 [Journal].
323. Iso *et al.*, 2002 [Journal].
324. Herrera, Arrevalo-Herrera, & Herrera, 1998 [Journal].
325. Barabino *et al.*, 2003 [Journal].
326. 2012, https://en.wikipedia.org/wiki/Phytosterol [Internet]; Ling & Jones, 1995.
327. Ling & Jones, 1995 [Journal].
328. 2012, https://en.wikipedia.org/wiki/Stigmasterol & https://en.wikipedia.org/wiki/Camp-esterol [Internet].
329. 2016, https://pubchem.ncbi.nlm.nih.gov/compound/5280794#section=Depositor-Supplied-Synonyms [Internet].
330. Awad *et al.*, 2003 & 1996 [Journals]; Bouic *et al.*, 1999 [Journal].

331. Berges *et al.*, 1995 [Journal].
332. Jourdain *et al.*, 2006 [Journal].
333. 2014, https://pubchem.ncbi.nlm.nih.gov/compound/160497 [Internet].
334. *Ibid.*
335. Singh *et al.*, 2012 [Journal].
336. Murugan *et al.*, 2009 [Journal].
337. Bertazzo *et al.*, in Watson, Preedy, & Zibadi, 2013 [Book].
338. Johnston & Gaas, 2006 [Journal].
339. Embi *et al.*, 2012 [Journal].
340. Farah *et al.*, 2012 [Journal].
341. Morris, 2012 [Journal].
342. Greger & Powers, 1992 [Journal]; Sheftel, 2000 [Book].
343. Voigt, Kamaruddin, & Wazir, 1993 [Journal].
344. Preza *et al.*, 2010 [Journal].
345. Abecia-Soria *et al.*, 2006 [Journal].
346. 2015, http://dietgrail.com/glutamic-acid/ [Internet].
347. 2015, http://wtb.tue.nl/woc/ptc/vanesch/pku/phenylalanine.html [Internet].
348. 2013, http://urticaria.thunderworksinc.com/pages/lowHistamine.htm [Internet].
349. Di Tomaso, Beltramo, & Piomelli, 1996 [Journal]: values obtained from samples of cocoa powder and chocolate following solvent extraction and three different kinds of chromatography (column, gas + mass spectrometry, & HPLC).
350. 2012, lipidlibrary.aocs.org [Internet].
351. De Laurentiis *et al.*, 2010 [Journal]; Luce *et al.*, 2014 [Journal].
352. Tessier *et al.*, 2003 [Journal].
353. di Tomaso, Beltramo, & Piomelli, 1996 [Journal].
354. Rondanelli *et al.*, 2009 [Journal].
355. Beltramo & Piomelli, 1998 [Journal].
356. *Ibid.*
357. Bertazzo *et al.*, in Watson, Preedy, & Zibadi, 2013 [Book]; Ziegleder *et al.*, 1992 [Journal].
358. Rusconi *et al.*, from Paoletti *et al.*, 2012 [Book].
359. Fuxe, Grobecker, & Jonsson, 1967 [Journal].
360. Berry, 2004 [Journal].
361. Broadley *et al.*, 2009 [Journal].
362. Shulgin & Shulgin, 2013 [Book].
363. Ott, 1996 [Book].
364. Sabelli *et al.*, 1978 [Journal].
365. Sabelli *et al.*, 1996 [Journal].
366. Paetsch & Greenshaw, 1993 [Journal].
367. Scott, Moffet, & Swash, 1977 [Journal].
368. 2012, https://en.wikipedia.org/wiki/Tyramine [Internet].
369. Zucchi *et al.*, 2006 [Journal].
370. Vickerstoff, 1998 [Book].
371. Jutel *et al.*, 2001 [Journal].

372. Borthwick *et al.*, 2012 [Journal].

373. Borthwick: personal correspondence, August 2012.

374. Cornacchia *et al.*, 2012 [Journal].

375. Cornacchia *et al.*, 2012 [Journal]; Borthwick & Da Costa, 2017 [Journal].

376. Stark & Hoffmann, 2005 [Journal].

377. Hoenicke & Gatermann, 2005 [Journal].

378. European Food Standards Agency, 2012 [Internet].

379. Hogervorst *et al.*, 2007 [Journal].

380. Farah, Zaibunissah, & Misnawi, 2012 [Journal].

381. Fuhr *et al.*, 2006 [Journal].

382. Borawska, in Sikorski, 2006 [Book].

383. Colombo, Pinorini-Godly, & Conti, in Paoletti *et al.*, 2012 [Book].

384. *Ibid.*

385. Hardwick *et al.*, 1991 [Journal].

386. Spencer *et al.*, 1994 [Journal].

387. Golf, Bender, & Grüttner, 1998 [Journal].

388. *Ibid.*

389. Forsleff *et al.*, 1999 [Journal].

390. Storey & Greger, 1987 [Journal].

391. Troost *et al.*, 2003 [Journal].

392. Kako, Kobayashi, & Yokogoshi, 2011 [Journal].

393. Bossard & Klinman, 1986 [Journal].

394. Indamar, Masurekar, & Bennett, 2010 [Journal].

395. Kyung & Fleming, 1997 [Journal].

396. Zavala-Sanchez *et al.*, 2002 [Journal]; Sakuma *et al.*, 1997 [Journal].

397. Tachibana & Yonei, 1985 [Journal]; Brossmer & Patscheke, 1975 [Journal].

398. Kaneko *et al.*, 1987 [Journal]; Kaneko, Kaji, & Matsuo, 1988 [Journal].

399. Nukamura *et al.*, 1999 [Journal].

400. Narasimhan *et al.*, 2004 [Journal].

401. Matsumoto, Adachi, & Suzuki, 2005 [Journal].

402. Reddy *et al.*, 2009 [Journal].

403. Young & Severson, 1994 [Journal].

404. 2018, https://pubchem.ncbi.nlm.nih.gov/compound/Pentadecane#section=Top & https://pubchem.ncbi.nlm.nih.gov/compound/25913#section=Top [Internet].

405. *Ibid.*

406. Young, 1994 [Book].

407. De Schawe *et al.*, 2018 [Journal].

408. Falade *et al.*, 2005 [Journal].

409. Wang *et al.*, 2014.

410. Becker *et al.*, 2013.

411. Loffredo & Violi, in Paoletti *et al.* (2012) [Book].

412. *Ibid.*

413. Wang *et al.*, 2014 [Journal].

414. Ohno *et al.*, 2009 [Journal].
415. Ramiro *et al.*, 2005 [Journal.
416. Moura-da-Silva *et al.*, 1996 [Journal].
417. Ramiro *et al.*, 2005 [Journal].
418. Carnesecchi *et al.*, 2002 [Journal].
419. Jenny *et al.*, 2009 [Journal].
420. Castell, Pérez-Cano, & Bisson, in Wasson *et al.*, 2013 [Book].
421. Becker *et al.*, 2013 [Journal].
422. Park *et al.*, 1979 [Journal].
423. Farhat *et al.*, 2014 [Journal].
424. DiFeliceantonio *et al.*, 2012 [Journal].
425. Abbey *et al.*, 2008 [Journal].
426. Yamada *et al.*, 2009 [Journal].
427. Graeff, Netto, & Zangrossi, 1998 [Journal].
428. Jalil *et al.*, 2008 [Journal].
429. Ruzaidi *et al.*, 2005 [Journal].
430. Ding *et al.*, 2006 [Journal].
431. Farhat *et al.*, 2014 [Journal].
432. Orozco *et al.*, 2003 [Journal].
433. Ramiro-Puig *et al.*, 2008 [Journal].
434. Ramiro-Puig & Castell, 2009; Pérez-Berezo *et al.*, 2009 [Journals].
435. Camps-Bossacoma *et al.*, 2017 [Journal].
436. Abri-Gil *et al.*, 2016 [Journal].
437. Amin, Koh, & Asmah, 2004 [Journal].
438. Castell, Pérez-Cano, & Bisson, in Wasson *et al.*, 2013 [Book].
439. Orozco *et al.*, 2003 [Journal].
440. Valavanidis, Vlachogianni, & Fiotakis, 2009 [Journal].
441. Giannandrea, 2009 [Journal].
442. Tomofuji *et al.*, 2009 [Journal].
443. Bahadorani & Hilliker, 2008 [Journal].
444. *Ibid.*
445. Grassi *et al.*, 2008 [Journal].
446. Allgrove *et al.*, 2011 [Journal].
447. Almoosawi *et al.*, 2010 [Journal].
448. Zhu *et al.*, 2005 [Journal].
449. Wirtz *et al.*, 2014 [Journal].
450. Martin *et al.*, 2009 [Journal].
451. Francis *et al.*, 2006 [Journal].
452. Visioli *et al.*, in Paoletti *et al.*, 2012 [Book].
453. Drake *et al.*, 2007 [Journal].
454. Massee *et al.*, 2015 [Journal].
455. Crichton, Elias, & Alkerwi, 2016 [Journal].
456. Moreira *et al.*, 2016 [Journal].

457. Grassi *et al.*, 2016 [Journal].
458. Castell, Pérez-Cano, & Bisson, in Watson *et al.*, 2013 [Book].
459. Meier, Noll, & Olokwu, 2017 [Journal].
460. Scholey & Owen, 2013 [Journal].
461. Rose, Koperski, & Golomb, 2010 [Journal].
462. Schuman, Gitlin, & Fairbanks, 1987 [Journal].
463. Brotchie & Parker, in Paoletti *et al.*, 2012 [Book].
464. Castell, Pérez-Cano, & Bisson, in Watson *et al.*, 2013 [Book].
465. Rusconi *et al.*, in Paoletti *et al.*, 2012 [Book].
466. Sathyapalan *et al.*, 2010 [Journal].
467. Chatzitoffis *et al.*, 2013 [Journal].
468. Maestripieri *et al.*, 2009 [Journal].
469. Felitti *et al.*, 1998 [Journal].
470. Ghazizadeh, Ambroggi, & Fields, 2014 [Internet]; Van Elzakker *et al.*, 2014 [Journal].
471. Eggleston & White, in Watson *et al.*, 2013 [Book].
472. *Ibid.*
473. *Ibid.*
474. Loffredo & Violi, in Paoletti *et al.*, 2012 [Book].
475. Wollgast, 2004 [Journal].
476. Baba *et al.*, 2007 [Journal].
477. Farouque *et al.*, 2006 [Journal].
478. Engler *et al.*, 2004 [Journal].
479. Muniyappa *et al.*, 2008 [Journal].
480. Faridi *et al.*, 2008 [Journal].
481. Taubert *et al.*, 2007 [Journal].
482. Flammer *et al.*, 2007 [Journal].
483. Wiswedel *et al.*, 2004 [Journal].
484. Schramm *et al.*, 2001 [Journal].
485. Wang-Polagruto *et al.*, 2006 [Journal].
486. Heiss *et al.*, 2005 [Journal].
487. Ried, Frank, & Stocks, 2009 [Journal].
488. Fisher *et al.*, 2003 [Journal].
489. Shiina *et al.*, 2009 [Journal].
490. Schnorr *et al.*, 2008 [Journal].
491. Monagas *et al.*, 2009 [Journal].
492. Wan *et al.*, 2001 [Journal].
493. Rein *et al.*, 2000 [Journal].
494. Pearson *et al.*, 2002, quoted in Wollgast, 2004 [Thesis].
495. Sies *et al.*, 2005 [Journal].
496. Zhu *et al.*, 2005 [Journal].
497. Balzer *et al.*, 2009 [Journal].
498. Hirano *et al.*, 2000 [Journal].
499. Fisher & Hollenberg, 2006 [Journal].

500. Mursu *et al.*, 2004 [Journal].
501. Hamed *et al.*, 2008 [Journal].
502. Fraga *et al.*, 2005 [Journal].
503. Baba *et al.*, 2007 [Journal].
504. Fisher *et al.*, 2003 [Journal].
505. Mathur *et al.*, 2002 [Journal].
506. Grassi *et al.*, 2005 [Journal].
507. Grassi *et al.*, 2008 [Journal].
508. Neukam *et al.*, 2007 [Journal].
509. Taubert, Rosen, & Schömig, 2007 [Journal].
510. Hooper *et al.*, 2012 [Journal].
511. Heinrich *et al.*, 2006 [Journal].
512. Williams, Tamburic, & Lally, 2009 [Journal].
513. Neukam *et al.*, 2007 [Journal].
514. Smit, 2011 [Book].
515. Allbright, in Szogyi, 1997 [Book].
516. De Gottardi *et al.*, 2012 [Journal].
517. Tzounis *et al.*, 2010 [Journal].
518. Müller-Lissner *et al.*, 2005 [Journal].
519. Taubert *et al.*, 2007 [Journal].
520. Erkkola *et al.*, 2012 [Journal].
521. Hodgson *et al.*, 2008 [Journal].
522. Lans, 2006 [Journal].
523. Pruijm *et al.*, 2013 [Journal].
524. Balcke *et al.*, 1989 [Journal].
525. Saftlas *et al.*, 2010 [Journal].
526. Triche *et al.*, 2008 [Journal].
527. Zellner *et al.*, 2004 [Journal].
528. Hormes & Rozin, 2009 [Journal].
529. Coe, in Szogyi, 1997 [Book].
530. Dean & Lue, 2005 [Journal].
531. Giannandrea, 2009 [Journal].
532. *Ibid.*
533. Orozco *et al.*, 2003 [Journal].
534. Rusconi *et al.*, in Paoletti *et al.*, 2012 [Book].
535. Bahadorani & Hilliker, 2008 [Journal].
536. Wollgast, 2004 [Journal]; Record *et al.*, 2003 [Journal].
537. Faridi *et al.*, 2008 [Journal].
538. Mullen *et al.*, 2009 [Journal].
539. Faridi *et al.*, 2008 [Journal].
540. Balcke *et al.*, 1989 [Journal].
541. Chalyk *et al.*, 2018 [Journal].
542. 2017, https://chronichives.com [Internet].

543. Smit, 2011 [Book].
544. Giannandrea, 2009 [Journal].
545. *Ibid.*
546. Erkkola *et al.*, 2012 [Journal]; Räikkönen *et al.*, 2004 [Journal].
547. Hodgson *et al.*, 2008 [Journal].
548. Wolz *et al.*, 2009 [Journal].
549. Wolz *et al.*, 2012 [Journal].
550. Nasser *et al.*, 2011 [Journal].
551. Rose, Koperski, & Golomb, 2010 [Journal]; Smeets *et al.*, 2006 [Journal].
552. Rankin *et al.*, 2005 [Journal].
553. Mounicou *et al.*, 2002 [Journal].

Mini-monographs

i. <u>Corozo Palm</u> *Attalea cohune*
ii. <u>Annatto</u> *Bixa orellana*
iii. <u>Popcorn Flower</u> *Bourreria huanita*
iv. <u>Cayenne</u> *Capsicum spp.*
v. <u>Pochote</u> *Ceiba aesculifolia ssp.parviflora*
vi. <u>Hand Flower</u> *Chiranthodendron pentadactylon*
vii. <u>Ear Flower</u> *Cymbopetalum penduliflorum*
viii. <u>Chupipe & N'ched</u> *Gonolobus spp.*
ix. <u>Magnolia</u> *Magnolia mexicana*
x. <u>Allspice</u> *Pimenta dioica*
xi. <u>Holy Leaf</u> *Piper auritum*
xii. <u>Frangipani</u> *Plumeria rubra*
xiii. <u>Marmalade Plum</u> *Pouteria sapota*
xiv. <u>Funeral Tree</u> *Quararibea funebris*
xv. <u>Wild Sarsaparilla</u> *Smilax spp.*
xvi. <u>Jaguar tree</u> *Theobroma bicolor*
xvii. <u>Vanilla</u> *Vanilla planifolia*

Attalea cohune (Liebm. ex Mart.), syn. *Orbignya guacuyule*, *Orbignya cohune*, *Cocos guacuyule*, *Attalea guacuyule*

Common names: Cohune palm, Corozo, Cayaco, Coco Corozo, Coco de aceite, Coquillo de aceite, Coquito, Guacoyul.[1]

Plant family: Arecaceae

Habit & habitat: Pacific coast of southern Mexico; high or median evergreen or deciduous forests. Up to 20m tall feather-leaved palm tree with a smooth trunk, a symmetrical crown of leaves. Chestnut-like round striated seed coats, fruits approx. 5–8cm long.[1,2]

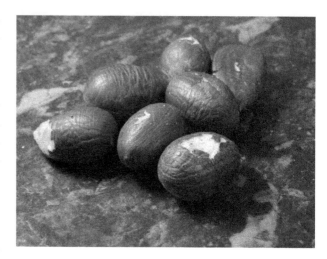

Cultivation: Needs full sun, tolerates littoral and sandy soil and high winds;[5] prefers deep, well-drained soil.[6]

Part used: Seeds.

Phytochemistry: Largely unknown. 70% oil, highly saturated with short- and medium-chain fatty acids, incl. lauric acid[3] (lauric acid 46%, myristic acid 15%, oleic acid 19%, palmitic acid 9.5%, caprylic acid 7.5%, capric acid 6.5%).[4]

Traditional use: "Heart of palm" from the <u>trunk</u> is commonly eaten as a delicacy; ten- to fifteen-year-old trees are cut four feet above ground, and the heart of the trunk between this cut and the first branches—the apical meristem and undeveloped leaves and bracts about 30cm tall and weighing 1–1.4kg—is tender, sweet, and edible.[6,7] In addition, the <u>leaves</u> are used for thatching, the <u>stems</u> to make flybrushes, and the <u>seeds</u> to make oil,[6] and as an essential part of the Oaxacan beverage, *tejate*. To make the oil, fallen fruits are collected from the ground, the endocarp is manually cracked open, and the kernels are mashed, then boiled over an open fire. After several hours, oil floats to the surface, is skimmed off, then heated separately to evaporate any remaining water.[6] Flour derived from fruit mesocarp of related South American species *Orbignya phalatera* is used in Brazilian folk medicine as an anodyne, laxative, anti-inflammatory for "rheumatism", as an anti-ulcer, anti-obesity, venotonic, and anti-tumour agent.[8]

Scientific data: There is no data for *Attalea cohune* (formerly known as *Orbignya guacuyle*), but there is some research data for the South American species *Orbignya speciosa* and *Orbignya phalatera*.

In vitro: *O. speciosa* fruit mesocarp ethanolic extract had a dose-dependent cytostatic effect on various tumour cell lines (lukaemic HL-60, K562, and K562-Lucena 1, and human breast cancer cell line MCF-7) at lower dosages than those which affected human lymphocytes.[9]

A polysaccharide isolated from *O. phalatera* fruit mesocarp enhanced phagocytosis and had anti-inflammatory activity.[10]

In vivo (non-human animals): 50mg/kg *O. phalatera* fruit mesocarp aqueous extract injected intraperitoneally into Wistar rats caused a minor increase in wound healing (fibroblast profusion and re-epithelialisation).[11] Similarly, intraperitoneal injection of *O. phalatera* fruit mesocarp aqueous extract at 50mg/kg in 25g/ml concentrations caused minor improvements in healing of colonic surgical anastomosis in Wistar rats, as measured by increased mononuclear cell activity on the third day after administration by comparison with the control group, though with no significant difference in outcome.[12] Intraperitoneal injection of the aqueous extract in mice at 10 and 20mg/kg increased peritoneal macrophage activity and MHC II expression, increasing the production of cytotoxic metabolites.[13] 500mg/kg of *O. phalatera* fruit mesocarp aqueous extract administered orally over several days had a significant anti-thrombotic effect in rats, increasing nitric oxide production and modestly elevating prothrombin and activated partial thromboplastin time by 12 and 13.9%, respectively.[8] Aqueous extracts of flour made from *O. phalatera* fruit administered to Sprague-Dawley rats on a high-iodine diet had significant anti-thyroid effects, which was replicated *in vitro* with anti-thyroid peroxidase activity on porcine thyroid slices.[14]

Summary of actions: Nutritive (high-calorie). Possibly: anti-thrombotic, anti-thyroid, gastroprotective, vulnerary, chemopreventive, immunomodulatory, anti-rheumatic, venotonic.

Indications: Uncertain. Possibly: *Internal*: Seeds: peptic or gastric ulceration, wound recovery, cardiovascular disease [([adjunct), cancer (adjunct or preventive), arthritic pain.

External: Seeds: varicose veins.

Cautions: None known.

Dose, preparation, and use with Cacao: The sole documented use of cohune palm nuts with Cacao is as an ingredient in *Tejate* (see Chapter 8 for full recipe). The seeds are boiled with corn (maize) kernels and wood ash; the cooked seeds are then ground on a metate with toasted aromatic *Quararibea funebris* flowers, to which are added toasted Cacao seeds and a toasted mamey (*Pouteria sapota*) seed, with a little water added to form a fatty paste, which is then ground into the cooked maize dough and used as the base for the beverage.

POSSIBLE USES (REQUIRE CONFIRMATION). THE FOLLOWING DOSES ARE ESTIMATED. *Internal*: Seeds: In decoction, 6–8g per dose, for the above indications; or a 1:3 tincture made with 25–30% ethanol (favouring water-soluble constituents), at 40–60ml per week.

External: Seeds: either whole fresh seed paste thinned with water, or a cream made from the expressed seed oil with 10% tincture and 15% aromatic water distilled from the whole seeds, applied to varicose veins twice daily.

References

1. Quattrocchi, U. (2017). *CRC World Dictionary of Palms: Common Names, Scientific Names, Eponyms, Synonyms, and Etymology*. USABoca Raton, FL: CRC Press.
2. Glassman, S. (1999). *A Taxonomic Treatment of the Palm Subtribe Attaleinae (Tribe Cocoeae)*. Chicago, USAIL: University of Illinois Press.

3. Shahidi, F. (ed.) (2006). *Nutraceutical and Specialty Lipids and their Co-Products*. USABoca Raton, FL: CRC Press.
4. Corozo Oil (*Attalea cohune*). *Espiritu del Campo*. http://espiritudelcampo.com/corozo.html [Accessed 24 November 2017].
5. *Attalea cohune*. *Azuero Earth Project*. http://azueroearthproject.org/trees/attalea-cohune/ [Accessed 24 November 2017].
6. McSweeney, K. (1995). The Cohune Palm (*Orbignya cohune*, Arecaceae) in Belize: A survey of uses. *Economic Botany, 49*(2): 162–171.
7. Soulé, J.-P. (1999). Cohune Palm Tree: The most important tree in the Mayan life. http://caske2000.org/survival/cohunepalm.htm [Accessed 25 November 2017].
8. Azevedo, A., Farias, J., Costa, G., Ferreira, S., Aragão-Filho, W., Sousa, P., Pinheiro, M., Maciel, M., Silva, L., Lopes, A., Barroqueiro, E., Borges, M., Guerra, R., & Nascimento, F. (2007). Anti-thrombotic effect of chronic oral treatment with *Orbignya phalatera* Mart. *Journal of Ethnopharmacology, 111*(1): 155–159.
9. Rennó, M., Barbosa, G., Zancan, P., Veiga, V., Alviano, C., Sola-Penna, M., Menezes, F., & Holandino, C. (2008). Crude ethanol extract from babassu (*Orbignya speciosa*): cytotoxicity on tumoral and non-tumoral cell lines. *Anais da Academia Brasileira de Ciencias, 80*(3): 467–476.
10. Da Silva, B., & Parente, J. (2001). An anti-inflammatory and immunomodulatory polysaccharide from *Orbignya phalatera*. *Fitoterapia. 72*(8): 887–893.
11. Martins, N., Malafaia, O., Ribas-Filho, J., Heibel, M., Baldez, R., Vasconcelos, P., Moreira, H., Mazza, M., Nassif, P., & Wallbach, T. (2006). Healing process in cutaneous surgical wounds in rats under the influence of *Orbignya phalerata* aqueous extract. *Acta Cirurgica Brasileira, 21*, Suppl. 3: 66–75.
12. Baldez, R., Malafaia, O., Czeczko, N., Martins, N., Ferreira, L., Ribas, C., Salles Júnior, G., Del Claro, R., Santos Lde, O., Graça Neto, L., & Araújo, L. (2006). Healing of colonic anastomosis with the use of aqueous extract of *Orbignya phalerata* (Babassu) in rats. *Acta Cirurgica Brasileira. 21*, Suppl. 2: 31–38.
13. Nascimento, F., Barroqueiro, E., Azevedo, A., Lopes, A., Ferreira, S., Silva, L., Maciel, M., Rodriguez, D., & Guerra, R. (2006). Macrophage activation induced by *Orbignya phalerata* Mart. *Journal of Ethnopharmacology, 103*(1): 53–58.
14. Gaitan, E., Cooksey, R., Legan, J., Lindsay, R., Ingbar, S., & Medeiros-Neto, G. (1994). Antithyroid effects *in vivo* and *in vitro* of babassu and mandioca: a staple food in goiter areas of Brazil. *European Journal of Endocrinology, 131*(2): 138–144.

Bixa orellana L.

Common names: Annatto, Achiote, Bija, Lipstick Plant, Colorau, Urucum, Orellana, Orleana.

Plant family: Bixaceae

Habit & habitat: Mexico down to northern south America. Small evergreen tree, fast-growing, up to 5m tall.

Cultivation: Soil type—well-drained, moist, alkaline to neutral pH, light (sandy) to medium (loamy). Requires high humidity. Frost tender, grows in full sun to semi-shade. Drought tolerant.[1,2]

Parts used: Seeds, leaves, branches and stems, bark, roots.

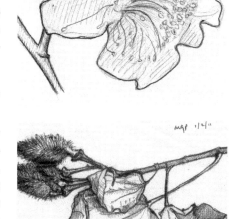

Phytochemistry (seeds): Carotenoids (bixin, 2–5% dry weight, norbixin, isobixin, beta-carotene, cryptoxanthin, lutein, zeaxanthin, crocetin); oily constituents e.g., geranylgeraniol, 1% dry weight; tannins, incl. ellagic acid; salicylic acid; threonine; tomentosic acid; amino acids, e.g., tryptophan and phenylalanine; 0.3–0.9% volatile compounds (bornyl acetate, ∝-caryophyllene, copaene, ∝-cubebene, (+)-cyclosativene, geranyl phenylacetate, 1-heptanetiol, 3-methylpyridine, 4-methylpyridine γ-elemene, β-humulene, isoledene, β-pinene, seline-6-en-4-ol, δ-selinene, (−)-spathulenol, and (+)-ylangene). Miscellaneous: cellulose, 40–45%, sugars, 3.5–5.5%, fixed oils 3%, 13–16% proteins.[3]

Traditional use: <u>Seeds</u>: Ground seeds used in traditional Cacao drinks. Culinary, as a food dye—the dye is present in the seed coat. Seeds are ground into a paste, or they may be soaked and rinsed with hot water to remove the pigment; the expressed seeds are then discarded, and the extract is evaporated, and the cooled extract is set into cakes and used for medicines and dye. Bitter, astringent, and purgative (in high doses). Regarded as "cold and dry in the third degree" by seventeenth-century European doctors, it was considered useful for toothache and "to strengthen the gums", against kidney stones, diarrhoea and dysentery, to slake thirst, reduce tumours and swellings, and as a stomachic and galactagogue.[16,17] Decoction traditionally employed as a febrifuge, and made into a syrup, against pharyngitis and bronchitis.[1] In South America, the seed decoction is also used to treat diarrhoea, and in anti-malarial formulae.[4] In Mexico, seed pulp is used for mouth cancer, and the whole seed used as a treatment for erectile dysfunction.[5] In the Philippines, seed paste is applied to burns to prevent scarring.[2] Dye made from seed coats is used as topical sunscreen and insect repellent in South America.[4]

In the West Indies, the seeds are used to treat diabetes.[4] Leaves: by infusion or decoction as a taenicide for worms (unspecified) in children, as a febrifuge, as an anti-emetic in the first trimester of pregnancy, and against dysentery and colic in West Indian and Chinese medicine.[2,3] Against heartburn and as a laxative in Brazilian medicine.[2] Roots: decoction is used as a diuretic, and to treat jaundice, "venereal disease", and asthma.[1] Bark decoction used to treat angina and asthma, and fresh sap applied to treat skin rashes of unspecified cause.[1] Stems/shoots infusion used as an aphrodisiac, and in the treatment of hepatitis.[2]

Scientific data: _In vitro_: _B. orellana_ seeds have anti-leishmanial, hypolipidaemic, anti-plasmodial (against _Plasmodium falciparum_ and _P. gallinaceum_), anti-gonorrhoeal, and antioxidant properties.[4] Isolated cis-bixin was selectively cytotoxic to various drug-resistant myeloma cell lines via oxidative enhancement.[11] Pre-incubation with _B. orellana_ leaf extract reduced histamine-induced endothelial cell permeability.[14]

   In vivo (non-human animals): Hypolipidaemic properties have been demonstrated in the mouse, and weak symptom-attenuating antivenin properties against _Bothrops atrox_ envenomation;[19] hypoglycaemic properties have been demonstrated in dogs, and hypotensive properties in rats.[4] Bixin isolated from _B. orellana_ inhibited cardiac fibrosis and inflammation following a high-fat diet in mice,[5] while isolated norbixin administered to mice orally over three months caused a reduction in markers of retinal damage similar to macular degeneration.[7] An acetone extract of whole _B. orellana_ seeds protected retinal cells from chemically induced cell death in live mice by non-antioxidant mechanisms.[9] Aqueous extract of _B. orellana_ seeds at daily doses of 400 and 800mg/kg both reduced fructose-induced hypertriglyceridemia by around 48%, and reduced ethanol-induced hypertriglyceridemia by approximately 34% and 62%, respectively.[10] _B. orellana_ seed essential oil administered intraperitoneally at 30mg/kg bodyweight halted progression of cutaneous leishmaniosis in infected mice.[8] _B. orellana_ seeds included as 0.1–0.2% of the diet of live rats prevented cyclophosphamide-induced molinaldehyde accumulation in rat brains, and a chloroform extract also prevented elevation of serum bilirubin and other markers of oxidative stress.[12] Oral administration of 150mg/kg aqueous extract of _B. orellana_ leaf for four consecutive days significantly attenuated acute histamine-induced paw swelling in rats.[15]

   In vivo (human): _B. orellana_ root extracts had anti-allergenic properties.[4] Rat and human studies show that both bixin and norbixin are well absorbed orally and subsequently found in both plasma and urine.[13]

Summary of actions: Seeds: hypolipidaemic, hypocholesterolaemic, hypotensive, diuretic; weakly anti-inflammatory and anti-allergenic; _possibly_ cardioprotective (anti-fibrotic), hepatoprotective, retinoprotective, neuroprotective, anti-leishmanial, cutaneous UV buffering.

Indications: Hypercholesterolaemia, hypertension.
   Possibly also: atherosclerosis-related erectile dysfunction; skin UV damage (to slow); macular degeneration; cardiac fibrosis (to prevent); type 2 diabetes mellitus. As an adjunctive treatment with other plants or drugs in: hepatitis; leishmaniosis; recovery from malaria; recovery from snakebite; recovery from anaphylaxis or inflammatory allergic reactions; lower respiratory tract and throat infections. In Cacao, as a galactagogue (?).

Cautions: Old seeds may cause headache, nausea, or gastric distress.[16] Known allergy.

Dose, preparation, and use with Cacao: Annatto paste may be used in Cacao drinks. To make this, the seeds are soaked in water and slowly cooked down over three days in a clay pot, stirring frequently, reduced to dryness, then moulded into logs.[18] Ground seed powder: _Internal_: tiny doses of 10–20mg daily vs. hypercholesterolaemia; larger quantities can be strongly diuretic. Dried fruits are ground into cocoa liquor with other spices, for use in chocolate drinks. _Topical_: possibly, burns, as a sunscreen and insect repellent *may stain skin).

References

1. http://pfaf.org/User/Plant.aspx?LatinName=Bixa+orellana [Accessed 14 September 2017].
2. http://rain-tree.com/annato.htm#.WdJnBmhSxhF [Accessed 2 October 2017].
3. Bown, D. (2002). _The Royal Horticultural Society New Encyclopaedia of Herbs and Their Uses_. London: Dorling Kindersley.
4. Vilar, D., Vilar, M., de Lima e Moura, T., Raffin, F., Rosa de Oliveira, Franco, C., Athayde-Filho, P., Diniz, M., & Barbosa-Filho, J. (2014). Traditional uses, chemical constituents, and biological activities of _Bixa orellana_ L.: A review. _Scientific World Journal, 857292_. https://ncbi.nlm.nih.gov/pubmed/25050404 [Accessed 17 April 2019].
5. 18 April 2008: Interview with Sr Mario Euan, herbalist and teacher at U-Yits-Ka'an School of Agriculture & Ecology, Mani, Yucatan Peninsula, Mexico. (See Appendix C, Interview 1.)
6. Xu, Z., & Kong, X. (2017). Bixin ameliorates high fat diet-induced cardiac injury in mice through inflammation and oxidative stress suppression. _Biomedicine and Pharmacotherapy, 89_: 991–1004.
7. Fontaine, V., Monteiro, E., Brazhnikova, E., Lesage, L., Balducci, C., Guibout, L., Feraille, L., Elena, P., Sahel, J., Veillet, S., & Lafont, R. (2016). Norbixin protects retinal pigmented epithelium cells and photoreceptors against A2E-mediated phototoxicity _in vitro_ and _in vivo_. _PLoS One, 11_(12): e0167793.
8. Monzote, L., García, M., Scull, R., Cuellar, A., & Setzer, W. (2014). Antileishmanial activity of the essential oil from Bixa orellana. _Phytotherapy Research, 28_(5): 753–758.
9. Tsuruma, K., Shimazaki, H., Nakashima, K., Yamauchi, M., Sugitani, S., Shimazawa, M., Linuma, M., & Hara, H. (2012). Annatto prevents retinal degeneration induced by endoplasmic reticulum stress _in vitro_ and _in vivo_. _Molecular Nutrition and Food Research, 56_(5): 713–724.
10. Ferreira, J., Sousa, D., Dantas, M., Fonseca, S., Menezes, D., Martins, A., & deQueiroz, M. (2013). Effects of Bixa orellana L. seeds on hyperlipidemia. _Phytotherapy Research, 27_(1): 144–147.
11. Tibodeau, J., Isham, C., & Bible, K. (2010). Annatto constituent cis-bixin has selective antimyeloma effects mediated by oxidative stress and associated with inhibition of thioredoxin and thioredoxin reductase. _Antioxidants and Redox Signalling, 13_(7): 987–997.
12. Oboh, G., Akomolafe, T., Adefegha, S., & Adetuyi, A. (2011). Inhibition of cyclophosphamide-induced oxidative stress in rat brain by polar and non-polar extracts of Annatto (Bixa orellana) seeds. _Experimental and Toxicologic Pathology, 63_(3): 257–262.
13. EFSA Panel on Food Additives and Nutrient Sources added to Food (ANS). (2016). The safety of annatto extracts (E 160b) as a food additive. http://onlinelibrary.wiley.com/doi/10.2903/j.efsa.2016.4544/full [Accessed 18 September 2017].
14. Yong, Y., Chiong, H., Somchit, M., & Ahmad, Z. (2015). Bixa orellana leaf extract suppresses histamine-induced endothelial hyperpermeability via the PLC-NO-cGMP signaling cascade. _BMC Complementary and Alternative Medicine, 15_: 356.

15. Yong, Y., Zakaria, Z., Kadir, A., Somchit, M., Ee Cheng Lian, G., & Ahmad, Z. (2013). Chemical constituents and antihistamine activity of Bixa orellana leaf extract. *BMC Complementary and Alternative Medicine, 13*: 32.

16. Stubbe, H. (1662). *The Indian Nectar, or, A discourse concerning chocolata [Etc.]* London: J.C. for Andrew Crook.

17. Hernández, F. (1615). *Quatro Libros de la Naturaleza, Y Virtudes de las Plantas, y animales, que estan recevidos en el uso de Medicina en la Nueva España, y la Methodo, y correction, y preparacion, que para administrarlas se requiere con lo que el Doctor Francisco Hernández escrobo en lengua Latina.* F. Ximenez (Trans.). www.wdl.org/en/item/7334/200m/#group=1&page=1 [Accessed 25 January 2012].

18. Trilling, S. (1999). *Seasons of My Heart: A Culinary Journey Through Oaxaca, Mexico.* New York: Ballantine.

19. Núñez, V., Otero, R., Barona, J., Saldarriaga, M., Osorio, R., Fonnegra, R., Jiménez, S., Díaz, A., & Quintana, J. (2004). Neutralization of the edema-forming, defibrinating and coagulant effects of Bothrops asper venom by extracts of plants used by healers in Colombia. *Brazilian Journal of Medical and Biological Research, 37*(7): 969–977.

Bourreria huanita (Lex.) Hemsl.

Common names: Esquisuchil, Huanita, Jasmin de Palo, Jasmin del Istmo, Guie-xoba (Zapotec),[2] Popcorn flower, Izquixochitl (Nahuatl), Ik'al te' (Tzotzil Maya), Muk'ta ch'it.[1]

Plant family: Boraginaceae

Habit & habitat: Tree up to 23m tall, smooth branches, alternate elliptical leaves, smooth on both sides. Stalked white flowers 4–12cm in size, in clusters. Distributed from Costa Rica to the south of Mexico (Oaxaca and Chiapas).[3]

Cultivation: Not frost tolerant, requires warmth (minimum 15–18°C) and humidity; indoor growing only outside zone 10. Full sun, well-drained but moist soil. Propagated by seed or cutting.

Parts used: Flowers, bark, leaves.

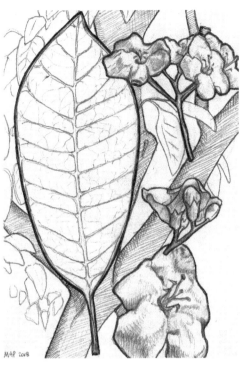

Phytochemistry: <u>Flowers</u>: Alkaloids, Polyphenols (incl. flavonoids, anthocyanins, tannins); Coumarins, Sesquiterpene lactones, saponins, triterpenoid sterols, p-hydroxybenzoic acid,[6] essential oil (incl. farnesyl cetone 8.38%, 2-hydroxy-phenylbenzoic acid, 8.37%; β-phenylethylsalicilate, 5.6%; 6, 10 dimethyl-2-unadecanone; heneicosane, 5.2%.)[9]

Traditional use: Dried flowers used to perfume and flavour Cacao drinks. Regarded as "cold and astringent" by European Galenical standards.[11] <u>Bark</u> was used as an anti-periodic (febrifuge for recurrent fever, e.g., malaria) and astringent.[1] The Mexica decocted *B. huanita* bark in combination with other herbs, salt, saltpetre, and ash and mixed the resulting liquid with honey to make a topical treatment for genital warts.[5] *B. huanita* <u>leaves</u> were used against fevers, and— in post-colonial medicine—colds.[4] *B. huanita* <u>flowers</u> were used in a multi-ingredient magico-medical Mexica prescription against "the fatigue of those who administer the republic"—an external wash, made from a spring water infusion of *Theobroma cacao* seeds and fruit, flowers of *B. huanita*, *Vanilla planifolia*, *Magnolia dealbata*, *Piper sanctum*, *Cymbopetalum penduliflorum*, bark of *Heamatoxylon brasiletto*, plus several different types of leaves, all to be mixed with mingled ocelot, wolf, jaguar, puma, and mountain cat blood, to "give the whole body the strength of a gladiator [and] … give impetus to the heart".[5] An infusion of *B. huanita* flowers was also part of a multi-ingredient oral prescription for badly injured people, presumably intended to relieve pain and accelerate recovery.[5] The Mexica used the flowers to treat dental pain, indigestion and slow bowel transit, and "chest ailments".[11] The flowers are used in contemporary Guatemalan folk medicine in infusion as a tranquilliser, analgesic, and against heart disease and high blood pressure; the infusion is also used, presumably topically, as an "antiseptic" against "skin complaints".[6] Other folk uses of unspecified plant parts include treating dysmenorrhoea, preventing abortion, and cancer prevention.[9]

Scientific data: *In vitro*: An 80% ethanolic extract of *B. huanita* bark had strong anti-leishmanial activity, with an IC_{50} of 6µg/ml; *B. huanita* leaf was also active, at 12µg/ml.[7] Ethanolic extract of *B. huanita* flowers also inhibited two pathogenic dermatophytic fungi, *Sporothrix schenckii* (cause of sporotrichosis) and *Fonsecaea pedrosoi* (cause of chromoblastomycosis), at MICs of 12.5µg/ml and 25µg/ml, respectively.[8]

In vivo (non-human animals): A dessicated hydroalcoholic solid extract (made with 70% ethanol) of unspecified parts of *B. huanita* administered orally to male mice prolonged pentobarbital-induced sleep at 300mg/kg, increased plus-maze exploration dose-dependently, reduced immobility dose-dependently in a tail-suspension test, but failed to increase locomotor activity in an open field test, reduce drug-induced seizures, alter memory retention, or block apomorphine-induced climbing behaviours. The extract was considered to have sedative, anxiolytic, and antidepressant activity, without negative effects on memory consolidation.[6]

Summary of actions: *Internal*: Flowers: hydroalcoholic extract is anxiolytic, antidepressant, sedative, and anodyne; possibly hypotensive. Bark: febrifuge; anti-malarial?, anti-leishmanial?

External: Flowers: ethanolic or non-polar extract as topical anti-fungal; ethanolic extract of bark as anti-leishmanial treatment, and possibly for warts.

Indications: *Internal*: Flowers: anxiety, depression, insomnia; toothache, dysmenorrhoea; hypertension?. Bark: possibly malaria and leishmaniasis.

Topical: Flowers: sporotrichosis, chromoblastomycosis. Bark: cutaneous leishmaniasis.

Cautions: None noted—insufficient information.

Dose, preparation, and use with Cacao: *Internal*: Flowers are dried and ground with cocoa liquor as a chocolate drink spice. THE FOLLOWING DOSES ARE ESTIMATED. Tincture, 60–80% ethanol, 1:3, approx. 20–40ml per week. Bark: unknown, presumably in decoction.

Topical: Flowers and bark may be made into an infused oil, ointment, or water-in-oil cream, or applied topically as 70–80% ethanolic tincture diluted in a suitable vehicle, e.g., aromatic water.

References

1. http://maya-ethnobotany.org/images-mayan-ethnobotanicals-medicinal-plants-tropical-agriculture-flower-spice-flavoring/cacao-flavoring-esquisuchil-bourreria-huanita-popcorn-flower-planted-by-hermano-pedro.php [Accessed 30 October 2017].
2. Campos Ríos, G. (2005). Revisión del género *Bourreria* P. Browne (Boraginaceae) en México. *Polibotánica, 19*: 39–103.
3. Helmsley, W. (1888). *Biologia Centrali-Americana; or Contributions to the Knowledge of the Fauna and Flora of Mexico and Central America.* London: R.H. Pouret and Dalau & Co.UK http://tropicos.org/Name/4001995?projectid=3 [Accessed 8 November 2017].

4. Cates, R., Thompson, A., Brabazon, H., McDonald, S., Lawrence, M., Williams, S., Penialillo, P., Soria, A., Espinoza, L., Martinez, J., Arbizu, D., Villagran, E., & Ancheta, F. (2014). Activities of Guatemalan medicinal plants against cancer cell lines and selected microbes: Evidence for their conservation. *Journal of Medicinal Plant Research, 8*(33): 1040–1050.

5. Badiano, J. (1552). *Libellus de Medicinalibus Indorum Herbis*. M. de la Cruz (Trans.). Mexico City: Fondo de Cultura Economica Instituto Mexicano del Seguro Social, 1996.

6. Holzmann, I., Cattani, D., Corso, M., Perondi, D., Zanella, S., Burger, C., Klein Júnior, L., Filho, V., Cruz, S., Torres, M., Cáceres, A., & de Souza, M. (2014). Psychopharmacological profile of hydroalcoholic extract and P-hydroxybenzoic acid obtained from *Bourreria huanita* (Boraginaceae) in mice. *Pharmacology & Pharmacy, 5*(11): 983–995.

7. Calderón, A., Romero, L. Ortega-Barría, E., Solís, P., Zacchino, S., Gimenez, A., Pinzón, R., Cáceres, A., Tamayo, G., Guerra, C., Espinosa, A., Correa, M., & Gupta, M. (2010). Screening of Latin American plants for antiparasitic activities against malaria, Chagas disease, and leishmaniasis. *Pharmaceutical Biology, 48*(5): 545–553.

8. Gaitán, I., Paz, A. Zacchino, S., Tamayo, G., Giménez, A., Pinzón, R., Cáceres, A., & Gupta, M. (2011). Subcutaneous antifungal screening of Latin American plant extracts against Sporothrix schenckii and Fonsecaea pedrosoi. *Pharmaceutical Biology, 49*(9): 907–919.

9. Cruz, M., Garicia, E., Letran, H., Gaitan, I., Medinilla, B., Orozco, R., Samayoa, M., & Caceres, A. (2010). Caracterizacion Quimica y Evaluacion de la Actividad Biologica de *Bourreria huanita* (Lllave & Lex.) Hemsl. *Revista Científica, 18*(1): 81–87.

10. Bennett, M. (2003). *Pulmonarias and the Borage Family*. LondonUK: B. T. Batsford.

11. Hernández, F. (1615). *Quatro Libros de la Naturaleza, Y Virtudes de las Plantas, y animales, que estan recevidos en el uso de Medicina en la Nueva España, y la Methodo, y correction, y preparacion, que para administrarlas se requiere con lo que el Doctor Francisco Hernández escrobo en lengua Latina*. F. Ximenez (Trans.). www.wdl.org/en/item/7334/200m/#group=1&page=1 [Accessed 25 January 2012].

Capsicum spp. L. *(C. annuum var. minimum, C. frutescens, C. baccatum, etc.)*

Common names: Chilli (Nahuatl), chilli pepper, Cayenne, Christmas pepper.

Plant family: Solanaceae

Habit & habitat: A small bush from Mesoamerica, cultivated since ancient times to yield both spicy and sweet varieties.

Cultivation: Perennial, seeds from August to October. Grows in light to heavy soils of variable pH, but prefers well-drained but moist soil and requires full sun.[2] Not frost-hardy, requires a minimum temperature of 4°C to grow.[1]

Parts used: Fruits, fresh or dried.

Phytochemistry: Capsaicinoids (incl. capsaicin, dihydrocapsaicin, and nordihydrocapsaicin), 0.3–0.4%; carotenoids, 0.2% (incl. capsanthin, β-carotene, β-cryptoxanthin, capsorubin); Flavonoids (incl. quercetin, luteolin, and apigenin glycosides); phenolic acids (incl. hydroxycinnamic and hydroxybenzoic acids); miscellaneous, incl. ascorbic acid, volatile oil.[4,5]

Traditional uses: Fresh or dried fruits used in traditional Cacao drinks. Dr Francisco Hernández,

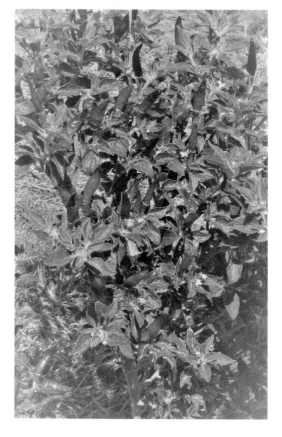

the seventeenth-century physician documented Mexico's medicinal flora, classified chilli as hot in the fourth and dry in the third degree, attributing it libido-enhancing, carminative, diuretic, emmenagogue, anti-catarrhal, and orexigenic (appetite-enhancing) properties, with the ability to remove "phlegmatic humours" from swollen joints, and alleviate sciatic and nervous pain. He cautioned that over-use could "overheat" the kidneys and "inflame the blood", giving rise to kidney and flank pain, and "frenzies".[3] Contemporary herbal medicine uses include internal use in fevers, poor circulation, asthma, and weak digestion, and external use for joint inflammation, muscle tension, sprains, chilblains, and neuralgic pain.[3] Internal uses are to improve circulation, increase diaphoresis (as a febrifuge in acute febrile illnesses), for colic and as a digestive stimulant; externally, as an anti-neuralgic and anodyne, for example, rubbed into gums to treat toothache.[4] Sluggish or weak digestion—use to increase appetite, and increase the tonic or strengthening power of herbal preparations.[6] To fortify digestion in delirium tremens (withdrawal in alcohol dependency); in combination with laxatives or stool softening agents in haemorrhoids; as a stimulant of vitality and poor circulation in elderly or debilitated persons.[7]

Scientific data: _In vitro_: Selected polyphenols from _Capsicum_ species inhibited the pathogenic bacteria _Staphylococcus aureus_ and _Pseudomonas aeruginosa_.[9] Isolated capsaicin has been demonstrated to reduce glutamate release in rat cortex by increasing neuronal calcineurin activation, reducing calcium ion entry.[10] Production of carcinogenic heterocyclic amines in cooked food was significantly reduced in the presence of capsaicin.[13] Capsaicin alters the expression of genes associated with cancer cell survival, growth, and spread, and is chemopreventive.[16] Whole _C. baccatum_ extracts inhibited lipopolysaccharide or interferon-gamma provoked macrophages from releasing of nitric oxide and TNF-α, suggesting anti-inflammatory effects; these effects were not dependent on capsaicin.[15]

In vivo (non-human animals): Capsaicin stimulates substance P release but with repeated applications depletes neuronal stores and desensitises the vanilloid receptors to which it binds, producing anti-neuralgic and anti-inflammatory effects by decreasing sensitivity (tachyphylaxis). Internally, capsaicin is gastroprotective and anti-ulcer; it also enhances gastric motility, and reduces gastric acid secretion in rats and cats. Administering oil suspension of _C. chinense_ fruits to rats caused a medium-term (seven days) increase and long-term (twenty-one days) decrease in immunoreactive astrocytes in the arcuate nucleus,[1] suggesting that ingestion of _Capsicum_ may affect the support of neurons in this area of the brain associated with hormonal and homeostatic regulation. Oral capsaicin has had favourable effects in rodent models of atherosclerosis, cardiac hypertrophy, metabolic syndrome, diabetes, non-alcoholic fatty liver, hypertension, and stroke risk.[20] _C. baccatum_ extracts inhibited inflammation induced by carrageenan, prostaglandin E2, and histamine in mice.[15] A 2% red chilli diet in diabetic rats did not affect blood sugar, but significantly increased insulin production.[18] Oral _C. frutescens_ administered to rats at 2.5, 5, and 10mg/kg bodyweight produced statistically significant ($p<0.05$) dose-dependent increases in the INR without anti-platelet activity, although the highest dose produced some signs of gastric erosion.[21]

In vivo (humans): A four-week study giving 14mg of mixed _Capsicum_ carotenoids per day to five volunteers found that erythrocyte carotenoid levels doubled during the study period.[17] In a six-year survey of 16,179 US adults, after adjusting for variables such as lifestyle, demographic, and medical issues, consumption of hot chilli peppers was associated with a 13% reduction in the risk of instant death, with a slight but non-significant reduction in the risk of cardiovascular mortality.[12] _Capsicum_ ingestion has also been shown to assist weight loss through capsaicin, which activates brown adipose tissue, triggers sympathetic nervous system response, and improves insulin response.[14] A 2009 Chinese survey of 8,433 adults aged 18–99 found that inclusion of chilli in the diet corresponded with less insulin resistance (measured by HOMA-IR) in both men and women; preference for hotter chilli corresponded with lower insulin resistance.[19] A lower incidence of thromboembolism has been noted in individuals who consume large amounts of hot _Capsicum_ species.[21] Topical capsaicin showed modest benefit over placebo in human double-blind clinical trials for neuropathic and osteoarthritic pain; more significant benefit was reported for lower back pain and pruritis.[5]

Summary of actions: _Internal_: Carminative, circulatory stimulant, gastroprotective, diaphoretic, insulinotropic, thermogenic, anticoagulant.

Topical: counter-irritant, anti-neuralgic, anti-pruritic.[5]

Indications: *Internal*: Poor peripheral circulation; atherosclerosis; high risk of thromboembolism, stroke, or heart attack; gastric ulcers; colic or flatulent dyspepsia; obesity; hyperglycaemia; sore throats.

Topical: Arthritic pain, lumbago; neuralgia, including sciatica, herpetic, and diabetic neuropathic pain; pruritis.[5]

Cautions: Avoid contact with eyes or sensitive areas, due to pain and irritation-causing properties. Massive overdose may cause vomiting, gastritis, and hypothermia; continual overdosing may cause gastritis, reno-, hepato- and neuro- toxicity. If inhaled, airway irritation will result.[8]

Dose, preparation, and use with Cacao: Powdered dried fruit ground into cocoa mass, with or without other spices, for use in Cacao-based beverages: a pinch per serving, or 2–6 Tabasco chillies per kg toasted and shelled Cacao.

Internal use: Dried fruits, 30–120mg t.d.s.; 1:20 tincture, 60% ethanol, 0.3–1ml per dose; 1:3 tincture, up to 3ml per week.

External use: Macerated oil of fresh or dried chillies, applied directly; cream containing 10–40mg of capsaicinoids per cm^2; or up to 5ml macerated oil or 1:3 tincture per 30g base cream.[5]

References

1. http://pfaf.org/User/Plant.aspx?LatinName=Capsicum+annuum [Accessed 16 October 2017].
2. Bown, D. (2002). *The Royal Horticultural Society New Encyclopaedia of Herbs and Their Uses.* London UK: Dorling Kindersley.
3. Hernández, F. (1615). *Quatro Libros de la Naturaleza, Y Virtudes de las Plantas, y animales, que estan recevidos en el uso de Medicina en la Nueva España, y la Methodo, y correction, y preparacion, que para administrarlas se requiere con lo que el Doctor Francisco Hernández escrobo en lengua Latina.* F. Ximenez (Trans.). www.wdl.org/en/item/7334/200m/#group=1&page=1 [Accessed 25 January 2012].
4. Williams, E. (2003). *Potter's Herbal Cyclopaedia.* Saffron Walden, UKUK: C. W. Daniel.
5. Bradley, P. (2006). *British Herbal Compendium—A Handbook of Scientific Information on Widely Used Plant Drugs.* Bournemouth, UK: British Herbal Medicine Association.
6. Grieve, M. (1931). *A Modern Herbal.* Twickenham, UK: Tiger.
7. Wickes Felter, H., & Lloyd, J. (1898). *King's American Dispensatory.* Published online by Henriette Kress, https://henriettes-herb.com/eclectic/kings/index.html [Accessed 26 October 2017].
8. Spinella, M. (2001). *The Psychopharmacology of Herbal Medicine.* Cambridge, MAUSA: Massachusetts Institute of Technology Press.
9. Mokhtar, M., Ginestra, G., Youcefi, F., Filocamo, A., Bisignano, C., & Riazi, A. (2017). Antimicrobial activity of selected polyphenols and capsaicinoids identified in pepper (Capsicum annuum L.) and their possible mode of interaction. *Current Microbiology, 74*(11): 1253–1260.
10. Lu, C., Lin, T., Hsie, T., Huang, S., & Wang, S. (2017). Capsaicin presynaptically inhibits glutamate release through the activation of TRPV1 and calcineurin in the hippocampus of rats. *Food & Function, 8*(5): 1859–1868.
11. Rycerz, K., Krawczyk, A., Jaworska-Adamu, J., Gołyński, M., Lutnicki, K., & Balicki, I. (2016). Immunoreactivity of arcuate nucleus astrocytes in rats after intragastric administration of habanero peppers (Capsicum Chinese Jacq.). *Polish Journal of Veterinary Sciences, 19*(4): 809–817.
12. Chopan, M., & Littenberg, B. (2017). The association of hot red chili pepper consumption and mortality: A large population-based cohort study. *PLoS One, 12*(1): e0169876.

13. Zeng, M., Zhang, M., He, Z., Qin, F., Tao, G., Zhang, S., Gao, Y., & Chen, J. (2017). Inhibitory profiles of chilli pepper and capsaicin on heterocyclic amine formation in roast beef patties. *Food Chemistry, 221*: 404–411.

14. Varghese, S., Kubatka, P., Rodrigo, L., Gazdikova, K., Caprnda, M., Fedotova, J., Zulli, A., Kruzliak, P., & Büsselberg, D. (2016). Chili pepper as a body weight-loss food. *International Journal of Food Sciences and Nutrition, 68*(4): 392–401.

15. Allemand, A., Leonardi, B., Zimmer, A., Moreno, S., Romão, P., & Gosmann, G. (2016). Red pepper (Capsicum baccatum) extracts present anti-inflammatory effects in vivo and inhibit the production of TNF-α and NO in vitro. *Journal of Medicinal Food, 19*(8): 759–767.

16. Clark, R., & Lee, S. (2016). Anticancer properties of capsaicin against human cancer. *Anticancer Research, 36*(3): 837–843.

17. Nishino, A., Ichihara, T., Takaha, T., Kuriki, T., Nihei, H., Kawamoto, K., Yasui, H., & Maoka, T. (2015). Accumulation of paprika carotenoids in human plasma and erythrocytes. *Journal of Oleo Science, 64*(10): 1135–1142.

18. Islam, M., & Choi, H. (2008). Dietary red chilli (Capsicum frutescens L.) is insulinotropic rather than hypoglycemic in type 2 diabetes model of rats. *Phytotherapy Research, 22*(8): 1025–1029.

19. Li, J., Wang, R., & Xiao, C. (2014). Association between chilli food habits with iron status and insulin resistance in a Chinese population. *Journal of Medicinal Food, 17*(4): 472–478.

20. McCarty, M., DiNicolantonio, J., & O'Keefe, J. (2015). Capsaicin may have important potential for promoting vascular and metabolic health. *Open Heart, 2*(1): e000262.

21. Ezekiel, J., & Oluwole, O. (2014). Effects of capsaicin on coagulation: Will this be the new blood thinner? *Clinical Medicine Research, 3*(5): 145–149.

Ceiba aesculifolia ssp. parviflora (H.B. & Kunth[3]) Britten & Baker[1] *(+ C. pentandra)*

Common names: Pochote, Ceiba, Pochote de Secas, Pochotl (Nahuatl);[1] Yax'che.[5]

Plant family: Malvaceae[3] (Bombaceae)[1]

Habit & habitat: Shorter than close relative *C. pentandra* (Kapok), grows up to 25m tall on dry plains and hillsides, up to 1,500m above sea level. Distinctive, straight cylindrical trunk covered with short, warty spines; branches high up the tree, distant, 5–8 leaflets, lanceolate. Whitish, bat-pollinated flowers, 3cm long; capsular fruit pods, oblong, 15–40cm long, filled with globular seeds embedded in silky cotton-like hairs.[4,6] Prefers arid conditions; rare species of low elevation in deciduous forests from Mexico to Costa Rica.[3] Seeds of *C. pentandra* were likely carried across the ocean millions of years ago, and colonised Africa.[7]

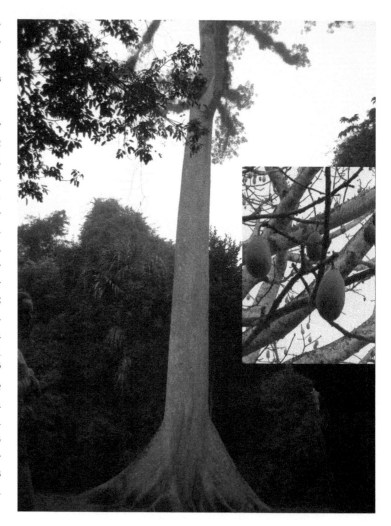

Cultivation: Propagated by seed, grows in light to heavy but well-drained soils, tolerates most pH's, dry or moist soil, and nutrient-poor ground. Needs full sun; drought-tolerant.

Parts used: Seeds, bark, leaves, flowers; *C. pentandra*: also gum (exudate).

Phytochemistry: *C. aesculifolia*: none recorded; the following applies to *C. pentandra*. <u>Seeds</u>: oils, 24% (including: unsaturated fatty acids—oleic 35–0%, Linoleic 29–42%; saturated fatty acids: palmitic 16–20%, stearic 2%, arachidic ≤1%, myristic ≤0.5%;[4] carbohydrates, incl. pentosans and diglycerides;[9,10] cyclopropanes, 2.4–5.6%;[9] phospholipids;[1] phenolics (incl. tannins, 15g/kg;[25] gossypol and esters, isoflavones[5] and flavonoids incl. quercetin)–.[9] <u>Bark</u>: phenolics (incl. tannins, ≤82%;

isoflavones, incl. vavain, vavain glucoside, 5-hydroxy-7,4',5'-trimethoxyisoflavone 3'-O-α-L-arabinofuranosyl(1->6)-β-D-glucopyranoside; flavan-3-ols: (+)-catechin);[11,14] glycosides, triterpenoid saponins,[26] sterols; hydrocyanic acid;[6] napthoquinones.[10] Leaves: mucilage,[6] caffeic acid,[9] volatile oil, saponins, alkaloids.[16] Flowers: sterols (incl. β-sitosterol-β-d-glucoside);[9] alkanes (incl. hentriacontane); flavonols (incl. kaempferol).[9] Roots: sesquiterpene lactones (including 8-formyl-7-hydroxy-5-isoproyl-2-methoxy-3-methyl-1,4-napthaquinone; 7-hydroxycadalene; 2,7-dimethoxy-5-isopropyl-3-methyl-8,1-naphthalene carbolactone; 2-hydroxy-5-isopropyl-7-methoxy-3-methyl-8,1-naphthalene carbolactone).[15]

Traditional uses: Seeds, roots, and flowers may be eaten as food; like the close relative *C. pentandra*, the downy fruit mesocarp is used to stuff pillows, start fires, insulate, and make cloth;[1,3] the wood is used for handicrafts or firewood, and the flowers are used as bait for catching deer.[1] Seeds are consumed by roasting the whole fruit then eating the seeds from the cooked seed pod, or boiling the extracted seeds in water.[1] The seeds of *C. aesculifolia* are eaten to increase sperm count and fertility in males.[2] Bark is infused in water and drunk on an empty stomach for several days to treat kidney disorders, "skin infections" (unspecified), and to reduce blood sugar levels (i.e., type 2 diabetes or prediabetes).[1] Fermented bark is used to treat sunstroke in Yucatan. Unspecified plant parts are used as a purgative and emetic, and to treat "digestive disorders" (also unspecified) in Mexico;[3] these uses appear to be interchangeable with the more common and commercially desirable species, *C. pentandra*. The bark of the latter species is also used as an emetic, and employed in India to treat dysentery, ascites, and anasarca,[4] as well as being used as an Ayahuasca additive in South America.[5] In Africa, the bark is used for similar purposes, as well as for dental pain, oedema, "heart trouble", and lung and skin troubles.[6] A fresh bark poultice, or juice, is used for topical treatment of cutaneous leishmaniasis in French Guiana, although the rationale could be symbolic—because the tree heals itself rapidly once cut, similar to the desired effect on skin lesions.[12] The leaves are used in African medicine as a poultice to treat solid tumours; fresh leaves pounded in water and taken as an infusion to treat fatigue and backache, and a decoction is used as an eyewash to treat conjunctivitis, and taken internally to treat gonorrhoea in West Africa.[6] A decoction of fresh leaves is used in Nigerian medicine to treat type 2 diabetes.[17] The flowers are used to treat constipation.[6] Roots are used in India to treat diabetes—specifically; fresh root sap[6] and the calcined root is administered in liquid to treat epilepsy in Burkina Faso, Africa.[8] Fruits: the unripe fruit pods of *C. pentandra* are used to treat vertigo and migraine in India.[10]

Scientific data: *In vitro*: *C. aesulifolia* bark has anti-bacterial, anti-diabetic (hypoglycaemic), and anti-inflammatory properties "similar to those reported for *Ceiba pentandra*",[1] to which all the following research pertains. *C. pentandra* bark methanolic extract has antioxidant activity and low cytotoxicity toward Vero cells, indicating low toxicity.[13] Isoflavones and (+)-catechin extracted from the bark weakly inhibited COX-1 but not COX-2 prostaglandin biosynthesis, suggesting possible anti-thrombotic but not anti-inflammatory activity.[14] Methanol extracts significantly increased glucose uptake by liver (56.57%) and skeletal muscle (94.19%) slices in hyperglycaemic solutions, and reduced glucose release by liver slices in a hypoglycaemic milieu by 33.94%, while a decoction exhibited anti-haemolytic effects which maximised at 77.57% at 100μg/mL.[19] However, an aqueous extract decreased activity of plasminogen activators in cultured human coronary aortic endothelial cells, inhibiting the secretion of fibrinolytic proteins, suggesting a lack of anti-thrombotic effect.[20] Petroleum ether, acetone, and ethanol bark extracts had significant cytotoxic activity against MCF-7 (oestrogen-receptor positive breast cancer cell line), Ehrlich ascites carcinoma (undifferentiated carcinoma cells), and B16F10 (murine melanoma) cells.[29] Ethanolic extract of *C. pentandra* <u>leaves</u> inhibited growth of *Bacillus subtilis* with a minimum inhibitory concentration of 0.5mg/ml, but was ineffective against other bacterial or fungal species tested.[16] A methanolic extract had strong radical scavenging activity in DPPH and ABTS, but not potassium ferricyanide reducing assays.[17] Aqueous and ethanolic extracts of dried leaves had antidrepanocytory (anti-sickling) effects in erythrocytes taken from sickle cell anaemia patients; the ethanolic extract was more potent than the aqueous extract.[18]

In vivo (<u>non-human animals</u>): Aqueous extract of *C. pentandra* <u>bark</u> administered to streptozotocin-induced diabetic rats as their drinking water over twenty-eight days (ad libitum) significantly reduced their plasma glucose levels without any signs of hepatotoxicity.[21] Likewise, both aqueous and ethanolic extracts of *C. pentandra* bark administered twice daily at 75 and 150mg/kg to streptozotocin-induced type 2 diabetic rats on a high-fat diet reduced hyperglycaemia up to 62% over nine days of treatment. The bark extracts also significantly improved oral glucose tolerance, pancreas weight, cholesterol and triglyceride levels, and reduced hepatic malonaldehyde while conserving glutathione; at the higher dose, the extracts outperformed the reference drug, 30mg/kg metformin.[27] A group of dexamethasone-induced insulin-resistant rats were orally dosed at 75 or 150mg/kg with a solid aqueous extract *C. pentandra* bark, significantly improving the test animals' glucose tolerance, plamsa lipid profiles, and oxidative status, without affecting their blood pressure or heart rate.[28] A measure of 400mg/kg of orally administered pre-dosed *C. pentandra* ethyl acetate stem bark extract protected rats against paracetamol-induced hepatotoxicity, significantly reducing elevation in liver enzymes, bilirubin, and the severity of histopathological lesions compared to the untreated group, only marginally less effectively than 100mg/kg oral silymarin. The same study found no acute toxicity from up to 2g/kg orally administered ethyl acetate solid extract in the rats.[26] Measures of 15 and 30mg/kg intraperitoneal doses of petroleum ether, acetone, and ethanolic extracts of *C. pentandra* bark given to mice with Ehrlich ascites carcinoma (undifferentiated cancer cell model) or Dalton's lymphoma ascites (T-cell lymphoma model) improved outcomes: all extracts caused significant improvement in Dalton's lymphoma ascites mice, with significant reduction in tumour volume and more than 50% reduction in tumour weight by the thirtieth day; in the Ehrlich ascites carcinoma model, only the petroleum ether and acetone extracts significantly improved survival time and retarded cancer progression symptoms (tumour-induced ascites-dependent bodyweight increase).[29] A toxicological study in mice found that the intravenous acute LD_{50} for <u>leaf</u> extracts was a huge dose of 5g/kg bodyweight, and a twenty-one-day graded dose for chronic toxicity ranging from 250 to 500mg/kg found no change in weight gain or haematological and serum biochemical parameters such as urea, liver enzymes, PCV, or bilirubin, indicating very low toxicity.[22] However, 5% raw or dried *C. pentandra* <u>seed</u> content in the diet of day-old broiler chickens caused a 20–58% decrease in weight gain over a four-week period compared to the control group, with a reduction in PCV and haemoglobin only partially reversed by nutrient supplementation,[23] and a separate study found that *C. pentandra* seed meal at 7, 14, or 21% of the diet caused lower bodyweight and reduced food intake at nine weeks in broiler chicks.[24]

Summary of actions: <u>Seeds</u>: pro-fertility (?—traditional use only); <u>Bark</u>: anti-diabetic, hypo-glycaemic, hepatoprotective, antioxidant, anti-tumour (anti-neoplastic), astringent. <u>Leaves</u>: possibly anti-diabetic, anti-sickling; anti-neoplastic (?—traditional use and research on bark extracts).

Indications: *Internal*: <u>Bark</u>: adjunctive treatment in type 2 diabetes, hypercholesterolaemia; possibly adjunctive treatment in breast cancer, lymphomas, or metastatic cancers; poly-drug use or hepatic impairment (to protect liver); acute or chronic diarrhoea (astringent). <u>Leaves</u>: adjunct in sickle cell anaemia and diabetes; traditional use in fatigue.

    Topical: <u>Leaves</u>: traditional—poultice for malignant tumours (adjunctive use only).

Cautions: <u>Seeds</u>—note toxicity in broiler chicks—do not over-consume. Occasional use should be safe. Leaves and bark appear to be safer. Avoid taking at the same time as iron supplements or other medicines (particularly alkaloid-containing drugs) due to the tannin content.

Dose, preparation, and use with Cacao: <u>Seeds</u> are toasted and combined with Cacao in traditional Cacao-based drink *Chocolatl* (see Chapter 8 for formula). THE FOLLOWING DOSES ARE ESTIMATED: *Internal*: <u>Bark</u>—for diabetes, a bark decoction of 5–15g dried bark in 1–2L water administered daily (adult dose); or finely powdered bark, 10—20g per day in divided doses as a cancer adjunct or for hepatoprotective purposes. <u>Leaves</u>: a handful of fresh leaves pounded in water and strained to treat fatigue (traditional formulation); tincture: 25–45% ethanol, 1:3, 30–140ml per week as adjunctive anti-diabetic or anti-sickling treatment.

    Topical: Fresh leaf poultice for solid tumours, pounded and applied; or, oil expressed from seeds may be used to make a paste with powdered dried leaves, and applied to a clean tumour surface, using a film of clean surgical gauze if there's an open wound, to avoid risk of infection.

References

1. Avendaño, A., Casas, A., Dávila, P., & Lira, R. (2006). Use forms, management and commercialization of "pochote" Ceiba aesculifolia (H.B. & K.) Britten & Baker f. subsp. parvifolia (Rose) P.E. Gibbs & Semir (Bombacaceae) in the Tehuacán Valley, Central Mexico. *Journal of Arid Environments, 67*: 15–35.
2. Monroy-Ortiz, C., & Castillo-España, P. (2007). *Plantas medicinales Utilizadas en el estad de Morelos*. 2nd edition. Cuernavaca, Mexico: Universidad Autonoma del Estado de Morelos.
3. Ceiba aesculifolia—Kunth (Britten & Baker). (2019). *Plants for a Future*. https://pfaf.org/User/Plant.aspx?LatinName=Ceiba+aesculifolia [Accessed 1 March 2019].
4. *CEIBA PENTANDRA (Linn.) Gaertn. BUBOI*. (2009). http://bpi.da.gov.ph/Publications/mp/pdf/b/buboi.pdf [Accessed 19 November 2009].
5. *Ceiba acuminata*. (2009). http://arboretum.arizona.edu/ethnobotany-heritage_trees.html [Accessed 19 November 2009].
6. Entry for Ceiba pentandra (Linn.) Gaertn. (family BOMBACACEAE). (2010). *Royal Botanic Gardens, Kew: Useful Plants of West Tropical Africa*. http://aluka.org/action/showMetadata?doi=10.5555/AL.AP.UPWTA.1_561&pgs=&cookieSet=1 [Accessed 27 January 2010].
7. Ocean currents carried kapok seeds from South America to Africa. (2010). National Science Foundation. http://sciencecentric.com/news/article.php?q=07061701 [Accessed 27 January 2010].

8. Kinda, P., Zerbo, P., Guenné, S., Compaoré, M., Ciobica, A., & Kiendrebeogo, M. (2017). Medicinal plants used for neuropsychiatric disorders treatment in the Hauts Bassins region of Burkina Faso. *Medicines, 4*(2): 32.

9. Ethnobotanical uses: *Ceiba pentandra* GAERTN. (BOMBACACEAE); Chemicals. (2009). *Dr. Duke's Phytochemical and Ethnobotanical Databases.* http://ars-grin.cov/cgi-bin/duke/farmacy2.pl [Accessed 19 November 2009].

10. Kishore, P., Reddy, M., Gunasekar, D., Caux, C., & Bodo, B. (2003). A new naphthoquinone from Ceiba pentandra. *Journal of Asian Natural Products Research, 5*(3): 227–230.

11. Ueda, H., Kaneda, N., Kawanishi, K., Alves, S., & Moriyasu, M. (2002). A new isoflavone glycoside from Ceiba pentandra (L.) Gaertner. *Chemical & Pharmaceutical Bulletin (Tokyo), 50*(3): 403–404.

12. Odonne, G., Berger, F., Stien, D., Grenand, P., & Bourdy, G. (2011). Treatment of leishmaniasis in the Oyapock basin (French Guiana): A K.A.P. survey and analysis of the evolution of phytotherapy knowledge amongst Wayãpi Indians. *Journal of Ethnopharmacology, 137*(3): 1228–1239.

13. Vieira, T., Said, A., Aboutabi, E., Azzam, M., & Creczynski-Pasa, T. (2009). Antioxidant activity of methanolic extract of Bombax ceiba. *Redox Report, 14*(1): 41–46.

14. Noreen, Y., el-Seedi, H., Perera, P., & Bohlin, L. (1998). Two new isoflavones from Ceiba pentandra and their effect on cyclooxygenase-catalyzed prostaglandin biosynthesis. *Journal of Natural Products, 61*(1): 8–12.

15. Rao, K., Sreeramulu, K., Gunasekar, D., & Ramesh, D. (1993). Two new sesquiterpene lactones from Ceiba pentandra. *Journal of Natural Products, 56*(12): 2041–2045.

16. Kubmarawa, D., Ajoku, G., Enwerem, N., & Okorie, D. (2007). Preliminary phytochemical and antimicrobial screening of 50 medicinal plants from Nigeria. *African Journal of Biotechnology, 6*(15): 1690–1696.

17. Oyedemi, S., Oyedemi, B., Ijeh, I., Ohanyerem, P., Coopoosamy, R., & Aiyegoro, O. (2017). Alpha-amylase inhibition and antioxidative capacity of some antidiabetic plants used by the traditional healers in Southeastern Nigeria. *Scientific World Journal*, Article ID: 3592491. https://hindawi.com/journals/tswj/2017/3592491/ [Accessed 3 March 2019].

18. Mpiana, P., Tshibangu, D., Shetonde, O., & Ngbolua, K. (2007). In vitro antidrepanocytary activity (anti-sickle cell anemia) of some Congolese plants. *Phytomedicine, 14*(2–3): 192–195.

19. Fofie, C., Wansi, S., Nguelefack-Mbuyo, E., Atsamo, A., Watcho, P., Kamanyi, A., Nole, T., & Nguelefack, T. (2014). In vitro anti-hyperglycemic and antioxidant properties of extracts from the stem bark of Ceiba pentandra. *Journal of Complementary and Integrative Medicine, 11*(3): 185–193.

20. Nsimba, M., Yamamoto, C., Lami, J., Hayakawa, Y., & Kaji, T. (2013). Effect of a Congolese herbal medicine used in sickle cell anemia on the expression of plasminogen activators in human coronary aortic endothelial cells culture. *Journal of Ethnopharmacology, 146*(2): 594–599.

21. Ladeji, O., Omekrah, I., & Solomon, M. (2003). Hypoglycemic properties of aqueous bark extract of Ceiba pentandra in streptozotocin-induced diabetic rats. *Journal of Ethnopharmacology, 84*(2–3): 139–142.

22. Sarkiyayi, S., Ibrahim, S., & Abubakar, M. (2009). Toxicological studies of *Ceiba pentandra* linn. *African Journal of Biochemistry Research, 3*(7): 279–281.

23. Thanu, K., Kadirvel, R., & Ayyaluswami, P. (1983). The effect of nutrient supplementation on the feeding value of kapok seed for poultry. *Animal Feed Science and Technology, 9*(4): 263–269.

24. Kategile, J. A., Ishengoma, M., & Katule, A. M. (1978). The use of kapok (*Ceiba pentandra*) seed cake as a source of protein in broiler rations. *Journal of the Science of Food and Agriculture, 29*(4). doi.org/10.1002/jsfa.2740290404 https://onlinelibrary.wiley.com/doi/abs/10.1002/jsfa.2740290404 [Accessed 4 March 2019].

25. Narahari, D., & Asha Rajini, R. (2003). Chemical composition and nutritive value of kapok seed meal for broiler chickens. *British Poultry Science, 44*(3): 505–509.
26. Bairwa, N., Sethiya, N., & Mishra, S. (2010). Protective effect of stem bark of Ceiba pentandra linn. Against paracetamol-induced hepatotoxicity in rats. *Pharmacognosy Research, 2*(1): 26–30.
27. Fofie, C., Katekhaye, S., Borse, S., Sharma, V., Nivsarkar, M., Nguelefack-Mbuyo, E., Kamanyi, A., Singh, V., & Nguelefack, T. (2019). Antidiabetic properties of aqueous and methanol extracts from the trunk bark of Ceiba pentandra in type 2 diabetic rat. *Journal of Cellular Biochemistry.* https://onlinelibrary.wiley.com/doi/abs/10.1002/jcb.28437 [Accessed 4 March 2019].
28. Fofié, C., Nguelefack-Mbuyo, E., Tsabang, N., Kamanyi, A., & Nguelefack, T. (2018). Hypoglycemic properties of the aqueous extract from the stem bark of Ceiba pentandra in dexamethasone-induced insulin resistant rats. *Evidence Based Complementary and Alternative Medicine.* https://hindawi.com/journals/ecam/2018/4234981/ [Accessed 4 March 2019].
29. Kumar, R., Kumar, N., Ramalingayya, G. V., Setty, M. M., Pai, K. S. R. (2016). Evaluation of Ceiba pentandra (L.) Gaertner bark extracts for in vitro cytotoxicity on cancer cells and in vivo antitumor activity in solid and liquid tumor models. *Cytotechnology, 68*(5): 1909–1923.

Chiranthodendron pentadactylon Larreat.

Common names: Flor de la Manita, Palo de Yaco, Mano de Leon, Hand Flower, Devil's Hand Flower, Macpalxochitl, Mapilxochitl (Nahuatl), Teyacua, Mapasuchil, Canak, Palo de tayyo, Ranac, Tayuyo, Papasuchil, Teyagua.[3]

Plant family: Sterculiaceac.

Habit & habitat: Grows in temperate zones in Mexico and Guatemala; also grows wild in Chiapas and Oaxaca. High humidity, 2000–3000 metres above sea level in "cloud forests".[3] Tree, twelve to

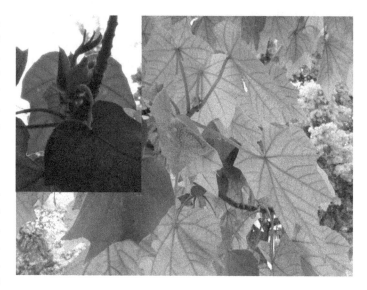

fifteen metres tall; has simple, alternate, three—to seven-lobed leaves, deeply five-lobed flowers with five distinctive, bright red stamens—hence the name of the plant.[1] Bat-pollinated, 3–4" oblong, five-lobed capsule-shaped fruit with black seeds.[17]

Cultivation: Flowers August–December. Seed rapidly loses viability in storage, becoming sterile after two months at 4°C,[13] so should be planted as soon as possible after harvest, soaking them in water for twelve to twenty-four hours beforehand. Likes well-drained moist soil of low to neutral pH in full sun. Prefers high humidity, tolerates light frost.[18]

Parts used: Flowers, leaves, and bark.

Phytochemistry: Flavonoids (incl. catechin, epicatechin, isoquercitrin, astragalin, tiliroside), Sterols,[9] Lectin.[14]

Traditional use: In contemporary folk medicine, the plant is regarded as being temperate, and having "cordial" (tonic, restorative) properties. The <u>flower</u> infusion is used to treat nervous problems, epilepsy, "heart issues", and dysentery.[1,3] *C. pentadactylon* flowers are combined with four other herbs—*Citrus sinensis* flowers, and aerial parts of *Passiflora incarnata*, *Ternstroemia pringlei*, and *Valeriana edulis*—"three fingers" of which should be boiled in a glass of water and drunk before each meal to treat insomnia. The <u>bark</u> and <u>leaves</u> form part of a magico-medical Mexica prescription against "pubic pain", in which an unguent is made from their expressed juice combined with the juice of *Datura meteloides*, brambles (*zarzas*), and another unknown herb, to be mixed with the blood of a swallow, a lizard, and a mouse, to which is added an obsidian blade, flint, and another stone, all warmed together.[2] More prosaically, the <u>leaves</u> were cooked with honey and applied to treat haemorrhoids, or a mixed infusion of flowers, leaves, and bark used as an ophthalmic wash and to treat chronic ulcers.[3] The leaves are also used as wraps for tamales in contemporary Mexico and Guatemala, as they are edible and impart their own flavour.[16]

Scientific data: *In vitro*: Ethanol and dichloromethane extracts of *C. pentadactylon* <u>flowers</u> inhibited replication of *Herpes simplex* virus type 1 and vesicular stomatitis viruses with minimal cellular toxicity, at 12.5–50µg/ml for the ethanol extract.[4] Aqueous flower extract also inhibited *Pseudomonas aeruginosa* replication at low concentrations, around 10µg/ml,[5] and solid extracts from the flowers made with methanol and water inhibited the replication of eight bacteria known to cause diarrhoea and dysentery (including *Escherichia coli*, four *Shigella* species, and two *Salmonella* species).[7] A methanol solid extract of the flowers also possessed significant anti-protozoal activity against *Entamoeba histolytica* at an IC_{50} of 2.5µg/ml, equipotent to the reference drug Emetine, and was somewhat effective against *Giardia lambla* (IC_{50} 44.2µg/ml).[8] The most active anti-amoebic and anti-giardial compound was (-)-epicatechin, with tiliroside being moderately anti-protozoan, but more anti-bacterial than the reference compound chloramphenicol.[15] Aqueous flower extract was also found to inhibit noradrenaline-induced contractions in isolated rat aortic smooth muscle, albeit with low potency.[6] *C. pentadactylon* whole <u>leaf</u> crude extract (equivalent to evaporated juice) had anti-bacterial activity against *Escherichia coli*, *Pseudomonas aeruginosa*, and *Salmonella typhimurium*, while an acetone extract did not inhibit *Salmonella*, but did inhibit *Staphylococcus aureus*; ethanolic extracts inhibited none of the tested bacteria.[12]

    In vivo (<u>non-human animals</u>): Methanolic and ethanolic solid extracts of *C. pentadactylon* <u>flowers</u> inhibited *Vibrio cholerae*-stimulated rat jejunal secretions, with the most active flavonoid fraction being epicatechin.[9] A *C. pentadactylon* extract* inhibited induced small intestinal hyperperistalsis in rats with similar efficacy to the reference drug Loperamide, and a methanolic flower extract effectively prevented cholera-toxin stimulated diarrhoea in mice with an IC_{50} of 351mg/kg.[15] *C. pentadactylon* <u>leaf</u> aqueous extract had no acute or sub-chronic toxicity—acute doses up to 6300mg/kg or dosing for twenty-eight days at 200mg/kg produced no symptoms of toxicity, nor were there any histopathological signs of organ damage, although all rats in the twenty-eight day group incrementally gained weight.[11]

Summary of actions: Anti-diarrhoeal, astringent, anti-amoebic, anti-protozoal, bacteriostatic; sedative, and anxiolytic (?), anabolic; topically antiviral.

Indications: *Internal*: <u>Flowers</u>: infectious diarrhoea, amoebiasis, giardiasis; anxiety, palpitations of nervous origin. <u>Leaves</u>: infectious diarrhoea, weight loss (to assist gain).

    Topical: <u>Flowers</u>: cream or non-polar extract for herpes simplex lesions; <u>leaf</u>: whole leaf juice against bacterial skin infections, ulcers; haemorrhoids; <u>leaves</u> and <u>bark</u> as a vulnerary wash.

Cautions: None noted. A very safe plant with low toxicity; flowers and leaves are edible.

Dose, preparation, and use with Cacao: *Internal*: <u>Flowers</u> are dried and ground with cocoa liquor as a chocolate drink spice; larger quantities may be used in unsweetened chocolate as an effective anti-dysenteric. THE FOLLOWING DOSES ARE ESTIMATED. Tincture, 25–40% ethanol, 1:3, approx. 20–40ml per week, or 5ml o.h. for acute doses. For aqueous infusion (tea), a handful of dried flowers per cup for anti-diarrhoeal action, less than that (1–2 tsp) for anxiety and palpitations. <u>Bark</u>: unknown, presumably in decoction. <u>Leaf</u>: similar dose to dried flowers, or cooked and eaten with food.

External: <u>Flowers</u> as infused oil or cream against Herpes simplex; <u>leaf</u> juice incorporated into a cream for bacterial skin infections, or whole dried leaf applied as a fine powder to wet ulcers; strong decoction of <u>leaf</u> and <u>bark</u> as a vulnerary wash.

*Note: abstract only—plant part or excipient unknown. The full article was unavailable unless purchased for an outrageous price, which I elected not to do.

References

1. Linares, E., Bye, R., & Flores, B. (1999). *Plantas Medicinales de Mexico—usos y remedios tradicionales.* Mexico City: Universidad Nacional Autonoma de Mexico, Instituto de Biologia.
2. Badiano, J. (1552). *Libellus de Medicinalibus Indorum Herbis.* M. de la Cruz (Trans.). Mexico: Fondo de Cultura Economica Instituto Mexicano del Seguro Social, 1996.
3. *Canak a sacred, edible and medicinal tree of Guatemala. A heritage from the Maya.* http://maya-ethnobotany.org/utilitarian-plant-fiber-medicinal-plant-mayan-ethnobotanicals-guatemala-el-salvador-honduras-mexico/images-photos-canak-chiranthodendron-pentadactylon-flowers-tree-leaves.php [Accessed 9 November 2017].
4. Abad, M., Bermejo, P., Villar, A., Palomino, S., & Carrasco, L. (1997). Antiviral activity of medicinal plant extracts. *Phytotherapy Research, 11*: 198–202.
5. Huerta, V., Mihalik, K., Crixell, S., & Vattem, D. (2008). Herbs, spices and medicinal plants used in Hispanic traditional medicine can decrease quorum sensing dependent virulence in *Pseudomonas aeruginosa. International Journal of Applied Research in Natural Products, 1*(2): 9–15.
6. Perusquia, M., Mendoza, S., Bye, R., Linares, E., & Mata, R. (1995). Vasoactive effects of aqueous extracts from five Mexican medicinal plants on isolated rat aorta. *Journal of Ethnopharmacology, 46*: 63–69.
7. Alanis, A., Calzada, F., Cervantes, A., Torres, J., & Ceballos, M. (2005). Antibacterial properties of some plants used in Mexican traditional medicine for the treatment of gastrointestinal disorders. *Journal of Ethnopharmacology, 100*: 153–157.
8. Calzada, F., Yepez-Mulia, L., & Aguilar, A. (2006). *In vitro* susceptibility of *Entamoeba histolytica* and *Giardia lambla* to plants used in Mexican traditional medicine for the treatment of gastrointestinal disorders. *Journal of Ethnopharmacology, 108*(3): 367–370.
9. Velazquez, C., Calzada, F., Esquivel, B., Barbosa, E., & Calzada, S. (2009). Antisecretory activity from the flowers of *Chirnathodendron pentadactylon* and its flavonoids on intestinal fluid accumulation induced by *Vibrio cholera* toxin in rats. *Journal of Ethnopharmacology, 126*(3): 455–458.
10. Calzada, F., Arista, R., & Pérez, H. (2010). Effect of plants used in Mexico to treat gastrointestinal disorders on charcoal-gum acacia-induced hyperperistalsis in rats. *Journal of Ethnopharmacology, 128*(1): 49–51.
11. González, E., Silva, C., Marin, B., Rodríguez, M., Hernández, A., & Navarro, B. (2014). Acute and sub chronic toxicity of *Chiranthodendron pentadactylon* leaves extracts in rats. *Planta Medica, 80*–P2B2.
12. Silva, C., González, E., Marin, B., Hernández, A., & Navarro, B. (2014). Antibacterial activity of *Chiranthodendron pentadactylon* leaves extracts. *Planta Medica, 80*–P2B51.

13. García-Franco, J., & Perales Rivera, H. (1990). Nota sobre la propagación y pérdida de viabilidad de las semillas de *Chiranthodendron pentadactylon* Larr. (Sterculiaceae). *Boletín de la Sociedad Botánica de México, 50*: 157–159, ref. 5.

14. Navarro, B., Ponce, J., Leticia, P., Rodriguez, V., & Hernández, A. (2012). Purification and characterization of a lectin from the hand flower tree (*Chiranthodendron pentadactylon*). *FEBS Journal, 279 Supp.* 1: 77.

15. Calzada, F., Juárez, T., García-Hernández, N., Valdes, M., Ávila, O., epez Mulia, L., & Velázquez, C. (2017). Antiprotozoal, antibacterial and antidiarrheal properties from the flowers of *Chiranthodendron pentadactylon* and isolated flavonoids. *Pharmacognosy Magazine, 13*(50): 240–244.

16. Photos Chiranthodendron pentadactylon flower canac manitas Aztec cacao chocolate flavoring medicine. *FLAAR*. http://maya-ethnobotany.org/images-mayan-ethnobotanicals-medicinal-plants-tropical-agriculture-flower-spice-flavoring/photos-chiranthodendron-pentadactylon-flower-canac-manitas-aztec-cacao-chocolate-flavoring-medicine.php [Accessed 13 November 2017].

17. The Devil's Hand Tree Chiranthodendron pentadactylon. https://gardenofeaden.blogspot.co.uk/2014/03/the-devils-hand-tree-chiranthodendron.html [Accessed 13 November 2017].

18. Devil's Hand Tree (Mexican Hand Tree) Chiranthodendron pentadactylon. Growing the seeds. http://strangewonderfulthings.com/tips170.htm [Accessed 13 November 2017].

19. Monroy-Ortiz, C., & Castillo-España, P. (2007). *Plantas medicinales Utilizadas en el estad de Morelos*. 2nd edition. Mexico: Universidad Autonoma del Estado de Morelos.

Cymbopetalum penduliflorum (Dunal) Baill.

Common names: Flor de Oreja, Orejuela, "Ear Flower", Muc' (Kek'chi),[15] Tzchiquin Itz, Hueinacaztli, Teonacaztli, Xochinacaztli (Nahuatl).[1]

Plant family: Annonaceae

Habit & habitat: Tropical lowland (wet) forests below 800m altitude in southern Mexico, Guatemala, Honduras, and Belize; tree up to 30 foot/13 metres high, bole 25cm+ diameter, pyramidal or spreading crown, deep green glossy semi-lanceolate leaves up to 10cm long; flowers March–June. Distinctive, large (up to 6cm across) greenish-yellow pendant flowers with thick leathery petals.[4,10]

Cultivation: Unknown.

Parts used: Dried flower petals.

Phytochemistry: Fat (27.6% dry weight);[6] resins; alkaloids, incl. the pyrrole alkaloid, funebrine, and the oxoaporphine alkaloid, liriodenine; flavonoids, incl. rhamnazin-3-O-rutinoside;[7] essential oil, containing tetracyclic triterpenoids, incl. ishwarone.[8]

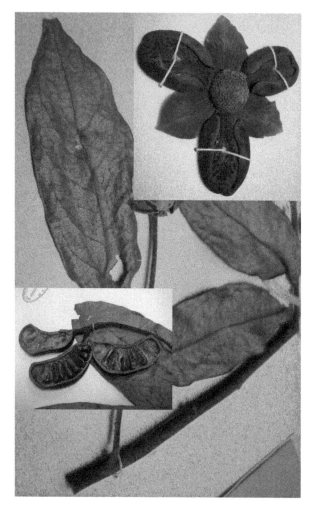

Note: Classified as an endangered species by the International Union for Conservation of Nature (IUCN) in 1998, though the tree's habitat range is larger than initially suspected.[11]

Traditional use: The Spanish chronicler and early ethnobotanist Fray Bernardino de Sahagun wrote of *C. peduliflorum* that the aromatic flowers added to chocolate drinks "inebriate like the mushrooms".[9] *C. peduliflorum* <u>flowers</u> formed part of a multi-ingredient magico-medical Mexica prescription, as an external wash against "the fatigue of those who administer the republic" (see *Bourreria huanita* monograph for details), as also for making a purely magical amulet "for travellers", where dried *C. penduliflorum* flowers were pulverised together with dried *Piper sanctum* and *Magnolia mexicana* flowers, *Vanilla planifolia* fermented seed pods, *Cyrtocarpa procera* bark, and three unknown plants, placed inside a *Xanthosmia sp.* flower, which was then enclosed in a whole *Talauma mexicana* flower and hung around the neck.[2] According to the seventeenth-century Spanish physician Francisco Hernández: "There is nothing else in the … markets of the

Indians more frequently found nor more highly prized than this flower."[12] Hernández described dried *C. penduliflorum* flowers as hot and dry in the fourth degree (similar to chillies, mustard, or garlic), and wrote that they thin phlegm, aid the heart, and in combination with toasted and de-seeded chillies are helpful in asthma; when added to chocolate, they make it more "thirst quenching" and "healthy".[5] Seventeenth-century English physician Henry Stubbe reported that *C. penduliflorum* flowers "improve chocolate far beyond its selfe" and aid digestion, "beget good blood", and have "cordial" properties—strengthening the "heart and vital spirits".[3]

Scientific data: <u>*In vitro*</u>: The alkaloid funebrine is also found in the chocolate spice *Quararibea funebris*,[13] but there is no research into its pharmacological properties; similarly, no pharmaceutical data exists for ishwarone, though it is a component of several medicinal plants. Liriodenine has some anti-microbial properties, being anti-fungal against pathogenic fungi *Candida albicans* and *Aspergillus niger* as well as several wood-rotting fungi, and inhibitory to *Staphylococcus aureus* (including methicillin-resistant *S. aureus*) with an IC_{50} of 2/3.13µg/ml. Liriodenine also has some anti-tumour activity against various cell lines (KA, A-549, HCT-8, and P-388, all at an IC_{50} <5µM, and L-1210, IC_{50} <10 µM) including melanoma, colon, lung, and breast cancer cell lines, via topoisomerase II inhibition and enhanced nitric oxide production, as well as complexing with metals such as copper and zinc to form cytotoxic topoisomerase I inhibitors. Liriodenine inhibits tracheal muscle spasm and platelet aggregation, has cardiac anti-arrhythmic properties and minimises cardiac ischaemia-reperfusion injury by elevating nitric oxide production. Liriodenine appears to possess sedative, anti-dopaminergic properties, protecting against dopamine-induced neurotoxicity.[14]

Summary of actions: Possibly: anxiolytic, anti-asthmatic, anti-arrhythmic, cardioprotective, sedative, anti-microbial vs. *Aspergillus niger*, *Candida albicans*, and *Staphylococcus aureus*; chemopreventive, possibly cytostatic.

Indications: Possibly: *Internal*: <u>Flowers</u>: anxiety, asthma, palpitations or cardiac arrhythmia; to assist recovery following myocardial infarction; adjunctive treatment of candidiasis and aspergillosis; cancer prevention. For asthma, cardiac recovery, and cancer prevention, administration with Cacao would be especially indicated.

Topical: <u>Flowers</u>: Apply as a fine dusting powder to sores or wet wounds, or to dry skin in the form of a cream (including polar and non-polar extract of dried flower petals) to treat *Staphylococcus aureus* skin infections, including MRSA.

Cautions: None known.

Dose, preparation, and use with Cacao: *Internal*: <u>Flowers</u>: dried petals are pulverised and ground into cocoa liquor for use in chocolate drinks. THE FOLLOWING DOSES ARE ESTIMATED. For medicinal purposes, half to one teaspoon of pulverised flower petals may be used, thrice daily; or a 1:3 tincture in 40% ethanol, at a dose of 20–50ml per week.

Topical: <u>Flowers</u>: finely sieved powder, as above; or, as a water-in-oil cream: an aromatic water distilled from dried petals may be made and subsequently cold-infused with dried flowers to extract polar constituents; the dried flowers may be macerated in oil to extract non-polar constituents, then the two extracts used to make a cream.

References

1. Coe, S., & Coe, M. (1996). *The True History of Chocolate*. London: Thames & Hudson.
2. Badiano, J. (1552). *Libellus de Medicinalibus Indorum Herbis*. M. de la Cruz (Trans.). Mexico: Fondo de Cultura Economica Instituto Mexicano del Seguro Social, 1996.
3. Stubbe, H. (1662). *The Indian Nectar, or, A Discourse concerning chocolata*. London: J.C. for Andrew Crook.
4. Popenoe, W. (1919). Batido and other Guatamalan beverages prepared from Cacao. *American Anthropologist, 21*(4): 403–409.
5. Hernández, F. (1615). *Quatro Libros de la Naturaleza, Y Virtudes de las Plantas, y animales, que estan recevidos en el uso de Medicina en la Nueva España, y la Methodo, y correction, y preparacion, que para administrarlas se requiere con lo que el Doctor Francisco Hernández escrobo en lengua Latina*. F. Ximenez (Trans.). www.wdl.org/en/item/7334/200m/#group=1&page=1 [Accessed 25 January 2012].
6. Johns, T., & Romeo, J. (1997). Functionality of food phytochemicals. In: *Recent Advances in Phytochemistry, Volume 31*. New YorkUSA: Springer Science and Business Media.
7. I. Studies leading towards the total synthesis of funebrine. II. Liriodenine and rhamnazin-3-o-rutinoside from *Cymbopetalum penduliflorum* (Dunal) Baill. (annonaceae). https://elibrary.ru/item.asp?id=5907838 [Accessed 17 November 2017].
8. Teng, L., & De Bardeleben, J. (1971). A novel tetracyclic sesquiterpene from the oil of orejuela of *Cymbopetalum penduliflorum* (Dunal.). *Experientia, 27*(1): 14–15.
9. Ott, J. (1996). *Pharmacotheon: Entheogenic Drugs, Their Plant Sources and History*. Washington, DCUSA: Natural Products Co.
10. *Cymbopetalum penduliflorum*. http://tropical.theferns.info/viewtropical.php?id=Cymbopetalum+penduliflorum [Accessed 21 November 2017].
11. Linsky, J. (2017). *Cymbopetalum penduliflorum*. *Global Trees Campaign*. http://globaltrees.org/threatened-trees/trees/cymbopetalum-mayanum/ [Accessed 21 November 2017].
12. Safford, W. (1910). The Sacred Ear-Flower of the Aztecs: Xochinacaztli. *Annual Reports of the Smithsonian Institute*: 427–431. http://samorini.it/doc1/alt_aut/sz/saf/saf_xoc.htm [Accessed 21 November 2017].
13. Dong, Y., Pai, N., Ablaza, S., Yu, S., Bolvig, S., Forsyth, D., & Le Quesne, P. (1999). Quararibea metabolites, 4. Total synthesis and conformational studies of (±)-Funebrine and (±)-Funebral. *Journal of Organic Chemistry, 64*(8): 2657–2666.
14. Chen, C., Wu, H., Chao, W., & Lee, C. (2013). Review on pharmacological activities of liriodenine. *African Journal of Pharmacy and Pharmacology, 7*(18): 1067–1070.
15. Hellmuth, N. (2013). Edible flowers in the Mayan diet. *Revue, 22*(4): 65–66.

Gonolobus spp. (Cav.) Schult.[7]
(*G. niger, G. barbatus;* + other species?)

Common names: Chupipe,[3] Cahuayote, Papullo, Papuyut, Chuchamber, Cuchamber, Cuchampera,[9] Cuauhchayot (Nahuatl),[11] Cuayote, Gallinita, Chinchayote (*G. niger*);[1] Tlallayotli (*G. nummularius*);[4] Tlallantlacacuitlapilli (Nahuatl);[16] N'ched (Zapotec) (*G. barbatus*).

Plant family: Apocynaceae (Asclepidaceae)[2]

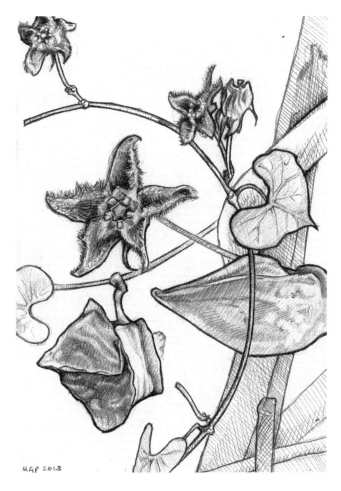

Habit & habitat: *G. niger* grows in the Veracruz region of Mexico, in dry forest and humid jungle, often over limestone.[9] It grows up to 2000 metres above sea level. A liana or climbing plant, thought to be a cross between the Frangipani (*Plumeria rubra*) and *Thevetia peruviana.* Thin, woody stems, opposite and ovate-elliptical leaves, clusters of 5–10 greenish flowers. Fruits September–November;[11] fruits are 10–12cm long and resemble small, four-sided or planed mangoes with angular "ribs". They are greenish when ripe, with white flesh,[5] but the core (where a mango stone would be) is filled with many seeds with a tuft of hair to assist wind dispersal. Flowers in May–September.[1]

Cultivation: Unknown. May prefer alkaline or chalky soil.

Parts used: Root,[2] seed husks,[3] fruit.[5]

Phytochemistry: Unknown. <u>All parts</u>: latex; <u>flower</u>: volatile oil–related species *G. barbatus*'s volatile oil is dominated by monoterpenoids, principally ocimene, with much lesser amounts of nitrogen-containing compounds such as benzylnitrite, benzenoids, and sesquiterpenoids.[14]

Traditional use: *G. niger* is principally used as a foaming agent in the contemporary Mexican *atole* of ancient origin called *Popo*. The fruits are eaten raw or fried with lemon and salt in Nicaragua and Costa Rica, or made into a sweet with cinnamon and sugar elsewhere in Central

America.[1] The semi-ripe fruit is made into a preserve by boiling it, throwing away the water, then re-boiling with sugar or *panela* until cooked;[11] seeds may be boiled or roasted and eaten.[15] All parts of the plant saving the fruit flesh are toxic, and to eat the fruits the ends are cut off and the latex is allowed to drain out before the flesh is scraped away from the skin.[9] The fresh roots are ground and used as the foaming agent in some regional variants of *Popo*; some *Popo* vendors use the ground skin or peel of the fruit.[3] The plant is said by some to be "cool" because ingesting excess fruit will cause diarrhoea, but other sources claim it is "warm" because the fruit flesh has a dry, astringent taste.[11] Hernández suggests that the root of the plant known as *tlallantlacacuitla-pilli* is "warm and moist", and half an ounce of powdered root taken with water, alone or mixed with *Pimienta dioica* seeds, helps urinary retention and "the kidneys and bladder"; a decoction of the roots, he avers, is sudorific and "relieves body pain".[16] A root decoction is used to treat gonorrhoea in contemporary Mexican folk medicine[10]—one glass taken three times daily.[11] The roots of the related species *G. nummularius* are used in contemporary Mexican ethnomedicine for "anti-microbial" properties in the (presumably) topical treatment of "ulcers".[4] The bark of related species *G. condurango* from Ecuador is used in treatments for cancer and chronic (second-ary and tertiary) syphilis.[7] The outer root bark of a *Gonolobus* species known locally as *N'ched* is used in the *atole* known as *Chaw Popox* in the Isthmus region of Oaxaca; *G. barbatus* appears to be the species in question, although this identification (made from my photos and drawing of the plant, above) has yet to be confirmed.

Scientific data: None. *In vitro*: Ethanolic extracts from related species *G. condurango* were dose-dependently cytotoxic to human cervical cancer cells (HeLa). The glycoside-A fraction specifi-cally caused DNA damage and accelerated cell senescence from 9–18 hours after exposure.[12] The ethanolic *G. condurango* whole plant extract had marked cytotoxicity to HeLa cells from concentrations of 75µg/ml, and it induced apoptosis by increasing ROS production and block-ing mitochondrial growth signals. Extracts were not cytotoxic to healthy liver cells (WRL-68) or mouse peripheral blood monocytes, but concentrations over 50µg/ml slowed cell proliferation. Higher concentrations had minor cytotoxicity against prostate cancer cells (PC3).[13]

Summary of actions: Uncertain. Possibly: *Internal*: <u>Roots</u>: diuretic, anti-inflammatory, febrifuge (traditional use); anti-neoplastic or cytostatic (*G. condurango*)?
   External: <u>Roots</u>: possibly: vulnerary, cicatrising.

Indications: Uncertain. Possibly: *Internal*: <u>Roots</u>: urinary retention (without mechanical obstruc-tion), UTIs, fibromyalgic pain (extrapolated from traditional uses); gonorrhoea (though must not be relied upon for this purpose); as an adjunct in cancers (to slow tumour growth). *External*: <u>Roots</u>: superficial ulceration.

Cautions: Uncertain. Latex is somewhat irritant and allegedly toxic. The plant is described as "poisonous",[1] so larger doses may cause diarrhoea and vomiting, though there are no incidents available on public record. The common name "Milkweed" is used to refer to related North American *Asclepias spp.* as well as some species of *Gonolobus*; while *Asclepias spp.* contain toxic cardiac glycosides, *Gonolobus spp.* do not,[17] so it's possible that some of its "poisonous" reputa-tion is through mis-identification.

Dose, preparation, and use with Cacao: *Internal*: Decorticated fresh inner root, or fresh skin of *G. niger* fruit is ground with toasted Cacao seeds[3] as a foaming agent.

Internal: <u>Roots</u>: Hernández recommends a heroic dose of 14–15g powdered root for urinary retention, taken in water, with or without some powdered Allspice (*Pimienta dioica*); for other purposes, three teaspoons of chopped dried root boiled in 1L water for 10–20 minutes, strained and drunk in divided doses (x3) throughout the day.

References

1. Gutierrez, L. (2014). *El Chupipe.* http://otromundoesposible.net/el-chupipe/ [Accessed 4 July 2018].
2. *Diccionario enciclopédico de la Gastronomía Mexicana* (2018). https://laroussecocina.mx/palabra/chupipi-o-chupipe/ [Accessed 4 July 2018].
3. 22 February 2011: Interview with Popo vendor, Acayuca, Veracruz, Mexico.
4. Monroy-Ortiz, C., & Castillo-España, P. (2007). *Plantas medicinales Utilizadas en el estad de Morelos.* 2nd edition. Mexico: Universidad Autonoma del Estado de Morelos.
5. Chocolate Popo: a Tasty Traditional Drink from Mexico (2018). http://extremechocolate.com/chocolate-popo-a-tasty-traditional-drink-from-mexico.html [Accessed 3 July 2018].
6. The Plant List (2010). *Kew Gardens, London UK* http://theplantlist.org/tpl/record/kew-2830118 [Accessed 28 July 2018].
7. Grieve, M. (1931). *A Modern Herbal.* Twickenham, UK: Tiger.
8. Gonolobus, an edible vine from Asclepiadaceae family (2011). *FLAAR,* Gauetamala. http://maya-ethnobotany.org/edible-nut-fruit-seed-tree-agroforestry-mayan-tropical-mayan-agriculture-diet-food-nutrition-health/cuchampera-gonolobus-asclepiadaceae-latex-vine.php [Accessed 30 July 2018].
9. Missouri Botanical Garden (2018). Flora Mesoamericana: *Gonolobus niger (Cav.) R. Br. Ex Schult.* http://www.tropicos.org/name/02609011?projectid=3 [Accessed 31 July 2018].
10. Gonzalez Stuart, A. (2004). Plants used in Mexican traditional medicine: Their application and effects in traditional healing practices. http://herbalsafety.utep.edu/wp-content/uploads/2016/09/Plants-Used-in-Mexican-Traditional-Medicine-July-04.pdf [Accessed 31 July 2018].
11. Alfaro, M., Oliva, V., Cruz, M., Olazcoaga, G., & Leon, A. (2001). *Catalogo de Plantas Utiles de la Sierra Norte de Puebla, Mexico.* Mexico City: Instituto de Biologia, UNAM.
12. Bishayee, K., Paul, A., Ghosh, S., Sikdar, S., Mukherjee, A ., Biswas, R., Boujedaini, N., & Khuda-Bukhsh, A. (2013). Condurango-glycoside-A fraction of *Gonolobus condurango* induces DNA damage associated senescence and apoptosis via ROS-dependent p53 signalling pathway in HeLa cells. *Molecular and Cellular Biochemistry, 382*(1–2): 173–183.
13. Bishayee, K., Mondal, J., Sikdar, S., & Khuda-Bukhsh, A. (2015). Condurango (*Gonolobus condurango*) extract activates fas receptor and depolarizes mitochondrial membrane potential to induce ROS-dependent apoptosis in cancer cells *in vitro. Pharmacopuncture, 18*(3): 32–41.
14. Jurgens, A., Dötterl, S., Liede-Schumann, S., & Meve, U. (2008). Chemical diversity of floral volatiles in Asclepiadoideae-Asclepiadeae (Apocynaceae). *Biochemical Systematics and Ecology, 36*: 842–852.
15. Juarez-Jaimes, V., Alvarado-Cardenas, L., & Villasenor, J. (2007). La familia *Apocynaceae sensu lato* en Mexico: diversidad y distribucion. *Revista Mexicana de Bioversidad, 78*: 459–482.

16. Hernández, F. (1943). *Historia de las Plantas de Nueva España*. I. Ochoterena (Ed.). Mexico City: Imprenta Universitaria. http://ibiologia.unam.mx/plantasnuevaespana/index.html [Accessed 6 August 2018].
17. Brower, L., Zandt Brower, J., & Corvino, J. (1967). Plant poisons in a terrestrial food chain. *Proceedings of the Natural Academy of Sciences of the United States of America, 57*(4): 893–898.

Magnolia mexicana DC. [Syn. (?) *Talauma mexicana; M. dealbata; M. (sp.?)*]

Common names: Three varieties sold as medicine in Mexico: Yolosúchil (*M. mexicana*), Magnolia (*M. dealbata*), Flor de Corazon (unknown species). Other names: Flor de Atole, Anonilla, Hierba de las Mataduras, Hualhua; Eloxochitl, Yolloxochitl (Nahuatl), Kuwi Xa'nat (Totonac), Guia-lacha-yati (Zapotec), Chocoijoyo (Zoque), Kul ak' (Lacandon Maya).[7]

Plant family: Magnoliaceae

Habit & habitat: Native to Mexico, grows in deciduous woodland, high altitude perennial forests, and southern tropical rain forests. In Mexico, mainly grows in north and north-eastern Chiapas, with populations in Oaxaca, Veracruz, and Puebla. The species is officially threatened by logging and deforestation.[8] It requires warm, moist environments 110–2900m above sea level. Tree up to 30m tall, with a rounded, compact canopy, greenish-grey bark with dark

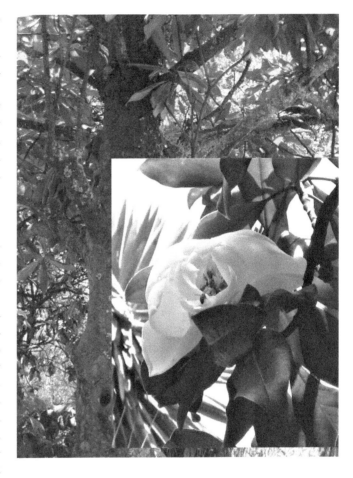

patches, deeply longitudinally furrowed and ribbed with leaf scars. Oblong to elliptical smooth shiny and leathery leaves, dark green underneath, 15–25cm long, 6.5–13cm wide. Flowers in March–July, distinctive, perfumed, with six thick white petals arranged in a spiral. Fruit is 10–15cm long, woody and red-ridged, looks like a custard apple; seeds are whitish with a red aril.[4,5,6,7]

Cultivation: Planted in autumn through to spring, requires full or at least partial sun and shelter in colder climates. Somewhat hardy, but requires temperatures above 5°C; flower buds may be frost-tender. Prefers dry, alkaline soils, tolerates wet and well-drained soil. If grown from seed, may take ten years to begin flowering; may also be propagated by cuttings or layering.[14]

Parts used: Flowers, bark, seeds.

Phytochemistry: Glycosides (incl. flavone glycoside quercitriol), alkaloids (incl. liriodenine, iso-quinolines such as talaumine), sesquiterpene lactones (incl. costunolide), sterols, essential oil, polyphenols[6] (incl. tannins; the quinone, 2-6-dimethoxy-1-4-benzoquinone[11]).

Traditional use: The Mexica name *Yolloxochitl* translates as "heart flower",[1] and the plant was traditionally used as a cordial—to restore emotional balance and alleviate symptoms such as palpitations.[6] Used as a spice with Cacao, and still used in contemporary Mexico to make *Atole de Magnolia*, *M. mexicana* <u>flowers</u> are "said to taste like ripe melon".[2] They are considered to have a warm or hot nature in Mesoamerican medicine.[10] The three "magnolias" sold in contemporary Mexico are different species: *Yolloxochitl* or yolosúchil (*M. mexicana?*) has a white, powerfully scented flower, which dries to a bright yellow colour, and retains a strong scent; *Flor de Corazon* has thicker petals, and dries to a scentless, hard, petrified-looking flower; and *Magnolia* (*M. dealbata?*) flowers dry to a mango-like hue with the appearance of thin slices of dried mango, with thinner petals and a delicate floral scent. *Yolloxochitl* was the variety used in Cacao-based drinks.[25] *M. mexicana* flowers (*yolloxochitl*, sold today as Yolosúchil), as well as *eloxochitl* (*M. dealbata*, sold today as Magnolia) were used in several magico-medical Mexica prescriptions, such as a preparation against fear or cowardice (see *Plumeria rubra* monograph, below), to prevent "losing one's mind" (see *Quararibea funebris* monograph, below) and "for the fatigue of those who administer the republic" (see *Bourreria huanita* monograph, above); they are also used in a purely magical formula to provide "help for travellers" (see *Cymbopetalum penduliflorum* monograph, above).[3] *M. mexicana* flowers were used to lower fever, and in treatments for paralysis, malaria, epilepsy, and gout.[6] According to seventeenth-century Spanish physician Francisco Hernández, they were used with Cacao to "comfort and cool the heart", and were of a "glutinous and astringent" nature, somewhat hot and dry. He recommended them to counter infectious diarrhoea and abdominal pain, against wind, and in combination with other herbs including *Piper sanctum* and *Vanilla planifolia* to "prevent sterility".[4,5] The flower may also have been used in combination with other plants as an anti-lithic "to clear the urinary passages".[4] Sixteenth-century Spanish physician Nicolas Monardes described use of fresh *M. mexicana* flower juice taken with Cacao as a remedy for melancholia, and advised that the best form of administration for treating diarrhoea is the toasted, pulverised dried flower given in water.[6] Another of Hernández's cotemporaries, the hermit Gregorio Lopez, commended the powdered flowers taken in wine against "flank pain", stomach pain, and urinary retention, and a decoction taken as an enema for bloody dysentery.[10] *M. mexicana* flowers are used in contemporary Mexican folk medicine for anxiety—4–5 thin slices of the flower infused in half a litre of water, and drunk in a divided dose (250ml, twice daily). Also used in combination with other herbs for insomnia and stress, palpitations with hypertension, heart disease, and "burning in the belly" (heartburn?).[4,5] A decoction of the flowers is used in combination with *Chiranthodendron pentadactylon* flowers to treat "cardiac rheumatism".[10] *M. mexicana* <u>seeds</u> and <u>bark</u> are reputed to strengthen the heart, the skeletal muscles, and the circulation.[4] The <u>bark</u> is used as a febrifuge and the <u>seeds</u> are used to treat paralysis in contemporary Mexican folk medicine,[7,8] while a syrup of the flowers is still used to prevent epilepsy.[8] The <u>bark</u> is also used as a tincture to treat the folk disease *susto* (fright), and, with other plants, to treat stomach pain, indigestion, head pain, dizziness, parasites, and *espanto* (a spiritual/physical folk sickness like *susto*, with some symptoms in common with hepatitis or renal failure).[10]

Scientific data: Like *Cymbopetalum penduliflorum*, *M. mexicana* contains the alkaloid liriodenine. What was written about this alkaloid in the *C. penduliflorum* monograph will therefore also apply here.

In vitro: Essential oil from related species *Magnolia grandiflora* leaves had anti-fungal activity, and anti-bacterial activity against *Staphylococcus aureus* and *Streptococcus pyogenes*.[12]

Ex vivo (non-human animals): A 1938 study of aqueous leaf extract showed reversible positively chronotropic and inotropic activity on frog hearts, and aqueous extracts of the flower had "digitalis-like" effects in rat hearts.[6] Hexane, dichloromethane, and ethanolic extracts of *M. mexicana* flowers had concentration-dependent relaxant effects on rat trachea, significant but less potent than theophylline, suggesting possible anti-asthmatic effects.[11] Aqueous extracts of aerial parts of *Magnolia grandiflora* induced concentration-dependent contraction of rat aortic rings; the authors suggested this may infer potential benefits for venous insufficiency.[13]

In vivo (non-human animals): Variable effects on blood pressure and heart rate depending on plant part and chemical fraction.[6] A 1956 experiment using hydroalcoholic tincture extract of unspecified plant parts in cats showed a "stimulant effect" on the "musculoskeletal system", "like digitalis". In 1982, an aqueous extract of dried leaf was found to be hypertensive in cats, while an ethanolic extract was hypotensive.[6]

In vivo (humans): Early experimentation with the <u>seeds</u> in 1891 showed they had beneficial effects in epilepsy, and according to a 1925 paper, a decoction of the <u>flowers</u> allegedly "promoted fertility" in women trying to conceive.[6] A clinical trial in 1938 showed that hydro- alcoholic extracts of <u>bark</u>, <u>leaves</u>, and <u>flowers</u> had positively inotropic, negatively chronotropic, and positively dromotropic action on the heart in mitral insufficiency, atherosclerosis, and cardiac hypertrophy.[6] These actions are typical of mild cardiac tonic plants such as Hawthorn (*Crataegus* sp.). Trials in 1977–80 using aqueous extracts of bark, leaves, and flowers "stimulated cardiac function" and "controlled cardiac disorders in adults".[6]

Summary of actions: *Internal*: <u>Flowers</u>: anxiolytic, anti-arrhythmic, cardiotonic, astringent, hypocholesterolaemic, hypotensive, antipyretic, anodyne; possibly anti-lithic (renal), anti-asthmatic, anti-seizure, neuroprotective. <u>Bark and seeds</u>: possibly: circulatory stimulant, anodyne, anti-inflammatory, antispasmodic, antipyretic, anxiolytic, neuroprotective.

External: <u>Flowers or leaves</u>: astringent and antimicrobial vs. dermatophytic fungi, *Staphylococcus aureus* and *Streptococcus pyogenes*.

Indications: *Internal*: <u>Flowers</u>: anxiety, palpitations, hypertension, hypercholesterolaemia, diarrhoea; possibly, heart failure, epilepsy, fevers, nephrolithiasis (prevention). <u>Bark</u>, possibly: vertigo, syncope, visceral pain.

Topical: <u>Leaves</u>: fungal skin infections, furunculosis, *Staphylococcal* skin infections.

Cautions: Uncertain. Hypothetical interaction with digitalis, anxiolytics, and sedatives, or anti-epileptic medications. Tannins may reduce the absorption of iron or other medications if ingested simultaneously, so should be taken apart from meals or any prescription medication.

Dose, preparation, and use with Cacao: *Internal*: <u>Flowers</u>: dried petals are pulverised and ground into cocoa liquor for use in chocolate drinks. THE FOLLOWING DOSES ARE ESTIMATED. By infusion, four to five slices of dried flower infused in 500mL boiling water for ten minutes, strained and drunk as 250ml, twice daily; estimated 2–6g in infusion each day. Or, a 1:3 tincture in 40% ethanol, at a dose of 20–50ml per week; higher doses for acute problems like diarrhoea or palpitations, 5–10ml per dose. <u>Bark</u>, 6g in decoction, daily; or 1:3 tincture in 40% ethanol, 20–50ml per week.

References

1. Coe, S., & Coe, M. (1996). *The True History of Chocolate*. London: Thames & Hudson.
2. Coe, S. (1994). *America's First Cuisines*. USA Austin, TX: University of Texas Press.
3. Badiano, J. (1552). *Libellus de Medicinalibus Indorum Herbis*. M. de la Cruz (Trans.). Mexico City: Fondo de Cultura Economica Instituto Mexicano del Seguro Social, 1996.
4. Linares, E., Bye, R., & Flores, B. (2000). *Plantas Medicinales de Mexico—usos y remedios tradicionales*. Mexico City: Universidad Nacional Autonoma de Mexico Instituto de Biologia.
5. Hernández, F. (1615). *Quatro Libros de la Naturaleza, Y Virtudes de las Plantas, y animales, que estan recevidos en el uso de Medicina en la Nueva España, y la Methodo, y correction, y preparacion, que para administrarlas se requiere con lo que el Doctor Francisco Hernández escrobo en lengua Latina*. F. Ximenez (Trans.). www.wdl.org/en/item/7334/200m/#group=1&page=1 [Accessed 25 January 2012].
6. Bucay, J. (2002). Uso tradicional e investigacion cientifica de *Talauma Mexicana* (D.C.) Don., o flor del corazon. *Revista Mexicana de Cardiologia, 13*(1): 31–38.
7. Yoloxóchitl (*Magnolia mexicana*). http://naturalista.mx/taxa/204973-Magnolia-mexicana [Accessed 13 January 2018].
8. Magnolia mexicana. The IUCN Red List of Threatened Species™ (2018). International Union for Conservation of Nature and Natural Resources. http://iucnredlist.org/details/193977/0 [Accessed 13 January 2018].
9. Magnolia is more than just beautiful: it is edible (seasoning for chocolate) and a respected medicinal plant; plus is very fragrant. (2018). https://maya-archaeology.org/cacao-cocoa-chocolate-seasoning-flavoring-ingredient-perfume-aromatheropy/magnolia-talauma-mexicana-medicinal-mayan-aztec-cacao-cocoa-chocolate-food-additive-flavor.php [Accessed 13 January 2018].
10. Atlas de las Plantas de la Medicina Tradicional Mexicana. (2009). *D.R. Biblioteca Digital de la Medicina Tradicional Mexicana*. http://www.medicinatradicionalmexicana.unam.mx/monografia.php?l=3&t=yolox%C3%B3chitl&id=7806 [Accessed 13 January 2018].
11. Sánchez-Recillas, A., Mantecón-Reyes, P., Castillo-España, P., Villalobos-Molina, R., Ibarra-Barajas, M., & Estrada-Soto, S. (2014). Tracheal relaxation of five medicinal plants used in Mexico for the treatment of several diseases. *Asian Pacific Journal of Tropical Medicine, 7*(3): 179–183.
12. Guerra-Boone, L., Alvarez-Román, R., Salazar-Aranda, R., Torres-Cirio, A., Rivas-Galindo, V., Waksman de Torres, N., González, G., & Pérez-López, L. (2013). Chemical compositions and antimicrobial and antioxidant activities of the essential oils from *Magnolia grandiflora, Chrysactinia mexicana*, and *Schinus molle* found in northeast Mexico. *Natural Products Communications, 8*(1): 135–138.

13. Ibarra-Alvarado, C., Rojas, A., Mendoza, S., Bah, M., Gutiérrez, D., Hernández-Sandoval, L., & Martínez, M. (2010). Vasoactive and antioxidant activities of plants used in Mexican traditional medicine for the treatment of cardiovascular diseases. *Pharmaceutical Biology, 48*(7): 732–739.
14. The Royal Horticultural Society. (2018). Magnolia. https://rhs.org.uk/advice/profile?PID=599 [Accessed 18 January 2018].
15. 23 September 2018: Interview with Sra Teresa Olivera, stallholder in mercado Benito Juarez, Oaxaca city, Oaxaca, Mexico.

Pimenta dioica (L.) Merr.[7]

Common names: Allspice, Pimiento Gordo, Jamaican pepper, Xocoxochitl (Nahuatl)[2]

Plant family: Myrtaceae[5]

Habit & habitat: An evergreen tree 6–12m tall, grows at 500–1300m above sea level. *P. dioica* has smooth, patchy outer bark, and yellowish inner bark; dark green leaves, 4–8cm long.[7] All parts of the plant are highly aromatic. Grows in deciduous and high altitude perennial forests in sub-temperate zones in Central America and the Carribean.[1,5] A dioecious plant, blooms in May–July with small creamy white flowers. Globular, brown seeds approx. 0.75cm diameter, with a rough coat and clove-like odour.[4]

Cultivation: Requires full sun, rich but well-drained and sandy soil; prefers alkaline or calcareous soils, and temperatures of 18–28°C. Propagated by cuttings in

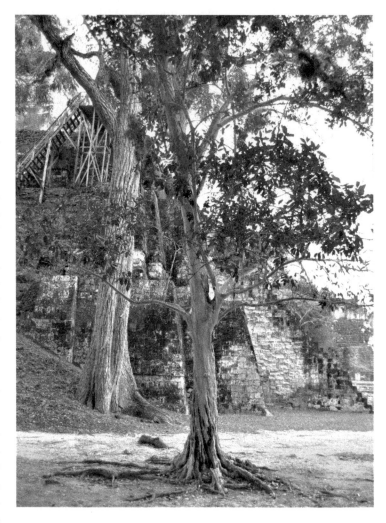

summer.[21] Moderately hardy but drought- and frost-tender, will be damaged in temperatures less than –2°C or if annual rainfall is below 1000mm.[22]

Parts used: Seeds, leaves.

Phytochemistry: Volatile oil, 3–4.5%,[4] [incl. eugenol (60–90%), methyl eugenol (4–10%), caryophyllene (3–5%)[14], thymol, pimentol, vanillin]; polyphenols [incl. tannins: pedunculagin,[7] vascalaginone, grandininol,[18] casuarinin, casuariin,[18] 1,2,3,6-tetra-O-galloylglucose, penta-O-galloylglucose; phenolic acids: syringic acid, gallic acid, ellagic acid, nilocitin, methyl gallate, methylflavogallate[18], ericifolin (eugenol 5-O-β-(6'- galloylglucopyranoside); polyphenolic glycosides: (2S)-3-(4-hydroxy-3-methoxyphenyl)-propane-1,2-diol 1-O-(6'-O-galloyl)-β-D-glucoside),[13] (4R)-,(4S)-terpineol 8-O-(60 -O-galloyl)-glucoside, (4R)-,(4S)-terpineol 8-O-[(200-O-galloyl)-

arabinosyl]-(1,6)-glucoside,[14] 2-hydroxy-3-methoxy-5-allyl)phenyl beta- d-(6-O-E- sinapoyl)gluco-pyranoside, (1′ R,5′ R)-5-(5-carboxymethyl-2-oxocyclopentyl)-3 Z -pentenyl beta-D-(6-O-galloyl) glucopyranoside, (S)-alpha-terpinyl [alpha-L-(2-O-galloyl)arabinofuranosyl]-(1-->6)-beta-D-glucopy-ranoside,(R)-alpha-terpinyl[alpha-L-(2-O-galloyl)arabinofuranosyl]-(1-->6)-beta-D-glucopyranoside,[17] 6-hydroxy-eugenol 4-O-(6′-O-galloyl)-beta-D-4C1-glucopyranoside, 3-(4-hydroxy-3-methoxyphenyl)-propane-1,2-diol-2-O-(2′,6′-di-O-galloyl)-beta-D-4C1-glucopyranoside[18]]; flavonoids: quercetin], Lig-nans, Terpenoids [incl. triterpenoid acids[8]].[13]

Traditional use: The dried <u>berries</u> are used as a spice in traditional Cacao beverages, and as a condiment. In contemporary Mexico, chocolate made with Allspice is recommended as a partu-rient for new mothers (first-time deliveries), alongside other herbs, although the Cacao content is kept low as too much chocolate is thought to increase inflammation during labour.[1] Dr Francisco Hernández, the seventeenth-century Spanish physician and chronicler, writes that *P. dioica* fruits are "bitter and sharp", hot and dry in the third degree (Galenical classification), almost black when ripe, and are cordial (antidepressant or enhancing vitality), emmenagogue, anti-emetic, diuretic, libido-enhancing, and carminative. He commends them in the treatment of bloody dysentery, and hypochondriac (flank) pain. He also mentions native use of an ambitious native medicine—impressive if it worked—a poultice applied to the shoulders made with *P. dioica*, an unspecified resin (Copal?), an unidentified substance called Colopatli, *Turbina corymbosa*, and a plant called Tetzitzicaztli, most likely a species of *Cnidoscolus*, to increase appetite, cure pains caused by "wind and cold" and treat "the swelling known as aneurism".[3] The seventeenth-century English physician Dr Henry Stubbe recommends Allspice berries, swallowed whole, as a carminative and digestive aid, and to freshen the breath; but, he says, once pulverised they create a "pretty violent heat", such that, in addition to the effects described by Hernández, they alleviate intestinal and renal colic, "consum[ing] cold and viscid humours".[2] In contemporary herbal medicine, the seeds are used in combination with other plants in treatment of diarrhoea, flatulence, and dyspepsia.[4] Allspice flannel poultices were used in Europe to treat neuralgia or rheumatism, following traditional use in Guatemala where crushed berries are applied to treat myalgia, bruising, and joint pain.[6,7] In Jamaica, Allspice tea is drunk to treat colds, dysmenor-rhoea, and hypertension, and in Costa Rica *P. dioica* is used to treat diabetes.[7] The plant has been incorporated into Indian Ayurvedic medicine, where it is used in preparations for respiratory congestion and toothache.[7]

Scientific data: <u>In vitro</u>: *P. dioica* berry essential oil produced 100% mortality in *Rhipicephalus microplus* tick larvae at concentrations above 1.25%, suggesting possibly Acaricidal utility in animal tick control.[15] Similarly, the essential oil had nematicidal activity against the pinewood nematode, *Bursaphelenchus* xylophilus;[19] whether it has similar activity against nematodes which are human pathogens is unknown. The essential oil also enhances trypsin activity,[4] suggesting it aids protein digestion but should be avoided in pancreatitis. Eugenol extracted from *P. dioica* essential oil is antimicrobial, specifically anti-fungal against *Candida albicans*, has anti-inflammatory activity via iCOX-2 and NF-KB pathways, and has anti-proliferative effects in HeLa (cervical cancer) cells with selective cytotoxicity.[7] Other compounds in *P. dioica* such as quercetin have antiviral, anti-cancer, and anti-inflammatory effects.[7] Ethyl acetate extracts of *P. dioica* fruits had strong radical-scavenging activity.[7] Powdered and lypophilised aqueous extract of *P. dioica* <u>berries</u> contained up to 35% polyphenols, of which ericifolin was found to be particularly anti-proliferative to prostate, breast, and pancreatic cancer cells.[7] Aqueous berry extract inhibited prostate tumour cell growth by 50% at concentrations of 40–85μg/ml, without affecting healthy cells.[12] Aqueous extract of *P. dioica* berries likewise had growth-inhibitory and cytotoxic effects on human breast cancer cells, failing to induce apoptosis but increasing markers of autophagy and inhibiting AKT/mTOR signalling, consequently enhancing the effectiveness of Rapamycin, a chemotherapeutic mTOR inhibitor.[10] *P. dioica* methanolic extract (plant part not specified) had selective-oestrogen receptor modifying effects, having antagonistic effects in MCF-7 breast cancer cells in the presence of oestradiol, suggesting possible chemopreventive effects in oestrogen-dependent breast cancer.[16] *P. dioica* extract, and principally the triterpene acids in the extract, activated bile acid receptor TGR5, associated with energy production, intestinal motility, and the pathogenesis or prevention of diabetes and obesity,[8] the activation of which diminishes monocyte-dependent inflammatory mediator production.[9] Ethyl acetate extracts of *P. dioica* fruits had concentration-dependent quorum-sensing inhibitory activity on *Chromobacterium* violaceum,[11] an occasionally pathogenic Gram-negative bacterium, suggesting potential utility in enteric bacterial infections. Polyphenols extracted from *P. dioica* <u>leaves</u> strongly inhibit replication of human Hep-G2 and HCT-116 cancer cells, with some effect on MCF-7 cells, implying potential utility in the chemoprevention or adjunctive treatment of liver, colon, and breast cancers, repectively.[7] Pedunculagin is the most cytotoxic against solid tumour cells, and induces macrophage and T-lymphocyte proliferation while inhibiting nitric oxide generation; grandinin stimulates T-lymphocytes most potently, while vascalaginone has the strongest macrophage-stimulating properties.[18]

In vivo (non-human animals): *P. dioica* aqueous extracts intravenously administered to anaesthetised rats at 30, 70, and 100mg/kg bodyweight had dose-dependent hypotensive, CNS depressant, analgesic, and hypothermic effects without affecting heart rate or body weight or causing other abnormalities. The ED50 was 53.94mg/kg. Aqueous extracts have stronger effects than ethanolic extracts, and CNS depression is dose-dependent; the hypotensive effect appears to be due to vasodilation, and is not mediated by effects on autonomic neurotransmitter (acetylcholine or adrenaline receptors).[7,20] Aqueous extracts of *P. dioica* berries administered at 150mg/kg bodyweight by oral gavage to athymic mice implanted with MDA-MB-231 human breast adenocarcinoma cells delayed tumour growth rate by 38% if the mice were pre-treated for two weeks, but only delayed tumour growth by 14% if administered post-implantation. By week seven post-implantation, only 25% of the untreated mice were still living; by comparison, 45% of the mice given only post-implantation treatment and 70% of the mice given pre- and post-implantation treatment were still living without loss of body weight, though their tumours continued to grow.[10] Similarly, athymic male mice implanted with LNCaP (androgen-sensitive prostate adenocarcinoma) cells had a 62.3% decrease in tumour volume and a 55% reduction in tumour growth without systemic toxicity when treated with aqueous extracts of *P. dioica* berries by daily gavage and intraperitoneal injection, respectively, at 100mg/kg bodyweight for 40–50 days following tumour cell implantation. Ericifolin was identified as the principal active constituent with anti-proliferative, pro-apoptotic, and anti-androgen receptor activities.[12]

Summary of actions: _Internal_: Carminative, diuretic; possibly hypotensive, anti-diabetic, anti-inflammatory, chemopreventive, and anti-proliferative, bacteriostatic (Gram-negative bacteria), antimicrobial, nematocidal, anodyne.

External: Analgesic, anti-inflammatory.

Indications: _Internal_: Flatulence and meteorism (bloating), pre-diabetes or diabetes mellitus, hypertension, infectious or post-antibiotic diarrhoea, candidiasis; possibly also nematode infestation, e.g., pinworms, trichuriasis, ascariasis; adjunctive treatment in prostate, pancreatic, liver, colon, and ER+ breast cancers.

External: Arthritic pain, myalgia or neuralgia.

Cautions: None noted. Allergy or dermal sensitivity/dermatitis are contraindications for internal and external use, respectively.

Dose, preparation, and use with Cacao: _Internal_: Dried berries are lightly toasted, pulverised, and ground into cocoa liquor for use in chocolate drinks. For carminative or chemopreventive use, ¼–½ a teaspoon of pulverised berries may be used, daily; or a 1:3 tincture in 60% ethanol, at a dose of 20–30ml per week. For acute problems such as worms or diarrhoea, higher doses may be necessary, e.g., ½ teaspoon powder thrice daily, or 5ml tincture thrice daily (105ml per week), or lower quantities in combination formulae with other plants. For experimental adjunctive treatment of cancers or hypotensive effects, based on animal models, and if used alone, larger doses of 6–12g per day may be necessary, taken as powdered herb or pressure-cooked decoction thereof.

External: Crushed fresh berries or leaves as a poultice; liniment made by macerating fresh or dried leaves in alcohol, or a tincture applied directly; or essential oil applied at maximum 2% concentration (owing to irritating properties of eugenol) in a suitable vehicle.

References

1. Monroy-Ortiz, C., & Castillo-España, P. (2007). _Plantas medicinales Utilizadas en el estad de Morelos._ 2nd edition. Mexico City: Universidad Autonoma del Estado de Morelos.
2. Stubbe, H. (1662). _The Indian Nectar, or, A Discourse concerning chocolata._ London: J.C. for Andrew Crook.
3. Hernández, F. (1615). _Quatro Libros de la Naturaleza, Y Virtudes de las Plantas, y animales, que estan recevidos en el uso de Medicina en la Nueva España, y la Methodo, y correction, y preparacion, que para administrarlas se requiere con lo que el Doctor Francisco Hernández escrobo en lengua Latina._ F. Ximenez (Trans.). www.wdl.org/en/item/7334/200m/#group=1&page=1 [Accessed 25 January 2012].
4. Williams, E. (2003). _Potter's Herbal Cyclopaedia._ Saffron Walden, UK: C. W. Daniel.
5. _Pimenta dioica._ Missouri Botanical Garden. http://missouribotanicalgarden.org/PlantFinder/PlantFinderDetails.aspx?kempercode=d449 [Accessed 18 January 2018].
6. University of California and Los Angeles. (2002). Spices: Exotic Flavors and Medicines. [Exhibition]. https://unitproj.library.ucla.edu/biomed/spice/index.cfm?displayID=1 [Accessed 18 January 2018].
7. Zhang, L., & Lokeshwar, B. (2012). Medicinal properties of the Jamaican pepper plant _Pimenta dioica_ and Allspice. _Current Drug Targets, 13_(4): 1900–1906.

8. Ladurner, A., Zehl, M., Grienke, U., Hofstadler, C., Faur, N., Pereira, F., Berry, D., Dirsch, V., & Rollinger, J. (2017). Allspice and clove as source of triterpene acids activating the G protein-coupled bile acid receptor TGR5. *Frontiers in Pharmacology, 17*(8): 468.

9. Duboc, H., Tache, Y., & Hofmann, A. (2014). The bile acid TGR5 membrane receptor: From basic research to clinical application. *Digestive and Liver Disease, 46*(4): 302–312.

10. Zhang, L., Shamaladevi, N., Jayaprakasha, G., Patil, B., & Lokeshwar, B. (2015). Polyphenol-rich extract of *Pimenta dioica* berries (Allspice) kills breast cancer cells by autophagy and delays growth of triple negative breast cancer in athymic mice. *Oncotarget, 6*(18): 16379–16395.

11. Vasavi, H., Arun, A., & Rekha, P. (2013). Inhibition of quorum sensing in *Chromobacterium violaceum* by *Syzygium cumini* L. and *Pimenta dioica* L. *Asian Pacific Journal of Tropical Biomedicine, 3*(12): 954–959.

12. Shamaladevi, N., Lyn, D., Shaaban, K., Zhang, L., Villate, S., Rohr, J., & Lokeshwar, B. (2013). Ericifolin: a novel antitumor compound from allspice that silences androgen receptor in prostate cancer. *Carcinogenesis, 34*(8): 1822–1832.

13. Yoshimura, M., Amakura, Y., & Yoshida, T. (2011). Polyphenolic compounds in clove and pimento and their antioxidative activities. *Bioscience, Biotechnology, and Biochemistry, 75*(11): 2207–2212.

14. Padmakumari, K., Sasidharan, I., & Sreekumar, M. (2011). Composition and antioxidant activity of essential oil of pimento (*Pimenta dioica* (L) Merr.) from Jamaica. *Natural Product Research, 25*(2): 152–160.

15. Martinez-Velazquez, M., Castillo-Herrera, G., Rosario-Cruz, R., Flores-Fernandez, J., Lopez-Ramirez, J., Hernández-Gutierrez, R., & Lugo-Cervantes, E. (2011). Acaricidal effect and chemical composition of essential oils extracted from *Cuminum cyminum, Pimenta dioica* and *Ocimum basilicum* against the cattle tick *Rhipicephalus (Boophilus) microplus* (Acari: Ixodidae). *Parasitology Research, 108*(2): 481–487.

16. Doyle, B., Frasor, J., Bellows, L., Locklear, T., Perez, A., Gomez-Laurito, J., & Mahady, G. (2009). Estrogenic effects of herbal medicines from Costa Rica used for the management of menopausal symptoms. *Menopause, 16*(4): 748–755.

17. Kikuzaki, H., Miyajima, Y., & Nakatani, N. (2008). Phenolic glycosides from berries of *Pimenta dioica*. *Journal of Natural Products, 71*(5): 861–865.

18. Marzouk, M., Moharram, F., Mohamed, M., Gamal-Eldeen, A., & Aboutabl, E. (2007). Anticancer and antioxidant tannins from *Pimenta dioica* leaves. *Zeitschrift fur Naturforschung, 62*(7): 526–536.

19. Park, I., Kim, J., Lee, S., & Shin, S. (2007). Nematicidal activity of plant essential oils and components From Ajowan (*Trachyspermum ammi*), Allspice (*Pimenta dioica*) and Litsea (*Litsea cubeba*) essential oils against pine wood nematode (*Bursaphelenchus xylophilus*). *Journal of Nematology, 39*(3): 275–279.

20. Suarez, A., Ulate, G., & Ciccio, J. (1997). Cardiovascular effects of ethanolic and aqueous extracts of *Pimenta dioica* in Sprague-Dawley rats. *Journal of Ethnopharmacology, 55*(2): 107–111.

21. Bown, D. (2002). *The Royal Horticultural Society New Encyclopaedia of Herbs and Their Uses.* LondonUK: Dorling Kindersley.

22. Allspice Cultivation. (2018). https://botanical-online.com/english/pimienta_dioica_cultivation.htm [Accessed 23 January 2018]

Piper auritum (Kunth.), syn. *Piper sanctum*

Common names: Hoja santa, Acuyo, Anisillo, Cordoncillo, Candela de Ixotte, Root beer plant, Mecaxochitl (Nahuatl)[1,6,7]

Plant family: Piperaceae.

Habit & habitat: Small, soft-wooded succulent herb up to 6m tall; single main stem with basal "prop" roots. Large, alternate leaves, up to 20cm wide and 30cm long; flower and fruit spike are opposite the leaves, up to 5mm thick and 25cm long; tiny, pale green flowers; fruits less than 1mm, pyramidal shape. Fruits and flowers throughout the year.[7] Crushed leaves smell like sarsaparilla or anise.[8]

Cultivation: Well-drained moist soil, prefers acid soils of light to medium texture (not clay). Propagated by seed and cutting.[7]

Parts used: Inflorescence (flower spikes), leaves.

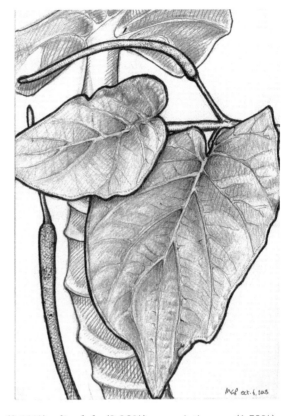

Phytochemistry: <u>Leaves:</u> polyphenols,[10] incl. flavonoids;[22] piperidine amides, incl. piperinel[22] essential oil [incl. ≤87% safrole;[6,8] plus β-caryophyllene (4.65%), germacrene (3.11%), linalol (2.29%), myristicene (1.59%), γ-terpinene (1.32–2.19%) terpinolene (1.11–1.87%), tetradecane (0.93%), β-pinene (0.74–1.45%) aromadendrene (0.68%), bicyclogermagrene (1.26%), α-terpinene & p-cimene (1.79%), l-linalool (0.66 %), cis-nerolidol (0.55–2.8%), and others];[8,18] aporphine alkaloids,[11] incl. 1,2,3-trimethoxy-4,5-dioxo-6a,7-dehydroaporphine;[22] aurantiamides I & II (phenylalanine-dipeptide derivatives);[12] ascorbic acid;[10] beta-carotene.[12] <u>Roots:</u> phenylpropanoids, incl. eugenol.[9]

Traditional use: *P. auritum* <u>flowers</u> formed part of a multi-ingredient magico-medical Mexica prescription, an external wash against "the fatigue of those who administer the republic" (see *Bourreria huanita* monograph for details), as also for making a purely magical amulet "for travellers" (see *Cymbopetalum penduliflorum* monograph for details).[4] The early European chronicler of Mexican plants, Dr Francisco Hernández, reported that *P. auritum* flowers were hot in the fourth and dry in the third degree, that they "gave Cacao an agreeable taste", assisted weight loss, colic, and "pain in the sides", and he ascribed emmenagogue, parturient, and diuretic properties to the flowers, commending them against "wind" and "poison". He also recommended them in combination with vanilla as a parturient.[2] The seventeenth-century Spanish physician Antonio de Ledesma commented that "mecasuchil" flowers had "a purgative quality" similar to senna (*Cassia angustifolia*).[3] The seventeenth-century English physician Henry Stubbe described *P. auritum* flowers as "cordial", hot in the first and dry in the second degree, "open[ing] obstructions [while] strengthen[ing] the body with a moderate adstriction", and a remedy for a "cold stomach and phlegmatic obstructions". Stubbe also commended a beverage made from toasted Cacao, maize, powdered *P. auritum* flowers and vanilla pods as being able to "refrigerate" as well as "provoke lust".[5] *P. auritum* <u>leaves</u> are used fresh in Mexican cooking for wrapping *tamales* or fish, and are an essential ingredient in Guatemalan *mole verde* sauce.[6] Other reported contemporary folk medicinal uses include fever, erysipelas, gout, angina, colic, headaches, and as a vulnerary;[8] it is also used to treat the folk-medical diagnosis of *susto* (fear).[22]

Scientific data: <u>*In vitro*</u>: Essential oil distilled from *P. auritum* <u>aerial parts</u> had anti-Leishmanial activity against four *Leishmania* species, particularly *L. donovani*, the cause of visceral leishmaniasis, with an IC_{50} of 22.3µg/ml against intracellular amastigotes (as compared to reference drug amphotericin B, with an IC_{50} of 0.03µg/ml). It was also notable that the essential oil had activity against *L. braziliensis*, which causes antimony-resistant mucocutaneous leishmaniasis.[8] Another study found moderate antileishmanial activity from whole *P. auritum* leaf extract, with an IC_{50} of 60µg/ml.[14] Fresh leaf extracts had very high antioxidant activity, which was lost on drying,[10] and full-spectrum leaf extracts significantly inhibited advanced glycation end product (AGE) formation.[13] In a study of 1:1 ethanolic extracts of sixteen Mexican spices and twenty-one chilli varieties, *P. auritum* had the highest activity against AGE formation, greater than that of isolated gallic acid, the reference compound. This suggests potential protective effects against diabetes and aging-related comorbidity.[22] A 10% ethanolic solution of *P. auritum* essential oil effectively inhibited the growth of various *Bacillus* species; although rarely a cause of human disease, the authors postulate uses for preserving archive materials from decay.[19] The essential oil of *P. auritum* also inhibits several bacteria which cause crop disease, such as *Xanthomonas alblineans* and *Acidovorax avenae* subsp.avenae.[18] Similarly, hexane extracts and essential oil of *P. auritum* moderately inhibited three saprophytic fungi which cause post-harvest decay in edible fruit crops (*Colletotrichum acutatum*, *C. gloeosporioides*, and *Botryodiplodia theobromae*.)[20] Ethanolic extracts of *P. auritum* at 0.33 and 3,3ml/L shows antispasmodic effects on isolated guinea pig ileal tissue smooth muscle, stimulating effects on rat uterine smooth muscle, and vasodilatory effects (relaxing vascular endothelial smooth muscle).[21]

<u>*In vivo*</u> (<u>non-human animals</u>): A hexane extract of *P. auritum* <u>leaf</u> orally administered to streptozotocin-induced diabetic Wistar rats at 200 and 400mg/kg over a twenty-eight-day period significantly decreased their blood glucose levels and fully normalised cholesterol levels, triglycerides, lipid peroxidation, pancreatic SOD, catalase, glutathione and glutathione peroxidase levels, liver and muscle glycogen levels, glycosylated haemoglobin, and AGE production, suggesting efficient inhibition of insulin resistance and prevention of diabetic co-morbidity.[15] Similar previous experiments revealed that pancreatic nitric oxide and iNOS were elevated in all animals consuming *P. auritum* hexane extract as compared to non-diabetic control animals and the diabetic rats, with significant increases in serum and pancreatic tissue insulin production in the diabetic animals,[16] and reduced renal glucose and thiobarbaturic acid elevation.[17] A 70% ethanolic extract of the leaf orally administered to Wistar rats forty-five minutes before sub-plantar injection of 1% carrageenan found that a dose of 863mg/kg was almost equivalent

to indomethacin in its anti-inflammatory activity, while the LD_{50} of the same extract was 1801.88mg/kg; however the lowest lethal dose was 955.98mg/kg, giving a much narrower therapeutic window—but this was very close to the lethal dose of the vehicle, ethanol. The authors noted that *P. auritum* has analgesic and anti-inflammatory activity, by inhibiting bradykinin formation and prostaglandin biosynthesis.[21] Freeze-dried aqueous and organic extracts of dried *P. auritum* leaf administered to adult male Webster mice by i.p. administration at doses of 1–500mg/kg had dose-dependent anxiolytic and anti-nociceptive effects. Aqueous extracts were the most potently anti-nociceptive and anxiolytic, with lower dose of 10mg/kg—perhaps equivalent to those achievable orally—having the greatest anxiolytic effects, comparable to diazepam; the aqueous extract was more potently analgesic, even at the lowest dose of 1mg/kg, than the reference compound, ibuprofen! Higher doses (200–500mg/kg) tended to produce decreased locomotion, with hexane extracts being the most sedative. The LD_{50} for the aqueous extract was at 3800mg/kg, ten times higher than the highest dose used in the experiment.[23]

Summary of actions: *Internal*: <u>Leaf</u> or <u>flower spike</u>, carminative; diuretic; hypoglycaemic, hypocholesterolaemic; anxiolytic, analgesic; anti-inflammatory; emmenagogue, parturient; antioxidant (fresh leaf only), AGE-inhibitor; anti-leishmanial.

    External: <u>Essential oil</u> as anti-leishmanial and antimicrobial; whole leaf to a lesser extent.

Indications: *Internal*: <u>Leaf</u> or <u>flower spike</u>: colic, water retention; adjuvant treatment of diabetes mellitus, particularly to prevent diabetic comorbidity; anxiety, headache, or mild pain syndromes; hypercholesterolaemia; angina; adjuvant to treatment of leishmaniasis, particularly visceral leishmaniasis.

    External: Whole <u>fresh leaf</u> preparations, or <u>essential oil</u>: leishmaniasis, localised (non-systemic) bacterial infections.

Cautions: Safrole, the principal constituent of *P. auritum* essential oil, is a weak hepatocarcinogen in rodents.[24] As *P. auritum* leaf contains many other constituents responsible for its antioxidant and potent anti-AGE effects, it's reasonable to assume that moderate and discontinuous whole leaf use as medicine or food flavouring is safe. However, the essential oil should be limited to external use for brief periods of time only, and never administered internally.

Dose, preparation, and use with Cacao: *Internal*: <u>Flower spikes</u>: dried inflorescences are pulverised and ground with toasted Cacao seeds for use in chocolate drinks.

    THE FOLLOWING DOSES ARE ESTIMATED: for medicinal purposes, the fresh or dried <u>leaf</u> should be preferred; dried and powdered aerial parts of the herb may be taken orally (e.g., with Cacao) at 2–4g daily. A hot water infusion of 1 tsp (approx. 1–3g) dried leaf taken thrice daily, or a 1:3 tincture in 40% ethanol, at a dose of 20–30ml per week. The preferred preparation may be a specific tincture, made in 96% ethanol using both fresh and dried *P. auritum* leaf. Ninety-six per cent ethanol should be poured over fresh leaves, macerating twice (using more fresh leaves the second time) to raise the water content, yielding a twice-infused specific tincture with an ethanol percentage of approximately 60%, before macerating a third time at 1:5 w/v with dried *P. auritum* leaves. This ensures a product which incorporates the far greater antioxidant properties of the fresh leaf, while not diluting the potency of the tincture (as making a "fresh-only" tincture often corresponds to a low dry weight ratio, e.g., 1:10).

External: <u>Leaves</u>: Fresh pasteurised leaf juice and macerated oil made into a water-in-oil cream; fresh leaf as a poultice; finely pulverised dried leaf, mixed with a carrier oil, for example, castor oil, and applied. <u>Essential oil</u> added to creams or used in a carrier oil, at no higher than 2% concentration, and to be used for limited time periods only.

References

1. Coe, S., & Coe, M. (1996). *The True History of Chocolate*. London: Thames & Hudson.
2. Hernández, F. (1615). *Quatro Libros de la Naturaleza, Y Virtudes de las Plantas, y animales, que estan recevidos en el uso de Medicina en la Nueva España, y la Methodo, y correction, y preparacion, que para administrarlas se requiere con lo que el Doctor Francisco Hernández escrobo en lengua Latina*. F. Ximenez (Trans.). www.wdl.org/en/item/7334/200m/#group=1&page=1 [Accessed 25 January 2012].
3. De Ledesma, A. C. (1631). *Curioso tratado de la naturaleza y calidad del chocolate, dividio en quarto partes*. E. Paltrinieri (Ed.). Edizioni dell'Orso, Alessandria, 1999.
4. Badiano, J. (1552). *Libellus de Medicinalibus Indorum Herbis*. M. de la Cruz (Trans.). Mexico City: Fondo de Cultura Economica Instituto Mexicano del Seguro Social, 1996.
5. Stubbe, H. (1662). *The Indian Nectar, or, A Discourse concerning chocolata [Etc.]*. London: J.C. for Andrew Crook.
6. Katzer, G. (2012). *Mexican Pepperleaf (Piper auritum Kunth)*. http://gernot-katzers-spice-pages.com/engl/Pipe_aur.html[Accessed 1 December 2017].
7. Narayanswamy, B. (2013). *Datasheet: Piper auritum*. https://cabi.org/isc/datasheet/41359 [Accessed 5 December 2017].
8. Monzote, l., García, M., Montalvo, A., Scull, R., & Miranda, M. (2010). Chemistry, cytotoxicity and antileishmanial activity of the essential oil from *Piper auritum*. *Memórias do Instituto Oswaldo Cruz, 105*(2). http://scielo.br/scielo.php?pid=S0074-02762010000200010&script=sci_arttext&tlng=es [Accessed 6 December 2017].
9. Nair, M., Sommerville, J., & Burke, B. (1989). Phenyl propenoids from roots of *Piper auritum*. *Phytochemistry, 28*(2): 654–655.
10. Conde-Hernández, L., & Guerrero-Beltrán, J. (2014). Total phenolics and antioxidant activity of *Piper auritum* and *Porophyllum ruderale*. *Food Chemistry, 142*: 455–460.
11. Hänsel, R., & Leuschke, A. (1975). Aporphine-type alkaloids from *Piper auritum*. *Lloydia, 38*(6): 529–530.
12. *Piper auritum (Piperaceae). Dr. Duke's Phytochemical and Ethnological Databases*. https://phytochem.nal.usda.gov/phytochem/plants/show/1519?part=&_ubiq=&ubiq=on [Accessed 7 December 2017].
13. Dzib-Guerra, W., Escalante-Erosa, F., García-Sosa, K., Derbré, S., Blanchard, P., Richomme, P., & Peña-Rodríguez, L. (2016). Anti-advanced glycation end-product and free radical scavenging activity of plants from the Yucatecan flora. *Pharmacognosy Research, 8*(4): 276–280.
14. Chinchilla-Carmona, M., Valerio-Campos, I., Sánchez-Porras, R., Bagnarello-Madrigal, V., Martínez-Esquivel, L., González-Paniagua, A., Alpizar-Cordero, J., Cordero-Villalobos, M., & Rodríguez-Chaves, D. (2014). Anti-leishmanial activity in plants from a biological reserve of Costa Rica. *Revista de Biologia Tropical, 62*(3): 1229–1240.
15. Gonzalez, A., Gutierrez, R., & Cotera, L. (2014). Antidiabetic activity of *Piper auritum* leaves in streptozotocin-induced diabetic rat, beneficial effect on advanced glycation endproduct. *Chinese Journal of Integrative Medicine*: 1–10. https://doi.org/10.1007/s11655-014-1753-2 [Accessed 7 December 2017].

16. Gutierrez, R. (2012). Effect of the hexane extract of *Piper auritum* on insulin release from β-cell and oxidative stress in streptozotocin-induced diabetic rat. *Pharmacognosy Magazine, 8*(32): 308–313.

17. Gonzalez, A., Gutierrez, R., & Cotera, L. (2012). Evaluation of the antioxidant and anti-glycation effects of the hexane extract from Piper auritum leaves in vitro and beneficial activity on oxidative stress and advanced glycation end-product-mediated renal injury in streptozotocin-treated diabetic rats. *Molecules, 17*(10): 11897–11919.

18. Sánchez, Y., Pino, O., Correa, T., Naranjo, E., & Iglesia, A. (2009). Estudio químico y microbiológico del aceite esencial de *Piper auritum* Kunth. (Caisimón de Anís). *Revista de Protección Vegetal, 24*(1). http://scielo.sld.cu/scielo.php?script=sci_arttext&pid=S1010-27522009000100006 [Accessed 6 December 2017].

19. Guiamet, O., Naranjo, J., Arenas, P., & de Saravia, S. (2008). Differential sensitivity of *Bacillus* sp. isolated from archive materials to plant extracts. *Pharmacology Online, 3*: 649–658.

20. Pineda, R., Vizcaíno, S., García, C., Gil, J., & Durango, D. (2012). Chemical compositiosn and antifungal activity of *Piper auritum* Kunth and *Piper holtonii* C. DC. Against phytopathogenic fungi. *Chilean Journal of Agricultural Research, 72*(4): 507–515.

21. Montalvo, R., & Parra, A. (1999). Evaluacion del efecto antiinflamatorio del extracto de *Piper auritum* H.B.K. y toxicidad aguga oral. *Revista Cubana de Plantas Medicinales*, 4(1). http://scielo.sld.cu/scielo.php?pid=S1028-47961999000100003&script=sci_arttext&tlng=en [Accessed 6 December 2017].

22. Gutierrez, R., Diaz, S., Reyes, I., & Gonzalez, A. (2010). Anti-glycation effect of spices and chilies used in traditional Mexican cuisine. *Journal of Natural Products, 3*: 95–102.

23. Estrada-Reyes, R., Martinez-Laurrabaquio, A., Suarez, D., & Araujo-Escalona, A. (2013). Neuropharmacological studies of *Piper auritum* Kunth (Piperaceae): antinociceptive and anxiolytic-like effects. *Journal of Medicinal Plants Research, 7*(23): 1718–1729.

24. Williams, G. (2010). Chemicals with carcinogenic activity in rodent liver. *Comprehensive Toxicology [2nd Edn.], 9*: 221–250.

Plumeria rubra f. typica, P.rubra f. acutifolia, P.rubra f. alba L. (Jasmine)

Common names: Frangipani, Flor de Mayo, Flor de Maiz Tostado, Flor del Cuervo, Caca-lasúchil, Cacaloxochitl (Mexica), Baak' Nik'te (Maya—*trans.* "bone flower"), Guie Chachi (Zapotec—*trans.* "brilliant flower").

Plant family: Apocynaceae.

Habit & habitat: Native to Mexico, spread to Ecuador, Peru, and Brasil, and distributed around the tropical and subtropical regions of the world. Grows between 30 and 1400m above sea level. Deciduous tree 3–9m tall, with alternate leaves, smooth and shiny on upper surface, hairy underneath; aromatic flowers grouped at the end of the branches: pink petals with purple, white, yellow, or red tints (*P. rubra f. typica*), or white flowers with a yellow centre (*P. rubra f. acutifolia*). *P. rubra f. acutifolia* also has almost white

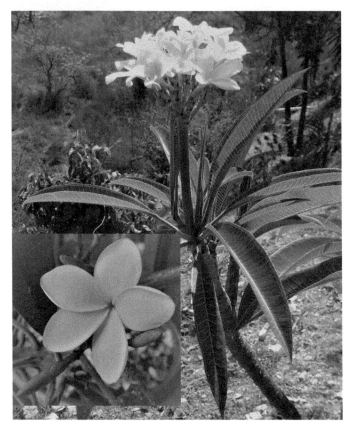

stems. Pollinated by hawkmoths. The fruit is a 15–30cm long brown pod filled with one-winged seeds for air dispersal. Dormant most of the year, flowers before the rainy season in May–July. Grows in tropical deciduous woodland and "hilly thickets" and "holm oak" woods.[1,3,6]

Cultivation: Likes full sun, dry conditions and sandy, light, well-drained soil. An equatorial plant, it is drought-resistant, but highly frost-sensitive. Easily propagated by cuttings.[2,3]

Parts used: Flowers, latex (sap), leaves, seed pods, fruit pulp, bark.

Phytochemistry: Latex in <u>bark</u> and <u>leaves</u>, with soluble proteins including the protease plumerin-R; iridoids (incl fulvoplumerin);[8] <u>leaves</u>, containing iridoids [incl. 6"-O-acetylplum-ieride-p-Z-coumarate, 6"-O-acetylplumieride-p-E-coumarate, plumieride, plumieride-p-Z-coumarate, plumieride, plumieride-p-Z-coumarate, plumieride-p-E-coumarate); and triterpenoids, (incl. stgmast-7-enol, lupeol carboxylic acid, lupeol acetate, ursolic acid).[13] <u>Flowers</u> containing flavone glycosides and flavonoids (incl. quercetin and kaempferol); essential oil, 0.04–0.07% (containing alcohols: geraniol, citronellol, farnesol, phenylethyl alchohol, aldehydes and ketones;Abenzyl esters, aliphatic alkanes, oxygenated monoterpenes, diterpenes, benzyl salicylate, benzyl benzoate); resin; iridoids;[14] fatty acids (alkanoic, lauric, palmitic and myristic acids).[13,14] Bark, containing alkaloids, glycosides, sterols, triterpenoids (incl.β-sitosterol-β-D-glucoside, lupeol nanoate, rubrinol glucoside, lupeol heptanoate); iridoid glycosides (incl. fulvoplumierin, plumieride coumarate, allamcin, allamandin); tannins and flavan-3-ol glycosides [incl. 2,5-dimethoxy-p-benzoquinone; (2R, 3S)-3,4′dihydroxy-7,3′,5′-trimethoxyflavan-5-O-β-D-glucopyranoside],[13] phenols, saponins;[8] plumericin, isoplumericin.[7] Roots, containing iridoid glycosides (fulvoplummierin, plumericin, isoplumerin, β-dihydroplumericin, β-dihydroplumericinic acid).[13]

Traditional use: *P. rubra* <u>flowers</u> mere used in a multi-ingredient magico-medical Mexica prescription against fear, timidity, or cowardice. The two-part prescription consisted of a drinkable potion, made by infusing the flowers of both varieties of *P. rubra* and four other unidentified herbs in river or stream water with some added kaolin ("whitened earth"); the second part of the prescription required that some of this potion be retained, further infused with *Laurus nobilis* leaf, mixed with fox and vixen blood and the "blood and excrement" of a species of native worm, swallow's excrement, and sea foam. This mixture could be further enriched "for those frightened by lightning or sparks" by the sap of a tree struck by lightning and flowers growing nearby; this paste was applied to the forehead and back of the neck. *P. rubra* flowers also formed part of the Mexica external wash against "the fatigue of those who administer the republic" (see *Bourreria huanita* monograph for details).[4] The Mexica also reportedly used the flowers to flavour Cacao beverages. *P. rubra* flowers also had a traditional reputation as an aphrodisiac.[2] Seventeenth-century Spanish physician Dr Francisco Hernández describes the <u>latex</u> as "cold and glutinous", and capable of taking away pain when applied to the chest; two drachms (7.5–8g) of fruit pulp may be used to "clean the stomach and intestines". Hernández also commends a decoction using two pounds (approx. 700g) of the pulverised <u>bark</u> in 16 quarts (18 litres) of water, reduced to a quarter of its volume (4.5 litres), to be taken in 6–8oz (170–230ml) doses morning and evening against "thick and phlegmatic humours", to dissolve "obstructions" causing pain in the stomach, liver, and spleen, in the early stages of dropsy, and "for those who have had great illnesses and cannot end their convalescence".[6] <u>Latex</u> and <u>flowers</u> are used topically in contemporary Mexican ethnomedicine against ringworm (*Tinea corporis*), verrucas, and to "draw out thorns"; as an eye wash (presumably flower infusion?), and to treat pelvic pain (manner unspecified).[6] In India, the latex is mixed with coconut oil and applied to treat herpes, scabies, and "ulcers".[13] A <u>bark</u> decoction is also used to treat internal bruising, rheumatism, and diarrhoea;[3,6] unspecified parts of the plant are used for toothache, and as an antispasmodic. In India, a decoction of 12–24g stem bark is used to treat dysentery.[13] For ear pain, the stems are roasted over a fire, and cotton balls are dipped in the <u>latex</u> which emerges and inserted into the affected ear;[3] in a more magico-medical contemporary use, the tenderest roasted branches may be applied as a poultice to the back at waist height to prevent having children.[6] The same latex may be cooked until fully coagulated, dried and pulverised, heated in a pan and then applied to stop bleeding; fresh (?) latex may be used to speed bone healing, by applying a cloth dipped in it to the affected part.[6] A <u>flower</u> infusion may be drunk as a galactagogue, and a decoction of 3–5 flowers in a litre of water is used as a douche for "vaginal diseases".[1] A decoction of flowers is used to treat diabetes.[13] Flowers, latex, and bark are all used in prescriptions as an expectorant against cough and in asthma.[6] <u>Leaves</u> have been used topically to treat ulcers, leprosy, and swelling.[3]

Scientific data: _In vitro_: Methanolic extract of _P. rubra_ <u>bark</u> was found to have an anthelmintic effect against earthworms (_Pherethima posthuma_)—the authors claim "It resembles anatomically and physiologically the round worm parasite of human being," in fact a completely different genus, _Ascaris_ spp. The concentration required to equal the efficacy of 15mg/ml piperazine was 25–50mg/ml.[8] An ethanolic extract of _P. rubra_ <u>leaves</u> inhibited growth of the _Fonsecaea pedrosoi_, the cause of chromoblastomycosis, a chronic subcutaneous mycotic infection, at ≥12.5µg/mL.[12] Leaf extracts also had varying effects on smooth muscle, contracting rat vas deferens, releasing guinea pig taenia caeci, and increasing rabbit ileal contraction; all these effects were in opposition to phentolamine, suggesting α-adrenergic activity. Methanolic leaf extracts also inhibited the Gram-positive bacteria _Bacillus subtilis_ and _Staphylococcus aureus_. Ethanolic leaf extract was also determined to have anti-mutagenic activity.[13] _P. rubra f. alba_ <u>flower</u> essential oil inhibited the same two bacteria, but also inhibited the fungal pathogens _Aspergillus niger_, _Candida albicans_, and _Penicillium chrysogenum_ with comparable efficacy to griseolfulvin, the reference anti-mycotic drug; a methanolic extract of the whole flower also inhibited _Escherichia coli_.[13] Meanwhile an ethanolic extract of _P. rubra f. acutifolia_ <u>bark</u> inhibited _Bacillus subtilis_, _Staphylococcus aureus_, _Enterococcus faecalis_, _Pseudomonas aeruginosa_, _Salmonella typhimurium_, _Aspergillus niger_, and _Candida albicans_.[13]

In vivo (non-human animals): _P. rubra_ <u>latex</u> administered intravenously to mice prevented ethanol-induced injury to gastric mucosa in a dose-dependent manner, with the strongest effect at 0.5mg/kg; mechanisms were determined to be primarily prostaglandin inhibition and antioxidant effects, with induction of nitric oxide, cyclic GMP, ATP-dependent potassium channels, and activation of vanilloid receptors as secondary mechanisms.[7] Real-world application of this information to the utility of _P. rubra_ latex is limited by the choice of an intravenous route of administration. Orally administered ethanolic extract of _P. rubra_ <u>bark</u> at doses of 250 and 500mg/kg had highly significant dose-dependent analgesic and anti-inflammatory activity in lab mice and rats, equalling or exceeding the reference drug, diclofenac; anti-inflammatory activity peaked at four hours after administration.[9] Hydro-ethanolic cold macerated 3:7 stem bark extract of _P. rubra_ was orally administered to streptozotocin-induced diabetic rats at 250 and 500mg/kg over a three-week period; in comparison to metformin and a non-diabetic control group, _Plumeria_ extract significantly reduced hyperglycaemia in the oral glucose tolerance test, the 500mg/kg dose being slightly less effective than metformin. Fasting blood glucose levels were controlled by metformin and _Plumeria_ 500mg/kg equally, and both doses of _Plumeria_ conserved diabetic rats' body weight as effectively as metformin. At the end of the test, both _Plumeria_ and metformin were found to have reduced blood total cholesterol, LDL, and triglycerides, and raised HDL; _Plumeria_ extracts had better effects on serum and liver peroxidase (lowered) and glutathione (raised) levels. However, on autopsy, pancreatic histology was found to be slightly better with metformin than the 500mg/kg dose of _Plumeria_ extract.[10] In rabbits injected with the pyretic agents typhoid vaccine or prostaglandin E1, orally administered methanolic extracts of _P. rubra_ bark at 100 and 200mg/kg normalised body temperature and had anti-pyretic effects comparable to paracetamol in the typhoid-vaccine model, and significantly reduced fever in the prostaglandin model, though not with the same potency as aspirin.[11]

Doses of 500mg/kg _P. rubra_ <u>leaf</u> extract had significant acute and chronic anti-inflammatory activity in rodents.[13] Doses of 200 and 400mg/kg of _P. rubra_ <u>leaf</u> ethanolic extract orally administered to mice with Ehrlich ascites carcinoma had better haematology (improved hae-moglobin, red and white blood cell counts), reduced tumour cell viability and volume in com-parison to the control group; 400mg/kg returned blood test parameters to "near normal". However, in contrast to i.v. 5-fluorouracil—which caused worsening of haematology results—there was no significant increase in lifespan with *P. rubra*. In a separate test, methanolic *P. rubra f. alba* leaf extract showed similar anti-cancer effects on Dalton lymphoma ascites. Chloroform and ethanolic extracts of the leaves had anti-ulcer effects in rats, and methanolic extracts at 100, 200, and 400mg/kg had dose-dependent hepatoprotective activity in rats comparable to silymarin.[13]

Other cited *in vivo* properties are: <u>flowers</u>, anxiolytic (ethanolic extract), antioxidant, hypo-lipidaemic, antiviral, anti-inflammatory (methanolic extract), anti-fertility (methanolic extract, female rats, reduced ovarian steroidogenic activity and dose-dependently delayed sexual maturation);[13] <u>leaf</u>, antibacterial; <u>seed pods</u>, antifertility—all extracts were abortifactient in female rats.[8,13]

Summary of Actions: *Internal*: <u>Bark</u>: analgesic, anti-inflammatory, anti-pyretic, hypoglycae-mic, anti-diabetic, hepatoprotective, antidiarrhoeal, antibacterial, anti-fungal, anthelmintic; possibly: anti-tussive, expectorant. <u>Flower</u>: anxiolytic, hypolidpidaemic, anti-inflammatory; possibly: anti-fertility (female), galactagogue, anti-tussive, expectorant. <u>Leaf</u>: anti-cancer; anti-inflammatory, α-adrenergic, hepatoprotective. <u>Latex</u>: anti-ulcer, mucoprotective.

External: <u>Bark</u>: antimicrobial (bacterial and fungal); anti-fertility? <u>Flower</u>: anti-fungal, anti-inflammatory, ophthalmic, antiviral; <u>essential oil</u>: antibacterial and anti-fungal. <u>Leaf</u>: anti-inflammatory, anti-ulcer, antibacterial (*S. aureus* and *B.subtilis*), anti-fungal (*F.pedrosoi*), anti-mutagenic. <u>Latex</u>: analgesic, vulnerary, antimicrobial, haemostatic.

Indications: *Internal*: <u>Bark</u>: diarrhoea and dysentery, abdominal pain, diabetes, arthritis; pos-sibly also cancer (adjunctive treatment, or as part of a combined plant-based protocol); asthma, hepatitis, roundworm/pinworm/threadworm infection, to reduce female fertility. <u>Flower</u>: anxiety, hypercholesterolaemia; possibly as a galactagogue, and against asthma. <u>Leaf</u>: possibly: cancer, hepatitis, peptic ulcer or gastritis. <u>Latex</u>: possibly: peptic ulceration.

External: <u>Flower</u>: bacterial or fungal skin infections; candidiasis, ringworm, possibly also blepharitis or conjunctivitis. <u>Essential oil</u>: vs. bacterial or fungal skin infections. <u>Leaf</u>: non-malignant skin cancers, ulcers, skin infections: *Staphylococcal* and chromoblastomycosis.

Cautions: Not for internal use in pregnancy, or by women who are attempting to conceive. Fresh latex may be somewhat caustic.

Dose, preparation, and use with Cacao: Fresh and dried flowers are used in Cacao drinks; a large volume of fresh flowers, with a much smaller quantity of the dried flowers are ground with Cacao seeds to incorporate them.

Internal: <u>Bark</u>: in decoction, dose range = 12–35g twice daily depending on bodyweight, drug sensitivity, and symptom severity. As a hydroalcoholic extract, 1:3 tincture in 40% ethanol, esti-mated 40–60ml per week, or 1:1 at 30ml per week; acute doses, 10–15ml in water thrice daily. <u>Flower</u>: By infusion or decoction, estimated a handful of fresh flowers or 3–6g dried per cup, thrice daily. Sixty per cent hydroalcoholic tincture, similar doses to bark tincture above.

External: <u>Flower</u>: for ophthalmic conditions, infusion made in boiling water and allowed to cool; made more concentrated for use as a vaginal douche or skin wash. A cream made from macerated oil combined with pasteurised fresh flower juice, or dried flowers infused into distilled aromatic water may be made, to which essential oil may be added.

<u>Essential oil</u> in cream, as above; or added to a vehicle such as almond oil or base cream at 2–10% (note that concentrations of essential oil above 2% may cause skin irritation).

<u>Leaf</u>: used to make a cream in process similar to flowers as above, or dried and applied to ulcers as a fine powder; or, fresh leaf juice or concentrated decoction directly applied; or, fresh or dried leaves used to make a poultice.

References

1. Monroy-Ortiz, C., & Castillo-España, P. (2007). *Plantas medicinales Utilizadas en el estad de Morelos. 2nd edition.* Mexico City: Universidad Autonoma del Estado de Morelos.
2. Flor de Mayo, Plumeria rubia, Plumeria obtusa, frangipani, is a known sacred Maya flower, but deserves further study to understand potential use as aphrodisiac. http://maya-ethnobotany.org/mayan-ethno-botany-tropical-agriculture-edible-flowers-medicinal-plants-flavoring-guatemala-mexico-belize/plumeria-rubia-flor-de-mayo-frangipani-cacao-balche-aphrodisiac-fragrance.php [Accessed 18 December 2017].
3. Shah, T. (2016). The truths behind the Temple Tree—*Plumeria rubra*. https://linkedin.com/pulse/truths-behind-temple-tree-plumeria-rubra-toral-shah [Accessed 18 December 2017].
4. Badiano, J. (1552). *Libellus de Medicinalibus Indorum Herbis.* M. de la Cruz (kTrans.). Mexico City: Fondo de Cultura Economica Instituto Mexicano del Seguro Social, 1996.
5. Hernández, F. (1615). *Quatro Libros de la Naturaleza, Y Virtudes de las Plantas, y animales, que estan recividos en el uso de Medicina en la Nueva España, y la Methodo, y correction, y preparacion, que para administrarlas se requiere con lo que el Doctor Francisco Hernández escrobo en lengua Latina.* F. Ximenez (Trans.). www.wdl.org/en/item/7334/200m/#group=1&page=1 [Accessed 25 January 2012].
6. da Silva, J., & Alba, M. (2004). Cacaloxóchitl, como planta medicinal y flor ornamental. *Tesina del Diplomado de Tlahui-Educa: Medicina Tradicional de México y sus Plantas Medicinales, 18*(2). http://tlahui.com/medic/medic18/cacalox1.htm [Accessed 18 December 2017].
7. Alencar, N., Pinheiro, R., Figueiredo, I., Luz, P., Freitas, L., de Souza, T., do Carmo, L., Marques, L., & Ramos, M. (2015). The preventive effect on ethanol-induced gastric lesions of the medicinal plant *Plumeria rubra*: Involvement of the latex proteins in the NO/cGMP/K_{ATP} signaling pathway. *Evidence Based Complementary and Alternative Medicine.* Published online 14 December. https://ncbi.nlm.nih.gov/pmc/articles/PMC4691623/ [Accessed 18 December 2017].
8. Srivastava, A., Gupta, A., & Rajendiran, A. (2017). Phytochemical screening and *in-vitro* anthelmintic activity of methanolic extract from the stem bark of *Plumeria rubra* Linn. *International Journal of Pharmaceutical Sciences and Research, 50*: 5336–5341. http://ijpSrcom/bft-article/phytochemical-screening-and-in-vitro-anthelmintic-activity-of-methanolic-extract-from-the-stem-bark-of-plumeria-rubra-linn/?view=fulltext [Accessed 18 December 2017].
9. Das, B., Ferdous, T., Mahmood, Q., Hannan, J., Bhattacharjee, R., & Das, B. (2013). Antinociceptive and anti-inflammatory activity of the bark extract of *Plumeria rubra* on laboratory animals. *European Journal of Medicinal Plants, 3*(1): 114–126.
10. Mondal, P., Das, S., Junejo, J., Borah, S., & Zaman, K. (2016). Evaluations of antidiabetic potential of the hydro-alcoholic extract of the stem bark of *Plumeria rubra* a traditionally used medicinal source in North-East India. *International Journal of Green Pharmacy, 10*(4): 252–260.

11. Khan, I., Aziz, A., Raza, M., Saleem, M., Bashir, S., & Alvi, A. (2015). Study pertaining to the hypothermic activity of *Plumeria rubra*, Linn. in PGE1 and TAB-vaccine induced pyrexia models in rabbits. *West Indian Medical Journal*. https://mona.uwi.edu/fms/wimj/article/2368 [Accessed 18 December 2017].

12. Gaitán, I., Paz, A. Zacchino, S., Tamayo, G., Giménez, A., Pinzón, R., Cáceres, A., & Gupta, M. (2011). Subcutaneous antifungal screening of Latin American plant extracts against Sporothrix schenckii and Fonsecaea pedrosoi. *Pharmaceutical Biology, 49*(9): 907–919.

13. Shinde, P., Patil, P., & Bairagi, V. (2014). Phytopharmacological review of *Plumeria* species. *Scholars Academic Journal of Pharmacy, 3*(2): 217–227.

14. Manisha, K., & Aher, A. (2016). Review on traditional medicinal plant: *Plumeria rubra*. *Journal of Medicinal Plants Studies, 4*(6): 204–207.

Pouteria sapota (Jacq.)

Common names: Mamey sapote, Zapote, Sapuyul, Marmalade plum.

Plant family: Sapotaceae.

Habit & habitat: Tree, fifteen to forty-five metres tall, native to Central America: Atlantic coast of Nicaragua, Belize, Honduras, Guatemala, and the Yucatan in Mexico. Naturally grows in higher altitude perennial forests.[1] Has a grooved trunk and dark pink, almond-scented inner bark, producing sticky white latex. Dense foliage, ovate-lanceolate leaves mostly at apex of

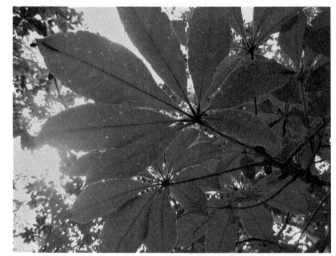

branches. Small flowers grow under new branches and along older branches without leaves. Fruits are elliptical-spherical, 8–20cm long and 500g to 3kg in weight, with reddish, rough, and brittle skin; flesh is dusky red, orange or greyish, with a slightly fibrous, somewhat granular texture.[3,4]

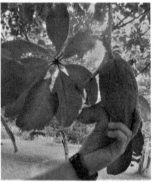

Cultivation: Seeds germinate after 40–70 days; mostly propagated by grafting. Seven years or more for a tree to begin fruiting (three—five years for grafts). Grows in moist, well-drained, loamy, clay or sandy soil of any pH, even very acid or saline soils. Requires full sun, and temperatures above 15°C, average range 25–33°C. Prefers higher rainfall—drought-sensitive. With no dry season, the tree fruits year-round.[3,4]

Parts used: Seeds, fruit, latex, bark, leaves.

Phytochemistry: Triterpenoids and flavonoids. Bark contains cyanogenic glycosides: lucumin;[3] fruit contains carotenoids (incl.β-carotene, lutein, violoxanthin, sapotexanthin,[6] cryptocapsin-5,6-epoxide, 3'deoxycapsanthin-5,8-epoxides),[8] polyphenols (incl. p-hydroxybenzoic acid, gallic acid, (+)-gallocatechin, (+)-catechin, (-)-epicatechin, (+)-catechin-3-0-gallate, myricitrin),[7] essential oil (incl. benzaldehyde, hexanal),[7] ascorbic acid and tocopherols.[5] Seeds containing cyanogenic glycosides (incl. lucumin), fixed oil (incl. palmitic, estearic, oleic and linoleic acids).[7] Leaves contain cyanogenic glycosides (incl. lucuminic acid, lucuminamide).[7]

Traditional use: Seeds used to treat dandruff and hair loss by crushing, then mixing the expressed oil with alcohol, and rubbing onto the affected area.[1] Seed oil is also used for muscle and joint pains,[3] and administered internally as a diuretic.[4] Seeds are also used as vulneraries, and ground dried seeds are used both raw and toasted as spices in Cacao drinks.[3] Crushed seed residue after oil extraction is used as a poultice to treat skin inflammation. Seed infusion is used as an eyewash, and powdered seed coat taken internally to help with kidney stones and arthritis, and to benefit the heart. The Mexica reportedly used it to treat epilepsy.[4] A leaf decoction is used to treat alcoholism;[1] a tea of leaves and bark is given to treat atherosclerosis and hypertension in Mexican folk medicine, and a bark decoction is used to allay coughs.[4] Fresh seeds have sedative or "stupefying" properties; latex is somewhat caustic and vesicant,[2] and may be used to treat fungal skin infections and for wart removal.[3,4] Fruit is eaten, and used to make sweets, or cooked as a vegetable when unripe.[3]

Scientific data: *In vitro*: methanol extracts of *P. sapota* stems have trypanocidal activity against the epimastigote form of *Trypanosoma* cruzi,[7] cause of Chagas's disease and trypanosomiasis. Other activities in the genus *Pouteria* include phagocyte modulation (aqueous and methanolic extracts of *P. cambodiana* stem bark); antimicrobial against *Staphylococcus aureus*, *Pseudomonas aeruginosa*, *Escherichia coli*, *Cladosporium sphaerospermum*, and *Bacillus cereus* (hexane, ethanol, aqueous, and methanolic extracts of *P. torta* leaves); antimicrobial against *Cladosporium cladosporioides*, *Cladosporium sphaerospermum*, and *Candida albicans* (hydroethanolic extracts of *P. psamophila* and *P. grandiflora* leaves); oestrogen antagonism at oestrogen receptor β (hexane extracts of *P. torta* leaves); and HIV inhibitory activity in MTT and recombinant virus assays (methanolic extracts of *P. viridis* leaves).[7]

In vivo (non-human animals): Other members of genus *Pouteria* had the following *in vivo* activities: anti-inflammatory and anti-nociceptive activities (ethanolic extract of *P. ramiflora* leaves); immunomodulatory to mouse macrophage phagocytosis and splenocyte proliferation (methanol extract of *P. cambodiana* stem bark); antimalarial activity against *Plasmodium berghei* in rats (hydroethanolic extract of *P. venosa* leaves).[7]

In vivo (human): Seed oil shown to be ineffective at promoting hair growth, but effectively prevents alopecia due to seborrhoeic dermatitis.[4]

Summary of actions: *Internal*: seeds possibly anodyne, anti-inflammatory, sedative, antispasmodic to smooth muscle, anti-tussive, diuretic, hypocholesterolaemic. Leaves and bark: possibly immunomodulatory, trypanocidal, anti-plasmodial, oestrogen modulating, anti-inflammatory, anodyne, hypocholesterolaemic, diuretic.

External: seeds ophthalmic, vulnerary, cutaneous anti-inflammatory. Leaves, possibly anti-candida, bacteriostatic. Seed oil anti-inflammatory—cutaneous and possibly musculoskeletal.

Indications: *Internal*: seeds, possibly: cough, hypercholesterolaemia, hypertension, anxiety with palpitations. Leaf and bark, possibly atherosclerosis, hypertension, trypanosomiasis or Chagas's disease, malaria, arthritic pain.

External: seed oil alopecia due to seborrhoeic dermatitis; arthritis; whole seed (decoction): conjunctivitis, blepharitis (powder): minor wounds and cuts. Fresh sap or latex: warts. Leaf: local *Candida albicans* or *Staphylococcus aureus* infection.

Cautions: seed, leaf, or bark overdose will cause cyanide poisoning. Pregnancy and breastfeeding. Latex allergy. Fresh sap or latex is vesicant—do not apply to sensitive skin.

Dosage: Toasted, pulverised seed is used in *tejate*, and other Cacao-based beverages, being ground into the cocoa liquor. ALL DOSES ARE ESTIMATED.

Internal: <u>Seed</u>: pulverised seed taken orally, 500mg twice daily; hydroalcoholic tincture, 1:3 at 25% ethanol (favouring polyphenols and glycosides), 20ml per week. <u>Bark and leaves</u>: in decoction, 2–3g two to three times daily; as a hydroalcoholic extract, 1:3 tincture in 25% ethanol, estimated 20–30ml per week.

External: <u>Seed</u>, seed coat pulverised and in infusion, ½ teaspoon per ½ teacupful of water, strained well and used as eye wash. Pulverised and sifted whole seed applied topically as a wound dressing to cuts and small wounds. <u>Seed oil</u>, used as ointment base or essential oil vehicle for anti-arthritic preparations, as for seborrhoeic dermatitis-related alopecia. <u>Leaf juice</u> or oil-in-water cream made with polar and non-polar constituents, for example using *P. sapota* seed fixed oil with infused heat-macerated leaves, plus pasteurised leaf juice or dried leaves steeped in aromatic water, or a CO_2 extract or similar. <u>Latex</u>, applied locally to warts.

References

1. Monroy-Ortiz, C., & Castillo-España, P. (2007). *Plantas medicinales Utilizadas en el estad de Morelos. 2nd edition*. Mexico City: Universidad Autonoma del Estado de Morelos.
2. (2010). http://worldagroforestry.org/af/treedb/index.php?keyword=Poison [Accessed 10 February 2010].
3. (2017). Neglected crops: 1492 from a different perspective ... Sapote (*Pouteria sapota*). http://fao.org/docrep/t0646e/T0646E0c.htm [Accessed 30 December 2017].
4. (2018). *Pouteria sapota*—(Jacq.) H. E.Moore & Stearn. *Plants for a Future*. http://pfaf.org/user/Plant.aspx?LatinName=Pouteria+sapota [Accessed 2 January 2018].
5. Yahia, E., Gutierrez-Orozco, F., & de Leon, C. (2011). Phytochemical and antioxidant characterization of mamey (*Pouteria sapota* Jacq. H. E. Moore & Stearn) fruit. *Food Research International*, 44(7): 2175–2181.
6. Murillo, E., McLean, R., Britton, G., Agocs, A., Nagy, V., & Deli, J. (2011). Sapotexanthin, an A-provitamin carotenoid from Red Mamey (*Pouteria sapota*). *Journal of Natural Products*, 74(2): 283–285.
7. Silva, C., Simeoni, L., & Silveira, D. (2009). Genus *Pouteria*: chemistry and biological activity. *Revista Brasileria de Farmacognosia*, 19(2): 501–509.
8. Guylas-Fekete, G., Murillo, E., Kurtan, T., Papp, T., Illyes, T., Drahos, L., Visy, J., Agocs, A., Turcsi, E., & Deli, J. (2013). Cryptocapsinepoxide-type carotenoids from red mamey, *Pouteria sapota*. *Journal of Natural Products*, 76(4): 607–614.

Quararibea funebris (La Llave) Vischer[12]

Common names: Rosita de Cacao, Molinillo, Batidor, Sapotillo, Madre de Cacao, Funeral Tree, Cacahuaxochitl, Xochicacauhuatl (Nahuatl), Majaz (Tzetzal Maya), Aj Maja'as (Itza Maya).[7]

Plant family: Malvaceae

Habit & habitat: A shrub or small tree with very aromatic flowers, reminiscent of vanilla or linden;[2] natural habitat is Mexico and Guatemala. Grows in warm, dry conditions.[6] Up to 20m tall, with a broad, depressed crown, leaves are large, smooth, and elliptical. Flowers after rain, white in colour with five curling petals and protuberant stamens.[7] Flowers bloom for only two or more weeks of the year, around March–August, during the rainy season.[7]

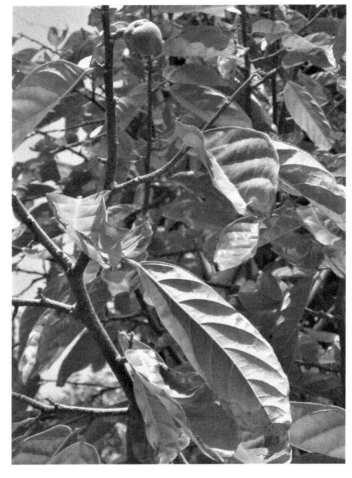

Cultivation: Semi-hardy, slow-growing; flowers after five to six years. Requires moist, well-drained soil and full sun; some-what frost tolerant but prefers temperatures above 15°C.[11]

Parts used: Flowers; root (?).

Phytochemistry: Alkaloids (incl. pyrrole alkaloid, funebrine,[1] funebral,[8] funebradiol[9]); proteins (incl. (2S,3S,4A)-γ-hydroxyisoleucine),[1] fatty acids (incl. linolenic and linoleic acids), sterols and steroidal glycosides (incl. B-sitosterol, stigmasterol, and glycosidic palmitic/oleic acid esters of these compounds);[2] volatile oil (incl. aminolactones: 3-hydroxy-4,5-dimethyl-2(5H)-furanone and a saturated analogue),[2] sugars (incl.glucose, fructose, sucrose); mucilage.

Traditional use: *Q. funebris* <u>flowers</u> were principally used to thicken, sweeten, and aromatise Cacao-based drinks.[6] In Mesoamerica they were also utilised in funeral rites and embalming, as the fragrance is very persistent, lasting decades or even centuries in dried flowers;[6,7] traditional chocolate whisks, or *molinillos*, are made using the wood of *Q. funebris*—hence one of the post-conquest names for the plant (*molinillo*). In addition to being a traditional Cacao spice, the flowers may also have been used to aromatise tobacco.[7] They were used in a Mexica prescription for "losing one's mind", against retardation, insanity, or schizophrenia: following the administration of an emetic decoction, possibly made from the root of a *Bidens* species, after a few days the patient was to drink the juice of fresh *Q. funebris* and *Magnolia mexicana* flowers, together with a preparation of their bark and roots (presumably a decoction), to "remove the bad humour in the chest". The third and fourth part of the prescription called for various animal products and precious stones to make a potion for drinking and lotion to be applied to the head.[3] According to seventeenth-century Spanish physician Francisco Hernández, a decoction of ½ an ounce of dried ground root of *cacahuaxochitl* (a traditional name of *Q. funebris*) was used to treat dysentery, but there is some dispute as to whether he is referring to this plant or not.[10] Other recorded traditional uses of the <u>flowers</u> include menstrual regulation, as an anti-pyretic, and against "fear".[2] Possible use as an entheogen—*Q. funebris* flowers appear alongside other entheogens such as *Nicotiana tabacum*, *Turbina corymbosa*, *Psilocybe aztecorum*, and *Heimia salicifolia* on the Mexica ("Aztec") statue of the love/ecstasy/flower god Xochipilli.[2,4,5] The Zapotecs in Oaxaca, Mexico also decocted the flowers as a cough remedy.

Scientific data: None. *Q. funebris* is a principal traditional Mesoamerican Cacao spice, second only in esteem to *Cymbopetalum penduliflorum*; but, despite being more accessible in markets and more commonly used in contemporary Mexico than *Cymbopetalum*, it is even less well researched. Both plants, too, contain the pyrrole alkaloid, funebrine. Although funebrine was isolated from *Q. funebris* more than three decades ago, the only published papers are technical studies of its structure and synthesis, but there is no publicly available pharmaceutical or medicinal research, just as there is none for the related compounds funebrine and funebradiol. It has been suggested that, given the known activity of γ-butyrolactone and other related compounds, the aminolactones in *Q. funebris* may be anticonvulsant and sedative, which accords with *Q. funebris*' traditional anxiolytic, antipsychotic and antispasmodic applications.[2]

Summary of actions: <u>flowers</u>, possibly: anxiolytic, antispasmodic, anti-tussive, anti-pyretic; antipsychotic, nootropic (?).

Indications: insufficient evidence. Possibly: anxiety, insomnia; spasmodic or irritable coughs; psychosis or dementia with fear or paranoia as a predominant symptom.

Cautions: None noted.

Dosage: Used in *pozonque*[7] and *tejate*, Cacao and maize-based drinks in contemporary Mexico. Toasted, pulverised flowers are used in *tejate*, being ground into the cocoa liquor. THE FOLLOWING DOSES ARE ESTIMATED.

Internal: <u>Flowers</u>: hot water infusion, 3–6g, thrice daily. Or 1:3 hydroethanolic tincture, 25–60% proof, 30–50ml per week; pulverised flowers, stamens, and corollas toasted briefly and separately (corollas require slightly more toasting than stamens)—approx. 0.5–3g per dose, thrice daily.

References

1. Raffauf, R., Zennie, T., Onan, K., & Le Quesne, P. (1984). Funebrine, a structurally novel pyrrole alkaloid, and other γ-hydroxyisoleucine-related metabolites of Quararibea funebris (llave) vischer (Bombacaceae). *Journal of Organic Chemistry, 49*(15): 2714–2718.
2. Raffauf, R., & Zennie, T. (1983). The phytochemistry of *Quararibea funebris*. *Botanical Museum Leaflets, Harvard University, 29*(2): 151–157.
3. Badiano, J. (1552). *Libellus de Medicinalibus Indorum Herbis*. M. de la Cruz (Trans.). Mexico City: Fondo de Cultura Economica Instituto Mexicano del Seguro Social, 1996.
4. Ott, J. (1996). *Pharmacotheon: Entheogenic drugs, their plant sources and history*. Washington, USADC: Natural Products Association.
5. *Quararibea funebris*—Rosita de Cacao and Drink of the Gods. https://toptropicals.com/html/toptropicals/plant_wk/quararibea.htm [Accessed 5 January 2018].
6. Schultes, R. (1957). The genus Quararibea in Mexico and the use of its flowers as a spice for chocolate. *Botanical Museum Leaflets, Harvard University, 17*(9): 247–264.
7. Rosita de cacao flowers, *Quararibea funebris*, funeral tree, molinillo is a major flavoring of cacao but can also be smoked! http://maya-ethnobotany.org/images-mayan-ethnobotanicals-medicinal-plants-tropical-agriculture-flower-spice-flavoring/rosita-de-cacao-flowers-quararibea-funebris-funeral-tree-molinillo-is-a-major-flavoring-of-cacao-but-can-also-be-smoked.php [Accessed 4 January 2018].
8. Zennie, T., Cassady, J., & Raffauf, R. (1986). Funebral, a new pyrrole lactone alkaloid from *Quararibea funebris*. *Journal of Natural Products, 49*(4): 695–698.
9. Zennie, T., & Cassady, J. (1990). Funebradiol, a new pyrrole lactone alkaloid from *Quararibea funebris* Flowers. *Journal of Natural Products, 53*(6): 1611–1614.
10. Hernández, F. (1615). *Quatro Libros de la Naturaleza, Y Virtudes de las Plantas, y animales, que estan recevidos en el uso de Medicina en la Nueva España, y la Methodo, y correction, y preparacion, que para administrarlas se requiere con lo que el Doctor Francisco Hernández escrobo en lengua Latina*. F. Ximenez (Trans.). www.wdl.org/en/item/7334/200m/#group=1&page=1 [Accessed 25 January 2012].
11. Topic: *Quararibea funebris*. http://tropicalfruitforum.com/index.php?topic=5296.0 [Accessed 8 January 2018].
12. Kew Gardens (2013). *The Plant List: A working list of all plant species*. http://theplantlist.org/tpl1.1/record/kew-2868348 [Accessed 8 January 2018].

Smilax spp. (S.aristolochiifolia, S.domingensis, S.spinosa, S.pringlei)

Common names: Cocolmeca, Cozol-mecatl (Nahuatl), Cocolmecatl, Cozolmeca, Colcameca, Olcacatzan, Tecuammaitl, Axquiote, Kok-Che (Mayan dialect), Zarzaparilla, Wild Sarsaparilla.[1,4,19]

Plant family: Smilaceae

Habit & habitat: Grows in temperate and semi-warm regions in Mexico, prefers moderately damp forests on the Atlantic slope, such as those in temperate mountainous areas and deciduous tropical forests.[2] Evergreen shrub, climber—can grow like a herb or woody vine; cylindrical stem with sparse hairs (*S. pringlei*).[2] Simple, lanceolate to ovate leaves, 5–9 veined, sparsely hairy. Tuberous rhizome;[1] small red berries with 2–3 seeds. Small flowers, dioecious.[3]

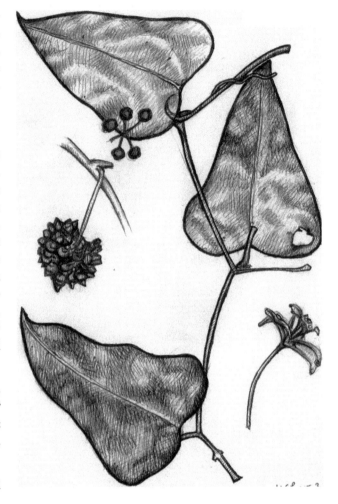

Cultivation: Grows in heavy or light, acid or alkaline but well-drained soil.[3] Frost-tender. Full sun to partial shade; propagated by seed sown in autumn, or by suckers in spring.[9]

Parts used: Fresh leaf and stem, dried root.

Phytochemistry: Steroidal saponins, incl. aglycones parillin, and sarsaponin and sarsaparilloside; phytosterols; flavonoids incl. quercetin and kaempferol; polyphenols; volatile oils.[8]

Traditional uses: Fresh young shoots and tender stems used in traditional Cacao drinks. Contemporary Mexican folk medicine use of *Smilax spp.* roots as infusion with other herbs, for weight loss. Traditional uses reported by Spanish colonists: *S. pringlei* dried root, identified as *cocolmeca* in Cuautla marketplaces, is used in combination with other plants for urinary tract problems: calculi, kidney inflammation, dysuria; also burning feet, painful shoulders, wounds and bruises, and melasma (hyperpigmentation of the skin, usually during pregnancy). It is used in other formulae for obesity, to enhance weight loss.[2] One Mexica magical formula calls for the ground root, mixed with five other roots and barks, to be put in a turkey head washed with urine as a talisman against scabies.[5] Regarded as a "blood cleanser" when used internally, *Smilax* species roots were traditionally regarded as anti-venereals against syphilis and gonorrhoea, and were used to help recovery from snakebite, for skin disorders, against weakness, and as a digestive tonic.[5,6] *Smilax* species roots are also considered to possess antipruritic, febrifuge, analgesic, and anti-rheumatic properties, are used in liver disease, and are considered specific for psoriasis in modern European herbal medicine.[1,3,6,9] Leaf: topical application vs. bloodshot eyes.[1]

Scientific data: Various Smilax species have been studied. *In vitro*, *S. regelii* root aqueous extract inhibited some fungal dermatophytes. Steroidal saponins from the roots of Asiatic Sarsaparilla species *S. glabra* have COX-2 inhibitory, anti-inflammatory activity.[10] Low concentrations of standardised aqueous extract of *S. glabra* roots inhibited migration and invasion of several cancer cell lines—HepG2 ( ), MDA-MB-231 ( ), and T24 ( ) *in vitro*.[11] *S. glabra* and *S. china* root extracts have pro-apoptotic and anti-proliferative activity against various liver, cervical, and breast cancer cell lines.[12,13,14] *S. china* root extract inhibited beta-amyloid and ischaemia-induced neuronal damage in cultured rat neurons.[16,17,18]

In vivo (non-human animals): *S. regelii* extract prevented carbon tetrachloride induced liver damage in rats.[6] Hypoglycaemic effects have been noted in mice following oral administration of root extract.[8] Oral *S. glabra* root extract at 400–800mg/kg bodyweight inhibited inflammation and normalised immune function in arthritic rats challenged with lipopolysaccharide injection or cyclophosphamide.[15] Standardised water extracts from *S. glabra* roots administered orally over a two-week period to young female nude mice previously inoculated with human breast adenocarcinoma cells significantly reduced the number of lung metastases in comparison with the control group.[11]

In vivo (humans): open (no placebo group) trials: improvements in psoriasis for daily *Smilax sp.* root decoction (15g in 1L) over two to three months; 2.4g *Smilax sp.* root standardised extract per day reduced serum urea in patients with nephritis; and standardised extracts of *S. ornata* equivalent to 30g dried root per day for several months proved superior to sulfones for the treatment of leprosy.[6]

Summary of actions: Anti-rheumatic, anti-inflammatory, depurative (trad. "blood cleanser") anti-psoriatic; possibly, anti-proliferative vs. liver, breast, and cervical cancers, neuroprotective.

Indications: Roots: psoriasis, chronic skin disorders, rheumatoid arthritis;[6] possible adjunct in long-term cancer prevention or management strategies.

Cautions: Theoretically, according to the German Commission E report, *Smilax* root species may increase elimination of digitalis glycosides and bismuth or other drugs when administered simultaneously, so should be used cautiously when taken for medicinal purposes.[6]

Dose, preparation, and use with Cacao: Young plant stems—most likely of Mexican Sarsaparillla, *S. aristolochiifolia*—are used interchangeably with *Aristolochia laxiflora* as a foaming agent for making *popo* in contemporary Oaxaca (see Chapter 8), and for making Sarsaparilla root beer.[4] To make *popo*, the fresh plant material is briefly toasted over hot ashes, then ground with corn to make a masa; Cacao paste and sugar are added, and the mixture is put in a sack and kneaded in water to yield a saponin-rich emulsion which is then whipped into a froth.[7] Cocolmeca was likely one of several pre-Colombian foaming agents for *cacahuatl* and other maize-free Cacao-based beverages.

References

1. Linares, E., Bye, R., & Flores, B. (1999). *Plantas Medicinales de Mexico: usos y remedios tradicionales.* Mexico City: Instituto de Biologia UNAM.
2. Monroy-Ortiz, C., & Castillo-Espana, P. (2007). *Plantas Medicinales Utilizadas en el Estad de Morelos. 2nd Edition.* Morelos, Mexico: Comision Nacional para el Conocimiento y Uso de la Bioversidad.
3. http://pfaf.org/user/Plant.aspx?LatinName=Smilax+aristolochiifolia [Accessed 24 August 2017].
4. https://laroussecocina.mx/diccionario/definicion/cocolmeca [Accessed 23 July 2017].
5. Badiano, J. (1552). *Libellus de Medicinalibus Indorum Herbis.* M. de la Cruz (Trans.). Mexico: Fondo de Cultura Economica Instituto Mexicano del Seguro Social, 1996.
6. Bone, K. (2003). *A Clinical Guide To Blending Liquid Herbs.* UKLondon: Churchill Livingstone.
7. Trilling, S. (1999). *Seasons of My Heart: A Culinary Journey Through Oaxaca, Mexico.* New York: Ballantine.
8. Williams, E. (2003). *Potter's Herbal Cyclopaedia.* Saffron Walden, UK: C. W. Daniel.
9. Bown, D. (2002). *The Royal Horticultural Society Encyclopedia of Herbs and their Uses.* London: Dorling Kindersley.
10. Shao, B., Guo, H., Cui, Y., Ye, M., Han, J., & Guo, D. (2007). Steroidal saponins from Smilax china and their anti-inflammatory activities. *Phytochemistry, 68*(5): 623–630.
11. She, T., Zhao, C., Feng, J., Wang, L., Qu, L., Fang, K., Cai, S., & Shou, C. (2015). Sarsaparilla (*Smilax glabra* rhizome) extract inhibits migration and invasion of cancer cells by suppressing TGF-β1 pathway. *PLoS One, 10*(3): e0118287.
12. She, T., Qu, L., Wang, L., Yang, X., Xu, S., Feng, J., Gao, Y., Zhao, C., Han, Y., Cai, S., & Shou, C. (2015). Sarsaparilla (Smilax glabra rhizome) extract inhibits cancer cell growth by S phase arrest, apoptosis, and autophagy via Redox-dependent ERK1/2 pathway. *Cancer Prevention Research (Philadelphia), 8*(5): 464 UK: Churchill Livingstone–474.
13. Sa, F., Gao, J., Fung, K., Zheng, Y., Lee, S., & Wang, Y. (2008). Anti-proliferative and pro-apoptotic effect of Smilax glabra Roxb. extract on hepatoma cell lines. *Chemico-Biological Interactions, 171*(1): 1–14.
14. Li, Y., Gan, G., Zhang, H., Wu, H., Li, C., Huang, Y., Liu, Y., & Liu, J. (2007). A flavonoid glycoside isolated from *Smilax china* L. rhizome *in vitro* anticancer effects on human cancer cell lines. *Journal of Ethnopharmacology, 113*(1): 115–124.
15. Jiang, J., & Xu, Q. (2003). Immunomodulatory activity of the aqueous extract from rhizome of *Smilax glabra* in the later phase of adjuvant-induced arthritis in rats. *Journal of Ethnopharmacology, 85*(1): 53–59.
16. Ban, J., Cho, S., Choi, S., Ju, H., Kim, J., Bae, K., Song, K., & Seong, Y. (2008). Neuroprotective effect of *Smilacis chinae* rhizome on NMDA-induced neurotoxicity *in vitro* and focal cerebral ischemia *in vivo. Journal of Pharmacological Sciences, 106*(1): 68–77.
17. Ban, J., Jeon, S., Bae, K., Song, K., & Seong, Y. (2006). Catechin and epicatechin from Smilacis chinae rhizome protect cultured rat cortical neurons against amyloid beta protein (25-35)-induced neurotoxicity through inhibition of cytosolic calcium elevation. *Life Sciences, 79*(24): 2251–2259.

18. Ban, J., Cho, S., Koh, S., Song, K., Bae, K., & Seong, Y. (2006). Protection of amyloid beta protein (25-35)-induced neurotoxicity by methanol extract of *Smilacis chinae* rhizome in cultured rat cortical neurons. *Journal of Ethnopharmacology, 106*(2): 230–237.
19. Gutierrez, L. (2014). El Chupipe. http://otromundoesposible.net/el-chupipe/ [Accessed 4 July 2018].

Theobroma bicolor (Hunb. & Bonpl.)[3]

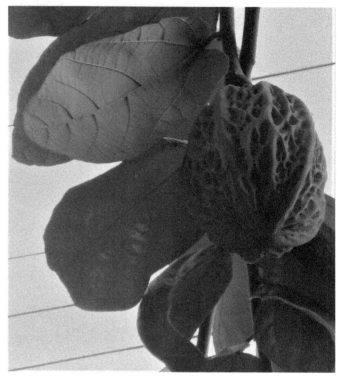

Common names: Pataxtle,[1] Cacao cimarrón,[2] Pataxte (Maya), Balamit, Balanté, Cacao Blanco, Pataste de Sapo, Patashte (Mexican common names), Mocambo, Nicaraguan Cacao, Peru Cocoa, Tiger Cocoa, Jaguar Cacao, Wild Cacao.[3]

Plant   family: Malvaceae (Sterculiaceae)

Habitat: Forests in humid regions of Central and South America. Requires mean annual temperatures from 25–30°C and 2000–3000+mm annual rainfall, up to 1000m above sea level.[3] Evergreen tree 25–30m tall; grey, fissured bark; alternate, simple cordate leaves, very large when the tree is immature but smaller on older trees. Unlike Cacao, flowers and fruit grow on the upper branches;[9] flowers are small, star-shaped, five-petalled pink or red with superior ovaries; fruit is oblong to ovoid, fatter and rounder than Cacao, green when unripe, turning yellow-brown when ripe, with a deeply grooved, ribbed and nerved hard pericarp. Unlike Cacao, fruit fall to the ground when ripe.[3,9]

Cultivation: Partial sun or shade, well-drained clay or loamy soil in tropical climates with moderately high humidity (see above).[3]

Parts used: Toasted or fermented seeds, fruit pulp.

Phytochemistry: Fruit pulp: polysaccharides, sugars (sucrose, glucose, fructose: higher sucrose, lower fructose and glucose than *T. cacao*),[4] organic acids (citric and malic acids), phenolics (<50% phenolic content of *T. cacao*;[4] incl. phenolic acids: salicylic, *trans*-cinnamic, sinapinic, chlorogenic, protocatechinic, gallic, quinic, p-hydroxybenzoic),[7] volatile compounds (incl. ethyl acetate, linalool, ethyl benzoate);[6] xanthine alkaloids: caffeine, ≤ 0.184mg/g; theophylline, ≤ 0.522mg/g; theobromine ≤ 1.468mg/g;[10] Class 1 chitinases.[4] Seeds: carbohydrates (total) 34.35% fresh weight,[3] proteins, 3.13—3.37% dry weight[3,4] (vs. 2.51% in *T. cacao*); lipids 25.48%[5]—33% dry weight[7] (vs. 57% in *T. cacao*; 96.5% triglycerides (of which: 1-stearyl-2,3 diolein 38.6%; 2-oleyl-1,3 distearin 25.4%, 1-palmito-2-oleyl-stearin 13.8%); 2.5% diglycerides;

1.7% free fatty acids (of which: stearic 42.3%, oleic 45.2%, palmitoleic 6%));[8] xanthine alkaloids: caffeine, ≤ 0.147mg/g; theophylline, ≤ 0.216mg/g; theobromine ≤ 1.710mg/g.[10]

Traditional use: Both pulp and seeds are used in foods and beverages. Fruit pulp is eaten on its own, made into beverages, or mixed with the red dye *achiote* made from Annatto (*Bixa Orellana*) (q.v.) and a little sugar to produce a common dessert. Toasted seeds mainly used as a Cacao substitute in *atoles* and beverages,[3] for which purpose they are regarded as a cheaper and inferior form of Cacao;[12] but they are sometimes eaten as a snack, or used in food, and appreciated in their own right. *T. bicolor* fruit and seeds have nutritive value and restorative properties, and in the post-conquest Yucatec Maya *Chilam Balam* books, *Balamte* (*T. bicolor*) is referred to as a tree in "the first level of heaven".[13] *T. bicolor* seeds are also fermented for several months by burying them in water-filled pits in Oaxaca, Mexico, and thereby transformed into a crumbly white bean with a black shell called *cacao blanco*, and used as a foaming agent in the regional *Chocolate Atole*.[11]

Scientific data: N/A. Almost unbelievably for a staple food plant, no tests have been carried out to determine or check for medicinal properties. The presence of the xanthine alkaloids, phenolics, and lipids in a similar profile to Cacao but with lower concentrations of xanthines and phenolics suggests similar but milder properties and effects to *Theobroma cacao*.

Summary of actions: Mild stimulant, restorative tonic; possibly anti-diabetic and cardioprotective actions like its relative, *Theobroma cacao,* but this requires experimental confirmation. Possible mild anti-asthmatic and bronchodilator (theophylline).

Indications: Exhaustion or fatigue with low mood; convalescence. May be suitable where Cacao is too stimulating or produces ADRs due to its higher alkaloid content. Note that *T. bicolor* fruit pulp contains more than double the theophylline of its seeds,[10] so may be more useful in asthma or drunk as a *refresco* in simple fatigue; the seeds, with their added macronutrient (fat and protein) content, may be more useful in convalescence.

Cautions: Allergy or xanthine sensitivity. Fruit pulp contains chitinases, known allergens also found in chestnuts and avocados.

Dose, preparation, and use with Cacao: Used both in place of and with Cacao. As a restorative or stimulating tonic for caffeine-sensitive persons, toasted seeds may be shelled and ground and used in beverages, in doses of 20–60g; the fruit pulp may be eaten raw, or blended with a little water to make a *refresco*. Both may be eaten as foods, and overdosage, though technically possible, is highly unlikely. Specially fermented seeds are used with toasted Cacao seeds to produce foam (see Chapters 2, 6, and 8).

References

1. 21 September 2018: Interview with restauranteur and chef Carmen Santiago, Teotitlan del Valle, Oaxaca, Mexico.
2. 2 October 2018: Interview with *Popo* vendor Doña Rosa Gregorio, Ojitlan, Oaxaca, Mexico.

3. Lim, T. (2012). Theobroma bicolor. *Edible Medicinal and Non-Medicinal Plants, volume 3: Fruits* (pp. 204–207). Dordrecht, the Netherlands: Springer.

4. Pérez-Mora, W., Jorrin-Novo, J., & Melgareio, L. (2018). Substantial equivalence analysis in fruits from three Theobroma species through chemical composition and protein profiling. *Food Chemistry, 240*: 496–504.

5. Furlán, A., & Bressani, R. (1999). Recursos vegetales con potencial de explotación agroindustrial de Guatemala. Caracterización química de la pulpa y la semilla de Theobroma bicolor. *Archivos latinoamericanos de nutricion, 49*(4): 373–378.

6. Quijano, C., & Pino, J. (2011). Analysis of volatile compounds of Cacao Maraco (*Theobroma bicolor* Humb. et Bonpl.) fruit. *Journal of Essential Oil Research, 21*(3): 211–215.

7. Torres, D., Assuncão, D., Mancini, P., Torres, R., & Mancini-Filho, J. (2002). Antioxidant activity of macambo (*Theobroma bicolor* L.) extracts. *European Journal of Lipid Science and Technology, 104*(5): 278–281.

8. Jee, M. (1984). Composition of the fat extracted from the seeds of Theobroma bicolor. *Journal of the American Oil Chemists' Society, 61*(4): 751–753.

9. (2015). http://maya-ethnobotany.org/cacao-cocoa-chocolate-recipes-cookbook-aztec-food-zapotec-mixtec-mayan-ethnobotanical/mayan-chocolate-cocoa-cacao-pataxte-theobroma-bicolor.php [Accessed 27 February 2019].

10. Duke, J. (1992). *Theobroma bicolor (Sterculiaceae)*. https://phytochem.nal.usda.gov/phytochem/plants/show/1998?et=P [Accessed 27 February 2019].

11. Kennedy, D. (2010). *Oaxaca al Gusto: An Infinite Gastronomy*. Austin, TXUSA: University of Texas Press; and 21 September 2018: Interview with restaurateur and chef Carmen Santiago, Teotitlan del Valle, Oaxaca, Mexico.

12. Coe, S. (1994). *America's First Cuisines*. Austin, TX: University of Texas Press.

13. Kufer, J., & McNeil, C. (2006). The Jaguar Tree (*Theobroma bicolor*). In: C. McNeil (Ed.), *Chocolate in Mesoamerica: A Cultural History of Cacao* (pp. 90–104). Gainesville, FLUSA: University Press of Florida.

Vanilla planifolia (Andrews)

Common names: Vanilla, Flor Negra, Tlilxochitl (Nahuatl),[1] Che'sib'ik (Q'eqchi Maya), Siisbik-k'aak (?—Maya dialect).[10]

Plant family: Orchidaceae[7]

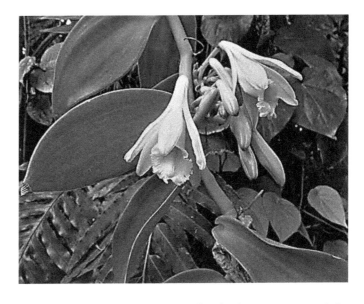

Habit & habitat: Grows in tropical lowlands, for example, the Gulf coast of Mexico,[1] Veracruz, Alta Verapaz, and Peten, as well as Izabal in Guatemala;[10] native to South America, West Indies, and Florida. A vine-like climbing orchid,[2] sticks to trees with long, whitish aerial roots. *V. planifolia* has 1–2cm thick zig-zag stems, fleshy pointed oblong leaves 8–25cm long, yellow-green flowers 5cm across,[7] and fleshy green pods which mature over eight to ten months, and become black, shrivelled, and highly aromatic after fermentation and drying.[8]

Cultivation: Meliponid bees, Vanilla's natural pollinators, are very inefficient, so for commercial purposes it is hand-pollinated.[2] Fruits take five to seven months to ripen. Requires well-drained, rich soil, bright, indirect sunlight, high humidity—80% or more—and prefers temperatures; between 26 and 30°C. Frost tender, minimum temperature is 16°C. Grown in loops rather than upright to maximise pod production. Propagated by 1.5–2m long cuttings, left coiled in a dry shady place for two to three weeks before planting.[7]

Parts used: Dried, fermented seed pod.

Phytochemistry: Essential oil (phenylpropanoids incl. vanillin (4-hydroxy-3- methoxy benzaldehyde), 1 to 3.5% dry weight whole bean, and 85% of all volatilesthe remainder constitute approximately 0.03–0.04% dry weight,[12] and include guaiacol,[12] vanillic acid, *p*-anisaldehyde, *p*-hydroxybenzoic acid, *p*-anisic acid, *p*-anisyl alcohol, *p*-cresol, *p*-coumaric acid, coumarin, glucovanillin, caproic acid, ferulic acid, piperonal, vitispiranes, eugenol, phenols, phenol ether, benzyl ether, bis-4-(β-d-glucopyranosyloxy)-benzyl-2-isopropyltartrate, bis-4-(β-d-glucopyranosyloxy)-benzyl-2-(2-butyl)tartrate); polyphenols: tannins, alkaloids,[23] resins,[11] lactones; carbohydrates, 25% dry weight; fats, 15% dry weight; vitamins, minerals, etc.[8]

Traditional use: Before use, Vanilla fruits (seed pods) are briefly scalded, fermented, then dried in the sun before "conditioning" for several months, which generates their characteristic aroma.[2] The fermented pods were principally used as a spice in Cacao drinks. Vanilla pods also featured in the magico-medicinal Mexica prescription body wash to treat "the fatigue of those who administer the republic" (see *Bourreria huanita* monograph for details).[3] According to the seventeenth-century Spanish physician Francisco Hernández, Vanilla combined with *Piper sanctum* effectively helped to expel the placenta, post-partum, or a stillborn child (intrauterine death); he described Vanilla as effective against "cold poisons" and "cold bites of poisonous animals".[5] Hernández's contemporary, Dr Juan de Cardenas, commended Vanilla as "having an advantage above all other spices in being … friendly to the heart".[6] The seventeenth-century English physician Henry Stubbe, following Hernández, recommended Vanilla "to strengthen the brain and the womb", as well as commending it in combination with *Bixa orellana* for diarrhoea and "weak stomachs", with *Piper sanctum* for "cold stomachs and phlegmatic obstructions" (e.g., stomach cramps, lack of appetite, expectoration of phlegm?), and with another unidentified native Mexican herb called Tepeyantli to treat coughs. He describes it as hot and dry in the third degree, and adds that, much like *Pimienta dioica*, it has cordial, carminative, emmenagogue, and parturient properties.[4] Other traditional medicinal uses of *V. planifolia* included treatment of fevers, spasms, dysmenorrhoea, and "hysteria".[11]

Scientific data: <u>*In vitro*</u>, ethanolic fresh leaf extracts from *V. planifolia* had significant bacteriostatic activity against *Escherichia coli* and *Proteus vulgaris*, with some activity against *Enterobacter aerogenes*, *Pseudomonas aeruginosa*, and *Streptococcus faecalis*, and low activity against *Salmonella typhi*.[23] Isolated vanillin has antimicrobial, antioxidant, anti-clastogenic, and anti-mutagenic properties,[8] preventing chromosome damage by X-rays and ultraviolet light, enhancing cisplatin cytotoxicity,[11] and inhibiting formation of non-small cell lung cancer stem cells at non-toxic doses by down-regulating transcription factors (NCI-H460 cell line).[8,14] Vanillin protected murine microglial BV-2 (dopaminergic) cells from LPS-induced inflammation, reducing expression of inducible nitric oxide, cyclooxygenase-2 and interleukins 1β and 6, demonstrating neuroprotective effects.[21] Vanillin interacts with the abnormal haemoglobin molecule in blood from people with sickle cell anaemia, causing a dose-dependent inhibition of deoxygenation-induced sickling, with no adverse effects on the cells.[18] Vanillin acts on sickle cell haemoglobin by reducing polymerisation, and alters the erythrocyte membrane permeability by inhibiting potassium chloride ion cotransporters and calcium-activated potassium channels in the cell membranes at concentrations between 0.3mM [IC_{50}] and 5mM (maximal).[15] Deoxygenated sickle cell erythrocytes are also abnormally permeable to cations, an effect which is partially and reversibly inhibited by tarantula venom toxin GsMTx-4 at 100µM, but irreversibly inhibited by vanillin at concentrations of 1000–5000 µM.[16]

<u>*In vivo*</u> (non-human animals): morphological muscle changes occurred in rats with damaged sciatic nerves given oral vanillin at doses of 150mg/kg. By comparison with untreated, injured rats, the vanillin group had greater vascularisation in the muscles (tibialis anterior and soleus), but increased inflammation evidenced by fibre atrophy and fascicular disorganisation (tibialis anterior).[13] On the other hand, vanillin orally and intra-peritoneally administered to rats at high concentration of 150 and 300mg/kg bodyweight produced no organ toxicity, though the 300mg/kg caused loss of consciousness. The researchers also noted that, while a 5% ethanol injection caused increased cell cycle arrest and apoptotic up-regulation in brain tissue, co-administration of vanillin abolished these effects, indicating neuroprotective properties.[17] Because vanillin is rapidly metabolised, oral administration of a vanillin prodrug significantly

increased the survival time of hypoxic sickle mice, while intraperitoneal injections of 7mg/kg also had significant effects.[19] Rats exposed to constant unpredictable mild stress exhibited symptoms of mild depression, assessed by immobility time in the forced swimming test and decreased sucrose consumption, which were reversed by either fluoxetine and inhalation of vanillin; vanillin inhalation also elevated 5-HT, noradrenaline, and dopamine levels more than fluoxetine in the rats' brains. The antidepressant effect of vanillin was abolished if the rats' olfactory bulbs were removed.[20] In a rat model of Parkinson's disease, intraperitoneal injections of vanillin at 5, 10, and 20mg/kg bodyweight dose-dependently and cumulatively reduced apomorphine-induced rotation and conserved tyrosine hydroxylase activity in the substantia nigra, showing anti-parkinsonian activity.[21] Vanillin decreased triglyceride levels in rats fed a high-fat diet, and increased insulin-stimulated glucose uptake.[11,24]

In vivo (humans): Vanillin inhibits erythrocyte sickling in sickle cell anaemia by penetrating erythrocytes and interacting with haemoglobin,[8,10] with oral doses of one to four grams of isolated vanillin per day being proposed for systemic anti-sickling activity[9] (equivalent to a minimum daily dosage of 28–29g whole vanilla!). In an eight-week double-blind placebo-controlled clinical trial with thirty participants, a daily dose of 1g vanillin was administered in divided doses of one 250mg capsule taken every six hours, after which the number of sickled erythrocytes declined from 81% to 61% in the _verum_ group, and the sickling time of blood taken from patients on vanillin was 1.6 times greater than blood taken from the control group, with 24.5% less shape variation in sickled blood cells. These results were indicative of reduced haemoglobin polymerisation and sickling tendency.[10] However, it has been pointed out that "Phenolic antioxidant compounds [such as vanillin] are not devoid of adverse reactions at high concentrations in biological systems," as they can sometimes enhance oxidative damage.[9] When Vanilla flavouring was added to nutritionally identical meals, those with added Vanilla were more satiating.[11,22]

Summary of actions: Antidepressant, bacteriostatic, neuroprotective, anti-sickling, hypolipidaemic, hypoglycaemic, appetite modifier (amphoteric—suppresses excess and increases deficiency), chemopreventive.

Indications: Possibly: sickle cell anaemia, depression, Parkinson's disease, type 2 diabetes mellitus, metabolic syndrome, infectious diarrhoea, cancer—adjunct to cisplatin or radiotherapy, or to prevent.

Cautions: Vanilla has been known to cause dermatitis. A syndrome called "vanillism" has been identified in workers packing and processing Vanilla, the symptoms of which are dermatitis, headaches, and insomnia.[11]

Dose, preparation, and use with Cacao: Traditionally, fermented pods were ground into cocoa mass for use in drinks. As the oral bioavailability of vanillin is poor, and the whole pod extract remains untested in sickle cell anaemia, a useful way of increasing bioavailability would be rectal administration via cocoa butter-based suppositories, made by double-infusing melted cocoa butter with chopped Vanilla pods at 1:10 (w/w), two to three times: one suppository inserted three times daily, with oral vanilla administered thrice daily as a tincture or the whole spice incorporated in Cacao-based drinks. In the event of a sickle cell crisis, two suppositories should be inserted immediately, and 2–3g Vanilla administered concomitantly in a drink containing 40g Cacao with a little Capsicum.

Tincture, 1:3, 60% ethanol: 20ml per week; acute doses: 5–10ml every hour. Powdered Vanilla pods: 0.25–0.5g thrice daily, acute dose 3–6g.

References

1. Coe, S., & Coe, M. (1996). *The True History of Chocolate*. London: Thames & Hudson.
2. Coe, S. (1994). *America's First Cuisines*. Austin, TXUSA: University of Texas Press.
3. Badiano, J. (1552). *Libellus de Medicinalibus Indorum Herbis*. M. de la Cruz (Trans.). Mexico City: Fondo de Cultura Economica Instituto Mexicano del Seguro Social, 1996.
4. Stubbe, H. (1662). *The Indian Nectar, or, A Discourse concerning chocolata*. London: J.C. for Andrew Crook.
5. Hernández, F. (1615). *Quatro Libros de la Naturaleza, Y Virtudes de las Plantas, y animales, que estan recevidos en el uso de Medicina en la Nueva España, y la Methodo, y correction, y preparacion, que para administrarlas se requiere con lo que el Doctor Francisco Hernández escrobo en lengua Latina*. M. de la Cruz (Trans.), 1996. www.wdl.org/en/item/7334/200m/#group=1&page=1 [Accessed 25 January 2012].
6. Grivetti, L. (2009). Medicinal chocolate in New Spain, Western Europe, and North America. In: Grivetti, L., & Shapiro, H. *Chocolate: History, Culture, and Heritage* (pp. 67-88). Hoboken, NJUSA: John Wiley & Sons.
7. Bown, D. (2002). *The Royal Horticultural Society New Encyclopaedia of Herbs and Their Uses*. London: Dorling Kindersley.
8. Menon, S., & Nayeem, N. (2013). *Vanilla Planifolia*: A review of a plant commonly used as flavouring agent. *International Journal of Pharmaceutical Sciences Review and Research*, 20(2): 225–228.
9. Okezie, A. (1992). Dietary management of sickle cell anaemia with vanillin. *Free Radical Research Communications*, 17(5): 349–350.
10. Fernandez Garcia, A., Cabal, C., Losada, J., Alvarez, E., Soler, C., & Otero, J. (2005). In vivo action of vanillin on delay time determined by magnetic relaxation. *Hemoglobin*, 29(3): 181–187.
11. (2009). Vanilla. *Wolters Kluwer Health*. https://www.drugs.com/npp/vanilla.html [Accessed 24 January 2018].
12. Zhang, S., & Mueller, C. (2012). Comparative analysis of volatiles in traditionally cured Bourbon and Ugandan vanilla bean (*Vanilla planifolia*) extracts. *Journal of Agricultural and Food Chemistry*, 60(42): 10433–10444.
13. Peretti, A., Antunes, J., Lovison, K., Kunz, R., Castor, L., Brancalhão, R., Bertolini, G., & Ribeiro, L. (2017). Action of vanillin (*Vanilla planifolia*) on the morphology of tibialis anterior and soleus muscles after nerve injury. *Einstein (Sao Paulo)*, 15(2): 186–191.
14. Srinual, S., Chanvorachote, P., & Pongrakhananon, V. (2017). Suppression of cancer stem-like phenotypes in NCI-H460 lung cancer cells by vanillin through an Akt-dependent pathway. *International Journal of Oncology*, 50(4): 1341–1351.
15. Hannemann, A., Cytlak, U., Gbotosho, O., Rees, D., Tewari, S., & Gibson, J. (2014). Effects of o-vanillin on K^+ transport of red blood cells from patients with sickle cell disease. *Blood Cells, Molecules & Diseases*, 53(1–2): 21–26.
16. Ma, Y., Rees, D., Gibson, J., & Ellory, J. (2012). The conductance of red blood cells from sickle cell patients: ion selectivity and inhibitors. *Journal of Physiology*, 590(9): 2095–2105.

17. Ho, K., Yazan, L., Ismail, N., & Ismail, M. (2011). Toxicology study of vanillin on rats via oral and intra-peritoneal administration. *Food and Chemical Toxicology, 49*(1): 25–30.

18. Abraham, D., Mehanna, A., Wireko, F., Whitney, J., Thomas, R., & Orringer, E. (1991). Vanillin, a potential agent for the treatment of sickle cell anemia. *Blood, 77*(6): 1334–1341.

19. Zhang, C., Li, X., Lian, L., Chen, Q., Abdulmalik, O., Vassilev, V., Lai, C., & Asakura, T. (2004). Anti-sickling effect of MX-1520, a prodrug of vanillin: an *in vivo* study using rodents. *British Journal of Haematology, 125*(6): 788–795.

20. Xu, J., Xu, H., Liu, Y., He, H., & Li, G. (2015). Vanillin-induced amelioration of depression-like behaviors in rats by modulating monoamine neurotransmitters in the brain. *Psychiatry Research, 225*(3): 509–514.

21. Yan, X., Liu, D. F., Zhang, X., Liu, D., Xu, S., Chen, G., Huang, B., Ren, W., Wang, W., Fu, S., & Liu, J. (2017). Vanillin protects dopaminergic neurons against inflammation-mediated cell death by inhibiting ERK1/2, P38 and the NF-κB signaling pathway. *International Journal of Molecular Sciences, 18*(2): E. 389.

22. Warwick, Z., Hall, W., Pappas, T., & Schiffman, S. (1993). Taste and smell sensations enhance the satiating effect of both a high-carbohydrate and a high-fat meal in humans. *Physiology and Behaviour, 53*(3): 553–563.

23. Shanmugavalli, N., Umashankar, V., & Raheem, A. (2009). Antimicrobial activity of *Vanilla planifolia*. *Indian Journal of Science and Technology, 2*(3): 37–40.

24. Park, S., Kim, D., & Kang, S. (2011). *Gastrodia elata* Blume water extracts improve insulin resistance by decreasing body fat in diet-induced obese rats: vanillin and 4-hydroxybenzaldehyde are the bioactive candidates. *European Journal of Nutrition, 50*(2): 107–118.

HONORARY MENTIONS

The following plants also have historical and ethnographic documentation of use as Cacao flavourings. I didn't have time to research all of these in any detail before publication, but the following should all be researched, monographed, and documented.

DOCUMENTED USE

- *Aristolochia laxiflora*: "Colcameca"—alternative foaming agent used in Popo. (Referenced by Trilling, 1999, pp.166 & 336 [Book].)
- *Clerodendrum ligustrinum*: Itsim-te, putative Classic Maya chocolate spice. (Referenced by Coe & Coe, 1996, p. 51 [Book]; Stuart, D., in McNeil, 2006, p. 199 [Book].)
- *Haematoxylum brasiletto*: Palo de Brasil—referenced by Maya Ethnobotany, http://maya-ethnobotany.org/dye-colorant-medicinal-plant-mayan-ethnobotanicals-guatemala-mexico/palo-de-brasil-tinto-haematoxylum-brasiletto-leguminosae.php [Accessed 4 March 2019].
- *Manilkara zapota*: Zapote, or Sapodilla, Piztle, Sapuyul (syn. *Lucuma mammosa, Archdelpha mammosa, Calocarpum mammosum*). Seeds used as flavouring in native Gautemalan or Mexican beverages; ground seeds also used in Ladino Maya *Posolli/Pozol* drink. (Referenced by Grivetti, in Grivetti & Shapiro, 2009, p. 108 [Book]; Popenoe, 1919 [Journal]; Coe, 1994, pp. 104 & 136 [Book].)

- *Philodendron pseudoradiatum*: Huacalxochitl, or Carry Crate Flower—listed by Diego Duran (referenced in Heyden's translation, 1994: p. 244, footnote 3, mentioned on http://maya-ethnobotany.org/images-mayan-ethnobotanicals-medicinal-plants-tropical-agriculture-flower-spice-flavoring/cymbopetalum-penduliflorum-orejuela-ear-flower-images.php [Accessed 4 March 2019]).
- *Pinus edulis:* Piñon Nuts. (Referenced by Grivetti, in Grivetti & Shapiro, 2009, p. 108 [Book].)

UNCERTAIN/PUTATIVE

- *Blomia prisca: Palo de Tzol*, in the Sapindaceae or Soap-berry family. "Dried berries used in Cacao, like Allspice"; also known as Palo de Tzol, Shi'lil, Xi'lil, Sijom. Tree; bitter seed in a skin; aromatic flowers, May–June. (Source: Boris, tour guide at Tikal, Guatemala—field notes, 2011. However, Don Reginaldo Chayax Huex, herbalist and director of the Asociacion Bio-Itza in San Jose, Peten, averred; according to him, the seeds of Palo de Tzol are disgustingly bitter and would ruin any beverage they were made with, so perhaps Boris was mistaken, or another part of the plant may be used, such as the outer seed coats, for example. See Appendix C, Interview 4 for the full conversation with Don Huex.)

Selected interviews

Translated by Marcos Patchett, Luciana Morera, Mohamed Awada,
and Magdalena Gutierrez

Author's note: *the six interviews transcribed below are a small selection from over twenty hours of audio recordings. Owing to space considerations, I have omitted many interesting conversations; the following interviews in particular contain extra material which is not alluded to in the main text of the book. The complete list of interviews is given at the end of this section.*

1. 18th April 2008, Mani, Yucatan Peninsula, Mexico. Interview with Sr Mario Euan, herbalist and teacher at U-Yits-Ka'an School of Agriculture & Ecology

Mario:	What's called traditional medicine are the secrets of the ancestors. I know because I was taught by my grandfather, my uncles, my father, they were … herbalists. Since I was twenty years old, I was taught to pick the medicinal plants in the mountains; I was shown animals for curing people, bugs [insects] for curing people, rocks and weeds from the field, to cure people; mainly, simple herbs. Trees, from the roots, bark, leaves, flowers, and fruits, all these things for specific ailments. If the illness needed leaves, we picked up leaves. If the illness required roots, we dug up roots, and used them for people. The thing is, if someone comes in with life, we pick them up [metaphorically help them]. However, if they are very critically ill, and almost dying, we don't compromise ourselves because they're already leaving [dying].
Me:	In your class … I think I understood—much of the time, it's important that people believe in the treatment. Because if somebody—because I didn't understand it all, but, if a person has doubts, it's more difficult because all the time it's "Where's my cure? Where's the solution?" And that's bad, because all the time in reality the solution is within them. And the herbs are only a method for assisting this process?
Mario:	Very good. Because the idea is that we cure ourselves with belief. If they want you to cure them you will cure them, with a rapid return to health, but if they go in with doubt … And modern medicine as well; perhaps they cure, perhaps not.

Me (interrupting):	One other, one other thing—
Mario:	[I'll say] this about doubts—we can't guarantee the health of that person, because the doubt is two-sided. I think if the person comes with their beliefs, they're going to say: "I want you to cure me." I go to apply the medicine—what cures more is the herbs, and the blessings of God.
Me:	Yes.
Mario:	He helps us to the greatest degree, to lift up the ill. When the ill is already on his feet [healthy], he shouldn't thank me—he should thank God that he is alive. The name of God is worshipped and glorified. For that person, who he lifts up, that's what I tell them—Don't give thanks to me, give thanks to God. He gave me life as well, I give you this medicine so you'll have more life.
Me (interrupting):	It's good to give thanks, it's good, but all people are instruments—
Mario:	Yes.
Me:	—to cure. So: chocolate drinks. Are there any such drinks here—or not? Because I think this isn't a region, here, where there are many chocolate drinks?
Mario:	There aren't.—Yes, there are some; but you buy them in the shops, ready-made.
Me:	Tablets.
Mario:	Exactly. Cacao isn't grown around here. They grow peanuts, but only for—
Me (interrupting):	Peanuts [*cacahuates*]?
Mario:	Peanuts. Very similar to Cacao.
Me:	Ah … It's another type, it's a relative?
Mario:	You buy them when you go to the movies, to the cinema, to watch or play football! You pick up a small packet of toasted nuts!
Me:	[Looks up in dictionary]—I understand, yes, peanuts, yes. So, people around here don't drink chocolate? Only from the shops?
Mario:	Yes, only the shops.
Me:	Very good. OK. Er … do you know any uses for chocolate? I talked two weeks ago with some very friendly ladies in the Witchcraft market [Sonora]—they have a herbal/medicinal stand, and they told me two uses, for me, very unique—one—Cacao with rosemary to avoid pregnancy, is, for me, new; and the other, Cacao with turkey egg for migraine. But, I understand, erm, "scientifically", chemically, because turkey—eggs—chemically help your body transform serotonin. Chocolate, Cacao, increases dopamine and serotonin. Serotonin is a part of the "cause" of migraine; there's an "explanation" for that. The other, I don't understand. But—I'm interested in the humoral properties—dry, moist, hot, cold; and the other man told me that Cacao has moist and hot properties. What do you believe?

Mario:	There are plants—that are used to refresh. Refreshing herbs. Herbs which have a refreshing power. To refresh; migraine, it's a change in the nerves. Heating of the head.
Me:	Yes, yes, yes. It's hot?
Mario:	Yes, it's hot. We pick refreshing herbs to be applied to reduce the pressure.
Me:	And Cacao, it has that power?
Mario:	Yes, it's cool, and it is—[interrupted]
Me:	You believe that Cacao is hot, or warm?
Mario:	Fresh [*fresca*].
Me:	*Fresca* is like cold?
Mario:	Exactly. It's like cold. For lowering the heat, or reducing the agitation. If there are people who seem agitated, or who seem hot—feverish—we seek refreshing herbs to lower the fever. There are people who suffer from being very cold, very cold, suffer from cough, or suffer from asthma; we give them hot herbs which reduce the cold that they have.
Me:	Cacao—it isn't good for asthma?
Mario:	No … it agitates the lungs, agitates phlegm; because for what you have in your lungs, it isn't good. Warm herbs are good for stopping asthma, and if possible with a little *Melipona* honey, they're warm honeys. So it warms [cooks] the phlegm, so it'll diminish, and can be spat out.
Me:	Thank you sir, it's interesting. Are there other herbs here which are used with Cacao, that you know of? The most common or most important here.
Mario:	Well, all of the herbs here; they're all important. What we're seeing here now is a lot of demand, kidney stones, gallstones, bladder stones, diabetes, and fungus. Yes—of the skin. They are things which, truly, aren't very big things; but—if the person doesn't know the herbs, then they will suffer. Or else the person stays hunched over from the stones in their kidneys, because if you're holding in the pain, you will stay hunched over. There are rich people who say, "I don't believe in herbs, I'm going to go get cut [have surgery]." They're cut; the stone is extracted. You have money, but a poor person—their wallet is hurt, their body is hurt, and they won't be able to go back to work as usual. Because a person who is a labourer, once they are cut [have surgery], they can't return to labouring, because the wound scars up and if he works hard perhaps he will reopen the wound.
Me:	So, without money here, they can't use—they can't have surgery?
Mario:	No—they can be cured with herbs. Then they won't hurt their wallet, they won't hurt their body, and they can carry on working as usual. But you know what, academic doctors, they can make good money. Traditional doctors, thank God, we only make the decoction and give it for them to take. In a few days, the stone will have gone down [descended].
Me:	Come down?
Mario:	With herbs.

Me: Very good. Because in England, those conditions—kidney stones, and diabetes ... herbalists, herb doctors—aren't allowed to treat them. It's illegal. But, a lot of the time, we have people that ask about them, "Can you give me a remedy?"; in that situation you have to write to their doctor to ask their permission, but, that's good, you can give herbs ...

Mario: Really, it's the law there? It's the law? Because here with us, that's how my grandparents were. When they see that someone is curing a person, they say, "You're taking my patient, you don't know anything." And they say, "Those who use medicine should know how to read and write to use it." There's no need to study [academically] if I have the experience of my grandparents. And the academic doctors, do they want to make fun of us, or what? We plant the illnesses in our body, harvest them, cause them ourselves and then suffer because of them. Academic doctors only buy from the pharmacy—whether he cures or not, there he is, taking the money [anyway].

Me: That's why this school is very important. Because your—all your experience— [is being passed on] to another generation.

Mario: [in agreement] Because there are already thirteen generations going through right now.

Me: Because now ... when modern medicine, chemicals, are more—not important, but more—

Mario: Expensive.

Me: Yes ...

Mario: Every year they raise the price of medicine.

Me: Yes.

Mario: And in turn, here, every year they plant botanical gardens, gardens of medicinal plants. It's very interesting.

Me: It's very interesting and it's very necessary. So ... erm ... Cacao—It's why I'm here! So, some plants that I believe are used with Cacao a lot, chilli? Historically annatto? Vanilla? And another, I don't know its name here—if it has any use here, but—*Hueynacaztli*? It's from Oaxaca, further from here ... but, vanilla, annatto ... You know ... around here—more local?

Mario: What is the ... green chilli, habanero chilli—they're abundant. Abundant. We use them as medicine, this chilli [whistles], the upright chilli [*chili parado*]; it grows like that, upright. Sometimes when I explain it to the students, they laugh because the upright chilli they say is a penis. The upright chilli hangs, but it doesn't hang upside down—it hangs upright. It's medicinal.

Me: OK. You use it in chocolate drinks?

Mario: No. We only use it like that.

Me: OK. What types of chillis are used in drinks?

Mario: None. They're only eaten. In food. In drinks: not at all.

Me: OK. Vanilla. Medicinal properties?

Mario:	Vanilla: no more than a flavouring, for a drink such as—such as *horchata*, they mix in vanilla—to give it flavour, but it's not used in medicine.
Me:	OK—annatto? Any uses?
Mario:	Annatto is useful—it's used as medicine. Primarily for infections, for throat infections. Secondly—for the people whose penis has taken a rest. It raises it [helps erections]. And annatto leaves, they're used in cough syrup.
Me:	And the properties of annatto, it's—cold, hot?
Mario:	Warm.
Me:	And—moist or dry?
Mario:	Er—moist.
Marcos:	And Cacao is a little cold and a little moist? How interesting.
Mario:	Mmm. Good. I think that we've reached the end.

2. 25th April 2008, No. 42 Calle 1 San Marco, San Cristobal de las Casas,
Chiapas, Mexico. Interview with herbalist Roberto Molina

Roberto: So—what would you like to ask? Well—I was talking to you about—well—
              the implications of time on the elements.

Marcos: Yes.

Roberto: On the natural elements. Ah, I was talking to you about the amount, about
              the element of time which … follows which is like a shine, and which also has
              several attributes like quantity, quality, and also has another element, in my
              view, which is magic.

              We could say that it's only [about] quantity or quality; however, either of
              the two creates magic. And I'm always thinking about Maya medicine as
              well. Or in—in helping, like [performing] a cure, always not to lose myself—
              so I don't lose myself in my mind, in my ideas. I always try to go back to
              basics—which are: the elements, time, and logic. And the basics for Maya
              medicine are nature—you can talk a lot about nature, but the basics are the
              elements. Nature—and the levels—it's how they lived life, as three levels.
              Like real life, the underworld, and the overworld. But this is very romanti-
              cised. But, it's more practical to think only—that these levels have no name,
              but they exist.

              So it could be like in a patient, it could be your—if you think on three levels,
              it could be your state of health, because a patient who comes to you with
              something wrong, still has a state of health, [but] at the same time, it could be
              your state of health, your disease state, and the mixture of these two [states],
              which is another, different state. So—to fix this, you can use time. So—on
              the same day that a patient is ill, there is a time of quality that you can make
              advantage of. Also, it's important to take the time of quantity [*es importante
              tomar el tiempo de cantidad*]. Or, how many times you're going to administer
              a plant, or how many times in one hour, how many times in one [period
              of] time, how many times in a day. But always it's very important to value
              quality over quantity.

              That—from my point of view—the global sickness, from which very few save
              themselves, very few in the communities, perhaps some [a few], but no longer
              [seldom]—the global sickness which we have is quantity. So, we have to strike
              a balance. And in general for each doctor, this ought to be somewhere to begin.
              We already know that each patient has an illness of quantity—in something—
              and we have to do the first thing—the first work, is this. Hundreds, hundreds,
              thousands of patients—you only have to control their quantity. Quantity—
              why? OK. It's a problem when you have a problem of quantity—with regard
              to, to eating, for example. It's a problem, but, when you have a problem of
              quantity with thinking—that's very strong. And you can't measure out por-
              tions of food very easily. But you can measure out portions of ideas, very easy.
              With media, with internet. So, this is very interesting. But in principle, it is not

being used well. And this is one of our jobs. Of all the people who have clear what the qualities of time are. Of quantity, and of quality.

So—for, for Cacao, which is a—which has—it's—hmm—OK. The virtues of Cacao—you know them, the nutritional virtues—and, what are its effects? More or less depending on who consumes it. But, if you want to get into magic, of the knowledge around Cacao—you must contextualise all of those values in quantity of time and quality of time. And when you have questions that you can't answer, you can help yourself with the elements, fire and water. And the elements not only as they are, they use where the elements come from, and the elements within the context of time. That is to say that fire of the daytime isn't the same as fire of the night. And, in that way, you can get very interesting answers about Cacao.

Marcos: For myself, one of my objectives is to put Cacao into European astrological language. Because all plants, this book has a—for example—lettuce. Lettuce is a plant of the Moon, and all plants can be put into, are ruled by a planet, and at times by a sign. Since this planet has an astrological meaning—it's easier to use astrology in medicine because *this* problem can be treated by *this* herb because it is a Moon herb. [Let's say] you have a sick person, with too much heat, too dry—lettuce is cool and moist so you can use it. For me it is so important to be able to classify Cacao in astrology because it is my tongue [language], I think, for all themes of time and the elements. It's something I use because—

Roberto: And lettuce is very good for sleep, right?

Marcos: Yes, also, the Moon is cool and moist and against Mars, which is hot and dry. The juice of the lettuce with rose oil on your head is for sleeping and to prevent headaches from heat. When you eat boiled lettuce, it's bitter, but it's good for indigestion, to reduce thirst—and a side effect is that it is forbidden for people with asthma [shortwinded] or those with some lung problems, or blood. Uff, it's fantastic. I want to put Cacao and other herbs used with it in this system and if possible to find the Mayan classifications. Because Maya astrology is really interesting to me because I know it is hard to find in books. Venus is maleficent—not maleficent but is a planet of war, but in European astrology it's a planet of peace, so the opposite. And it is the planet of sweets, friendly, agreeable, and here, I believe Venus is used to decide when to go into war and is a bit maleficent—I don't know very well. The qualities are in opposition; and when Cacao is drunk here [it] is traditionally bitter and spicy; and in Europe is sweet, and tasty. It's interesting to me, I don't know— very interesting. And values in religion, I don't know at the moment, it's all [just] ideas.

Roberto: Another really interesting thing I was telling you about before—you need to go to Mexico city. There, in the airport, there's a place where you—they— well, they have a Oaxacan shop. And they want to sell a new idea of Cacao. So there they have some types of spices, they take the Cacao, they mix it up and you bite into it, you can ask for whatever amount you want. I was in shock there … almost—why? I went because I said to myself—these shops, chocolate [shops]—have no interest in—they have products like—very—yes, like different, but they also have Cacao. And they offer it to you with lots of sugar—again—but I said, it's not possible. I mean, for someone to think of Cacao without sugar. Well! But, I asked them for Cacao without any sugar. They put it into a machine they have there, Mexican, special—

Marcos: —in the airport?

Roberto: In the airport, yes. They put it [the Cacao] in the machine—and I just walked around. From five metres I could smell the aroma of Cacao. Very strong! From five metres away the smell reached me. I went to see, there was my Cacao, one kilo only. When it came out, the Cacao was like a—a very liquid texture—

Marcos: Because without sugar in the machine—it's not a tablet, it's more liquid?

Roberto: —Aha—and it was pure Cacao. And I told the lady there, no, no, no! Without milk, without water! [She said,] "Nothing else! Only Cacao!" And it became liquid.

Marcos: It was very liquid? Or a bit solid?

Roberto: More liquid than solid—that's to say, it fell [poured] like this, shhhhhh … it stayed sticky. It was like a volcano! And this is something marvellous. You must watch when they grind it. Why when it's ground? Because that transformation is very, very, very special. So I think it's very important to experiment with different types of heat, different times, different ways of grinding, everything. And no—but it is, er—Benjamin [Roberto's expatriate European neighbour, who prepares his own drinking chocolate from Cacao beans] said that metal is no good for Cacao.

Marcos: Yes, yes—I think that's true.

Roberto: Yes—I think it's true. But—it depends how it's used, it depends on the time—the amount of time—and I think that because it was so immediate—

Marcos: Yes, it's hot, and in contact with the metal for a long time, it's bad, but very brief contact is quite—it's not very hot—

Roberto: Yes. I think not. There isn't a problem. My tongue, my mouth—it's very sensitive, and I can tell when food has been affected by metal.

Marcos: Yes. OK.

Roberto: So—this Cacao—nothing happened—very good.

Marcos: Yes? This type—this liquid in the airport? Yes?

Roberto: From the airport. Very good it was too.

* * *

Roberto: So I think it's important to specify—why? Because all the books, all that is written in Europe about the ancient cultures of Mexico or Mesoamerica, are a bit confused. For example, if we talk about health. If we talk about health in Europe, we are talking about a very similar global system.

Marcos: Yes.

Roberto:	But it isn't global—but, well, let's say it's global, OK. If we're talking about health care—and health care is provided more by the government. If we're talking about health in Mexico, there's also health care which is provided by the government. But there is another health care [system] which isn't state health care, it isn't given by the state—it's personal health. These are the systems of health in Mexico when we talk about the *mestizos* [mixed race]. But in Mexico, there's also an indigenous population, who are Mexicans too. This population is very different. In fact, health for the indigenous people, isn't—yes!—there is a part, a very small part, that has to do with the community. But health is something very personal. What's more, health is part of politics, of economics—like Cacao. It's the same, but for us—no! One thing is, for my average citizen [*mestizo*]; one thing is—your health; another thing is your economy. A very different other thing is the politics—
Marcos:	In the Maya world—
Roberto:	In the indigenous world—
Marcos:	It's the same—it's one part—your body is part of the larger body of the world.
Roberto:	Exactly. And, to say for example—but that's it, that's it, your body is the same, it's very pretty, it's very poetic—but in practice, it's that—to grow Cacao, there is a ceremony—beforehand—there's a party—because it's come to the part of the cycle when they're going to start planting the seeds. And this is very practical; it's like—like you would have done as well. Before you began university, you took a journey, you had a party. And this is the same thing they do. And it begins there—like that—the ceremony. And the authorities also take part in this party, the farmers take part, the religious authorities, the political authorities; everyone joins in. So—you're going to say something; can you pause it? I need to speak to someone.

* * *

Roberto:	So, it's important—when we talk about—Chinese medicine? I don't know China, but I think that we're talking about a part of Chinese medicine, or of ancient Chinese medicine. So I think that this is very important—about Cacao or about Maya medicine. One part of Maya medicine is still alive today; but another part isn't. And this is very important to clarify. One part of Maya medicine is used in Mexico by some Mexicans in some regions, but it isn't Mexican medicine or Mayan medicine, because there are Mayan regions where they don't use Mayan medicine.
Marcos:	[It's] diffuse?
Roberto:	Right. It's very, very diffuse [unclear]. And the books—because it's a bit complicated to explain, and because it must be questioned—there isn't a written knowledge in Mexico either. People prefer not to put it down [in writing]. Because they want to put down something very clear.
Marcos:	OK—because when it's written, some things are—it's like, set in stone and if it's a tradition of several very valuable parts, to set it down [in print,

	inaccurately]—it isn't right—it isn't good, because there are several different

inaccurately]—it isn't right—it isn't good, because there are several different parts. So, if I write—you think that in this book—about how to use Cacao—and other herbs—examples would be better? Or what—what do you think?

Roberto: OK—from my point of view it would be better to put down a little bit of history. Like how Cacao was used in the field of medicine, in economics, yes; and afterwards, how it was developed. And afterwards you could give an example, of a drink, for instance. Like this drink from its point of origin, its evolution until after the Spanish came, and its development today. Because they're also very different. And—OK—the evolution of the beverage by the *mestizos*, perhaps? How it has been evolved in regions inhabited by indigenous people?

Marcos: It would be good to compare the different kinds of uses, the different qualities. It's my intention to include a few modern drinks such as *Tejate, atole, Pozol* and all the drinks with—the recipes, the formulas—the indigenous ones—and—but—more sugar, Cinnamon—but they're modern, Spanish, as well. Yes—it would be good to compare contemporary uses with those of indigenous communities and *mestizos*. Yes.

Roberto: Because the indigenous people also drink *atole*, for example, today. And the young and the old drink Cacao on its own.

* * *

Roberto: There isn't a household where they make everything … it also depends on the region, and what we were talking about, the plants in that place … and also this—we have to say we're coming [announce our arrival].

Marcos: That's good.

Roberto: Perhaps Erasto [Roberto's brother]—he travels in all the communities a lot—he's already done this. So, I think he—you [should] go to see him, but not in the place which is different—but you can see the two [locations], and that will be very interesting. But he … he's constantly working on this all day. It's his work. To learn, and then, to teach. Learn it, teach it. And right now he's where he wants to be, living in Palenque because it's closer to—it's more the climate for Cacao. So they grow Cacao.

* * *

Roberto: For example, one very curative thing is—salt. Sea salt. Why? Because it contains all the minerals. It contains gold and silver as well. And it's very good for health, and for me, it's the same as water, but not in its mineral content; water collects all the energy of the earth, of the minerals, all these energies, carries it, and when you take showers you can absorb them—not the minerals—but, [I mean] you can absorb the energy of the water. And I have been working with this energy. So, and it's very simple, how do you absorb the energy? It's very simple; just like when you walk past a very good-looking girl. She's very pretty. Then—if you– if you really concentrate on the girl, even if you only see her for an instant, it's a feeling. If you've made a connection before that encounter, or something, if you think that somehow you've seen her before or something like that, it's stronger. If you take her image, and you put [visualise] yourself with her, and you can keep yourself with her [in your mind] it's a much stronger experience; so, it's the same with these qualities of water. But you don't know who this girl is; perhaps she's an assassin. You don't know it. OK. It's the same with water. You don't know exactly what all this water you're washing yourself with, has [contains]. But it's passing over your body. If you realise, if you give credence to the fact that right now, you are bathing, but, also, you are having an experience of contact with the water like you were saying, in this way, certainly, your experience of bathing will be improved. If you concentrate on the water, it will be much better. And if you think about it, even though it's not certain that the water contains minerals, and you can imagine those, how should you think of them? Because you can't see them. It's easy. You can think of them as temperatures, as colours, smells, and you take [absorb] them. So I've begun, for instance, to work with giving the properties of gold to water, a very bright gold colour, and with a concentration exercise I put it into my body. And the other day, I got a lot of money. [Laughs].

Good. Like that—you can also, for example, when I've very low energy, the colour red is very strong, and gives a lot of energy, it's the colour of blood. It gives a lot of health. I imagine that I'm taking the colours from the water into my body. And truthfully, no, I can't say for certain, but I'm convinced that I experience a better shower, and that it does affect my health. I don't know how, but it certainly has an effect. I take a conscious shower, no more showers like "shhhhh" [mimes eyes shut, half-asleep], and similarly, now I can, when I'm in other countries where the water is different, I can feel the difference. And I can't say that one is better than the other, but this is for certain: water which hasn't had a lot of contact with metals, hasn't been processed much, is fresher. And healthier.

Marcos:	Better for—conducting? Conducting properties?
Roberto:	This is very important for—I think—for drinks; very, very important.
Marcos:	—A good type of water? Fresh? Living water? Interesting—very interesting. Because I'm interested that here in Mexico, I'm interested in the power of emotions. Water in Europe—[in relation to] chemistry and astrology—is element of emotions, it's of the subconscious, it's emotional not intellectual, it is deeper and is the element of … but here … [loud water sound]
Roberto:	The combination of water and elements is very good. I think it's possible to talk about lots of other things as well, but the combination of elemental water and oxygen is the work we have. Because these are the elements are getting really bad. Water and oxygen.
Marcos:	They're bad?!

Roberto: On the planet [i.e., on a global level].

Marcos: Ah, OK.

Roberto: They're getting really bad. I mean we're always in an era [*O sea cada vez esta-mos en una era*], so just imagine if you met your grandfather, or your great-grandparents, [and you told them] that they sell bottled water. How do they [get away with] sell[ing] water in bottles? Water—I mean, no—it's not for sale. Before, [perhaps] a long time ago—for millions of years. We are in an age where there is already a very serious water problem, to the point where you have to buy it in bottles. It's not only a distribution issue. The industry, I'm sure, has a secret; they know that a long time ago water became something very precious, and as a test, they are selling it as a product. But really, the problem isn't the distribution, the problem is the water, as an element. So—and the other problem is oxygen. Yes, now we're in a warming period talking about rising temperatures, but I think this is somewhat to hide the two real problems: water and oxygen. So in the future, we're going to be able to buy oxygen—don't you think?

* * *

Roberto: Yes, oxygen will be the next element which will be sold as a product like this, because already in the cities the oxygen quality is very bad. So I think that these two elements work a lot in everything, including food. It's also very interesting that these are exactly the elements which distribute health to the brain. So, to say that there's a shortage of oxygen and water in the world is to say that in the world, we have problems with the brain. Meaning that already people can't think well. Everyone, everyone is already not thinking well. Yes, yes, quantitively, we can think a lot, but perhaps not with much quality. Because the principal element of the brain is oxygen, but this is dis-tributed by water and salt; so, it's logical; but it's these things which, in my opinion, denote the change of the age. In many cultures, it's said that there is [i.e., we are in] a change of era. And, if we look at it in a very scientific man-ner, the scientists also say that there are changes in science. But I think that these changes, in whichever culture, whatever level, whatever—including economics—will come from these two elements.

* * *

Roberto: I think that—this sickness produced by the lack of water and oxygen is—on many levels, but one very important thing which is affected is concentration and the sense of being focused. That's to say that already people can't focus, or concentrate.

* * *

Marcos:	The method of curing with water—you can take an infusion, if you have an emotional connection or a recent connection with another person, you can take it, and affect the other person. Is that right?
Roberto:	Er—well—we're talking about levels again, no? If we're talking about a particular patient, there are levels. These levels could be more easily described as channels. So—there are different channels. If I have it, I am thinking of a patient, I can focus on them on different levels. If my patient isn't concentrating, if they don't have a focus on what I believe, my medical beliefs, I lose a level. Because I can't work on this level. Yes, I can work [on this level], but only at a particular time or in special cases.
Marcos:	When there is a strong emotional connection?
Roberto:	No! I can work when there is a special event. That's to say, there are three—patient, doctor, and astrology. We can say "the stars". If the patient—there's no emotional connection, no mental connection, neither is there any trust. So, only one channel can be seen, the stars. At one particular moment. But if not, this is lost, this level, so I must look for another level, and another level. But, for example, as I've told you, when there is a quality of shared time, such as that which you were saying for example an emotional connection; there, there is a connection. Your patient goes, but this connection persists, in you, and in your patients.
Marcos:	How can you tell if there is such a connection?
Roberto:	There are three levels. Once again. Three levels. There is a physical level. If you touch your patient; if you sometimes touch something and there is electricity; like that, this you can say, when you say there is electricity, or your patient produces electricity in your chair, or produces something, it's a very easy way of telling whether there's a positive or negative connection. Mental—something mental, that's to say that they understand perfectly what you want to explain. Or you understand perfectly that which they want to explain to you. An emotional connection, you will feel "here" or something. So—if you want to be clearer about this connection, you can make little charts of questions. Do you feel good with me? But—questions like this, very, very interesting questions. For example, you can do this with your questions as well—how do you feel with your parents, for instance? And—good, why? And now you can begin to see other relationships; your patient won't even realise it, and you can identify all of the connections. And afterwards, you can round it off, you can grade the connection, then you can say, OK. I had a small emotional connection but no physical connection, and also she had a connection with me but this person is 100% disconnected from their surroundings. So, finally, you say to yourself I have this level of connection, so you make a decision. I can work at a distance, or not.
Marcos:	And for working at a distance, one of these types are good—physical, mental, emotional, any of these are good? You can use water?

Roberto: OK. Why can you work at a distance? You have your feelings, emotions, thoughts that you can transmit. Sometimes, you can't transmit them while you're talking either—for example, when we're quarrelling with our partner, no? We have a lot of things we want to transmit, but we can't transmit them while talking. Even though we are talking the same language, even though we want to feel attraction, yet there are little things which can't be [expressed]. But there are things which you transmit, without talking, as well, with your partner. So, it's the same, there are things which you can transmit at a distance, and things which you can't. But because we don't have proof of this knowledge yet, the only way is to try it; it's the only way! You must—try it for yourself! And you take a tea, a herb which your patient needs—if it isn't bad for you—[laughs]—it's very good, you can take it—and you're going to try to pass on [its virtues] by concentrating hard. There is—you visualise— that this work is good for him. A—to will [*desear*] it. OK. This visualisation is converted into a desire [*desear*]; and this feeling, of desire, is a very profound feeling. It's the thing that makes things happen—for example, in a very big corporation, we say to ourselves, we have this primary objective, we have this, and this, now we have this objective, now we have this product, we're going to have a new product in the world, it's this, and then, you have it on a screen; and you say, this is the new product. And we say: we're going to make this! It's not a probability—it's a certainty. That is a big wish. To do something, to develop something. This feeling is—it's the same feeling you can use to work at a distance. A true wish for that thing to happen.

Marcos: To achieve an objective—that's what you want to do?

Roberto: No. OK. There's a difference between "wanting" a car, and wishing for a car, when it's the mind, when it's your whole head—a car, a car, a car. It's the same with a woman. Sometimes, you say to yourself that it's not about this person or that idea. It's very deep. It's more than a wish. It's bigger than that. So, that's what you can do to work at a distance.

Marcos: So emotional? To work at a distance?

Roberto: Right. You need to get to that state. And you said the same thing I did. My friend and I have a connection; and it's the same thing I began to tell you about, it's a —you have to evaluate—"test?"—the connection. When it's possible, or not. But you need to be very, very—we could say, very, very cold, very calculating; unsentimental. We talked about a feeling, but you must have a very clear awareness, if it's a person, you have to be very scientific about it—with this person, or not; if now, or not now; with these plants you don't have to be as clear about everything, as she did, as clear as she was [talking about a friend of mine we discussed off the record, who worked some candle magic for a family member]. Even though she was very emotional, she was still perfectly clear about what she had to do. The photo, the candle—all of it, she was clear. All of it. And the continuous connection. Very, very, very important. And, usually, the first and easiest experiences like this are with your family or close people, because there is already a—

Marcos: Stronger—

Roberto: —connection. Precisely. But you can also create this sort of connection with anybody. With your worst enemy, you can produce it. If you—because you're seeing it as a way to help, as a doctor, you are not very concentrated on anything. Yes, a concentration—"to be in focus". And connected.

Marcos: I only see ten to twelve patients every week, and that's why I don't have a very strong emotional connection …

Roberto: For you, it's like—you can see it as hot or cold water. You put it into a very large space, very large [*Lo pones en un lugar muy largo*]. You could be [like] hot water if you have a connection, but if he doesn't have water—a connection—he could be [like] the cold water. But you have to conduct it, it's not enough for them to be that way. You have to conduct it, to distribute it. So there is a tube, a medium, very long, because, really, we don't know about it. If we knew about it perfectly, it would be very easy, but we don't know it. So this tube, for the water to mix, if it were hot, it's much quicker. For both. Or if they both were cold.

Marcos: Yes, the difference between hot and cold is emotional—

Roberto: No, also physical, your humour, your odour—the smell of a person—

Marcos: Smell?

Roberto: It's very physical. It's not emotional, the physical appearance, it's physical, not emotional. It's strength—when you have a patient, if it is very strong, you don't have to touch him, you are already seeing, which is strong, and that is physical. So well, then this has to mix. It doesn't matter if he, if there is no connection. Because you still—if you believe you can—it [the connection] is hot [active, strong]. If you believe you can, you will. But that's on you. Sometimes it's very easy, but when it's not, you can [still do it]. Now, very importantly— there's the rest, too; nature, their family, the stars. Sometimes you have the intention, and the other person as well, but the rest is saying no. And there's that, I call it, listening to life. What I mean is, we listen to it all, but not what life wants—there's what you want, what I want, and what life wants.

Marcos: This is why I like astrology; it's sometimes a [useful] situation map.

Roberto: Exactly, it's a map. It's very good.

3. 26th January 2011. Interview with "Cacao shaman" Keith Wilson and his assistants, San Marcos La Laguna, Lake Atitlan, Guatemala

Keith:	… and it's easier to pour out of the bottles than out of here, so …
Marcos:	So that's just your pre-prepared beans, ground—finely ground, and mixed with water?
Keith:	Yeah—yeah, I'll go through this a little bit more when I get out there, it's pretty simple.
Marcos:	OK.
Keith:	Erm—when I make it for myself, you know, cardamom, vanilla, even a little coconut milk—
Marcos:	OK. Nice.… but this is just pure Cacao, no additives?
Keith:	Nope. Nothin' in it.
Ama (assistant):	Little LSD.
[laughter]	
Keith:	[rolling eyes] Ohhh, yeah! I've actually been asked that—"Did you put mush-rooms in the Cacao?"
Marcos:	[laughing] Well, it is historically valid … but … yeah …
Keith:	Yes, it is, historically … [rhetorically, distracted, to one of the "cooks" stirring the pot of Cacao:] Where are we going next?—This one.
Guy (attendee):	How long have you been doing the ceremonies for?
Keith:	Five years.
Marcos:	What was it you said about the bacteria, the mould on the shells? Because that was really—
Keith:	OK—
Marcos:	—interesting.
Keith:	You've got, erm—typical scenario, you've got Cacao being dried on the ground in the tropics, in a rainforest, coastal environment, where it rains all year, and so, the Cacao being on the ground, it rains, and the Cacao gets rinsed with barnyard tea.
Marcos:	[laughing]
Keith:	We're talkin' the real story here … And then it dries, and eventually, when the Cacao dries enough to be collected, it's put in *costals, costales*—
Marcos:	When you say *costales* are they like the collecting boxes, you mean, with the …?
Keith:	Gunny sacks!
Marcos:	A'ight.
Keith:	Yeah. [To male assistant:] Just the other one, now that's ready to roll. This has got all the mud in it. —OK: let me get an idea how many people are here.… As you can tell I'm in busy mode, I got a reporter here writing a book on me, and somebody else that's here to do a videography, a documentary on me, so—it's a little busy!
River (attendee):	You're writing a book?
Marcos:	Yeah, on Cacao, on the history and medicinal uses of it—I'm not a reporter, I'm a herbalist. But I'm kind of in reporter mode …

River:	Did you know this was here?
Marcos:	Yeah, yeah, yeah, that's why I came here, 'cos I met a guy I work with in Neal's Yard in London, and he kind of knew of Keith, so he said you've got to go here.
River [To Keith]:	There might be a few more people coming down from the Pyramids [Los Pyramides, hostel/New Age centre in San Marcos]—I talked to the Pyramids people and like five people, maybe, said they were thinking of coming. And that might circulate some more.
Keith:	Or less.
River:	—or less.
Keith:	They all move—the Pyramids people, move—
River:	Together.
Keith:	Together, yeah. The Pyramids people they move together, and if some kind of word goes through, that—whatever—none of 'em come. And then the next batch, Pyramids people, I'll have a dozen or more.
River:	Right.… So it's either a bunch today or a bunch this weekend.
Keith:	Usually the Pyramids people get the idea that Sunday is not the day to come.

* * *

Keith:	It's all been measured when I make it, each person has ten ounces of water and two ounces of chocolate [= 284g water, i.e., approx. 300ml to 57g Cacao]. So we're startin' with two thirds of that; two thirds of twelve would be eight [oz of water + Cacao, i.e., approx. 200ml water to 43g Cacao]. So that's where we're startin'.
Marcos:	OK. And that's pure Cacao?
Moses (assistant):	Yeah, so we start with, like, the blocks—shit, that I've just added to the hot water—
Keith:	Don't worry about it, that's close to—
Moses:	Close to everyone else's? About two ounces—
Keith:	Yeah. Couple of ounces—about one per cent! Haha. [… much discussion about who gets what …]
Moses:	So—I'm adding water to mix it to make it, like, smooth—we begin with ten ounces of water [drowned out by chatter] … eight ounces so that way people who may be more sensitive to it can adjust it.
Marcos:	Well it's weird, with Cacao, some days I can drink three or four cups of the, er, proper strong chocolate, some days just one cup can give me a headache or something. That's rare, but it happens.
Moses:	… yeah …
Marcos:	… and I read Keith's blurb on it, and he said sometimes that's because you've got [issues that] you're not expressing, or you're [holding back], and that kind of fits.

Moses: There's also, like you know, what's going on with your diet; like, if I eat a full meal and then drink this,—

Keith
[shouting over]: River, can you reach the chillies?

Moses: —it's not gonna—it's not no good, it's just not gonna have much effect.

Keith
[shouting over]: They should be! Shelf, near the door—

Moses: —and you don't want to do it if you have a fully empty stomach, 'cos, like, it'll cause nausea, so it's kind of like—

Marcos: —a balance—

Moses: —[inaudible] eat more lightly;—then we do again like half hour, an hour, together, a third dose for those who want it.

Marcos: OK. So there's one dose now, and then possibly a second dose in an hour?— Yeah, 'cos I'd probably do a second dose like three hours later!

Moses: Part of the reason we, like—it takes twenty or thirty minutes to get going really well, depending on your level of sensitivity; like, sometimes I do it even quicker 'cos I've been working on it for a little while—

Ama (assistant): —is this for serving? River, are these for serving?

Moses: —but also, it kinda [obscured by nearby conversation] hours, if you waited three hours and took a third dose you could be [flying] for like another two or three after that—so I mean, yeah, it totally depends, I usually try and cap my intake after a certain time, otherwise, sometimes I'm like, I can't sleep 'cos my body's too wired—

Marcos: [laughing] I getcha …

* * *

Marcos: This is really good stuff, I made it in London; I made it with *panela*, but what I'm really interested in is old school beverages made with traditional plants—because obviously *panela* isn't Hispanic, cinnamon's imported from Sri Lanka, sugar is a post-Hispanic addition. I want to make it—I made just the plain chocolate, I made it with *Quararibea*—*Rosita de Cacao* from Oaxaca, there are lots of spices here in Guatemala, but I still haven't come across the spices I really want to find, and I really want to experiment and find out what each one does when you combine.

Moses: I find that you really need to sort of experiment with all of these other chocolates that go into these organic food stores and buy their best stuff, like David Willstop [?] and all that. Honestly today, I haven't had anything that tastes as potent as the stuff that we have here.

Marcos: Well, it sounds like the process he does (A) finding the right beans and (B) sort of intuiting and sort of checking each bean, like there's no replacement. You can't get that with the factory-made stuff. Oh, that's another thing he said, er, in bulk—yeah, well—what he said [inaudible—too much background noise]

Moses:	I know he says too there's a huge variance between a really good quality—like organic, fairtrade, raw, stuff in that whole category. There's big variance in what actually has a good use in terms of spiritual and making a personal difference. So you can have 8% Ecuadorian [inaudible] it has the same grade, but it doesn't have the same compounds that affect consciousness or health.
Marcos:	It's like, if you grow the same plant in a different part of the world, the chemistry will be different. So there's that physical material aspect, and there's also the history of slavery and how it's arrived at the place it's arrived at.
Moses:	And also variety too, those countries are still using mostly hybridised varieties to get their … stuff.
Marcos:	This is so cool! … It's just, it's just really cool, 'cos a lot of this stuff is stuff that I've, I mean I've done lots of research and I know what I think, and a lot of it is, I have my intuition and then in this sort of wacky New Agey way, I kind of know that I think this is true, but it helps to kind of know if other people think this is true … [inaudible]

* * *

Marcos:	Let me get that from you again—[indistinct]—so the key thing is the toasting?
Keith:	Well—the light toast gets rid of a lot of that: bacteria and moulds which are normal on traditionally ground dried Cacao.
Marcos:	Do you also—I mean, this is just—from the other fermented, historically based—fermentation by-products themselves will probably contribute to the effects of the Cacao.
Keith:	Yes; and also, as I understand it, after fermentation ends, it's an enzymatic process going on inside the beans, and that continues until well after they dry. So—now—most of the Cacao that I get is coming from a coastal area, so I do an additional drying in the sun, 'cos here I'm at several thousand feet higher altitude, generally have much better sun and much dryer air, and if I take about forty per cent of the Cacao that I buy, and just throw it in a container, I get another layer of mould on it, 'cos it isn't dry enough.
Marcos:	Ah—sudden question that just popped into my head, just flew out—
Keith:	It'll come back …
Marcos:	Yes—erm, that sounds, er—that was it! About the, just about the raw people: do you know whether the beans that they advocate are raw in the sense that they just take them out of the fruit, and scrape the pulp off and dry them, or have they been fermented?
Keith:	Most of them are fermented. Some of 'em aren't. 'Cos some of the raw people are such jerks, they don't want to do anything with it, even peel them!
Marcos:	That's kind of insane. [thinks briefly] I kind of get it though …
Keith:	Well, well we're working out of a belief-system driven thing,—
Marcos:	—an ideology, yeah—

Keith:	—yeah, rather than something that is driven by another level of knowing. But, you know, that's OK, because Cacao is—I have a little thing in my business, Cacao can help with that level of insanity.
Marcos:	[laughs]
Keith:	Where they really believe that the way to get proper information about the world and your environment is from your rational mind!
Marcos:	Hmm. That's a disease I've got …
Keith:	Well, that's a contemporary addiction.
Marcos:	I'm kind of trying to percolate it from the top down. Do you know what I mean? Like—[laughs]
Keith:	Yeah. So the first step in working with that addiction is heart opening. And that's the step about Cacao.
Marcos:	I had two readings this week, a tarot reading and my friend—er, new friend! Her name temporarily escapes me, I keep thinking Kirsten but that's not her name—anyway she did a reading on me last night, she does chakra readings, and my heart thing was blocked.
Keith:	That's the one.
Marcos:	Which is probably why—
Keith:	OK—[…] have to start integrating with the group …
Marcos:	What's that?
Anna:	It's chilli—
Marcos:	Oh! Brilliant!
Ama:	Just so if you need it for accelerating it.
Marcos:	Is it very strong chilli? [tastes it] Ah, it's alright.
Anna:	*Muy bien.*
River:	There's more out there too if you need to have more.
Ama:	Cool. That's in the door, and then when we need a refill.
Marcos [tasting the chocolate]:	Oh, this is good! [laughs]

4. 11th February 2011. Interview with Sr. Reginaldo Chayax Huex, herbalist and director of the Asociacion Bio-Itza, San Jose, Peten, West Guatemala

[About *Palo de Tzol*, and *Pimienta dioica* (Pimienta, Allspice):]

Mr Huex: Very good, Marcos, I believe that this information is very important because, today I see that you brought the photograph that you took yourself, at the moment when you recognised the tree. Then the tree comes [flowers] now, in this month of March, they begin to bloom. It flowers and makes a fruit, that big. They ripen and redden; they take on a red colour when they are ripe. And that you can have a lot of juice, juice inside, and suck one, like a very sweet honey. Wherever it is the birds, the monkeys, and the spider monkeys eat it; it makes a good meal.

Marcos: Is it OK for humans too?

Mr Huex: Yes—for people, it's very tasty. And not only this, there are several trees that make fruit. So in this month of March there are many trees that give fruit. They flower, [then] the fruits ripen in May or June.

Marcos: And when they're ripe, are they red?

Mr Huex: Reds, yes. They are red.

Marcos: And the fruits have medicinal properties, or other parts of the tree?

Mr Huex: No, they do not have this medicinal properties, and they're not—they're—

Marcos: To eat, yes. The guide yesterday told me that some ladies dry the fruits, and use them in Cacao drinks.

Mr Huex: No—where was that lady from?—is she from here? Here in the Peten?

Marcos: I don't know—they told me that some local ladies from this region—near Tikal—used it.

Mr Huex: Well, the truth is that the seed of this is bitter.

Marcos: The seed. Ah—do you use seeds for drinks?

Mr Huex: No, the seed is bitter; you can't make drinks [from it]. Because it's bitter.

Marcos: It's very bitter?

Mr Huex: Yes—very bitter. Now the sweet part is the water [juice] beneath the shell, and around the seed [i.e., the fruit]. The seed alone, the one that comes out, the one that is born [the pip], is bitter.

Marcos: OK. And does it have medicinal properties? For worms or similar?

Mr Huex: It doesn't have medicinal properties. The red [berries]—Pft! That's why the animals, like the spider monkey, the monkey, or the lowland paca only suck the water [juice]. They don't chew the seed, because it's very bitter. The seed—do you know the *cahuey*?

Marcos: The *cahuey*?

Mr Huex: The *cahuey*, do you know it? Well, the seed has the appearance of coffee. The seeds.

Marcos: Café ?

Mr Huex: *Ca-huey*. It's the seed [of the fruit] … This is what the seed looks like. The seed is like that, only bigger. Inside it has a very bitter pip. So they are covered

	with flesh that when ripe, can be pure water [juice]; [you can] break the shell, suck! You suck the honey [sweet juice], but the seed is bitter.
Marcos:	OK. This is *Palo de Tzol*?
Mr Huex:	That's *Palo de Tzol* …
Marcos:	This part is fruit, inside?
Mr Huex:	This part is the seed; here is the flesh, and then you break the shell, suck everything it has here.
Marcos:	And the seed …
Mr Huex:	The seed is bitter!
Marcos:	This part?
Mr Huex:	It's that part, right! Very bitter! Then it's weird or strange that you're telling me they told you that you can drink it, no, no, no—no way! One [seed] is bitter, so what would that be like? In even higher quantities it's even more bitter.
Marcos:	Yes? One?
Mr Huex:	One is bitter. And when it's ground up, it's even more bitter. [clicks tongue]
Marcos:	OK, thanks. Are there other plants here that you know?
Mr Huex:	I only know—I don't know if this is the one mentioned here, *Flor de Mayo*. This is a flower, but only for ornaments. For decorating, to put …
Marcos:	Oh—you don't know—are they not medicinal?
Mr Huex:	They're not medicinal.
	[Note: they are, but clearly aren't used for this purpose in the Peten. See monograph on *Plumeria rubra* in Appendix B].
Marcos:	OK. And Allspice?
Mr Huex:	Allspice is like that, it's a very delicious tea, which has [medicinal] qualities; the dose to make tea [infusion] is three little leaves, that you can decoct and make a very nice tea; it's relaxing. You come wet from the mountain, or from walking in the mountains, you get wet, you got caught in the rain, your temperature lowers—
Marcos:	Decreased your temperature?
Mr Huex:	Yes—your temperature lowers, you get a bit cold, you get three leaves of allspice tea and you cook them hot—and you'll sleep very well, yes, it's relaxing …
Marcos:	Ah, yes. Good, thank you.
Mr Huex:	And at the same time, it's medicinal. That's the way it is, it's medicinal.
Marcos:	What properties does it have?
Mr Huex:	It's very important in medicine, because it's very good for colic pain. So, for medicinal purposes, you use five leaves per litre of water. Boil it, then you can chill it in a bottle so that you drink it in the morning, and at midday, so that it takes away the stomach pains. Or another, very important use: when you're walking in the mountains, you get tooth pain, you have toothache—you grab the most tender, the most recent leaves, the youngest two leaves, and you chew. You can chew it, you leave it—
Marcos:	Right—
Mr Huex:	You leave it, leave it—

Marcos:	Mmm-hm. Near the [source of the] pain.
Mr Huex:	Fifteen minutes there. It has a lot of anaesthesia; it has a lot of mint [*sic*].
Marcos:	The seeds have the same properties?
Mr Huex:	The seed has the same property; [they're] even a little stronger than the leaves.
Marcos:	Stronger? Oh—and that's why you can use the seeds for sore tooth pain, and colic, and—
Mr Huex:	Right. This one I am telling you about is for when one is walking in the forest. When you have the seed, you can go down [from the mountains], and put it to dry, and you can keep it. When you have internal pains, you decoct ten seeds per glass of water.
Marcos:	Thanks. How long do you need to boil it? Five minutes?
Mr Huex:	About ten minutes. Ten minutes to extract everything—
Marcos:	And—boiling water, or—
Mr Huex:	Boiling water—with low heat. Not much fire. When it starts to boil, you go to the fire, and lower it, so it's slow, slow.
Marcos:	Do you need to cover it too?
Mr Huex:	Exactly. So that no steam is released—exactly! For any need or problem when the tree doesn't have any leaves or fruits, [you can use] the bark. You peel it, and you can—with a piece of about fifteen centimetres [long], you can make a tea with a glass of water, that has the same effects.
Marcos:	But, it's not as strong as the leaves—
Mr Huex:	No, no—that's why it's bigger, the dose. You know about Allspice?
Marcos:	Yes, but it's more for cooking, it's like the Basil is an herb originally from Europe but here it has more uses for medicine. It's very interesting because there's another species of Basil that grows in India—its name is Holy Basil, and for them it is a very important herb, as the name suggests, and it's interesting because the uses are similar—for fatigue, to take infusion—
Mr Huex:	Very good for nausea [mimics vomiting]
Marcos:	Cough?
Mr Huex:	No, vomiting. Here we have pepper, basil, oregano, and yucca for curing mumps.
Marcos:	But do you know this plant? I have a picture …

* * *

[about *Piper sanctum* (Hoja Santa, Root Beer Plant):]

Mr Huex:	It's very important, because it also contains a lot, a lot of menthol, a lot—
Marcos:	Phlegm?
Mr Huex:	—It's very good because it has a lot of menthol.
Marcos:	I understand—how do you say … [gestures to face, sniffles—miming catarrh]
Mr Huex:	Yes—it's very good for that; and it's very good for fever.
Marcos:	[An] infusion—of the leaves?
Mr Huex:	The leaves—[the] tender [ones]—the little tip—where the flower comes out, the tender part of the branch.

Marcos:	OK—I understand.
Mr Huex:	There's also some here.
Marcos:	Here?
Mr Huex:	Yes!
Marcos:	Ah good! Because I don't know what part the ancients used in drinks.
Mr Huex:	Want us to go see it?
Marcos:	Yes! Perfect.

* * *

[about *Piper sanctum*:]

Marcos:	Can I take a picture?
Mr Huex:	Sure!
Marcos:	What's the smell? Can I chew it? Mm—it's fine!
Mr Huex:	Very good! This is for the flu. And it's very good for the fever, they get these off like this, great—little ones, a bit of cattle fat [tallow?] or beef fat is used. And it's applied all over here—then you stick [the leaf] on the chest.
Marcos:	Ah, I understand. For coughs, too?
Mr Huex:	No—it's for fever. Now for coughing, it's decocted, and it's drunk.
Marcos:	At the same time?
Mr Huex:	No, no, no. The fever is one [use]; the fever is what I just told you about.
Marcos:	OK—to put it—
Mr Huex:	To put on like a poultice.
Marcos:	I need—I do not know how to say—hit it? [i.e., bruise the herb]
Mr Huex:	No, no, no—so, the whole [leaf], just cover one in beef fat, [from] the cattle here, and stick it on—
Marcos:	Back—
Mr Huex:	On the back, [over the] lungs—and, good! Now for the cough, [we do] this: for coughs, all that is taken, peeled, peel as well as that, it is decocted; then it's decocted, decocted all of this, like this—
Marcos:	The parts of the skin?
Mr Huex:	The skin, right. All this; that's decocted, the inner parts of the stem. Like the one we already ate. That's what you decoct, and you drink for a fit of coughs.
Marcos:	Yes? I need it now!
Mr Huex:	At the same time, it's a typical dish. Yes. At the same time, you can look for a fish, or a pound of meat—pork, *tepezquintle* [spotted paca], any kind of meat, make the ingredients, add all the ingredients to the meat, and then put it [the leaf] here. And then another one goes here; covering the fish, or the meat.
Marcos:	Oh, very good, to infuse—
Mr Huex:	Aha, correct. Wrap it with this [leaf]. Then put it in a—in a frying pan or in a pot, with a slow fire, let it cook slowly. About twenty minutes later, open the pot or the pan, it's very good. And you get to eat a very tasty meal. Since it is medicinal, and it is—

Marcos:	Also, nutritional.
Mr Huex:	Correct.
Marcos:	Very good. Therefore, this medicine is hot and dry, and removes phlegm.
Mr Huex:	Aha, this one in Itza is called *Obele*. Of Santa Maria.
Marcos:	Does this have seeds too? Produce seeds?
Mr Huex:	It produces seeds—because it's called—this is the flower.
Marcos:	Those are the flowers? … Because I don't know if the elders used the leaves in Cacao drinks; I do not know but I think they use the seeds, because it seems like the seeds mix better with the taste of the chocolate. The seeds have the same properties?
Mr Huex:	Yes.
Mr Huex:	This means that they are ancient plants—

* * *

Marcos:	—very old?
Mr Huex:	Very old.
Marcos:	Yes. —This Basil plant grows here for a long time? [i.e., is it indigenous?]
Mr Huex:	Yes. This, I've known this plant since my childhood, and there it is still. This is native here, from this place. There are other types which have a flower like the colour of that, that is a similar colour to the one they bring here from the West, but it's not from here, no, no …
Marcos:	This species—
Mr Huex:	This is from here.
Marcos:	And the other one is medicinal too?
Mr Huex:	It's medicinal but it's more—it's less potent than this one. This is the best there is, because it's native here. Here it rains, there is summer, then it dies, and when the rain falls, it comes back up. And it's very good for nausea. The leaves are decocted and drunk, to resolve [nausea]. And our grandparents, they did eye drops or "Eye Mo" for the eyes in their day; only this little seed. They took the little seed, and put it in the eye.
Marcos:	To clean them?
Mr Huex:	To clean them! When one has bad eyesight, one's eyes hurt, you put in the seed; after five minutes, it starts coming out with the trash, or the bad [stuff in the eye]—
Marcos:	Yes. They remove everything. Yes.
Mr Huex:	Everything that's the cause, that's bad for the sight, it takes everything out.
Marcos:	It's interesting—
Mr Huex:	And—at the same time, you can make some rice porridge, grab a bunch of spinach with it [this herb], and it's a good—
Marcos:	Good smell.
Mr Huex:	Good dish too! [laughs] A good flavour.

Marcos:	A midwife near Chisec told me that she uses Basil, I think too—because in the books, in the herbalists in my country, the ancient herbalists, the Western Basil, is used for children when the woman is pregnant, I do not know how you say, but—expel—
Mr Huex:	To clean up! Yes, yes, yes. Here, no, here there's only this one [for that purpose], and, at the same time, you can cook it, and make an *atole*, pour a bit of water of Basil [an infusion], very tasty—it can be done.
Marcos:	Aha! Use in *atole*? You think it's—I don't know, it's my imagination, but do they use this plant with Cacao in drinks, or not?
Mr Huex:	I don't know, I don't believe I've ever seen it. It's medicinal, and—
Marcos:	And—in *atole*—
Mr Huex:	[For] *atole*, it's decocted, and the water is poured in the *atole*. It's very tasty, because it also takes out the gases [carminative]—that's Basil.
Marcos:	It's one of my plants—
Mr Huex:	Favourite?
Marcos:	Yes.
Mr Huex:	And this part [the leaves], too, does the same work that the seed does. And this one has one—when it grows, it's there, it comes, it grows a little bit more, and it's folded, like so.
Marcos:	Yes, yes. What's this plant called?
Mr Huex:	That's what we call *cura ojo*, or *cura vista* [Eye Healer]. Because this is [a variety that] grows here, it grows a little bit more, but it grows in this shape, like an *empanada*, like a doubling, like that. And it absorbs the night dew, the coldness of the night, it becomes empowered here, it grows a little bit more, and it stays in this form. And the cold night comes, it folds together, and that too is [used as] an eyewash.
Marcos:	Ah! Yes, yes, yes—I understand—to clean the eyes.
Mr Huex:	These are two very important classes. It's just that our grandparents were very botanical [i.e., knowledgeable about plants].
Marcos:	It's very interesting, the uses of plants in the very old books of my country are similar in some ways.

* * *

Marcos:	And this is *Mano de Coco* [coconut hand]?
Mr Huex:	More commonly known as a *Mano de Lagarto* [lizard hand]; it's very good for malaria.
Marcos:	Right now I have a medicine that they use for malaria, herbal medicine; but it uses one plant from China and the other from South America. The plant from South America is Cinchona, the plant from China is Sweet Wormwood, I don't know exactly what it is, a kind of *Artemisia*; but it's a plant like that.
Mr Huex:	Allspice, there it is—

Marcos:	Oh, yes I see it; and you have the other tree, the tree *Arbol de las Manitas, Manita de Leon*? That one? You sure it is the same?
Mr Huex:	Yes.
Marcos:	One moment [searches for photo in camera]. Ah! Here it is. It's the same?
Mr Huex:	Yes, it is the same.
Marcos:	Sure?
Mr Huex:	Yes, yes…. Only there, when they are already very high, the leaves are very small—
Marcos:	OK—aah, it's one—
Mr Huex:	It's a liana. There, look.
Marcos:	OK. I do not think it's the same—I need to look … Oh, well, OK.
Mr Huex:	So where there's a big tree, it goes up in the tree.
Marcos:	Yes, I understand. I believe that—
Mr Huex:	Green, like that; they grow upward like that. It hugs the trees.
Marcos:	Yes, I understand. Just a moment … Here! It's a bit confusing because this is a tree, it's not a liana. This part is a—
Mr Huex:	That's right.
Marcos:	Yes. But it's not this one, right? I don't think it's this one.
Mr Huex:	Just look to see how this one has already fallen. There, when they separate it remove the liana from the tree], when there is no tree they stay up by themselves, and then they let themselves fall.
Marcos:	Yes? Because it would not be a tree, because this is a tree, and this part is a very small part. [In] the picture [it] seems bigger, but it isn't. That's the flower.
Mr Huex:	Aha! That's it! It's the same! This is the flower. Yes, the flower grows like this. It will flower soon. Aha, there will be a flower, [it] will be red, and there comes the big flower.
Marcos:	Yes? But this flower is—Because the leaves are completely different, it's a different tree, I think.
Mr Huex:	*Mano de Leon*, you say?
Marcos:	*Arbol de las Manitas*, or other names are—*Mano de Leon*.
Mr Huex:	We know it, because there is one that they call *Corazon de Leon*.
Marcos:	This?
Mr Huex:	That's the one!
Marcos:	It's small?
Mr Huex:	Aha—it grows very small.
Marcos:	Is it a tree?
Mr Huex:	It's a tree—it's a *Matoche*. *Matoche* does not grow much, trees like this …
Marcos:	Because I think it's a different plant, because this flower is so big. It's not—I think the flowers of this would be –
Mr Huex:	It's a flower, like that. Then the seed comes out.
Marcos:	I think, it seems in my photos …

Mr Huex:	No—it's totally different. Because we call it *Mano de Leon*, and there's a tree—not here, but in the forest there is, that's called *Mano de Leon*, that's a tree. But the flower is white. Not this one; it's another type.
	[… I ask about Magnolia from photos]
Mr Huex:	It's different to see a picture! It's hard to see them, to know them, because a photograph is different—
Marcos:	Yes, I understand, it's difficult.… Oh! Guava! Do you know some medicinal uses of this?
Mr Huex:	Yes! That's very medicinal, good for the rear end, or a lot of diarrhoea.
Marcos:	Ah. Which part?
Mr Huex:	You can use the flesh [of the fruit] or the bark, or it could be the fruit's skin/shell. But when it's this immature, not ripe. Not ripe, it has to be immature. And the leaf is for diarrhoea, [and] to heal wounds. [To treat] an infection, you can decoct the leaf, and then wash it [the infected area—washed with the decoction]. And the same little leaf, tender as it is, they dry it well, it dries well, and then you crush it very finely, and put it [the powder] on top of a wound—
Marcos:	Dust from the dried leaves?
Mr Huex:	Yes, like that. They are a very healing [vulnerary] medicine.
Marcos:	[*Cicatrizante.*] I like this word.
Mr Huex:	Moreover, you can make a jelly from the ripe fruit.
Marcos:	Jelly?
Mr Huex:	Yes. Ripe [fruit], remove the skin, and, grind the seed a little bit, make a jelly, put in a little honey, and that's a good jelly.
Marcos:	Oh, I understand. The jelly is for food only?
Mr Huex:	It's just to eat, sort of like ice cream.
Marcos:	OK. Do the fruits have medicinal uses too?
Mr Huex:	The ripe fruit is to eat, for pleasure [only].
Marcos:	Do you have a Mayan—Itza name, for this?
Mr Huex:	Yes. *Pi'chi.*
Marcos:	Thanks. Ah—Ceiba. Or—*Ya'axche.*
Mr Huex:	Ceiba! *Ya'axche.*
Marcos:	Ceiba. Yes. Some medicinal uses of this?
Mr Huex:	In the first place, it's a sacred tree, because according to our local history, from our grandparents, or our ancestors, it was the first tree in life. And moreover, it's very medicinal, because when it's tender or young, it has many thorns. And when a baby is born, that has a lot coming out of it [i.e., a lot of bad humours, secretions, or poor health] when born, or many infections, then you take nine thorns from the ceiba tree, and decoct them, then bathe the baby [with that liquid], on Fridays. Nine Fridays is the treatment for these [infections/bad humours] to be removed.
Marcos:	Friday? Only Friday?
Mr Huex:	Only on Friday.

Marcos:	OK—and is it important what time of day? In the morning, at night?
Mr Huex:	Since it's Friday—there's no schedule. [laughs] It's like the Basil—Basil in Itza is *Kekeltun*.
Marcos:	*Kekeltun*. Ceiba in Itza is *Ya'axche*? It's *Ya'axche*. Good. And Ceiba thorns, immature, and—yes, the seeds have medicinal uses?
Mr Huex:	No! Of the Ceiba, no.
Marcos:	And the flowers?
Mr Huex:	Neither. Only the thorns.
Marcos:	OK. There are other medicinal uses?
Mr Huex:	No. On the contrary—it's a very beautiful tree, but we value it a lot, that's why we do not hurt it [i.e., don't use it for medicine so much].
Marcos:	… Yes, because the seeds of Ceiba—in the Cacao drinks—in some of the writings of the Catholic priests, say that the Mexicas, near the conquest, use the seeds of the Ceiba in the Cacao drinks. Interesting, because it is a lost use.
Mr Huex:	Aha, because we barely use it [for medicine].
Marcos:	Very good. I think I have a lot here.
Mr Huex:	There's a lot here; like this. We also call this [plant] *Santa Maria*, but we say [*chal che?*]. It's the same as the one over there that has more flowers. This is another plant like Basil [that's] very old. And this is much used by midwives; before the baby is born, to avoid problems [during birth], [they] decoct the leaf and give it to the mother to have a fast delivery.
Marcos:	But before, three months before the birth?
Mr Huex:	No, right away when the baby is going to be born. Then, for four days after the baby was born, they continue to drink for cleanliness [i.e., to fully expel the placenta and "clean the womb"]. A very old plant.
Marcos:	Very good.

5. 13th February 2011. Interview with Mr. Ca'al, a resident of San Luis, Peten, West Guatemala

Mr Ca'al:	[describing a doll or poppet used for the ritual cure of *susto*, or "fright", a folk illness]…. you make this yourself. The head is made, the hands, the arms are made [unintelligible] and the eyes, [are made] of corn. Or the teeth [are made] of corn. And you have to cut some nails and put nails on its little fingers. And you dry some cornflakes and put them on like this. Don't attach it! [?] And I don't know how many times, so the back won't dry more [?—*Y no se cuantas veces, para atrás no secar mas.*] And they look at it, and one leaves without turning around to look at it [again]. It's powerful, and it heals.
Marcos:	It cures, it's used for *susto*?
Mr Ca'al:	[When the patient begins] to eat, [you know] it's starting to work.
Marcos:	It's different. That's why, for *susto*, you drink—
Mr Ca'al:	You don't drink [i.e., it's not a beverage]. I'm going to cut a little bit off its tail. [unintelligible] a little and [unintelligible] smoke again, the smoke going downwards removes it from the bed. It seems like witchcraft! It isn't witchcraft!
Marcos:	Yes. It's one method, and *susto* caused by—other causes—you use corn? You [were] saying?
Mr Ca'al:	No.
Marcos:	My Spanish is very bad.
Mr Ca'al:	Aha.
Marcos:	What do you use? Use a river, water from—
Mr Ca'al:	Wax with [*yequito*], a doll. A wax doll. And you add eyes and a nose …
Marcos:	OK. Yes. … I don't know what a doll [*muñeco*] is …
Mrs Veronica Ca'al:	Doll [is] a man, a boy, yes in wax.
Mr Ca'al:	Wax like—Plasticine?—wax. Wax [to make a] doll.
Marcos:	Ah! I understand—yes—and take this doll and look at it, about your eyes. —Three times?
Mr Ca'al:	Six or seven attempts. She has to walk away, and not turn around to see. Then the child begins to eat.
Marcos:	Because this disease, *susto*, is not a disease that … It doesn't exist in other countries, other parts of the world; it exists, already, but it's not—
Mr Ca'al:	Well—it's not a disease? It has no effect?
Marcos:	Erm—I don't know, it's a disease, *susto*, and there are other diseases here, that aren't known in other parts of the world. I don't know if they exist, I think they exist in other ways, and they have other methods of treatment.
Mr Ca'al:	When a person is scared, the Mayas check the pulse. Very weak. That child has sickness.
Marcos:	*Susto*—it's always a disease in children, is it [ever found in] adults?

Mr Ca'al:	Yes—of children. But if it isn't treated, you see the young girl, and she has anaemia, and [unintelligible]. And there's another, another thing that the Mayans knew. For example, a person—a nail, metal, causes tetanus and we Mayans, we have a different name for it, but we cure it. It is *soña*. *Soña*, what the—pfft—we take out a scorpion—[…]
Marcos:	I forgot, I'm very tired—*alacran*—?
Mr Ca'al:	Animal. Tiny.
Mrs Veronica Ca'al:	It's an animal—something like a scorpion. It's not a scorpion, but that's the same family.
Marcos:	Ah! Scorpion. Yes, similar.
Mr Ca'al:	And—when a pain moves like this, that pain is—if the pain [unintelligible] then the Mayas do [unintelligible]

* * *

Mr Ca'al:	When one scorpion—ah! [mimes a scorpion sting] Yes?
Marcos:	Yes.
Mr Ca'al:	There's one [method]—[you use] this machete, and it works.
Marcos:	What do you do with the machete? Cut it?
Mr Ca'al:	No. —Also, the animal—where's the animal? [mimes looking for scorpion on the ground] [You take] the dead animal, the organs—the insides—
Marcos:	Yes. And what do you do with the machete?
Mr Ca'al:	That which has the defect [or injury/harm], in a manner of speaking that person is made [into/like] that animal. We were sailing on the river one time with about ten, maybe eight men, fishing with a harpoon; but I didn't hit the fish with the point of the iron harpoon, I hit another guy, here on the ankle— in the water. And what could he do about it? Nothing! They picked up a machete too. So let's go! We had alcohol. Little measures of alcohol.
Marcos:	Ah—to disinfect it. Yes.
Mr Ca'al:	But—there was a wound, and the pain was increasing.
Marcos:	Yes, yes—infection.
Mr Ca'al:	Infection. One [type of infection] like that, we call *kinamo*. We gave him pills, and we set off. We walked for about an hour and the man couldn't take it anymore, he would shout: aah! Aah!
Marcos:	Very painful.
Mr Ca'al:	Painful. And as we had caught several fish, there was a small fish and I said to him, don't look at it. And I grabbed it from the pile [of fish], I took out the fish and said to the other guy—give me your foot. And I grabbed the fish, I eviscerated it—
Marcos:	What kind of fish?
Mr Ca'al:	Two-banded sea bream [*mojarra*]. So I handed over a handkerchief, filled with the organs of the fish. But, because there was a little bit of alcohol left,

	everybody drank a little bit. But we didn't watch what he was doing, we just listened. We continued walking with the cart below. After ten minutes, he was asleep.
Marcos:	Wow. To take—what part to take? Is it [the] liquid [from] inside the fish? You applied the organs of the fish [externally]?
Mr Ca'al:	Only the organs. The healer is the fish. Extract the organs and put them in a handkerchief …
Marcos:	And what does he take [i.e., ingest]?
Mr Ca'al:	Nothing. But we gave him a little liquor, too.
Marcos:	Only alcohol.
Mr Ca'al:	[politely ending the interview] I'll be going to sleep myself in a few minutes.
Marcos:	Thanks. Interesting.

*6. 14th February 2011. Interview with Don Mateo Poptchu,
Mayan spiritual guide, San Luis, Peten, West Guatemala*

Don Mateo: Whoever wants to tell the future, can do so as [unintelligible]; the correct wood [plant material] needs to be used for divination. One takes a fist[ful of seeds] like that … but he [the client] asks me, he has to ask what day is today on the calendar, he counts and then grabs a fist[ful of beans] like that but without counting even one [i.e., without noting the number of seeds]. I remove four at a time. You have to count the days when it comes out, if I get three, because one is not going to count, I just keep them in my fist. If the three times are exact [i.e., round numbers], then they can be taken out there. [Note: See Barbara Tedlock's book, *Time and the Highland Maya*, for details of this sortilege-based divinatory process, and how it lines up with the traditional calendar.]

Marcos: The number of days, is the number of seeds you use?

Don Mateo: More, more, more, even, I grab a bunch like that, enough beans. Aha. That's how you do a reading [divination].

Marcos: And how do you take the answer from this?

Don Mateo: Depending on what comes out, it points to which *nawal* it is. The *nawal* is like the stars of our birth.

Marcos: It's like there's a calendar that you use, [to arrive at] the answer.

Don Mateo: Yes, yes, aha. It's drawn three times exactly, because one doesn't just count them out of the fist [once], [unintelligible], it's done three times to be exact, [so that] the question is [answered] exact[ly].

Marcos: And the seeds that you use, are *Palo de* …?

Don Mateo: They are *Palo de*—several, [names several plants in Mopan]. Aya, I have mine.

Daniela: You have a book of this information, or only—

Don Mateo: Only in the head, everything in the forehead [in one's mind], aha. Sure, I barely use it [the book] because it's hard to find, here in the western region, because [Quiche, Tenango?, Txaltenango?]—only those people use it.

Marcos: How many years do I need to learn this, is it many years?

Don Mateo: No—few days, some—fifteen, twenty days.

Marcos: Yes? OK.

Don Mateo: Good, then, come on, let's get on with the Cacao questions, yes?

Marcos: Yes! Cacao has uses in some rituals in any way?

Don Mateo: Good, Cacao is used in any activity, in any ritual. Because it's what our grandparents used, from the beginning of the world, where creation began. In any activity they use Cacao in sowing, beginning things, when they go to the mountain, they use only Cacao. It's all that the first generation used to do work.

Marcos: It's like a drink?

Don Mateo: It's a drink.

Marcos: The seeds are used in divination, or similar?

Don Mateo: Not that, no!

Marcos:	Or just for ritual drinks?
Don Mateo:	That's like what my mother made yesterday, because that's how they use it. In other words, the village, here, passing the Mopan, but it was well used before, and when there's an activity or sowing, or any work whatsoever, they prepare the Cacao. I look for an elder [important] lady, she prepares it, makes it, then once it's made ready, all the people drink it when they wake up. And for ceremonies, the same, too. When there's a ceremony—I witnessed it recently, here, in the village. They say that the seeds can also be used for their aroma when they're toasted; they perfume [the area]. That's very useful, since Cacao is used here for any activity. But what's happening [now] is that Cacao is hardly used here any more, as a professional here in Poptun says: where's the Cacao, where's the *Pozol*, where's our *Pinole*? Mmmhm! Today we drink these sodas and many things, and now there are diseases. On the other hand, we didn't have diseases when we only drank Cacao, since it's the cure [for illnesses] on earth. It grows and gives the fruit without need for fertilisers. Then my mother-in-law says that she doesn't stop drinking Cacao because she is already used to it, but only to drink it. So they prepare it as they like, but they peel it [remove the husks?] to drink. The Cacao that is activated [fermented?] is also used for bread, and the Titsi group does that as well. It's made even when there is no activity, but when they have some ceremonies, that's what's used.
Marcos:	It's all the time. Cacao has a significance in—does it have a special significance in some rituals or in general?
Don Mateo:	Almost none! Almost none!—Not there, because it is not found there. It's used only for drinks.
Marcos:	Really? OK—I heard there are some rituals that use Cacao drinks. And are there special Cacao drinks that are only made for different rituals or different months?
Don Mateo:	No—no. Well, they're used, but—as I'll repeat for you—for the most part, the majority of those of us who serve Cacao, we only serve it because we grow it [ourselves]. It's like, because we live here, we grow Cacao, so [naturally] we cut and dry it. [But] nowadays, here, nobody knows Cacao [anymore], they only buy it second-hand [i.e., ready-made]. Before, we used to plant Cacao, coffee—now there's barely any left. Now I'm going to repeat it, they hardly use it anymore. When there used to be a wedding before, there would be Cacao, or for any other activity, Cacao would be made first. But right now, no; right now, now it's—a soda, [unintelligible] …
Ms Ca'al:	Because it's older. It was used in colonial times, they used it as currency. Hey, people exchanged this [Cacao] for some work or in exchange for products, or money.
Marcos:	But today some—reports—describe that in some regions of Guatemala, there are specific drinks made with Cacao, they are not taken, only used in rituals at different times of the year. But no—

Don Mateo:	Well yes, as I will repeat each department, each region, each group has different customs—
Daniela:	Like in [inaudible]
Marcos:	But here in Maya Mopan, it's not—
Ms Ca'al:	Only twenty-five, twenty-fourth of August. Traditional heritage, more than anything; the *patronal* [feast day of the local patron saint], and the [commemoration of] the unification of the town.
Don Mateo:	But there are a lot of villages like here in [Chicimuna], I don't remember where I saw it, not just one or two—only in the enduring tradition of the *patronal*. On the other hand, in another place, there are saints which are celebrated every month or two. There they celebrate and on another they do not celebrate, and they do not use Cacao. It's different here—
Marcos:	OK. Thank you. Your whole name is Don Mateo—
Don Mateo:	Pop!
Marcos:	Don Mateo Pop?
Don Mateo:	Aha! T—C—H—U. It's the last [name].
Marcos:	Don Mateo Pop Tchu?
Don Mateo:	Aha.
Marcos:	Thanks. And what is your title, in Mopan?
Don Mateo:	Ah! [unintelligible—mix of Mayan and Spanish]
Marcos:	Is that in Kek'chi?
Don Mateo:	In Kek'chi.
Marcos:	OK. Your title is—as the title of your work as a spiritual guide?
Don Mateo:	Ah, yes, as a spiritual guide, I've been working there for fourteen years.
Marcos:	And how do you start doing it [meaning, how did you begin?]
Don Mateo:	[DM thinks I'm still asking about Cacao:] In other words, it is done in a spiritual manner. So, I [need to] go to the villages, not here anymore; the elders, I've seen it there. In every ritual activity, Cacao comes first. If there's no Cacao, there's no ritual—aha—Cacao is first. It's everywhere where you go, the rituals, or to bless the home. It is used a lot, [unintelligible] Cacao.
Marcos:	OK. But, for you, how did you become a spiritual guide? For you—do you want to do?—how do you start?
Don Mateo:	Ah! That is, when I went to receive, I went to a course. Aha, then. To start with, you have to learn the twenty days calendar. For those twenty days, you have the calendar. That is, two hundred and twenty-six. The calendar of [unintelligible—solar or annual, every day calendar] has three hundred [days], but our calendar has two hundred and twenty-six … Aha—so we learn there and they gave me those beans when we have to do fortune telling.
Marcos:	The method of fortune telling.
Don Mateo:	Aha, aha, yes. They gave me that, and they showed me how to do it. There I learned.
Ms Ca'al:	[aside, to me] What do you want to do? Do you [want anything] to drink?
Don Mateo:	Then I started there, they saw me and they named me as a spiritual guide. In the villages we go out [are called on?] a lot, I go out then, when I'm called,

	to do the ritual there, and a prayer for the home, or for, as they say, to ask permission for nature to begin something [a cleansing ritual?—*pedir permiso para la naturaleza para botar*], to plant, that's the first thing that the—but it's not done here anymore, it's no longer done.
Marcos:	But—people consult for weddings, for health … for—all manner of things?
Don Mateo:	Oh, yes!
Marcos:	It's very interesting, it's like astrology in my country, horary astrology, there is a type of astrology when I answer questions. It is a bit similar.
Don Mateo:	Yes, because a guy told me that either there in Japan, or in—you have to ask permission from God, from nature. The Japanese over there, when they make watches, first they ask God to do well what they are going to do in the day. Then they ask God, and everything they do is perfect.
Marcos:	[to Danielle] Did you understand that?
Danielle:	In [Japan], yeah?
Marcos:	They—what? In Japan, they …?
Danielle:	They do not [inaudible]
Marcos:	Yes—it's a bit similar, astrology is more about—from this moment.… that job is interesting. Yes, what is your title in Kek'chi? Title of the work, of the spiritual guide? As it is said in Kek'chi?
Don Mateo:	*Ka'molb'e.*
Danielle:	[laughs] Well …
	[back and forth trying to pronounce]
Marcos:	Can you write it? Well, OK. It's a title, the best translation is spiritual guidance. Well, and before each divination do you need to pray?
Don Mateo:	Oh yes. That is why first, we ask God in heaven who protected us. Then we pray to God, the grandparents—you have to pray.
Marcos:	Well, thank you very much. I think it's all, it's very complete, divination, that's why these situations would be for all kinds of problems.
Don Mateo:	Oh yes, aha. Because according to what is counted and taken out in a divination, which depends on the problem, what will come or what's already happened, you have to set out from [i.e., begin] there. Because as some said—I don't know if [or] who [*no se si quien*]: "Because trees don't talk, they don't criticise"; the tree grows and the fruit is not sinful. So you have to speak precisely; that's how they did it.
Danielle:	[in English] I think the time he's taking has to be exact.
Marcos:	[not fully understanding] Ah, yes, I understand, it's [for] agriculture. And by saying it, this is information is in books, or is it divination, do I need to verify it with a divination process or do I receive information in the knowledge? It's from the calendar?
Don Mateo:	No, you have all you need. There's no book.
Sra Ca'al:	Aah—the *nawal*, that one [too]?
Don Mateo:	Ah—yes the *nawals* are in a book, it's useful; but [the book itself] isn't for making divinations.

Ms Ca'al:	It's only for looking up the *nawal*, you can do that, if you'd like? You do it, when you do a reading for someone, you ask for their birth date and everything. He'll tell you what it says—[about] who you are and everything.
Marcos:	Yes, no problem. Is it only your birthday?
Ms Ca'al:	He's going to tell you …
Don Mateo:	This is the Maya calendar!
Marcos:	Ah! Very good!
Don Mateo:	[You can] buy it in Guatemala.
Marcos:	Every year is a little different, no?
Don Mateo:	Ah, yes, aha!
Ms Ca'al:	Who wants to go first? Who wants to give their date of birth?
Marcos:	OK, date of birth, March 31, 1978.
Don Mateo:	You were born on the day—thirty-first of March. Eight *ahmak* is the day of birth; *ahmak* is the day … *ah'mak* is … it's the sinner [*pecador*]. [laughs] Oh, sinner.
Ms Ca'al:	Oh, you commit many sins. It's the day I was born, [too].
Don Mateo:	Aha, March 31. And he was conceived on the thirteenth [*anil*]. That is where the seed was when he was conceived—
Ms Ca'al:	It's the day of conception.
Don Mateo:	The seed—
Mrs Ca'al:	From the moment you were conceived, you were in sin!
Don Mateo:	Then, your work. This in the [*ak'pak*]—The [*ak'pak*] means that it is in the net—I do not know how I—how to say it to you. You, sometimes, do not know your own mood [*humor*]. [unintelligible].
Ms Ca'al:	It's a person who is a bit—not like that, but they like to cheat. Something like—
Don Mateo:	A … if a person is talking, he is going to interrupt you—it's not—you are going to say it is not true, he is going to interrupt you.
Ms Ca'al:	In other words, this is something like that … mmm, as I was saying—they call this kind of person a trickster. A bit unlawful. A bit like, at the very least, I can't fully trust you then because I don't know if it, what you tell me is true or—like, it's not very sincere.
Marcos:	Ah, OK. He's not very sincere.

[Don Mateo and Mrs Ca'al converse in Mopan]

Don Mateo:	What's your name, let me look at my calendar …
Ms Ca'al:	He says that according to him, from your birth he sees something to do with love—a sinful person, he sees it like that.
Marcos:	[looks up *pecador* in the disctionary] AHH! It's very bad, I don't like it. [everyone laughs] Trap [*trampa*]?
Don Mateo:	Trap is your job. It's how you work.
Marcos:	[after looking up *trampa* in the dictionary] Trap? OK.

Ms Ca'al:	You know that when they told me which one was mine, there was another boy with me. I was in love—but he—I knew he had a wife, and he said no, I don't have a wife. But I could well imagine what he was looking for. And the man was [unintelligible]—and I told him, oh yes, you have three women, one [of them] in the United States, you have so many children, you're someone who likes the good life … and he said, no, no I don't want [that]!
Marcos:	So, sinner is my personality, or is it?
Ms Ca'al:	You live according to your worldview at any [given] moment.
Marcos:	OK, sinner. And [*engendaron*] conception?
Don Mateo:	When you were conceived, when your mom was pregnant …
Ms Ca'al:	From the moment of sperm entry …
Marcos:	Ah! Conception. They begot, they are begot …
Ms Ca'al:	Begotten, or at the moment of conception.
Marcos:	Both. OK, sinner, I can see it. But I don't lie, never, if possible, never lie—sin, yes. But trap—trap, means …?
Don Mateo:	In your work … I work—what you're doing now …
Marcos:	But like in my work, I work with medicinal plants. In what way is that cheating?
Don Mateo:	Not sometimes in words, or when one is talking. There are some people like that, but not everyone. Not all people [with the same birth date] … Here is the meaning. The *ahmak*—with age, it purifies the spirit of the living and the dead.
Marcos:	Oh well, it's not that bad.
Don Mateo:	And it's the day we commemorate or give tribute to the deceased. "Sins for our sins." [Ms Ca'al laughs—they speak Mopan.] Everything has something negative and positive.
Danielle:	I think it's similar to Native Americans like they have—for example I'm a wolf, but they have a negative and a positive.
Marcos:	Ah OK. Because in English astrology I am Scorpio [rising]. And it's a sign that I can be very bad, but their job is to identify and take the bad from others too, and I can embody it in a very bad way with envy or in a way to take the negativity of others. It is a—choice—as it is said? It's a choice. But the sinner—I can see that!
Ms Ca'al:	Choosing—choosing is looking for the good and bad of a person.
Marcos:	But it's not completely bad, then.
Don Mateo:	Well, yes, there are people who—not all *nawals* or people are the same. Because depending on how they arrive, the thirteens [*los treces*], how the thirteens [*los treces*] are counted. If they are threes [i.e., born on the day three *ah'mak*], it could be very strong, then they could be as I described, then they really are cheaters, or they like to sin. According to the numbers. [speaks Mayan]
Marcos:	And what does the trap mean, about work?
Don Mateo:	That is to say—

Ms Ca'al:	The use of the *ah'mak*, is to say of him and his wife, that more than anything, he's a sinner. He is a sinner.
Marcos:	Is it the same?
Don Mateo:	The [*ak'pak*] is your job. But maybe, as you say, in your work you go around, finding out about these rural things. But also, when it's low [i.e., dishonest], not everybody does that. But here one—one doesn't know girls. You like it—[unintelligible]—you like to interrupt …
Ms Ca'al:	[unintelligible] they talk. There was a girl who came here, and [unintelligible]
Don Mateo:	But not everyone …
Ms Ca'al:	Everybody is attracted to different things.
Marcos:	I have a friend who was born on the same day as me, a school friend. We're very different. Like me, he now works with patients, he is an osteo—he works to repair patients who have bone pain, osteopathy. So, yes, like me he deals with patients. It's interesting … […]
Don Mateo:	Thirty, and here thirteen. No, six here, six here, twelve. Thirteen.
Marcos:	Movements for all parts of the body.
Don Mateo:	Aha, aha. Because it moves. They derived the thirteen movements from this.
Marcos:	And the divination, what do the numbers with the feet mean? Are they levels? Characteristics? For example, for example—an eight sinner, is it different from a sinner of ten in some way? Or only …
Don Mateo:	Oh, yes, because it's not the same. It has to be quite positive and negative. When you have more negativity, that's what makes you do what you want to do. But this is quite positive, because positivity is lawful, and negativity is almost unlawful.
Marcos:	And the eight, is it lawful? Unlawful? Each number has different qualities? And my number, eight?
Don Mateo:	The eight is almost—
Marcos:	Between the two. OK.
Don Mateo:	It's already higher. More …
Marcos:	More good? OK, I understand.
Don Mateo:	It's equal in the state of its [goodness and badness]—if I look at it—yes, it's the same [amount of each]. Two *anil* … [*sic*]
Danielle:	And the birthday days, are they very different, for example, the day of birth on August 2 is quite different from the one on August 1?
Don Mateo:	He was born on the second of August, right? It's his birthday?
Danielle:	I don't know when it is …
Don Mateo:	Ahhh, it's not very accurate … well, that's why, if it's August 2nd, it's the [unintelligible], you have wisdom. If it's August 1, it's the idea. You're saying or recording what you hear and you do not know what you are going to make of it, so you keep it in mind. Then you would be the recipient of science.

Marcos: I need to ask, starting at thirteen, my work number: what's that? What is cheating: three or thirteen?

Don Mateo: It's like when a spider makes a trap, he catches animals; and when he says a verse, he catches a fish with the net –

Marcos: But is my work number bad or is it good?

Don Mateo: No, it's fine. It's like—it's not bad. As I said today, if you are not cheating, you're working to understand the culture, [then] that's good.

Marcos: Well, it's not bad.

Full list of interviews

1. 9th April 2008, Mexico City. Mercado de Sonora, 'Esperancita'—herb stall
2. 9th April 2008, Mexico City. Mercado de Sonora, *Santeria* herb stall 'El Elefante'
3. 12th April 2008, Puyucatengo, Mexico: interview with herbalist Tomas Villanueva
4. 18th April 2008, Mani, Yucatan Peninsula, Mexico: Interview with Sr. Mario Euan, herbalist & teacher at U-Yits-Ka'an school of Agriculture & Ecology.
5. 20th April 2008, Hacienda la Luz, Comalcalco, Tabasco. Commentary/Interviews with tour guide Claudia.
6. 25th April 2008, No. 42 Calle 1 San Marco, San Cristobal de las Casas, Chiapas, Mexico. Interview with herbalist Roberto Molina.
7. Thursday 1st May 2008, Interview with a stallholder selling ingredients for *tejate* & *chocolate atole, Mercado 20 de Noviembre*, Oaxaca City, Oaxaca, Mexico.
8. Thursday 1st May 2008, Interview with stallholder selling medicinal herbs and magical supplies, *Mercado 20 de Noviembre*, Oaxaca City, Oaxaca, Mexico.
9. Friday 2nd May 2008, Interview with Sra Lupita Juarez, Organic Produce Market, Oaxaca City, Oaxaca, Mexico.
10. Friday 2nd May 2008, Interview with stallholder selling medicinal herbs and magical supplies, *Mercado Benito Juarez*, Oaxaca City, Oaxaca, Mexico.
11. 26th January 2011, Interview with Señora Lopreto, *panecito* and *pinole* maker, San Antonio Suchitequepez, Guatemala (with my guide and Cacao expert, Juan-Pablo Porres Esquina).
12. 26th January 2011, At Cacao farmer Don Ramiro's Finca, San Antonio Suchitequepez, Guatemala.
13. 20th January 2011, Interview with Sra Claudia Leon, chocolate tablet maker, San Antonio Suchitequepez, Guatemala.
14. Weds 26th Jan 2011. Interview with 'Cacao shaman' Keith Wilson, & introduction to Cacao Ceremony, San Marcos La Laguna, Lake Atitlan, Guatemala.
15. Sat 29th Jan 2011. Interview with Ignacio Cac Sacul, President of the Cacao Grower's Association, Cahabon, Alta Verapaz, North Guatemala.
16. Sat 29th Jan 2011. Interview with Don Juan Francisco, Cohoban Cacao Grower's Association technical advisor & independent Cacao farmer, Alta Verapaz, North Guatemala
17. Mon 31st Jan 2011. Interview with Doña Rosalia, local chocolate maker & vendor, Alta Verapaz, North Guatemala
18. Thu 3rd Feb 2011. Interview with Kek'chi curandero, Don Antonio Xoc, Ya'al Pemech, Alta Verapaz, North Guatemala. Interpreted [into Spanish] by Sr. Oswaldo Che'pan.
19. Fri 4th Feb 2011. Interview with Comadrona Dona Ca'al, Rex'hua, Alta Verapaz, North Guatemala.
20. Fri 11th Feb 2011. Interview with Sr. Reginaldo Chayax Huex, herbalist & director of the Asociacion Bio-Itza, San Jose, Peten, West Guatemala.
21. Sun 13th Feb 2011. Interview with Sr. Ca'al, San Luis, Peten, West Guatemala.
22. Sun 13th Feb 2011. Interview with curandero Don Angel Chiac, San Luis, Peten, West Guatemala.

23. 14th Feb 2011, Interview with Don Mateo Poptchu, Mayan spiritual guide, San Luis, Peten, West Guatemala.

24. 18th Feb 2011, Interview with vendor of Cal [Lime, for cooking] at Ocotlan market, Oaxaca, Mexico.

25. 22nd Feb 2011, Interview with vendor of Popo [local Cacao-based drink] in Acayucan, Veracruz, Mexico.

26. 21st September 2018, Interview with Carina Santiago, chef and owner of Tierra Antigua restaurant, with her student, Kalisa Wells. Teotitlán del Valle, Oaxaca, México.

27. 23rd September 2018, Interview with Sra. Teresa Olivera, stallholder in Mercado Benito Juarez, Oaxaca City, Oaxaca, Mexico.

28. Weds 26th September 2018, Interview with Sra. Anna Maria Garcia Vásquez, maker and vendor of *bu'pu*, with her husband Roberto, in Juchitan de Zaragoza, Oaxaca, Mexico.

29. Friday 28th September 2018, Interview with Sra. Delfina Valverde, maker of Chaw Popox, San Mateo de Mar, Oaxaca, Mexico.

30. Sunday 30th September 2018, Interview with Sr. Jose Antonio, medicinal herb vendor, Tuxtepec, Oaxaca, Mexico.

31. Tuesday 2nd October 2018, Interview with Doña Rosa Gregorio, vendor of *popo*, Tuxtepec & Ojitlan, Oaxaca, Mexico.

32. Monday 8th October 2018, Interview with Doña Maria Eugenia Navarrete Matei, maker of *popo*, Hueyapan de Ocampo, Veracruz, Mexico.

33. Friday 12th October 2018, Interview with agronomist Rosia Torres Torres, Tapachula, Chiapas, Mexico.

34. Sunday 14th October 2018, Interview with stallholder Señora Ernestina Tawal, San Antonio Suchitequepez, Guatemala.

35. Thursday 18th October 2018, Interview with stallholder Señora Claudia Maribel Ya'teni, Coban, Alta Verapaz, Guatemala.

Experiences

1. Chocolate for PTSD: a therapeutic experiment

This is a brief account of an unofficial experiment conducted sometime in 2016, on a lunch break at the Park Clinic, a complementary medicine clinic formerly run by Middlesex University. I was the clinical supervisor for the Western Herbal Medicine BSc and MSc courses.

We were in the run-up to the final clinical examinations, which is always a time when students start to have breakdowns of various sorts. One of my class told me about some severe PTSD issues he was having. He and his sister grew up in a war-torn country; they not only witnessed, but were forced to participate in various atrocities as children. After moving to the UK, he was OK for a few years, but his PTSD symptoms began when some close family members drowned while attempting to flee his homeland and come to the UK. Shortly after this, he began to experience crippling anxiety attacks, nightmares, vivid flashbacks, palpitations, and uncontrollable outbursts of aggression, made worse by stress—such as upcoming examinations. I suggested a herbal prescription to help reduce his general anxiety level and the frequency of the panic attacks, and asked if he would like to participate in an experiment with chocolate to see whether it could help—there were no guarantees, but the information I had about its traditional use and pharmacology suggested that it might. A week or two later, his symptoms had calmed down a bit, and he came into clinic without having his usual morning coffee, and after only a light breakfast, as I'd requested.

I had brought in some of my home-prepared tablets of Guatemalan *criollo* Cacao *fermentado*, made with a blend of spices (*Vanilla planifolia*, *Pimienta dioica*, *Quararibea funebris*, *Bixa orellana*, *Magnolia dealbata*, *Capsicum frutescens*). I'd also brought a molinillo and a ceramic, wide-mouthed jug for making the chocolate. I weighed out 40g of the Cacao, added a little bit of maple syrup, poured on boiling water, frothed it—no foaming agent, so a light cappuccino-style froth—and gave him the dose. He drank it approximately half an hour before lunch break. At lunchtime, we went into one of the empty clinic rooms; he sat on one side of the desk, I sat on the other. I explained my plan, which was to use some guided meditation, Keith Wilson style (see Appendix C, Interview 14), along with an adapted version of an NLP visualisation I'd picked up several years earlier from a practitioner called Olive Hickmott in a therapists' workshop at Neal's Yard Therapy Rooms in Covent Garden. I was also going to incorporate some basic principles I'd gleaned from reading about PTSD and the "reconsolidation window" (see Chapter 5 for discussion) when traumatic memories are recalled, and the response to trauma can be modified. He could feel the effects of the Cacao, so we began.

I asked him to close his eyes, and take three deep breaths—one to relax physically, two to relax mentally, and three to relax emotionally. I then asked him to visualise a huge whirlpool with a giant charcoal tablet at the bottom of it in the distance, and with every out breath any stress and negativity was leaving his body and being sucked into the whirlpool; and above our heads was a huge ball of golden light, and with every in breath, the body would fill up with golden light. Darkness out, light in. We continued that for five to ten minutes, until he felt more relaxed. Then I asked him to see in his mind's eye a traumatic event—something which recurred in his nightmares—but as a still photograph, that he was outside of, so it couldn't touch or harm him; at any time he could change the image. Then I asked him to alter the image in any way he wanted, so as to make it absurd, or harmless. At this point he began to sweat, very visibly; I asked if he was OK, he said "Yes." We then did more of the golden light/whirlpool visualisation, then ended the session.

He said, "It was very strange—it felt like my heart was unplugged." I asked him to explain this; he said normally, if he ever thought about any of the things that had happened to him, he could feel his adrenaline levels rise—sweating, starting to panic, and extreme palpitations; but this time, while he felt stressed, the palpitations just didn't happen, as if he was slightly removed from the stress. As homework, I asked him to take chocolate in the same way once a week or so—no more than that—and repeat the visualisation on his own; I recommended using "Wille's Supreme Cacao" cooking chocolate, as it's made from 100% single estate Cacao beans with no added sugar or fat—in my experience it's high quality, and the closest commercial analogue of home-made Cacao tablets. A week or so later, he hadn't tried the visualisation excercise again, but had notably less panic and PTSD symptoms.

With the exams and so on I didn't see him very often after that, and didn't follow up with him again until recently, almost three years later, for the purpose of writing this account. Unfortunately, the ultimate outcome wasn't good. While he had experienced some improvement after that first session with me, when he tried it himself at home on his own, the symptoms got worse; he also tried replicating the technique with his sister, playing the role of therapist himself, and her symptoms also got worse. He continued taking the initial herbal prescription, as that helped his anxiety, but understandably never tried the chocolate again.

My thoughts on the outcome are as follows:

The initial improvement could have been a "placebo" effect—a genuine therapeutic effect which had nothing to do with the chocolate, but rather to his trust in me and hope in the process. However, the "heart unplugged" sensation was very interesting, given Cacao's traditional heart-related symbolism as described in Chapter 9 (which we hadn't discussed), the recorded adrenaline-blunting property of whole Cacao in humans (Wirtz et al., 2014 [Journal]), and perhaps the observation that epicatechin in Cacao binds to δ-opioid receptors in the heart itself (Panneerselvam et al., 2010 [Journal].)

It was foolish of me to advise him to try repeating the procedure on his own at home; in MDMA therapy for PTSD, for example, they wouldn't just hand the drug out after one session and say "Off you go mate, have a crack at it yourself." I'm also not a qualified psychotherapist, so while I'd got some information, it's likely that similar techniques in the hands of an experienced psychotherapist—such as the PTSD reprogramming used in Human Givens therapy, which involves visualising fast-forwarding and rewinding a traumatic event under controlled conditions until it no longer provokes a response—may have been more effective. Nevertheless, he did experience some improvement after the first session, before attempting to replicate it at home. The main issue could be one of monitoring and oversight: a third party is needed to help moderate and control the process, to act as a "container" for the subject. The other factor could be the chocolate dosage and quality: Willie's Cacao is excellent, but (with much due respect) doesn't hold a candle to the home-made stuff, and the dosage used was likely to have been lower, too. But I suspect that the main issue was the dangers of DIY therapy. A drowning man makes a poor swimming instructor.

My take-home suggestions for any actual psychotherapists who want to experiment with chocolate in this way:

• Use an established PTSD re-programming technique, such as Human Givens therapy.
• Use home-prepared Cacao, made from *criollo* Mexican or Guatemalan Cacao; average adult dose of 40g taken in 60–240ml hot water, with a little sweetening. (See Chapter 8 for preparation instructions.) Appropriate spices may include *Quararibea funebris* and *Magnolia mexicana* (see Appendix B for details—*Quararibea* may have anxiolytic properties, *Magnolia* reduces palpitations and cardiac excitability).
• On the day of a session, the subject should not have taken any other form of caffeine, and only eaten very lightly so that they will get the full effect of the drug. The dose should be given approximately thirty minutes before the start of the session—note that caffeine peaks in the bloodstream at thirty minutes, theobromine and many of the flavanols at two hours after ingestion.
• Advise the patient *not* to attempt the same visualisation on their own, and not to attempt repeating the process with anyone else!

2. Psychedelic Chocolate

Obligatory Disclaimer: This article is published for educational purposes only. I do not endorse the use of illegal substances; the following events took place before enaction of the UK Psychoactive Substances Act in 2016.

I do, however, question the integrity of any legislation which outlaws the use of non-toxic psychoactive substances, fails to differentiate between many different types of psychoactive substance, recognises no value in recreational or therapeutic use of non-commercial psychoactive substances, yet upholds the legal status of two of the most deadly, therapeutically useless (in their present forms) and addictive psychoactive substances known to man on the basis of familiarity, precedent, and profit. I advocate the universal decriminalisation of all psychoactive substances with the provision of accurate dosage and safety information at point of sale, so that their use may be more readily monitored and controlled, their purity and safety increased, the allure of the forbidden diminished, addicts detected sooner and referred to appropriate support services, criminal control of the illegal drugs market can be dismantled, and the unfortunate, expensive, and ultimately counterproductive penalisation of users abolished.

I ran a simple market stall a few times every year, selling chocolate drinks, from around 2011–2017. The stalls were up in my hometown of Bingley, and, later, in nearby Shipley, in the "Shipley Alternative" indoor market. I started them with my step-mum Caron, who has a background in catering and always wanted to do a stall; when we began, I'd be on one half of the table, selling a few of my "unusual" or "interesting" chocolate drinks, and Caron would be on the other half, selling rather more cakes and biscuits and jams. She now runs a small business making excellent chocolate candy. When we moved to the Shipley Alternative market, we both got separate tables indoors—luxury! In the early days at that market, I did quite a decent trade, and decided to try making some "Psychedelic Chocolate", containing a low dose of the psychoactive, LSA-containing Morning Glory (*Turbina corymbosa*) seeds. Magic Mushrooms (*Psilocybe sp.*) would have been more historically authentic, but they're illegal, whereas Morning Glory seeds were legal at the time. (Sadly, since then, the UK Psychoactive Substances Act of 2016 has outlawed all naturally occurring or synthetic psychoactive substances other than alcohol and tobacco—two of the most objectively harmful ones!—caffeine, and medicinal drugs).

There's no evidence that Morning Glory seeds were used with Cacao in pre-Colombian Mesoamerica, although Morning Glory seeds are similar enough in effect to the mushrooms that Cacao may have been used as a potentiator (see Chapter 7 for discussion). Lysergic acid amide (LSA), the principal psychoactive constituent in Morning Glory seeds, is a naturally occurring psychedelic compound with similar activity to its much more potent synthetic cousin, lysergic acid dimethylamide (LSD). My market-mate Debbie, who periodically ran a stall next to mine selling antiques and bric-a-brac (my favourite kind of stall), being a fellow nonconformist and aficionado of mind-altering substances was quite interested in trying it, and was bringing a crew of friends with her. So I had to make a decent job of it.

Like LSD, LSA is denatured (broken down) by heat, so the seeds needed to be extracted in cool or room-temperature water. The only issue is that the chocolate drinks, being made from tablets, required warm water—so, I'd have to dissolve the Cacao tablets in a little hot water, add cool water to bring the temperature down, then add the cold-water extract of the plant. At the time I was making my chocolate drinks very thick, as I thought this was necessary for foam production (it isn't)—I was using 20g Cacao to 30ml water, served in heavy cast-iron green tea cups, to give the small serving sizes a bit of "heft" in keeping with their powerful, layered flavour, and so that people didn't feel short-changed at £5 a pop. Incidentally, the cups were glazed on the inside, so the surface in contact with the liquid was non-reactive—an important consideration for polyphenol-rich drugs. (Now I use 120ml water per 20g, which allows for just the same foaming action, with a milder, less concentrated taste, and more volume). This small volume serving meant that by the time I'd added a splash (say, 5ml) of boiling water to dissolve the Cacao, and enough cool water (say, 10ml) to bring down the temperature, I only had 10ml left to play with: nowhere near an active dose of a simple cold-water seed infusion. So, in order to get anything like enough of the LSA-containing infusion into each dose, I made individual servings of 40g Cacao (made with 60ml water in total), use 10–15ml boiling water to melt and stir the Cacao, then add the remaining 45–50ml cool liquid in the form of the Morning Glory seed infusion. This risked denaturing some of the LSA, but I guessed that the extra volume of seed infusion would be advantageous, as if the liquid was added quickly the temperature would be lowered quickly, too.

I made the Morning Glory seed infusion the night before, grinding the seeds to a coarse powder to increase their surface area, putting them in a 1L plastic bottle, filling it with water from the cold tap, shaking it well and leaving it to stand overnight (whenever I walked past it, or it occurred to me, I'd give it a little shake to help the infusion along). Dosage information is scant, with online forums suggesting an infusion of ten seeds as a threshold dose for antidepressant effects, up to around 150 seeds for a very potent psychedelic effect. The seeds must be infused, as ingesting the powdered seed allegedly causes nausea—the drug itself may cause mild nausea though, due to activation of serotonin receptors in the stomach, so this may simply be due to ingesting more of the active compounds when the whole seed is eaten. If this happens, half a teaspoon of powdered dried ginger (*Zingiber officinale*) taken by mouth, or just one or two puffs of smoked *Cannabis sativa* leaf (a well-balanced outdoor-grown variety, not an unnecessarily potent "skunk"-type hydroponic cultivar) are sufficient to quell it. The ginger, being taken orally, takes around twenty to thirty minutes to work, the effect of the smoked cannabis is pretty much instantaneous; on the other hand, the second plant is often illegal. As I'd be selling the "spiked" chocolate at a market, I erred on the side of caution: I can't remember exactly what amount I used, but I calculated the dose to be around an infusion of ten to twenty seeds per serving.

In the event, Debbie and her friends all bought a cup. To prepare each cup, I broke up 40g Cacao tablets into a jug, poured on 15ml or so of boiling water and stirred to dissolve the Cacao; then I filtered some of the Morning Glory seed infusion using a clean square of muslin and a sieve, and added 45ml of that liquid to the jug, with two or three teaspoons of maple syrup. Then I frothed it well with the molinillo, and served it up. After the market, Debbie's feedback was "We taxi'd up to the runway, but never took off"—noting that she and her friends felt some euphoria, and the beginnings of a "trip", but nothing more. They all felt happy, but had hoped for a little more. I noted that Debbie's pupils were very dilated—this phenomenon, known as mydriasis, is indicative of the LSA working, like LSD, as drugs which strongly affect serotonin receptors in the brain are known to cause this phenomenon.

Given the very small amount of infusion used in each dose, I speculated that the mild MAO-inhibitory effects of the Cacao (see Chapters 4 and 5 for discussion) had augmented the probably sub-threshold effects of the extract somewhat. My thoughts now are that, should this experiment be repeated (in a jurisdiction where Morning Glory seeds are still legal), a larger volume of liquid per serving would solve the "sub-active dose" issue. A single serving could be prepared with 40g Cacao and 30–40ml boiling water to dissolve it, 30–40ml cold water to cool it down, and 160ml of a filtered cold-water extract made with 100–120 *Turbina corymbosa* seeds per 160ml water (i.e., 100+ seeds per dose), and two or three teaspoons of maple syrup. If necessary, a second, follow-up dose could be taken after sixty to ninety minutes, made using half the quantities (20g Cacao + 15–20ml hot water, 15–20ml cold water, 80ml Morning Glory seed cold infusion, and sweetening).

3. Chocolate for Hobos

When I was doing market stalls a few times a year I was making large quantities, so I always had excess stock at the end of the year—of the real, potent stuff. So for three years, on the winter solstice, I'd take any home-made drinking chocolate I had left over and trundle round central

London, making chocolate drinks for homeless people. I'd pack everything I needed into a wheelie bag—three or four thermoses of hot water, a jug, a molinillo, my supplies of chocolate, maple syrup, weighing scales, and paper cups—and meet whichever friends or volunteers I'd coerced into accompanying me at Seven Dials in Covent Garden around 10pm. Then we'd make some chocolate for ourselves—a good strong 40g dose—and set off in search of rough sleepers.

Invariably, I found that as I felt the chocolate start to have its effect on me—suddenly feeling rather nice—we'd find the first homeless crew, who at that time of night were beginning to hunker down in doorways, arches, and backstreets. The first year, my old school room-mate Simon and a friend of his accompanied me, and they're both built like the proverbial brick outhouse (tall, fit, and good at martial arts), which was reassuring, although they both went home at midnight. I carried on for a bit, and ended up serving chocolate to a pair of homeless crackheads (literally—they were on the pipe as I was making the chocolate) in a backstreet doorway at 1am. The crack smokers turned out to be very friendly—one of them gave me a Chinese "Kung Hei Fat Choi" (Happy New Year) keyring, which I still have. They were also arguing the pros and cons of immigration on the basis of its positive or negative effects on the country ("They come over here, looking for jobs …"), which I found very amusing given the circumstances, though I decided not to share my thoughts on the matter.

It turns out that homeless people are just as diverse as everybody else: some loved it, some didn't. Some particularly memorable encounters were with a Spanish man sleeping rough in Trafalgar Square, who was so grateful for getting "real chocolate" which reminded him of the drinking chocolate from his childhood in Spain. A crew of homeless people sitting in a doorway on Charing Cross Road: one old lady, very drunk, took a sip and instantly vomited—she apologised profusely, but said "It's too strong, not what I was expecting"; but another man on the same step drank his whole cup, and his eyes were bright with pleasure, and he kept saying "It's the real thing, that"—displaying the same thought-clarifying, resuscitatory effect that real Cacao has on me. Probably my favourite memory is a homeless lady outside McDonalds on Charing Cross Road who sipped it, then clutched my arm, and asked "Where can I get this?" I had to tell her she couldn't, but the closest thing was probably "Willy's Supreme Cacao" cooking chocolate, which was available in Waitrose. I sincerely hope that she and her friends all went to Waitrose to buy chocolate. I laugh every time I think of the scandalised horror of upper middle-class shoppers purchasing organic wild-caught smoked salmon and stone-ground ciabatta or whatnot encountering a mob of vagrants hunting for real chocolate. To paraphrase Terence McKenna, psychoactive drugs are all about dissolving boundaries.

Mexican and Guatemalan Cacao suppliers and growers

The organisations below are those who I encountered on my travels. I'm sure there are others, just as deserving. But it was AMCO who gave me the greatest support, linking me with various experts (such as my friend and Cacao supplier J-P), farmers and organisations, even if they seemed somehow to have got the impression that I was a buyer for an international organisation (although I did say I was an author doing research)—this certainly opened doors for me, although a few people were rather disappointed when I arrived, having expected a rich chocolate tycoon, but receiving instead a financially challenged author. The representatives of APROCAV, particularly, were very keen—one might even say desperate—to find an international market: I was presented with an official plea from local growers and Cacao-vendors looking for an international market, pictured overleaf. I hope readers who are searching for authentic Guatemalan *criollo* Cacao will consider ordering from them.

Mexico

AMCO: *Agroindustrias Unidas de Cacao S.A. de C.V.*
Carretera Huixtla-Tapachula Km.253.5, C:P: 30680 Tuzantan, Chiapas.
http://agroindustriascacao.com/ [Accessed 18 April 2019]
Contact: branch manager, Maria del Rocio Torres Torres maria.torres@ecomtrading.com

Guatemala

Asociacion de Productores de Cacao de Alta Verapaz (APROCAV): Cahabón, Alta Verapaz, Guatemala.
Contact: President Ignacio Cac Sacul aprocavjd@gmail.com
   (Next pages: their appeal for international buyers.)

***

Plus, a fantastic restaurant run by an ethnobotanist, serving indigenous food, cooked with traditional ingredients, many home-grown. Fully vegan and vegetarian options available. Also produce their own chocolate. If you're in Coban, definitely worth a visit.

Café Xkape Koban, Diagonal 4, 5-1, Zona 2, Cobán, Alta Verapaz. Tel: (502) 7951 4152
Xkape.koban@gmail.com
https://facebook.com/xkape.koban

Señor:

Lic.Marcos

Nosotros, los miembros del comité de chocolate, todos somos mayores de edad quien nos identificamos con nuestra cedula de vecindad, residimos en el caserío san Cristóbal sacta del municipio de cahabon, departamento de alta Verapaz ante ustedes respetuosamente.

EXPONEMOS

Nosotras las mujeres productoras de chocolate, que estamos viendo que nos hace falta las herramientas y recursos económicos para trabajar por que nosotras las mujeres queremos que nuestros productos sea de buena calidad y comprable y tenemos deseo para vender nuestro producto en los diferentes lugares para el desarrollo de nuestra familia, por eso nos fijamos ante ustedes, sabemos que son buenas personas que han ayudado a personas que están casos de recursos económicos.

Por ellos les SOLOCITAMOS: que nos donen un capital de semilla y herramientas de trabajo.

Esperamos que nuestra petición sea concedida favorablemente, para realizar en realidad nuestro trabajo y así saldremos bien en el trabajo, y les agradecemos sus finas atenciones y la comprensión de nuestras necesidades que tenemos actualmente.

Cahabon 28 de enero de 2011

Candelaria choc sub   0-16 30 342

Maria de Jesús Tzalám caal   0-16 33,307

osaria Cac Sacul   0-16 32,923

osefina Cac Cac   2093 5 3988 1612

Luisa Cac sacul   0-16 23.540

Candelaria Tec   0-16 26457

Maria Elena pop Tec   0-16 34809

Elizabeth Guadalupe xuc choj   0-16

Paulina Sub coc   0-16 - 27,553

Elvira Maquin sub

Aurelia Sub Pop

BIBLIOGRAPHY

Books

Aguilar-Moreno, M. (2006). The Good and Evil of Chocolate in Colonial Mexico. In: C. McNeil (Ed.), *Chocolate in Mesoamerica: A Cultural History of Cacao* (pp. 273–288). Gainesville, FL: University Press of Florida.

Allbright, B. (1997). Trends in chocolate. In: A. Szogyi (Ed.), *Chocolate, Food of the Gods* (pp. 137–144). Westford, CT: Greenwood Press.

Armstrong, K. (2006). *The Great Transformation: The World in the Time of Buddha, Socrates, Confucius and Jeremiah*. London: Atlantic.

Badiano, J. (1552). *Libellus de Medicinalibus Indorum Herbis*. M. de la Cruz (Trans.). Mexico City: Fondo de Cultura Economica Instituto Mexicano del Seguro Social, 1996.

Bales, K. (2000). *Slavery: Commodities and Disposable People in the Modern World*. London: Channel 4 Television.

Barrera, L., & Aliphat, M. (2006). The Itza Maya control over Cacao. In: C. McNeil (Ed.), *Chocolate in Mesoamerica: a Cultural History of Cacao* (pp. 289–306). Gainesville, FL: University Press of Florida.

Beckett, S. (2000). *The Science of Chocolate*. Cambridge: The Royal Society of Chemistry.

Bensky, D., & Gamble, A. (1993). *Chinese Herbal Medicine Materia Medica*. Washington, DC: Eastland Press. [Revised].

Berdan, F., & Anawalt, P. (1997). *The Essential Codex Mendoza*. Berkeley, CA: University of California Press.

Bernaert, H., Blondeel, I., Allegaert, L., & Lohmuller, T. (2012). Industrial treatment of cocoa in chocolate production: health implications. In: R. Paoletti, A. Poli, A. Conti, & F. Visioli (Eds.), *Chocolate and Health* (pp. 17–31). Milan, Italy: Springer-Verlag.

Bertazzo, A., Comai, S., Mangiarini, F., & Chen, S. (2013). Composition of Cacao beans. In: R. Watson, V. Preedy, & S. Zibadi (Eds.), *Chocolate in Health and Nutrition. Nutrition and Health, Volume 7*. Totowa, NJ: Humana Press.

Blackmore, S., & Troscianko, E. (2018). *Consciousness: An Introduction*. Abingdon, UK: Routledge.

Bletter, N., & Daly, D. (2006). Cacao and its relatives in South America. An overview of taxonomy, ecology, biogeography, chemistry, and ethnobotany. In: C. McNeil (Ed.), *Chocolate in Mesoamerica: A Cultural History of Cacao* (pp. 31–68). Gainesville, FL: University Press of Florida.

Bonatti, G. (1994). *Liber Astronomiae, Part I*. R. Zoller (Trans.), R. Hand (Ed.). WV, USA: Golden Hind Press.

Bone, K. (2003). *A Clinical Guide to Blending Liquid Herbs*. Maryland Heights, MO: Churchill Livingstone.

Bone, K. (2014). The microcirculation: a new frontier in cardiovascular phytotherapy. In: H. Brice-Ytsma, & F. Watkins (Eds.), *Herbal Exchanges* (pp. 153–163). London: Strathmore Publishing.

Boone, E. (2007). *Cycles of Time and Meaning in the Mexican Books of Fate*. Austin, TX: University of Texas Press.

Borawska, M. (2007). Mood Food. In: Z. Sikorski (Ed.), *Chemical and Functional Properties of Food Components* [3rd edition] (pp. 427–438). Boca Raton, FL: CRC Press.

Bown, D. (2002). *The Royal Horticultural Society Encyclopaedia of Herbs and Their Uses*. London: Dorling Kindersley.

Bozarth, E. (Ed.) (1987). *Methods of Assessing the Reinforcing Properties of Abused Drugs*. KY: Springer-Verlag.

Brian, T. (1655). *The pisse-prophet, or, Certain pisse-pot lectures : wherein are newly discovered the old fallacies, deceit, and jugling of the pis-pot science used by all those (whether quacks, and empiricks, or other methodical physicians) who pretend knowledge of diseases by the urine in giving judgement of the same*. London: R. Thrale.

Brice-Ytsma, H., & Watkins, F. (Eds.) (2014). *Herbal Exchanges*. London: Strathmore Publishing.

Briggs, M. (2008). *Chocolate: The Tasty Treat with a Dark Secret*. Leicester, UK: Abbeydale Press.

Cabezon, B., Barriga, P., & Grivetti, L. (2009). Chocolate and sinful behaviours. In: L. Grivetti, & H. Shapiro (Eds.), *Chocolate: History, Culture, and Heritage* (pp. 37–48). Hoboken, NJ: John Wiley & Sons.

Carper, J. (1988). *The Food Pharmacy: Dramatic New Evidence that Food Is Your Best Medicine*. London: Pocket Books.

Castell, M., Pérez-Cano, F., & Bisson, J.-F. (2013). Clinical benefits of cocoa: An overview. In: R. Watson, V. Preedy, & S. Zibadi (Eds.), *Nutrition and Health, Volume 7: Chocolate in Health and Nutrition* (pp. 265–275). New York: Springer, Humana Press.

Cheak, A. (2018). Thigh of iron, thigh of gold: On alchemy, astrology, and animated statues. In: A. Coppock & D. Schulke (Eds.), *The Celestial Art: Essays on Astrological Magic* (pp. 225–245). Richmond Vista, CA, USA: Three Hands Press.

Chevalier, J., & Bain, A. (2002). *The Hot and the Cold: Ills of Humans and Maize in Native Mexico*. Toronto, Canada: University of Toronto Press.

Coe, M. (2005). *The Maya* [7th edition]. London: Thames & Hudson.

Coe, S. (1994). *America's First Cuisines*. Austin, TX: University of Texas Press.

Coe, S. (1997). Cacao: Gift of the New World. In: A. Szogyi (Ed.), *Chocolate, Food of the Gods* (pp. 147–153). Westford, CT: Greenwood Press.

Coe, S., & Coe, M. (1996). *The True History of Chocolate*. London: Thames & Hudson.

Colombo, M., Pinorini-Godly, M., & Conti, A. (2012). Botany and pharmacognosy of the Cacao tree. In: R. Paoletti, A. Poli, A. Conti, & F. Visioli (Eds.), *Chocolate and Health* (pp. 41–62). Milan, Italy: Springer-Verlag.

Cotterell, A. (Ed.) (2000). *Encyclopedia of World Mythology*. Bath, UK: Parragon.

Culpeper, N. (1653). *The English Physician—Enlarged*. Ware, UK: Wordsworth Reference, 2007.

Culpeper, N. (1655). *Astrological Judgment of Diseases from the Decumbiture of the Sick*. Abingdon, MD: Astrology Classics, 2003.

Cummins, A. (2018). The azured vault: Astrological magic in seventeenth-century England. In: A. Coppock & D. Schulke (Eds.), *The Celestial Art: Essays on Astrological Magic* (pp. 191–224). Richmond Vista, CA, USA: Three Hands Press.

Diaz del Castillo, B. (1632). *The Discovery and Conquest of Mexico 1517–1521*. A. Maudslay (Trans.). London: Routledge.

Dreiss, M., & Greenhill, S. (2008). *Chocolate: Pathway to the Gods*. Tucson, AZ: University of Arizona Press.

Dunning, P., & Fox, C. (2009). Base metal chocolate pots in North America. In: L. Grivetti & H. Shapiro (Eds.), *Chocolate: History, Culture, and Heritage* (pp. 723–730). Hoboken, NJ: John Wiley & Sons.

Ebadi, M., Wszolek, Z., & Pfeiffer, R. (2005). *Parkinson's Disease*. Boca Raton, FL: CRC Press.

Eggleston, K., & White, T. (2013). Chocolate and pain tolerance. In: R. Watson, V. Preedy, & S. Zibadi (Eds.), *Nutrition and Health, Volume 7: Chocolate in Health and Nutrition* (pp. 437–447). New York: Springer, Humana Press.

Elliott, C. (1997). Curing irrationality with chocolate addiction. In: A. Szogyi (Ed.), *Chocolate, Food of the Gods* (pp. 19–33). Westford, CT: Greenwood Press.

Evans, W. (2002). *Trease and Evans Pharmacognosy* [15th edition]. London: W. B. Saunders.

Faust, B., & López, J. (2006). Cacao in the Yukatek Maya healing ceremonies of Don Pedro Ucán Itza. In: C. McNeil (Ed.), *Chocolate in Mesoamerica: A Cultural History of Cacao* (pp. 408–428). Gainesville, FL: University Press of Florida.

Feng, G., & English, J. (Trans.) (1989). *The Complete Tao Te Ching*. London: Vintage.

Freidel, D., Schele, L., & Parker, J. (1993). *Maya Cosmos: Three Thousand Years on the Shaman's Path*. New York: Harper Collins.

Fulder, S. (1993). *The Book of Ginseng*. Rochester, VT: Healing Arts Press.

Fyne, R. (1997). Candy, Cheka, and Controversy: The propaganda failure of Alexander Tarasov-Rodionov's 1922 novel *Chocolate*. In: A. Szogyi (Ed.), *Chocolate, Food of the Gods* (pp. 59–66). Westford, CT: Greenwood Press.

Galli, C. (2012). Cocoa, chocolate and blood lipids. In: R. Paoletti, A. Poli, A. Conti, & F. Visioli (Eds.), *Chocolate and Health* (pp. 127–135). Milan, Italy: Springer-Verlag.

Gay, J., & Clark, F. (2009). Making Colonial Era chocolate: The colonial Williamsburg experience. In: L. Grivetti & H. Shapiro (Eds.), *Chocolate: History, Culture, and Heritage* (pp. 635–645). Hoboken, NJ: John Wiley & Sons.

Gerard, J. (1597). *Gerard's Herbal: John Gerard's Historie of Plants*. M. Woodward (Ed.). Canterbury, UK: Tiger, 1998.

Gettings, F. (1990). *The Arkana Dictionary of Astrology*. London: Penguin Arkana.

Greer, J. M., & Warnock, C. (Trans.) (2010). *The Picatrix: Liber Atratus Edition*. Phoenix, Arizona, USA: Adocentyn Press.

Griggs, B. (1997). *Green Pharmacy: The History and Evolution of Western Herbal Medicine*. Vermont, Canada: Healing Arts Press.

Grivetti, L. (2009). Medicinal chocolate in New Spain, Western Europe, and North America. In: L. Grivetti & H. Shapiro (Eds.), *Chocolate: History, Culture, and Heritage* (pp. 67–88). Hoboken, NJ: John Wiley & Sons.

Grivetti, L., & Cabezon, B. (2009). Ancient gods and Christian celebrations. In: L. Grivetti & H. Shapiro (Eds.), *Chocolate: History, Culture, and Heritage* (pp. 27–35). Hoboken, NJ: John Wiley & Sons.

Haertzen, C., & Hickey, J. (1987). Addiction Research Center Inventory (ARCI): Measurement of euphoria and other drug effects. In: M. Bozarth (Ed.), *Methods of Assessing the Reinforcing Properties of Abused Drugs* (pp. 489–524). New York: Springer.

Haertzen, C., & Hickey, J. (1987). *Methods of Assessing the Reinforcing Properties of Abused Drugs*. New York: Springer-Verlag.

Hamnett, B. (1999). *A Concise History of Mexico*. Cambridge: Cambridge University Press.

Hanks, P. (Ed.) (1989). *The Collins Pocket Dictionary*. Wrotham, UK: William Collins.

Henderson, J., & Joyce, R. (2006). Brewing distinction: The development of Cacao beverages in formative Mesoamerica. In: C. McNeil (Ed.), *Chocolate in Mesoamerica: A Cultural History of Cacao* (pp. 140–153). Gainesville, FL: University Press of Florida.

Hobbs, C. (1986). *Medicinal Mushrooms: An exploration of Tradition, Healing, and Culture*. Oregon, USA: Botanica Press.

Hughes, W. (1672). *The American Physitian; or, a treatise of the roots, plants, trees, shrubs, fruit, herbs etc. growing in the English plantations in America [...] Whereunto is added a discourse of the cacao-nut-tree, and the use of its fruit; with all the ways of making of chocolate*. London: William Cook.

Illes, J. (2004). *The Element Encyclopaedia of 5000 Spells*. London: Element/HarperCollins.

Joneja, J. (1998). *Dietary Management of Food Allergies & Intolerances: A Comprehensive Guide*. Vancouver, British Columbia, Canada: J. A. Hall Publications.

Junius, M. (1979). *The Practical Handbook of Plant Alchemy*. Rochester, VT: Healing Arts Press.

Kaptchuk, T. (2000). *The Web that Has No Weaver: Understanding Chinese Medicine*. Lincolnwood, IL: Contemporary Publishing.

Kennedy, D. (2010). *Oaxaca al Gusto: An Infinite Gastronomy*. Austin, TX: University of Texas Press.

Khan, N., & Nicod, N. (2012). Biomarkers of cocoa consumption. In: R. Paoletti, A. Poli, A. Conti, & F. Visioli (Eds.), *Chocolate and Health* Milan, Italy: Springer-Verlag.

Kohl, J., & Francoeur, R. (1995). *The Scent of Eros: Mysteries of Odor in Human Sexuality*. Lincoln, NE, USA: Author's Choice Press.

Kufer, J., & McNeil, C. (2006). The Jaguar Tree (*Theobroma bicolor* Bonpl.). In: C. McNeil (Ed.), *Chocolate in Mesoamerica: A Cultural History of Cacao* (pp. 90–104). Gainesville, FL: University Press of Florida.

de Ledesma, A. C. (1631). *Curioso tratado de la naturaleza y calidad del chocolate, dividio en quarto partes*. E. Paltrinieri (Ed.). Alessandria, Italy: Edizioni dell'Orso, 1999.

Lekatsas, B. (1997). Inside the Pastilles of the Marquis de Sade. In: A. Szogyi (Ed.), *Chocolate, Food of the Gods* (pp. 99–107). Westford, CT: Greenwood Press.

León-Portilla, M. (1992). *Fifteen Poets of the Aztec World*. Norman, OK: University of Oklahoma Press.

Linares, E., Bye, R., & Flores, B. (2000). *Plantas Medicinales de Mexico—usos y remedios tradicionales*. Mexico City: Universidad Nacional Autonoma de Mexico Instituto de Biologia.

Loffredo, L., & Violi. F. (2012). Polyphenolic antioxidants and health. In: R. Paoletti, A. Poli, A. Conti, & F. Visioli (Eds.), *Chocolate and Health* (pp. 77–85). Milan, Italy: Springer-Verlag.

Mann, C. (2005). *Ancient Americans*. London: Granta.

Martin, S. (2006). Cacao in ancient Maya religion: First Fruit from the Maize Tree and other tales from the underworld. In: C. McNeil (Ed.), *Chocolate in Mesoamerica: A Cultural History of Cacao* (pp. 54–183). Gainesville, FL: University Press of Florida.

Martin, S. (2012). *Opium Fiend: A 21st Century Slave to a 19th Century Addiction*. New York: Villard.

Mazariegos, O. (Ed.) (2006). *Kakaw: Chocolate in Guatemalan Culture*. Museo Popol Vuh, Guatemala City, Guatemala: Universidad Francisco Marroquin.

McGee, H. (1984). *On Food and Cooking*. New York: Simon & Schuster.

McIntosh, A., Kubena, K., & Landmann, W. (1997). Chocolate and loneliness among the elderly. In: A. Szogyi (Ed.), *Chocolate, Food of the Gods* (pp. 3–17). Westford, CT: Greenwood Press.

McNeil, C. (2006a). Introduction. In: C. McNeil (Ed.), *Chocolate in Mesoamerica: A Cultural History of Cacao* (pp. 1–28). Gainesville, USA: University Press of Florida.

McNeil, C. (2006b). Traditional Cacao use in modern Mesoamerica. In: C. McNeil (Ed.), *Chocolate in Mesoamerica: A Cultural History of Cacao* (pp. 341–366). Gainesville, FL: University Press of Florida.

McTaggart, L. (2001). *The Field*. London: Element.

Milbrath, S. (1999). *Star Gods of the Maya: Astronomy in Art, Folklore, and Calendars*. Austin, TX: University of Texas Press.

Miller, M., & Taube, K. (1993). *An Illustrated Dictionary of The Gods and Symbols of Ancient Mexico and the Maya*. London: Thames & Hudson.

Mills, S. (1991). *The Essential Book of Herbal Medicine*. St. Ives, UK: Penguin Arkana.

Molinari, E., & Callus, E. (2012). Psychological drivers of chocolate consumption. In: R. Paoletti, A. Poli, A. Conti, & F. Visioli (Eds.), *Chocolate and Health* (pp. 137–146). Milan, Italy: Springer-Verlag.

Moermann, D. (2002). *Meaning, Medicine, and the "Placebo Effect"*. New York: Cambridge University Press.

Monroy-Ortiz, C., & Castillo-España, P. (2007). *Plantas medicinales Utilizadas en el estad de Morelos* [2nd edition]. Cuernavaca, Mexico: Universidad Autonoma del Estado de Morelos.

Moore, L. (2017). *Lady Fanshawe's Receipt Book*. London: Atlantic.

Morrison, M., & Tweedy, K. (2000). Estrogen and depression in aging women. In: M. Morrison (Ed.), *Hormones, Gender and the Aging Brain* (pp. 84–113). Cambridge: Cambridge University Press.

Moss, M. (2013). *Salt, Sugar, Fat: How the Food Giants Hooked Us*. New York: Random House.

Noriega, E., & González, N. (2009). History of Cacao and chocolate in Cuban literature, games, music and culinary arts. In: L. Grivetti & H. Shapiro (Eds.), *Chocolate: History, Culture, and Heritage* (pp. 523–542). Hoboken, NJ: John Wiley & Sons.

Ogata, N., Gómez-Pompa, A., & Taube, K. (2006). The domestication and distribution of *Theobroma cacao* L. in the neotropics. In: C. McNeil (Ed.), *Chocolate in Mesoamerica: A Cultural History of Cacao* (pp. 69–89). Gainesville, FL: University Press of Florida.

Ott, J. (1985). *The Cacahuatl Eater: Ruminations of an Unabashed Chocolate Addict*. Washington, DC: Natural Products Co.

Ott, J. (1996). *Pharmacotheon: Entheogenic Drugs, Their Plant Sources and History*. Washington, DC: Natural Products Co.

Oxford Concise Colour Medical Dictionary [3rd edition]. (2002). Oxford: Oxford University Press.

Paracelsus (1656). *The Archidoxes of Magic*. R. Turner (Trans.). Maine, USA: Ibis Press, 2004.

Parker, G., & Brotchie, H. (2012). Chocolate and mood. In: R. Paoletti, A. Poli, A. Conti, & F. Visioli (Eds.), *Chocolate and Health* (pp. 147–153). Milan, Italy: Springer-Verlag.

Parkinson, J. (1640). *Theatrum Botanicum: The Theater of Plants*. Delhi, India: Facsimile Publisher, 2018.

Pech, J. (2010). *The Chocolate Therapist: A User's Guide to the Extraordinary Health Benefits of Chocolate*. Hoboken, NJ: John Wiley & Sons.

Pendell, D. (2002). *Pharmakodynamis: Stimulating Plants, Potions, and Herbcraft: Excitantia and Empathogenica*. Berkeley, CA: North Atlantic.

Persoone, D. (2008). *Cacao: Expedition in Mexico*. Dereume, Belgium: Françoise Blouard.

Pizzorno, J., & Murray, M. (Eds.) (1993). *Textbook of Natural Medicine* [3rd Edition]. St. Louis, MO: Churchill Livingstone Elsevier.

Prasad, C. (2005). Food-derived neuroactive cyclic dipeptides. In: H. Lieberman, R. Kanarek, & C. Prasad (Eds.), *Nutritional Neuroscience* (pp. 331–340). London: CRC Press, Taylor & Francis.

Pratchett, T. (1992). *Lords and Ladies*. London: Victor Gollancz.

Qurra, I. (2005). *De Imaginibus*. C. Warnock (Ed. & Trans.). USA: Renaissance Astrology.

Radin, D. (2018). *Real Magic*. New York: Harmony.

van Ree, J. (1998). Drug use and addiction: human research. In: R. Niesink, R. Jaspers, L. Kornet, & J. van Ree (Eds.), *Drugs of Abuse and Addiction: Neurobehavioral Toxicology* (pp. 191–244). Boca Raton, FL: CRC Press.

Reents-Budet, D., & McNeil, C. (2006). The social context of Kakaw drinking among the ancient Maya. In: C. McNeil (Ed.), *Chocolate in Mesoamerica: A Cultural History of Cacao* (pp. 202–223). Gainesville, FL: University Press of Florida.

Reston, G. (2003). *Los Mayas—Genios de la Ciencia y la Astrologia*. Buenos Aires: Grijalbo.

Robert, H. (1957). *Les Vertus Thérapeutiques du Chocolat*. Paris: Editions Artulen.

Robson, V. (1923). *The Fixed Stars and Constellations in Astrology*. Bel Air, MD: Astrology Classics, 2005.

Rudgley, R. (1998). *The Encyclopaedia of Psychoactive Substances*. London: Abacus.

Rusconi, M., Rossi, M., Moccetti, T., & Conti, A. (2012). Acute vascular effects of chocolate in healthy human volunteers. In: R. Paoletti, A. Poli, A. Conti, & F. Visioli (Eds.), *Chocolate and Health* (pp. 87–102). Milan, Italy: Springer-Verlag.

Sahagún, B. (1829). *Historia General de las Cosas de Nueva España*. Bustamante, C. (Trans.). La Vergne, TN: BiblioBazaar LLC, 2010.

Saunders, N. (1993). *E for Ecstasy*. London: Neal's Yard Desktop Publishing Studio.

Saunders, N. (1996). *Ecstasy Reconsidered*. Exeter, UK: BPC Wheatons.

Schultes, R., & Hofmann, A. (1992). *Plants of the Gods: Their Sacred, Healing, and Hallucinogenic Powers*. Rochester, VT: Healing Arts Press.

Sheftel, V. (2000). *Indirect Food Additives and Polymers: Migration and Toxicology*. Boca Raton, FL: Lewis Publishers.

Sheldrake, R. (2009). *Morphic Resonance: The Nature of Formative Causation*. Rochester, VT: Park Street Press.

Shulgin, A., & Shulgin, A. (2013). *PIHKAL: A Chemical Love Story*. Berkeley, CA: Transform Press.

Smit, H. (2011). Theobromine and the pharmacology of cocoa. In: B. Fredholm (Ed.), *Handbook of Experimental Pharmacology 200* (pp. 201–234). Berlin: Springer-Verlag.

Spinella, M. (2001). *The Psychopharmacology of Herbal Medicine*. Cambridge, MA: MIT Press.

Starr, L., Starr, E., & Szogyi, A. (1997). Locus of control and chocolate perceptions. In: A. Szogyi (Ed.), *Chocolate, Food of the Gods* (pp. 11–17). Westford, CT: Greenwood Press.

Steinbrenner, L. (2006). Cacao in Greater Nicoya: Ethnohistory and a unique tradition. In: C. McNeil (Ed.), *Chocolate in Mesoamerica: A Cultural History of Cacao* (pp. 253–270). Gainesville, FL: University Press of Florida.

Stubbe, H. (1662). *The Indian Nectar, or, A Discourse concerning chocolata*. London: J. C. for Andrew Crook.

Sudano, I., Flammer, A., Noll, G., & Corti, R. (2012). Vascular and platelet effects of cocoa. In: R. Paoletti, A. Poli, A. Conti, & F. Visioli (Eds.), *Chocolate and Health*. Milan, Italy: Springer-Verlag.

Szogyi, A. (1997). Chocolatissimo! In: A. Szogyi (Ed.), *Chocolate, Food of the Gods* (pp. 197–203). Westford, CT: Greenwood Press.

Taubes, G. (2017). *The Case Against Sugar*. London: Portobello Press.

Tedlock, B. (1992). *Time and the Highland Maya* [Revised Edition]. Albuquerque, NM: University of New Mexico Press.

Tedlock, D. (Trans.) (1996). *Popol Vuh: The Definitive Edition of the Mayan Book of the Dawn of Life and the Glories of Gods and Kings* [2nd Edition]. New York: Touchstone.

Telly, C. (1997). Chocolate—its quality and flavour (Which is the world's best chocolate?). In: A. Szogyi (Ed.), *Chocolate, Food of the Gods*. Westford, CT: Greenwood Press.

Tobyn, G. (1997). *Culpeper's Medicine: A Practice of Western Holistic Medicine*. Shaftesbury, UK: Element.

Traister, B. (2001). *The Notorious Astrological Physician of London: Works and Days of Simon Forman*. Chicago, IL: University of Chicago Press.

Trilling, S. (1999). *Seasons of My Heart: A Culinary Journey Through Oaxaca, Mexico*. New York: Ballantine.

Trotter, R., & Chavira, J. (1997). *Curanderismo: Mexican American Folk Healing* [2nd Edition]. Athens, GA: University of Georgia Press.

Ullmann, J. (1997). Location factors in cocoa growing and the chocolate industry. In: A. Szogyi (Ed.), *Chocolate, Food of the Gods* (pp. 183–195). Westford, CT: Greenwood Press.

Vail, G. (2009). Cacao use in Yucatán among the pre-Hispanic Maya. In: L. Grivetti & H. Shapiro, H. (Eds.), *Chocolate: History, Culture, and Heritage* (pp. 3–15). Hoboken, NJ: John Wiley & Sons.

Van der Kolk, B. (2014). *The Body Keeps the Score: Mind, Brain and Body in the Transformation of Trauma*. London: Penguin, Random House.

Visioli, F., Bernardini, E., Poli, A., & Paoletti, R. (2012). Chocolate and health: a brief review of the evidence. In: R. Paoletti, A. Poli, A. Conti, & F. Visioli (Eds.), *Chocolate and Health* (pp. 63–75). Milan, Italy: Springer-Verlag.

Wagner, R. (2001). *The History of Coffee in Guatemala*. Bogota, Colombia: Villegas Asociados.

Warnock, C. (2005). *Kyranides: On the Occult Virtues of Plants, Animals, & Stones, Hermetic & Talismanic Magic* (Trans.). USA: Renaissance Astrology Facsimile Editions.

Wasson, R. (1980). *The Wondrous Mushroom: Mycolatry in Mesoamerica*. St. Louis, MO: McGraw-Hill.

Whitfield, P. (2001). *Astrology: A History*. New York: Harry N. Abrams.

Williams, E. (Ed.) (2003). *Potter's Herbal Cyclopaedia*. Saffron Walden, UK: C. W. Daniel.

Wilson, P. (2012). Chocolate as medicine: a changing framework of evidence throughout history. In: R. Paoletti, A. Poli, A. Conti, & F. Visioli, F. (Eds.), *Chocolate and Health* (pp. 1–16). Milan, Italy: Springer-Verlag.

Wilson, P., & Hurst, J. (2012). *Chocolate as Medicine: A Quest Over the Centuries*. Cambridge: The Royal Society of Chemistry.

Withering, W. (1785). *Practical Remarks on Dropsy, and Other Diseases*. London: G. G. J. & J. Robinson.

Wolfe, D., & Holdstock, S. (2005). *Naked Chocolate*. Great Yarmouth, UK: Rawcreation.

Wood, V. (1990). *Mens Sana in Thingummy Doodah*. London: Methuen.

Young, A. (1994). *The Chocolate Tree*. Washington, DC: Smithsonian Iinstitution Scholarly Press.

Yuker, H. (1997). Perceived attributes of chocolate. In: A. Szogyi (Ed.), *Chocolate, Food of the Gods* (pp. 35–43). Westford, CT: Greenwood Press.

Ziegleder, D. (2009). Flavour development in cocoa and chocolate. In: S. Beckett (Ed.), *Industrial Chocolate Manufacture and Use*. Oxford: Blackwell Publishing.

Journals, periodicals, and academic papers

Abbey, M., Patil, V., Vause, C., & Durham, P. (2008). Repression of calcitonin gene-related peptide expression in trigeminal neurons by a Theobroma cacao extract. *Journal of Ethnopharmacology, 115*(2): 238–248.

Abecia-Soria, L., Pezoa-García, N., & Amaya-Farfan, J. (2006). Soluble albumin and biological value of protein in cocoa (*Theobroma cacao* L.) beans as a function of roasting. *Time Journal of Food Science, 70*(4): S294–S298.

Abril-Gil, M., Massot-Cladera, M., Pérez-Cano, F., Castellote, C., Franch, A., & Castell, M. (2012). A diet enriched with cocoa prevents IgE synthesis in rat allergy model. *Pharmacology Research, 65*(6): 603–608.

Abril-Gil, M., Pérez-Cano, F., Franch, A., & Castell, M. (2016). Effect of a cocoa-enriched diet on immune response and anaphylaxis in a food allergy model in brown Norway rats. *Journal of Nutritional Biochemistry, 27*: 317–326.

Aikpokpodion, P., & Dongo, L. (2010). Effects of fermentation intensity on polyphenols and antioxidant capacity of cocoa beans. *International Journal of Sustainable Crop Production, 5*(4): 66–70.

Airaksinen, M., Ho, B., An, R., & Taylor, D. (1978). Major pharmacological effects of 6-methoxytetrahydro-beta-carboline, a drug elevating the tissue 5-hydroxytryptamine level. *Europe PMC, 8*(1): 42–46.

Airaksinen, M., & Kari, I. (1981). Beta-carbolines, psychoactive compounds in the mammalian body. Part I: Occurrence, origin and metabolism. *Medical Biology, 59*(1): 21–34.

Airaksinen, M., Saano, V., Steidel, E., Juvonen, H., Huhtikangas, A., & Gynther, J. (1984). Binding of β-carbolines and tetrahydroisoquinolines by opiate receptors of the β-type. *Acta Pharmacologica et Toxicologica, 55*(5): 380–385.

Akatsu, S. (1917). The resistance of spirochetes to the action of hexamethylenetetramine derivatives and mercurial and arsenic compounds. *Journal of Experimental Medicine, 25*(3): 363–373.

Akita, M., Kuwahara, M., Itoh, F., Nakano, Y., Osakabe, N., Kurosawa, T., & Tsubone, H. (2008). Effects of cacao liquor polyphenols on cardiovascular and autonomic nervous functions in hypercholesterolaemic rabbits. *Basic Clinical Pharmacology & Toxicology, 103*(6): 581–587.

Alanis, A., Calzada, F., Cervantes, A., Torres, J., & Ceballos, M. (2005). Antibacterial properties of some plants used in Mexican traditional medicine for the treatment of gastrointestinal disorders. *Journal of Ethnopharmacology, 100*: 153–157.

Alcocer, P., & Neurath, J. (2004). La eficacia de la magia en los ritos coras y huicholes. *Arqueologia Mexicana, 12*(69): 48–53.

Allgrove, J., Farrell, E., Gleeson, M., Williamson, G., & Cooper, K. (2011). Regular dark chocolate consumption's reduction of oxidative stress and increase of free-fatty-acid mobilization in response to prolonged cycling. *International Journal of Sport Nutrition and Exercise Metabolism, 21*(2): 113–123.

Almoosawi, S., Fyfe, L., Ho, C., & Al-Dujaili, E. (2010). The effect of polyphenol-rich dark chocolate on fasting capillary whole blood glucose, total cholesterol, blood pressure and glucocorticoids in healthy overweight and obese subjects. *British Journal of Nutrition, 103*(6): 842–850.

Amin, I., Koh, B., & Asmah, R. (2004). Effect of cacao liquor extract on tumor marker enzymes during chemical hepatocarcinogenesis in rats. *Journal of Medicinal Food, 7*(1): 7–12.

Amoroso, T., & Workman, M. (2016). Treating posttraumatic stress disorder with MDMA-assisted psychotherapy: A preliminary meta-analysis and comparison to prolonged exposure therapy. *Journal of Psychopharmacology, 30*(7): 595–600.

D'Andrea, G., D'Amico, D., Bussone, G., Bolner, A., Aguggia, M., Saracco, M., Galloni, E., De Riva, V., Colavito, D., Leon, A., Rosteghin, V., & Perini, F. (2013). The role of tyrosine metabolism in the pathogenesis of chronic migraine. *Cephalalgia, 33*(11): 932–937.

Anonymous. (1975). Ancient Aztec cures worked, although the *picitl* didn't know why. *Chemical and Engineering News, 53*(50): 32–33.

Aremu, C., & Abara, A. (1992). Hydrocyanate, oxalate, phytate, calcium and zinc in selected brands of Nigerian cocoa beverage. *Plant Foods for Human Nutrition, 42*(3): 231–237.

Arlorio, M., Locatelli, M., Travaglia, F., Coïsson, J., Del Grosso, E., Minassi, A., Appendino, G., & Martelli, A. (2008). Roasting impact on the contents of clovamide (N-caffeoyl-L-DOPA) and the antioxidant activity of cocoa beans (Theobroma cacao L.). *Food Chemistry, 106*(3): 967–975.

Ascherio, A., Chen, H., Weisskopf, M., O'Reilly, E., McCullough, M., Calle, E., Schwarzschild, M., & Thun, M. (2006). Pesticide exposure and risk for Parkinson's disease. *Annals of Neurology, 60*(2): 197–203.

Austin, A. (2004). La magia y la adivinacion en la tradicion Mesoamericana. *Arqueología Mexicana, 12*(69): 20–29.

Awad, A., Chen, Y., Fink, C., & Hennessey, T. (1996). Beta-sitosterol inhibits HT-29 human colon cancer cell growth and alters membrane lipids. *Anticancer Research, 16*(5A): 2797–2804.

Awad, A., Roy, R., & Fink, C. (2003). Beta-sitosterol, a plant sterol, induces apoptosis and activates key caspases in MDA-MB-231 human breast cancer cells. *Oncology Reports, 10*(2): 497–500.

Ayvaz, G., Balos Törüner, F., Karakoç, A., Yetkin, I., Cakir, N., & Arslan, M. (2002). Acute and chronic effects of different concentrations of free fatty acids on the insulin secreting function of islets. *Diabetes & Metabolism, 28*(6 Pt 2, 3): S7–12; discussion 3S108–112.

Baba, S., Osakabe, N., Kato, Y., Natsume, M., Yasuda, A., Kido, T., Fukuda, K., Muto, Y., & Kondo, K. (2007). Continuous intake of polyphenolic compounds containing cocoa powder reduces LDL oxidative susceptibility and has beneficial effects on plasma HDL-cholesterol concentrations in humans. *American Journal of Clinical Nutrition, 85*(3): 709–717.

Bagdas, D., Cinkilic, N., Ozboluk, H., Ozyigit, M., & Gurun, M. (2012). Antihyperalgesic activity of chlorogenic acid in experimental neuropathic pain. *Journal of Natural Medicine, 67*(4): 698–704.

Baggott, M., Childs, E., Hart, A., de Bruin, E., Palmer, A., Wilkinson, J., & de Wit, H. (2013). Psychopharmacology of theobromine in healthy volunteers. *Psychopharmacology, 228*(1): 109–118.

Bahadorani, S., & Hilliker, A. (2008). Cocoa confers life span extension in Drosophila melanogaster. *Nutrition Research, 28*(6): 377–382.

Baharum, Z., Akim, A., Taufiq-Yap, Y., Hamid, R., & Kasran, R. (2014). In vitro antioxidant and antiproliferative activities of methanolic plant part extracts of Theobroma cacao. *Molecules, 19*(11): 18317–18331.

Balcke, P., Zazgornik, J., Sunder-Plassmann, G., Kiss, A., Hauser, A., Gremmel, F., Derfler, K., Stockenhuber, F., & Schmidt, P. (1989). Transient hyperoxaluria after ingestion of chocolate as a high risk factor for calcium oxalate calculi. *Nephron, 51*(1): 32–34.

Balzer, J., Rassaf, T., Heiss, C., Kleinbongard, P., Lauer, T., Merx, M., Heussen, N., Gross, H., Keen, C., Schroeter, H., & Kelm, M. (2009). Sustained benefits in vascular function through flavanol-containing cocoa in medicated diabetic patients: a double-masked, randomized, controlled trial. *Leukemia Research, 33*(6): 823–828.

Ban, J., Cho, S., Choi, S., Ju, H., Kim, J., Bae, K., Song, K., & Seong, Y. (2008). Neuroprotective effect of *Smilacis chinae* rhizome on NMDA-induced neurotoxicity *in vitro* and focal cerebral ischemia *in vivo*. *Journal of Pharmacological Sciences, 106*(1): 68–77.

Ban, J., Cho, S., Koh, S., Song, K., Bae, K., & Seong, Y. (2006). Protection of amyloid beta protein (25–35)-induced neurotoxicity by methanol extract of *Smilacis chinae* rhizome in cultured rat cortical neurons. *Journal of Ethnopharmacology, 106*(2): 230–237.

Ban, J., Jeon, S., Bae, K., Song, K., & Seong, Y. (2006). Catechin and epicatechin from Smilacis chinae rhizome protect cultured rat cortical neurons against amyloid beta protein (25–35)-induced neurotoxicity through inhibition of cytosolic calcium elevation. *Life Sciences, 79*(24): 2251–2259.

Barabino, S., Rolando, M., Camicione, P., Ravera, G., Zanardi, S., Giuffrida, S., & Calabria, G. (2003). Systemic linoleic and gamma-linoleic acid therapy in dry eye syndrome with an inflammatory component. *Cornea, 22*(2): 97–101.

Barnes, P. (2013). Theophylline: new perspectives for an old drug. *American Journal of Respiratory and Critical Care Medicine, 167*: 813–818.

Baskerville, T., & Douglas, A. (2010). Dopamine and oxytocin interactions underlying behaviors: potential contributions to behavioral disorders. *CNS Neuroscience & Therapeutics, 16*(3): e92–123.

Battaglia, G., Brooks, B., Kulsakdinun, C., & De Souza, E. (1988). Pharmacologic profile of MDMA (3,4-methylenedioxymethamphetamine) at various brain recognition sites. *European Journal of Pharmacology, 149*(1–2): 159–163.

Beltramo, M., & Piomelli, D. (1998). Reply: Trick or treat from food endocannabinoids? *Nature, 396*: 636–637.

Berges, R., Windeler, J., Trampisch, H., & Senge, T. (1995). Randomised, placebo-controlled, double-blind clinical trial of beta-sitosterol in patients with benign prostatic hyperplasia. Beta-sitosterol Study Group. *Lancet, 345*(8964): 1529–1532.

Berry, M. (2004). Mammalian central nervous system trace amines. Pharmacologic amphetamines, physiologic neuromodulators. *Journal of Neurochemistry, 90*(2): 257–271.

Bershad, A., Miller, M., Baggott, M., & de Wit, H. (2016). The effects of MDMA on socio-emotional processing: Does MDMA differ from other stimulants? *Journal of Psychopharmacology, 30*(12): 1248–1258.

Bifulco, M., Capuzno, M., Marasco, M., & Pisanti, S. (2014). The basis of the modern medical hygiene in the medieval Medical School of Salerno. *Journal of Maternal-Fetal & Neonatal Medicine, 28*(14): 1691–1693.

Bingham, S., McNeil, N., & Cummings, J. (1981). The diet of individuals: a study of a randomly-chosen cross section of British adults in a Cambridgeshire village. *British Journal of Nutrition, 45*(1): 23–35.

Bisson, J., Guardia-Llorens, M., Hidalgo, S., Rozan, P., & Messaoudi, M. (2008). Protective effect of Acticoa powder, a cocoa polyphenolic extract, on prostate carcinogenesis in Wistar-Unilever rats. *European Journal of Cancer Prevention, 17*(1): 54–61.

Bisson, J., Hidalgo, S., Rozan, P., & Messaoudi, M. (2007). Therapeutic effect of ACTICOA powder, a cocoa polyphenolic extract, on experimentally induced prostate hyperplasia in Wistar-Unilever rats. *Journal of Medicinal Food, 10*(4): 628–635.

Bjelakovic, G., Nikolova, D., Simonetti, R., & Gluud, C. (2004). Antioxidant supplements for prevention of gastrointestinal cancers: a systematic review and meta-analysis. *Lancet, 364*(9441): 1219–1228.

Bobermin, L., Quincozes-Santos, A., Guerra, M., Leite, M., Souza, D., Gonçalves, C., & Gottfried, C. (2012). Resveratrol prevents ammonia toxicity in astroglial cells. *PLoS One, 7*(12): e52164.

Bode, L., Bunzel, D., Huch, M., Cho, G., Ruhland, D., Bunzel, M., Bub, A., Franz, C., & Kulling, S. (2013). In vivo and in vitro metabolism of trans-resveratrol by human gut microbiota. *American Journal of Clinical Nutrition, 97*(2): 295–309.

Bodor, N., & Farag, H. (1983). Improved delivery through biological membranes. A redox chemical drug-delivery system and its use for brain-specific delivery of phenylethylamine. *Journal of Medicinal Chemistry, 26*(3): 313–318.

Bohon, C., & Stice, E. (2012). Negative affect and neural response to palatable food intake in bulimia nervosa. *Appetite, 58*(3): 964–970.

Bollheimer, L., Volkert, D., Bertsch, T., Sieber, C., & Büttner, R. (2012). [Reversal of aging and lifespan elongation : Current biomedical key publications and the implications for geriatrics.] [Article in German.] *Zeitschrift für Gerontologie und Geriatrie, 46*(6): 563–568.

Bonvehí, J., & Coll, F. (2000). Evaluation of purine alkaloids and diketopiperazines contents in processed cocoa powder. *European Food Research and Technology, 210*: 189–195.

Borah, A., Paul, R., Mazumder, M., & Bhattacharjee, N. (2013). Contribution of β-phenethylamine, a component of chocolate and wine, to dopaminergic neurodegeneration: implications for the pathogenesis of Parkinson's disease. *Neuroscience Bulletin, 29*(5): 655–660.

Borthwick, A., & Da Costa, N. (2017). 2,5-diketopiperazines in food and beverages: Taste and bioactivity. *Critical Reviews in Food Science and Nutrition, 57*(4): 718–742.

Borthwick, A., Liddle, J., Davies, D., Exall, A., Hamlett, C., Hickey, D., Mason, A., Smith, I., Nerozzi, F., Peace, S., Pollard, D., Sollis, S., Allen, M., Woollard, P., Pullen, M., Westfall, T., & Stanislaus, D. (2012). Pyridyl-2,5-diketopiperazines as potent, selective, and orally bioavailable oxytocin antagonists: Synthesis, pharmacokinetics, and in vivo potency. *Journal of Medicinal Chemistry, 55*(2): 783–796.

Bossard, M., & Klinman, J. (1986). Mechanism-based inhibition of dopamine beta-monooxygenase by aldehydes and amides. *Journal of Biological Chemistry, 261*(35): 16421–16427.

Bouic, P., Clark, A., Lamprecht, J., Freestone, M., Pool, E., Liebenberg, R., Kotze, D., & van Jaarsveld, P. (1999). The effects of B-sitosterol (BSS) and B-sitosterol glucoside (BSSG) mixture on selected immune parameters of marathon runners: inhibition of post marathon immune suppression and inflammation. *International Journal of Sports Medicine, 20*(4): 258–262.

Bowen, C., Negus, S., Kelly, M., & Mello, N. (2002). The effects of heroin on prolactin levels in male rhesus monkeys: use of cumulative dosing procedures. *Psychoneuroimmunology, 27*(3): 319–336.

Bray, G., & Bellanger, T. (2006). Epidemiology, trends, and morbidities of obesity and the metabolic syndrome. *Endocrine, 29*(1): 109–117.

Broadley, K., Akhtar, M., Herbert, A., Fehler, M., Jones, E., Davies, W., Kidd, E., & Ford, W. (2009). Effects of dietary amines on the gut and its vasculature. *British Journal of Nutrition, 101*(11): 1645–1652.

Brossmer, R., & Patscheke, H. (1975). 2-phenylethanol and some of its amphiphilic derivatives as inhibitors of platelet aggregation. Structure-activity relationship. *Arzneimittel-Forschung, 25*(11): 1697–1702.

Bucay, J. (2002). Uso tradicional e investigacion cientifica de *Talauma Mexicana* (D.C.) Don., o flor del corazon. *Revista Mexicana de Cardiologia, 13*(1): 31–38.

Buijsse, B., Feskens, E., Kok, F., & Kromhout, D. (2006). Cocoa intake, blood pressure, and cardiovascular mortality. The Zutphen Elderly Study. *Archives of Internal Medicine, 166*(4): 411–417.

Buijsse, B., Weikert, C., Drogan, D., Bergmann, M., & Boeing, H. (2010). Chocolate consumption in relation to blood pressure and risk of cardiovascular disease in German adults. *European Heart Journal, 31*(13): 1616–1623.

Buitrago-Lopez, A., Sanderson, J., Johnson, L., Warnakula, S., Wood, A., Di Angelantonio, E., & Franco, O. (2011). Chocolate consumption and cardiometabolic disorders: systematic review and meta-analysis. *British Medical Journal, 343*: d4488.

Burgos-Morón, E., Calderón-Montaño, J., Orta, M., Pastor, N., Pérez-Guerrero, C., Austin, C., Mateos, S., & López-Lázaro, M. (2012). The coffee constituent chlorogenic acid induces cellular DNA damage and formation of topoisomerase I- and II-DNA complexes in cells. *Journal of Agricultural and Food Chemistry, 60*(30): 7384–7391.

Buydens-Branchey, L., Branchey, M., McMakin, D., & Hibbeln, J. (2003). Polyunsaturated fatty acid status and relapse vulnerability in cocaine addicts. *Psychiatry Research, 120*(1): 29–35.

Calzada, F., Juárez, T., García-Hernández, N., Valdes, M., Ávila, O., epez Mulia, L., & Velázquez, C. (2017). Antiprotozoal, antibacterial and antidiarrheal properties from the flowers of *Chiranthodendron pentadactylon* and isolated flavonoids. *Pharmacognosy Magazine, 13*(50): 240–244.

Calzada, F., Yepez-Mulia, L., & Aguilar, A. (2006). *In vitro* susceptibility of *Entamoeba histolytica* and *Giardia lambla* to plants used in Mexican traditional medicine for the treatment of gastrointestinal disorders. *Journal of Ethnopharmacology, 108*(3): 367–370.

Camps-Bossacoma, M., Pérez-Cano, F., Franch, A., & Castell, M. (2017). Gut microbiota in a rat oral sensitisation model: Effect of a cocoa-enriched diet. *Oxidative Medicine and Cellular Longevity*. Article ID 7417505, 12 pages.

Cano, M., Aguilar, A., & Hernández, J. (2013). Lipid-lowering effect of maize-based traditional Mexican food on a metabolic syndrome model in rats. *Lipids in Health and Disease, 12*(35). Open access online: https://lipidworld.biomedcentral.com/articles/10.1186/1476-511X-12-35 [Accessed 15 February 2019].

Cao, R., Peng, W., Wang, Z., & Xu, A. (2007). Beta-carboline alkaloids: biochemical and pharmacological functions. *Current Medicinal Chemistry, 14*(4): 479–500.

Carlson, H., Wasser, H., & Reidelberger, R. (1985). Beer-induced prolactin secretion: a clinical and laboratory study of the role of salsolinol. *Journal of Clinical Endocrinology and Metabolism, 60*(4): 673–677.

Carnésecchi, S., Schneider, Y., Lazarus, S., Coehlo, D., Gossé, F., & Raul, F. (2002). Flavanols and procyanidins of cocoa and chocolate inhibit growth and polyamine biosynthesis of human colonic cancer cells. *Cancer Letters, 175*(2): 147–155.

Carod-Artal, F. (2015). Hallucinogenic drugs in pre-Colombian Mesomerican cultures. *Neurologia, 30*(1): 42–49.

Carr, J., & Lovering, T. (2000). Mu and delta opioid receptor regulation of pro-opiomelanocortin peptide secretion from the rat neurointermediate pituitary in vitro. *Neuropeptides, 34*(1): 69–75.

Carrera-Lanestosa, A., Moguel-Ordóñez, Y., & Segura-Campos, M. (2017). *Stevia rebaudiana* Bertoni: A natural alternative for treating diseases associated with metabolic syndrome. *Journal of Medicinal Food, 20*(10): 933–943.

Chalyk, N., Klochkov, V., Sommereux, L., Bandaletova, T., Kyle, N., & Petyaev, I. (2018). Continuous dark chocolate consumption affects human facial skin surface by stimulating corneocyte desquamation and promoting bacterial colonization. *Journal of Clinical and Aesthetic Dermatology, 11*(9): 37–41.

Chatzitoffis, A., Nordström, P., Hellström, C., Arver, S., Åsberg, M., & Jokinen, J. (2013). CSF 5-HIAA, cortisol and DHEAS levels in suicide attempters. *European Neuropsychopharmacology, 23*(10): 1280–1287.

Check, J., Katsoff, D., Kaplan, H., Liss, J., & Boimel, P. (2008). A disorder of sympathomimetic amines leading to increased vascular permeability may be the etiologic factor in various treatment refractory health problems in women. *Medical Hypotheses, 70*(3): 671–677.

Chen, C., Wu, H., Chao, W., & Lee, C. (2013). Review on pharmacological activities of liriodenine. *African Journal of Pharmacy and Pharmacology, 7*(18): 1067–1070.

Chen, W., Wang, D., Wang, L., Bei, D., Wang, J., See, W., Mallery, S., Stoner, G., & Liu, Z. (2012). Pharmacokinetics of protocatechuic acid in mouse and its quantification in human plasma using LC-tandem mass spectrometry. *Journal of Chromatography B. Analytical Technologies in the Biomedical and Life Sciences, 908*: 39–44.

Cho, E., Lee, K., & Lee, H. (2008). Cocoa procyanidins protect PC12 cells from hydrogen-peroxide-induced apoptosis by inhibiting activation of p38 MAPK and JNK. *Mutation Research, 640*(1–2): 123–130.

Cho, H., Kang, H., Kim, Y., Lee, D., Kwon, H., Kim, Y., & Park, H. (2012). Inhibition of platelet aggregation by chlorogenic acid via cAMP and cGMP-dependent manner. *Blood Coagulation & Fibrinolysis, 23*(7): 629–635.

Choi, S., & Diehl, A. (2008). Hepatic triglyceride synthesis and non-alcoholic fatty liver disease. *Current Opinion in Lipidology, 19*(3): 295–300.

Chopan, M., & Littenberg, B. (2017). The association of hot red chili pepper consumption and mortality: A large population-based cohort study. *PLoS One, 12*(1): e0169876.

Ciftci, O., Disli, O., & Timurkaan, N. (2012). Protective effects of protocatechuic acid on TCDD-induced oxidative and histopathological damage in the heart tissue of rats. *Toxicology and Industrial Health.* Apr 10. [Epub ahead of print.] https://journals.sagepub.com/doi/abs/10.1177/0748233712442735 [Accessed 17 March 2019].

Cimini, A., Gentile, R., D'Angelo, B., Benedetti, E., Cristiano, L., Avantaggiati, M., Giordano, A., Ferri, C., & Desideri, G. (2013). Cocoa powder triggers neuroprotective and preventive effects in a human Alzheimer's disease model by modulating BDNF signaling pathway. *Journal of Cellular Biochemistry, 114*(10): 2209–2220.

Cinkilic, N., Cetintas, S., Zorlu, T., Vatan, O., Yilmaz, D., Cavas, T., Tunc, S., Ozkan, L., & Bilaloglu, R. (2013). Radioprotection by two phenolic compounds: Chlorogenic and quinic acid, on X-ray induced DNA damage in human blood lymphocytes in vitro. *Food and Chemical Toxicology, 53*: 359–363.

Clandinin, M., Cook, S., Konard, S., & French, M. (2000). The effect of palmitic acid on lipoprotein cholesterol levels. *International Journal of Food Sciences and Nutrition, 51*: S61–71.

Clark, R., & Lee, S. (2016). Anticancer properties of capsaicin against human cancer. *Anticancer Research, 36*(3): 837–843.

Coban, S., Yildiz, F., Terzi, A., Al, B., Ozgor, D., Ara, C., Polat, A., & Esrefoglu, M. (2010). The effect of caffeic acid phenethyl ester (CAPE) against cholestatic liver injury in rats. *Journal of Surgical Research, 159*(2): 674–679.

Colantuoni, C., Schwenker, J., McCarthy, J., Rada, P., Ladenheim, B., Cadet, J.-L., Schwartz, J., Moran, H., & Hoebel, G. (2001). Excessive sugar intake alters binding to dopamine and mu-opioid receptors in the brain. *Neuroreport: 'Motivation, Emotion, Feeding, Drinking', 12*(16): 3549–3552.

Collins, J., Prohaska, J., & Knutson, M. (2010). Metabolic crossroads of iron and copper. *Nutrition Review, 68*(3):133–147.

Copeland, R., Legget, Y., Kanaan, Y., Taylor, R., & Tizabi, Y. (2005). Neuroprotective effects of nicotine against salsolinol-induced cytotoxicity: implications for Parkinson's disease. *Neurotoxicity Research, 8*(3–4): 289–293.

Copetti, M., Iamanaka, B., Mororó, R., Pereira, J., Frisvad, J., & Taniwaki, M. (2012). The effect of cocoa fermentation and weak organic acids on growth and ochratoxin A production by Aspergillus species. *International Journal of Food and Microbiology, 155*(3): 158–164.

Cordero, M., Alcocer-Gómez, E., Cano-García, F., Sánchez-Domínguez, B., Fernández-Riejo, P., Moreno Fernández, A., Fernández-Rodríguez, A., & De Miguel, M. (2014). Clinical symptoms in fibromyalgia are associated to overweight and lipid profile. *Rheumatology International, 34*(3): 419–422.

Cornacchia, C., Cacciatore, I., Baldassarre, L., Mollica, A., Feliciani, F., & Pinnen F. (2012). 2,5-diketopiperazines as neuroprotective agents. *Mini Reviews in Medicinal Chemistry, 12*(1): 2–12.

Cortés, P. (2004). La magia de la palabra en el ritual de los bacabes. *Arqueologia Mexicana, 12*(69): 34–39.

Costa de Miranda, R., Paiva, E., Cadena, S., Brandt, A., & Vilela, R. (2016). Polyphenol-rich foods alleviate pain and ameliorate quality of life in fibromyalgic women. *International Journal for Vitamin and Nutrition Research, 21*: 1–10.

Crichton, G., Elias, M., & Alkerwi, A. (2016). Chocolate intake is associated with better cognitive function: The Maine-Syracuse Longitudinal Study. *Appetite, 100*: 126–132.

Curran, H., Nutt, D., & deWit, H. (2018). Psychedelics and related drugs: therapeutic possibilities, mechanisms and regulation. *Psychopharmacology, 235*(2): 373–375.

Dahiya, S., Karpe, R., Hegde, A., & Sharma, R. (2005). Lead, cadmium and nickel in chocolates and candies from suburban areas of Mumbai, India. *Journal of Food Composition and Analysis, 18*(6): 517–522.

Das, B., Ferdous, T., Mahmood, Q., Hannan, J., Bhattacharjee, R., & Das, B. K. (2013). Antinociceptive and anti-inflammatory activity of the bark extract of *Plumeria rubra* on laboratory animals. *European Journal of Medicinal Plants, 3*(1): 114–126.

Davison, K., Coates, M., Buckley, J., & Howe, P. (2008). Effect of cocoa flavanols and exercise on cardiometabolic risk factors in overweight and obese subjects. *International Journal of Obesity, 32*(8): 1289–1296.

Davinelli, S., Corbi, G., Righetti, S., Sears, B., Olarte, H., Grassi, D., & Scapagnini, G. (2018). Cardio-protection by cocoa polyphenols and ω-3 fatty acids: A disease-prevention perspective on aging-associated cardiovascular risk. *Journal of Medicinal Food, 21*(10): 1060–1069.

Dean, R., & Lue, T. (2005). Physiology of penile erection and pathophysiology of erectile dysfunction. *Urologic Clinics of North America, 32*(4): 379–v.

Ding, E., Hutfless, S., Ding, X., & Girotra, S. (2006). Chocolate and prevention of cardiovascular disease: a systematic review. *Nutrition & Metabolism (London), 3*: 2.

Djoussé, L., Hopkins, P., Arnett, D., Pankow, J., Borecki, I., North, K., & Ellison, R. (2010). Chocolate consumption is inversely associated with calcified atherosclerotic plaque in the coronary arteries: the NHLBI Family Heart Study. *Indian Journal of Pharmacology, 42*(6): 334–337.

Djoussé, L., Hopkins, P., North, K., Pankow, J., Arnett, D., & Ellison, R. (September 2010). Chocolate consumption is inversely associated with prevalent coronary heart disease: the National Heart, Lung, and Blood Institute Family Heart Study. *Clinical Nutrition, 30*(2): 182–187.

Drago, F. (1990). Behavioural effects of prolactin. *Current Topics in Neuroendocrinology, 10*: 263–289.

Drake, R., Felbaum, D., Huntley, C., Reed, A., Matthews, L., & Raudenbush, B. (2007). Effects of chocolate consumption on enhancing cognitive performance. *Appetite, 49*(1): 288.

Drewnowski, A. (1992). Food preferences and the opioid peptide system. *Trends in Food Science and Technology, 3*: 97–99.

Drewnowski, A., Krahn, D., Demitrack, M., Nairn, K., & Gosnell, B. (1992). Taste responses and preferences for sweet high-fat foods: evidence for opioid involvement. *Physiology & Behaviour, 51*(2): 371–379.

Drexler, S., Merz, C., Hamacher-Dang, T., Tegenthoff, M., & Wolf, O. (2015). Effects of cortisol on reconsolidation of reactivated fear memories. *Neuropsychopharmacology, 40*: 3036–3043.

Dubuis, E., Wortley, M., Grace, M., Maher, S., Adcock, J., Birrell, M., & Belvisi, M. (2014). Theophylline inhibits the cough reflex through a novel mechanism of action. *Journal of Allergy and Clinical Immunology, S0091-6749, 13*: 1781–1788.

Dzib-Guerra, W., Escalante-Erosa, F., García-Sosa, K., Derbré, S., Blanchard, P., Richomme, P., & Peña-Rodríguez, L. (2016). Anti-advanced glycation end-product and free radical scavenging activity of plants from the Yucatecan flora. *Pharmacognosy Research, 8*(4): 276–280.

Eby, G., & Eby, K. (2010). Magnesium for treatment-resistant depression: a review and hypothesis. *Medical Hypotheses, 74*(4): 649–660.

Edmond, J. (2001). Essential polyunsaturated fatty acids and the barrier to the brain: the components of a model for transport. *Journal of Molecular Neuroscience, 16*(2–3): 181–193; discussion: 215–221.

Elwers, S., Zambrano, A., Rohsius, C., & Lieberei, R. (2009). Differences between the content of phenolic compounds in Criollo, Forastero and Trinitario cocoa seed (*Theobroma cacao* L.). *European Food Research and Technology, 229*: 937–948.

van Elzakker, M., Dahlgren, M., Davis, F., Dubois, S., & Shin, L. (2014). From Pavlov to PTSD: The extinction of conditioned fear in rodents, humans, and anxiety disorders. *Neurobiology of Learning and Memory, 113*: 3–18.

Embi, A., Scherlag, B., Embi, P., Menes, M., & Po, S. (2012). Targeted cellular ionic calcium chelation by oxalates: Implications for the treatment of tumour cells. *Cancer Cell International, 12*(1): 51.

Engler, M., Engler, M., Chen, C., Malloy, M., Browne, A., Chiu, E., Kwak, H., Milbury, P., Paul, S., Blumberg, J., & Mietus-Snyder, M. (2004). Flavonoid-rich dark chocolate improves endothelial function and increases plasma epicatechin concentrations in healthy adults. *Journal of the American College of Nutrition, 23*(3): 197–204.

Epel, E., Blackburn, E., Lin, J., Dhabhar, F., Adler, N., Morrow, J., & Cawthorn, R. (2004). Accelerated telomere shortening in response to life stress. *Proceedings of the National Academy of Sciences of the United States of America, 73*(1): 16–22.

Erkkola, M., Nwaru, B., Kaila, M., Kronberg-Kippilä, C., Ilonen, J., Simell, O., Veijola, R., Knip, M., & Virtanen, S. (2012). Risk of asthma and allergic outcomes in the offspring in relation to maternal food consumption during pregnancy: a Finnish birth cohort study. *Pediatrica Allergy and Immunology, 23*(2): 186–194.

Ertel, S. (2009). Appraisal of Shawn Carlson's Renowned Astrology Tests. *Journal of Scientific Exploration, 23*(2): 125–137.

Esch, T., & Stefano, G. (2005). The Neurobiology of Love. *Neuroendocrinology Letters, 26*(3): 175–190.

Eskandari, N., Bastan, R., & Peachell, P. (2013). Regulation of human skin mast cell histamine release by PDE inhibitors. *Allergologia et Immunopathologia (Madr)*. Pt.ii: S0301-0546, *13*: 240–241.

Espinoza, J., Takami, A., Trung, L., Kato, S., & Nakao, S. (2012). Resveratrol prevents EBV transformation and inhibits the outgrowth of EBV-immortalized human B cells. *PLoS One, 7*(12): e51306.

Estrada-Reyes, R., Martinez-Laurrabaquio, A., Suarez, D., & Araujo-Escalona, A. (2013). Neuropharmacological studies of *Piper auritum* Kunth (Piperaceae): antinociceptive and anxiolytic-like effects. *Journal of Medicinal Plants Research, 7*(23): 1718–1729.

Evrensel, A., & Ceylan, M. (2015). The gut-brain axis: the missing link in depression. *Clinical Psychopharmacology and Neuroscience, 13*(3): 239–244.

Exton, M., Bindert, A., Krüger, T., Scheller, F., Hartmann, U., & Schedlowski, M. (1999). Cardiovascular and endocrine alterations after masturbation-induced orgasm in women. *Psychosomatic Medicine, 61*(3): 280–289.

Ezekiel, J., & Oluwole, O. (2014). Effects of capsaicin on coagulation: Will this be the new blood thinner? *Clinical Medicine Research, 3*(5): 145–149.

Fagetti, A. (2017). Periplos nocturnos: las plantas sagradas de los mazatecos. *Plantas Sagradas. Artes de Mexico, 127*: 28–36.

Falade, O., Otemuyiwa, I., Oladipo, A., Oyedapo, O., Akinpelu, B., & Adewusi, S. (2005). The chemical composition and membrane stability activity of some herbs used in local therapy for anemia. *Journal of Ethnopharmacology, 31; 102*(1): 15–22.

Fallarini, S., Miglio, G., Paoletti, T., Minassi, A., Amoruso, A., Bardelli, C., Brunelleschi, S., & Lombardi, G. (2009). Clovamide and rosmarinic acid induce neuroprotective effects in in vtiro models of neuronal death. *British Journal of Pharmacology, 157*(6): 1072–1084.

Fan, L., Wang, K., Cheng, B., Wang, C., & Dang, X. (2006). Anti-apoptotic and neuroprotective effects of tetramethylpyrazine following spinal cord ischemia in rabbits. *BMC Neuroscience, 7*(1): 48.

Farah, D., Zaibunnisa, A., & Misnawi, J. (2012). Optimization of cocoa beans roasting process using Response Surface Methodology based on concentration of pyrazine and acrylamide. *International Food Research Journal, 19*(4): 1355–1359.

Farah, I., Lewis, V., Ayensu, W., & Cameron, J. (2012). Therapeutic implications of the Warburg effect: role of oxalates and acetates on the differential survival of mrc-5 and a549 cell lines. *Biomedical Sciences Instrumentation, 48*: 119–125.

Farhat, G., Drummond, S., Fyfe, L., & Al-Dujalili, E. (2014). Dark chocolate: an obesity paradox or a culprit for weight gain? *Phytotherapy Research, 28*: 791–797.

Faridi, Z., Njivke, V., Dutta, S., Ali, A., & Katz, D. (2008). Acute dark chocolate and cocoa ingestion and endothelial function: a randomized controlled crossover trial. *American Journal of Clinical Nutrition, 88*(1): 58–56.

Farouque, H., Leung, M., Hope, S., Baldi, M., Schechter, C., Cameron, J., & Meredith, I. (2006). Acute and chronic effects of flavanol-rich cocoa on vascular function in subjects with coronary artery disease: a randomized double-blind placebo-controlled study. *Clinical Science (London)*, *111*(1): 71–80.

di Feliceantonio, A., Mabrouk, O., Kennedy, R., & Berridge, K. (2012). Enkephalin surges in dorsal neostriatum as a signal to eat. *Current Biology, 22*(20): 1918–1924.

Felitti, V., Anda, R., Nordenberg, D., Williamson, D., Spitz, A., Edwards, V., Koss, M., & Marks, J. (1998). Relationship of childhood abuse and household dysfunction to many of the leading causes of death in adults. *American Journal of Preventive Medicine, 14*(4): 245–258.

Fernandez Garcia, A., Cabal, C., Losada, J., Alvarez, E., Soler, C., & Otero, J. (2005). *In vivo* action of vanillin on delay time determined by magnetic relaxation. *Hemoglobin, 29*(3): 181–187.

Ferreira, J., Sousa, D., Dantas, M., Fonseca, S., Menezes, D., Martins, A., & deQueiroz, M. (2013). Effects of Bixa orellana L. seeds on hyperlipidemia. *Phytotherapy Research, 27*(1): 144–147.

Firth, A., & Smith, W. (1964). The anti-anaphylactic activity of theophylline and some related xanthine derivatives. *Journal of Pharmacy and Pharmacology, 16*(3): 183–188.

Fisher, H. (1998). Lust, attraction and attachment in mammalian reproduction. *Human Nature, 9*(1): 23–52.

Fisher, H., Aron, A., & Brown, L. (2005). Romantic love: an fMRI study of a neural mechanism for mate choice. *Journal of Comparative Neurology, 493*(1): 58–62.

Fisher, H., Aron, A., Mashek, D., Li, H., & Brown, L. (2002). Defining the brain systems of lust, romantic attraction, and attachment. *Archives of Sexual Behaviour, 31*(5): 413–419.

Fisher, N., & Hollenberg, N. (2006). Aging and vascular responses to flavanol-rich cocoa. *Journal of Hypertension, 24*(8): 1575–1580.

Fisher, N., Hughes, M., Gerhard-Herman, M., & Hollenberg, N. (2003). Flavanol-rich cocoa induces nitric-oxide-dependent vasodilation in healthy humans. *Journal of Hypertension, 21*(12): 2281–2286.

Flammer, A., Hermann, F., Sudano, I., Spieker, L., Hermann, M., Cooper, K., Serafini, M., Lüscher, T., Ruschitzka, F., Noll, G., & Corti, R. (2007). Dark chocolate improves coronary vasomotion and reduces platelet reactivity. *Circulation, 116*(21): 2376–2382.

Fontaine, V., Monteiro, E., Brazhnikova, E., Lesage, L., Balducci, C., Guibout, L., Feraille, L., Elena, P., Sahel, J., Veillet, S., & Lafont, R. (2016). Norbixin protects retinal pigmented epithelium cells and photoreceptors against A2E-mediated phototoxicity *in vitro* and *in vivo*. *PLoS One, 11*(12): e0167793.

Forsleff, L., Schauss, A., Bier, I., & Stuart, S. (1999). Evidence of functional zinc deficiency in Parkinson's disease. *Journal of Alternative and Complementary Medicine, 5*(1): 57–64.

Fraga, C., Actis-Goretta, L., Ottaviani, J., Carrasquedo, F., Lotito, S., Lazarus, S., Schmitz, H., & Keen, C. (2005). Regular consumption of a flavanol-rich chocolate can improve oxidant stress in young soccer players. *Clinical and Developmental Immunology, 12*(1): 11–17.

Francis, S., Head, K., Morris, P., & Macdonald, I. (2006). The effect of flavanol-rich cocoa on the fMRI response to a cognitive task in healthy young people. *Journal of Cardiovascular Pharmacology, 47*, Suppl. 2: S215–220.

Fredholm, B., Bättig, K., Holmén, J., Nehlig, A., & Zvartau, E. (1999). Actions of caffeine in the brain with special reference to factors that contribute to its widespread use. *Pharmacological Reviews, 51*(1): 83–133.

Fricker, G., Kromp, T., Wendel, A., Blume, A., Zirkel, J., Rebmann, H., Setzer, C., Quinkert, R.-O., Martin, F., & Müller-Goymann, C. (2010). Phospholipids and lipid-based formulations in oral drug delivery. *Pharmaceutical Research, 27*(8): 1469–1486.

Fuhr, U., Boettcher, M., Kinzig-Schippers, M., Weyer, A., Jetter, A., Lazar, A., Taubert, D., Tomalik-Scharte, D., Pournara, P., Jakob, V., Harlfinger, S., Klaassen, T., Berkessel, A., Angerer, J., Sörgel, F., & Schömig, E. (2006). Toxicokinetics of acrylamide in humans after ingestion of a defined dose in a test meal to improve risk assessment for acrylamide carcinogenicity. *Cancer Epidemiology Biomarkers & Prevention, 15*(2): 266–271.

Fukushima, T., Tan, X., Luo, Y., & Kanda, H. (2011). Serum vitamins and heavy metals in blood and urine, and the correlations among them in Parkinson's disease patients in China. *Neuroepidemiology, 36*(4): 240–244.

Fulton, J., Plewig, G., & Kligman, A. (1969). Effect of chocolate on acne vulgaris. *Journal of the American Medical Association, 210*(11): 2071–2074.

Fung, V., Cameron, T., Hughes, T., Kirby, P., & Dunkel, V. (1988). Mutagenic activity of some coffee flavor ingredients. *Mutation Research, 204*(2): 219–228.

Fuxe, K., Grobecker, H., & Jonsson, J. (1968). The effect of β-phenylethylamine on central and peripheral monoamine-containing neurons. *European Journal of Pharmacology, 2*(3): 202–207.

Galland, L. (2014). The gut microbiome and the brain. *Journal of Medicinal Food, 17*(12): 1261–1272.

Galleano, M., Oteiza, P., & Fraga, C. (2009). Cocoa, chocolate and cardiovascular disease. *Journal of Cardiovascular Pharmacology, 54*(6): 483–490.

Gambini, J., López-Grueso, R., Olaso-González, G., Inglés, M., Abdelazid, K., El Alami, M., Bonet-Costa, V., Borrás, C., & Viña, J. (2013). Resveratrol: Distribución, propeiedades y perspectivas. *Revista Española de Geriatria Gerontologia, 48*(2): 79–88.

de la Garza, M. (2017). Umbrales hacia "otros mundos": Plantas sagradas nahuas y mayas. *Plantas Sagradas. Artes de Mexico, 127*: 16–27. Mexico City: Artes de Mexico y del Mundo, S.A. de C.V.

Geracitano, R., Federici, M., Prisco, S., Bernardi, G., & Mercuri, N. (2004). Inhibitory effects of trace amines on rat midbrain dopaminergic neurons. *Neuropharmacology, 46*(6): 807–814.

Giannandrea, F. (2009). Correlation analysis of cocoa consumption data with worldwide incidence rates of testicular cancer and hypospadias. *International Journal of Environmental Research and Public Health, 6*(2): 568–578.

Girish, K., Kemparaju, K., Nagaraju, S., & Vishwanath, B. (2009). Hyaluronidase inhibitors: a biological and therapeutic perspective. *Current Medicinal Chemistry, 16*(18): 2261–2288.

Giuliano, C., Robbins, T., Nathan, P., Bullmore, E., & Everitt, B. (2012). Inhibition of opioid transmission at the μ-opioid receptor prevents both food seeking and binge-like eating. *Neuropsychopharmacology, 37*(12): 2643–2652.

Glockner, J. (2017). Crónica de una Incomprensión. *Artes de Mexico (Plantas Sagradas), 127*: 8–15.

Gluck, M., Geliebter, A., Hung, J., & Yahav, E. (2004). Cortisol, hunger, and desire to binge eat following a cold stress test in obese women with binge eating disorder. *Psychosomatic Medicine, 66*(6): 876–881.

Goadsby, P. (2012). Pathophysiology of migraine. *Annals of Indian Academy of Neurology, 15*(Suppl. 1): S15–S22.

Golf, S., Bender, S., & Grüttner, J. (1998). On the significance of magnesium in extreme physical stress. *Cardiovascular Drugs and Therapy, 12*(2) (Suppl.): 197–202.

Gomez-Zorita, S., Tréguer, K., Mercader, J., & Carpéné, C. (2013). Resveratrol directly affects in vitro lipolysis and glucose transport in human fat cells. *Journal of Physiology and Biochemistry, 69*(3): 585–593.

Gordon, I., Zagoory-Sharon, O., Leckman, J., & Feldman, R. (2010). Prolactin, oxytocin, and the development of paternal behaviour across the first six months of fatherhood. *Hormones and Behaviour, 58*(3): 513–518.

de Gottardi, A., Berzigotti, A., Seijo, S., D'Amico, M., Thormann, W., Abraldes, J., García-Pagán, J., & Bosch, J. (2012). Postprandial effects of dark chocolate on portal hypertension in patients with cirrhosis: results of a phase 2, double-blind, randomized controlled trial. *American Journal of Clinical Nutrition*, 96(3): 584–590.

Goya, L., Martín, M., Sarriá, B., Ramos, S., Mateos, R., & Bravo, L. (2016). Effect of cocoa and its flavonoids on biomarkers of inflammation: Studies of cell culture, animals and humans. *Nutrients*, 8(4): 212.

Graeff, F., Netto, C., & Zangrossi, H. (1998). The elevated T-maze as an experimental model of anxiety. *Neuroscience & Biobehavioural Reviews*, 23(2): 237–246.

Grassi, D., Lippi, C., Necozione, S., Desideri, G., & Ferri, C. (2005). Short-term administration of dark chocolate is followed by a significant increase in insulin sensitivity and a decrease in blood pressure in healthy persons. *American Journal of Clinical Nutrition*, 81(3): 611–614.

Grassi, D., Lippi, C., Necozione, S., Desideri, G., & Ferri, C. (2008). Blood pressure is reduced and insulin sensitivity increased in glucose-intolerant, hypertensive subjects after 15 days of consuming high-polyphenol dark chocolate. *Journal of Nutrition*, 139(9): 1671–1676.

Grassi, D., Socci. V., Tempesta, D., Ferri, C., De Gennaro, L., Desideri, G., & Ferrara, M. (2016). Flavanol-rich chocolate acutely improves arterial function and working memory performance counteracting the effects of sleep deprivation in healthy individuals. *Journal of Hypertension*, 34(7): 1298–1308.

Grassin-Delyle, S., Abrial, C., Fayad-Kobeissi, S., Brollo, M., Faisy, C., Alvarez, J., Naline, E., & Devillier, P. (2013). The expression and relaxant effect of bitter taste receptors in human bronchi. *Respiratory Research*, 22(14): 134.

Graulich, M. (2004). Moctezuma II y el fin del imperio azteca. *Arqueología Mexicana*, 12(69): 70–75.

Greger, J., & Powers, C. (1992). Assessment of exposure to parenteral and oral aluminum with and without citrate using a desferrioxamine test in rats. *Toxicology*, 76(2): 119–132.

Gröber, U., Schmidt, J., & Kisters, K. (2015). Magnesium in prevention and therapy. *Nutrients*, 7(9): 8199–8226.

Grofe, M. (2007). The recipe for rebirth: Cacao as fish in the mythology and symbolism of the ancient Maya. [Thesis: Department of Native American Studies, University of California at Davis.] www.famsi.org/research/grofe/GrofeRecipeForRebirth.pdf [Accessed 4 April 2019].

Grome, J., & Stefanovich, V. (1986). Differential effects of methylxanthines on local cerebral blood flow and glucose utilization in the conscious rat. *Naunyn-Schmiedebergs Archives of Pharmacology*, 333(2): 172–177.

Gu, L., House, S., Wu, X., Ou, B., & Prior, R. (2006). Procyanidin and catechin contents and antioxidant capacity of cocoa and chocolate products. *Journal of Agricultural and Food Chemistry*, 54(11): 4057–4061.

Guan, S., Zhang, X., Ge, D., Liu, T., Ma, X., & Cui, Z. (2011). Protocatechuic acid promotes the neuronal differentiation and facilitates survival of phenotypes differentiated from cultured neural stem and progenitor cells. *European Journal of Pharmacology*, 670(2–3): 471–478.

Gutierrez, R., Diaz, S., Reyes, I., & Gonzalez, A. (2010). Anti-glycation effect of spices and chiles used in traditional Mexican cuisine. *Journal of Natural Products*, 3: 95–102.

Hadaway, P., Alexander, B., Coambs, R., & Beyerstein, B. (1979). The effect of housing and gender on preference for morphine-sucrose solutions in rats. *Psychopharmacology (Berlin)*, 66(1): 87–91.

Hamed, M., Gambert, S., Bliden, K., Bailon, O., Singla, A., Antonino, M., Hamed, F., Tantry, U., & Gurbel, P. (2008). Dark chocolate effect on platelet activity, C-reactive protein and lipid profile: a pilot study. *Southern Medical Journal*, 101(12): 1203–1208.

Hanhineva, K., Törrönen, R., Bondia-Pons, I., Pekkinen, J., Kolehmainen, M., Mykkänen, H., & Poutanen, K. (2010). Impact of dietary polyphenols on carbohydrate metabolism. *Internationl Journal of Molecular Sciences, 11*(4): 1365–1402.

Hanington, E. (1967). Preliminary report on tyramine headache. *British Medical Journal, 2*(5551): 550–551.

Hänsel, R., & Leuschke, A. (1975). Aporphine-type alkaloids from *Piper auritum. Lloydia, 38*(6): 529–530.

Hardwick, L., Jones, M., Brautbar, N., & Lee, D. (1991). Magnesium absorption: Mechanisms and the influence of vitamin D, calcium and phosphate. *Journal of Nutrition, 121*(1): 13–23.

Hardy, S., Langelier, Y., & Prentki, M. (2000). Oleate activates phosphatidylinositol 3-kinase and promotes proliferation and reduces apoptosis of MDA-MB-231 breast cancer cells, whereas palmitate has opposite effects. *Cancer Research, 60*(22): 6353–6358.

Hashizume, T., Onodera, Y., Shida, R., Isobe, E., Suzuki, S., Sawai, K., Kasuya, E., & Nagy, G. (2009). Characteristics of prolactin-releasing response to salsolinol (SAL) and thyrotropin-releasing hormone (TRH) in ruminants. *Domestic Animal Endocrinology, 36*(2): 99–104.

Haskell, C., Dodd, F., Wightman, E., & Kennedy, D. (2013). Behavioural effects of compounds co-consumed in dietary forms of caffeinated plants. *Nutrition Research Reviews, 26*(1): 49–70.

Hawkes, C. (1992). Endorphins: the basis of pleasure? *Journal of Neurology, Neurosurgery & Psychiatry, 55*(4): 247–250.

Hays-Gilpin, K., & Hill, J. (1999). The flower world in material culture: An iconographic complex in the Southwest and Mesoamerica. *Journal of Anthropological Research, 55*(1): 1–37.

Heinrich, U., Neukam, K., Tronnier, H., Sies, H., & Stahl, W. (2006). Long-term ingestion of high flavanol cocoa provides photoprotection against UV-induced erythema and improves skin condition in women. *Journal of Nutrition, 136*(6): 1565–1569.

Heinzen, E., Booth, R., & Pollack, G. (2005). Neuronal nitric oxide modulates morphine antinociceptive tolerance by enhancing constitutive activity of the mu-opioid receptor. *Biochemical Pharmacology, 69*(4): 679–688.

Heiss, C., Kleinbongard, P., Dejam, A., Perré, S., Schroeter, H., Sies, H., & Kelm, M. (2005). Acute consumption of flavanol-rich cocoa and the reversal of endothelial dysfunction in smokers. *Journal of the American College of Cardiology, 46*(7): 1276–1283.

Hensel, A., Deters, A., Müller, G., Stark, T., Wittschier, N., & Hofmann, T. (2007). Occurrence of N-phenylpropenoyl-L-amino acid amides in different herbal drugs and their influence on human keratinocytes, on human liver cells and on adhesion of Helicobacter pylori to the human stomach. *Planta Medica, 73*(2): 142–150.

Heo, H., & Lee, C. (2005). Epicatechin and catechin in cocoa inhibit amyloid beta protein induced apoptosis. *Journal of Agricultural and Food Chemistry, 53*(5): 1445–1448.

Heptinstall, S., May, J., Fox, S., Kwik-Uribe, C., & Zhao, L. (2006). Cocoa flavanols and platelet and leukocyte function: recent in vitro and ex vivo studies in healthy adults. *Journal of Cardiovascular Pharmacology, 47*, Suppl. 2: S197–205; discussion: S206–209.

Herraiz, T. (2000). Tetrahydro-β-carbolines, potential neuroactive alkaloids, in chocolate and cocoa. *Journal of Agricultural and Food Chemistry, 48*(10): 4900–4904.

Herraiz, T., & Galisteo, J. (2003). Tetrahydro-beta-carboline alkaloids occur in fruits and fruit juices. Activity as antioxidants and radical scevengers. *Journal of Agricultural and Food Chemistry, 51*(24): 7156–7161.

Herrera, J., Arevalo-Herrera, M., & Herrera, S. (1998). Prevention of preeclampsia by linoleic acid and calcium supplementation: a randomized controlled trial. *Obstetrics & Gynecology, 91*(4): 585–590.

Hervera, A., Negrete, R., Leánez, S., Martín-Campos, J., & Pol, O. (2011). Peripheral effects of morphine and expression of μ-opioid receptors in the dorsal root ganglia during neuropathic pain: nitric oxide signalling. *Molecular Pain, 7*: 25.

Hetherington, M., & MacDiarmid, J. (1993). "Chocolate addiction": a preliminary study of its description and its relationship to problem eating. *Appetite, 21*(3): 233–246.

Heyden, D. (1975). An interpretation of the cave underneath the Pyramid of the Sun in Teotihuacan, Mexico. *American Antiquity, 40*(2): 131–147.

Hipólito, L., Martí-Prats, L., Sánchez-Catalán, M., Polache, A., & Granero, L. (2011). Induction of conditioned place preference and dopamine release by salsolinol in posterior VTA of rats: Involvement of μ-opioid receptors. *Neurochemistry International, 59*(5): 559–562.

Hirano, R., Osakabe, N., Iwamoto, A., Matsumoto, A., Natsume, M., Takizawa, T., Igarashi, O., Itakura, H., & Kondo, K. (2000). Antioxidant effects of polyphenols in chocolate on low-density lipoprotein both in vitro and ex vivo. *Journal of Nutritional Science and Vitaminology (Tokyo), 46*(4): 199–204.

Ho, H., Chang, C., Ho, W., Liao, S., Lin, W., & Wang, C. (2013). Gallic acid inhibits gastric cancer cells metastasis and invasive growth via increased expression of RhoB, downregulation of AKT/small GTPase signals and inhibition of NF-κB activity. *Toxicology and Applied Pharmacology, 266*(1): 76–85.

Ho, K., Yazan, L., Ismail, N., & Ismail, M. (2011). Toxicology study of vanillin on rats via oral and intra-peritoneal administration. *Food and Chemical Toxicology, 49*(1): 25–30.

Hodgson, J., Devine, A., Burke, V., Dick, I., & Prince, R. (2008). Chocolate consumption and bone density in older women. *American Journal of Clinical Nutrition, 87*(1): 175–180.

Hoenicke, K., & Gatermann, R. (2005). Studies on the stability of acrylamide in food during storage. *Journal of AOAC International, 88*(1): 268–273.

Hogervorst, J., Schouten, L., Konings, E., Goldbohm, R., & Van Den Brandt, P. (2007). A prospective study of dietary acrylamide intake and the risk of endometrial, ovarian and breast cancer. *Cancer Epidemiology Biomarkers & Prevention, 16*(11): 2304–2313.

Hollenberg, K. (2006). Vascular action of cocoa flavanols in humans: the roots of the story. *Journal of Cardiovascular Pharmacology, 47*, Suppl. 2: S99–102; discussion: S119–121.

Hollenberg, N., Fisher, N., & McCullough, M. (2009). Flavanols, the Kuna, cocoa consumption, and nitric oxide. *Journal of the American Society of Hypertension, 3*(2): 10.1016.

Holt, R., Lazarus, S., Sullards, M., Zhu, Q., Schramm, D., Hammerstone, J., Fraga, C., Schmitz, H., & Keen, C. (2002). Procyanidin dimer B2 [epicatechin-(4beta-8)-epicatechin] in human plasma after the consumption of a flavanol-rich cocoa. *American Journal of Clinical Nutrition, 76*(4): 798–804.

Holzmann, I., Cattani, D., Corso, M., Perondi, D., Zanella, S., Burger, C., Klein Júnior, L., Filho, V., Cruz, S., Torres, M., Cáceres, A., & de Souza, M. (2014). Psychopharmacological profile of hydroalcoholic extract and P-hydroxybenzoic acid obtained from *Bourreria huanita* (Boraginaceae) in mice. *Pharmacology & Pharmacy, 5*(11): 983–995.

Hooper, L., Kay, C., Abdelhamid, A., Kroon, P., Cohn, J., Rimm, E., & Cassidy, A. (2012). Effects of chocolate, cocoa, and flavan-3-ols on cardiovascular health: a systematic review and meta-analysis of randomized trials. *American Journal of Clinical Nutrition, 95*(3): 740–751.

Horman, I., Brambilla, E., & Stalder, R. (1981). Evidence against the reported antithiamine effect of caffeic and chlorogenic acids. *International Journal for Vitamin and Nutrition Research, 51*(4): 385–390.

Hormes, J., & Rozin, P. (2009). Perimenstrual chocolate craving. What happens after menopause? *Appetite, 53*(2): 256–259.

Hossain, S., Aoshima, H., Koda, H., & Kiso, Y. (2003). Effects of coffee components on the response of GABA(A) receptors expressed in Xenopus oocytes. *Journal of Agricultural and Food Chemistry, 51*(26): 7568–7575.

Hosseinzadeh, S., Poorsaadati, S., Radkani, B., & Forootan, M. (2011). Psychological disorders in patients with chronic constipation. *Gastroenterology and Hepatology from Bed to Bench, 4*(3): 159–163.

Huang, Y., Jin, M., Pi, R., Zhang, J., Chen, M., Ouyang, Y., Liu, A., Chao, X., Liu, P., Liu, J., Ramassamy, C., & Qin, J. (2013). Protective effects of caffeic acid and caffeic acid phenethyl ester against acrolein-induced neurotoxicity in HT22 mouse hippocampal cells. *Neuroscience Letters, 535*: 146–151.

Hurst, W., Glinski, J., Miller, K., Apgar, J., Davey, M., & Stuart, D. (2008). Survey of the trans-resveratrol and trans-piceid content of cocoa-containing and chocolate products. *Journal of Agricultural and Food Chemistry, 56*(18): 8374–8378.

Ichikawa, M., Yoshida, J., Ide, N., Sasaoka, T., Yamaguchi, H., & Ono, K. (2006). Tetrahydro-β-carboline derivatives in aged garlic extract show antioxidant properties. *Journal of Nutrition, 136*(3): S726–S731.

Inamdar, A., Masurekar, P., & Bennett, J. (2010). Neurotoxicity of fungal volatile organic compounds in Drosophila melanogaster. *Toxicological Sciences, 117*(2): 418–426.

Iso, H., Sato, S., Umemura, U., Kudo, M., Koike, K., Kitamura, A., Imano, H., Okamura, T., Naito, Y., & Shimamoto, T. (2002). Linoleic acid, other fatty acids, and the risk of stroke. *Stroke, 33*(8): 2086–2093.

Itoh, Y., Kawamata, Y., Harada, M., Kobayashi, M., Fujii, R., Fukusumi, S., Ogi, K., Hosoya, M., Tanaka, Y., Uejima, H., Tanaka, H., Maruyama, M., Satoh, R., Okubo, S., Kizawa, H., Komatsu, H., Matsumura, F., Noguchi, Y., Shinohara, T., Hinuma, S., Fujisawa, Y., & Fujino, M. (2003). Free fatty acids regulate insulin secretion from pancreatic beta cells through GPR40. *Nature, 422*(6928): 173–176.

Jaffé, W. (2015). Nutritional and functional components of non centrifugal cane sugar: A compilation of the data from the analytical literature. *Journal of Food Composition and Analysis, 43*: 194–202.

Jalil, A., Ismail, A., Pei, C., Hamid, M., & Kamaruddin, S. (2008). Effects of cocoa extract on glucometabolism, oxidative stress, and antioxidant enzymes in obese-diabetic (Ob-db) rats. *Journal of Agricultural and Food Chemistry, 56*(17): 7877–7884.

Jati, M., Jinap, S., Jamilah, B., & Nazamid, S. (2004). Effect of polyphenol concentration on pyrazine formation during cocoa liquor roasting. *Food Chemistry, 85*(1): 73–80.

Jayanthi, R., & Subash, P. (2010). Antioxidant effect of caffeic acid on oxytetracycline induced lipid peroxidation in albino rats. *Indian Journal of Clinical Biochemistry, 25*(4): 371–375.

Jenny, M., Santer, E., Klein, A., Ledochowski, M., Schennach, H., Ueberall, F., & Fuchs, D. (2009). Cacao extracts suppress tryptophan degradation of mitogen-stimulated peripheral blood mononuclear cells. *Journal of Ethnopharmacology, 122*(2): 261–267.

Jiang, J., & Xu, Q. (2003). Immunomodulatory activity of the aqueous extract from rhizome of *Smilax glabra* in the later phase of adjuvant-induced arthritis in rats. *Journal of Ethnopharmacology, 85*(1): 53–59.

Johnston, C., & Gaas, C. (2006). Vinegar: Medicinal uses and antiglycemic effect. *Medscape General Medicine, 8*(2): 61.

Jourdain, C., Tenca, G., Deguercy, A., Troplin, P., & Poelman, D. (2006). In-vitro effects of polyphenols from cocoa and beta-sitosterol on the growth of human prostate cancer and normal cells. *European Journal of Cancer Prevention, 15*(4): 353–361.

Jutel, M., Watanabe, T., Klunker, S., Akdis, M., Thomet, O., Malolepszy, J., Zak-Nejmark, T., Koga, R., Kobayashi, T., Blaser, K., & Akdis, C. (2001). Histamine regulates T-cell and antibody responses by differential expression of H1 and H2 receptors. *Nature, 413*: 420–425.

Kabara, J., Swieczkowski, D., Conley, A., & Truant, J. (1972). Fatty acids and derivatives as antimicrobial agents. *Antimicrobial Agents and Chemotherapy, 2*(1): 23–28.

Kako, H., Kobayashi, Y., & Yokogoshi, H. (2011). Effects of n-hexanal on dopamine release in the striatum of living rats. *European Journal of Pharmacology, 651*(1–3): 77–82.

Kamatenesi-Mugisha, M., & Oryem-Origa, H. (2005). Traditional herbal remedies used in the management of sexual impotence and erectile dysfunction in western Uganda. *African Health Sciences, 5*(1): 40–49.

Kanbak, G., Canbek, M., Oğlakçı, A., Kartkaya, K., Sentürk, H., Bayramoğlu, G., Bal, C., Göl, B., & Ozmen, A. (2012). Preventive role of gallic acid on alcohol dependent and cysteine protease-mediated pancreas injury. *Molecular Biology Reports, 39*(12): 10249–10255.

Kaneko, T., Honda, S., Nakano, S., & Matsuo, M. (1987). Lethal effects of a linoleic acid hydroperoxide and its autoxidation products, unsaturated aliphatic aldehydes, on human diploid fibroblasts. *Chemico-Biological Interactions, 63*(2): 127–137.

Kaneko, T., Kaji, K., & Matsuo, M. (1988). Cytotoxicities of a linoleic acid hydroperoxide and its related aliphatic aldehydes toward cultured human umbilical vein endothelial cells. *Chemico-Biological Interactions, 67*(3–4): 295–304.

Kang, J. (2007). Salsolinol, a tetrahydroisoquinoline catechol neurotoxin, induces human Cu, Zn-superoxidie dismutase modificaiton. *Journal of Biochemistry and Molecular Biology, 40*(5): 684–689.

Kang, N., Lee, K., Lee, D., Rogozin, E., Bode, A., Lee, H., & Dong, Z. (2008). Cocoa procyanidins suppress transformation by inhibiting mitogen-activated protein kinase kinase. *Journal of Biological Chemistry, 283*(30): 20664–20673.

Kao, T., Ou, Y., Kuo, J., Chen, W., Liao, S., Wu, C., Chen, C., Ling, N., Zhang, Y., & Peng, W. (2006). Neuroprotection by tetramethylpyrazine against ischemic brain injury in rats. *Neurochemistry International, 48*(3): 166–176.

Karadag˘, A., Balta, I., Saricaog˘lu, H., Kiliç, S., Kelekçi, K., Yildirim, M., Arica, D., Öztürk, S., Karaman, G., Çerman, A., Bilgili, S., Turan, E., Demirci, M., Uzunçakmak, T., Güvenç, S., Ataseven, A., Ferahbas¸, A., Aksoy, B., Çölgeçen, E., Ekiz, Ö., Demir, F., Bilgiç, Ö., Çakmak, S., Uçmak, D., Özug˘uz, P., Konkuralp, Y., Ermertcan, A., Gökdemir, G., Bas¸kan, E., Alyamaç, G., & S¸anli, H. (2019). The effect of personal, familial, and environmental characteristics on acne vulgaris: a prospective, multicenter, case controlled study. *Giornale Italiano di Dermatologia e Venereologia, 154*(2): 177–185.

Karakeci, A., Firdolas, F., Ozan, T., Unus, I., Ogras, M., & Orhan, I. (2013). Second pathways in the pathophysiology of ischemic priapism and treatment alternatives. *Urology, 82*(3): 625–629.

Kart, A., Cigremis, Y., Karaman, M., & Ozen, H. (2010). Caffeic acid phenethyl ester (CAPE) ameliorates cisplatin-induced hepatotoxicity in rabbit. *Experimental and Toxicologic Pathology, 62*(1): 45–52.

Kemparaju, K., & Girish, K. (2006). Snake venom hyaluronidase: a therapeutic target. *Cell Biochemistry & Function, 24*(1): 7–12.

Kenny, T., Keen, C., Jones, P., Kung, H., Schmitz, H., & Gershwin, M. (2004). Cocoa procyanidins inhibit proliferation and angiogenic signals in human dermal microvascular endothelial cells following stimulation by low-level H2O2. *Experimental Biology and Medicine (Maywood), 229*(8): 765–771.

Kenny, T., Keen, C., Schmitz, H., & Gershwin, M. (2007). Immune effects of cocoa procyanidin oligomers on peripheral blood mononuclear cells. *Experimental Biology and Medicine (Maywood), 232*(2): 293–300.

Khalil, M., Marcelletti, J., Katz, L., Katz, D., & Pope, L. (2000). Topical application of docosanol- or stearic acid-containing creams reduces severity of phenol burn wounds in mice. *Contact Dermatitis, 43*(2): 79–81.

Kim, K., Bae, O., Lim, K., Noh, J., Kang, S., Chung, K., & Chung, J. (2012). Novel antiplatelet activity of protocatechuic acid through the inhibition of high shear stress-induced platelet aggregation. *Journal of Pharmacology and Experimental Therapeutics, 343*(3): 704–711.

Kim, Y., & Je, Y. (2016). Flavonoid intake and mortality from cardiovascular disease and all causes: A meta-analysis of prospective cohort studies. *The FASEB Journal, 30*(1), Suppl.: 294.

Knaup, B., Oehme, A., Valotis, A., & Schreier, P. (2009). Anthocyanins as lipoxygenase inhibitors. *Molecular Nutrition & Food Research, 53*(5): 617–624.

Koch, C. (2018). What is consciousness? *Scientific American, 318*(6): 60–64.

Koli, R., Erlund, I., Jula, A., Marniemi, J., Mattila, P., & Alfthan, G. (2010). Bioavailability of various polyphenols from a diet containing moderate amounts of berries. *Journal of Agricultural & Food Chemistry, 58*(7): 3927–3932.

Kosman, V., Stankevich, N., Makarov, V., & Tikhonov, V. (2007). Biologically active substances in grated cocoa and cocoa butter. [Article in Russian.] *Voprosy Pitaniia, 76*(3): 62–67.

Kristinsson, J., Snaedal, J., Tórsdóttir, G., & Jóhannesson, T. (2012). Ceruloplasmin and iron in Alzheimer's disease and Parkinson's disease: a synopsis of recent studies. *Neuropsychiatric Disease and Treatment, 8*: 515–521.

Kruger, T., Exton, M., Pawlak, C., von zur Mühlen, A., Hartmann, U., & Schedlowski, M. (1998). Neuroendocrine and cardiovascular response to sexual arousal and orgasm in men. *Psychoneuroendocrinology, 23*(4): 401–411.

Kumar, K., Vani, M., Wang, S., Liao, J., Hsu, L., Yang, H., & Hseu, Y. (2013). In vitro and in vivo studies disclosed the depigmenting effects of gallic acid: A novel skin lightening agent for hyperpigmentary skin diseases. *Biofactors, 39*(3): 259–270.

Kurek, M., Czerwionka-Szaflarska, M., Doroszewska, G., & Przybilla, B. (1996). Les exorphines provenant de la caséine du lait de vache provoquent des réactions urticariennes pseudo-allergiques chez les enfants sains. *Revue Française d'Allergologie et d'Immunologie Clinique, 36*(2): 191–196.

Kyung, K., & Fleming, H. (1997). Antimicrobial activity of sulfur compounds derived from cabbage. *Journal of Food Protection, 60*(1): 67–71.

Lam, S., Velikov, K., & Velev, D. (2014). Pickering stabilization of foams and emulsions with particles of biological origin. *Current Opinion in Colloid & Interface Science, 19*(5): 490–500.

Lannuzel, A., Höglinger, G., Champy, P., Michel, P., Hirsch, E., & Ruberg, M. (2006). Is atypical parkinsonism in the Caribbean caused by the consumption of Annonacae? *Journal of Neural Transmission (Supplement), 70*: 153–157.

Lans, A. (2006). Ethnomedicines used in Trinidad and Tobago for urinary problems and diabetes mellitus. *Journal of Ethnobiology and Ethnomedicine, 2*: 45.

Larsen, C., & Grattan, D. (2012). Prolactin, neurogenesis, and maternal behaviours. *Brain, Behaviour, and Immunity, 26*(2): 201–209.

de Laurentiis, A., Fernandez-Solari, J., Mohn, C., Burdet, B., Zorrilla-Zubilete, M., & Rettori, V. (2010). The hypothalamic endocannabinoid system participates in the secretion of oxytocin and tumor necrosis factor-alpha induced by lipopolysaccharide. *Journal of Neuroimmunology, 221*(1–2): 32–41.

Lee, D., Lin, X., Paskaleva, E., Liu, Y., Puttamadappa, S., Thornber, C., Drake, J., Habulin, M., Shekhtman, A., & Canki, M. (2009). Palmitic acid is a novel CD4 fusion inhibitor that blocks HIV entry and infection. *AIDS Research and Human Retroviruses, 25*(12): 1231–1241.

Lee, K., Kim, Y., Lee, H., & Lee, C. (2003). Cocoa has more phenolic phytochemicals and a higher antioxidant capacity than teas and red wine. *Journal of Agricultural and Food Chemistry, 51*(25): 7292–7295.

Lee, K., Kundu, J., Kim, S., Chun, K., Lee, H., & Surh, Y. (2006). Cocoa polyphenols inhibit phorbol ester-induced superoxide anion formation in cultured HL-60 cells and expression of cyclooxygenase-2 and activation of NF-kappaB and MAPKs in mouse skin in vivo. *Journal of Nutrition, 136*(5): 1150–1155.

Lelo, A., Birkett, D., Robson, R., & Miners, J. (1986). Comparative pharmacokinetics of caffeine and its primary demethylated metabolites paraxanthine, theobromine and theophylline in man. *British Journal of Clinical Pharmacology, 22*(2): 177–182.

Lende, A., Kshirsagar, A., Deshpande, A., Muley, M., Patil, R., Bafna, P., & Naik, S. (2011). Anti-inflammatory and analgesic activity of protocatechuic acid in rats and mice. *Inflammopharmacology, 19*(5): 255–263.

Li, G., Rivas, P., Bedolla, R., Thapa, D., Reddick, R., Ghosh, R., & Kumar, A. (2013). Dietary resveratrol prevents development of high-grade prostatic intraepithelial neoplastic lesions: Involvement of SIRT1/S6K axis. *Cancer Prevention Research (Philadelphia), 6*(1): 27–39.

Li, M., Wang, X., Shi, J., Li, Y., Yang, N., Zhai, S., & Dang, S. (2015). Caffeic acid phenethyl ester inhibits liver fibrosis in rats. *World Journal of Gastroenterology, 21*(13): 3893–3903.

Li, Y., Gan, G., Zhang, H., Wu, H., Li, C., Huang, Y., Liu, Y., & Liu, J. (2007). A flavonoid glycoside isolated from *Smilax china* L. rhizome *in vitro* anticancer effects on human cancer cell lines. *Journal of Ethnopharmacology, 113*(1): 115–124.

Lim, J., Mietus-Snyder, M., Valente, A., Schwarz, J., & Lustig, R. (2010). The role of fructose in the pathogenesis of NAFLD and the metabolic syndrome. *Nature Reviews Gastroenterology and Hepatology, 7*: 251–264.

Ling, W., & Jones, P. (1995). Dietary phytosterols: a review of metabolism, benefits and side effects. *Life Sciences, 57*(3): 195–206.

Lippi, G., Mattiuzzi, C., & Cervellin, G. (2014). Chocolate and migraine: the history of an ambiguous association. *Acta Bio-medica, 85*(3): 216–221.

Liu, P., Liang, H., Xia, Q., Li, P., Kong, H., Lei, P., Wang, S., & Tu, Z. (2013). Resveratrol induces apoptosis of pancreatic cancer cells by inhibiting miR-21 regulation of BCL-2 expression. *Clinical and Translational Oncology, 15*(9): 741–746.

Liu, Z., Li, Y., & Yang, R. (2012). Effects of resveratrol on vascular endothelial growth factor expression in osteosarcoma cells and cell proliferation. *Oncology Letters, 4*(4): 837–839.

Lohsiriwat, S., Puengna, N., & Leelakusolvong, S. (2006). Effect of caffeine on lower esophageal sphincter pressure in Thai healthy volunteers. *Diseases of the Esophagus, 19*(3): 183–188.

Lopresti, A. (2017). Salvia (sage): A review of its potential cognitive-enhancing and protective effects. *Drugs in R&D, 17*(1): 53–64.

Louis, E., & Zheng, W. (2010). Beta-carboline alkaloids and essential tremor: exploring the environmental determinants of one of the most prevalent neurological diseases. *Scientific World Journal, 10*: 1783–1794.

Lucas, I., & Kolodziej, H. (2013). In vitro antileishmanial activity of resveratrol originates from its cytotoxic potential against host cells. *Planta Medica, 79*(1): 20–26.

Luce, V., Fernandez Solari, J., Rettori, V., & De Laurentiis, A. (2014). The inhibitory effect of anandamide on oxytocin and vasopressin secretion from neurohypophysis is mediated by nitric oxide. *Regulatory Peptides, 188*: 31–39.

Macht, M., & Dettmer, D. (2006). Everyday mood and emotions after eating a chocolate bar or an apple. *Appetite, 46*(3): 332–336.

Maestripieri, D., Hoffman, C., Anderson, G., Carter, S., & Higley, J. (2009). Mother-infant interactions in free-ranging rhesus macaques: Relationships between physiological and behavioural variables. *Physiology and Behaviour, 96*(4): 613–619.

Mansour, H., & Tawfik, S. (2012). Early treatment of radiation-induced heart damage in rats by caffeic acid phenethyl ester. *European Journal of Pharmacology, 692*(1–3): 46–51.

Mao, T., Van de Water, J., Keen, C., Schmitz, H., & Gershwin, M. (2002). Effect of cocoa flavanols and their related oligomers on the secretion of interleukin-5 in peripheral blood mononuclear cells. *Journal of Medicinal Food, 5*(1): 7–22.

Mao, T., Van de Water, J., Keen, C., Schmitz, H., & Gershwin, M. (2003). Cocoa flavonols and procyanidins promote transforming growth factor-beta1 homeostasis in peripheral blood mononuclear cells. *Experimental Biology and Medicine (Maywood), 228*(1): 93–99.

Mariani, S., Ventriglia, M., Simonelli, I., Donno, S., Bucossi, S., Vernieri, F., Melgari, J., Pasqualetti, P., Rossini, P., & Squitti, R. (2013). Fe and Cu do not differ in Parkinson's disease: A replication study plus meta-analysis. *Neurobiology of Aging, 34*(2): 632–633.

Marseglia, A., Palla, G., & Caligiani, A. (2014). Presence and variation of γ-aminobutyric acid and other free amino acids in cocoa beans from different geographical origins. *Food Research International, 63*, Part C: 360–366.

Martin, F., Antille, N., Rezzi, S., & Kochhar, S. (2012). Everyday eating experiences of chocolate and non-chocolate snacks impact postprandial anxiety, energy and emotional state. *Nutrients, 4*(6): 554–567.

Martin, F., Rezzi, S., Peré-Trepat, E., Kamlage, B., Collino, S., Leibold, E., Kastler, J., Rein, D., Fay, L., & Kochhar, S. (2009). Metabolic effects of dark chocolate consumption on energy, gut microbiota, and stress-related metabolism in free-living subjects. *Journal of Proteome Research, 8*(12): 5568–5579.

Marzouk, M., Moharram, F., Mohamed, M., Gamal-Eldeen, A., & Aboutabl, E. (2007). Anticancer and antioxidant tannins from *Pimenta dioica* leaves. *Zeitschrift fur Naturforschung, 62*(7): 526–536.

Masella, R., Santangelo, C., D'Archivio, M., Li Volti, G., Giovannini, C., & Galvano, F. (2012). Protocatechuic acid and human disease prevention: biological activities and molecular mechanisms. *Current Medicinal Chemistry, 19*(18): 2901–2917.

Massee, L., Ried, K., Pase, M., Travica, N., Yoganathan, J., Scholey, A., Macpherson, H., Kennedy, G., Sali, A., & Pipingas, A. (2015). The acute and sub-chronic effects of cocoa flavanols on mood, cognitive and cardiovascular health in young healthy adults: a randomized, controlled trial. *Frontiers in Pharmacology, 20*(6): 93.

Massolt, E., van Haard, P., Rehfeld, J., Posthuma, E., van der Veer, E., & Schweitzer, D. (2010). Appetite suppression through smelling of dark chocolate correlates with changes in ghrelin in young women. *Regulatory Peptides, 161*(1–3): 81–86.

Mastroiacovo, D., Kwik-Uribe, C., Grassi, D., Necozione, S., Raffaele, A., Pistacchio, L., Righetti, R., Bocale, R., Carmela Lechiara, M., Marini, C., Ferri, C., & Desideri, G. (2014). Cocoa flavanol consumption improves cognitive function, blood pressure control, and metabolic profile in elderly subjects: the Cocoa, Cognition, and Aging (CoCoA) Study—a randomized controlled trial. *American Journal of Clinical Nutrition, 101*(3): 538–548.

Mathur, S., Devaraj, S., Grundy, S., & Jialal, I. (2002). Cocoa products decrease low density lipoprotein oxidative susceptibility but do not affect biomarkers of inflammation in humans. *Journal of Nutrition, 132*(12): 3663–3667.

Matsumoto, H., Adachi, S., & Suzuki, Y. (2005). [Estrogenic activity of ultraviolet absorbers and the related compounds]. [Article in Japanese.] *Yakugaku Zasshi, 125*(8): 643–652.

Matsumura, Y., Nakagawa, Y., Mikome, K., Yamamoto, H., & Osakabe, N. (2014). Enhancement of energy expenditure following a single oral dose of flavan-3-ols associated with an increase in catecholamine secretion. *PLOS One, 9*(11): e112180.

Mattson, M., & Wan, R. (2005). Beneficial effects of intermittent fasting and caloric restriction on the cardiovascular and cerebrovascular systems. *Journal of Nutritional Biochemistry, 16*(3): 129–137.

McCarty, M., DiNicolantonio, J., & O'Keefe, J. (2015). Capsaicin may have important potential for promoting vascular and metabolic health. *Open Heart, 2*(1): e000262.

McGuire, P. (2000). Long term psychiatric and cognitive effects of MDMA use. *Toxicology Letters 112–113*: 153–156.

McPartland, J. (2008). Expression of the endocannabinoid system in fibroblasts and myofascial tissues. *Journal of Bodywork and Movement Therapies, 12*(2): 169–182.

Meier, B., Noll, S., & Molokwu, O. (2017). The sweet life: The effect of mindful chocolate consumption on mood. *Appetite, 108*: 21–27.

Meinhardt, L., Rincones, J., Bailey, B., Aime, M., Griffith, G., Zhang, D., & Pereira, G. (2008). *Moniliophthora perniciosa*, the causal agent of witches' broom disease of cacao: what's new from this old foe? *Molecular Plant Pathology, 9*(5): 577–588.

Mellor, D., & Naumovski, N. (2016). Effect of cocoa in diabetes: the potential of the pancreas and liver as key target organs, more than an antioxidant effect? *International Journal of Food Science and Technology, 51*(4): 829–841.

Melzig, M., Putscher, I., Henklein, P., & Haber, H. (2000). In vitro pharmacological activity of the tetrahydroisoquinoline salsolinol present in products from Theobroma cacao L. like cocoa and chocolate. *Journal of Ethnopharmacology, 73*(1–2): 153–159.

Menon, S., & Nayeem, N. (2013). *Vanilla Planifolia*: a review of a plant commonly used as flavouring agent [*sic*]. *International Journal of Pharmaceutical Sciences Review and Research, 20*(2): 225–228.

Merchant, A., Curhan, G., Rimm, E., Willett, W., & Fawzi, W. (2005). Intake of n-6 and n-3 fatty acids and fish and risk of community-acquired pneumonia in US men. *American Journal of Clinical Nutrition, 82*(3): 668–674.

Messerli, F. (2012). Chocolate consumption, cognitive function, and Nobel laureates. *New England Journal of Medicine, 367*(16): 1562–1564.

Migliori, M., Cantaluppi, V., Mannari, C., Bertelli, A., Medica, D., Quercia, A., Navarro, V., Scatena, A., Giovannini, L., Biancone, L., & Panichi, V. (2015). Caffeic acid, a phenol found in white wine, modulates endothelial nitric oxide production and protects from oxidative stress-associated endothelial cell injury. *PLoS One, 10*(4): e0117530. https://journals.plos.org/plosone/article?id=10.1371/journal.pone.0117530 [Accessed 18 March 2019].

Miller, E., Pastor-Barriuso, R., Dalal, D., Riemersma, R., Appel, L., & Guallar, E. (2005). Meta-analysis: High-dosage vitamin E supplementation may increase all-cause mortality. *Annals of Internal Medicine, 142*(1): 37–46.

Miller, K., Hurst, W., Payne, M., Stuart, D., Apgar, J., Sweigart, D., & Ou, B. (2008). Impact of alkalization on the antioxidant and flavanol content of commercial cocoa powders. *Journal of Agricultural and Food Chemistry, 56*(18): 8527–8533.

Min, S., Yang, H., Seo, S., Shin, S., Chung, M., Kim, J., Lee, S., Lee, H., & Lee, K. (2013). Cocoa polyphenols suppress adipogenesis in vitro and obesity in vivo by targeting insulin receptor. *International Journal of Obesity (London), 37*(4): 584–592.

Miner, M., Seftel, A., Nehra, A., Ganz, P., Kloner, A., Montorsi, P., Vlachopoulos, C., Ramsey, M., Sigman, M., Tilkemeier, P., & Jackson, G. (2012). Prognostic utility of erectile dysfunction for cardiovascular disease in younger men and those with diabetes. *American Heart Journal, 164*(1): 21–28.

Misztal, T., Tomaszewska-Zaremba, D., Górski, K., & Romanowicz, K. (2010). Opioid-salsolinol relationship in the control of prolactin release during lactation. *Neuroscience, 170*(4): 1165–1171.

Miyake, Y., Tanaka, K., Fukushima, W., Sasaki, S., Kiyohara, C., Tsuboi, Y., Yamada, T., Oeda, T., Miki, T., Kawamura, N., Sakae, N., Fukuyama, H., Hirota, Y., & Nagai, M. (2011). Dietary intake of metals and risk of Parkinson's disease: a case-control study in Japan. *Journal of the Neurological Sciences, 306*(1–2): 98–102.

Modell, B., & Darlison, M. (2008). Global epidemiology of haemoglobin disorders and derived service indicators. *Bulletin of the World Health Organization, 86*(6): 417–496.

Møller, S. (1992). Serotonin, carbohydrates, and atypical depression. *Pharmacology & Toxicology, 71*, Suppl. 1: 61–71.

Momtazi-Borojeni, A., Esmaeili, S., Abdollahi, E., & Sahebkar, A. (2017). A review on the pharmacology and toxicology of steviol glycosides extracted from Stevia rebaudiana. *Current Pharmaceutical Design, 23*(11): 1016–1622.

Monagas, M., Khan, N., Andres-Lacueva, C., Casas, R., Urpí-Sardà, M., Llorach, R., Lamuela-Raventós, R., & Estruch, R. (2009). Effect of cocoa powder on the modulation of inflammatory biomarkers in patients at high risk of cardiovascular disease. *American Journal of Clinical Nutrition, 90*(5): 1144–1150.

Mondal, P., Das, S., Junejo, J., Borah, S., & Zaman, K. (2016). Evaluations of antidiabetic potential of the hydro-alcoholic extract of the stem bark of *Plumeria rubra* a traditionally used medicinal source in North-East India. *International Journal of Green Pharmacy, 10*(4): 252–260.

Montalvo, R., & Parra, A. (1999). Evaluacion del efecto antiinflamatorio del extracto de *Piper auritum* H.B.K. y toxicidad aguga oral. *Revista Cubana de Plantas Medicinales, 4*(1): 11–14. http://scielo.sld.cu/scielo.php?pid=S1028-47961999000100003&script=sci_arttext&tlng=en [Accessed 6 December 2017].

Monteleone, P., Brambilla, F., Bortolotti, F., Ferraro, C., & Maj, M. (1998). Plasma prolactin response to d-fenfluramine is blunted in bulimic patients with frequent binge episodes. *Psychological Medicine, 28*(4): 975–983.

de Montellano, B. (2004). Magia medicinal azteca. *Arqueologia Mexicana, 12*(69): 30–33.

Montomayor, J., Lachenaud, P., da Silva e Mota, J., Loor, R., Kuhn, D., Brown, J., & Schnell, R. (2008). Geographic and genetic population differentiation of the Amazonian chocolate tree. *PLoS One, 3*(10): e3311. doi: 10.1371/journal.pone.0003311.

Moreira, A., Diógenes, M., de Mendonça, A., Lunet, N., & Barros, H. (2016). Chocolate consumption is associated with a lower risk of cognitive decline. *Journal of Alzheimer's Disease, 53*(1): 85–93.

Morgan, M., McFie, L., Fleetwood, L., & Robinson, J. (2002). Ecstasy (MDMA): are the psychological problems associated with its use reversed by prolonged abstinence? *Psychopharmacology, 159*(3): 294–303.

Morris, D. (2012). Effects of oral lactate consumption on metabolism and exercise performance. *Current Sports Medicine Reports, 11*(4): 185–188.

Motegi, T., Katayama, M., Uzuka, Y., & Okamura, Y. (2013). Evaluation of anticancer effects and enhanced doxorubicin cytotoxicity of xanthine derivatives using canine hemangiosarcoma cell lines. *Research in Veterinary Science, 95*(2): 600–605.

Mounicou, S., Szpunar, J., Lobinski, R., Andrey, D., & Blake, C. (2002). Bioavailability of cadmium and lead in cocoa: comparison of extraction procedures prior to size-exclusion fast-flow liquid chromatography with inductively coupled plasma mass spectrometric detection (SEC-ICP-MS). *Journal of Analytical Atomic Spectrometry, 17*: 880–886.

Moura-da-Silva, A., Laing, G., Paine, M., Dennison, J., Politi, V., Crampton, J., & Theakston, R. (1996). Processing of pro-tumor necrosis factor-α by venom metalloproteinases: A hypothesis explaining local tissue damage following snake bite. *European Journal of Immunology, 26*(9): 2000–2005.

Mravec, B. (2006). Salsolinol, a derivate of dopamine, is a possible modulator of catecholaminergic transmission: a review of recent developments. *Physiological Research, 55*: 353–364.

Mubarak, A., Bondonno, C., Liu, A., Considine, M., Rich, L., Mas, E., Croft, K., & Hodgson, J. (2012). Acute effects of chlorogenic acid on nitric oxide status, endothelial function, and blood pressure in healthy volunteers: a randomized trial. *Journal of Agricultural and Food Chemistry, 60*(36): 9130–9136.

Mullen, W., Borges, G., Donovan, J., Edwards, C., Serafini, M., Lean, M., & Crozier, A. (2009). Milk decreases urinary excretion but not plasma pharmacokinetics of cocoa flavan-3-ol metabolites in humans. *American Journal of Clinical Nutrition, 89*(6): 1784–1791.

Müller-Lissner, S., Kaatz, V., Brandt, W., Keller, J., & Layer, P. (2005). The perceived effect of various foods and beverages on stool consistency. *European Journal of Gastroenterology & Hepatology, 17*(1): 109–112.

Muniyappa, R., Hall, G., Kolodziej, T., Karne, R., Crandon, S., & Quon, M. (2008). Cocoa consumption for 2 wk enhances insulin-mediated vasodilatation without improving blood pressure or insulin resistance in essential hypertension. *American Journal of Clinical Nutrition, 88*(6): 1685–1696.

Murphy, K., Chronopoulos, A., Singh, I., Francis, M., Moriarty, H., Pike, M., Turner, A., Mann, N., & Sinclair, A. (2003). Dietary flavanols and procyanidin oligomers from cocoa (Theobroma cacao) inhibit platelet function. *American Journal of Clinical Nutrition, 77*(6): 1466–1473.

Mursu, J., Voutilainen, S., Nurmi, T., Rissanen, T., Virtanen, J., Kaikkonen, J., Nyyssönen, K., & Salonen, J. (2004). Dark chocolate consumption increases HDL cholesterol concentration and chocolate fatty acids may inhibit lipid peroxidation in healthy humans. *Free Radical Biology and Medicine, 37*(9): 1351–1359.

Murugan, V., Mukherjee, K., Maiti, K., & Mukherjee, P. (2009). Enhanced oral bioavailability and antioxidant profile of ellagic acid by phospholipids. *Journal of Agricultural and Food Chemistry, 57*(11): 4559–4565.

Nabavi, S. M., Habtemariam, S., Nabavi, S. F., Sureda, A., Daglia, M., Moghaddam, A., & Amani, M. (2013). Protective effect of gallic acid isolated from Peltiphyllum peltatum against sodium fluoride-induced oxidative stress in rat's kidney. *Molecular and Cellular Biochemistry, 372*(1–2): 233–239.

Nakamura, Y., Suganuma, E., Matsuo, T., Okamoto, S., Sato, K., & Ohtsuki, K. (1999). 2,4-nonadienal and benzaldehyde bioantimutagens in Fushimi sweet pepper (Fushimi-Togarashi). *Journal of Agricultural and Food Chemistry, 47*(2): 544–549.

Nakano, M., Yamamoto, T., Okamura, H., Tsuda, A., & Kowatari, Y. (2012). Effects of oral supplementation with pyrroloquinoline quinone on stress, fatigue, and sleep. *Functional Foods in Health & Disease, 2*(8): 307–324.

Naoi, M., Maruyama, W., & Nagy, G. (2004). Dopamine-derived salsolinol derivatives as endogenous monoamine oxidase inhibitors: occurrence, metabolism and function in human brains. *Neurotoxicology, 25*(1–2): 193–204.

Narasimhan, B., Belsare, D., Pharande, D., Mourya, V., & Dhake, A. (2004). Esters, amides and substituted derivatives of cinnamic acid: synthesis, antimicrobial activity and QSAR investigations. *European Journal of Medicinal Chemistry, 39*(10): 827–834.

do Nascimento, S., Pena, P., Brum, D., Imazaki, F., Tucci, M., & Efraim, P. (2013). Behavior of Salmonella during fermentation, drying and storage of cocoa beans. *International Journal of Food Microbiology, 167*(3): 363–368.

Nasser, J., Bradley, L., Leitzsch, J., Chohan, O., Fasulo, K., Haller, J., Jaeger, K., Szulanczyk, B., & Del Parigi, A. (2011). Psychoactive effects of tasting chocolate and desire for more chocolate. *Physiology & Behaviour, 104*(1): 117–121.

Neukam, K., Stahl, W., Tronnier, H., Sies, H., & Heinrich, U. (2007). Consumption of flavanol-rich cocoa acutely increases microcirculation in human skin. *European Journal of Nutrition, 46*(1): 53–56.

Nishino, A., Ichihara, T., Takaha, T., Kuriki, T., Nihei, H., Kawamoto, K., Yasui, H., & Maoka, T. (2015). Accumulation of paprika carotenoids in human plasma and erythrocytes. *Journal of Oleo Science, 64*(10): 1135–1142.

Norling, L., Ly, L., & Dalli, J. (2017). Resolving inflammation by using nutrition therapy: roles for specialized proresolving mediators. *Current Opinion in Clinical Nutrition and Metabolic Care, 20*(2): 145–152.

Núñez, V., Otero, R., Barona, J., Saldarriaga, M., Osorio, R., Fonnegra, R., Jiménez, S., Díaz, A., & Quintana, J. (2004). Neutralization of the edema-forming, defibrinating and coagulant effects of Bothrops asper venom by extracts of plants used by healers in Colombia. *Brazilian Journal of Medical and Biological Research, 37*(7): 969–977.

Oboh, G., Agunloye, O., Akinyemi, A., Ademiluyi, A., & Adefegha, S. (2013). Comparative study on the inhibitory effect of caffeic and chlorogenic acids on key enzymes linked to Alzheimer's disease and some pro-oxidant induced oxidative stress in rats' brain—in vitro. *Neurochemical Research, 38*(2): 413–419.

Ogawa, M., Takano, K., Kawabe, K., Moriyama, M., Ihara, H., & Nakamura, Y. (2013). Theophylline potentiates lipopolysaccharide-induced NO production in cultured astrocytes. *Neurochemical Research, 39*(1): 107–116.

Ohno, M., Sakamoto, K., Ishizuka, K., & Fujita, S. (2009). Crude cacao *theobroma cacao* extract reduces mutagenicity induced by benzo[a]pyrene through inhibition of CYP1A activity *in vitro. Phytotherapy Research, 23*(8): 1134–1139.

Okiyama, K., Smith, D., Gennarelli, T., Simon, R., Leach, M., & McIntosh, T. (1995). The sodium channel blocker and glutamate release inhibitor BW1003C87 and magnesium attenuate regional cerebral edema following experimental brain injury in the rat. *Journal of Neurochemistry, 64*(2): 802–809.

Oktar, S., Aydin, M., Yönden, Z., Alçin, E., Ilhan, S., & Nacar, A. (2010). Effects of caffeic acid phenethyl ester on isoproterenol-induced myocardial infarction in rats. *Anantolian Journal of Cardiology, 10*(4): 298–302.

de Oliveira, M., Santos, M., & Côni, A. (1975). Analgesic activity of dimeric proanthocyanidins—preliminary experiments. *Arquivos de Instituto Biologico (Sao Paulo), 42*: 145–150.

de Orellana, M. (2017). Visionary nature. *Artes de Mexico: Plantas Sagradas, 127*: 65. Mexico City: Artes de Mexico y del Mundo, S.A. de C.V.

Orozco, T., Wang, J., & Keen, C. (2003). Chronic consumption of a flavanol- and procyanindin-rich diet is associated with reduced levels of 8-hydroxy-2′-deoxyguanosine in rat testes. *Journal of Nutritional Biochemistry, 14*(2): 104–110.

Osakabe, N., Baba, S., Yasuda, A., Iwamoto, T., Kamiyama, M., Takizawa, T., Itakura H., & Kondo, K. (2009). Daily cocoa intake reduces the susceptibility of low-density lipoprotein to oxidation as demonstrated in healthy human volunteers. *Free Radical Research, 34*(1): 93–99.

Osakabe, N., Sanbongi, C., Yamagishi, M., Takizawa, T., & Osawa, T. (1998). Effects of polyphenol substances derived from Theobroma cacao on gastric mucosal lesion induced by ethanol. *Bioscience, Biotechnology & Biochemistry, 62*(8): 1535–1538.

Ott, V., Finlayson, G., Lehnert, H., Heitmann, B., Heinrichs, M., Born, J., & Hallschmid, M. (2013). Oxytocin reduces reward-driven food intake in humans. *Diabetes, 62*(10): 3418–3425.

Ozgocmen, S., Ozyurt, H., Sogut, S., & Akyol, O. (2005). Current concepts in the pathophysiology of fibromyalgia: the potential role of oxidative stress and nitric oxide. *Rheumatology International, 26*(7): 585–597.

Paetsch, P., & Greenshaw, A. (1993). 2-phenylethylamine-induced changes in catecholamine receptor density: implications for antidepressant drug action. *Neurochemistry Research, 18*(9): 1015–1022.

Pang, C., Zheng, Z., Shi, L., Sheng, Y., Wei, H., Wang, Z., & Ji, L. (2016). Caffeic acid prevents acetaminophen-induced liver injury by activating the Keap1-Nrf2 antioxidative defense system. *Free Radical Biology and Medicine, 91*: 236–246.

Pang, P., Shan, J., & Chiu, K. (1996). Tetramethylpyrazine, a calcium antagonist. *Planta Medica, 62*(5): 431–435.

Panneerselvam, M., Tsutsumi, Y., Bonds, J., Horikawa, Y., Saldana, M., Dalton, N., Head, B., Patel, P., Roth, D., & Patel, H. (2010). Dark chocolate receptors: epicatechin-induced cardiac protection is dependent on δ-opioid receptor stimulation. *American Journal of Physiology—Heart and Circulatory, 299*(5): H1604–H1609.

Pari, L., & Karthikesan, K. (2007). Protective role of caffeic acid against alcohol-induced biochemical changes in rats. *Fundamental and Clinical Pharmacology, 21*(4): 355–361.

Park, C., Stankiewicz, Z., Rayman, M., & Hauschild, A. (1979). Inhibitory effect of cocoa powder on the growth of a variety of bacteria in different media. *Canadian Journal of Microbiology, 25*(2): 233–235.

Park, J. (2005). Quantitation of clovamide-type phenylpropenoic acid amides in cells and plasma using high-performance liquid chromatography with a coulometric electrochemical detector. *Journal of Agricultural and Food Chemistry, 53*: 8135–8140.

Park, J. (2007). Caffedymine from cocoa has COX inhibitory activity suppressing the expression of a platelet activation marker, P-selectin. *Journal of Agricultural and Food Chemistry, 55*: 2171–2175.

Park, J., & Schoene, N. (2006). Clovamide-type phenylpropenoic acid amides, N-coumaroyldopamine and N-caffeoyldopamine, inhibit platelet-leukocyte interactions via suppressing P-selectin expression. *Journal of Pharmacology and Experimental Therapeutics, 317*(2): 813–819.

Parker, G., Parker, I., & Brotchie, H. (2006). Mood state effects of chocolate. *Journal of Affective Disorders, 92*(2–3): 149–159.

Parrott, A. (2001). Human psychopharmacology of Ecstasy (MDMA): a review of 15 years of empirical research. *Human Psychopharmacology, 16*(8): 557–577.

Parrott, A., Montgomery, C., Wetherell, M., Downey, L., Stough, C., & Scholey, A. (2014). MDMA, cortisol, and heightened stress in recreational ecstasy users. *Behavioural Pharmacology, 25*(5–6): 458–472.

Parsons, G., Keeney, P., & Patton, S. (1969). Identification and quantitative analysis of phospholipids in cocoa beans. *Journal of Food Science, 34*(6): 497–499.

Pase, M., Scholey, A., Pipingas, A., Kras, M., Nolidin, K., Gibbs, A., Wesnes, K., & Stough, C. (2013). Cocoa polyphenols enhance positive mood states but not cognitive performance: a randomized, placebo-controlled trial. *Journal of Psychopharmacology, 27*(5): 451–458.

Passie, T., Seifert, J., Schneider, U., & Emrich, H. (2002). The pharmacology of psilocybin. *Addiction Biology, 7*(4): 357–364.

Pastore, P., Favaro, G., Badocco, D., Tapparo, A., Cavalli, S., & Saccani, G. (2005). Determination of biogenic amines in chocolate by ion chromatographic separation and pulsed integrated amperometric detection with implemented wave-form at Au disposable electrode. *Journal of Chromatography A, 1098*(1–2): 111–115.

Peciña, S., Schulkin, J., & Berridge, K. (2006). Nucleus accumbens corticotropin-releasing factor increases cue-triggered motivation for sucrose reward: paradoxical positive incentive effects in stress? *BMC Biology, 4*: 8.

Pérez-Berezo, T., Ramiro-Puig, E., Pérez-Cano, F., Castellote, C., Permanyer, J., Franch, A., & Castell, M. (2009). Influence of a cocoa-enriched diet on specific immune response in ovalbumin-sensitized rats. *Molecular Nutrition & Food Research, 53*(3): 389–397.

Petta, S., Marchesini, G., Caracausi, L., Macaluso, F., Cammà, C., Ciminnisi, S., Cabibi, D., Porcasi, R., Craxì, A., & Di Marco, V. (2013). Industrial, not fruit fructose intake is associated with the severity of liver fibrosis in genotype 1 chronic hepatitis C patients. *Journal of Hepatology, 59*(6): 1169–1176.

Polache, A., & Granero, L. (2013). Salsolinol and ethanol-derived excitation of dopamine mesolimbic neurons: new insights. *Frontiers in Behavioural Neuroscience, 7*, Article 74: 1–2.

Popenoe, W. (1919). Batido and other Guatemalan beverages prepared from Cacao. *American Anthropological Association, 21*(4): 403–409.

Poulsen, M., Vestergaard, P., Clasen, B., Radko, Y., Christensen, L., Stødkilde-Jørgensen, H., Møller, N., Jessen, N., Pedersen, S., & Jørgensen, J. (2013). High-dose resveratrol supplementation in obese men: an investigator-initiated, randomized, placebo-controlled clinical trial of substrate metabolism, insulin sensitivity, and body composition. *Diabetes, 62*(4): 1186–1195.

Preza, A., Jaramillo, M., Puebla, A., Mateos, J., Hernández, R., & Lugo, E. (2010). Antitumor activity against murine lymphoma L5178Y model of proteins from cacao (Theobroma cacao L.) seeds in relation with in vitro antioxidant activity. *BMC Complementary and Alternative Medicine, 10*: 61.

Price, L., Ricaurte, G., Krystal, J., & Heniger, G. (1989). Neuroendocrine and mood responses to intravenous L-tryptophan in 3,4-methylenedioxymethamphetamine (MDMA) users: preliminary observations. *Archives of General Psychiatry, 46*(1): 20–22.

Pruijm, M., Hofmann, L., Charollais-Thoenig, J., Forni, V., Maillard, M., Coristine, A., Stuber, M., Burnier, M., & Vogt, B. (2013). Effect of dark chocolate on renal tissue oxygenation as measured by BOLD-MRI in healthy volunteers. *Clinical Nephrology, 80*(3): 211–217.

Quertemont, E., & Didone, V. (2006). Role of acetaldehyde in mediating the pharmacological and behavioral effects of alcohol. *Alcohol Research and Health, 29*(4): 258–265.

Quinlan, P., Lane, J., & Aspinall, L. (1997). Effects of hot tea, coffee and water ingestion on physiological responses and mood: the role of caffeine, water and beverage type. *Psychopharmacology (Berl), 134*(2): 164–173.

Quoc Trung, L., Espinoza, J., Takami, A., & Nakao, S. (2013). Resveratrol induces cell cycle arrest and apoptosis in malignant NK cells via JAK2/STAT3 pathway inhibition. *PLoS One, 8*(1): e55183.

Radojčić, I., Delonga, K., Mazor, S., Dragović-Uzelac, V., Carić, M., & Vorkapić-Furač, J. (2009). Polyphenolic content and composition and antioxidative activity of different cocoa liquors. *Czech Journal of Food Sciences, 27*(5): 330–337.

Raffauf, R., & Zennie, T. (1983). The phytochemistry of *Quararibea funebris*. *Botanical Museum Leaflets, Harvard University, 29*(2): 151–157.

Räikkönen, K., Pesonen, A., Järvenpää, A., & Strandberg, T. (2004). Sweet babies: chocolate consumption during pregnancy and infant temperament at six months. *Early Human Development, 76*(2): 139–145.

Ramiro, E., Franch, A., Castellote, C., Pérez-Cano, F., Permanyer, J., Izquierdo-Pulido, M., & Castell, M. (2005). Flavonoids from Theobroma cacao down-regulate inflammatory mediators. *Journal of Agricultural and Food Chemistry, 53*(22): 8506–8511.

Ramiro-Puig, E., Casadesús, G., Lee, H., Zhu, X., McShea, A., Perry, G., Pérez-Cano, F., Smith, M., & Castell, M. (2009). Neuroprotective effect of cocoa flavonoids on in vitro oxidative stress. *European Journal of Nutrition, 48*(1): 54–61.

Ramiro-Puig, E., & Castell, M. (2009). Cocoa: antioxidant and immunomodulator. *British Journal of Nutrition, 101*(7): 931–940.

Ramiro-Puig, E., Perez-Cano, F., Ramos-Romero, S., Perez-Berezo, T., Castellote, C., Permanyer, J., Franch, A., Izquierdo-Pulido, M., & Castell, M. (2008). Intestinal immune system of young rats influenced by cocoa-enriched diet. *Journal of Nutritional Biochemistry, 19*(8): 555–565.

Rankin, C., Nriagu, J., Aggarwal, J., Arowolo, T., Adebayo, K., & Flegal, A. R. (2005). Lead contamination in cocoa and cocoa products: isotopic evidence of global contamination. *Environmental Health Perspectives, 113*(10): 1344–1348.

Rawson, R. (2013). Current research on the epidemiology, medical and psychiatric effects, and treatment of methamphetamine use. *Journal of Food and Drug Analysis, 21*(4): S77–S81.

Raynor, K., Kong, H., Chen, Y., Yasuda, K., Yu, L., Bell, G., & Reisine, T. (1994). Pharmacological characterization of the cloned kappa-, delta-, and mu-opioid receptors. *Molecular Pharmacology, 45*(2): 330–334.

Raza, M., Alorainy, M., & Algasham, A. (2007). Evaluation of ambrein and epicoprostanol for their antioxidant properties: protection against adriamycin-induced free radical toxicity. *Food and Chemical Toxicology, 45*(9): 1614–1619.

Record, I., McInerney, J., Noakes, M., & Bird, A. (2003). Chocolate consumption, fecal water antioxidant activity, and hydroxyl radical production. *Nutrition and Cancer, 47*(2): 131–135.

Reddy, P., Rao, R., Shashidhar, J., Sastry, B., Rao, J., & Babu, K. (2009). Phytochemical investigation of labdane diterpenes from the rhizomes of Hedychium spicatum and their cytotoxic activity. *Bioorganic and Medicinal Chemistry Letters, 19*(21): 6078–6081.

Redovniković, I., Delonga, K., Mazor, S., Dragović-Uzelac, V., Carić, M., & Vorkapić-Furač, J. (2009). Polyphenolic content and composition and antioxidative activity of different cocoa liquors. *Czech Journal of Food Sciences, 27*(5): 330–337.

Reiche, E., Nunes, S., & Morimoto, H. (2004). Stress, depression, the immune system, and cancer. *Lancet Oncology, 5*(10): 617–625.

Rein, D., Paglieroni, T., Wun, T., Pearson, D., Schmitz, H., Gosselin, R., & Keen, C. (2000). Cocoa inhibits platelet activation and function. *American Journal of Clinical Nutrition, 72*(1): 30–35.

Reuter, S., Gupta, S., Chaturvedi, M., & Aggarwal, B. (2010). Oxidative stress, inflammation, and cancer: How are they linked? *Free Radical Biology and Medicine, 49*(11): 1603–1616.

Ried, K., Frank, O., & Stocks, N. (2009). Dark chocolate or tomato extract for prehypertension: a randomised controlled trial. *BMC Complementary and Alternative Medicine, 9*: 22.

Rios, L., Bennett, R., Lazarus, S., Rémésy, C., Scalbert, A., & Williamson, G. (2002). Cocoa procyanidins are stable during gastric transit in humans. *American Journal of Clinical Nutrition, 76*(5): 1106–1110.

Rios, L., Gonthier, M., Rémésy, C., Mila, I., Lapierre, C., Lazarus, S., Williamson, G., & Scalbert, A. (2003). Chocolate intake increases urinary excretion of polyphenol-derived phenolic acids in healthy human subjects. *American Journal of Clinical Nutrition, 77*(4): 912–918.

Ristow, M., & Schmeisser, K. (2014). Mitohormesis: Promoting health and lifespan by increased levels of reactive oxygen species (ROS). *Dose Response, 12*(2): 288–341.

Robledo, P., Mendizabal, V., Ortuño, J., De La Torre, R., Kieffer, B., & Maldonado, R. (2004). The rewarding properties of MDMA are preserved in mice lacking μ-opioid receptors. *European Journal of Neuroscience, 20*(3): 853–858.

Rodríguez-Arias, M., Valverde, O., Daza-Losada, M., Blanco-Gandía, M., Aguilar, M., & Miñarro, J. (2013). Assessment of the abuse potential of MDMA in the conditioned place preference paradigm: Role of CB1 receptors. *Progress in Neuro-Psychopharmacology and Biological Psychiatry, 47*: 77–84.

Romero-Luna, H., Hernández-Sánchez, H., & Dávila-Ortiz, G. (2017). Traditional fermented beverages from Mexico as a potential probiotic source. *Annals of Microbiology, 67*(9): 577–586.

Rondanelli, M., Opizzi, A., Solerte, S., Trotti, R., Klersy, C., & Cazzola, R. (2009). Administration of a dietary supplement (*N*-oleyl-phosphatidylethanolamine and epigallocatechin-3-gallate formula) enhances compliance with diet in healthy overweight subjects: a randomized controlled trial. *British Journal of Nutrition, 101*: 457–464.

Rose, D. (1997). Effects of dietary fatty acids on breast and prostate cancers: evidence from in vitro experiments and animal studies. *American Journal of Clinical Nutrition, 66*(6 Suppl.): 1513S–1522S.

Rose, F., Hodak, M., & Bernholc, J. (2011). Mechanism of copper(II)-induced misfolding of Parkinson's disease protein. *Scientific Reports, 1*(11): (5 pages).

Rose, N., Koperski, S., & Golomb, B. (2010). Mood food: chocolate and depressive symptoms in a cross-sectional analysis. *Archives of Internal Medicine, 170*(8): 699–703.

Rosen, R., Brown, C., Heiman, J., Leiblum, S., Meston, C., Shabsigh, R., Ferguson, D., & D'Agostino, R. (2000). The female sexual function index (FSFI): a multidimensional self-report instrument for the assessment of female sexual function. *Journal of Sex and Marital Therapy, 26*(2): 191–208.

Roura, E., Andrés-Lacueva, C., Estruch, R., Mata Bilbao, M., Izquierdo-Pulido, M., & Lamuela-Raventós, R. (2008). The effects of milk as a food matrix for polyphenols on the excretion profile of cocoa (-)-epicatechin metabolites in healthy human subjects. *British Journal of Nutrition, 100*(4): 846–851.

Roura, E., Andrés-Lacueva, C., Estruch, R., Mata Bilbao, M., Izquierdo-Pulido, M., Waterhouse, A., & Lamuela-Raventós, R. (2007). Milk does not affect the bioavailability of cocoa powder flavonoid in healthy human. *Annals of Nutrition and Metabolism, 51*(6): 493–498.

Ruzaidi, A., Amin, I., Nawalyah, A., Hamid, M., & Faizul, H. (2005). The effect of Malaysian cocoa extract on glucose levels and lipid profiles in diabetic rats. *Journal of Ethnopharmacology, 98*(1–2): 55–60.

Sa, F., Gao, J., Fung, K., Zheng, Y., Lee, S., & Wang, Y. (2008). Anti-proliferative and pro-apoptotic effect of Smilax glabra Roxb. extract on hepatoma cell lines. *Chemico-Biological Interactions, 171*(1): 1–14.

Sabelli, H., Borison, R., Diamond, B., Havdala, H., & Narasimhachari, M. (1978). Phenylethylamine and brain function. *Biochemical Pharmacology, 27*(13): 1707–1711.

Sabelli, H., Fink, P., Fawcett, J., & Tom, C. (1996). Sustained antidepressant effect of PEA replacement. *Journal of Neuropsychiatry and Clinical Neurosciences, 8*(2): 168–171.

Sadaf, H., Raza, S., & Hassan, S. (2017). Role of gut microbiota against calcium oxalate. *Microbial Pathogenesis, 109*: 287–291.

Saftlas, A., Triche, E., Beydoun, H., & Bracken, M. (2010). Does chocolate intake during pregnancy reduce the risks of preeclampsia and gestational hypertension? *Annals of Epidemiology, 20*(8): 584–591.

Sakagami, H., Kawano, M., Thet, M., Hashimoto, K., Satoh, K., Kanamoto, T., Terakubo, S., Nakashima, H., Haishima, Y., Maeda, Y., & Sakurai, K. (2011). Anti-HIV and immunomodulation activities of cacao mass lignin-carbohydrate complex. *In Vivo, 25*(2): 229–236.

Sakagami, H., Satoh, K., Fukamachi, H., Ikarashi, T., Shimizu, A., Yano, K., Kanamoto, T., Terakubo, S., Nakashima, H., Hasegawa, H., Nomura, A., Utsumi, K., Yamamoto, M., Maeda, Y., & Osawa, K. (2008). Anti-HIV and vitamin C-synergized radical scavenging activity of cacao husk lignin fractions. *In Vivo, 22*(3): 327–332.

Sakaguchi, M., Hiramatsu, Y., Takada, H., Yamamura, M., Hioki, K., Saito, K., & Yamamoto, M. (1984). Effect of dietary unsaturated and saturated fats on azoxymethane-induced colon carcinogenesis in rats. *Cancer Research, 44*(4): 1472–1477.

Sakuma, S., Fujimoto, Y., Tagano, S., Tsunomori, M., Nishida, H., & Fujita, T. (1997). Effects of non-anal, *trans*-2-nonenal and 4-hydroxy-2,3-*trans*-nonenal on cyclooxygenase and 12-lipoxygenase metabolism of arachidonic acid in rabbit platelets. *Journal of Pharmacy and Pharmacology, 49*(2): 150–153.

Salonia, A., Fabbri, F., Zanni, G., Scavini, M., Fantini, G., Briganti, A., Naspro, R., Parazzini, F., Gori, E., Rigatti, P., & Montorsi, F. (2006). Chocolate and women's sexual health: An intriguing correlation. *Journal of Sexual Medicine, 3*(3): 476–482.

Sampeck, K. (2016). Cacao biology: chocolate culture, a superfood. *ReVista: Harvard Review of Latin America, 16*(1): 3–9.

Sanbongi, C., Suzuki, N., & Sakane, T. (1997). Polyphenols in chocolate, which have antioxidant activity, modulate immune functions in humans in vitro. *Cellular Immunology, 177*(2): 129–136.

Sanchez, A., Reeser, J., Lau, H., Yahiku, P., Willard, R., McMillan, P., Cho, S., Magie, A., & Register, U. (1973). Role of sugars in human neutrophilic phagocytosis. *American Journal of Clinical Nutrition, 26*(11): 1180–1184.

Santos, H., & da Silva, G. (2018). To what extent does cinnamon administration improve the glycemic and lipid profiles? *Clinical Nutrition ESPEN, 27*: 1–9.

Sarris, J., Stough, C., Wahid, Z., Murray, G., Teschke, R., Savage, K., Dowell, A., Ng, C., & Schweitzer, I. (2013). Kava in the treatment of generalized anxiety disorder: a double-blind, randomized, placebo-controlled study. *Journal of Clinical Psychopharmacology, 33*(5): 643–648.

Sasaki, T., Fujii, K., Yoshida, K., Shimura, H., Sasahira, T., Ohmori, H., & Kuniyasu, H. (2006). Peritoneal metastasis inhibition by linoleic acid with activation of PPARgamma in human gastrointestinal cancer cells. *Virchows Archiv: An International Journal of Pathology, 448*(4): 422–427.

Sathe, R., Komisaruk, B., Ladas, A., & Godbole, S. (2001). Naltrexone-induced augmentation of sexual response in men. *Archives of Medical Research, 32*(3): 221–226.

Sathyapalan, T., Beckett, S., Rigby, A., Mellor, D., & Atkin, S. (2010). High cocoa polyphenol rich chocolate may reduce the burden of the symptoms in chronic fatigue syndrome. *Nutrition Journal, 9*: 55.

Scazzocchio, B., Varì, R., Filesi, C., D'Archivio, M., Santangelo, C., Giovannini, C., Iacovelli, A., Silecchia, G., Li Volti, G., Galvano, F., & Masella, R. (2011). Cyanidin-3-O-β-glucoside and protocatechuic acid exert insulin-like effects by upregulating PPARγ activity in human omental adipocytes. *Diabetes, 60*(9): 2234–2244.

de Schawe, C., Kessler, M., Hensen, I., & Tscharntke, T. (2018). Abundance and diversity of flower visitors on wild and cultivated cacao (*Theobroma cacao* L.) in Bolivia. *Agroforestry Systems, 92*(1): 117–125.

Schiavi, R., Schreiner-Engel, P., Mandeli, J., Schanzer, H., & Cohen, E. (1990). Healthy aging and male sexual function. *American Journal of Psychiatry, 147*(6): 766–771.

Schifano, F., & Magni, G. (1994). MDMA ("ecstasy") abuse: psychopathological features and craving for chocolate: a case series. *Biological Psychiatry, 36*(11): 763–767.

Schlesinger, N. (2010). Diagnosing and treating gout: a review to aid primary care physicians. *Postgraduate Medical Journal, 122*(2): 157–161.

Schnorr, O., Brossette, T., Momma, T., Kleinbongard, P., Keen, C., Schroeter, H., & Sies, H. (2008). Cocoa flavanols lower vascular arginase activity in human endothelial cells in vitro and in erythrocytes in vivo. *Archives of Biochemistry and Biophysics, 476*(2): 211–215.

Scholey, A., & Owen, L. (2013). Effects of chocolate on cognitive function and mood: a systematic review. *Nutritional Review, 71*(10): 665–681.

Schramm, D., Karim, M., Schrader, H., Holt, R., Kirkpatrick, N., Polagruto, J., Ensunsa, J., Schmitz, H., & Keen, C. (2003). Food effects on the absorption and pharmacokinetics of cocoa flavanols. *Life Sciences, 73*(7): 857–869.

Schramm, D., Wang, J., Holt, R., Ensunsa, J., Gonsalves, J., Lazarus, S., Schmitz, H., German, J., & Keen, C. (2001). Chocolate procyanidins decrease the leukotriene-prostacyclin ratio in humans and human aortic endothelial cells. *American Journal of Clinical Nutrition, 73*(1): 36–40.

Schuier, M., Sies, H., Illek, B., & Fischer, H. (2005). Cocoa-related flavonoids inhibit CFTR-mediated chloride transport across T84 human colon epithelia. *Journal of Nutrition, 135*(10): 2320–2325.

Schuman, M., Gitlin, M., & Fairbanks, L. (1987). Sweets, chocolate, and atypical depressive traits. *Journal of Nervous and Mental Disease, 175*(8): 491–495.

Scorticati, C., Mohn, C., De Laurentiis, A., Vissio, P., Solari, J., Seilicovich, A., McCann, S., & Rettori, V. (2003). The effect of anandamide on prolactin secretion is modulated by estrogen. *Proceedings of the National Academy of Sciences of the United States of America, 100*(4): 2134–2139.

Scott, D., Moffett, A., & Swash, M. (1977). Effects of oral amines on the EEG. *Journal of Neurology, Neurosurgery, and Psychiatry, 40*(2): 179–185.

Seale, S., Feng, Q., Agarwal, A., & El-Alfy, A. (2012). Neurobehavioral and transcriptional effects of acrylamide in juvenile rats. *Pharmacology Biochemistry and Behavior, 101*(1): 77–84.

Serra, A., Macià, A., Rubió, L., Anglès, N., Ortega, N., Morelló, J., Romero, M., & Motilva, M. (2013). Distribution of procyanidins and their metabolites in rat plasma and tissues in relation to ingestion of procyanidin-enriched or procyanidin-rich cocoa creams. *European Journal of Nutrition, 52*(3): 1029–1038.

Shacter, E., & Weitzman, S. (2002). Chronic inflammation and cancer. *Oncology (Williston Park, NY), 16*(2): 217–226, 229; discussion: 230–232.

Shamaladevi, N., Lyn, D., Shaaban, K., Zhang, L., Villate, S., Rohr, J., & Lokeshwar, B. (2013). Ericifolin: a novel antitumor compound from allspice that silences androgen receptor in prostate cancer. *Carcinogenesis, 34*(8): 1822–1832.

Shanmugavalli, N., Umashankar, V., & Raheem (2009). Antimicrobial activity of *Vanilla planifolia*. *Indian Journal of Science and Technology, 2*(3): 37–40.

Shao, B., Guo, H., Cui, Y., Ye, M., Han, J., & Guo, D. (2007). Steroidal saponins from Smilax china and their anti-inflammatory activities. *Phytochemistry, 68*(5): 623–630.

She, T., Qu, L., Wang, L., Yang, X., Xu, S., Feng, J., Gao, Y., Zhao, C., Han, Y., Cai, S., & Shou, C. (2015). Sarsaparilla (Smilax glabra rhizome) extract inhibits cancer cell growth by S phase arrest, apoptosis, and autophagy via redox-dependent ERK1/2 pathway. *Cancer Prevention Research (Philadelphia), 8*(5): 464–474.

She, T., Zhao, C., Feng, J., Wang, L., Qu, L., Fang, K., Cai, S., & Shou, C. (2015). Sarsaparilla (*Smilax glabra* rhizome) extract inhibits migration and invasion of cancer cells by suppressing TGF-β1 pathway. *PLoS One, 10*(3): e0118287.

Shelley, A., & Coscaron, S. (2001). Simuliid blackflies (Diptera: Simuliidae) and ceratopogonid midges (Diptera: Ceratopogonidae) as vectors of *Mansonella ozzardi* (Nematoda: Onchocercidae) in northern Argentina. *Memorias do Instituto Oswaldo Cruz, 96*(4): 451–458.

Shen, M., Wu, R., Zhao, L., Li, J., Guo, H., Fan, R., Cui, Y., Wang, Y., Yue, S., & Pei, J. (2012). Resveratrol attenuates ischemia/reperfusion injury in neonatal cardiomyocytes and its underlying mechanism. *PLoS One, 7*(12): e51223.

Sheth, S., Jajoo, S., Kaur, T., Mukherjea, D., Sheehan, K., Rybak, L., & Ramkumar, V. (2012). Resveratrol reduces prostate cancer growth and metastasis by inhibiting the Akt/MicroRNA-21 pathway. *PLoS One, 12*: e51655.

Shi, H., Dong, L., Jiang, J., Zhao, J., Zhao, G., Dang, X., Lu, X., & Jia, M. (2013). Chlorogenic acid reduces liver inflammation and fibrosis through inhibition of toll-like receptor 4 signaling pathway. *Toxicology, 303*(1): 107–114.

Shiina, Y., Funabashi, N., Lee, K., Murayama, T., Nakamura, K., Wakatsuki, Y., Daimon, M., & Komuro, I. (2009). Acute effect of oral flavonoid-rich dark chocolate intake on coronary circulation, as compared with non-flavonoid white chocolate, by transthoracic Doppler echocardiography in healthy adults. *International Journal of Cardiology, 131*(3): 424–429.

Shimoyama, A., Santin, J., Machado, I., de Oliveira, E., Silva, A., de Melo, I., Mancini-Filho, J., & Farsky, S. (2013). Antiulcerogenic activity of chlorogenic acid in different models of gastric ulcer. *Naunyn-Schmiedeberg's Archives of Pharmacology, 386*(1): 5–14.

Shinde, P., Patil, P., & Bairagi, V. (2014). Phytopharmacological review of *Plumeria* species. *Scholars Academic Journal of Pharmacy, 3*(2): 217–227.

Sies, H., Schewe, T., Heiss, C., & Kelm, M. (2005). Cocoa polyphenols and inflammatory mediators. *American Journal of Clinical Nutrition, 81*(1 Suppl.): 304S–312S.

Silva, C., Simeoni, L., & Silveira, D. (2009). Genus *Pouteria*: chemistry and biological activity. *Revista Brasileria de Farmacognosia, 19*(2): 501–509.

Simons, E., Becker, A., Simons, K., & Gillespie, C. (1985). The bronchodilator effect and pharmaco-kinetics of theobromine in young patients with asthma. *Journal of Allergy and Clinical Immunology, 76*(5): 703–707.

Singh, D., Rawat, M., Semalty, A., & Semalty, M. (2012). Quercetin-phospholipid complex: an amorphous pharmaceutical system in herbal drug delivery. *Current Drug Discovery Technologies, 9*(1): 17–24.

Singh, J., Reddy, S., & Kundukulam, J. (2011). Risk factors for gout and prevention: a systematic review of the literature. *Current Opinion in Rheumatology, 23*(2): 192–202.

Sinha, R. (2008). Chronic stress, drug use, and vulnerability to addiction. *Annals of the New York Academy of Sciences, 1141*: 105–130.

Slattery, M., & West, D. (1993). Smoking, alcohol, coffee, tea, caffeine, and theobromine: risk of prostate cancer in Utah (United States). *Cancer Causes & Control, 4*(6): 559–563.

Smeets, P., de Graaf, C., Stafleu, A., van Osch, M., Nievelstein, R., & der Grond, J. (2006). Effect of satiety on brain activation during chocolate tasting in men and women. *American Journal of Clinical Nutrition, 86*(6): 1297–1305.

Smit, H., & Blackburn, R. (2005). Reinforcing effects of caffeine and theobromine as found in chocolate. *Psychopharmacology (Berl), 181*(1): 101–106.

Smit, H., Gaffan, E., & Rogers, P. (2004). Methylxanthines are the psycho-pharmacologically active constituents of chocolate. *Psychopharmacology (Berl), 176*(3–4): 412–419.

Soaje, M., & Dreis, R. (2004). Involvement of opioid receptor subtypes in both stimulatory and inhibitory effects of the opioid peptides on prolactin secretion during pregnancy. *Cellular and Molecular Neurobiology, 24*(2): 193–204.

Sokolov, A., Pavlova, M., Klosterhalfen, S., & Enck, P. (2013). Chocolate and the brain: Neurobiological impact of cocoa flavanols on cognition and behavior. *Neuroscience and Biobehavioural Reviews, 37*(10 Pt. 2): 2445–2453.

Song, G., Gao, Y., Di, Y., Pan, L., Zhou, Y., & Ye, J. (2006). High-fat feeding reduces endothelium-dependent vasodilation in rats: differential mechanisms for saturated and unsaturated fatty acids? *Clinical and Experimental Pharmacology and Physiology, 33*(8): 708–713.

Sotelo, A., & Alvarez, R. (1991). Chemical composition of wild Theobroma species and their comparison to the Cacao bean. *Journal of Agricultural and Food Chemistry, 39*: 1940–1943.

Spencer, H., Fuller, H., Norris, C., & Williams, D. (1994). Effect of magnesium on the intestinal absorption of calcium in man. *Journal of the American College of Nutrition, 13*(5): 485–492.

Spencer, J., Schroeter, H., Shenoy, B., Srai, S., Debnam, E., & Rice-Evans, C. (2001). Epicatechin is the primary bioavailable form of the procyanidin dimers B2 and B5 after transfer across the small intestine. *Biochemical and Biophysical Research Communications, 285*(3): 588–593.

Spiegel, D. (2016). Psilocybin-assisted psychotherapy for dying cancer patients—aiding the final trip. *Journal of Psychopharmacology, 30*(12): 1215–1217.

Srinual, S., Chanvorachote, P., & Pongrakhananon, V. (2017). Suppression of cancer stem-like phenotypes in NCI-H460 lung cancer cells by vanillin through an Akt-dependent pathway. *International Journal of Oncology, 50*(4): 1341–1351.

Stammel, W., Thomas, H., Staib, W., & Kühn-Velten, W. (1991). Tetrahydroisoquinoline alkaloids mimic direct but not receptor-mediated inhibitory effects of estrogens and phytoestrogens on testicular endocrine function. Possible significance for Leydig cell insufficiency in alcohol addiction. *Life Sciences, 49*(18): 1319–1329.

Stanhope, K., Schwarz, J., Keim, N., Griffen, S., Bremer, A., Graham, J., Hatcher, B., Cox, C., Dyachenko, A., Zhang, W., McGahan, J., Seibert, A., Krauss, R., Chiu, S., Schaefer, E., Ai, M., Otokozawa, S., Nakajima, K., Nakano, T., Beysen, C., Hellerstein, M., Berglund, L., & Havel, P. (2009). Consuming fructose-sweetened, not glucose-sweetened, beverages increases visceral adiposity and lipids and decreases insulin sensitivity in overweight/obese humans. *Journal of Clinical Investigation, 119*(5): 1322–1334.

Stark, T., & Hofmann, T. (2005). Structures, sensory activity, and dose/response functions of 2,5-diketopiperazines in roasted cocoa nibs (Theobroma cacao). *Journal of Agricultural and Food Chemistry, 53*(18): 7222–7231.

Stark, T., Lang, R., Keller, D., Hensel, A., & Hofmann, T. (2008). Absorption of N-phenylpropenoyl-L-amino acids in healthy humans by oral administration of cocoa (Theobroma cacao). *Molecular Nutrition and Food Research, 52*(10): 1201–1214.

Stefano, G., & Kream, R. (2011). Reciprocal regulation of cellular nitric oxide formation by nitric oxide synthase and nitrite reductases. *Medical Science Monitor, 17*(10): RA221–226.

Sterger, K. (2010). Crosses, flowers and toads: Maya bloodletting iconography in Yaxchilan lintels 24, 25 and 26. [Thesis—Department of Humanities, Classics, and Comparative Literature, Brigham Young University.] https://scribd.com/document/71503199/Crosses-Flowers-And-Toads-Maya-Blodletting-Iconography [Accessed 4 April 2019].

Stone, J. (2011). Glutamatergic antipsychotic drugs: A new dawn in the treatment of schizophrenia? *Therapeutic Advances in Psychopharmacology, 1*(1): 5–18.

Storey, M., & Greger, J. (1987). Iron, zinc and copper interactions: chronic versus acute responses of rats. *Journal of Nutrition, 117*(8): 1134–1142.

Strandberg, T., Strandberg, A., Pitkälä, K., Salomaa, V., Tilvis, R., & Miettinen, T. (2008). Chocolate, well-being and health among elderly men. *European Journal of Clinical Nutrition, 62*(2): 247–253.

Stross, B. (2011). Food, foam and fermentation in Mesoamerica: Bubbles and the sacred state of inebriation. *Food, Culture & Society, 14*(4): 477–501.

Sueishi, Y., & Hori, M. (2012). Nitric oxide scavenging rates of solubilized resveratrol and flavonoids. *Nitric Oxide, 29C*: 25–29.

Sugimoto, N., Miwa, S., Hitomi, Y., Nakamura, H., Tsuchiya, H., & Yachie, A. (2014). Theobromine, the primary methylxanthine found in Theobroma cacao, prevents malignant glioblastoma proliferation by negatively regulating phosphodiesterase-4, extracellular signal-regulated kinase, Akt/mammalian target of rapamycin kinase, and nuclear factor-kappa B. *Nutrition and Cancer, 66*(3): 419–423.

Sylvester, P., Ip, M., & Briski, K. (1993). Effects of specific fatty acids on prolactin-induced NB2 lymphoma cell proliferation. *Life Sciences, 52*(24): 1977–1984.

Szabo, I., Pallag, A., & Blidar, C.-F. (2009). The antimicrobial activity of the *Cnicus benedictus* L. extracts. *Analele Universitatii din Oradea, Fascicula Biologie, XVI*(1): 126–128.

Tachibana, A., & Yonei, S. (1985). Inhibition of excision repair of DNA in u.v.-irradiated Escherichia coli by phenethyl alcohol. *International Journal of Radiation Biology and Related Studies in Physics, Chemistry, and Medicine, 47*(6): 663–671.

Taha, S. (1992). Effect of ambrein on smooth muscle responses to various agonists. *Journal of Ethnopharmacology, 60*(1): 19–26.

Taha, S., Islam, M., & Ageel, A. (1995). Effect of ambrein, a major constituent of ambergris, on masculine sexual behavior in rats. *Archives Internationales de Pharmacodynamie et de Therapie, 329*(2): 283–294.

Takahashi, M., Fukunaga, H., Kaneto, H., Fukudome, S., & Yoshikawa, M. (2000). Behavioral and pharmacological studies on gluten exorphin A5, a newly isolated bioactive food protein fragment, in mice. *Japanese Journal of Pharmacology, 84*(3): 259–265.

Tapia, P. (2006). Sublethal mitochondrial stress with an attendant stoichiometric augmentation of reactive oxygen species may precipitate many of the beneficial alterations in cellular physiology produced by caloric restriction, intermittent fasting, exercise and dietary phytonutrients: "Mitohormesis" for health and vitality. *Medical Hypotheses, 66*(4): 832–843.

Taubert, D., Roesen, R., Lehmann, C., Jung, N., & Schömig, E. (2007). Effects of low habitual cocoa intake on blood pressure and bioactive nitric oxide: a randomized controlled trial. *Journal of the American Medical Association, 298*(1): 49–60.

Taubert, D., Roesen, R., & Schömig, E. (2007). Effect of cocoa and tea intake on blood pressure: a meta-analysis. *Archives of Internal Medicine, 167*(7): 626–634.

Tavakoli, J., Miar, S., Zadehzare, M., & Akbari, H. (2012). Evaluation of effectiveness of herbal medication in cancer care: A review study. *Iranian Journal of Cancer Prevention, 5*(3): 144–156.

Teixeira, P., Thomazella, D., & Pereira, G. (2015). Time for chocolate: current understanding and new perspectives on Cacao Witches' Broom disease research. *PLoS Pathogens, 11*(10): e1005130. https://doi.org/10.1371/journal.ppat.1005130

Teraoka, M., Nakaso, K., Kusumoto, C., Katano, S., Tajima, N., Yamashita, A., Zushi, T., Ito, S., & Matsura, T. (2012). Cytoprotective effect of chlorogenic acid against α-synuclein-related toxicity in catecholaminergic PC12 cells. *Journal of Clinical Biochemistry and Nutrition, 51*(2): 122–127.

Tessier, J., Thurner, B., Jüngling, E., Lückhoff, A., & Fischer, Y. (2003). Impairment of glucose metabolism in hearts from rats treated with endotoxin. *Cardiovascular Research, 60*(1): 119–130.

Tholstrup, T. (2005). Influence of stearic acid on hemostatic risk factors in humans. *Lipids, 40*(12): 1229–1235.

Thompson, R., Ruch, W., & Hasenöhrl, R. (2004). Enhanced cognitive performance and cheerful mood by standardized extracts of *Piper methysticum* (Kava-kava). *Human Psychopharmacology: Clinical and Experimental, 19*(4): 243–250.

Tohda, C., Kuboyama, T., & Komatsu, K. (2005). Search for natural products related to regeneration of the neuronal network. *Neurosignals, 14*(1–2): 34–45.

Tohda, C., Nakamura, N., Komatsu, K., & Hattori, M. (1999). Trigonelline-induced neurite outgrowth in human neuroblastoma SK-N-SH cells. *Biological & Pharmaceutical Bulletin, 22*(7): 679–682.

Tomas-Barberan, F., Cienfuegos-Jovellanos, E., Marín, A., Muguerza, B., Gil-Izquierdo, A., Cerda, B., Zafrilla, P., Morillas, J., Mulero, J., Ibarra, A., Pasamar, M., Ramón, D., & Espín, J. (2007). A new process to develop a cocoa powder with higher flavonoid monomer content and enhanced bioavailability in healthy humans. *Journal of Agricultural and Food Chemistry, 55*(10): 3926–3935.

di Tomaso, E., Beltramo, M., & Piomelli, D. (1996). Scientific correspondence: brain cannabinoids in chocolate. *Nature, 22*(382): 677–678.

Tomé-Carneiro, J., Gonzálvez, M., Larrosa, M., Yáñez-Gascón, M., García-Almagro, F., Ruiz-Ros, J., Tomás-Barberán, F., García-Conesa, M., & Espín, J. (2013). Grape resveratrol increases serum adiponectin and downregulates inflammatory genes in peripheral blood mononuclear cells: a triple-blind, placebo-controlled, one-year clinical trial in patients with stable coronary artery disease. *Cardiovascular Drugs and Therapy, 27*(1): 37–48.

Tomofuji, T., Ekuni, D., Irie, K., Azuma, T., Endo, Y., Tamaki, N., Sanbe, T., Murakami, J., Yamamoto, T., & Morita, M. (2009). Preventive effects of a cocoa-enriched diet on gingival oxidative stress in experimental periodontitis. *Journal of Periodontology, 80*(11): 1799–1808.

Triche, E., Grosso, L., Belanger, K., Darefsky, A., Benowitz, N., & Bracken, M. (2008). Chocolate consumption in pregnancy and reduced likelihood of preeclampsia. *Epidemiology, 19*(3): 459–464.

Troost, F., Brummer, R., Dainty, J., Hoogewerff, J., Bull, V., & Saris, W. (2003). Iron supplements inhibit zinc but not copper absorption *in vivo* in ileostomy subjects. *American Journal of Clinical Nutrition, 78*(5): 1018–1023.

Tryon, M., DeCant, R., & Laugero, K. (2013). Having your cake and eating it too: a habit of comfort food may link chronic social stress exposure and acute stress-induced cortisol hyporesponsiveness. *Physiology & Behaviour, 10*(114–115): 32–37.

Tsai, S., & Yin, M. (2012). Anti-glycative and anti-inflammatory effects of protocatechuic acid in brain of mice treated by D-galactose. *Food and Chemical Toxicology, 50*(9): 198–205.

Tsuruma, K., Shimazaki, H., Nakashima, K., Yamauchi, M., Sugitani, S., Shimazawa, M., Linuma, M., & Hara, H. (2012). Annatto prevents retinal degeneration induced by endoplasmic reticulum stress *in vitro* and *in vivo*. *Molecular Nutrition and Food Research, 56*(5): 713–724.

Turcotte, A., Scott, P., & Tague, B. (2013). Analysis of cocoa products for ochratoxin A and aflatoxins. *Mycotoxin Research, 29*(3): 193–201.

Tzounis, X., Rodriguez-Mateos, A., Vulevic, J., Gibson, G., Kwik-Uribe, C., & Spencer, J. (2010). Prebiotic evaluation of cocoa-derived flavanols in healthy humans by using a randomized, controlled, double-blind, crossover intervention study. *American Journal of Clinical Nutrition, 93*(1): 62–72.

Ulloth, J., Casiano, C., & De Leon, M. (2003). Palmitic and stearic fatty acids induce caspase-dependent and independent cell death in nerve growth factor differentiated PC12 cells. *Journal of Neurochemistry, 84*(4): 655–668.

Usmani, O., Belvisi, M., Patel, H., Crispino, N., Birrell, M., Korbonits, M., Korbonits, D., & Barnes, P. (2005). Theobromine inhibits sensory nerve activation and cough. *FASEB Journal, 19*(2): 231–233.

Valavanidis, A., Vlachogianni, T., & Fiotakis, C. (2009). 8-hydroxy-2'-deoxyguanosine (8-OHdG): A critical biomarker of oxidative stress and carcinogenesis. *Journal of Environmental Science & Health. Part C: Environmental Carcinogenesis & Ecotoxicology Reviews, 27*(2): 120–139.

Valle, R. (2017). La leyenda del toloache. *Artes de Mexico: Plantas Sagradas, 127*: 82–83. Mexico City: Artes de Mexico y del Mundo, S.A. de C.V.

Vauzour, D., Ravaioli, G., Vafeiadou, K., Rodriguez-Mateos, A., Angeloni, C., & Spencer, J. (2008). Peroxynitrite induced formation of the neurotoxins 5-S-cysteinyl-dopamine and DHBT-1: Implications for Parkinson's disease and protection by polyphenols. *Archives of Biochemistry and Biophysics, 476*(2): 145–151.

Velazquez, C., Calzada, F., Esquivel, B., Barbosa, E., & Calzada, S. (2009). Antisecretory activity from the flowers of *Chirnathodendron pentadactylon* and its flavonoids on intestinal fluid accumulation induced by *Vibrio cholera* toxin in rats. *Journal of Ethnopharmacology, 126*(3): 455–458.

Verstraeten, S., Oteiza, P., & Fraga, C. (2004). Membrane effects of cocoa procyanidins in liposomes and Jurkat T cells. *Biological Research, 37*(2): 293–300.

Vilar, D., Vilar, M., de Lima e Moura, T., Raffin, F., Rosa de Oliveira, M., Franco, C., Athayde-Filho, P., Diniz, M., & Barbosa-Filho, J. (2014). Traditional uses, chemical constituents, and biological activities of *Bixa orellana* L.: A review. *Scientific World Journal*, 2014, June 23: ID 857292, 11 pp.

Vinceti, M., Pellacani, G., Malagoli, C., Bassissi, S., Sieri, S., Bonvicini, F., Krogh, V., & Seidenari, S. (2005). A population-based case-control study of diet and melanoma risk in northern Italy. *Public Health Nutrition, 8*(8): 1307–1314.

Voigt, J., Kamaruddin, S., & Wazir, S. (1993). The major seed proteins of *Theobroma cacao L. Food Chemistry, 47*: 145–151.

Wahby, A., Mahdy, E., El-Mezayn, H., Salama, W., Ebrahim, N., Abdel-Aty, A., & Fahmy, A. (2012). Role of hyaluronidase inhibitors in the neutralization of toxicity of Egyptian horned viper *Cerastes cerastes* venom. *Journal of Genetic Engineering and Biotechnology, 10*(2): 213–219.

Wan, Y., Vinson, J., Etherton, T., Proch, J., Lazarus, S., & Kris-Etherton, P. (2001). Effects of cocoa powder and dark chocolate on LDL oxidative susceptibility and prostaglandin concentrations in humans. *American Journal of Clinical Nutrition, 74*(5): 596–602.

Wang, D., Cheng, X., Yu, S., Qiu, L., Lian, X., Guo, X., Hu, Y., Lu, S., Yang, G., & Liu, H. (2018). Data mining: Seasonal and temperature fluctuations in thyroid-stimulating hormone. *Clinical Biochemistry, 60*: 59–63.

Wang, G., Yao, J., Jing, H., Zhang, F., Lin, M., Shi, L., Wu, H., Gao, D., Liu, K., & Tian, X. (2012). Suppression of the p66shc adapter protein by protocatechuic acid prevents the development of lung injury induced by intestinal ischemia reperfusion in mice. *Journal of Trauma and Acute Care Surgery, 73*(5): 1130–1137.

Wang, H., Huang, P., Lie, T., Li, J., Hutz, R., Li, K., & Shi, F. (2010). Reproductive toxicity of acrylamide-treated male rats. *Reproductive Toxicology, 29*(2): 225–230.

Wang, J., Schramm, D., Holt, R., Ensunsa, J., Fraga, C., Schmitz, H., & Keen, C. (2000). A dose-response effect from chocolate consumption on plasma epicatechin and oxidative damage. *Journal of Nutrition, 130*(8 Suppl.): 2115S–2119S.

Wang, J., Varghese, M., Ono, K., Yamada, M., Levine, S., Tzavaras, N., Gong, B., Hurst, W., Blitzer, R., & Pasinetti, G. (2014). Cocoa extracts reduce oligomerization of amyloid-β: implications for cognitive improvement in Alzheimer's disease. *Journal of Alzheimer's Disease, 41*(2): 643–650.

Wang, Z., Liang, C., Li, G., Yu, C., & Yin, M. (2007). Stearic acid protects primary cultured cortical neurons against oxidative stress. *Acta Pharmacologica Sinica, 28*(3): 315–326.

Wang-Polagruto, J., Villablanca, A., Polagruto, J., Lee, L., Holt, R., Schrader, H., Ensunsa, J., Steinberg, F., Schmitz, H., & Keen, C. (2009). Chronic consumption of flavanol-rich cocoa improves endothelial function and decreases vascular cell adhesion molecule in hypercholesterolemic postmenopausal women. *Breast Cancer Research and Treatment, 117*(1): 111–119.

Warnotte, C., Nenquin, M., & Henquin, J. (1999). Unbound rather than total concentration and saturation rather than unsaturation determine the potency of fatty acids on insulin secretion. *Molecular and Cellular Endocrinology, 153*(1–2): 147–153.

Willeit, M., Praschak-Rieder, N., Neumeister, A., Zill, P., Leisch, F., Stastny, J., Hilger, E., Thierry, N., Konstantinidis, A., Winkler, D., Fuchs, K., Sieghart, W., Aschauer, H., Ackenheil, M., Bondy, B., & Kasper, S. (2003). A polymorphism (5-HTTLPR) in the serotonin transporter promoter gene is associated with DSM-IV depression subtypes in seasonal affective disorder. *Molecular Psychiatry, 8*: 942–946.

Williams, S., Tamburic, S., & Lally, C. (2009). Eating chocolate can significantly protect the skin from UV light. *Letters in Applied Microbiology, 49*(3): 354–360.

Winick-Ng, W., Leri, F., & Kalisch, B. (2012). Nitric oxide and histone deacetylases modulate cocaine-induced mu-opioid receptor levels in PC12 cells. *BMC Pharmacology and Toxicology, 13*: 11.

Wirtz, P., Känel, R., Meister, R., Arpagaus, A., Treichler, S., Kuebler, U., Huberk, S., & Ehlert, U. (2014). Research correspondence: Dark chocolate intake buffers stress reactivity in humans. *Journal of the American College of Cardiology, 63*(21): 2297–2299.

Wiswedel, I., Hirsch, D., Kropf, S., Gruening, M., Pfister, E., Schewe, T., & Sies, H. (2004). Flavanol-rich cocoa drink lowers plasma F(2)-isoprostane concentrations in humans. *Free Radical Biology and Medicine, 37*(3): 411–412.

Wojcicki, J., & Heyman, M. (2012). Reducing childhood obesity by eliminating 100% fruit juice. *American Journal of Public Health, 102*(9): 1630–1633.

Wollgast, J. (2004). The contents and effects of polyphenols in chocolate. [Dissertation for obtaining the degree of doctor, Faculty of Agricultural and Nutritional Sciences, Home Economics, and Environmental Management, University of Giessen, Germany.] Giessen, Germany: Justus Liebig University.

Wolz, M., Kaminsky, A., Löhle, M., Koch, R., Storch, A., & Reichmann, H. (2009). Chocolate consumption is increased in Parkinson's disease: Results from a self-questionnaire study. *Journal of Neurology, 256*(3): 488–492.

Wolz, M., Schleiffer, C., Klingelhöfer, L., Schneider, C., Proft, F., Schwanebeck, U., Reichmann, H., Riederer, P., & Storch, A. (2012). Comparison of chocolate to cacao-free white chocolate in Parkinson's disease: a single-dose, investigator-blinded, placebo-controlled, crossover trial. *Journal of Neurology, 259*(11): 2447–2451.

Wu, Y., & Liu, F. (2012). Targeting mTOR: Evaluating the therapeutic potential of resveratrol for cancer treatment. *Anticancer Agents in Medicinal Chemistry, 13*(7): 1032–1038.

Xie, G., Krnjević, K., & Ye, J. (2013). Salsolinol modulation of dopamine neurons. *Frontiers in Behavioural Neuroscience, 7*, Article 52: 1–7.

Xu, J., Xu, H., Liu, Y., He, H., & Li, G. (2015). Vanillin-induced amelioration of depression-like behaviors in rats by modulating monoamine neurotransmitters in the brain. *Psychiatry Research, 225*(3): 509–514.

Xu, Z., & Kong, X. (2017). Bixin ameliorates high fat diet-induced cardiac injury in mice through inflammation and oxidative stress suppression. *Biomedicine and Pharmacotherapy, 89*: 991–1004.

Xue, X., Lin, L., Xiao, F., Pi, T., Lai, Y., & Luo, H. (2011). [Neurotrophic effects of protocatechuic acid on neurite outgrowth and survival in cultured cerebral cortical neurons of newborn rat.] [Article in Chinese.] *Zhong Yao Cai, 34*(4): 567–572.

Yamada, T., Yamada, Y., Okano, Y., Terashima, T., & Yokogoshi, H. (2009). Anxiolytic effects of short- and long-term administration of cacao mass on rat elevated T-maze test. *Journal of Nutritional Biochemistry, 20*(12): 948–955.

Yamagishi, M., Natsume, M., Osakabe, N., Nakamura, H., Furukawa, F., Imazawa, T., Nishikawa, A., & Hirose, M. (2002). Effects of cacao liquor proanthocyanidins on PhIP-induced mutagenesis in vitro, and in vivo mammary and pancreatic tumorigenesis in female Sprague–Dawley rats. *Cancer Letters, 185*(2): 123–130.

Yamagishi, M., Natsume, M., Osakabe, N., Okazaki, K., Furukawa, F., Imazawa, T., Nishikawa, A., & Hirose, M. (2003). Chemoprevention of lung carcinogenesis by cacao liquor proanthocyanidins in a male rat multi-organ carcinogenesis model. *Cancer Letters, 191*(1): 49–57.

Yamashita, Y., Kumabe, T., Cho, Y., Watanabe, M., Kawagishi, J., Yoshimoto, T., Fujino, T., Kang, M., & Yamamoto, T. (2000). Fatty acid induced glioma cell growth is mediated by the acyl-CoA synthetase 5 gene located on chromosome 10q25.1-q25.2, a region frequently deleted in malignant gliomas. *Oncogene, 19*(51): 5919–5925.

Yan, X., Liu, D. F., Zhang, X., Liu, D., Xu, S., Chen, G., Huang, B., Ren, W., Wang, W., Fu, S., & Liu, J. (2017). Vanillin protects dopaminergic neurons against inflammation-mediated cell death by inhibiting ERK1/2, P38 and the NF-κB signaling pathway. *International Journal of Molecular Sciences, 18*(2): E.389.

Yanovski, S. (2003). Sugar and fat: cravings and aversions. *Journal of Nutrition, 133*(3): 835S–837S.

Yasuda, A., Takano, H., Osakabe, N., Sanbongi, C., Fukuda, K., Natsume, M., Yanagisawa, R., Inoue, K., Kato, Y., Osawa, T., & Yoshikawa, T. (2008). Cacao liquor proanthocyanidins inhibit lung injury induced by diesel exhaust particles. *International Journal of Immunopathology & Pharmacology, 21*(2): 279–288.

Yazawa, K., Kihara, T., Shen, H., Shimmyo, Y., Niidome, T., & Sugimoto, H. (2006). Distinct mechanisms underlie distinct polyphenol-induced neuroprotection. *FEBS Letters, 580*(28–29): 6623–6628.

Yi, H., Akao, Y., Maruyama, W., Chen, K., Shih, J., & Naoi, M. (2006). Type A monoamine oxidase is the target of an endogenous dopaminergic neurotoxin, N-methyl(R)salsolinol, leading to apoptosis in SH-SY5Y cells. *Journal of Neurochemistry, 96*(2): 541–549.

Yoon, C., Chung, S., Lee, S. W., Park, Y., Lee, S. K., & Park, M. (2012). Gallic acid, a natural polyphenolic acid, induces apoptosis and inhibits proinflammatory gene expressions in rheumatoid arthritis fibroblast-like synoviocytes. *Joint Bone Spine, 80*(3): 274–279.

Young, A., & Severson, D. (1994). Comparative analysis of steam distilled floral oils of cacao cultivars (*Theobroma cacao* L., Sterculiaceae) and attraction of flying insects: Implications for a *Theobroma* pollination syndrome. *Journal of Chemical Ecology, 20*(10): 2687–2703.

Yu, G., Maskray, V., Jackson, S., Swift, C., & Tiplady, B. (1991). A comparison of the central nervous system effects of caffeine and theophylline in elderly subjects. *British Journal of Clinical Pharmacology, 32*(3): 341–345.

Yu, H., Inoguchi, T., Kakimoto, M., Nakashima, N., Imamura, M., Hashimoto, T., Umeda, F., & Nawata, H. (2001). Saturated non-esterified fatty acids stimulate de novo diacylglycerol synthesis and protein kinase c activity in cultured aortic smooth muscle cells. *Diabetologia, 44*(5): 614–620.

Yu, Y., Wang, R., Chen, C., Du, X., Ruan, L., Sun, J., Li, J., Zhang, L., O'Donnell, J., Pan, J., & Xu, Y. (2013). Antidepressant-like effect of trans-resveratrol in chronic stress model: Behavioral and neurochemical evidences. *Journal of Psychiatric Research, 47*(3): 315–322.

Yuan, H., Zhang, W., Li, H., Chen, C., Liu, H., & Li, Z. (2013). Neuroprotective effects of resveratrol on embryonic dorsal root ganglion neurons with neurotoxicity induced by ethanol. *Food and Chemical Toxicology, 55C*: 192–201.

Zaru, A., Maccioni, P., Colombo, G., & Gessa, G. (2013). The dopamine β-hydroxylase inhibitor, nepicastat, suppresses chocolate self-administration and reinstatement of chocolate seeking in rats. *British Journal of Nutrition, 110*(8): 1524–1533.

Zavala-Sánchez, M., Pérez-Gutiérrez, S., Perez-González, C., Sánchez-Saldivar, D., & Arias-García, L. (2002). Antidiarrhoeal activity of nonanal, an aldehyde isolated from *Artemisia ludoviciana*. *Pharmaceutical Biology, 40*(4): 263–268.

Zelber-Sagi, S., Ratizu, V., & Oren, R. (2011). Nutrition and physical activity in NAFLD: An overview of the epidemiological evidence. *World Journal of Gastroenterology, 17*(29): 3377–3389.

Zellner, D., Garriga-Trillo, A., Centeno, S., & Wadsworth, E. (2004). Chocolate craving and the menstrual cycle. *Appetite, 42*(1): 119–121.

Zhang, F., Wang, Y., Liu, H., Lu, Y., Wu, Q., Liu, J., & Shi, J. (2012). Resveratrol produces neurotrophic effects on cultured dopaminergic neurons through prompting astroglial BDNF and GDNF release. *Evidence Based Complementary and Alternative Medicine*, Article ID 937605, 7 pages. http://dx.doi.org/10.1155/2012/937605

Zhang, L., Deng, M., & Zhou, S. (2011). Tetramethylpyrazine inhibits hypoxia-induced pulmonary vascular leakage in rats via the ROS-HIF-VEGF pathway. *Pharmacology, 87*(5–6): 265–273.

Zhang, L., & Lokeshwar, B. (2012). Medicinal properties of the Jamaican pepper plant *Pimenta dioica* and Allspice. *Current Drug Targets, 13*(4): 1900–1906.

Zhang, L., Shamaladevi, N., Jayaprakasha, G., Patil, B., & Lokeshwar, B. (2015). Polyphenol-rich extract of *Pimenta dioica* berries (Allspice) kills breast cancer cells by autophagy and delays growth of triple negative breast cancer in athymic mice. *Oncotarget, 6*(18): 16379–16395.

Zhang, M., Zhou, X., & Zhou, K. (2013). Resveratrol inhibits human nasopharyngeal carcinoma cell growth via blocking pAkt/p70S6K signaling pathways. *International Journal of Molecular Medicine*, *31*(3): 621–627.

Zhang, S., & Mueller, C. (2012). Comparative analysis of volatiles in traditionally cured Bourbon and Ugandan vanilla bean (*Vanilla planifolia*) extracts. *Journal of Agricultural and Food Chemistry*, *60*(42): 10433–10444.

Zhu, Q., Hammerstone, J., Lazarus, S., Schmitz, H., & Keen, C. (2003). Stabilizing effect of ascorbic acid on flavan-3-ols and dimeric procyanidins from cocoa. *Journal of Agricultural and Food Chemistry*, *51*(3): 828–833.

Zhu, Q., Schramm, D., Gross, H., Holt, R., Kim, S., Yamaguchi, T., Kwik-Uribe, C., & Keen, C. (2005). Influence of cocoa flavanols and procyanidins on free radical-induced human erythrocyte hemolysis. *Clinical and Developmental Immunology*, *12*(1): 27–34.

Ziegleder, G., Stojacic, E., & Stumpf, B. (1992). The occurrence of beta-phenylethylamine and its derivatives in cocoa and cocoa products. *Zeitschrift für Lebensmittel-Untersuchung und Forschung*, *195*(3): 235–238.

Zioudrou, A., Streaty, R., & Klee, W. (1979). Opioid peptides derived from food proteins. The exorphins. *Journal of Biological Chemistry*, 254: 2446–2449.

Zoumas, B., Kreiser, W., & Martin, R. (1980). Theobromine and caffeine content of chocolate products. *Journal of Food Science*, *45*(2): 314–316.

Zucchi, R., Chiellini, G., Scanlan, T., & Grandy, D. (2006). Trace amine-associated receptors and their ligands. *British Journal of Pharmacology*, *149*(8): 967–978.

Zumbé, A. (1998). Polyphenols in cocoa: are there health benefits? *BNF Nutrition Bulletin*, *23*(83): 94–102.

Internet and podcasts

Alencar, N., Pinheiro, R., Figueiredo, I., Luz, P., Freitas, L., de Souza, T., do Carmo, L., Marques, L., & Ramos, M. (2015). The preventive effect on ethanol-induced gastric lesions of the medicinal plant *Plumeria rubra*: Involvement of the latex proteins in the NO/cGMP/K_{ATP} signaling pathway. *Evidence Based Complementary and Alternative Medicine*. Published online 14 December 2015. https://ncbi.nlm.nih.gov/pmc/articles/PMC4691623/ [Accessed 18 December 2017].

Alexander, B. (2010). Addiction: The view from Rat Park. http://brucekalexander.com/articles-speeches/rat-park/148-addiction-the-view-from-rat-park [Accessed 26 March 2017].

Asprey, D. (2016). Harvard scientists compare chocolate to Viagra! *Bulletproof Blog*. https://blog.bulletproof.com/harvard-scientists-compare-blood-flow-from-chocolate-to-viagra/ Bulletproof 360 Inc. [Accessed 2 February 2017].

Bardelli, C., Zeng, H., Locatelli, M., Amoruso, A., Coisson, J., Travaglia, F., Arlorio, M., Brunelleschi, S. (2011). Anti-inflammatory properties of clovamide and *Theobroma cacao* phenolic extracts in human monocytes: evaluation of respiratory burst, cytokine release, NF-κ B activation and PPARγ. *35th National Congress of the Italian Pharmacological Society*. Bologna, 14–17 September. http://cong35.sifweb.org/congresso_abs_view.php?id=44 [Accessed 22 August 2012].

Bassett, M. (2008). Aztec concepts of the human body (1). http://mexicolore.co.uk/aztecs/home/aztec-concepts-of-the-human-body-1 [Accessed 19 January 2019].

Becker, K., Gesiler, S., Ueberall, F., Fuchs, D., & Gostner, J. (2013). Immunomodulatory properties of cacao extracts—potential consequences for medical applications. *Frontiers in Pharmacology*. https://doi.org/10.3389/fphar.2013.00154 [Accessed 4 March 2019].

Berry, K. (2009). Understanding chemical dependence from an acupuncture and from an acupuncture and traditional Chinese medicine perspective [PowerPoint presentation]. *EuroNADA Conference.* http://nada-acupuncture.ch/pdf/09euronada-k_berry-dependency_tcm_perspective.pdf [Accessed 7 April 2019].

Blake, W. (1790). The marriage of Heaven and Hell. *Bartleby.com.* https://bartleby.com/235/253.html [Accessed 4 April 2019].

"Bodhipaksa". (2007). Krishnamurti: "It is no measure of health to be well adjusted to a profoundly sick society." *Wildmind Meditation.* https://wildmind.org/blogs/quote-of-the-month/krishnamurti-measure-of-health [Accessed 7 April 2019].

Byrne, P. (2013). Dog walker finds smelly lump of whale vomit on beach that's worth £100,000. *Daily Mirror.* https://mirror.co.uk/news/uk-news/dog-walker-finds-lump-of-whale-1564302 [Accessed 23 February 2019].

Cano, V. (2009). The legend of chocolate. *Stories from the Americas.* http://storiesfromtheamericas.blogspot.com/2009/01/legend-of-chocolate.html [Accessed 11 December 2018].

Chiarini, G. (2013). Emulsification and Foaming. http://world-gourmet-society.com/en/blog/culinary-guru-corner/49-emulsification-and-foaming [Accessed 15 February 2018].

"Chris". (2006). Chocolate on the brain: Is chocolate an antidepressant? http://scienceblogs.com/mixingmemory/2006/06/chocolate_on_the_brain_is_choc.php [Accessed 6 February 2010].

Cornejo, O., Muh-Ching, Y., Dominguez, V., Andrews, M., Sockell, A., Møller, E., Livingstone, D., Stack, C., Romero, A., Umaharan, P., Royaert, S., Tawari, N., Ng, P., Schnell, R., Phillips, W., Mockaitis, K., Bustamante, C., & Motamayor, J. (2017). Genomic insights into the domestication of the chocolate tree, *Theobroma cacao* L. *bioRxiv: The Preprint Server for Biology.* doi: https://doi.org/10.1101/223438 https://biorxiv.org/content/early/2017/11/22/223438 [Accessed 16 August 2018].

Davrieux, F., Assemat, S., Sukha, D., Portillo, E., Boulanger, R., Bastianelli, D., & Cros, E. (2005). Genotype characterization of cocoa into genetic groups through caffeine and theobromine content predicted by near infra red spectroscopy. [Conference paper: 12th International Conference on Near Infrared Spectroscopy, 9–15 April 2005, Auckland, New Zealand.] Available from: https://researchgate.net/publication/264464012_genotype_characterization_of_cocoa_into_genetic_groups_through_caffeine_and_theobromine_content_predicted_by_nirs [Accessed 25 February 2016]

Dharmananda, S. (2001). Are Aristolochia plants dangerous? *Institute for Traditional Medicine Online.* http://itmonline.org/arts/aristolochia.htm [Accessed 19 February 2018].

Dharmananda, S. (2012). Ligustrazine: Key component of the Chinese herb chuanxiong. *Institute for Traditional Medicine Online.* http://itmonline.org/arts/ligustrazine.htm [Accessed 2 September 2012].

Duke, J. (1983). *Theobroma cacao* L. Excerpt from online article: http://hort.purdue.edu/newcrop/duke_energy/theobroma_cacao.html [Accessed 21 August 2012].

European Food Standards Agency (2012). A Rolling Programme of Surveys on Process Contaminants in UK Retail Foods. Acrylamide & Furan: Survey 4. *European Food Standards Agency information sheet.* No. 2/12, April 2012. www.food.gov.uk/multimedia/pdfs/acrylamide-furan-survey.pdf [Accessed 18 August 2013].

Franciotti, K. (2016). Magic mushroom drug helps people with cancer face death. *New Scientist.* https://newscientist.com/article/2114789-magic-mushroom-drug-helps-people-with-cancer-face-death/ [Accessed 16 September 2018].

Fraser, P. (2018). A Supplement to Clarke's Dictionary of Practical Materia Medica: Chocolatum. http://hominf.org/remedy/chocolat.htm [Accessed 15 March 2018].

Ghazizadeh, A., Ambroggi, F., & Fields, H. (2014). Ventromedial prefrontal cortex shapes responses of nucleus accumbens shell neurons to suppress unreinforced actions. *Neuroscience 2010: F100 Research. Open for Science.* http://f1000research.com/posters/698 14 December 2010 [Accessed 24 April 2016].

Goldhill, O. (2016). Scientists say your "mind" isn't confined to your brain, or even your body. *Quartz.* https://qz.com/866352/scientists-say-your-mind-isnt-confined-to-your-brain-or-even-your-body/ [Accessed 10 December 2018].

Gonzalez, A., Gutierrez, R., & Cotera, L. (2014). Antidiabetic activity of *Piper auritum* leaves in streptozotocin-induced diabetic rat, beneficial effect on advanced glycation endproduct. *Chinese Journal of Integrative Medicine*, pp. 1 –10. https://doi.org/10.1007/s11655-014-1753-2 [Accessed 7 December 2017].

de Gortari, Y. (2012). El metate: como se usa el metate utensilios Mexicanos. https://youtube.com/watch?v=MqJuyOHx2OM#action=share [Accessed 16 August 2018].

"H. T." (2013). Diabetes in Mexico: eating themselves to death. *Economist*, 10 April 2013. http://economist.com/blogs/americasview/2013/04/diabetes-mexico [Accessed 2 May 2017].

Hernández, F. (1615). *Quatro Libros de la Naturaleza, y Virtudes de las Plantas y animales que estan recevidos en el uso de Medicina en la Nueva Espana, Etc.* F. Ximenez (Trans.) www.wdl.org/en/item/7334/zoom/#group=1&page=1 [Accessed 25 January 2012].

Hill, C., & MacDonald, J. (2008). Insects and ticks > biting midges. *Purdue University: Medical Entomology.* https://extension.entm.purdue.edu/publichealth/insects/bitingmidge.html [Accessed 13 August 2018].

Holton, K. (2016). The role of diet in the treatment of fibromyalgia. *Pain Management, 6*(4). https://doi.org/10.2217/pmt-2016-0019 [Accessed 2 May 2017].

Ji, S. (2012a). Can wheat drive more than your digestive system crazy? *GreenMedInfo.* www.greenmedinfo.com/blog/can-wheat-drive-more-your-digestive-system-crazy [Accessed 6 April 2012].

Ji, S. (2012b). Do hidden opiates in our food explain food addictions? *GreenMedInfo.* http://www.greenmedinfo.com/blog/do-hidden-opiates-our-food-explain-food-addictions1?page=2 [Accessed 29 May 2014].

Lawley, R. (2013a). Aflatoxins. http://foodsafetywatch.org/factsheets/aflatoxins/ [Accessed 3 August 2017].

Lawley, R. (2013b). Ochratoxins. http://foodsafetywatch.org/factsheets/aflatoxins/ [Accessed 3 August 2017].

Leggett, D. (2017). Qi nutrition. Chocolate: good or bad? http://meridianpress.net/articles/chocolate-good-or-bad.html [Accessed 11 August 2017].

Mach, D., hosted by White, G. (2018). Talking "The Mirror of Magic" and Kurt Seligmann. *Rune Soup* [Podcast]. 10 October.

Marlow, K. (2013). What is consciousness? *Psychology Today.* http://psychologytoday.com/us/blog/the-superhuman-mind/201303/what-is-consciousness [Accessed 10 December 2018].

McManamy, J. (2011). Your second-favourite organ may be the key player. http://mcmanweb.com/love_lust.html [Accessed 18 January 2013].

Miller, D. (2017). Are dark chocolate and cacao really healthy? *Grow youthful: health at any age.* https://growyouthful.com/tips/cacao-chocolate-cocoa.php [Accessed 1 April 2019].

"Moe" (2014). As above, so below. *Gnostic Warrior.* https://gnosticwarrior.com/as-above-so-below-4.html [Accessed 4 April 2019].

Morrison, C. (2012). The GP who gave up fruit and veg to cure her aches and pains. *Daily Mail.* http://dailymail.co.uk/health/article-2174474/The-GP-gave-fruit-veg-cure-aches-pains.html (updated 17 July 2012) [Accessed 2 August 2017].

Pepling, R. (2003). Soap bubbles. *Science & Technology,* 81(17): 34. American Chemical Society. https://pubs.acs.org/cen/whatstuff/stuff/8117sci3.html [Accessed 16 February 2018].

Safford, W. (1910). The sacred ear-flower of the Aztecs: Xochinacaztli. In: Annual Report of the Board of Regents of the Smithsonian Institution (pp. 427–431). Washington, DC: Washington Government Printing Office. https://library.si.edu/digital-library/book/annualreportof-bo1910smits [Accessed 12 March 2019].

Sedghi, A. (2015). I should cocoa: which country spends the most on chocolate? *The Guardian.* https://theguardian.com/news/datablog/2015/jul/19/which-country-spends-the-most-on-chocolate-bars [Accessed 20 August 2018].

Da Silva, J., & Alba, M. (2004). Cacaloxóchitl, como planta medicinal y flor ornamental. *Tesina del Diplomado de Tlahui-Educa: Medicina Tradicional de México y sus Plantas Medicinales, 18*(2). http://tlahui.com/medic/medic18/cacalox1.htm [Accessed 18 December 2017].

Sims, M. (2010). What is neuroscience telling us about supporting families? [PowerPoint presentation.] www.une.edu.au/staff/msims7 [Accessed 18 May 2013].

Soto, M. (2005). La ruta del cacao Maya hacia el mundo. www.huixtlaweb.com/cuentos/ruta_del_cacao.html [Accessed 2 February 2011].

Spade, P. (2019). William of Ockham. *Stanford Encyclopaedia of Philosophy.* https://plato.stanford.edu/entries/ockham/#OckhRazo [Accessed 7 April 2019].

Thomson, T. (2012). Science briefs: the fear factor and chocolate abuse. *The Manitoban.* http://themanitoban.com/20/12/10/science-brief-the-fear-factor-and-chocolate-abuse/12021/ [Accessed 20 February 2013].

Tice, R. (1997). Trigonelline: Review of toxicological literature. *Integrated Laboratory Systems.* https://ntp.niehs.nih.gov/ntp/htdocs/chem_background/exsumpdf/trigonelline_508.pdf [Accessed 10 April 2019].

Tilburt, J., & Kaptchuk, T. (2008). Herbal medicine research and global health: an ethical analysis. *Bulletin of the World Health Organization, 86*(8): 577–656. http://who.int/bulletin/volumes/86/8/07-042820/en/ [Accessed 5 October 2018].

University of California and Los Angeles (2002). Spices: Exotic Flavors and Medicines. [Exhibition.] https://unitproj.library.ucla.edu/biomed/spice/index.cfm?displayID=1 [Accessed 18 January 2018].

Wilson, G. (2012). The Great Porn Experiment. *TedX,* Glasgow. 16 May. http://youtube.com/watch?v=wSF82AwSDiU [Accessed 18 January 2013].

(1975). Aztec medicine had effective remedies. *Chemical & Engineering News Archive, 53*(50): 32–33. https://pubs.acs.org/doi/abs/10.1021/cen-v053n050.p032 [Accessed 7 November 2018].

(1997). Ochratoxin A: Group 2B. *International Agency for Research on Cancer (IARC)—Summaries & Evaluations, 6*: 489. http://inchem.org/documents/iarc/vol56/13-ochra.html [Accessed 10 August 2017].

(2009). Scopolamine in Colombia. *Expat Chronicles.* http://expat-chronicles.com/2009/10/scopolamine-in-colombia/ [Accessed 16 September 2018].

(2012). Anandamide. lipidlibrary.aocs.org [Accessed 20 August 2012].

(2012). Campesterol. *Wikipedia.* https://en.wikipedia.org/wiki/Campesterol [Accessed 30 November 2012].

(2012). Phytosterol. *Wikipedia.* https://en.wikipedia.org/wiki/Phytosterol [Accessed 30 November 2012].

(2012). Stigmasterol. *Wikipedia*. https://en.wikipedia.org/wiki/Stigmasterol [Accessed 30 November 2012].

(2012). Tyramine. *Wikipedia*. https://en.wikipedia.org/wiki/Tyramine [Accessed 15 June 2012].

(2012). Oleic Acid (Compound). *PubChem*. https://pubchem.ncbi.nlm.nih.gov/compound/445639 [Accessed 5 December 2012].

(2012). Stigmasterol (Compound). *PubChem*. https://pubchem.ncbi.nlm.nih.gov/compound/5280794 [Accessed 3 March 2016].

(2013). *British Heart Foundation*. http://extras.bhf.org/heartstats [Accessed 14 August 2013].

(2013). Gallic Acid. *Wikipedia*. http://en.wikipedia.org/wiki/Gallic_acid [Accessed 12 February 2013].

(2013). Caco. *Wiktionary*. http://en.m.wiktionary.org/wiki/caco#Latin [Accessed 22 November 2013].

(2018). *British Heart Foundation*. https://giftshop.bhf.org.uk/dechox [Accessed 24 August 2018].

(2013). *Website of the International Chronic Urticaria Society*. http://urticaria.thunderworksinc.com/pages/lowhistamine.htm [Accessed 22 February 2013].

(2014). The Adverse Childhood Experiences (ACE) Study. *Centers for Disease Control and Prevention*. http://cdc.gov/violenceprevention/acestudy/ [Accessed 17 September 2014].

(2014). Cycloartane. *PubChem*. https://pubchem.ncbi.nlm.nih.gov/compound/160497 [Accessed 16 August 2014].

(2015). Glutamic acid content of foods. http://dietgrail.com/glutamic-acid/ [Accessed 12 August 2015].

(2015). Phenylalanine content in grams per 100 grams product. http://wtb.tue.nl/woc/ptc/vanesch/pku/phenylalanine.html [Accessed 12 August 2015].

(2016). EFSA Panel on Food Additives and Nutrient Sources Added to Food (ANS). *European Food Safety Authority*. https://efsa.europa.eu [Accessed date not recorded in 2016].

(2016). Health Concerns About Dairy Products. *The Physicians' Committee for Responsible Medicine*. http://pcrm.org/health/diets/vegdiets/health-concerns-about-dairy-products [Accessed 27 April 2017].

(2016). Salsolinol (Compound). *PubChem*. https://pubchem.ncbi.nlm.nih.gov/compound/Salsolinol#section=Biological-Test-Results [Accessed 18 February 2016].

(2017). Cacao (Qiaokeli). https://whiterabbitinstituteofhealing.com/herbs/cacao/ [Accessed 11 August 2017].

(2017). Canak a sacred, edible and medicinal tree of Guatemala. A heritage from the Maya. *FLAAR*. http://maya-ethnobotany.org/utilitarian-plant-fiber-medicinal-plant-mayan-ethnobotanicals-guatemala-el-salvador-honduras-mexico/images-photos-canak-chiranthodendron-pentadactylon-flowers-tree-leaves.php [Accessed 9 November 2017].

(2017). Flor de Mayo, Plumeria rubia, Plumeria obtusa, frangipani, is a known sacred Maya flower, but deserves further study to understand potential use as aphrodisiac. *FLAAR*. http://maya-ethnobotany.org/mayan-ethno-botany-tropical-agriculture-edible-flowers-medicinal-plants-flavoring-guatemala-mexico-belize/plumeria-rubia-flor-de-mayo-frangipani-cacao-balche-aphrodisiac-fragrance.php [Accessed 18 December 2017].

(2017). International Chronic Urticaria Society: Histamine Restricted Diet. *International Chronic Urticaria Society*. https://chronichives.com/useful-information/histamine-restricted-diet/ [Accessed 10 July 2017].

(2017). Neglected crops: 1492 from a different perspective … Sapote (*Pouteria sapota*). http://fao.org/docrep/t0646e/T0646E0c.htm [Accessed 30 December 2017].

(2018). About Ghirardelli. https://ghirardelli.com/about-ghirardelli?storeId=11003&langId=-1 [Accessed 20 August 2018].

(2018). *Ceratopogonidae.* http://faculty.ucr.edu/~legneref/medical/ceratopogonidaemed.htm [Accessed 13 August 2018].

(2018). Cacao: *Theobroam cacao* L. *Encyclopaedia of Life: Smithsonian National Museum of Natural History.* http://eol.org/pages/484592/details#morphology [Accessed 9 August 2018].

(2018). Pentadecane (Compound). *PubChem.* https://pubchem.ncbi.nlm.nih.gov/compound/Pentadecane#section=Top [Accessed 13 August 2018].

(2018). 1-Pentadecene (Compound). *PubChem.* https://pubchem.ncbi.nlm.nih.gov/compound/25913#section=Top [Accessed 13 August 2018].

(2018). Plants of the World online: *Theobroma cacao* L. *Kew Science.* http://powo.science.kew.org/taxon/urn:lsid:ipni.org:names:320783-2 [Accessed 9 August 2018].

(2018). *Pouteria sapota*—(Jacq.) H. E. Moore & Stearn. *Plants for a Future.* http://pfaf.org/user/Plant.aspx?LatinName=Pouteria+sapota [Accessed 2 January 2018].

(2018). *Theobroma cacao,* the food of the gods. *Barry Callebaut.* https://barry-callebaut.com/about-us/media/press-kit/history-chocolate/theobroma-cacao-food-gods [Accessed 16 August 2018].

(2018). *Theobroma cacao*: cacao. *Encyclopedia of Life,* ref. *Missouri Botanical Garden.* http://www.eol.org/pages/484592/details#morphology [Accessed 9 August 2018].

(2019). About Bourneville. *Cadbury.* https://cadbury.co.uk/about-bournville [Accessed 8 February 2019].

(2019). Cocoa powder for mares with low milk production [Forum]. *Horse & Hound.* https://forums.horseandhound.co.uk/threads/cocoa-powder-for-mares-with-low-milk-production.266749/ [Accessed 20 March 2019].

(2019). Kidney pattern differentiation in Chinese medicine. *Sacred Lotus Chinese Medicine.* https://sacredlotus.com/go/diagnosis-chinese-medicine/get/zang-fu-kidney-patterns-tcm [Accessed 4 February 2019].

(2019). World Health Rankings. https://worldlifeexpectancy.com/mexico-life-expectancy [Accessed 16 February 2019].

(2019). Oleic Acid. *Wikipedia.* https://en.wikipedia.org/wiki/Oleic_acid [Accessed 10 April 2019].

(2019). Palmitic Acid. *Wikipedia.* https://en.wikipedia.org/wiki/Palmitic_acid [Accessed 10 April 2019].

(2019). Stearic Acid. *Wikipedia.* https://en.wikipedia.org/wiki/Stearic_acid [Accessed 10 April 2019].

ACKNOWLEDGEMENTS

'Nequamaquam nos homines sumus, sed partes hominis;
Ox omnibus aliquid fieri potest, idque non magnum;
Ex singulis fere nihil.
[We are not whole men, but parts of men;
From all of us together something might be made, and that not much;
From each of us individually nothing].'

(*from* Robert Burton's *Anatomy of Melancholy*, 1621)

For all who have helped and encouraged me to complete this book, thank you!

For practical and psychological assistance, emergency aid, and friendship: Wendy Chung, Melanie Dymond, Lynne Hulka, and Vagelis Dimitriou; mum (I promise I'll take a spare credit card next time) and dad.

For major assistance, generosity, hospitality, and life support in Guatemala and Mexico, and ongoing supply: Juan-Pablo Porres Esquina, and Alejandra Martinez Porres Esquina.

Susana Trilling, for her helpful advice, connections, and contacts; Verónica Caal, for helping a lot and knowing everybody; Maribel Omaña Mendez and Arnaud, for your hospitality and good company; Lupita Juarez, for being super friendly and helpful; Roberto Molina, for fantastic accommodation and information; Veronica Juarez at UNAM herbario, for friendly help and assistance; Emmanuel Cruz Canela, for photographic assistance; Crispina Navarro Gomez and family in Ocotlán, for their generosity; Don Placido Castiliano, for the tour; Mario Gonzalez, for unconventional use of an oil drum; Rocio Remedios of Teotihuacan (*los dioses van con tuyo*); Alfredo Ramirez Rosario, for keeping an eye open for monkey balls; Esteban and his mother at Hotel Don Juan Metalbatz in Coban, for hospitality and friendliness; Casa de los Amigos, Mexico City, for being a great place to stay.

All my interviewees, for their time and generosity: Reginaldo Chayax Huex of Asociacion Bio-Itza, San José, Peten; Carina Santiago and her student, Kalisa Wells; Keith Wilson; Doña Rosa Gregorio and Roberto Gregorio; Señora Anna Maria Garcia Vasquez and Roberto Vasquez; Mario Euan; Juan Francisco Tzir; Ignacio Cac Sacul; Don Mateo Poptchu; Don Angel Chiac; Doña Juana Ca'al; Don Antonio Xoc; Señora Teresa Olivera; Tomas Villanueva; Doña Rosalia of Lanquin; Señora Lopreto and her daughter; Doña Maria Eugenia Navarrete Matei and her mother; Señora Aurelia Pop; Señora Delfina Valverde; Señora Rosia Torres Torres and Jorge

695

Perez Leon; Señora Claudia Maribel Ya'teni; Don Ramiro; Señora Ernestina Tawal; José Antonio; Claudia at Hacienda la Luz in Tabasco.

James and Jennifer Maloney, for hosting a leaky traveller; Heidi Nygård; Omar Ramirez Casas, for culinary counsel and cultural connoisseurship; Bridget Price, Victoria Masters, and Victoria Gervasi for connections and suggestions; Vincent James, for tarot and friendship; Kiralee, for the chakra readings; Rae, for the sneaky channelling; Maya Adar; Julissa in San Antonio Suchitequepez, for the fried breakfasts; Daniela, the accidental American in San Luís, Peten, for translation and orientation; Eric Pecay, Rex'hua taxista extraordinaire; Erdi Debesai, for research assistance; Luciana Morera, for translation services; Dr Celia Bell of Middlesex University, for advice and support; and Chantal Coady of Rococo Chocolates, for an interested ear, connections, and suggestions.

Jon Backus, for the best kind of distraction, and Dana Brickenstein, for good company; Charles James Walker; Gabriel Ovando Flores (*que rico*); Simon "Zippy" Irwin for minder duties; Mr and Mrs Grimmer, for much walking despite knee trouble; and last but certainly not least, Zoe Webber: we should totally use the bogs in McDonald's more regularly.

Special thanks to Alan Borthwick, PhD, for personal correspondence about his research on 2,5-diketopiperazines.

Author inspiration: Jonathan Ott, for his book on chocolate.

Finally, thanks to my publisher, Olly Rathbone—for your sins, much appreciated; and Mel McDougall, for the support! And all my wonderful former students, colleagues and clients who have been supportive and interested.

INDEX